Ultrasound of Fetal Syndromes

Ultrasound of Fetal Syndromes

Second Edition

BERYL R. BENACERRAF, M.D.

Clinical Professor of Obstetrics,
Gynecology and Reproductive
Biology
Clinical Professor of Radiology
Harvard Medical School
Brigham and Women's Hospital
Massachusetts General Hospital
Boston, Massachusetts

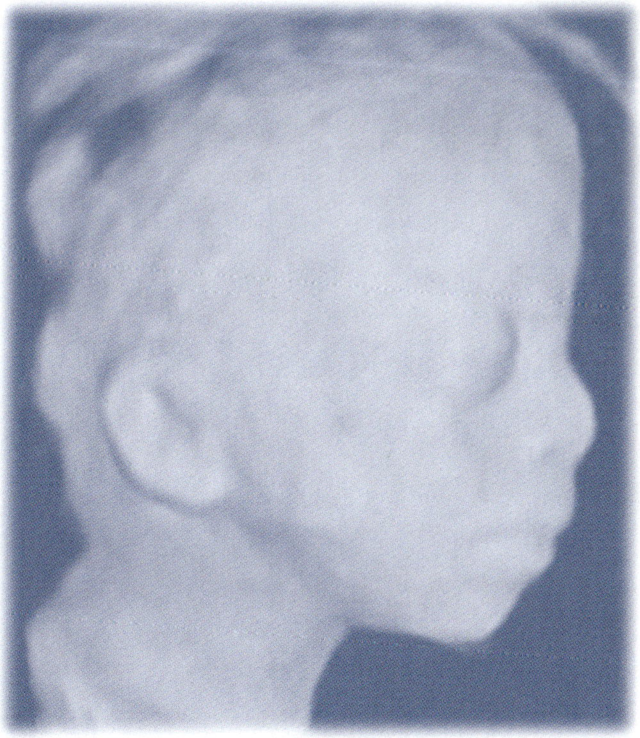

CHURCHILL
LIVINGSTONE
ELSEVIER

CHURCHILL
LIVINGSTONE
ELSEVIER

1600 John F. Kennedy Blvd.
Ste 1800
Philadelphia, PA 19103-2899

ULTRASOUND OF FETAL SYNDROMES, SECOND EDITION ISBN: 978-0-443-06641-2

Library of Congress Cataloging-in-Publication Data
Benacerraf, Beryl R.
Ultrasound of fetal syndromes/Beryl Benacerraf.—2nd ed.
p. ; cm.
Includes bibliographical references and index.
ISBN 978-0-443-06641-2
1. Fetus—Ultrasonic imaging. 2. Fetus—Abnormalities—Diagnosis. 3. Fetus—Diseases—Diagnosis. 4. Prenatal diagnosis. I. Title.
[DNLM: 1. Fetal Diseases—ultrasonography. 2. Abnormalities—ultrasonography. 3. Diagnosis, Differential. 4. Fetus—abnormalities. 5. Ultrasonography, Prenatal. WQ 211 B456u 2007]
RG628.3.U58B46 2007
618.3′207543—dc22

2007005669

Acquisitions Editor: Todd Hummel
Developmental Editor: Colleen McGonigal
Project Manager: Bryan Hayward
Design Direction: Ellen Zanolle

Printed in Canada

Last digit is the print number: 9 8 7 6 5 4 3 2 1

This book is dedicated to
my parents Baruj and Annette Benacerraf,
who always stimulated me to strive for the highest standards;
to my husband, Peter Libby, who gave me love,
encouragement, and support throughout my life;
and to my children, Oliver and Brigitte Libby,
whose achievement and promise make me proud.

List of Contributors

Bryann Bromley, M.D.

Associate Clinical Professor of Obstetrics and Gynecology and Reproductive Biology
Department of Obstetrics and Gynecology
Massachusetts General Hospital, Harvard Medical School and
Brigham and Women's Hospital, Harvard Medical School
Boston, Massachusetts

Diagnostic Ultrasound Associates, PC
Boston, Massachusetts

Thomas D. Shipp, M.D.

Associate Professor of Obstetrics and Gynecology and Reproductive Biology
Department of Obstetrics and Gynecology
Brigham and Women's Hospital, Harvard Medical School
Boston, Massachusetts

Diagnostic Ultrasound Associates, PC
Boston, Massachusetts

Preface

This book is a reference for practitioners providing prenatal diagnosis. When a fetal malformation, such as cleft lip and palate, is identified sonographically, parents typically want to know the prognosis for the fetus, the likelihood of other abnormalities, the need for further studies, and the risk of recurrence in future pregnancies. To answer these questions, most sonologists and practitioners dealing with prenatal diagnosis have extrapolated information from books on pediatric diagnosis, without any reference to sonographic prenatal diagnosis. Some books, such as Jones' *Smith's Recognizable Patterns of Human Malformations,* have been extremely useful for those of us in the field of prenatal diagnosis. However, they have not provided pertinent information about sonographic findings in fetuses with syndromes. The second edition of this text includes 20 additional syndromes and 12 new differential diagnostic headings compared with the first edition, as well up updates of all the syndromes and their references. More than 70% of the images in this book are new since the last edition and include a large variety of three-dimensional illustrations. The final two chapters are written by my colleagues, Dr. Bryann Bromley and Dr. Thomas D. Shipp.

It is with the prenatal diagnostician in mind that this book was written. The discussion of each syndrome includes a concise summary with sonographic images to support a prenatal diagnosis. Furthermore, there is a differential diagnosis section that includes each of the syndromes, organized by diagnosis of a common feature and cross-referenced with the main text. Finally, there are two additional chapters, one addressing abnormalities of twins and the other discussing the common borderline abnormalities that parents, sonologists, and counselors encounter. These borderline findings include anomalies that are found in both normal and aneuploid fetuses.

This book is not a textbook on ultrasound, of which there are many excellent offerings. Rather, it is intended as a reference book that one can consult to look up a specific abnormality (e.g., cleft lip and palate, club feet) and identify the possible associated abnormalities that could lead to the diagnosis of a particular syndrome. Examples of each syndrome having the particular finding in question (e.g., cleft lip and palate, club feet) are discussed and illustrated. If two findings are present in the same fetus, one can arrive at a diagnosis of the most likely syndromes that encompass these two findings.

This book can be used not only by sonographers and sonologists but also by genetic counselors and other personnel who help parents deal with the sonographic evaluation of their unborn child. Various abnormalities are presented, both by organ system and by differential diagnosis. The template for each anomaly is designed to include a brief description of the anomaly, the sonographic findings, the earliest sonographic diagnosis available, and information regarding prognosis.

It is hoped that this book will be as useful to practitioners of prenatal diagnosis as many genetics and dysmorphology books have been for pediatricians and geneticists.

Beryl Benacerraf, M.D.

Acknowledgment

*I would like to thank my beloved cat, Misha,
who sat on my lap lovingly and unconditionally,
encouraging me during the entire writing of this book.*

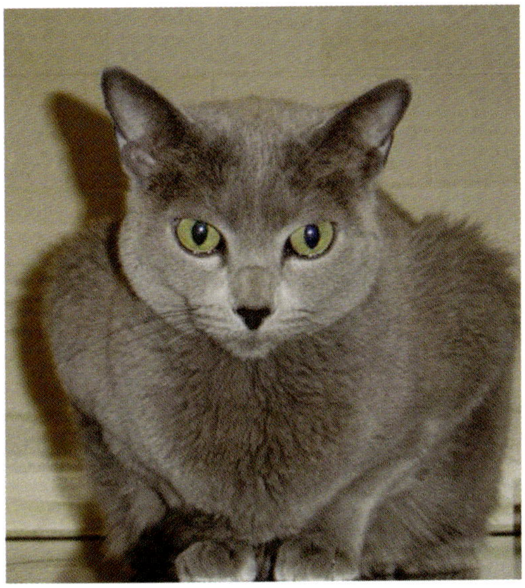

Contents

1 Differential Diagnoses 1

2 SYNDROMES 129

3 Sonographic Fetal Findings with Borderline Significance—The Grey Zone in Fetal Diagnosis 571

4 Fetal Anomalies and Syndromes Associated with Monochorianic Twins 603

1 Differential Diagnoses

CATARACT

OCULAR ABNORMALITIES

Coloboma

Congenital Aniridia

Microphthalmia (see p. 169)

ENZYMATIC DISORDERS

Glucose-6-Phosphate Dehydrogenase (G6PD) Deficiency

Homocystinuria

GROWTH ABNORMALITIES

Smith-Lemli-Opitz Syndrome: Autosomal recessive syndrome featuring microcephaly, mental retardation, and genital and renal anomalies (occasional) (see p. 140)

FACIAL AND BRAIN ABNORMALITIES

Branchio-Oculo-Facial Syndrome: Autosomal dominant disorder characterized by mental retardation, growth deficiency, ocular defects, and clefting of the upper lip (occasional) (see p. 149)

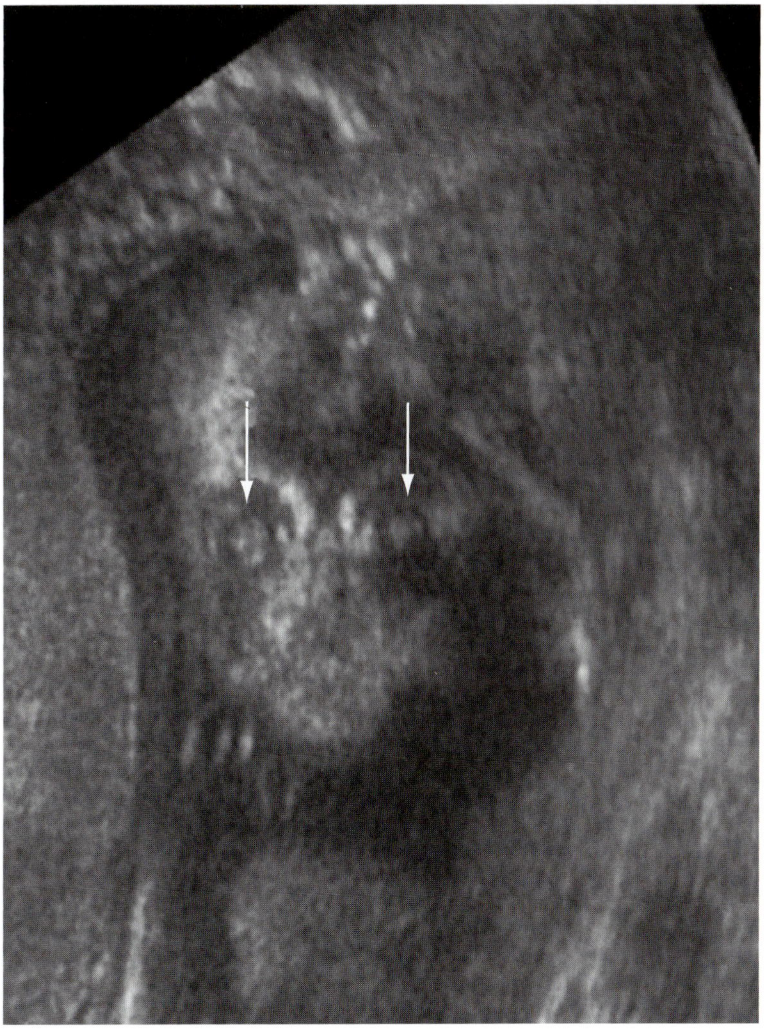

FIGURE 1-1 Coronal view through the fetal face of an early second-trimester fetus with trisomy 13. Note bilateral cataracts indicated by the echogenic lens of the eye *(arrows)*.

Hallermann-Streiff Syndrome: Disorder characterized by brachycephaly with frontal and parietal bossing, microphthalmia, cataracts, and depressed nasal bridge

Neu-Laxova Syndrome: Autosomal recessive condition characterized by microcephaly, lissencephaly, exophthalmos, severe intrauterine growth restriction (IUGR), swollen subcutaneous tissues, and ichthyosis (see p. 211)

Stickler Syndrome: Autosomal dominant syndrome characterized by ocular defects, cleft palate, micrognathia/hypoplasia of the mandible, and early orthopedic degenerative abnormalities (see p. 181)

Walker-Warburg Syndrome: Autosomal recessive condition characterized by severe congenital oculocerebral abnormalities, including lissencephaly, hydrocephalus, encephalocele, microcephaly, microphthalmia, and cataracts (see p. 217)

LIMB AND SKELETAL ABNORMALITIES

Chondrodysplasia Punctata: Heterogeneous group of bone dysplasias characterized by asymmetric limb shortening and abnormal early calcification of the proximal and distal epiphyses (see p. 266)

Hypochondroplasia: Autosomal dominant skeletal dysplasia characterized by moderate limb shortening; resembles achondroplasia but is less severe (occasional) (see p. 274)

Kniest Syndrome: Autosomal dominant condition characterized by kyphoscoliosis, platyspondyly, and shortened tubular long bones (occasional) (see p. 281)

Roberts Syndrome: Autosomal recessive condition characterized by severe shortening of the limbs (pseudothalidomide syndrome) and facial anomalies (occasional) (see p. 247)

OTHER SYNDROMES AND SEQUENCES

Arthrogryposis: Sequence of neurologic, muscular, and connective tissue disorders leading to fetal joint contractures and rigidity, as well as decreased activity (occasional) (see p. 362)

Cerebro-Oculo-Facio-Skeletal (COFS) Syndrome: Autosomal recessive condition characterized by joint contractures of all the extremities, with severe facial and brain abnormalities (see p. 374)

Marfan Syndrome: Autosomal dominant connective tissue disorder characterized by tall stature, long limbs, pectus deformities, congenital heart defects, and ocular anomalies (occasional) (see p. 344)

TERATOGENS

Clomiphene (Clomid) (see p. 437)

Cortisone (see p. 437)

Progestin (see p. 437)

Rubella (see p. 449)

Toxoplasmosis (see p. 452)

Valproic acid (see p. 436)

Varicella (see p. 456)

Warfarin (Coumadin) (see p. 435)

MICROPHTHALMIA/ANOPHTHALMIA (Unilateral or Bilateral)

FACIAL AND BRAIN ABNORMALITIES

Branchio-Oculo-Facial Syndrome: Autosomal dominant disorder characterized by mental retardation, growth deficiency, ocular defects, and clefting of the upper lip (see p. 149)

Fraser Syndrome: Autosomal recessive syndrome featuring cryptophthalmos, syndactyly, and genital, renal, and tracheal anomalies (see p. 160)

Goldenhar Syndrome: Asymmetry of the face and ears in conjunction with vertebral anomalies of the upper spine (see p. 162)

Hydrolethalus: Autosomal recessive disorder characterized by hydrocephalus, polydactyly, heart defects, and polyhydramnios (see p. 194)

Meckel-Gruber Syndrome: Autosomal recessive condition characterized by posterior encephalocele, postaxial polydactyly, and polycystic kidneys (see p. 199)

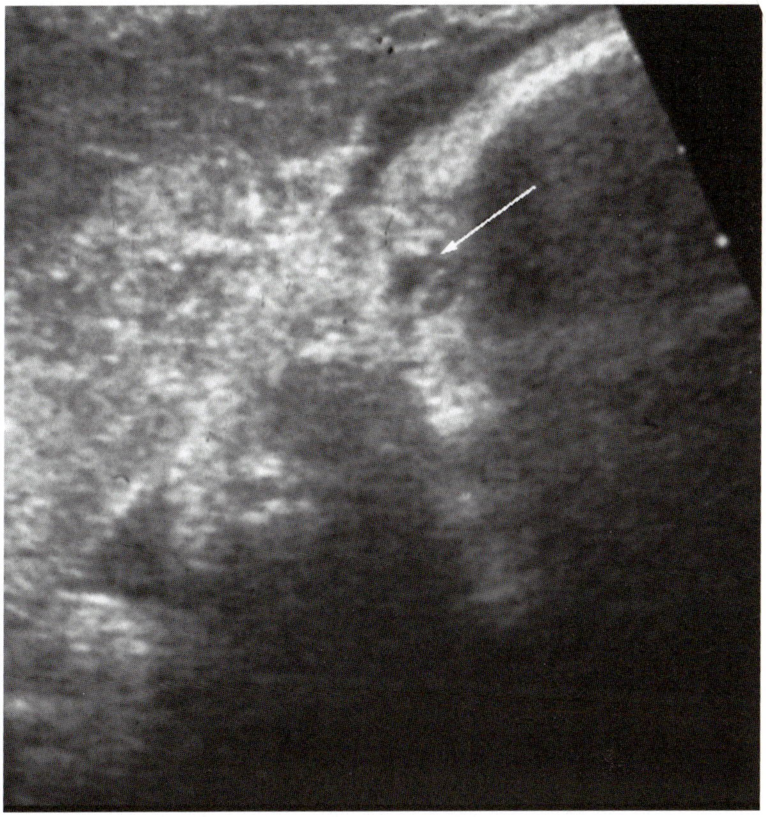

FIGURE 1-2 Modified coronal view of a third-trimester fetus with microphthalmia shows a small orbit *(arrow)*.

Median Cleft Face: Midline facial defects resulting in hypertelorism and bifid or broad nasal bridge (occasional) (see p. 165)

Neu-Laxova Syndrome: Autosomal recessive condition characterized by microcephaly, lissencephaly, exophthalmos, severe IUGR, swollen subcutaneous tissues, and ichthyosis (see p. 211)

Walker-Warburg Syndrome: Autosomal recessive condition characterized by severe congenital oculocerebral abnormalities, including lissencephaly, hydrocephalus, encephalocele, microcephaly, microphthalmia, and cataracts (see p. 217)

LIMB AND SKELETAL ABNORMALITIES

Chondrodysplasia Punctata: Heterogeneous group of bone dysplasias characterized by asymmetric limb shortening and abnormal early calcification of the proximal and distal epiphyses (occasional) (see p. 266)

Fanconi Anemia: Autosomal recessive condition characterized by radial hypoplasia, absent thumbs, and tendency for leukemia (occasional) (see p. 229)

Roberts Syndrome: Autosomal recessive condition characterized by severe shortening of the limbs (pseudothalidomide syndrome) and facial anomalies (occasional) (see p. 247)

CHROMOSOMAL ANOMALIES

Triploidy: Occurring as a result of a complete extra set of chromosomes, this is a lethal abnormality characterized by severe early-onset IUGR as well as multiple anomalies of practically all organ systems (see p. 473)

Trisomy 9: Occurring as a result of an extra chromosome 9, this is a severe abnormality characterized by multiple anomalies of practically all organ systems (see p. 478)

Trisomy 13 (Patau Syndrome): Occurring as a result of an extra chromosome 13, this is a severe abnormality characterized by multiple anomalies of the central nervous system, face, heart, and extremities (see p. 483)

Trisomy 18 (Edwards Syndrome): Occurring as a result of an extra chromosome 18, this is a severe abnormality characterized by IUGR and multiple anomalies of the central nervous system, face, heart, and extremities (see p. 490)

OTHER SYNDROMES AND SEQUENCES

Cerebro-Oculo-Facio-Skeletal (COFS) Syndrome: Autosomal recessive condition characterized by joint contractures of all the extremities, with severe facial and brain abnormalities (see p. 374)

CHARGE Association: **C**oloboma of the iris, **h**eart defect, choanal **a**tresia, intrauterine growth **r**estriction, **g**enital anomalies, and **e**ar anomalies (occasional) (see p. 376)

Fryns Syndrome: Autosomal recessive condition characterized by diaphragmatic defects, digital and facial abnormalities, and brain anomalies (occasional) (see p. 325)

Proteus Syndrome: Asymmetric focal overgrowth, subcutaneous tumors, and hemihypertrophy (occasional) (see p. 352)

TERATOGENS

Alcohol (see p. 438)

Phenylephrine (see p. 439)

TORCH (**t**oxoplasmosis, **o**ther infections, **ru**bella, **c**ytomegalovirus infection, and **h**erpes simplex) infections (rubella and varicella) (see p. 441)

HYPOTELORISM/CYCLOPIA (Extreme)

FACIAL AND BRAIN ABNORMALITIES

Cleft Lip and Palate (see p. 154)

Septo-Optic Dysplasia: Disorder characterized by absence of the septum pellucidum and hypoplasia of the optic nerves, commonly associated with agenesis of the corpus callosum (occasional) (see p. 214)

CRANIOSYNOSTOSIS

Crouzon Syndrome: Autosomal dominant condition characterized by craniosynostosis of the coronal sutures, midface hypoplasia, and ocular proptosis (see p. 313)

CHROMOSOMAL ANOMALIES

Trisomy 13 (Patau Syndrome): Occurring as a result of an extra chromosome 13, this is a severe abnormality characterized by multiple anomalies of the central nervous system, face, heart, and extremities (see p. 483)

OTHER SYNDROMES AND SEQUENCES

Holoprosencephaly sequence (see p. 386)

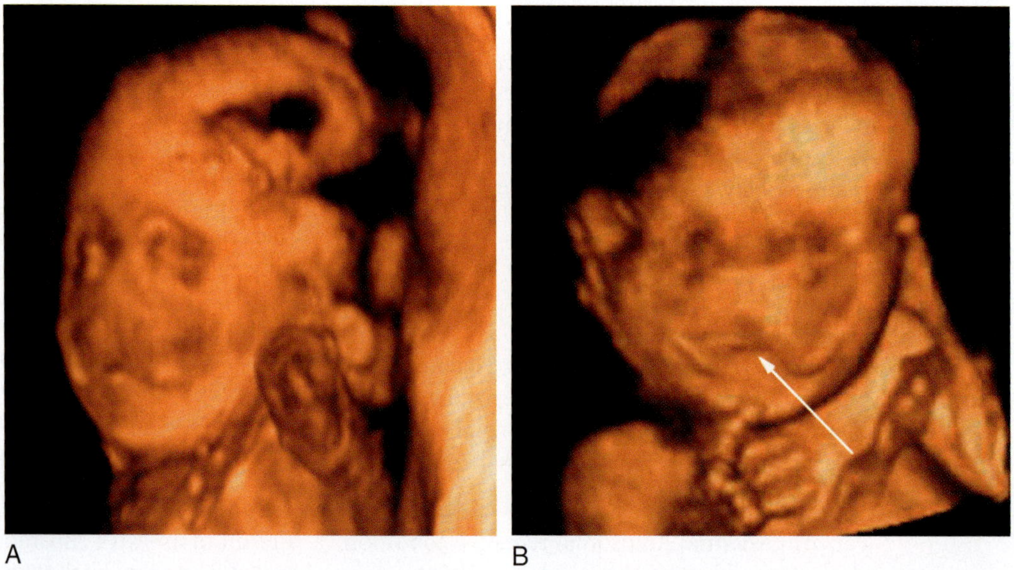

FIGURE 1-3 (A, B) Two views of the fetal face of a second-trimester fetus with trisomy 13 using three-dimensional surface rendering. Note hypotelorism and nasal hypoplasia. Midline facial cleft is seen *(arrow)*.

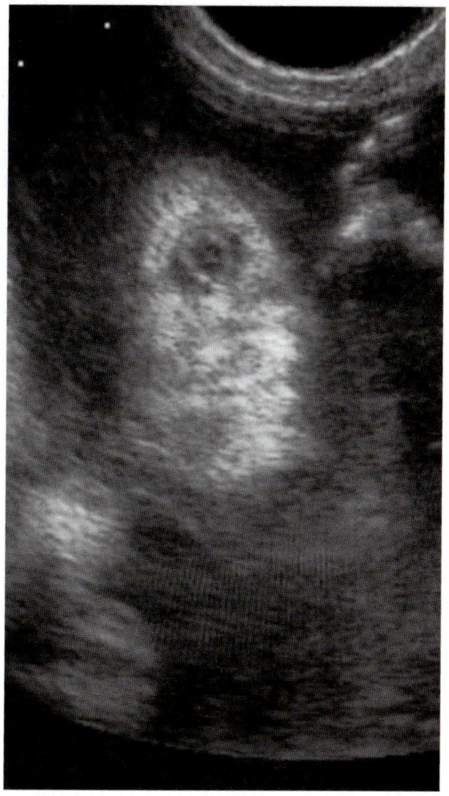

FIGURE 1-4 Coronal frontal view through the fetal face shows a single orbit in a fetus that has cyclopia with holoprosencephaly.

HYPERTELORISM

GROWTH ABNORMALITIES

Noonan Syndrome: Phenotypically, a Turner-like syndrome featuring short stature, webbed neck, cardiac abnormalities, and normal karyotype (see p. 131)

FACIAL AND BRAIN ABNORMALITIES

Encephalocele (Anterior)

Fraser Syndrome: Autosomal recessive syndrome featuring cryptophthalmos; syndactyly; and genital, renal, and tracheal anomalies (occasional) (see p. 160)

Gorlin Syndrome: Autosomal dominant syndrome characterized by macrocephaly, facial abnormalities, and multiple tumors (occasional) (see p. 192)

Median Cleft Face: Midline facial defects resulting in hypertelorism and bifid or broad nasal bridge (see p. 165)

Neu-Laxova Syndrome: Autosomal recessive condition characterized by microcephaly, lissencephaly, exophthalmos, severe IUGR, swollen subcutaneous tissues, and ichthyosis (see p. 211)

Smith-Lemli-Opitz Syndrome: Autosomal recessive syndrome featuring microcephaly, mental retardation, and genital and renal anomalies (occasional) (see p. 140)

LIMB AND SKELETAL ABNORMALITIES

Atelosteogenesis, Type I: Lethal skeletal dysplasia characterized by severe limb shortening and deficient ossification of the bones, resulting in micromelic dwarfism (see p. 260)

Camptomelic Dysplasia: Short-limbed skeletal dysplasia characterized by bowing of the long bones, particularly in the lower extremities; bell-shaped, narrow chest; and facial anomalies (see p. 262)

Chondrodysplasia Punctata: Heterogeneous group of bone dysplasias characterized by asymmetric limb shortening and abnormal early calcification of the proximal and distal epiphyses (see p. 266)

Cleidocranial Dysostosis: Autosomal dominant skeletal disorder characterized by hypoplasia, absence of the clavicle, and ossification abnormalities of the skull (see p. 268)

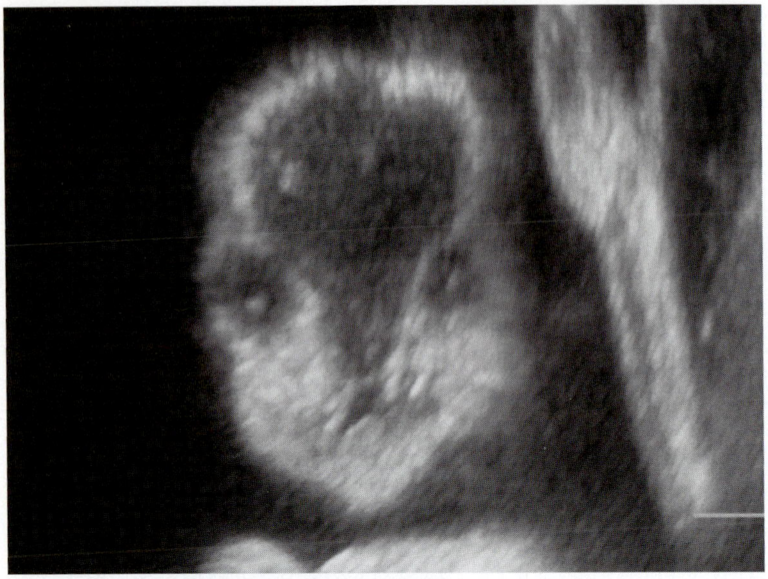

FIGURE 1-5 **Coronal view through the fetal face of a fetus that has severe hypertelorism with median cleft face syndrome.**

Larsen Syndrome: Condition characterized by abnormal facies and spinal and limb abnormalities, including dislocations and hyperextensions at the joints (see p. 242)

Multiple Pterygium Syndrome: Autosomal recessive condition characterized by multiple contractures and webbing across the joints, cystic hygromata, and facial defects (see p. 244)

Roberts Syndrome: Autosomal recessive condition characterized by severe shortening of the limbs (pseudothalidomide syndrome) and facial anomalies (see p. 247)

CRANIOSYNOSTOSIS

Apert Syndrome: Craniosynostosis, acrocephaly, and syndactyly (see p. 304)

Crouzon Syndrome: Autosomal dominant condition characterized by craniosynostosis of the coronal sutures, midface hypoplasia, and ocular proptosis (see p. 313)

Pfeiffer Syndrome: Acrocephalic skull, craniosynostosis (particularly of the coronal and sagittal sutures), and syndactyly of hands and feet (see p. 316)

CHROMOSOMAL ANOMALIES

Deletion 5p (Cri du Chat Syndrome): Abnormality of the chromosome 5, characterized by microcephaly, hypertelorism, micrognathia, hydrops, and growth delay (see p. 457)

Deletion 4p (Wolf-Hirschhorn Syndrome): Abnormality of chromosome 4 , characterized by IUGR, facial dysmorphology, cardiac defects, and hypospadias (see p. 459)

Deletion 11q (Jacobsen Syndrome): Deletion of the distal long arm of chromosome 11, characterized by multiple anomalies of practically all the organ systems (see p. 464)

Tetrasomy 12p (Pallister-Killian Syndrome): Mosaic aneuploidy characterized by multiple congenital abnormalities of the central nervous system, face, heart, and many other organs (see p. 471)

Triploidy: Occurring as a result of a complete extra set of chromosomes, this is a lethal abnormality characterized by severe early-onset IUGR as well as multiple anomalies of practically all organ systems (see p. 473)

Trisomy 10: Rare abnormality with only those individuals with mosaic trisomy 10 surviving to infancy. Abnormalities include IUGR and anomalies of the face, heart, hands, and feet (see p. 480)

Trisomy 18 (Edwards Syndrome): Occurring as a result of an extra chromosome 18, this is a severe abnormality characterized by IUGR and multiple anomalies of the central nervous system, face, heart, and extremities (see p. 490)

OTHER SYNDROMES AND SEQUENCES

CHARGE Association: **C**oloboma of the iris, **h**eart defect, choanal **a**tresia, intrauterine growth **r**estriction, **g**enital anomalies, and **e**ar anomalies (occasional) (see p. 376)

Opitz Syndrome: Disorder characterized by ocular hypertelorism, micrognathia, and, in males, hypospadias (see p. 399)

Pena Shokeir Syndrome: Autosomal recessive condition characterized by IUGR, multiple joint contractures, facial anomalies, and pulmonary hypoplasia; also known as fetal akinesia/hypokinesia sequence or neurogenic arthrogryposis (see p. 402)

TERATOGENS

Carbamazepine (Tegretol) (see p. 436)

Hydantoin (see p. 436)

Phenantoin (see p. 436)

CHOANAL ATRESIA

FACIAL AND BRAIN ABNORMALITIES

Cerebrocostomandibular Syndrome: Autosomal recessive condition characterized by severe micrognathia, cleft palate, and vertebral body abnormalities associated with defective costal development (occasional) (see p. 152)

Treacher Collins Syndrome: Autosomal dominant syndrome characterized by facial and ear abnormalities (see p. 184)

LIMB AND SKELETAL ABNORMALITIES

Ectrodactyly-Ectodermal Dysplasia-Clefting (EEC) Syndrome: Autosomal dominant condition characterized by labial clefting and ectrodactyly (lobster-claw deformities of the limbs), as well as genitourinary tract anomalies (occasional) (see p. 225)

CRANIOSYNOSTOSIS

Antley-Bixler Syndrome: Disorder characterized by craniosynostosis, resulting in severe brachycephaly, midfacial hypoplasia, multiple skeletal fusions, and contractures (see p. 303)

Pfeiffer Syndrome: Acrocephalic skull, craniosynostosis (particularly of the coronal and sagittal sutures), and syndactyly of hands and feet (occasional) (see p. 316)

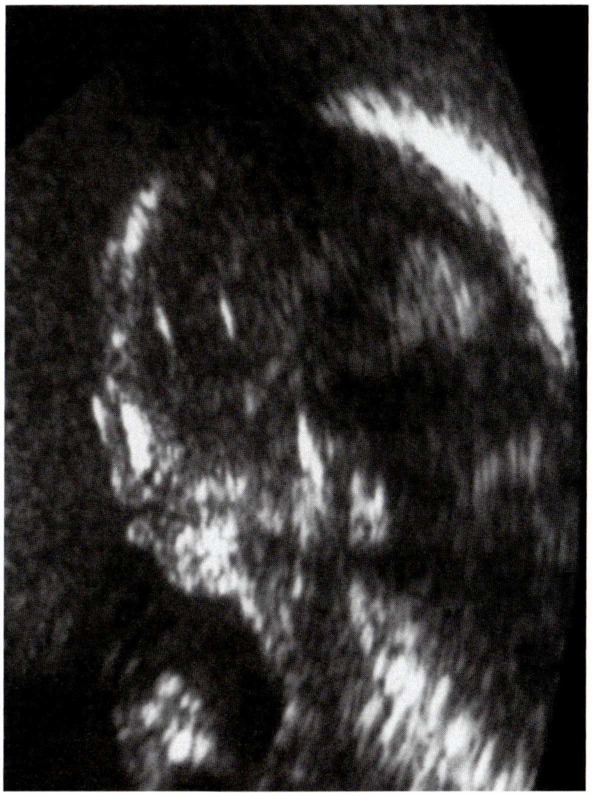

FIGURE 1-6 Profile view of the fetal face at 20 weeks shows severe micrognathia as well as choanal atresia in a fetus that has severe Treacher Collins syndrome.

OTHER SYNDROMES AND SEQUENCES

CHARGE Association: Coloboma of the iris, **h**eart defect, choanal **a**tresia, intrauterine growth **r**estriction, **g**enital anomalies, and **e**ar anomalies (see p. 376)

TERATOGENS

Warfarin (Coumadin) (see p. 435)

MICROGNATHIA

GROWTH ABNORMALITIES

Cerebrocostomandibular Syndrome: Autosomal recessive condition characterized by severe micrognathia, cleft palate, and vertebral body abnormalities associated with defective costal development (see p. 152)

Cornelia de Lange Syndrome: Facial and limb malformations, growth restriction, and mental developmental delay (see p. 129)

Russell-Silver Syndrome: Asymmetric growth restriction of the skeleton in conjunction with a normal-size head and short stature (see p. 136)

Seckel Syndrome: Autosomal recessive syndrome characterized by severe IUGR with microcephaly and severely abnormal profile (see p. 138)

Smith-Lemli-Opitz Syndrome: Autosomal recessive syndrome featuring microcephaly, mental retardation, and genital and renal anomalies (see p. 140)

FACIAL AND BRAIN ABNORMALITIES

Cerebrocostomandibular Syndrome: Autosomal recessive condition characterized by micrognathia, abnormal ribs, and narrow chest (see p. 152)

Goldenhar Syndrome: Asymmetry of the face and ears in conjunction with vertebral anomalies of the upper spine (see p. 162)

Hydrolethalus: Autosomal recessive disorder characterized by hydrocephalus, polydactyly, heart defects, and polyhydramnios (see p. 194)

Joubert Syndrome: Autosomal recessive syndrome characterized by dysmorphic facial features and agenesis of the cerebellar vermis (see p. 197)

Meckel-Gruber Syndrome: Autosomal recessive condition characterized by posterior encephalocele, postaxial polydactyly, and polycystic kidneys (see p. 199)

Nager Syndrome: Acrofacial dysostosis syndrome similar to Treacher Collins syndrome, characterized primarily by mandibular hypoplasia, malformed ears, and abnormal radial ray (see p. 171)

Neu-Laxova Syndrome: Autosomal recessive condition characterized by microcephaly, lissencephaly, exophthalmos, severe IUGR, swollen subcutaneous tissues, and ichthyosis (see p. 211)

Oral-Facial-Digital Syndrome, Type II (Mohr Syndrome): Autosomal recessive syndrome characterized by short stature; deafness; and facial, hand, and foot abnormalities (see p. 175)

Pierre Robin Syndrome: Hypoplasia of the mandible and cleft palate (see p. 177)

Shprintzen Syndrome: Autosomal dominant syndrome characterized by short stature, mild mental retardation, micrognathia, and cardiac and limb abnormalities (see p. 179)

Stickler Syndrome: Autosomal dominant syndrome characterized by ocular defects, cleft palate, micrognathia/hypoplasia of the mandible, and early orthopedic degenerative abnormalities (see p. 181)

Treacher Collins Syndrome: Autosomal dominant syndrome characterized by facial and ear abnormalities (see p. 184)

LIMB AND SKELETAL ABNORMALITIES

Achondrogenesis: Lethal skeletal dysplasia characterized by extreme hypoplasia of the bones, micromelia, decreased ossification of the bones (particularly those of the skull and spine), and hydrops (see p. 253)

Atelosteogenesis, Type I: Lethal skeletal dysplasia characterized by severe limb shortening and deficient ossification of the bones, resulting in micromelic dwarfism (see p. 260)

Camptomelic Dysplasia: Short-limbed skeletal dysplasia characterized by bowing of the long

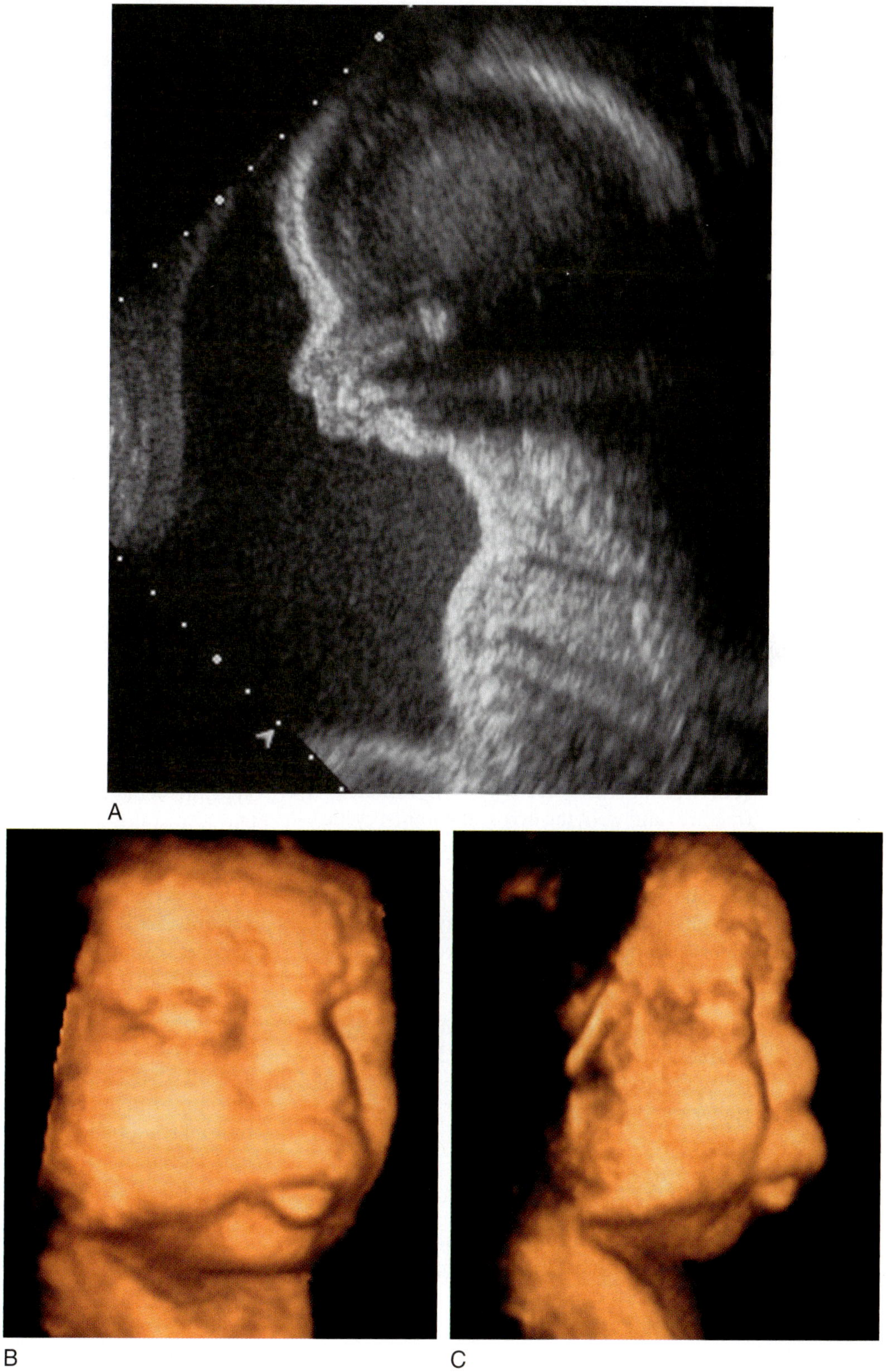

FIGURE 1-7 (**A**) Longitudinal profile view of a second-trimester fetus with severe micrognathia. (**B, C**) Two three-dimensional surface views of a severely dysmorphic third-trimester fetus with micrognathia.

bones, particularly in the lower extremities; bell-shaped, narrow chest; and facial anomalies (see p. 262)

Cleidocranial Dysostosis: Autosomal dominant skeletal disorder characterized by hypoplasia, absence of the clavicle, and ossification abnormalities of the skull (occasional) (see p. 268)

Diastrophic Dysplasia: Skeletal dysplasia characterized by micromelia, club feet, hand abnormalities (hitchhiker thumb), and kyphoscoliosis (see p. 270)

Ectrodactyly–Ectodermal Dysplasia–Clefting (EEC) Syndrome: Autosomal dominant condition characterized by labial clefting, ectrodactyly (lobster-claw deformities of the limbs), and genitourinary tract anomalies (occasional) (see p. 225)

Femoral Hypoplasia–Unusual Facies Syndrome: Syndrome characterized by short lower limbs, especially hypoplastic femurs, and facial abnormalities; may be part of a spectrum of abnormalities that includes caudal regression syndrome (see p. 231)

Multiple Pterygium Syndrome: Autosomal recessive condition characterized by multiple contractures and webbing across the joints, cystic hygromata, and facial defects (see p. 244)

Roberts Syndrome: Autosomal recessive condition characterized by severe shortening of the limbs (pseudothalidomide syndrome) and facial anomalies (see p. 247)

Thrombocytopenia–Absent Radius (TAR) Syndrome: Autosomal recessive syndrome characterized by radial aplasia and thrombocytopenia (occasional) (see p. 251)

CRANIOSYNOSTOSIS

Antley-Bixler Syndrome: Disorder characterized by craniosynostosis, resulting in severe brachycephaly, midfacial hypoplasia, multiple skeletal fusions, and contractures (see p. 303)

Carpenter Syndrome: Autosomal recessive condition characterized by acrocephaly, syndactyly, and preaxial polydactyly (see p. 310)

Crouzon Syndrome: Autosomal dominant condition characterized by craniosynostosis of the coronal sutures, midface hypoplasia, and ocular proptosis (see p. 313)

CHROMOSOMAL ANOMALIES

Deletion 4p (Wolf-Hirschhorn Syndrome): Abnormality of chromosome 4 characterized by IUGR, facial dysmorphology, cardiac defects, and hypospadias (see p. 459)

Deletion 5p (Cri du Chat Syndrome): Abnormality of chromosome 5 characterized by microcephaly, hypertelorism, micrognathia, hydrops, and growth delay (see p. 457)

Deletion 11q (Jacobsen Syndrome): Deletion of the distal long arm of chromosome 11 characterized by multiple anomalies of practically all organ systems (see p. 464)

DiGeorge Syndrome: Also known as velocardiofacial syndrome or Shprintzen syndrome, this disorder results from a deletion of chromosome 22q11.2 and is characterized by cardiac abnormalities involving largely the great vessels, facial abnormalities, hypocalcemia, and hypoplasia of the thymus (see p. 466)

Triploidy: Occurring as a result of a complete extra set of chromosomes, this is a lethal abnormality characterized by severe early-onset IUGR as well as multiple anomalies of practically all organ systems (see p. 473)

Trisomy 9: Occurring as a result of an extra chromosome 9, this is a severe abnormality characterized by multiple anomalies of practically all organ systems (see p. 478)

Trisomy 10: Rare abnormality with only those patients with mosaic trisomy 10 surviving to infancy. Abnormalities include IUGR and face, heart, hand, and foot anomalies (see p. 480)

Trisomy 18 (Edwards Syndrome): Occurring as a result of an extra chromosome 18, this is a severe abnormality characterized by IUGR and multiple anomalies of the central nervous system, face, heart, and extremities (see p. 490)

OTHER SYNDROMES AND SEQUENCES

Amniotic Band Syndrome: Condition caused by premature rupture of the amnion, resulting in an asymmetric, destructive fetal process whereby the fetus becomes adherent to, intertwined with, and tethered by the fibrous bands; associated with diverse anomalies (see p. 356)

Cerebro-Oculo-Facio-Skeletal (COFS) Syndrome: Autosomal recessive condition characterized by joint contractures of all the extremities, with severe facial and brain abnormalities (see p. 374)

CHARGE Association: Coloboma of the iris, **h**eart defect, choanal **a**tresia, intrauterine growth **r**estriction, **g**enital anomalies, and **e**ar anomalies (occasional) (see p. 376)

Fryns Syndrome: Autosomal recessive condition characterized by diaphragmatic defects, digital and facial abnormalities, and brain anomalies (see p. 325)

Infantile Polycystic Kidney Disease (see p. 329)

MURCS Association: **Mü**llerian duct aplasia, **r**enal aplasia, **c**ervicothoracic **s**omite dysplasia (occasional) (see p. 398)

Opitz Syndrome: Disorder characterized by ocular hypertelorism, micrognathia, and, in males, hypospadias (see p. 399)

Pena Shokeir Syndrome: Autosomal recessive condition characterized by IUGR, multiple joint contractures, and facial anomalies, and pulmonary hypoplasia; also known as fetal akinesia/hypokinesia sequence or neurogenic arthrogryposis syndrome (see p. 402)

TERATOGENS

Alcohol (see p. 438)

Aminopterin (see p. 438)

Amitriptyline (see p. 437)

Methotrexate (see p. 435)

Valproic acid (see p. 436)

FACIAL ASYMMETRY

FACIAL AND BRAIN ABNORMALITIES

Aicardi Syndrome: Rare X-linked syndrome characterized by agenesis of the corpus callosum, interhemispheric cyst, chorioretinal abnormalities, and infantile seizures (orbits) (see p. 188)

Fraser Syndrome: Autosomal recessive syndrome featuring cryptophthalmos; syndactyly; and genital, renal, and tracheal anomalies (see p. 160)

Goldenhar Syndrome: Asymmetry of the face and ears in conjunction with vertebral anomalies of the upper spine (see p. 162)

Oral-Facial-Digital Syndrome, Type I: X-linked dominant condition (lethal in males), OFD1 is one of nine syndromes (OFD1–OFD9) that include median cleft lip and palate, hypertelorism, micrognathia, and digital anomalies (see p. 174)

CRANIOSYNOSTOSIS

Saethre-Chotzen Syndrome: Autosomal dominant syndrome characterized by facial asymmetry, craniosynostosis of the coronal sutures, and digital abnormalities of the hands and feet (may be caused by unilateral coronal synostosis) (see p. 320)

Klippel-Feil Sequence: Abnormal cervical vertebrae, webbed neck, and facial asymmetry (see p. 394)

NASAL BONE HYPOPLASIA (Otherwise Normal Nose)

LIMB AND SKELETAL ABNORMALITIES

Cleidocranial Dysostosis: Autosomal dominant skeletal disorder characterized by hypoplasia, absence of the clavicle, and ossification abnormalities of the skull (occasional) (see p. 268)

CHROMOSOMAL ANOMALIES

Deletion 5p (Cri du Chat Syndrome): Abnormality of chromosome 5 characterized by microcephaly, hypertelorism, micrognathia, hydrops, and growth delay (see p. 457)

Trisomy 21 (Down Syndrome): Occurring as a result of an extra chromosome 21, this abnormality is characterized by nuchal fold thickening, short long-bones, abnormal nasal bone, heart defects, and other anomalies. Twenty-five percent of fetuses with Down syndrome do not display any sonographic abnormalities or markers (see p. 496)

FACIAL AND BRAIN ABNORMALITIES

Cleft Lip and Palate (see p. 154)

LIMB AND SKELETAL ABNORMALITIES

Achondroplasia: Autosomal dominant condition with rhizomelic limb shortening (nonlethal, heterozygous type usually is not apparent until late in the second trimester) (see p. 257)

Atelosteogenesis, Type I: Lethal skeletal dysplasia with severe limb shortening and deficient ossification of bones, resulting in micromelic dwarfism (see p. 260)

Camptomelic Dysplasia: Short-limbed skeletal dysplasia with bowing of the long bones, particularly in the lower extremities; bell-shaped, narrow chest; and facial anomalies (occasional) (see p. 262)

Chondrodysplasia Punctata: Heterogeneous group of bone dysplasias characterized by asymmetric limb shortening and abnormal early calcification of the proximal and distal epiphyses (see p. 266)

Cleidocranial Dysostosis: Autosomal dominant skeletal disorder characterized by hypoplasia, absence of the clavicle, and ossification abnormalities of the skull (occasional) (see p. 268)

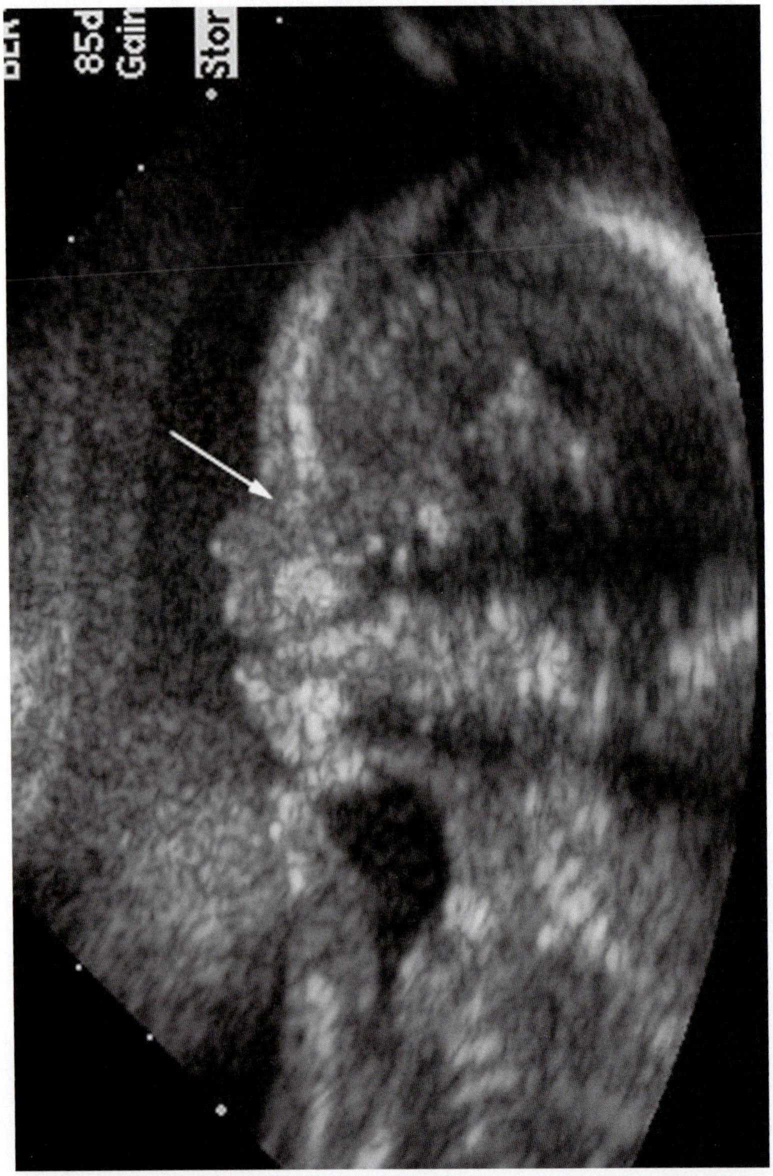

FIGURE 1-8 Profile view of a second-trimester fetus with Down syndrome shows absence of nasal bone ossification *(arrow)*.

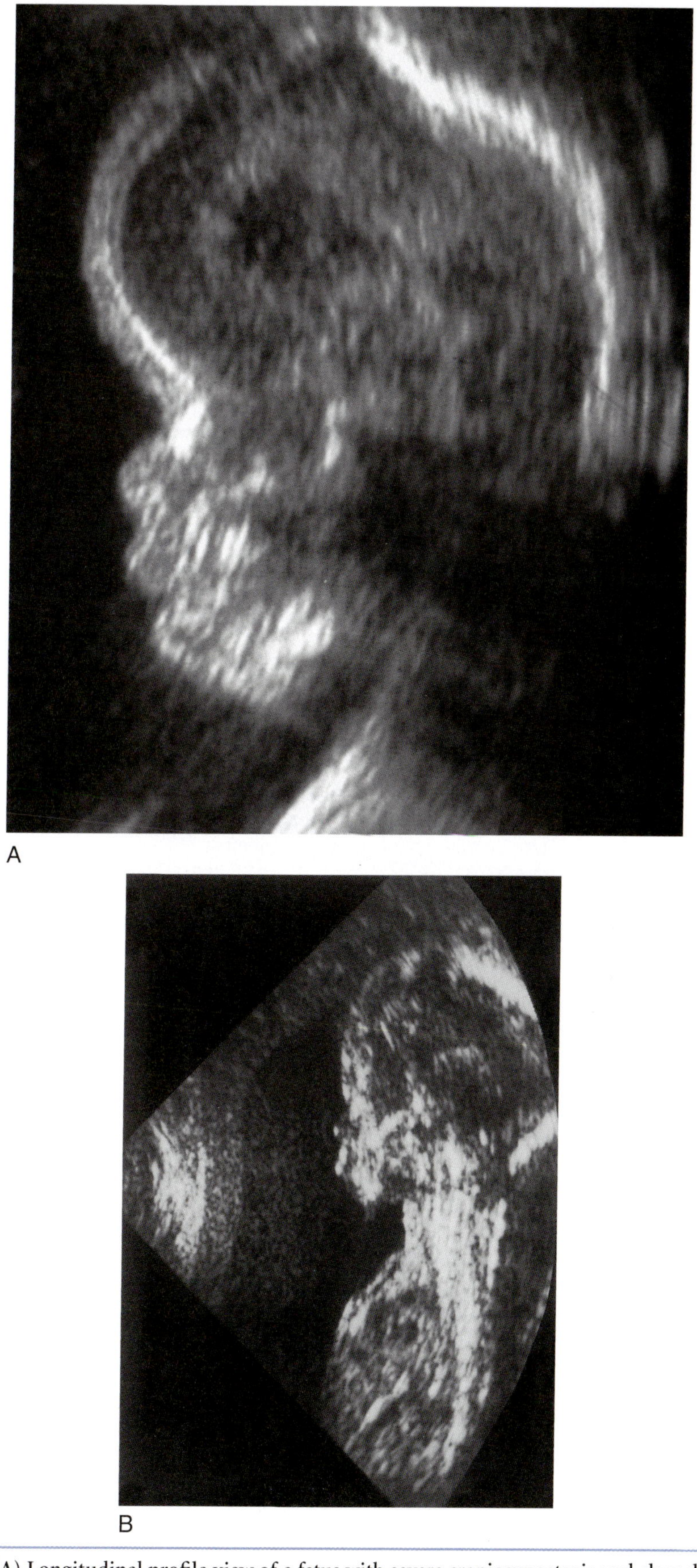

FIGURE 1-9 (A) Longitudinal profile view of a fetus with severe craniosynostosis and cloverleaf-shaped skull. Note the steep angle made by the nasal bridge and the forehead, as well as the severe acrocephaly and brachycephaly. (B) Longitudinal view of a second-trimester fetus whose mother was taking multiple medications for a seizure disorder. Note the midface hypoplasia, which gives the impression of a protruding chin.

Freeman-Sheldon (Whistling Face) Syndrome: Autosomal dominant condition characterized by unusual facial features and skeletal anomalies, such as flexion deformities of the joints (see p. 237)

Larsen Syndrome: Condition characterized by abnormal facies and spine and limb abnormalities, including dislocations and hyperextensions at the joints (see p. 242)

Thanatophoric Dysplasia: Most common skeletal dysplasia; characterized by narrow chest; short ribs; short, bowed long bones; and flat vertebral bodies (see p. 294)

CRANIOSYNOSTOSIS

Antley-Bixler Syndrome: Disorder characterized by craniosynostosis, resulting in severe brachycephaly, midfacial hypoplasia, multiple skeletal fusions, and contractures (see p. 303)

Apert Syndrome: Craniosynostosis, acrocephaly, and syndactyly (see p. 304)

Carpenter Syndrome: Autosomal recessive condition with acrocephaly, syndactyly, and preaxial polydactyly (see p. 310)

Pfeiffer Syndrome: Acrocephalic skull, craniosynostosis (particularly of the coronal and sagittal sutures), and syndactyly of hands and feet (see p. 316)

CHROMOSOMAL ANOMALIES

Deletion 11q (Jacobsen Syndrome): Deletion of the distal long arm of chromosome 11 characterized by multiple anomalies of practically all organ systems (see p. 464)

Trisomy 13 (Patau Syndrome): Occurring as a result of an extra chromosome 13, this is a severe abnormality characterized by multiple anomalies of the central nervous system, face, heart, and extremities (see p. 483)

Trisomy 21 (Down Syndrome): Occurring as a result of an extra chromosome 21, this abnormality is characterized by nuchal fold thickening, short long-bones, abnormal nasal bone, heart defects, and other anomalies. Twenty-five percent of fetuses with Down syndrome do not display any sonographic abnormalities or markers (see p. 496)

OTHER SYNDROMES AND SEQUENCES

CHARGE Association: **C**oloboma of the iris, **h**eart defect, choanal **a**tresia, intrauterine growth **r**estriction, **g**enital anomalies, and **e**ar anomalies (see p. 376)

Holoprosencephaly Sequence (see p. 386)

Pena Shokeir Syndrome: Autosomal recessive condition with IUGR, multiple joint contractures, facial anomalies, and pulmonary hypoplasia; also known as fetal akinesia/hypokinesia sequence or neurogenic arthrogryposis syndrome (see p. 402)

TERATOGENS

Alcohol (see p. 438)

Carbamazepine (Tegretol) (see p. 436)

Cyclophosphamide (see p. 435)

Hydantoin (see p. 436)

Phenantoin (see p. 436)

Valproic acid (see p. 436)

Warfarin (Coumadin) (see p. 435)

FACIAL CLEFT

GROWTH ABNORMALITIES

Smith-Lemli-Opitz Syndrome: Autosomal recessive syndrome featuring microcephaly, mental retardation, and genital and renal anomalies (occasional palate) (see p. 140)

FACIAL AND BRAIN ABNORMALITIES

Branchio-Oculo-Facial Syndrome: Autosomal dominant disorder characterized by mental retardation, growth deficiency, ocular defects, and clefting of the upper lip (pseudo or incomplete cleft lip) (see p. 149)

Fraser Syndrome: Autosomal recessive syndrome featuring cryptophthalmos, syndactyly, and genital, renal, and tracheal anomalies (occasional) (see p. 160)

Goldenhar Syndrome: Asymmetry of the face and ears in conjunction with vertebral anomalies of the upper spine (occasional) (see p. 162)

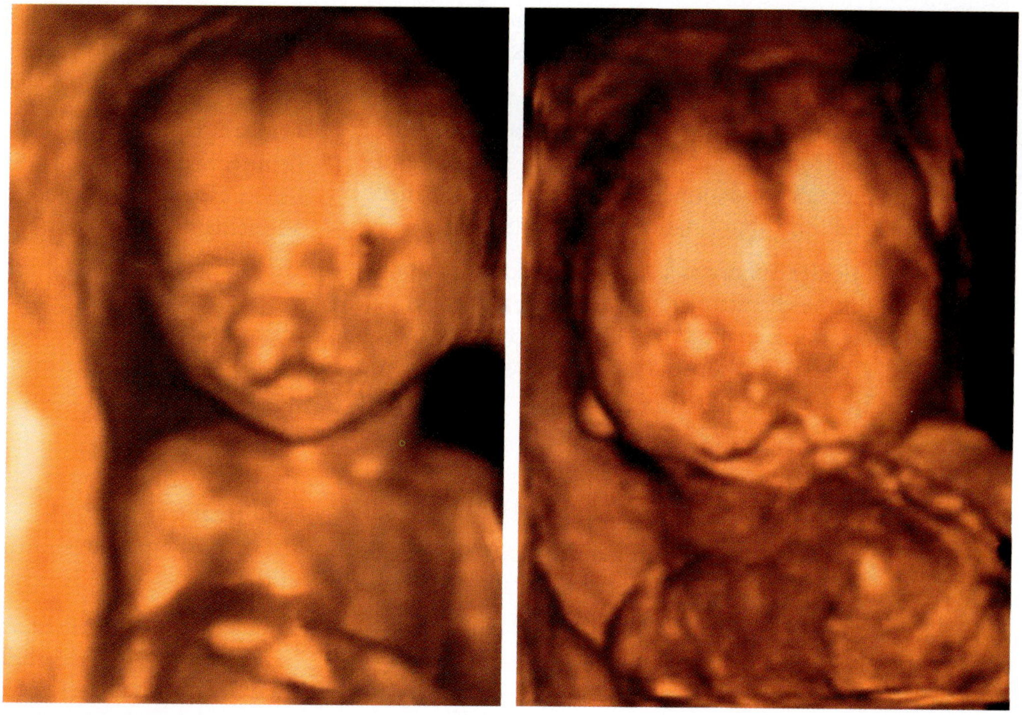

FIGURE 1-10 Three-dimensional surface rendering view of two different fetuses with unilateral complete cleft lip and palate.

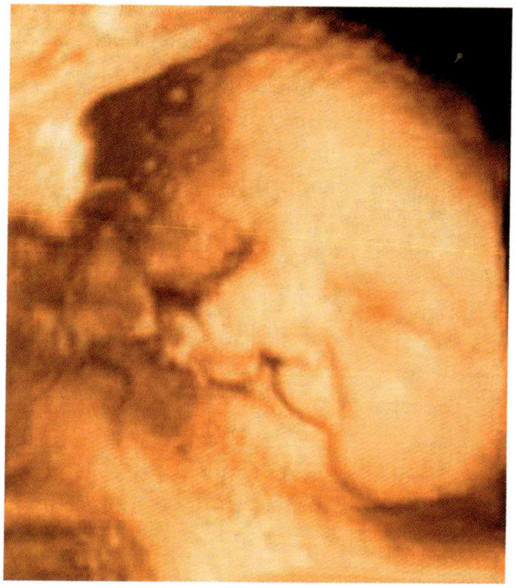

FIGURE 1-11 Third-trimester fetus with bilateral cleft lip and palate. Note extension of the labial cleft into nostril area.

Gorlin Syndrome: Autosomal dominant syndrome characterized by macrocephaly, facial abnormalities, and multiple tumors (see p. 192)

Hydrolethalus: Autosomal recessive disorder characterized by hydrocephalus, polydactyly, heart defects, and polyhydramnios (see p. 194)

Meckel-Gruber Syndrome: Autosomal recessive condition characterized by posterior encephalocele, postaxial polydactyly, and polycystic kidneys (palate) (see p. 199)

Nager Syndrome: Acrofacial dysostosis syndrome similar to Treacher Collins syndrome; characterized primarily by mandibular hypoplasia, malformed ears, and abnormal radial ray (frequent palate and occasional lip) (see p. 171)

Neu-Laxova Syndrome: Autosomal recessive condition characterized by microcephaly, lissencephaly, exophthalmos, severe IUGR, swollen subcutaneous tissues, and ichthyosis (occasional) (see p. 211)

Oral-Facial-Digital Syndrome, Type I: X-linked dominant condition (lethal in males), OFD1 is one of nine syndromes (OFD1–OFD9) that include median cleft lip and palate, hypertelorism, micrognathia, and digital anomalies (see p. 174)

Oral-Facial-Digital Syndrome, Type II (Mohr Syndrome): Autosomal recessive syndrome characterized by short stature; deafness; and facial, hand, and foot abnormalities (see p. 175)

Pierre Robin Syndrome: Hypoplasia of the mandible and cleft palate (see p. 177)

Septo-Optic Dysplasia: Disorder characterized by absence of the septum pellucidum and hypoplasia of the optic nerves, commonly associated with agenesis of the corpus callosum (occasional) (see p. 214)

Shprintzen Syndrome: Autosomal dominant syndrome characterized by short stature, mild mental retardation, micrognathia, and cardiac and limb abnormalities (see p. 179)

Stickler Syndrome: Autosomal dominant syndrome characterized by ocular defects, cleft palate, micrognathia/hypoplasia of the mandible, and early orthopedic degenerative abnormalities (palate) (see p. 181)

Treacher Collins Syndrome: Autosomal dominant syndrome characterized by facial and ear abnormalities (palate) (see p. 184)

Van der Woude Syndrome: Dominant labial clefting syndrome characterized by pits in the lower lip and variable cleft lip and palate (see p. 186)

Walker-Warburg Syndrome: Autosomal recessive condition characterized by severe, congenital oculocerebral abnormalities, including lissencephaly, hydrocephalus, encephalocele, microcephaly, microphthalmia, and cataracts (occasional) (see p. 217)

LIMB AND SKELETAL ABNORMALITIES

Adams-Oliver Syndrome: Disorder characterized by terminal transverse defects of the upper and lower extremities, as well as denuded areas on the scalp with or without an underlying bony skull (bone) defect (occasional) (see p. 223)

Camptomelic Dysplasia: Short-limbed skeletal dysplasia characterized by bowing of the long bones, particularly in the lower extremities; bell-shaped, narrow chest; and facial anomalies (palate) (see p. 262)

Chondrodysplasia Punctata: Heterogeneous group of bone dysplasias characterized by asymmetric limb shortening and abnormal early calcification of the proximal and distal epiphyses (see p. 266)

Cleidocranial dysostosis: Autosomal dominant skeletal disorder characterized by hypoplasia, absence of the clavicle, and ossification abnormalities of the skull (occasional palate only) (see p. 268)

Diastrophic Dysplasia: Skeletal dysplasia characterized by micromelia, clubbed feet, hand abnormalities (hitchhiker thumb), and kyphoscoliosis (palate) (see p. 270)

Ectrodactyly–Ectodermal Dysplasia–Clefting (EEC) Syndrome: Autosomal dominant condition characterized by labial clefting and ectrodactyly (lobster-claw deformities of the limbs), as well as genitourinary tract anomalies (see p. 225)

Femoral Hypoplasia–Unusual Facies Syndrome: Syndrome characterized by short lower limbs, especially hypoplastic femurs, and facial abnormalities; may be part of a spectrum of abnormalities that includes caudal regression syndrome (palate only) (see p. 231)

Kniest Syndrome: Autosomal dominant condition characterized by kyphoscoliosis, platyspondyly, and shortened tubular long bones (palate) (see p. 281)

Larsen Syndrome: Condition characterized by abnormal facies and spine and limb abnormalities, including dislocations and hyperextensions at the joints (see p. 242)

Majewski Syndrome (Short Rib–Polydactyly Syndrome, Type II): Autosomal recessive skeletal dysplasia characterized by short ribs, narrow thorax, polydactyly, and median facial cleft (see p. 283)

Multiple Pterygium Syndrome: Autosomal recessive condition characterized by multiple contractures and webbing across the joints, cystic hygromata, and facial defects (palate) (see p. 244)

Roberts Syndrome: Autosomal recessive condition characterized by severe shortening of the limbs (pseudothalidomide syndrome) and facial anomalies (see p. 247)

Thrombocytopenia–Absent Radius (TAR) Syndrome: Autosomal recessive syndrome characterized by radial aplasia and thrombocytopenia (palate) (see p. 251)

CRANIOSYNOSTOSIS

Crouzon Syndrome: Autosomal dominant condition characterized by craniosynostosis of the coronal sutures, midface hypoplasia, and ocular proptosis (occasional) (see p. 313)

CHROMOSOMAL ANOMALIES

Deletion 4p (Wolf-Hirschhorn Syndrome): Abnormality of chromosome 4 characterized by IUGR, facial dysmorphology, cardiac defects, and hypospadias (see p. 459)

Deletion 11q (Jacobsen Syndrome): Deletion of the distal long arm of chromosome 11 characterized by multiple anomalies of practically all organ systems (occasional) (see p. 464)

DiGeorge Syndrome: Also known as velocardiofacial syndrome or Shprintzen syndrome, this disorder results from a deletion of chromosome 22q11.2 and is characterized by cardiac abnormalities involving largely the great vessels, facial abnormalities, hypocalcemia, and hypoplasia of the thymus (see p. 466)

Trisomy 9: Occurring as a result of an extra chromosome 9, this is a severe abnormality characterized by multiple anomalies of practically all organ systems (see p. 478)

Trisomy 10: Rare abnormality with only those patients with mosaic trisomy 10 surviving to infancy. Abnormalities include IUGR and face, heart, hand, and foot anomalies (see p. 480)

Trisomy 13 (Patau Syndrome): Occurring as a result of an extra chromosome 13, this is a severe abnormality characterized by multiple anomalies of the central nervous system, face, heart, and extremities (see p. 483)

Trisomy 18 (Edwards Syndrome): Occurring as a result of an extra chromosome 18, this is a severe abnormality characterized by IUGR and multiple anomalies of the central nervous system, face, heart, and extremities (occasional) (see p. 490)

Trisomy 22: Occurring as a result of an extra chromosome 22, this is a lethal abnormality characterized by multiple anomalies of the heart, face, extremities, and gastrointestinal and genitourinary systems (see p. 509)

OTHER SYNDROMES AND SEQUENCES

Amniotic Band Syndrome: Condition caused by premature rupture of the amnion, resulting in an asymmetric destructive fetal process whereby the fetus becomes adherent to, intertwined with, and tethered by the fibrous bands; associated with diverse anomalies (see p. 356)

Arthrogryposis: Sequence of neurologic, muscular, and connective tissue disorders leading to fetal joint contractures and rigidity, as well as decreased activity (occasional) (see p. 362)

Caudal Regression Syndrome/Sirenomelia: Although of different etiologies, these two syndromes are similar: disruption of the caudal portion of the neural tube, absence or dysplasia of the sacrum, and renal and lower extremity anomalies (occasional) (see p. 370)

CHARGE Association: Coloboma of the iris, **h**eart defect, choanal **a**tresia, intrauterine growth **r**estriction, **g**enital and **e**ar anomalies (occasional) (see p. 376)

Fryns Syndrome: Autosomal recessive condition characterized by diaphragmatic defects, digital and facial abnormalities, and brain anomalies (see p. 325)

Jarcho-Levin Syndrome (Spondylothoracic Dysplasia): Most common among Puerto Ricans; characterized by vertebral defects resulting in very short thorax and spine and protuberant abdomen (occasional palate) (see p. 332)

Holoprosencephaly (see p. 386)

Klippel-Feil Sequence: Abnormal cervical vertebrae, webbed neck, and facial asymmetry (occasional palate) (see p. 394)

Marfan Syndrome: Autosomal dominant connective tissue disorder with tall stature, long limbs, pectus deformities, congenital heart defects, and ocular anomalies (occasional palate) (see p. 344)

MURCS Association: Müllerian duct aplasia, **r**enal aplasia, **c**ervicothoracic **s**omite dysplasia (occasional) (see p. 398)

Opitz Syndrome: Disorder characterized by ocular hypertelorism, micrognathia, and, in males, hypospadias (see p. 399)

Pena Shokeir Syndrome: Autosomal recessive condition characterized by IUGR, multiple joint contractures, facial anomalies, and pulmonary hypoplasia; also known as fetal akinesia/hypokinesia sequence or neurogenic arthrogryposis (occasional palate) (see p. 402)

Pentalogy of Cantrell: Combination of five anomalies: ectopia cordis, omphalocele, disruption of distal sternum, anterior diaphragm, and diaphragmatic pericardium (occasional) (see p. 405)

TERATOGENS

Alcohol (see p. 438)

Aminopterin (Antifolate) (see p. 438)

Carbamazepine (Tegretol) (see p. 436)

Codeine (see p. 439)

Cortisone (see p. 437)

Ethosuximide (see p. 436)

Fluphenazine (see p. 438)

Hydantoin (see p. 436)

Hyperthermia (see p. 439)

Imipramine (see p. 438)

Metronidazole (Flagyl) (see p. 434)

Phenantoin (see p. 436)

Quinine (see p. 434)

Radiation (see p. 439)

Valproic acid (see p. 436)

EAR ANOMALIES

GROWTH ABNORMALITIES

Noonan Syndrome: Phenotypically Turner-like, with short stature, webbed neck, cardiac abnormalities, and normal karyotype (low-set ears) (see p. 131)

FACIAL AND BRAIN ABNORMALITIES

Branchio-Oculo-Facial Syndrome: Autosomal dominant disorder characterized by mental retardation, growth deficiency, ocular defects, and clefting of the upper lip (occasional) (see p. 149)

Fraser Syndrome: Autosomal recessive syndrome featuring cryptophthalmos; syndactyly; and genital, renal, and tracheal anomalies (see p. 160)

Goldenhar Syndrome: Asymmetry of the face and ears with vertebral anomalies of the upper spine (see p. 162)

Hydrolethalus: Autosomal recessive disorder characterized by hydrocephalus, polydactyly, heart defects, and polyhydramnios (low-set ears) (see p. 194)

Nager Syndrome: Acrofacial dysostosis syndrome similar to Treacher Collins syndrome; primarily mandibular hypoplasia, malformed ears, and abnormal radial ray (low-set ears) (see p. 171)

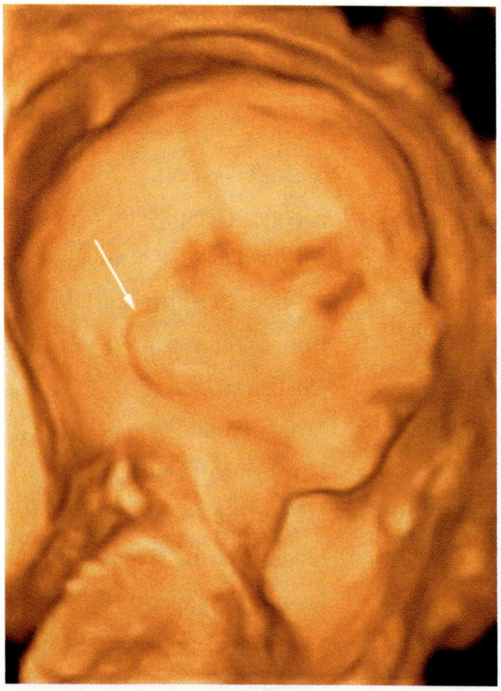

FIGURE 1-12 Three-dimensional surface rendering of a second-trimester fetus with micrognathia and low-set ears *(arrow)*.

Shprintzen Syndrome: Autosomal dominant syndrome characterized by short stature, mild mental retardation, micrognathia, and cardiac and limb abnormalities (see p. 179)

Treacher Collins Syndrome: Autosomal dominant syndrome characterized by facial and ear abnormalities (see p. 184)

LIMB AND SKELETAL ABNORMALITIES

Ectrodactyly–Ectodermal Dysplasia–Clefting (EEC) Syndrome: Autosomal dominant condition characterized by labial clefting and ectrodactyly (lobster-claw deformities of the limbs), as well as genitourinary tract anomalies (see p. 225)

Femoral Hypoplasia–Unusual Facies Syndrome: Syndrome characterized by short lower limbs, especially hypoplastic femurs, and facial abnormalities; may be part of a spectrum of abnormalities that includes caudal regression syndrome (low-set ears) (see p. 231)

CRANIOSYNOSTOSIS

Carpenter Syndrome: Autosomal recessive condition characterized by acrocephaly, syndactyly, and preaxial polydactyly (low-set ears) (see p. 310)

CHROMOSOMAL ANOMALIES

Deletion 11q (Jacobsen Syndrome): Deletion of the distal long arm of chromosome 11 characterized by multiple anomalies of practically all organ systems (see p. 464)

Tetrasomy 12p (Pallister-Killian Syndrome): Mosaic aneuploidy characterized by multiple congenital abnormalities of the central nervous system, face, heart, and many other organs (low-set ears) (see p. 471)

Trisomy 18 (Edwards Syndrome): Occurring as a result of an extra chromosome 18, this is a severe abnormality characterized by IUGR and multiple anomalies of the central nervous system, face, heart, and extremities (low-set ears) (see p. 490)

Trisomy 21 (Down Syndrome): Occurring as a result of an extra chromosome 21, this abnormality is characterized by nuchal fold thickening, short long-bones, abnormal nasal bone, heart defects, and other anomalies. Twenty-five percent of fetuses with Down syndrome do not display any sonographic abnormalities or markers (small ears) (see p. 496)

OTHER SYNDROMES AND SEQUENCES

CHARGE Association: **C**oloboma of the iris, **h**eart defect, choanal **a**tresia, intrauterine growth **r**estriction, **g**enital anomalies, and **e**ar anomalies (see p. 376)

Fryns Syndrome: Autosomal recessive condition characterized by diaphragmatic defects, digital and facial abnormalities, and brain anomalies (see p. 325)

Klippel-Feil Syndrome: Abnormal cervical vertebrae, webbed neck, and facial asymmetry (low-set ears) (see p. 394)

MURCS Association: **Mü**llerian duct aplasia, **r**enal aplasia, **c**ervicothoracic **s**omite dysplasia (see p. 398)

TERATOGENS

Alcohol (see p. 438)

Aminopterin (low-set ears) (see p. 438)

Chlorpropamide (see p. 439)

Estrogen (see p. 437)

Methotrexate (low-set ears) (see p. 435)

Phenantoin (low-set ears) (see p. 436)

Phenylephrine (see p. 439)

Trimethadione (low-set ears) (see p. 436)

Valproic acid (low-set ears) (see p. 436)

ABNORMAL HEAD SHAPE

STRAWBERRY

Trisomy 18 (Edwards syndrome) (see p. 490)

LEMON

Open neural tube defect (NTD)

CLOVERLEAF

Thanatophoric Dysplasia: Most common skeletal dysplasia, with narrow chest; short ribs; short, bowed long bones; and flat vertebral bodies (sec p. 294)

Crouzon Syndrome: Autosomal dominant condition characterized by craniosynostosis of the coronal sutures, midface hypoplasia, and ocular proptosis (see p. 313)

Pfeiffer Syndrome: Acrocephalic skull, craniosynostosis (particularly of the coronal and sagittal sutures), and syndactyly of hands and feet (see p. 316)

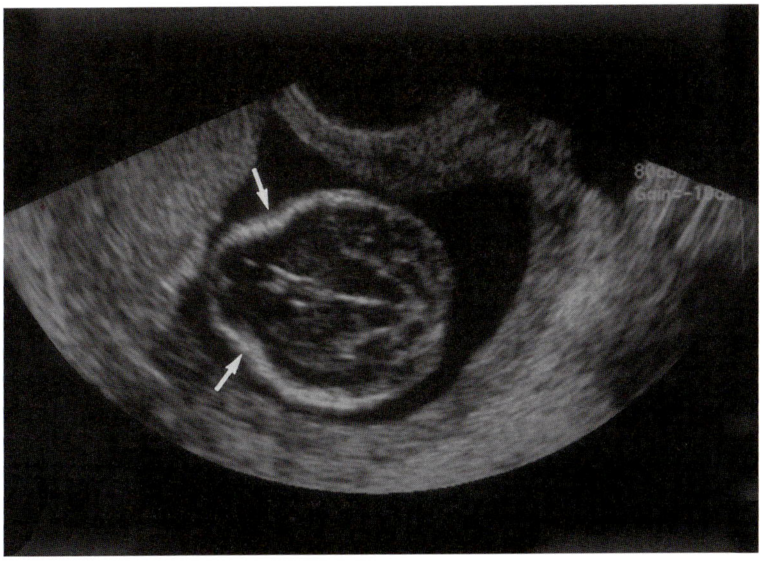

FIGURE 1-13 Transverse view through the fetal head shows a lemon-shaped deformity of the frontal bones *(arrows)* that is consistent with an open neural tube defect. Note that the cerebellum has a banana-like shape and is wrapping around the brainstem.

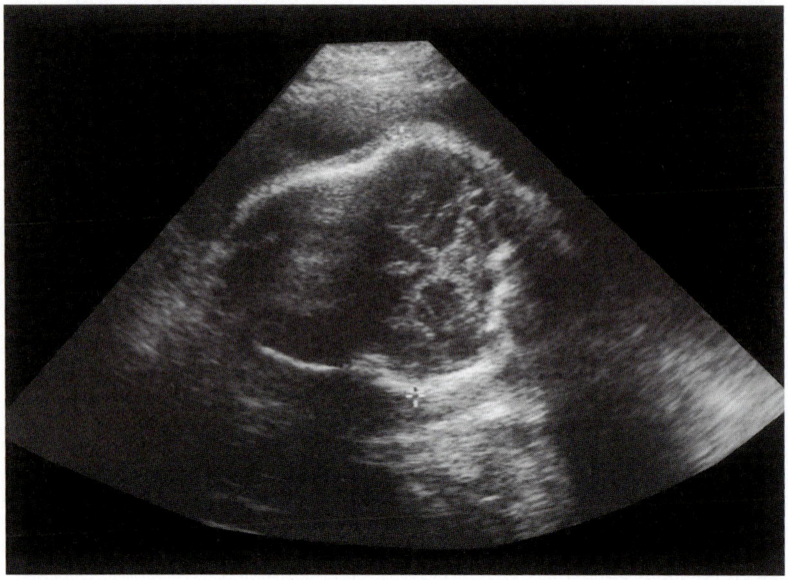

FIGURE 1-14 Coronal view through the head of a fetus with a cloverleaf-shaped head.

CRANIOSYNOSTOSIS

Antley-Bixler Syndrome: Disorder characterized by craniosynostosis, resulting in severe brachycephaly, midfacial hypoplasia, multiple skeletal fusions, and contractures (see p. 303)

Apert Syndrome: Craniosynostosis, acrocephaly, and syndactyly (acrocephaly and brachycephaly) (see p. 304)

Carpenter Syndrome: Autosomal recessive condition with acrocephaly, syndactyly, preaxial polydactyly (acrocephaly and brachycephaly) (see p. 310)

Crouzon Syndrome: Autosomal dominant condition characterized by craniosynostosis of the coronal sutures, midface hypoplasia, and ocular proptosis (occasional cloverleaf) (see p. 313)

Pfeiffer Syndrome: Acrocephalic skull, craniosynostosis (particularly of the coronal and sagittal sutures), and syndactyly of hands and feet (occasional cloverleaf) (see p. 316)

Saethre-Chotzen Syndrome: Autosomal dominant syndrome characterized by facial asymmetry, craniosynostosis of the coronal sutures, and digital abnormalities of the hands and feet (see p. 320)

Roberts Syndrome: Autosomal recessive condition characterized by severe shortening of the limbs (pseudothalidomide syndrome) and facial anomalies (occasional craniosynostosis) (see p. 247)

Proteus Syndrome: Asymmetric focal overgrowth, subcutaneous tumors, and hemihypertrophy (occasional craniosynostosis) (see p. 352)

FRONTAL BOSSING

Gorlin Syndrome: Autosomal dominant syndrome characterized by macrocephaly, facial abnormalities, and multiple tumors (see p. 192)

Russell-Silver Syndrome: Asymmetric growth restriction of the skeleton in conjunction with a normal-size head and short stature (see p. 136)

Achondroplasia: Autosomal dominant condition characterized by rhizomelic limb shortening (nonlethal, heterozygous type usually is not apparent until late in the second trimester) (see p. 257)

TRIGONOCEPHALY

Deletion 11q (Jacobsen Syndrome): Deletion of the distal long arm of chromosome 11 characterized by multiple anomalies of practically all organ systems (see p. 464)

SKULL ASYMMETRY

Deletion 4p (Wolf-Hirschhorn Syndrome): Abnormality of chromosome 4 characterized by

IUGR, facial dysmorphology, cardiac defects, and hypospadias (see p. 459)

Amniotic Band Syndrome: Condition caused by premature rupture of the amnion, resulting in an asymmetric destructive fetal process whereby the fetus becomes adherent to, intertwined with, and tethered by the fibrous bands; associated with diverse anomalies (see p. 356)

BRACHYCEPHALY

Cornelia de Lange Syndrome: Facial and limb malformations, growth restriction, and mental developmental delay (see p. 129)

Chondrodysplasia Punctata (Rhizomelic Type)**:** Heterogeneous group of bone dysplasias characterized by asymmetric limb shortening and abnormal early calcification of the proximal and distal epiphyses (see p. 266)

Trisomy 21 (Down Syndrome): Occurring as a result of an extra chromosome 21, this abnormality is characterized by nuchal fold thickening, short long-bones, abnormal nasal bone, heart defects, and other anomalies. Twenty-five percent of fetuses with Down syndrome do not display any sonographic abnormalities or markers (see p. 496)

FLUID COLLECTIONS IN THE HEAD

BILATERAL

Choroid Plexus Cyst: Fluid collection within choroid plexus

Porencephalic Cyst: Communicating with lateral ventricles

Ventriculomegaly: Fluid collection around the choroid plexus, with choroid plexus in a dependent position

UNILATERAL

Supratentorial

Arachnoid Cyst: Abutting meninges

Arteriovenous Malformation: As demonstrated by Doppler flow studies

Bleed: Complex mass, often involving the ventricle and changing over time

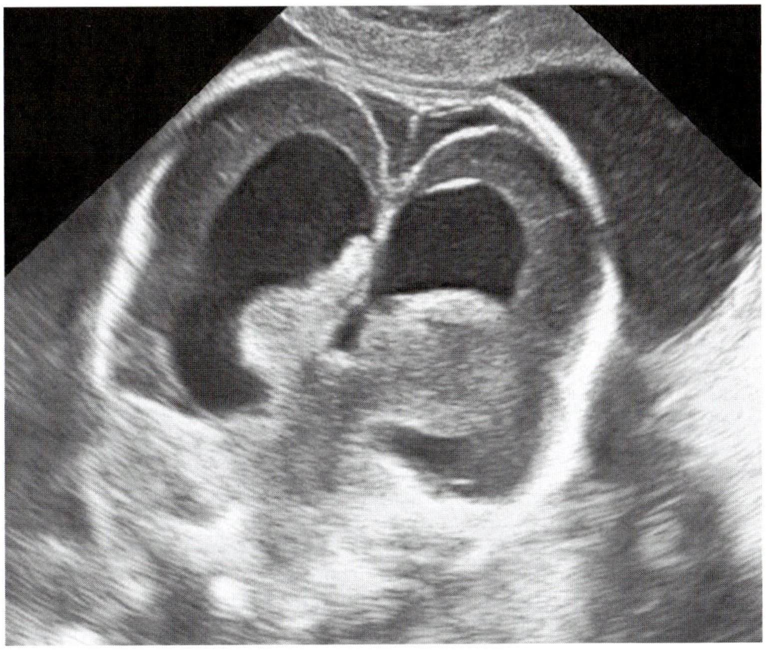

FIGURE 1-15 Coronal view of the fetal brain shows moderate ventriculomegaly at 20 weeks. Note asymmetry of the choroid plexus.

Porencephalic Cyst: Communicating with lateral ventricles

Schizencephaly: Disorganized fluid collections

Tumor: Usually a complex mass, with solid areas

Infratentorial

Arachnoid Cyst: Cyst compressing the cerebellum against the brainstem, with vermis remaining intact

Dandy-Walker Cyst: Cyst separating two hypoplastic cerebellar hemispheres, with absent vermis

Dandy-Walker Variant: Near-normal cerebellar hemispheric shape associated with a keyhole connection of the fourth ventricle with the cisterna magna, as well as hypoplastic vermis

Mega Cisterna Magna: Normal-looking cerebellum with large cisterna magna

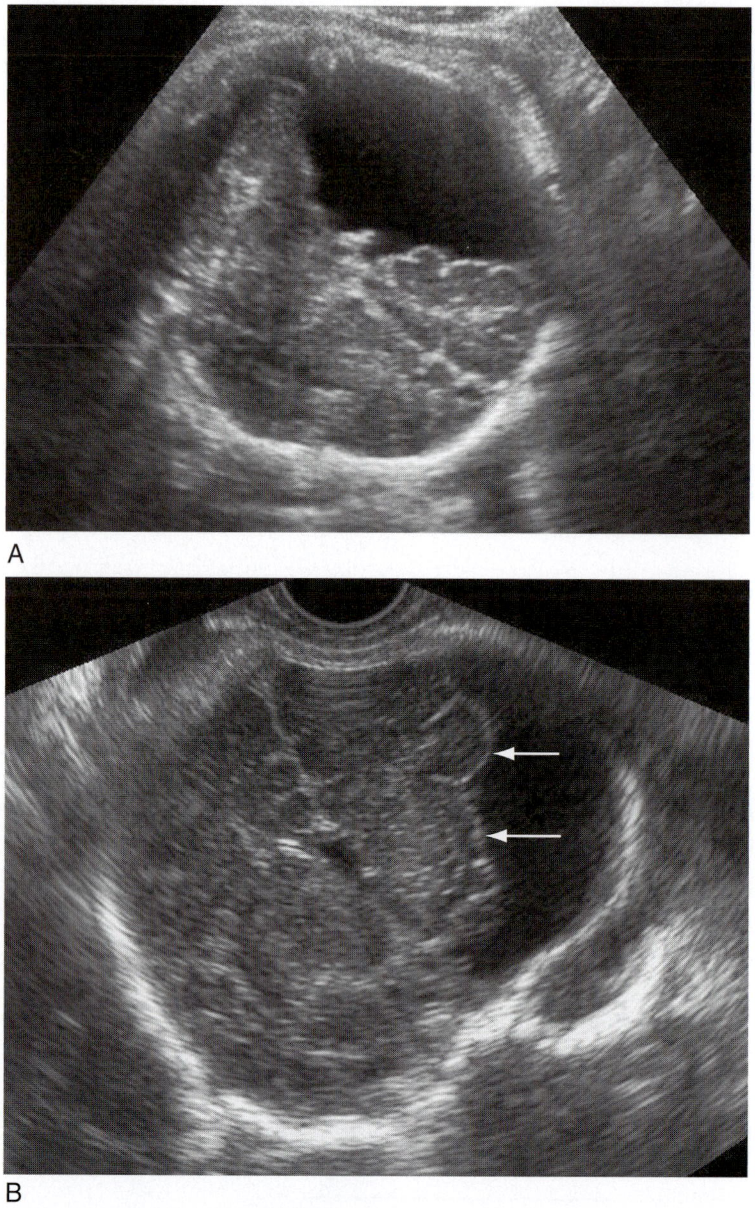

FIGURE 1-16 (A) Transverse view through the fetal head of a third-trimester fetus with a large arachnoid cyst at the base of the skull. (B) Coronal view of the same fetal head with the arachnoid cyst elevating the fetal brain away from the base of the skull *(arrows)*.

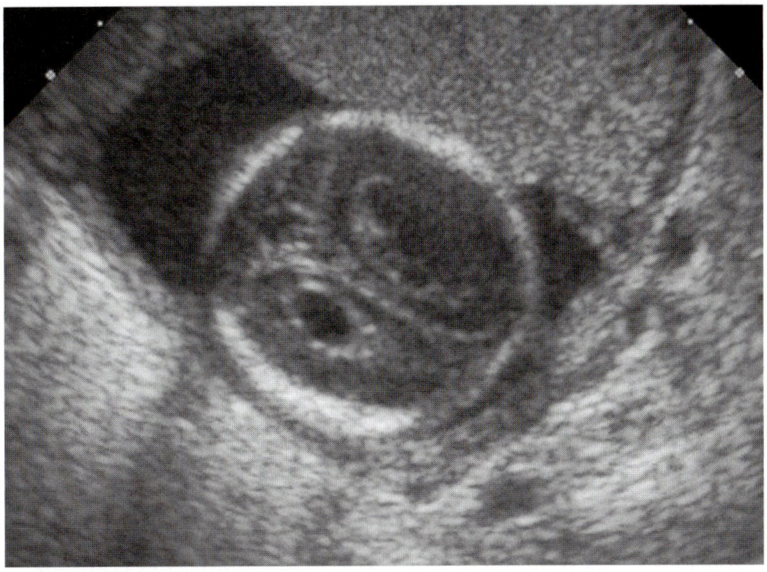

FIGURE 1-17 Early second-trimester fetus with bilateral choroid plexus cysts.

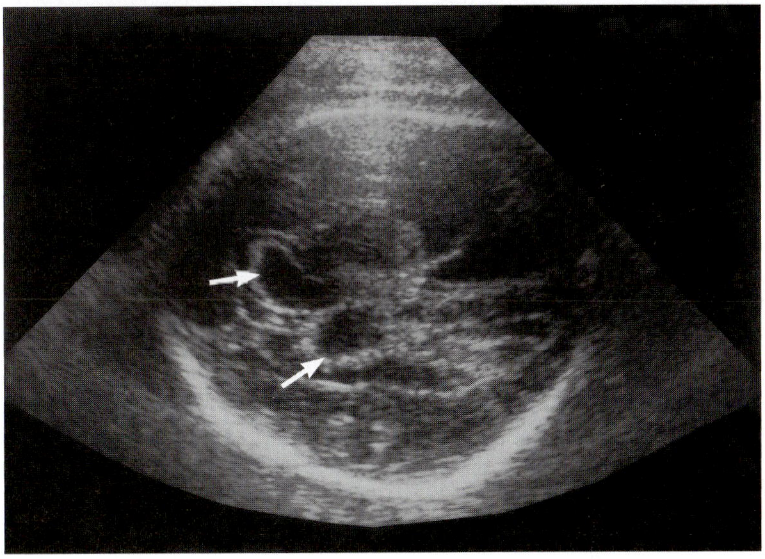

FIGURE 1-18 Oblique view through the fetal head shows several cystic areas *(arrows)* originating from one side, with some distortion of the ventricular system. This fetus had undergone a large, intracranial bleed in utero.

Central

Aneurysm of Vein of Galen: As demonstrated by Doppler studies

Arachnoid Cyst

Enlarged Third Ventricle: With agenesis of corpus callosum

Holoprosencephaly: Fused thalami, monoventricle, and facial anomalies (see p. 386)

Hydranencephaly: Total destruction of supratentorial brain

Interhemispheric Cyst: Associated with agenesis of corpus callosum

Septo-Optic Dysplasia: Disorder characterized by absence of septum pellucidum and hypoplasia of the optic nerves, commonly associated with agenesis of the corpus callosum (see p. 214)

INTRACRANIAL CYST

Aicardi Syndrome: Rare X-linked syndrome characterized by agenesis of the corpus callosum, interhemispheric cyst, chorioretinal abnormalities and infantile seizures (interhemispheric cyst) (see p. 188)

Oral-Facial-Digital Syndrome, Type I: X-linked dominant condition (lethal in males), OFD1 is one of nine syndromes (OFD1-OFD9) that include median cleft lip and palate, hypertelorism, micrognathia, and digital anomalies (porencephalic cyst) (see p. 174)

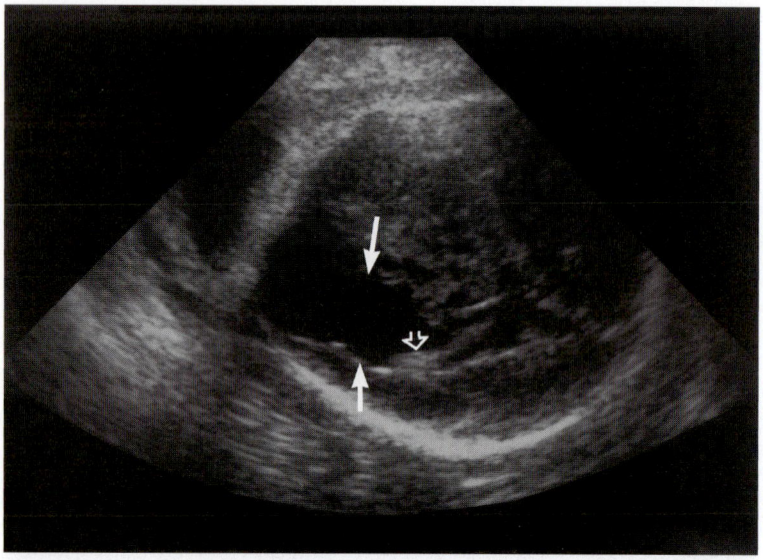

A

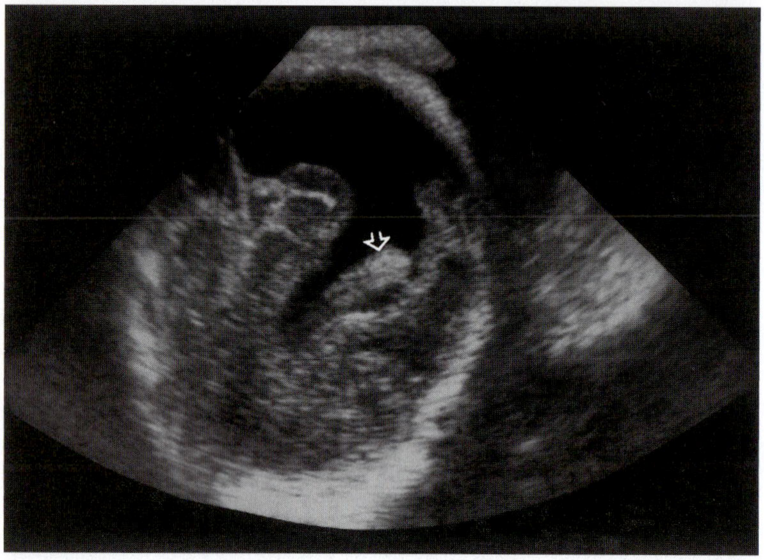

B

FIGURE 1-19 Porencephalic cyst. Transabdominal (A) and transvaginal (B) views of a fetus with a large, porencephalic cyst involving the occipital region of the brain. The cyst *(solid arrows)* is communicating with the lateral ventricles. Open arrow indicates choroid plexus.

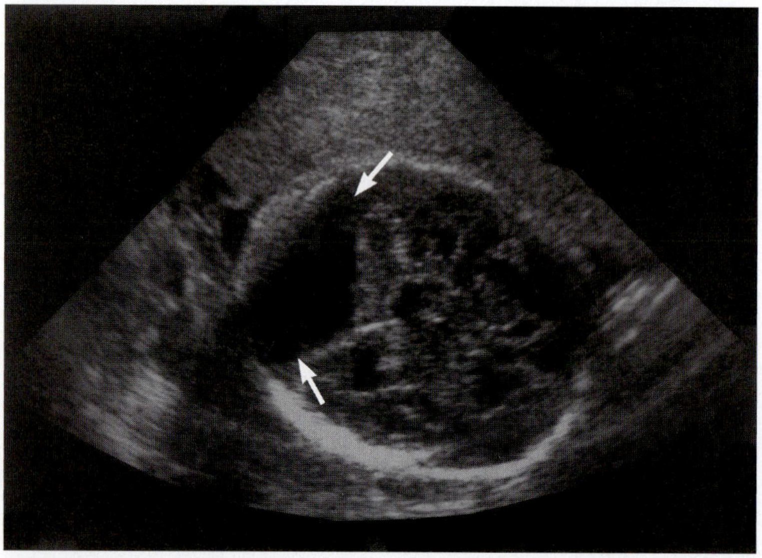

FIGURE 1-20 Transverse view through the posterior fossa of a fetus shows a large, arachnoid cyst *(arrows)* that is displacing the cerebellum against the brainstem.

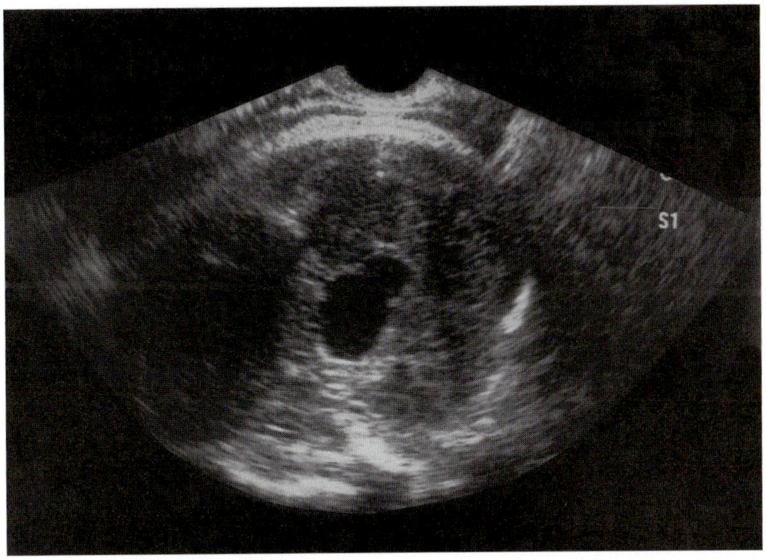

A

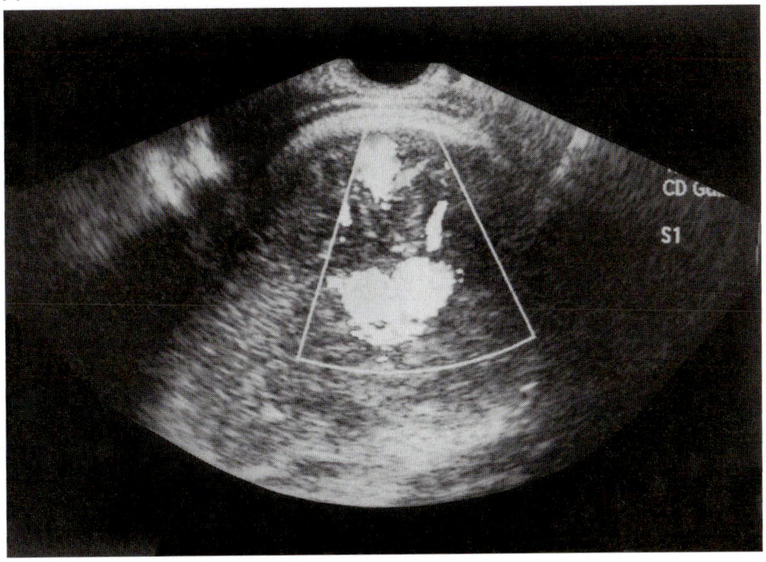

B

FIGURE 1-21 (A) Aneurysm of the vein of Galen. Oblique view through the fetal head shows a fluid collection centrally located in the fetal head. (B) Color Doppler image reveals that the lesion is a vessel—an aneurysm of the vein of Galen—which was confirmed at birth.

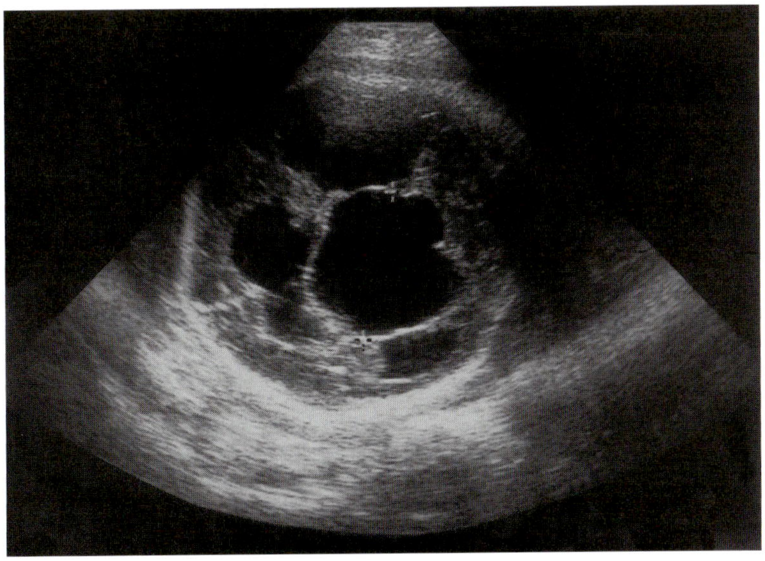

FIGURE 1-22 Arachnoid cyst. Transverse view through the head of a fetus with a large, centrally located, arachnoid cyst. The cyst (shown by electronic calipers) is occluding the ventricular system. Fluid collections around the cyst indicate the dilated lateral ventricular system.

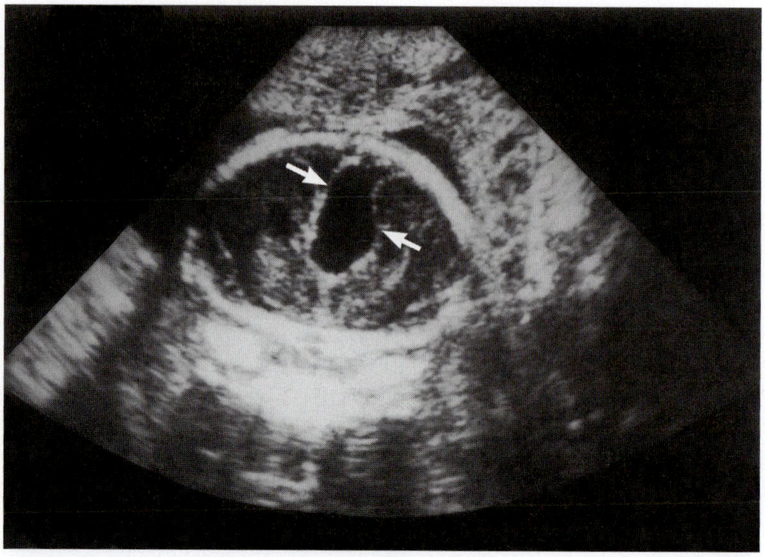
A

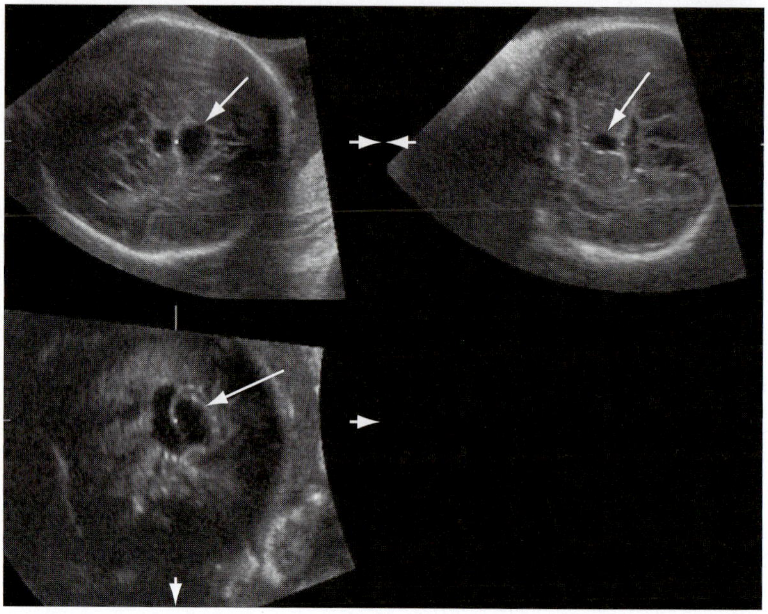
B

FIGURE 1-23 (A) Interhemispheric cyst. Transvaginal view of a second-trimester fetus with agenesis of the corpus callosum shows a cyst *(arrows)* adjacent to the falx. This lesion was found to be an interhemispheric cyst. (B) Multiplanar display of a fetal head in the third trimester shows an interhemispheric cyst *(arrows)* associated with agenesis of the corpus callosum. Note the appearance of the septate cyst seen in several planes simultaneously.

Oral-Facial-Digital Syndrome, Type II (Mohr Syndrome): Autosomal recessive syndrome characterized by short stature; deafness; and facial, hand, and foot abnormalities (arachnoid cyst–occasional) (see p. 175)

Septo-Optic Dysplasia: Disorder characterized by absence of the septum pellucidum and hypoplasia of the optic nerves, commonly associated with agenesis of the corpus callosum (see p. 214)

Trisomy 18 (Choroid Plexus Cyst) (see p. 490)

VENTRICULOMEGALY

FACIAL AND BRAIN ABNORMALITIES

Aicardi Syndrome: Rare X-linked syndrome characterized by agenesis of the corpus callosum, interhemispheric cyst, chorioretinal abnormalities, and infantile seizures (see p. 188)

Cerebrocostomandibular Syndrome: Autosomal recessive condition characterized by severe micrognathia, cleft palate, and vertebral body abnormalities associated with defective costal development (occasional) (see p. 152)

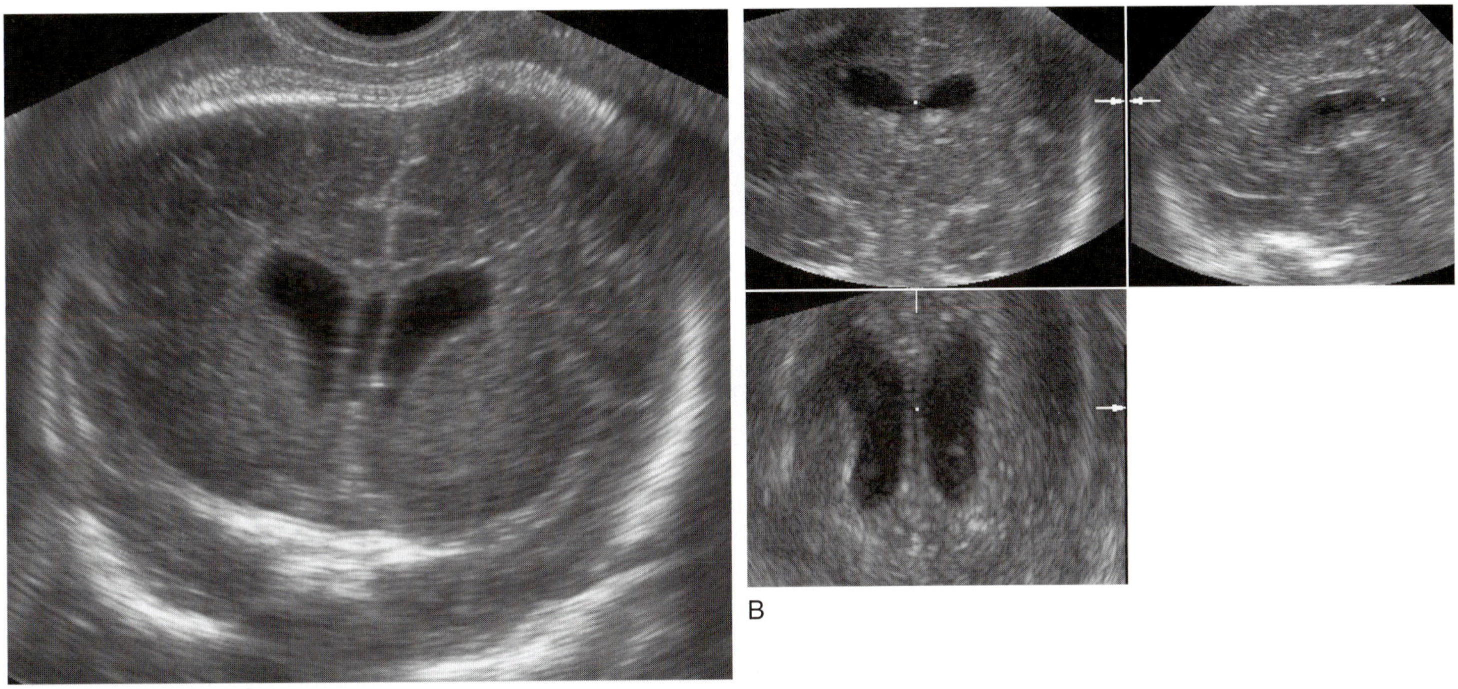

A

B

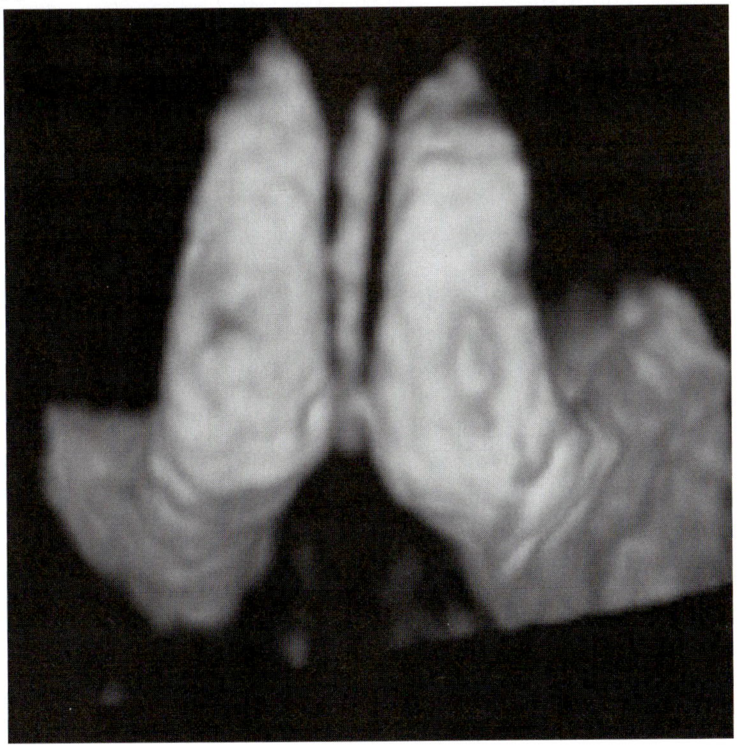

C

FIGURE 1-24 (A) Coronal view of a third-trimester fetus with mild ventriculomegaly shows mildly dilated frontal horns. (B) Three-dimensional volume imaging shows mildly dilated ventricles in the three orthogonal planes simultaneously. Note the intact corpus callosum in the B plane. (C) Same ventricular system using inverse mode three-dimensional imaging. Note the cast of the entire ventricular system.

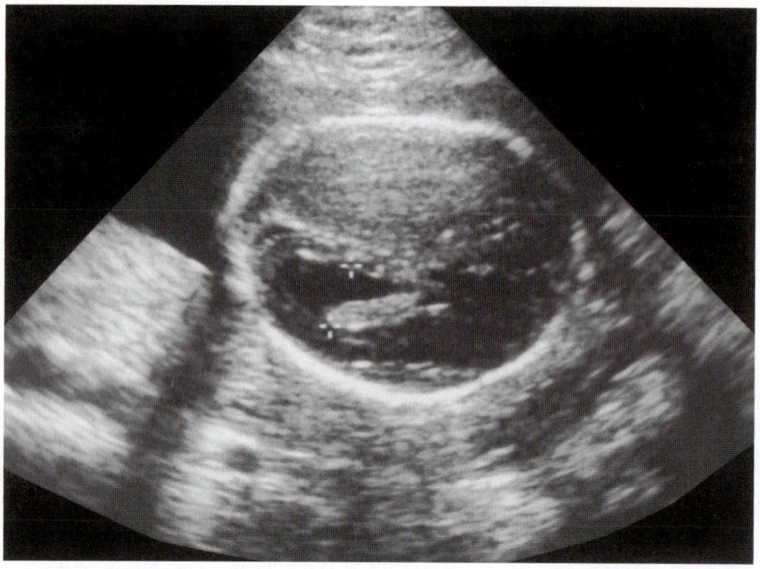

FIGURE 1-25 Transverse view through the fetal head shows evidence of mild ventriculomegaly. The calipers indicate a lateral ventricular width of 11 mm. Note slight displacement of the choroid plexus laterally. This fetus had Miller-Dieker syndrome.

Fraser Syndrome: Autosomal recessive syndrome featuring cryptophthalmos; syndactyly; and genital, renal, and tracheal anomalies (occasional) (see p. 160)

Goldenhar Syndrome: Asymmetry of the face and ears in conjunction with vertebral anomalies of the upper spine (occasional) (see p. 162)

Gorlin Syndrome: Autosomal dominant syndrome characterized by macrocephaly, facial abnormalities, and multiple tumors (see p. 192)

Hydrolethalus: Autosomal recessive disorder characterized by hydrocephalus, polydactyly, heart defects, and polyhydramnios (see p. 194)

Joubert Syndrome: Autosomal recessive syndrome characterized by dysmorphic facial features and agenesis of the cerebellar vermis (see p. 197)

Meckel-Gruber Syndrome: Autosomal recessive condition characterized by posterior encephalocele, postaxial polydactyly, and polycystic kidneys (see p. 199)

Miller-Dieker Syndrome: Lissencephaly, type I; characterized by complete absence of gyri of the brain, microcephaly, and severe mental retardation (see p. 208)

Neu-Laxova Syndrome: Autosomal recessive condition characterized by microcephaly, lissencephaly, exophthalmos, severe IUGR, swollen subcutaneous tissues, and ichthyosis (occasional) (see p. 211)

Oral-Facial-Digital Syndrome, Type I: X-linked dominant condition (lethal in males), OFD1 is one of nine syndromes (OFD1–OFD9) that include median cleft lip and palate, hypertelorism, micrognathia, and digital anomalies (see p. 174)

Oral-Facial-Digital Syndrome, Type II (Mohr Syndrome): Autosomal recessive syndrome characterized by short stature; deafness; and facial, hand, and foot abnormalities (occasional) (see p. 175)

Septo-Optic Dysplasia: Disorder characterized by absence of the septum pellucidum and hypoplasia of the optic nerves, commonly associated with agenesis of the corpus callosum (see p. 214)

Smith-Lemli-Opitz Syndrome: Autosomal recessive syndrome featuring microcephaly, mental retardation, and genital and renal anomalies (occasional) (see p. 140)

Spinal Dysraphism (see p. 418)

Walker-Warburg Syndrome: Autosomal recessive condition characterized by severe, congenital, oculocerebral abnormalities, including lissencephaly, hydrocephalus, encephalocele, microcephaly, microphthalmia, and cataracts (see p. 217)

X-Linked Hydrocephalus (see p. 221)

LIMB AND SKELETAL ABNORMALITIES

Achondroplasia (Homozygous and Heterozygous)**:** Autosomal dominant condition with rhizomelic limb shortening (nonlethal, heterozygous type usually is not apparent until late in the second trimester) (occasional) (see p. 257)

Camptomelic Dysplasia: Short-limbed skeletal dysplasia with bowing of the long bones, particularly in the lower extremities; bell-shaped, narrow chest; and facial anomalies (occasional) (see p. 262)

Chondrodysplasia Punctata (Rhizomelic): Heterogeneous group of bone dysplasias with asymmetric limb shortening and abnormal early calcification of the proximal and distal epiphyses (see p. 266)

Fanconi Anemia: Autosomal recessive condition characterized by radial hypoplasia, absent thumbs, and tendency for leukemia (occasional) (see p. 229)

Metatropic Dysplasia: Short-limbed skeletal dysplasia characterized by progressive, severe kyphoscoliosis, narrow chest, and metaphyseal flaring (occasional) (see p. 285)

Multiple Pterygium Syndrome: Autosomal recessive condition characterized by multiple contractures and webbing across the joints, cystic hygromata, and facial defects (occasional) (see p. 244)

Osteopetrosis: Autosomal recessive condition characterized by diffuse skeletal sclerosis and resulting in increased bone density, fractures, ventriculomegaly, and shortened long bones (see p. 287)

Roberts Syndrome: Autosomal recessive condition characterized by severe shortening of the limbs (pseudothalidomide syndrome) and facial anomalies (occasional) (see p. 247)

Thanatophoric Dysplasia: Most common skeletal dysplasia; narrow chest; short ribs; short, bowed long bones; and flat vertebral bodies (see p. 294)

CRANIOSYNOSTOSIS

Antley-Bixler Syndrome: Disorder characterized by craniosynostosis, resulting in severe brachycephaly, midfacial hypoplasia, multiple skeletal fusions, and contractures (occasional) (see p. 303)

Apert Syndrome: Craniosynostosis, acrocephaly, and syndactyly (see p. 304)

Crouzon Syndrome: Autosomal dominant condition characterized by craniosynostosis of the coronal sutures, midface hypoplasia, and ocular proptosis (occasional) (see p. 313)

Pfeiffer Syndrome: Acrocephalic skull, craniosynostosis (particularly of the coronal and sagittal sutures), and syndactyly of hands and feet (occasional) (see p. 316)

CHROMOSOMAL ANOMALIES

Deletion 5p (Cri du Chat Syndrome): Abnormality of chromosome 5 characterized by microcephaly, hypertelorism, micrognathia, hydrops, and growth delay (see p. 457)

Deletion 11q (Jacobsen Syndrome): Deletion of the distal long arm of chromosome 11 characterized by multiple anomalies of practically all organ systems (occasional) (see p. 464)

Tetrasomy 12p (Pallister-Killian Syndrome): Mosaic aneuploidy characterized by multiple congenital abnormalities of the central nervous system, face, heart, and many other organs (see p. 471)

Triploidy: Occurring as a result of a complete extra set of chromosomes, this is a lethal abnormality characterized by severe early-onset IUGR and multiple anomalies of practically all organ systems (see p. 473)

Trisomy 9: Occurring as a result of an extra chromosome 9, this is a severe abnormality characterized by multiple anomalies of practically all organ systems (see p. 478)

Trisomy 13 (Patau Syndrome): Occurring as a result of an extra chromosome 13, this is a severe abnormality characterized by multiple anomalies of the central nervous system, face, heart, and extremities (see p. 483)

Trisomy 18 (Edwards Syndrome): Occurring as a result of an extra chromosome 18, this is a severe abnormality characterized by IUGR and multiple anomalies of the central nervous system, face, heart, and extremities (occasional) (see p. 490)

Trisomy 21 (Down Syndrome): Occurring as a result of an extra chromosome 21, this abnormality is characterized by nuchal fold thickening, short long-bones, abnormal nasal bone, heart defects, and other anomalies. Twenty-five percent of fetuses with Down syndrome do not display any sonographic abnormalities or markers (see p. 496)

OTHER SYNDROMES AND SEQUENCES

Arthrogryposis: Sequence of neurologic, muscular, and connective tissue disorders leading to fetal joint contractures, rigidity, and decreased activity (see p. 362)

CHARGE Association: **C**oloboma of the iris, **h**eart defect, choanal **a**tresia, intrauterine growth restriction, genital and ear anomalies (occasional) (see p. 376)

Fryns Syndrome: Autosomal recessive condition characterized by diaphragmatic defects, digital and facial abnormalities, and brain anomalies (see p. 325)

Opitz Syndrome: Disorder characterized by ocular hypertelorism, micrognathia, and, in males, hypospadias (occasional) (see p. 399)

Renal Agenesis (occasional) (see p. 412)

TERATOGENS

Aminopterin (see p. 438)

Carbon monoxide (see p. 438)

Chlorpheniramine (see p. 439)

Codeine (see p. 439)

Cortisone (see p. 437)

Cytomegalovirus (see p. 441)

Ethosuximide (see p. 436)

Progestin (see p. 437)

Quinine (see p. 434)

Toxoplasmosis (see p. 452)

Varicella (see p. 456)

MACROCEPHALY

GROWTH ABNORMALITIES

Beckwith-Wiedemann Syndrome: Gigantism in utero in conjunction with macroglossia, omphalocele, and renal anomalies (see p. 142)

Maternal diabetes (see p. 146)

FACIAL AND BRAIN ABNORMALITIES

Gorlin Syndrome: Autosomal dominant syndrome with macrocephaly, facial abnormalities, multiple tumors (see p. 192)

Intracranial Mass (tumor, intracranial bleed, cyst)

Normal Variants

Ventriculomegaly

X-linked Hydrocephalus (see p. 221)

LIMB AND SKELETAL ABNORMALITIES

Achondrogenesis: Lethal skeletal dysplasia characterized by extreme hypoplasia of the bones, micromelia, decreased ossification of the bones (particularly those of the skull and spine), and hydrops (see p. 253)

Achondroplasia: Autosomal dominant condition characterized by rhizomelic limb shortening (nonlethal, heterozygous type usually is not apparent until late in the second trimester) (see p. 257)

Camptomelic Dysplasia: Short-limbed skeletal dysplasia characterized by bowing of the long bones, particularly in the lower extremities; bell-shaped, narrow chest; and facial anomalies (see p. 262)

Metatropic Dysplasia: Short-limbed skeletal dysplasia characterized by progressive, severe kyphoscoliosis, narrow chest, and metaphyseal flaring (see p. 285)

OTHER SYNDROMES AND SEQUENCES

Holoprosencephaly (see p. 386)

MICROCEPHALY

GROWTH ABNORMALITIES

Cornelia de Lange Syndrome: Facial/limb anomalies, growth restriction, and mental developmental delay (see p. 129)

Seckel Syndrome: Autosomal recessive syndrome characterized by severe IUGR with microcephaly and severely abnormal profile (see p. 138)

Smith-Lemli-Opitz Syndrome: Autosomal recessive syndrome featuring microcephaly, mental retardation, and genital and renal anomalies (see p. 140)

FACIAL AND BRAIN ABNORMALITIES

Branchio-Oculo-Facial Syndrome: Autosomal dominant disorder characterized by mental retardation, growth deficiency, ocular defects, and clefting of the upper lip (occasional) (see p. 149)

Cerebrocostomandibular Syndrome: Autosomal recessive condition characterized by severe micrognathia, cleft palate, and vertebral body abnormalities associated with defective costal development (occasional) (see p. 152)

Fraser Syndrome: Autosomal recessive syndrome featuring cryptophthalmos, syndactyly, and genital, renal, and tracheal anomalies (occasional) (see p. 160)

Holoprosencephaly (see p. 386)

Lissencephaly: Smooth brain syndromes

Meckel-Gruber Syndrome: Autosomal recessive condition characterized by posterior encephalocele, postaxial polydactyly, and polycystic kidneys (see p. 199)

Miller-Dieker Syndrome: Lissencephaly, type I; characterized by complete absence of gyri of the brain, microcephaly, and severe mental retardation (see p. 208)

Neu-Laxova Syndrome: Autosomal recessive condition characterized by microcephaly, lissencephaly, exophthalmos, severe IUGR, swollen subcutaneous tissues, and ichthyosis (see p. 211)

Neural Tube Defects (see p. 40)

Oral-Facial-Digital Syndrome, Type II (Mohr Syndrome): Autosomal recessive syndrome characterized by short stature; deafness; and facial, hand, and foot abnormalities (occasional) (see p. 175)

Shprintzen Syndrome: Autosomal dominant syndrome characterized by short stature, mild mental retardation, micrognathia, and cardiac and limb abnormalities (see p. 179)

Walker-Warburg Syndrome: Autosomal recessive condition with severe, congenital, oculocerebral abnormalities, including lissencephaly, hydrocephalus, encephalocele, microcephaly, microphthalmia, and cataracts (see p. 217)

LIMB AND SKELETAL ABNORMALITIES

Adams-Oliver Syndrome: Disorder characterized by terminal transverse defects of the upper and lower extremities, as well as denuded areas on the scalp with or without an underlying bony skull (bone) defect (occasional) (see p. 223)

Chondrodysplasia Punctata (Rhizomelic Type)**:** Heterogeneous group of bone dysplasias characterized by asymmetric limb shortening and abnormal early calcification of the proximal and distal epiphyses (see p. 266)

Fanconi Anemia: Autosomal recessive condition characterized by radial hypoplasia, absent thumbs, and tendency for leukemia (occasional) (see p. 229)

Freeman-Sheldon (Whistling Face) Syndrome: Autosomal dominant condition characterized by unusual facial features and skeletal anomalies, such as flexion deformities of the joints (see p. 237)

Multiple Pterygium Syndrome: Autosomal recessive condition characterized by multiple contractures and webbing across the joints, cystic hygromata, and facial defects (occasional) (see p. 244)

Roberts Syndrome: Autosomal recessive condition with severe shortening of the limbs (pseudothalidomide syndrome) and facial anomalies (see p. 247)

CHROMOSOMAL ANOMALIES

Deletion 4p (Wolf-Hirschhorn Syndrome): Abnormality of chromosome 4 characterized by IUGR, facial dysmorphology, cardiac defects, and hypospadias (see p. 459)

Deletion 5p (Cri du Chat Syndrome): Abnormality of chromosome 5 characterized by microcephaly, hypertelorism, micrognathia, hydrops, and growth delay (see p. 457)

Deletion 11q (Jacobsen Syndrome): Deletion of the distal long arm of chromosome 11 characterized by multiple anomalies of practically all organ systems (see p. 464)

DiGeorge Syndrome: Also known as velocardiofacial syndrome or Shprintzen syndrome, this disorder results from a deletion of chromosome 22q11.2 and is characterized by cardiac abnormalities involving largely the great vessels, facial abnormalities, hypocalcemia, and hypoplasia of the thymus (see p. 466)

Trisomy 9: Occurring as a result of an extra chromosome 9, this is a severe abnormality characterized by multiple anomalies of practically all organ systems (see p. 478)

Trisomy 13 (Patau Syndrome): Occurring as a result of an extra chromosome 13, this is a severe abnormality characterized by multiple anomalies of the central nervous system, face, heart, and extremities (see p. 483)

OTHER SYNDROMES AND SEQUENCES

Arthrogryposis: Sequence of neurologic, muscular, and connective tissue disorders leading to fetal joint contractures and rigidity, as well as decreased activity (occasional) (see p. 362)

Cerebro-Oculo-Facio-Skeletal (COFS) Syndrome: Autosomal recessive condition characterized by joint contractures of all the extremities, with severe facial and brain abnormalities (see p. 374)

Genetic Syndromes, Such as Primary Microcephaly

Holoprosencephaly (see p. 386)

Neural Tube Defects Associated with Arnold-Chiari Syndrome, Type II Malformations (see p. 40)

TERATOGENS

Alcohol (see p. 438)

Aminopterin (see p. 438)

Chlordiazepoxide (Librium) (see p. 437)

Chlorpropamide (see p. 439)

Clomiphene (see p. 437)

Cytomegalovirus (see p. 441)

Folic acid metabolism disorders

Hydantoin (occasional) (see p. 436)

Hyperthermia (see p. 439)

Methotrexate (see p. 435)

Phenantoin (see p. 436)

Phenylketonuria (PKU) syndrome (see p. 438)

Radiation (see p. 439)

Rubella (see p. 449)

Toxoplasmosis (see p. 452)

Trimethadione (see p. 436)

Valproic acid (see p. 436)

Varicella (see p. 456)

AGENESIS OF THE CORPUS CALLOSUM

FACIAL AND BRAIN ABNORMALITIES

Aicardi Syndrome: Rare X-linked syndrome characterized by agenesis of the corpus callosum, interhemispheric cyst, chorioretinal abnormalities, and infantile seizures (see p. 188)

Cerebrocostomandibular Syndrome: Autosomal recessive condition characterized by severe micrognathia, cleft palate, and vertebral body abnormalities associated with defective costal development (occasional) (see p. 152)

Gorlin Syndrome: Autosomal dominant syndrome characterized by macrocephaly, facial abnormalities, and multiple tumors (occasional) (see p. 192)

Meckel-Gruber Syndrome: Autosomal recessive condition characterized by posterior encephalocele, postaxial polydactyly, and polycystic kidneys (see p. 199)

Median Cleft Face: Midline facial defects resulting in hypertelorism and bifid or broad nose (occasional) (see p. 165)

Miller-Dieker Syndrome: Lissencephaly, type I; characterized by complete absence of gyri of the brain, microcephaly, and severe mental retardation (see p. 208)

Neu-Laxova Syndrome: Autosomal recessive condition characterized by microcephaly, lissencephaly, exophthalmos, severe IUGR, swollen subcutaneous tissues, and ichthyosis (see p. 211)

Oral-Facial-Digital Syndrome, Type I: X-linked dominant condition (lethal in males), OFD1 is

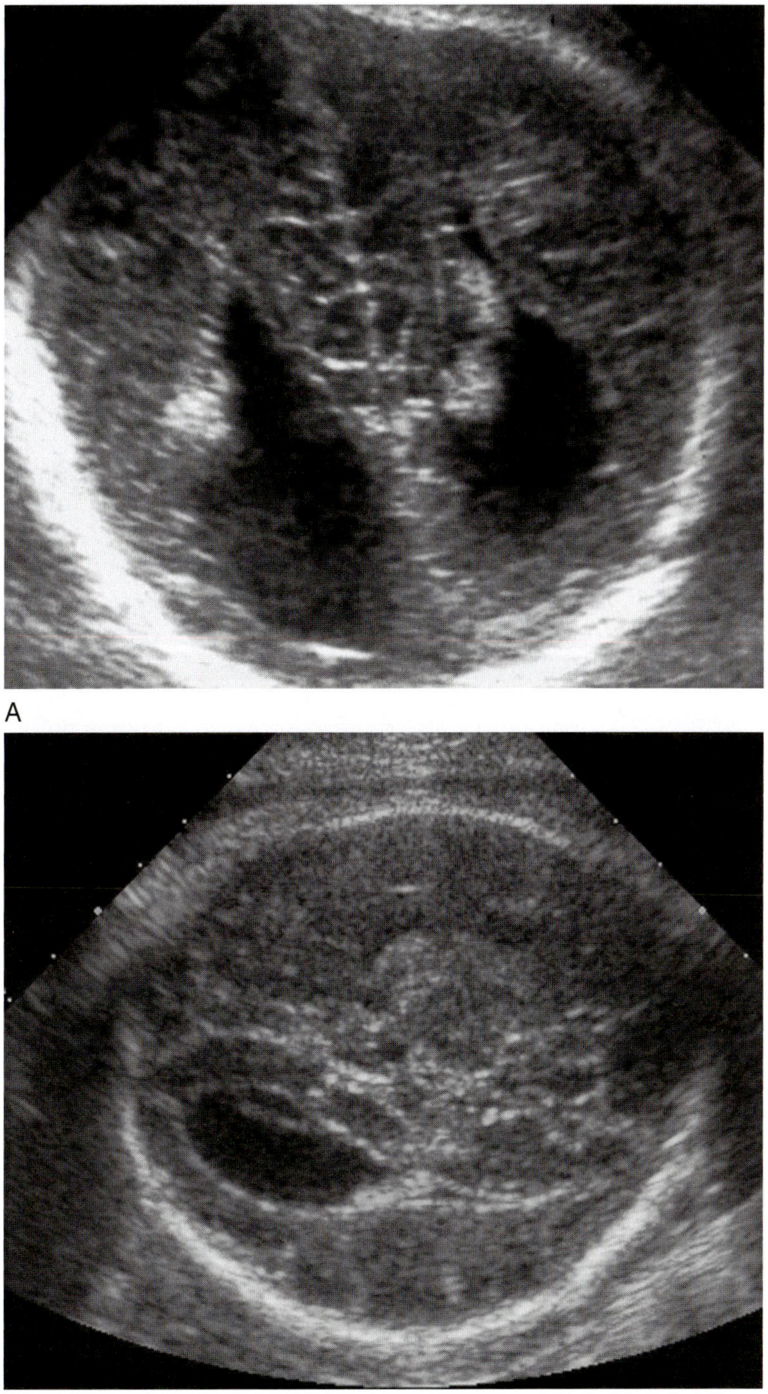

FIGURE 1-26 **(A) Third-trimester fetus with agenesis of the corpus callosum. Note colpocephaly indicated by the teardrop-shaped occipital horns of the lateral ventricles. (B) Dilated occipital horns of a different fetus with agenesis of the corpus callosum. Note characteristic colpocephaly (bulbous dilation of the occipital horns) associated with this condition.**

one of nine syndromes (OFD1–OFD9) that include median cleft lip and palate, hypertelorism, micrognathia, and digital anomalies (see p. 174)

Septo-Optic Dysplasia: Disorder characterized by absence of the septum pellucidum and hypoplasia of the optic nerves, commonly associated with agenesis of the corpus callosum (see p. 214)

Smith-Lemli-Opitz Syndrome: Autosomal recessive syndrome featuring microcephaly, mental retardation, and genital and renal anomalies (occasional) (see p. 140)

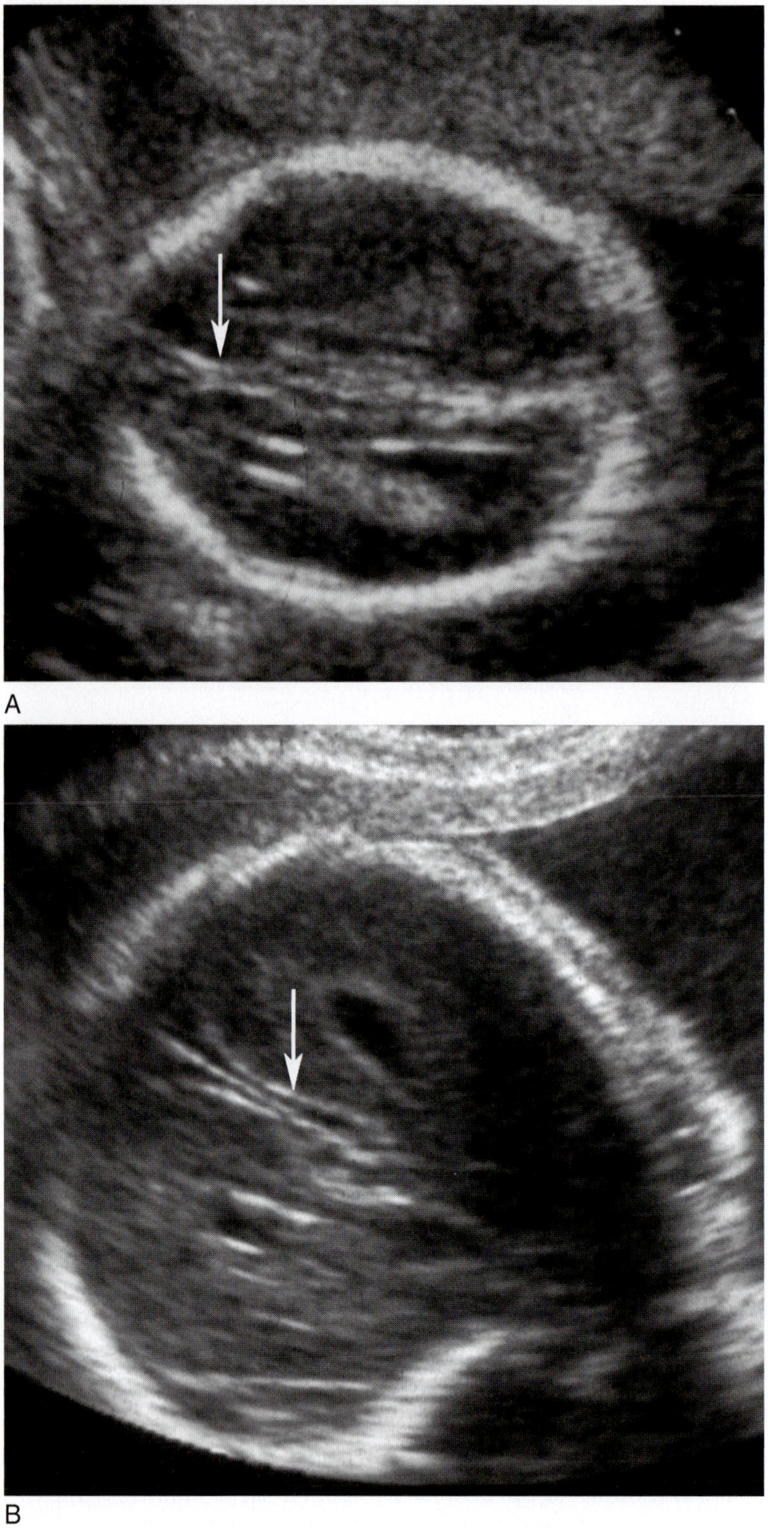

FIGURE 1-27 Axial (A) and coronal (B) views through the fetal head of an early second-trimester fetus with agenesis of the corpus callosum. Note absence of the cavum septum pellucidum *(arrow)*, resulting in abnormal separation between the two frontal horns. There is no evidence of ventriculomegaly at this early stage.

Walker-Warburg Syndrome: Autosomal recessive condition characterized by severe, congenital, oculocerebral abnormalities, including lissencephaly, hydrocephalus, encephalocele, microcephaly, microphthalmia, and cataracts (see p. 217)

LIMB AND SKELETAL ABNORMALITIES

Fanconi Anemia: Autosomal recessive condition characterized by radial hypoplasia, absent thumbs, and tendency for leukemia (occasional) (see p. 229)

Thanatophoric Dysplasia: Most common skeletal dysplasia; narrow chest; short ribs; short, bowed long bones; and flat vertebral bodies (occasional) (see p. 294)

CRANIOSYNOSTOSIS

Apert Syndrome: Craniosynostosis, acrocephaly, and syndactyly (see p. 304)

Crouzon Syndrome: Autosomal dominant condition characterized by craniosynostosis of the coronal sutures, midface hypoplasia, and ocular proptosis (occasional) (see p. 313)

CHROMOSOMAL ANOMALIES

Deletion 4p (Wolf-Hirschhorn Syndrome): Abnormality of chromosome 4 characterized by IUGR, facial dysmorphology, cardiac defects, and hypospadias (see p. 459)

Triploidy: Occurring as a result of a complete extra set of chromosomes, this is a lethal abnormality characterized by severe early-onset IUGR and multiple anomalies of practically all organ systems (see p. 473)

Trisomy 13 (Patau Syndrome): Occurring as a result of an extra chromosome 13, this is a severe abnormality characterized by multiple anomalies of the central nervous system, face, heart, and extremities (see p. 483)

Trisomy 18 (Edwards Syndrome): Occurring as a result of an extra chromosome 18, this is a severe abnormality characterized by IUGR and multiple anomalies of the central nervous system, face, heart, and extremities (see p. 490)

OTHER SYNDROMES AND SEQUENCES

Arthrogryposis: Sequence of neurologic, muscular, and connective tissue disorders leading to fetal joint contractures and rigidity, as well as decreased activity (see p. 362)

Cerebro-Oculo-Facio-Skeletal (COFS) Syndrome: Autosomal recessive condition characterized by joint contractures of all the extremities, with severe facial and brain abnormalities (see p. 374)

Fryns Syndrome: Autosomal recessive condition characterized by diaphragmatic defects, digital and facial abnormalities, and brain anomalies (see p. 325)

Holoprosencephaly (see p. 386)

Opitz Syndrome: Disorder characterized by ocular hypertelorism, micrognathia, and, in males, hypospadias (occasional) (see p. 399)

DANDY-WALKER CYST OR VERMIAN HYPOPLASIA

GROWTH ABNORMALITIES

Smith-Lemli-Opitz Syndrome: Autosomal recessive syndrome featuring microcephaly, mental retardation, and genital and renal anomalies (occasional) (see p. 140)

FACIAL AND BRAIN ABNORMALITIES

Aicardi Syndrome: Rare X-linked syndrome characterized by agenesis of the corpus callosum, interhemispheric cyst, chorioretinal abnormalities, and infantile seizures (occasional) (see p. 188)

Joubert Syndrome: Autosomal recessive syndrome characterized by dysmorphic facial features and agenesis of the cerebellar vermis (see p. 197)

Meckel-Gruber Syndrome: Autosomal recessive condition characterized by posterior encephalocele, postaxial polydactyly, and polycystic kidneys (see p. 199)

Neu-Laxova Syndrome: Autosomal recessive condition characterized by microcephaly, lissencephaly, exophthalmos, severe IUGR, swollen subcutaneous tissues, and ichthyosis (see p. 211)

Oral-Facial-Digital Syndrome, Type I: X-linked dominant condition (lethal in males), OFD1 is one of nine syndromes (OFD1–OFD9) that include median cleft lip and palate, hypertelorism, micrognathia, and digital anomalies (see p. 174)

Oral-Facial-Digital Syndrome, Type II (Mohr Syndrome): Autosomal recessive syndrome characterized by short stature; deafness; and facial, hand, and foot abnormalities (occasional) (see p. 175)

Walker-Warburg Syndrome: Autosomal recessive condition with severe congenital

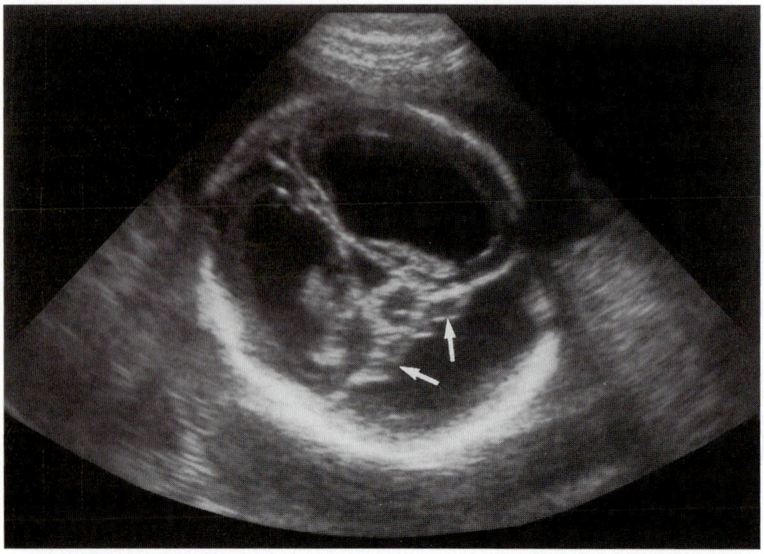

FIGURE 1-28 Coronal view through the fetal head shows marked bilateral ventriculomegaly. The posterior fossa has a large fluid collection, and the cerebellar hemispheres *(arrows)* are extremely small. This fetus had a Dandy-Walker cyst.

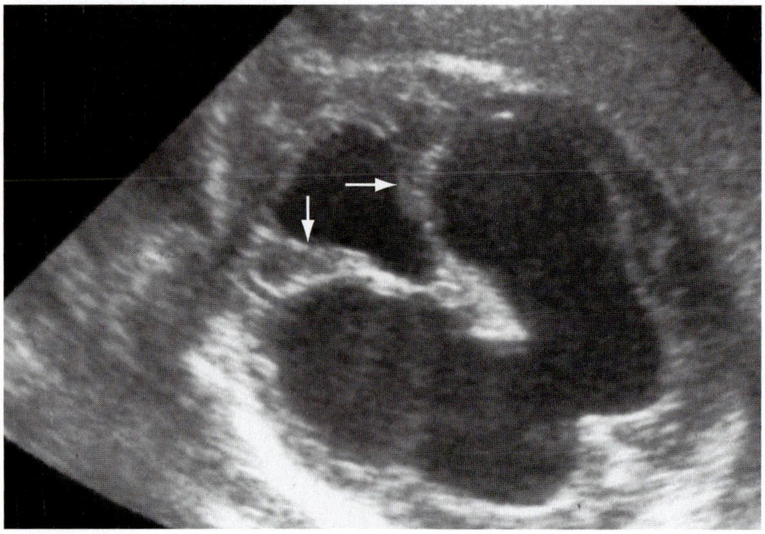

FIGURE 1-29 Transverse view through the fetal head shows bilateral ventriculomegaly and a cyst in the posterior fossa, consistent with a Dandy-Walker cyst. Note that the cerebellar hemispheres *(arrows)* are compressed along the tentorium and that the cerebellar vermis is absent.

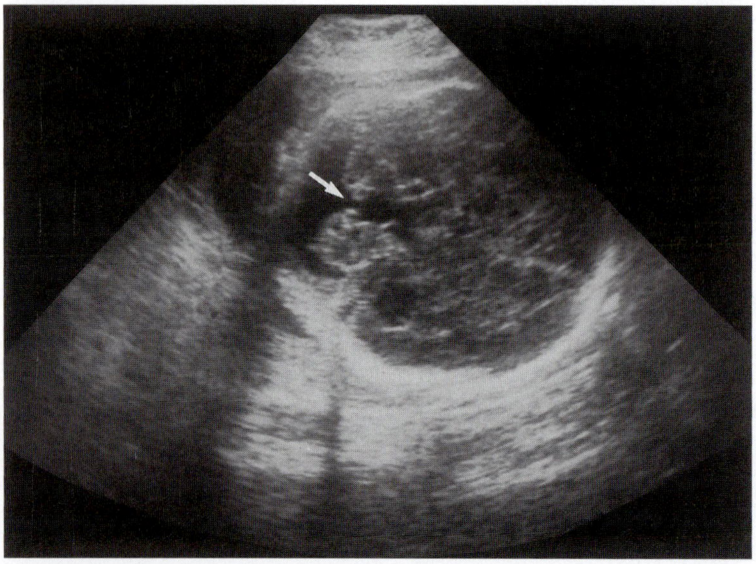

FIGURE 1-30 Transverse view through the posterior fossa of a fetus with a variant of Dandy-Walker cyst. Note the communication between the fourth ventricle and the cisterna magna *(arrow)*. The cerebellar hemispheres are not as hypoplastic as those seen in a true Dandy-Walker cyst.

oculocerebral abnormalities, including lissencephaly, hydrocephalus, encephalocele, microcephaly, microphthalmia, and cataracts (see p. 217)

LIMB AND SKELETAL ABNORMALITIES

Ellis-van Creveld Syndrome: Autosomal recessive skeletal dysplasia characterized by disproportionately short extremities, narrow chest, polydactyly, and heart defects (occasional) (see p. 272)

Majewski Syndrome (Short Rib–Polydactyly Syndrome, Type II): Autosomal recessive skeletal dysplasia characterized by short ribs, narrow thorax, polydactyly, and median facial cleft (occasional) (see p. 283)

Thrombocytopenia–absent radius (TAR) Syndrome: Autosomal recessive syndrome characterized by radial aplasia and thrombocytopenia (occasional) (see p. 251)

CHROMOSOMAL ANOMALIES

Deletion 5p (Cri du Chat Syndrome): Abnormality of chromosome 5 characterized by microcephaly, hypertelorism, micrognathia, hydrops, and growth delay (see p. 457)

Deletion 4p (Wolf-Hirschhorn Syndrome): Abnormality of chromosome 4 characterized by IUGR, facial dysmorphology, cardiac defects, and hypospadias (see p. 459)

Tetrasomy 12p (Pallister-Killian Syndrome): Mosaic aneuploidy characterized by multiple congenital abnormalities of the central nervous system, face, heart, and many other organs (see p. 471)

Triploidy: Occurring as a result of a complete extra set of chromosomes, this is a lethal abnormality characterized by severe early-onset IUGR and multiple anomalies of practically all organ systems (see p. 473)

Trisomy 9: Occurring as a result of an extra chromosome 9, this is a severe abnormality characterized by multiple anomalies of practically all organ systems (see p. 478)

Trisomy 18 (Edwards Syndrome): Occurring as a result of an extra chromosome 18, this is a severe abnormality characterized by IUGR and multiple anomalies of the central nervous system, face, heart, and extremities (see p. 490)

OTHER SYNDROMES AND SEQUENCES

Arthrogryposis: Sequence of neurologic, muscular, and connective tissue disorders leading to fetal joint contractures and rigidity, as well as decreased activity (see p. 362)

CHARGE Association: Coloboma of the iris, **h**eart defect, choanal **a**tresia, intrauterine growth **r**estriction, **g**enital anomalies, and **e**ar anomalies (occasional) (see p. 376)

Fryns Syndrome: Autosomal recessive condition characterized by diaphragmatic defects, digital and facial abnormalities, and brain anomalies (see p. 325)

MURCS Association: Müllerian duct aplasia, **r**enal aplasia, **c**ervicothoracic **s**omite dysplasia (occasional) (see p. 398)

Opitz Syndrome: Disorder characterized by ocular hypertelorism, micrognathia, and, in males, hypospadias (occasional) (see p. 399)

ECHOGENIC MASS IN THE HEAD

BLOOD

Intracranial bleed

CALCIUM

Intracranial calcifications

COMBINATION

Intracranial tumor, such as a teratoma

FAT

Lipoma of the corpus callosum

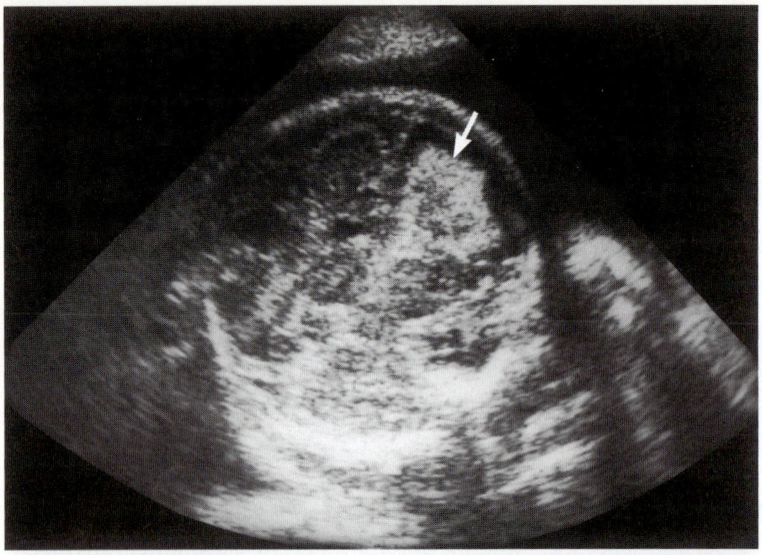

FIGURE 1-31 Coronal view through the head of a fetus that has just undergone an intracranial hemorrhage shows an echogenic area *(arrow)* that corresponds to the area of fresh hemorrhage.

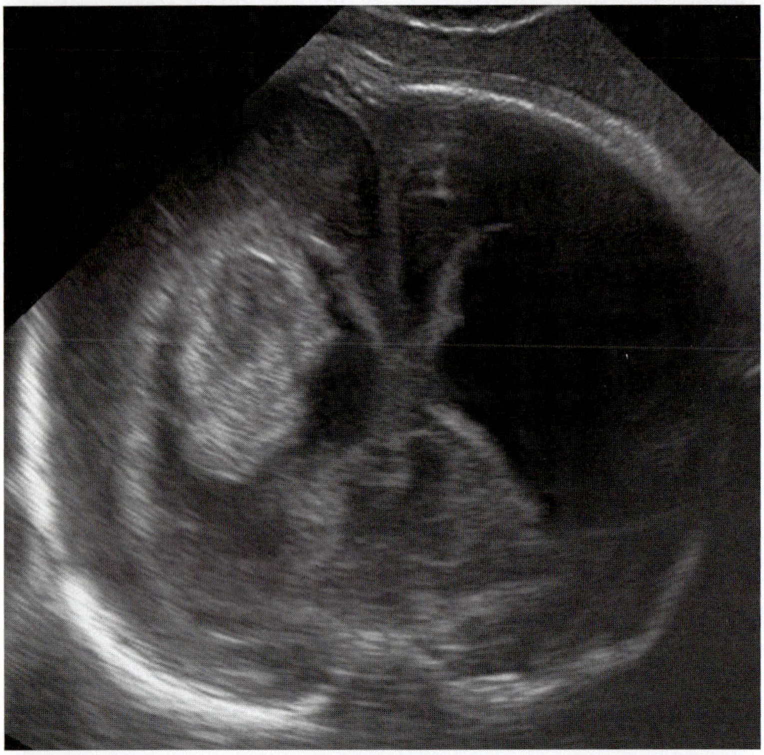

A

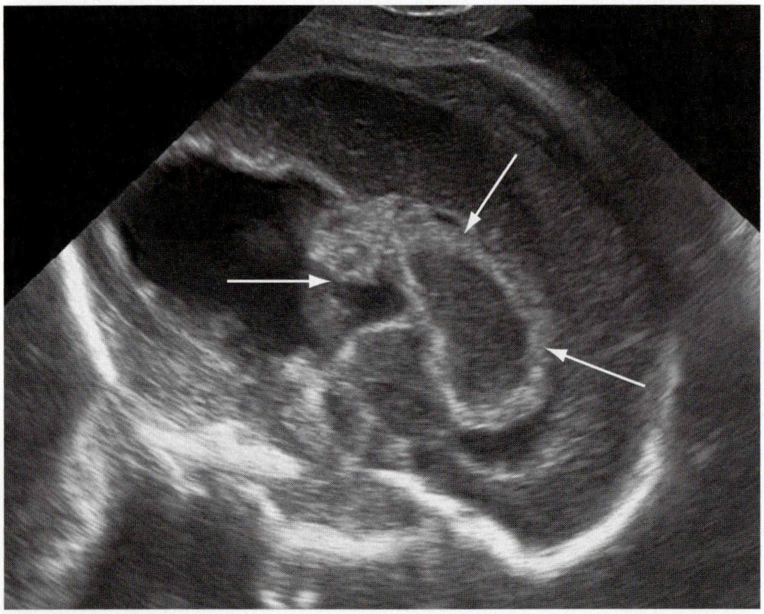

B

FIGURE 1-32 Transverse (A) and longitudinal (B) views of the fetal head in the third trimester show evidence of intracranial bleed. Note bilateral ventriculomegaly and echogenic mass on one side, consistent with an intraventricular clot *(arrows)*.

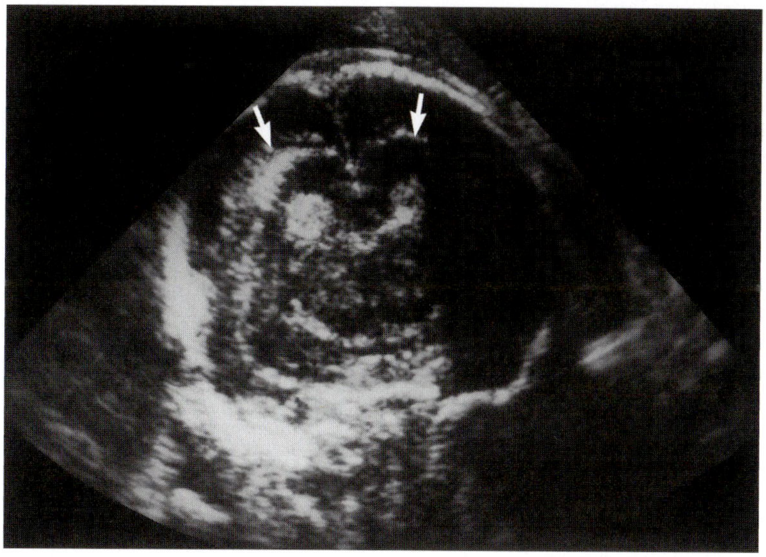

FIGURE 1-33 Coronal view through the fetal head of a fetus with a viral infection shows numerous calcium deposits *(arrows)* throughout the brain parenchyma.

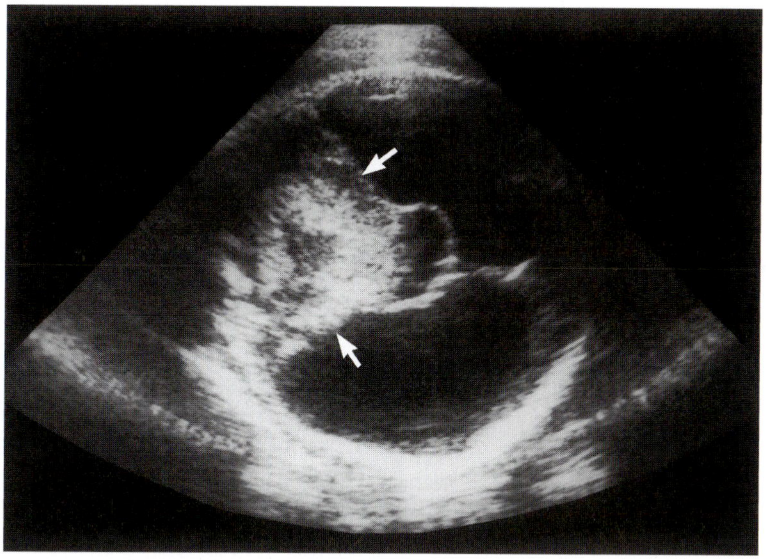

FIGURE 1-34 Intracranial tumor. View of the posterior aspect of the fetal head shows that the entire posterior fossa is filled with a large echogenic mass *(arrows)*. There is severe bilateral ventriculomegaly. The mass was a posterior fossa teratoma.

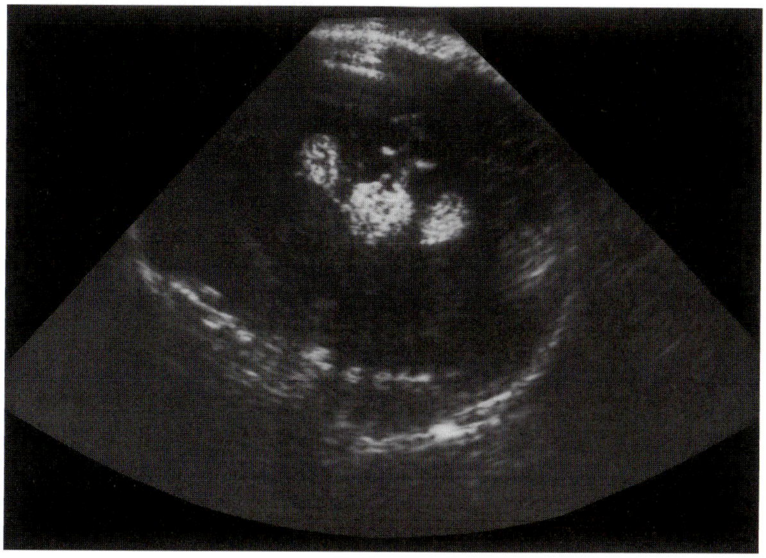

FIGURE 1-35 Lipoma of the corpus callosum. Transvaginal coronal view of the head of a third-trimester fetus shows a central echogenic mass with bilateral extension into the lateral ventricles. This was a lipoma of the corpus callosum, with partial agenesis of the corpus callosum.

HOLOPROSENCEPHALY

FACIAL AND BRAIN ABNORMALITIES

Shprintzen Syndrome: Autosomal dominant syndrome characterized by short stature, mild mental retardation, micrognathia, and cardiac and limb abnormalities (occasional) (see p. 179)

Smith-Lemli-Opitz Syndrome: Autosomal recessive syndrome featuring microcephaly, mental retardation, and genital and renal anomalies (occasional) (see p. 140)

LIMB AND SKELETAL ABNORMALITIES

Ectrodactyly–Ectodermal Dysplasia–Clefting (EEC) Syndrome: Autosomal dominant condition characterized by labial clefting, ectrodactyly (lobster-claw deformities of the limbs), and genitourinary tract anomalies (occasional) (see p. 225)

CHROMOSOMAL ANOMALIES

Triploidy: Occurring as a result of a complete extra set of chromosomes, this is a lethal abnormality characterized by severe early-onset IUGR and multiple anomalies of practically all organ systems (see p. 473)

Trisomy 13 (Patau Syndrome): Occurring as a result of an extra chromosome 13, this is a severe abnormality characterized by multiple anomalies of the central nervous system, face, heart, and extremities (see p. 483)

TERATOGEN

Hydantoin (occasional) (see p. 436)

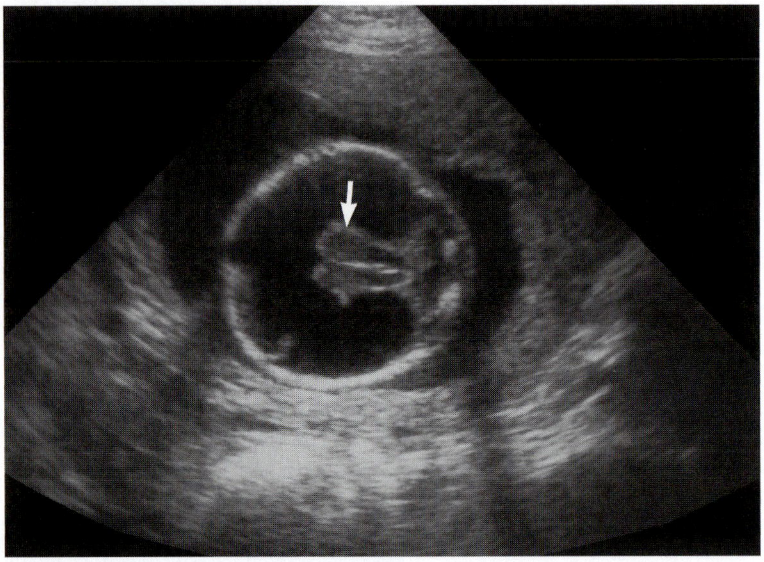

FIGURE 1-36 Coronal view through the head of a fetus with trisomy 13 and holoprosencephaly. Note the fused thalami *(arrow)*.

NEURAL TUBE DEFECT

FACIAL AND BRAIN ABNORMALITIES

Cerebrocostomandibular Syndrome: Autosomal recessive condition characterized by severe micrognathia, cleft palate, and vertebral body abnormalities associated with defective costal development (occasional) (see p. 152)

Fraser Syndrome: Autosomal recessive syndrome featuring cryptophthalmos, syndactyly, and genital, renal, and tracheal anomalies (occasional) (see p. 160)

Hydrolethalus: Autosomal recessive disorder characterized by hydrocephalus, polydactyly, heart defects, and polyhydramnios (see p. 194)

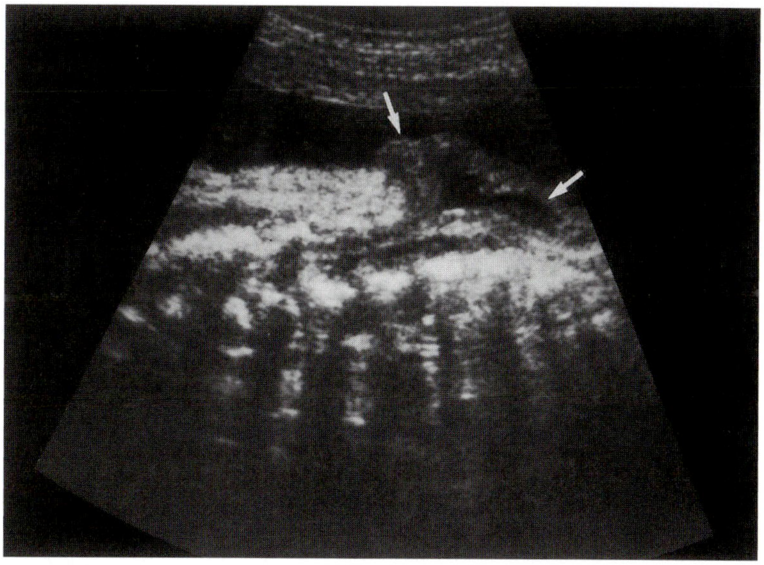

FIGURE 1-37 Magnified view of a lumbar neural tube defect *(arrows)*.

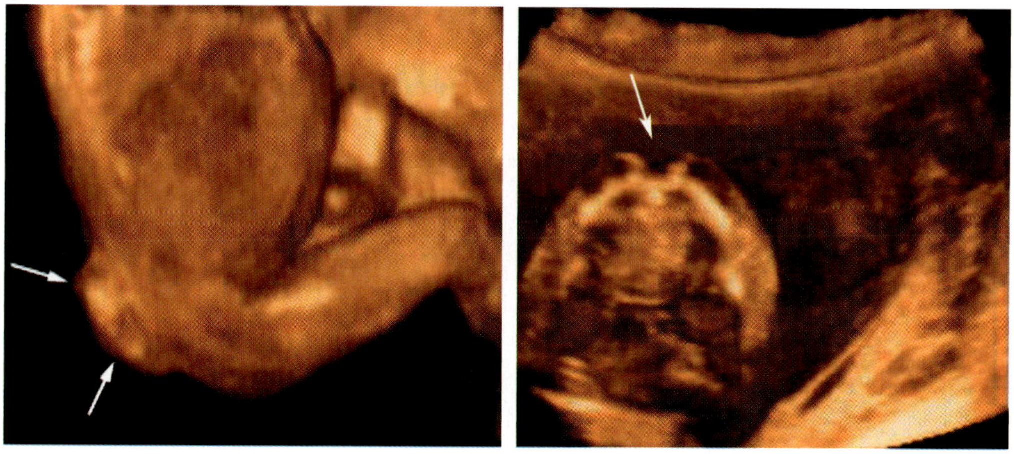

FIGURE 1-38 (A) Three-dimensional surface rendering of a neural tube defect involving the lower lumbar spine *(arrows)*. (B) Coronal view through the fetal lower spine shows the opening *(arrow)* at the level of the posterior elements, consistent with an open neural tube defect.

Joubert Syndrome: Autosomal recessive syndrome characterized by dysmorphic facial features and agenesis of the cerebellar vermis (encephalocele) (see p. 197)

Meckel-Gruber Syndrome: Autosomal recessive condition characterized by posterior encephalocele, postaxial polydactyly, and polycystic kidneys (encephalocele) (see p. 199)

Median Cleft Face: Midline facial defects resulting in hypertelorism and bifid or broad nasal bridge (see p. 165)

Microcephaly (see p. 205)

Neu-Laxova Syndrome: Autosomal recessive condition characterized by microcephaly, lissencephaly, exophthalmos, severe IUGR, swollen subcutaneous tissues, and ichthyosis (occasional) (see p. 211)

Oral-Facial-Digital Syndrome, Type II (Mohr Syndrome): Autosomal recessive syndrome characterized by short stature; deafness; and facial, hand, and foot abnormalities (occasional) (see p. 175)

Walker-Warburg Syndrome: Autosomal recessive condition characterized by severe congenital oculocerebral abnormalities, including lissencephaly, hydrocephalus, encephalocele, microcephaly, microphthalmia, and cataracts (encephalocele) (see p. 217)

LIMB AND SKELETAL ABNORMALITIES

Adams-Oliver Syndrome: Disorder characterized by terminal transverse defects of the upper and lower extremities, as well as denuded areas on the scalp with or without an underlying bony skull (bone) defect (occasional encephalocele or acrania) (see p. 223)

Roberts Syndrome: Autosomal recessive condition characterized by severe shortening of the limbs (pseudothalidomide syndrome) and facial anomalies (occasional encephalocele) (see p. 247)

CHROMOSOMAL ANOMALIES

Deletion 5p (Cri du Chat Syndrome): Abnormality of chromosome 5 characterized by microcephaly, hypertelorism, micrognathia, hydrops, and growth delay (encephalocele) (see p. 457)

Triploidy: Occurring as a result of a complete extra set of chromosomes, this is a lethal abnormality characterized by severe early-onset IUGR and multiple anomalies of practically all organ systems (see p. 473)

Trisomy 9: Occurring as a result of an extra chromosome 9, this is a severe abnormality characterized by multiple anomalies of practically all organ systems (see p. 478)

Trisomy 13 (Patau Syndrome): Occurring as a result of an extra chromosome 13, this is a severe abnormality characterized by multiple anomalies of the central nervous system, face, heart, and extremities (see p. 483)

Trisomy 18 (Edwards Syndrome): Occurring as a result of an extra chromosome 18, this is a severe abnormality characterized by IUGR and multiple anomalies of the central nervous system, face, heart, and extremities (occasional) (see p. 490)

OTHER SYNDROMES AND SEQUENCES

Amniotic Band Syndrome: Condition caused by premature rupture of the amnion, resulting in an asymmetric, destructive fetal process whereby the fetus becomes adherent to, intertwined with, and tethered by the fibrous bands; associated with diverse anomalies (asymmetric) (see p. 356)

Caudal Regression Syndrome/Sirenomelia: Although of different etiologies, these two syndromes are similar; characterized by disruption of the caudal portion of the neural tube, absence or dysplasia of the sacrum, and renal and lower extremity anomalies (occasional) (see p. 370)

Cloacal Exstrophy Sequence: Complex disorder characterized by a combination of defects that include omphalocele, imperforate anus, cloacal exstrophy, spinal defects, and genital abnormalities (see p. 382)

Jarcho-Levin Syndrome (Spondylothoracic Dysplasia): Disorder occurring most commonly among Puerto Ricans; characterized by vertebral defects resulting in a very short thorax and spine and a protuberant abdomen (occasional) (see p. 332)

Pentalogy of Cantrell: Combination of five anomalies: ectopia cordis, omphalocele, disruption of the distal sternum, anterior diaphragm, and diaphragmatic pericardium (occasional) (see p. 405)

Renal Agenesis (occasional) (see p. 412)

VATER Association: **V**ertebral defects, **a**nal atresia, **t**racheoesophageal fistula, **e**sophageal atresia, and **r**adial and renal dysplasias (occasional) (see p. 429)

TERATOGENS

Aminopterin (see p. 438)

Carbamazepine (Tegretol) (see p. 436)

Clomiphene (Clomid) (see p. 437)

Cocaine (see p. 439)

Cytarabine (see p. 435)

Dextroamphetamine (see p. 439)

Hyperthermia (see p. 439)

Imipramine (see p. 438)

Methotrexate (see p. 435)

Progestin (see p. 437)

Radiation (see p. 439)

Valproic acid (see p. 436)

Warfarin (Coumadin) (see p. 435)

SHORT SPINE

FACIAL AND BRAIN ABNORMALITIES

Iniencephaly/anencephaly (see p. 418)

OTHER SYNDROMES AND SEQUENCES

Caudal Regression Syndrome/Sirenomelia: Although of different etiologies, these two syndromes are similar; characterized by disruption of the caudal portion of the neural tube, absence or dysplasia of the sacrum, and renal and lower extremity anomalies (see p. 370)

Jarcho-Levin Syndrome (Spondylothoracic Dysplasia): Disorder occurring most commonly among Puerto Ricans; characterized by vertebral defects resulting in a very short thorax and spine and a protuberant abdomen (see p. 332)

Klippel-Feil Syndrome: Abnormal cervical vertebrae, webbed neck, and facial asymmetry (neck) (see p. 394)

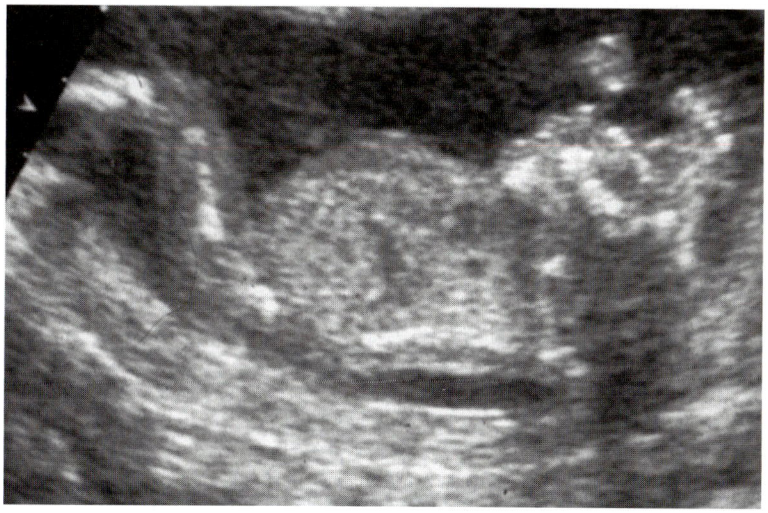

FIGURE 1-39 First-trimester fetus with iniencephaly. Note the short spine and anencephaly making the ventral aspect of this fetus longer than the length of the spine.

VERTEBRAL BODY SEGMENTAL ABNORMALITIES (Other than Platyspondyly)

GROWTH ABNORMALITIES

Noonan Syndrome: Phenotypically, a Turner-like syndrome featuring short stature, webbed neck, cardiac abnormalities, and normal karyotype (see p. 131)

FACIAL AND BRAIN ABNORMALITIES

Aicardi Syndrome: Rare X-linked syndrome characterized by agenesis of the corpus callosum, interhemispheric cyst, chorioretinal abnormalities, and infantile seizures (occasional) (see p. 188)

Cerebrocostomandibular Syndrome: Autosomal recessive condition characterized by severe micrognathia, cleft palate, and vertebral body abnormalities associated with defective costal development (see p. 152)

Goldenhar Syndrome: Asymmetry of the face and ears in conjunction with vertebral anomalies of the upper spine (see p. 162)

Gorlin Syndrome: Autosomal dominant syndrome characterized by macrocephaly, facial abnormalities, and multiple tumors (see p. 192)

Oral-Facial-Digital Syndrome, Type II (Mohr Syndrome): Autosomal recessive syndrome characterized by short stature; deafness; and facial, hand, and foot abnormalities (occasional) (see p. 175)

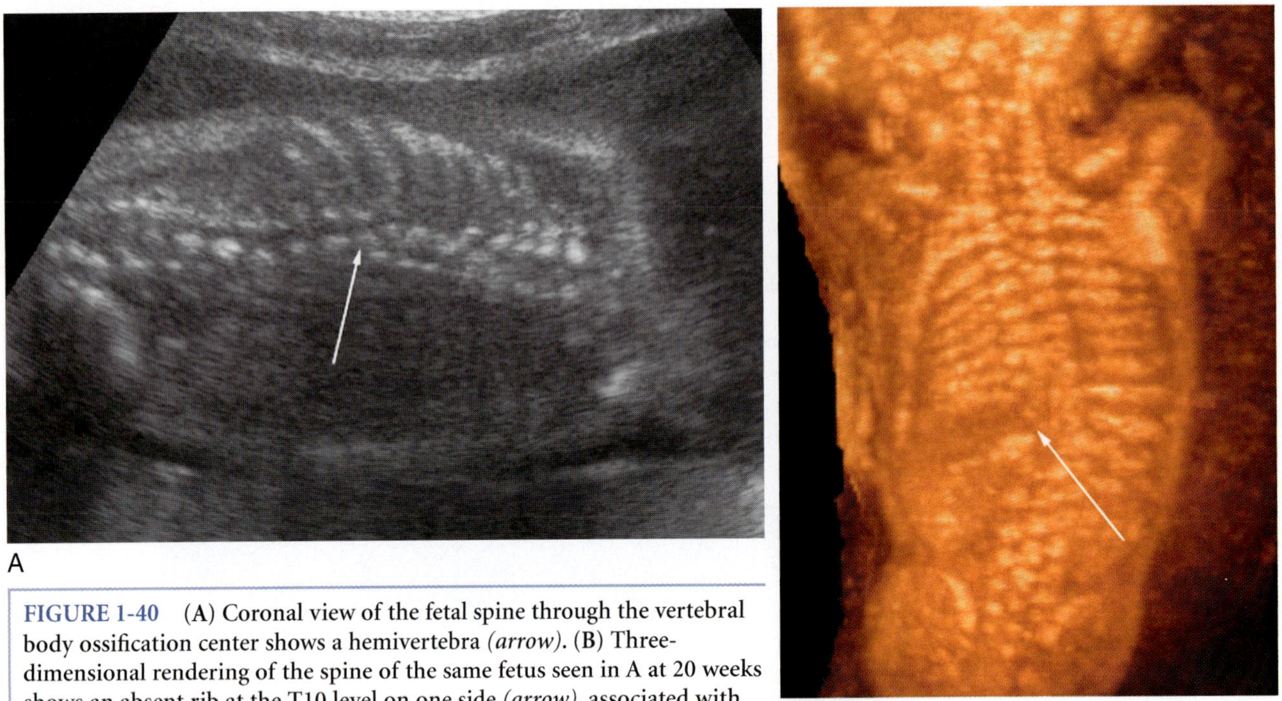

A

B

FIGURE 1-40 (A) Coronal view of the fetal spine through the vertebral body ossification center shows a hemivertebra *(arrow)*. (B) Three-dimensional rendering of the spine of the same fetus seen in A at 20 weeks shows an absent rib at the T10 level on one side *(arrow)*, associated with the vertebral body abnormality.

LIMB AND SKELETAL ABNORMALITIES

Atelosteogenesis, Type I: Lethal skeletal dysplasia characterized by severe limb shortening and deficient ossification of the bones, resulting in micromelic dwarfism (see p. 260)

Chondrodysplasia Punctata (Nonrhizomelic Type)**:** Heterogeneous group of bone dysplasias characterized by asymmetric limb shortening and abnormal early calcification of the proximal and distal epiphyses (kyphoscoliosis and vertebral body anomalies) (see p. 266)

Femoral Hypoplasia–Unusual Facies Syndrome: Syndrome characterized by short lower limbs, especially hypoplastic femurs, and facial abnormalities; may be part of a spectrum of abnormalities that includes caudal regression syndrome (sacral dysplasia) (see p. 231)

Freeman-Sheldon (Whistling Face) Syndrome: Autosomal dominant condition characterized by unusual facial features and skeletal anomalies, such as flexion deformities of the joints (kyphoscoliosis) (see p. 237)

Larsen Syndrome: Condition characterized by abnormal facies and spine and limb abnormalities, including dislocations and hyperextensions at the joints (see p. 242)

Multiple Pterygium Syndrome: Autosomal recessive condition characterized by multiple contractures and webbing across the joints, cystic hygromata, and facial defects (occasional) (see p. 244)

CRANIOSYNOSTOSIS

Apert Syndrome: Craniosynostosis, acrocephaly, and syndactyly (C5–6) (see p. 304)

Pfeiffer Syndrome: Acrocephalic skull, craniosynostosis (particularly of the coronal and sagittal sutures), and syndactyly of hands and feet (occasional) (see p. 316)

OTHER SYNDROMES AND SEQUENCES

Caudal Regression Syndrome/Sirenomelia: Although of different etiologies, these two syndromes are similar; characterized by disruption of the caudal portion of the neural tube, absence or dysplasia of the sacrum, and renal and lower extremity anomalies (see p. 370)

CHARGE Association: **C**oloboma of the iris, **h**eart defect, choanal **a**tresia, intrauterine growth **r**estriction, **g**enital anomalies, and **e**ar anomalies (occasional) (see p. 376)

Cloacal Exstrophy Sequence: Complex disorder characterized by a combination of defects that include omphalocele, imperforate anus, cloacal exstrophy, spinal defects, and genital abnormalities (see p. 382)

Jarcho-Levin Syndrome (Spondylothoracic Dysplasia): Disorder occurring most commonly among Puerto Ricans; characterized by vertebral defects resulting in a very short thorax and spine and a protuberant abdomen (see p. 332)

Klippel-Feil Syndrome: Abnormal cervical vertebrae, webbed neck, and facial asymmetry (cervical) (see p. 394)

Marfan Syndrome: Autosomal dominant connective tissue disorder characterized by tall stature, long limbs, pectus deformities, congenital heart defects, and ocular anomalies (occasional) (see p. 344)

MURCS Association: **M**üllerian duct aplasia, **r**enal aplasia, **c**ervicothoracic **s**omite dysplasia (C5–T1) (see p. 398)

Renal Agenesis (occasional) (see p. 412)

VATER Association: **V**ertebral defects, **a**nal atresia, **t**racheoesophageal fistula, **e**sophageal atresia, and **r**adial and renal dysplasias (see p. 429)

TERATOGENS

Oral contraceptives (see p. 437)

Quinine (see p. 434)

Thalidomide (see p. 437)

Warfarin (Coumadin) (see p. 435)

PLATYSPONDYLY

LIMB AND SKELETAL ABNORMALITIES

Atelosteogenesis, Type I: Lethal skeletal dysplasia characterized by severe limb shortening and deficient ossification of the bones, resulting in micromelic dwarfism (see p. 260)

Kniest Syndrome: Autosomal dominant condition characterized by kyphoscoliosis, platyspondyly, and shortened tubular long bones (see p. 281)

Metatropic Dysplasia: Short-limbed skeletal dysplasia characterized by progressive, severe kyphoscoliosis, narrow chest, and metaphyseal flaring (see p. 285)

Spondyloepiphyseal Dysplasia Congenita: Autosomal dominant, heterogeneous group of disorders characterized by a short spine with platyspondyly, which results in kyphoscoliosis and lordosis (see p. 291)

Thanatophoric Dysplasia: Most common skeletal dysplasia; characterized by narrow chest; short ribs; short, bowed long bones; and flat vertebral bodies (see p. 294)

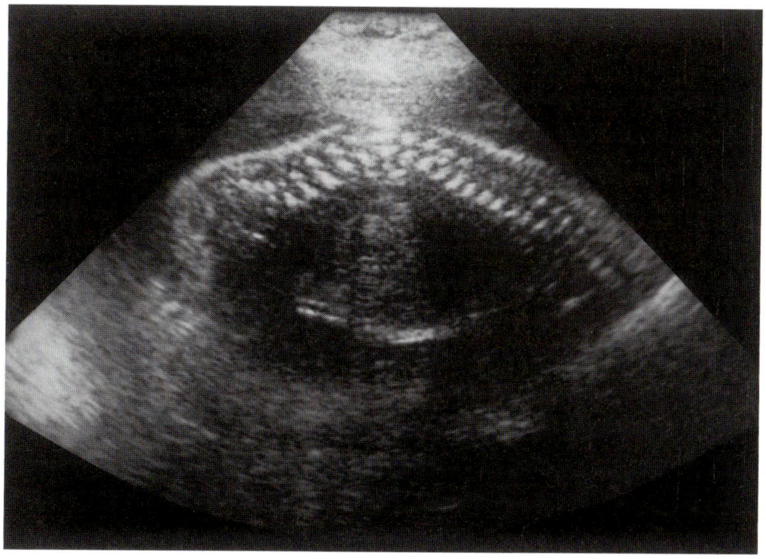

FIGURE 1-41 Longitudinal view of the spine of a fetus with thanatophoric dysplasia shows a slight kyphosis of the spine secondary to platyspondyly of the vertebral bodies.

RIB ABNORMALITIES

OTHER SYNDROMES AND SEQUENCES

Jarcho-Levin Syndrome: Most common among Puerto Ricans; characterized by vertebral defects resulting in a very short thorax and spine and a protuberant abdomen (see p. 332)

Klippel-Feil Syndrome: Abnormal cervical vertebrae, webbed neck, and facial asymmetry (see p. 394)

MURCS Association: **Mü**llerian duct aplasia, **r**enal aplasia, **c**ervicothoracic **s**omite dysplasia (occasional) (see p. 398)

Spondylocostal Dysostosis: Mild form of Jarcho-Levin syndrome (see p. 332)

Spondylothoracic Dysostosis: Form of Jarcho-Levin syndrome with varying degrees of severity within a family (see p. 332)

VATER Association: **V**ertebral defects, **a**nal atresia, **t**racheoesophageal fistula, **e**sophageal atresia, and **r**adial and renal dysplasias (see p. 429)

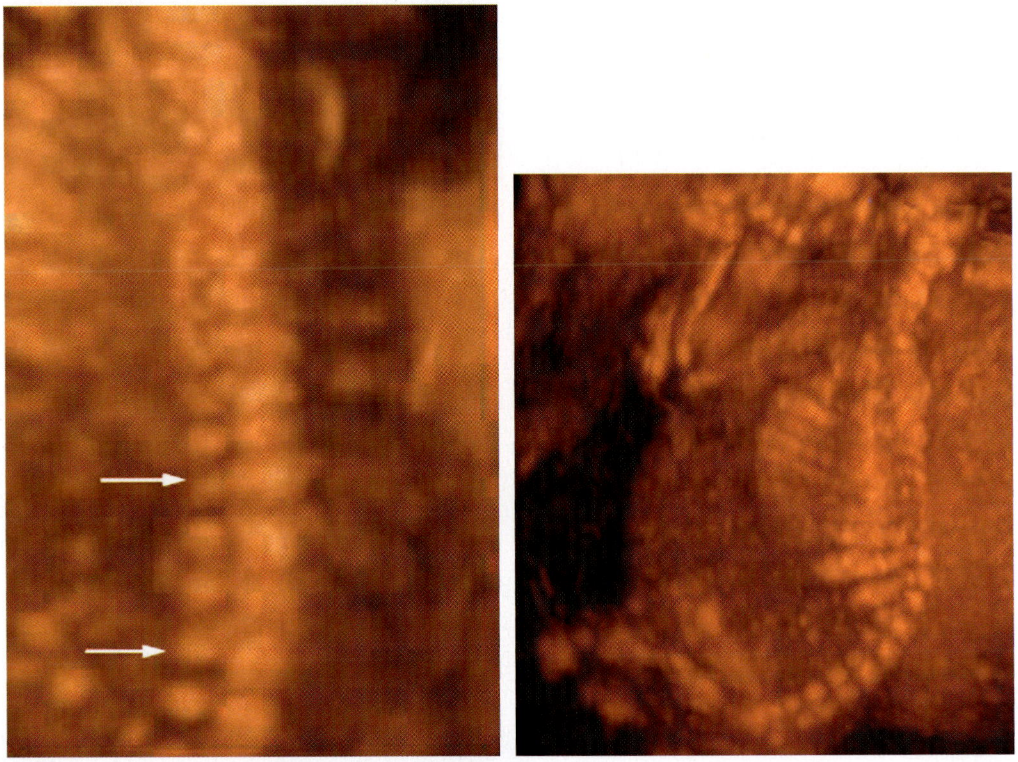

A B

FIGURE 1-42 (A) Three-dimensional surface rendering of the fetal skeleton (sagittal view) shows the small and flat vertebral body ossification centers, consistent with platyspondyly *(arrows)*, associated with thanatophoric dysplasia. (B) Second-trimester fetus with platyspondyly seen using a skeletal rendering mode. Note the kyphotic deformity of the fetal spine resulting from the platyspondyly.

MASS ON SURFACE OF THE FETUS

Amniotic Band Syndrome: Condition caused by premature rupture of the amnion, resulting in an asymmetric, destructive fetal process whereby the fetus becomes adherent to, intertwined with, and tethered by the fibrous bands; associated with diverse anomalies (see p. 356)

Anterior Abdominal Wall Defect: (see differential diagnosis for this condition) (see p. 52)

Cloacal Exstrophy Sequence: Complex disorder characterized by a combination of defects that include omphalocele, imperforate anus, cloacal exstrophy, spinal defects, and genital abnormalities (see p. 382)

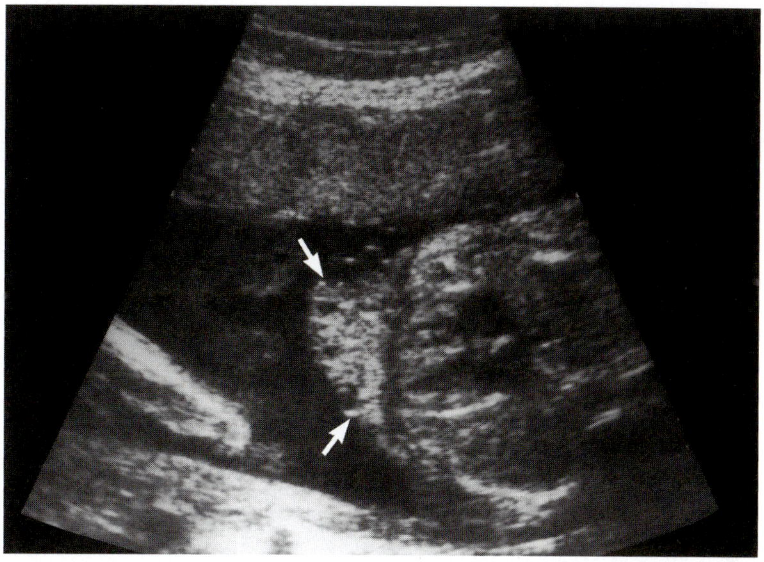

FIGURE 1-43 Transverse view through the fetal anterior chest shows an irregular solid mass *(arrows)* originating from the region of the sternum. Note the four-chamber view of the heart, directly underneath the mass. This was a hamartoma of the sternum.

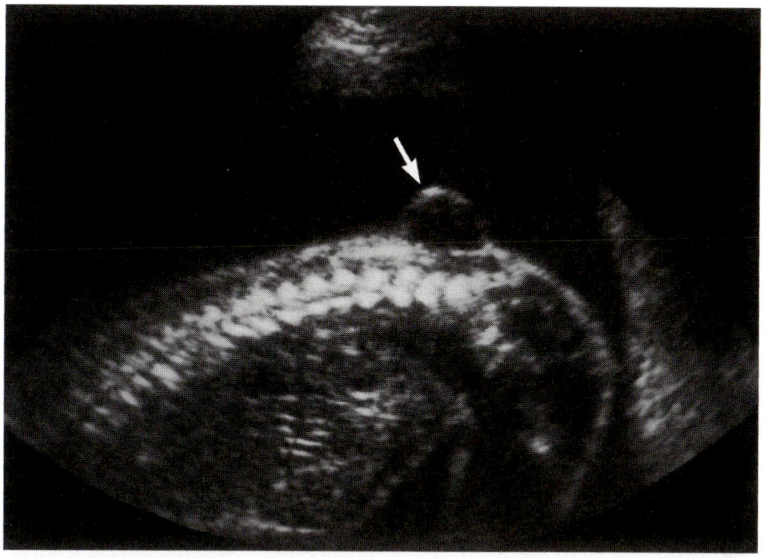

A

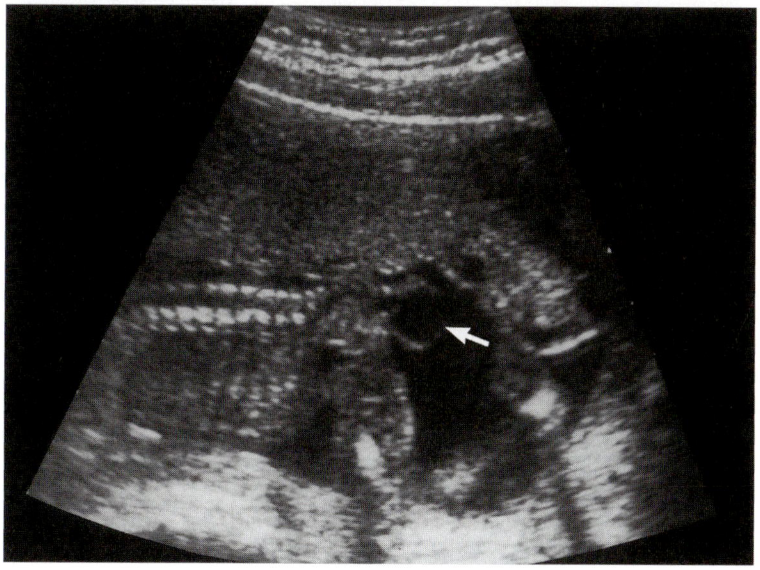

B

FIGURE 1-44 (A) Lumbar neural tube defect *(arrow)* is seen as a lucent bubble off the back of the fetus. (B) Small, cystic, sacrococcygeal teratoma originating from the fetal buttock. The appearance of the mass *(arrow)* is similar to the neural tube defect seen in *A*. However, this mass is away from the spine and involves a different area of the fetal body.

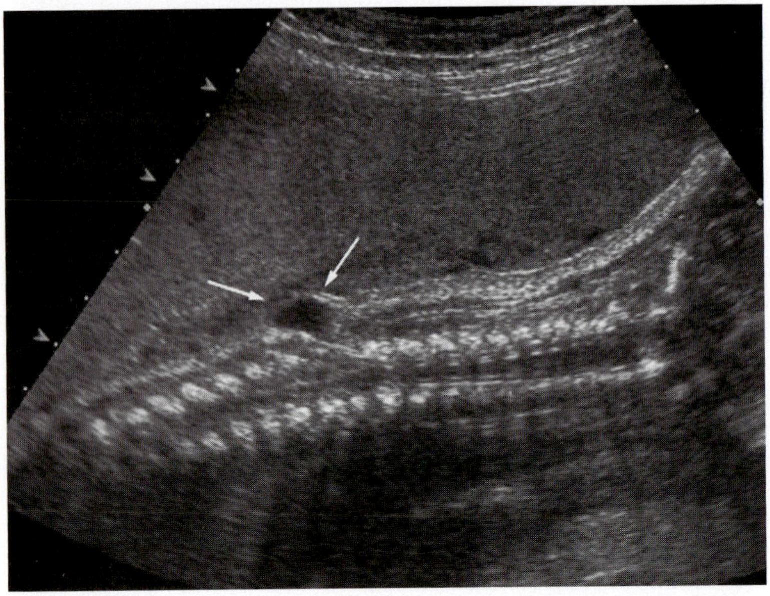

FIGURE 1-45 Neural tube defect in the thoracic spine as evidenced by the small cyst *(arrows)* protruding from the midspine posteriorly.

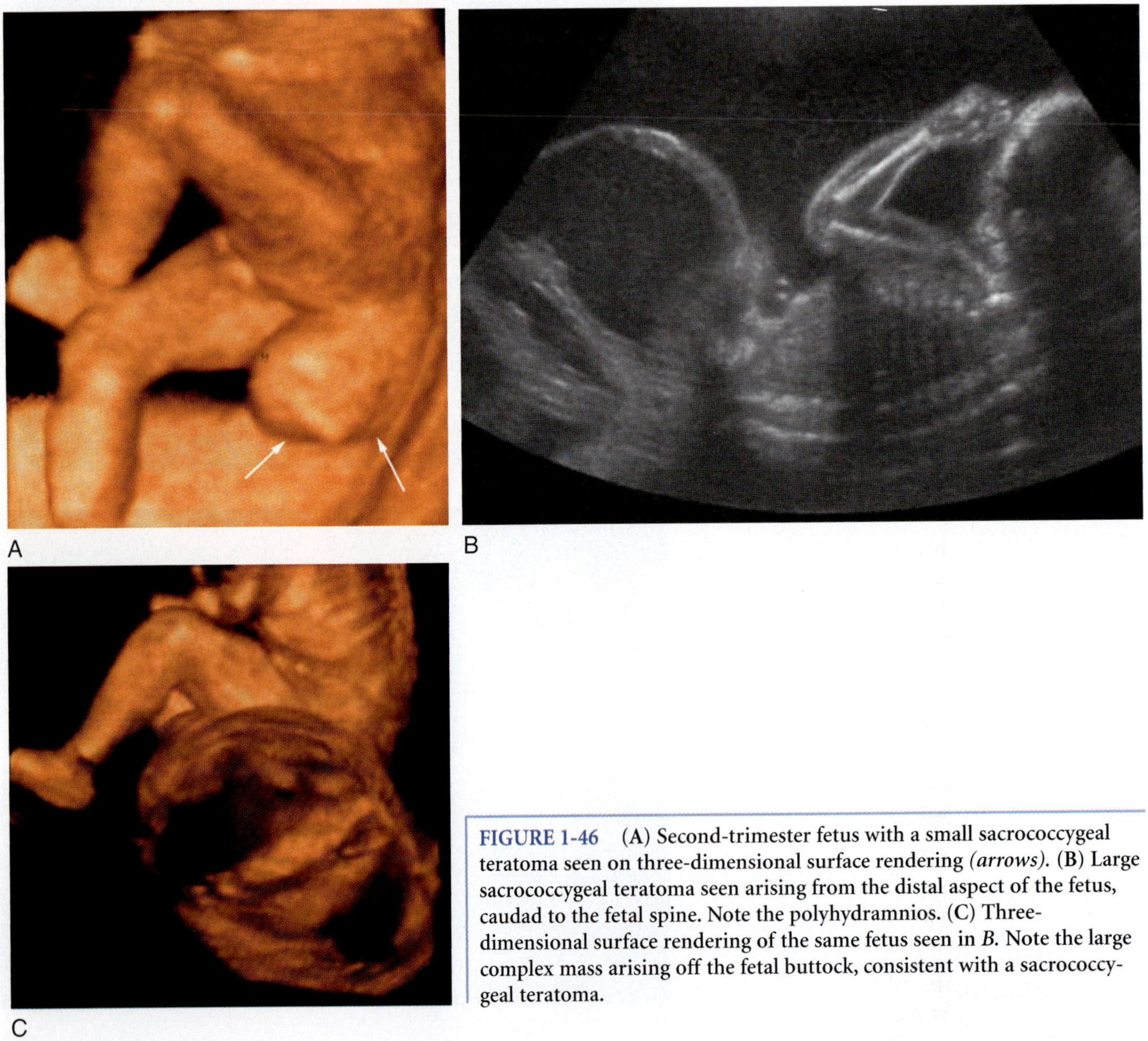

FIGURE 1-46 (A) Second-trimester fetus with a small sacrococcygeal teratoma seen on three-dimensional surface rendering *(arrows)*. (B) Large sacrococcygeal teratoma seen arising from the distal aspect of the fetus, caudad to the fetal spine. Note the polyhydramnios. (C) Three-dimensional surface rendering of the same fetus seen in *B*. Note the large complex mass arising off the fetal buttock, consistent with a sacrococcygeal teratoma.

Cystic Hygroma: (see differential diagnosis for Nuchal Thickening/Cystic Hygroma) (see p. 515)

Encephalocele

Hamartoma (e.g., of the sternum)

Hemangioma or Lymphangioma: Possibilities include Proteus syndrome (see p. 352) and Klippel-Trenaunay-Weber syndrome (see p. 519)

Neural Tube Defect (see p. 418)

NUCHAL MEMBRANE

Amniotic Band Syndrome: Condition caused by premature rupture of the amnion, resulting in an asymmetric, destructive fetal process whereby the fetus becomes adherent to, intertwined with, and tethered by the fibrous bands; associated with diverse anomalies (intracranial structures usually are abnormal) (see p. 356)

Encephalocele

Hair (late third trimester, floats with ballottement)

Nuchal Cord (use Doppler)

Nuchal Cystic Hygroma or Thickening (see p. 50): Condition associated with normal

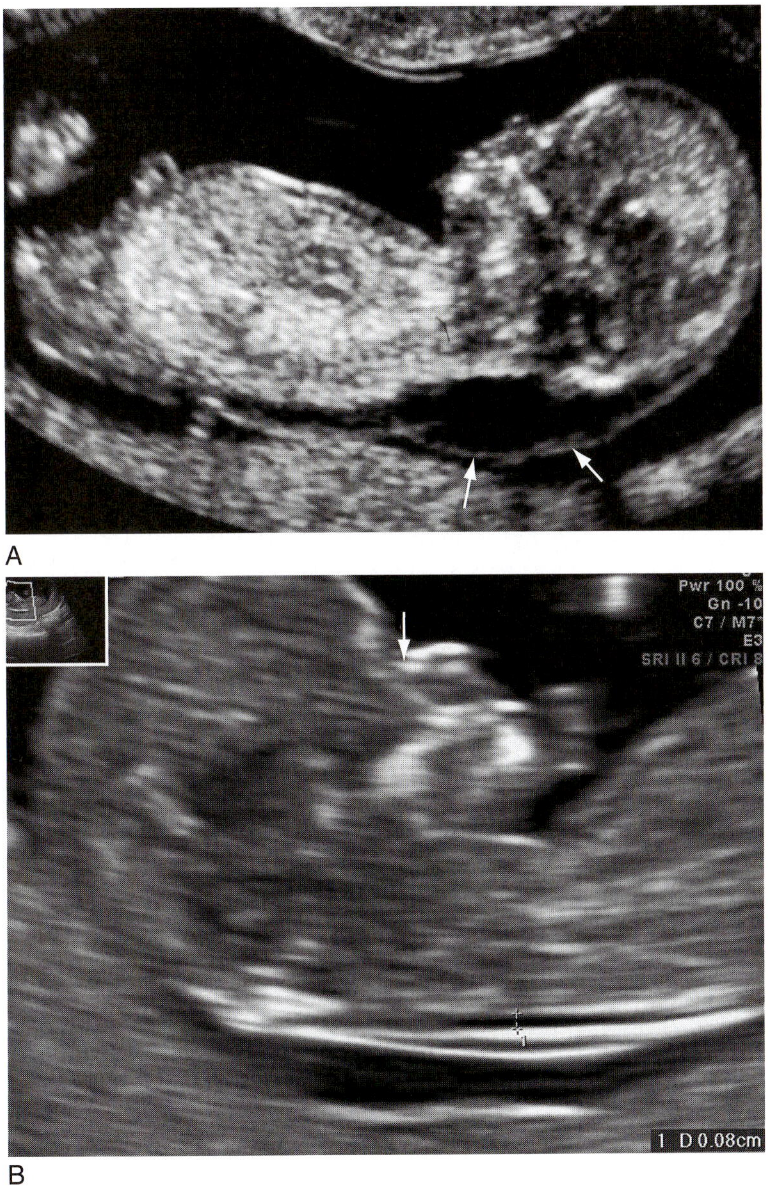

FIGURE 1-47 (A) Second-trimester fetus with a thickened nuchal translucency extending all the way around the fetus, both posteriorly *(arrows)* and anteriorly. The extent of nuchal thickening suggests a cystic hygroma. This finding is associated with a high risk of chromosomal abnormality. (B) Normal nuchal translucency measurement of a first-trimester fetus with normal karyotype. Note that the nasal bone is visible *(arrow)*.

intracranial findings. If associated with hydrops, it carries a poor prognosis, with >80% risk of abnormal karyotype. If isolated, it is associated with 12%-20% risk of abnormal karyotype.

NUCHAL THICKENING/CYSTIC HYGROMA (First and/or Second Trimesters)

GROWTH ABNORMALITIES

Cornelia de Lange Syndrome: Facial/limb anomalies, growth restriction, and mental developmental delay (see p. 129)

Noonan Syndrome: Phenotypically, a Turner-like syndrome featuring short stature, webbed neck, cardiac abnormalities, and normal karyotype (see p. 131)

Perlman Syndrome: Autosomal recessive fetal overgrowth syndrome characterized by macrosomia, bilaterally enlarged kidneys, renal tumors, and other visceromegaly associated with polyhydramnios (see p. 147)

Smith-Lemli-Opitz Syndrome: Autosomal recessive syndrome featuring microcephaly, mental retardation, and genital and renal anomalies (see p. 140)

FACIAL AND BRAIN ABNORMALITIES

Cerebrocostomandibular Syndrome: Autosomal recessive condition characterized by severe micrognathia, cleft palate, and vertebral body abnormalities associated with defective costal development (see p. 152)

Hydrolethalus: Autosomal recessive disorder characterized by hydrocephalus, polydactyly, heart defects, and polyhydramnios (see p. 194)

Joubert Syndrome: Autosomal recessive syndrome characterized by dysmorphic facial features and agenesis of the cerebellar vermis (see p. 197)

LIMB AND SKELETAL ABNORMALITIES

Achondrogenesis: Lethal skeletal dysplasia with extreme hypoplasia of the bones, micromelia, decreased ossification of the bones (particularly those of the skull and spine), and hydrops (see p. 253)

Achondroplasia: Autosomal dominant condition with rhizomelic limb shortening (nonlethal, heterozygous type usually is not apparent until late in the second trimester) (occasional) (see p. 257)

Camptomelic Dysplasia: Short-limbed skeletal dysplasia with bowing of the long bones, particularly in the lower extremities; bell-shaped, narrow chest; and facial anomalies (occasional) (see p. 262)

Ectrodactyly–Ectodermal Dysplasia–Clefting (EEC) Syndrome: Autosomal dominant condition with labial clefting, ectrodactyly (lobster-claw deformities of the limbs), and genitourinary tract anomalies (occasional) (see p. 225)

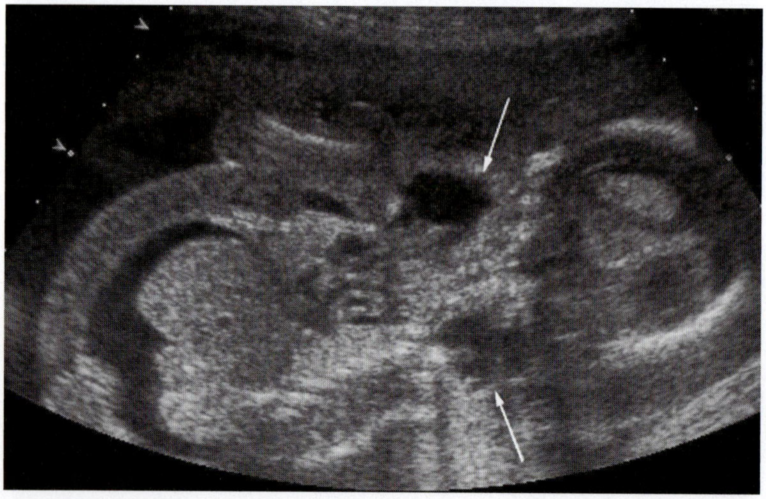

FIGURE 1-48 Second-trimester fetus with severe hydrops, consistent with lymphangiectasia. Note the bilateral cystic hygromas along the fetal neck *(arrows)*, extensive skin edema along the chest and belly, and ascites.

Ellis-van Creveld Syndrome: Autosomal recessive skeletal dysplasia characterized by disproportionately short extremities, narrow chest, polydactyly, and heart defects (see p. 272)

Fanconi Anemia: Autosomal recessive condition characterized by radial hypoplasia, absent thumbs, and tendency for leukemia (see p. 229)

Holt-Oram Syndrome: Autosomal dominant condition characterized by upper extremity abnormalities, such as radial hypoplasia, and heart defects (see p. 238)

Hypophosphatasia: Autosomal recessive condition characterized by severe demineralization of the bones and congenital deficiency of alkaline phosphatase (see p. 275)

Jeune Thoracic Dystrophy (Asphyxiating Thoracic Dysplasia): Autosomal recessive skeletal dysplasia characterized by very narrow chest with short ribs, moderately short long-bones, and sporadic polydactyly (occasional) (see p. 278)

Multiple Pterygium Syndrome: Autosomal recessive condition characterized by multiple contractures and webbing across the joints, cystic hygromata, and facial defects (see p. 244)

Roberts Syndrome: Autosomal recessive condition characterized by severe shortening of the limbs (pseudothalidomide syndrome) and facial anomalies (occasional) (see p. 247)

Thanatophoric Dysplasia: Most common skeletal dysplasia; characterized by narrow chest; short ribs; short, bowed long bones; and flat vertebral bodies (occasional) (see p. 294)

CRANIOSYNOSTOSIS

Apert Syndrome: Craniosynostosis, acrocephaly, and syndactyly (see p. 304)

CHROMOSOMAL ANOMALIES

Deletion 5p (Cri du Chat Syndrome): Abnormality of chromosome 5 characterized by microcephaly, hypertelorism, micrognathia, hydrops, and growth delay (see p. 457)

Deletion 11q (Jacobsen Syndrome): Deletion of the distal long arm of chromosome 11 characterized by multiple anomalies of practically all organ systems (see p. 464)

DiGeorge Syndrome: Also known as velocardiofacial syndrome or Shprintzen syndrome, this disorder results from a deletion of chromosome 22q11.2 and is characterized by cardiac abnormalities involving largely the great vessels, facial abnormalities, hypocalcemia, and hypoplasia of the thymus (see p. 466)

Tetrasomy 12p (Pallister-Killian Syndrome): Mosaic aneuploidy characterized by multiple congenital abnormalities of the central nervous system, face, heart, and many other organs (see p. 471)

Triploidy: Occurring as a result of a complete extra set of chromosomes, this is a lethal abnormality characterized by severe early-onset IUGR and multiple anomalies of practically all organ systems (see p. 473)

Trisomy 9: Occurring as a result of an extra chromosome 9, this is a severe abnormality characterized by multiple anomalies of practically all organ systems (see p. 478)

Trisomy 10: Rare abnormality with only those patients with mosaic trisomy 10 surviving to infancy. Abnormalities include IUGR and face, heart, hand, and foot anomalies (see p. 480)

Trisomy 13 (Patau Syndrome): Occurring as a result of an extra chromosome 13, this is a severe abnormality characterized by multiple anomalies of the central nervous system, face, heart, and extremities (see p. 483)

Trisomy 18 (Edwards Syndrome): Occurring as a result of an extra chromosome 18, this is a severe abnormality characterized by IUGR and multiple anomalies of the central nervous system, face, heart, and extremities (see p. 490)

Trisomy 21 (Down Syndrome): Occurring as a result of an extra chromosome 21, this abnormality is characterized by nuchal fold thickening, short long-bones, abnormal nasal bone, heart defects, and other anomalies. Twenty-five percent of fetuses with Down syndrome do not display any sonographic abnormalities or markers (see p. 496)

Trisomy 22 (occasional)**:** Occurring as a result of an extra chromosome 22, this is a lethal abnormality characterized by multiple anomalies of the heart, face, extremities, and gastrointestinal and genitourinary systems (see p. 509)

XO syndrome (Turner Syndrome): Occurring as a result of a single X chromosome (XO), Turner syndrome is characterized primarily in early pregnancy by large cystic hygromata, lymphangiectasia, and heart defects. Affected infants who survive gestation may represent Turner mosaic individuals (see p. 510)

OTHER SYNDROMES AND SEQUENCES

Arthrogryposis: Sequence of neurologic, muscular, and connective tissue disorders leading to fetal joint contractures and rigidity, as well as decreased activity (see p. 362)

Cardiosplenic Syndromes (Asplenia/Polysplenia): Defects in lateralization of normal body asymmetry, including severe heart defects and anomalies of the intrathoracic and intraabdominal viscera (see p. 365)

Caudal Regression Syndrome/Sirenomelia: Although of different etiologies, these two syndromes are similar; characterized by disruption of the caudal portion of the neural tube, absence or dysplasia of the sacrum, and renal and lower extremity anomalies (see p. 370)

CHARGE Association: Coloboma of the iris, **h**eart defect, choanal **a**tresia, intrauterine growth **r**estriction, **g**enital anomalies, and **e**ar anomalies (occasional) (see p. 376)

Congenital Adrenal Hyperplasia: Characterized by a deficiency of one of the enzymes of cortisol biosynthesis (usually 21-hydroxylase deficiency), resulting in defective cortisol synthesis. Consequent overproduction and accumulation of cortisol precursors causes excessive production of androgens, leading to virilization of female fetuses (see p. 378)

Congenital High Airway Obstruction Syndrome: Group of disorders characterized by complete obstruction of the upper airway, secondary to either laryngeal or glottic atresia and leading to massive enlargement of the lungs (see p. 380)

Fryns Syndrome: Autosomal recessive condition with diaphragmatic defects, digital and facial abnormalities, and brain anomalies (see p. 325)

Holoprosencephaly Sequence (see p. 386)

Jarcho-Levin Syndrome (Spondylothoracic Dysplasia): Most common among Puerto Ricans; characterized by vertebral defects resulting in a very short thorax and spine and a protuberant abdomen (see p. 332)

Osteogenesis Imperfecta: Heterogeneous group of conditions characterized by severe osseous fragility, decreased ossification, and multiple fractures (see p. 345)

Pentalogy of Cantrell: Combination of five anomalies: ectopia cordis, omphalocele, disruption of the distal sternum, anterior diaphragm, and diaphragmatic pericardium (see p. 405)

TERATOGEN

Parvovirus (see p. 446)

ANTERIOR ABDOMINAL WALL DEFECTS

Bladder Exstrophy

Cord Lesion

Gastroschisis

Omphalocele (see differential diagnosis for this condition) (see p. 55)

Urachal Cyst

OTHER SYNDROMES AND SEQUENCES

Amniotic Band Syndrome: Condition caused by premature rupture of the amnion, resulting in an asymmetric, destructive fetal process whereby the fetus becomes adherent to, intertwined with, and tethered by the fibrous bands; associated with diverse anomalies (see p. 356)

Cloacal Exstrophy Sequence: Complex disorder characterized by a combination of defects that include omphalocele, imperforate anus, cloacal exstrophy, spinal defects, and genital abnormalities (see p. 382)

Limb–Body Wall Complex (see p. 361)

Pentalogy of Cantrell: Combination of five anomalies: ectopia cordis, omphalocele, disruption of the distal sternum, anterior diaphragm, and diaphragmatic pericardium (see p. 405)

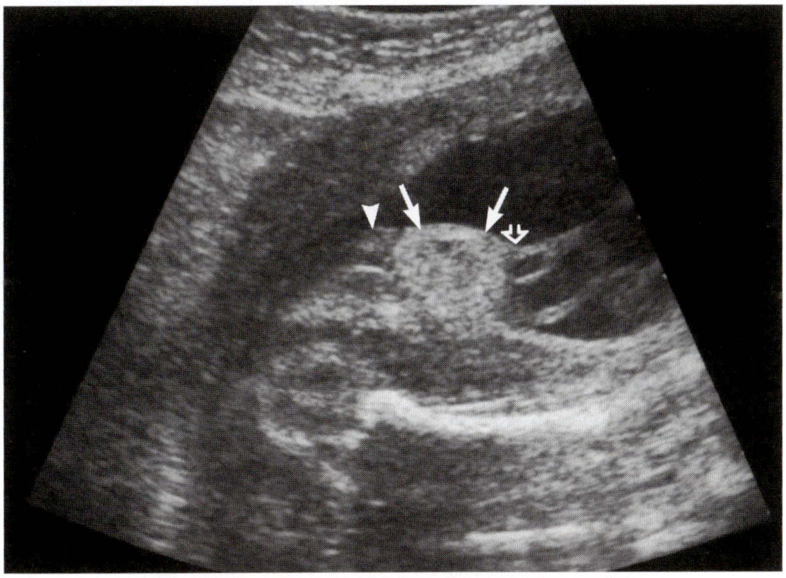

A

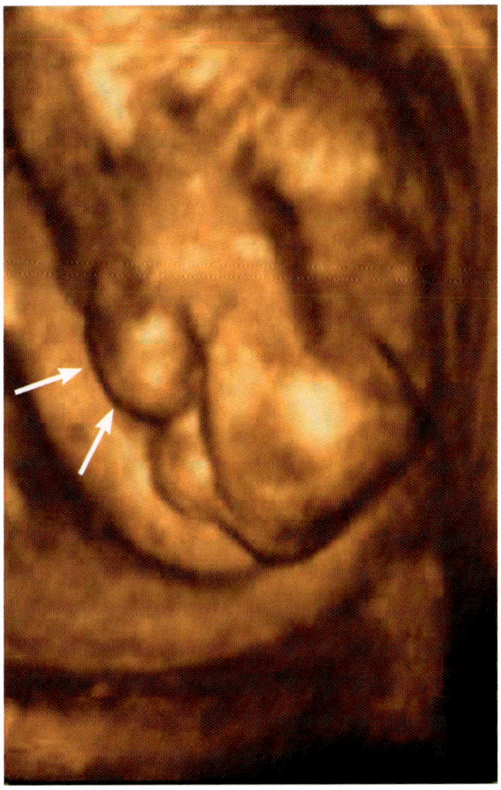

B

FIGURE 1-49 (A) Oblique view through the perineum of a fetus with cloacal exstrophy reveals a mass *(solid arrows)* originating just below the level of the insertion of the cord *(open arrow)*. A portion of the fetal genitalia *(arrowhead)* is visible just beneath the mass. (B) Surface rendering of the lower portion of the fetal body shows the fetal buttock. The rounded mass on the anterior abdominal wall inferiorly indicates bladder exstrophy *(arrows)*.

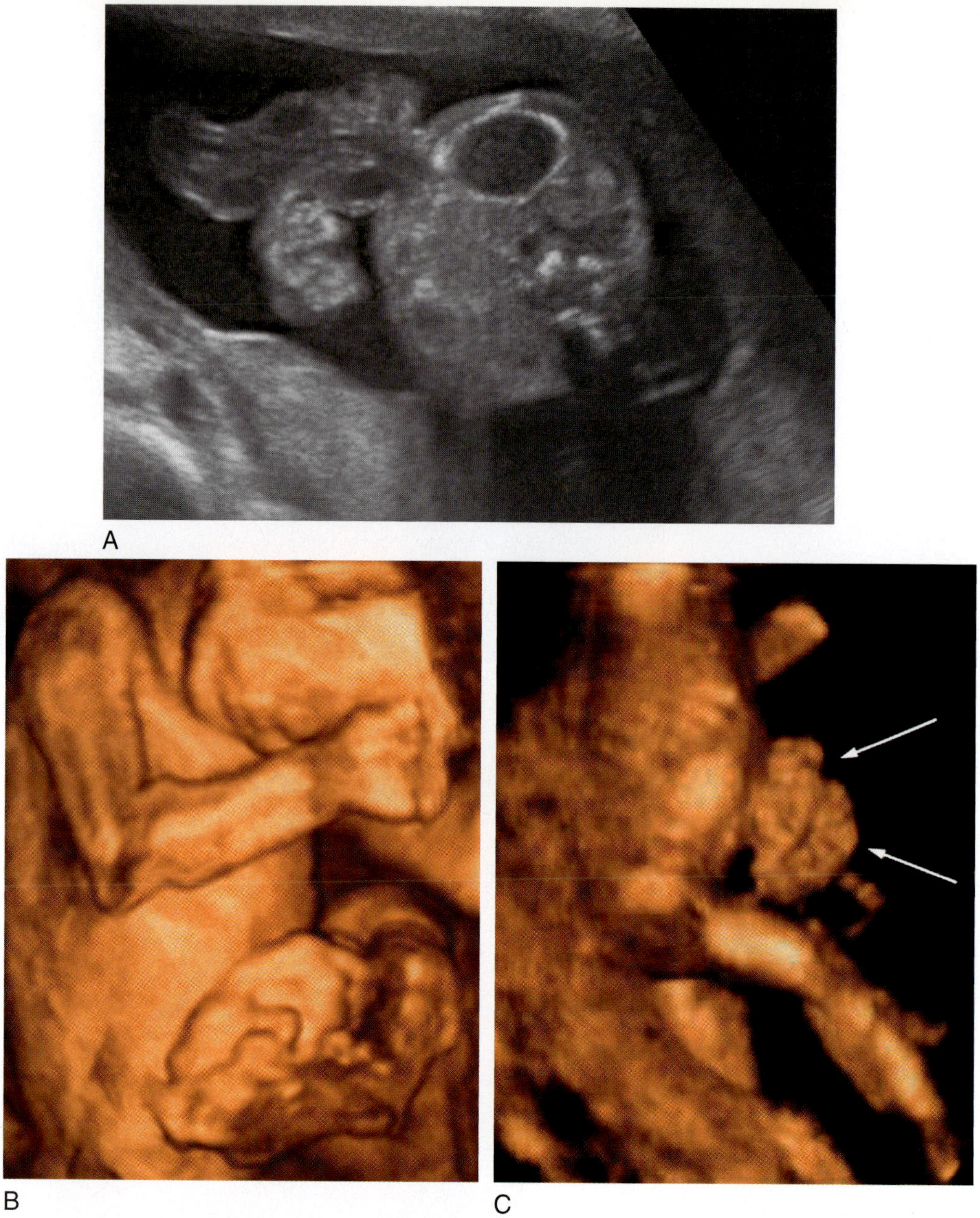

FIGURE 1-50 Gastroschisis. (A) Transverse view through the fetal anterior abdominal wall shows an intraabdominal dilated loop of bowel and multiple loops floating free in the amniotic fluid, next to the insertion of the umbilical cord. (B) Three-dimensional surface rendering of the same fetus seen in *A* shows gastroschisis on the surface of the fetal abdomen. (C) Three-dimensional surface rendering of a younger fetus with a large gastroschisis. Note the large mass emanating from the anterior abdominal wall *(arrows)*.

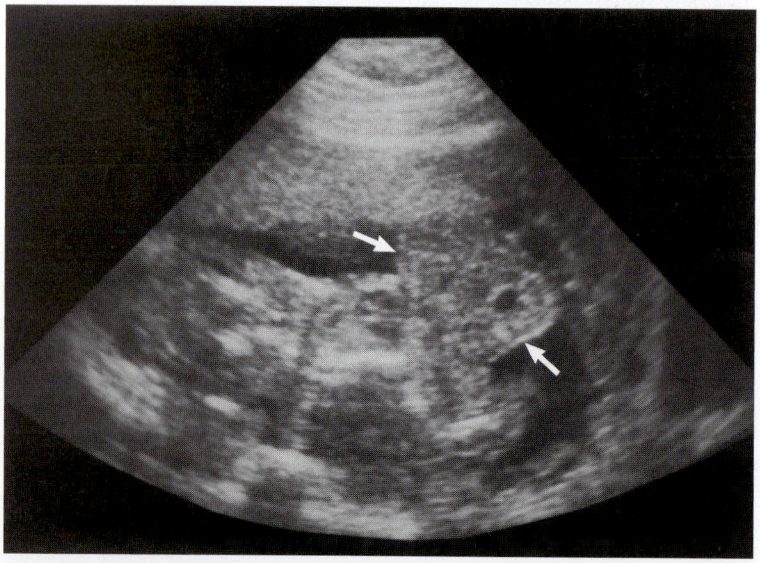

FIGURE 1-51 Longitudinal view of a first-trimester fetus with limb–body wall complex. A huge defect of the anterior abdominal wall *(arrows)* is visible, with some distortion of the fetal body beneath it.

OMPHALOCELE

GROWTH ABNORMALITIES

Beckwith-Wiedemann Syndrome: Gigantism in utero in conjunction with macroglossia, omphalocele, and renal anomalies (see p. 142)

FACIAL AND BRAIN ABNORMALITIES

Cerebrocostomandibular Syndrome: Autosomal recessive condition characterized by severe micrognathia, cleft palate, and vertebral body abnormalities associated with defective costal development (occasional) (see p. 152)

Shprintzen Syndrome: Autosomal dominant syndrome characterized by short stature, mild mental retardation, micrognathia, and cardiac and limb abnormalities (occasional) (see p. 179)

CRANIOSYNOSTOSIS

Carpenter Syndrome: Autosomal recessive condition characterized by acrocephaly, syndactyly, and preaxial polydactyly (acrocephalosyndactyly, type II) (see p. 310)

CHROMOSOMAL ANOMALIES

Tetrasomy 12p (Pallister-Killian Syndrome): Mosaic aneuploidy characterized by multiple congenital abnormalities of the central nervous system, face, heart, and many other organs (see p. 471)

Triploidy: Occurring as a result of a complete extra set of chromosomes, this is a lethal abnormality characterized by severe early-onset IUGR and multiple anomalies of practically all organ systems (see p. 473)

Trisomy 13 (Patau Syndrome): Occurring as a result of an extra chromosome 13, this is a severe abnormality characterized by multiple anomalies of the central nervous system, face, heart, and extremities (see p. 483)

Trisomy 18 (Edwards Syndrome): Occurring as a result of an extra chromosome 18, this is a severe abnormality characterized by IUGR and multiple anomalies of the central nervous system, face, heart, and extremities (see p. 490)

OTHER SYNDROMES AND SEQUENCES

Amniotic Band Syndrome: Condition caused by premature rupture of the amnion, resulting in an asymmetric, destructive fetal process whereby the fetus becomes adherent to, intertwined with, and tethered by the fibrous bands; associated with diverse anomalies (see p. 356)

CHARGE Association: Coloboma of the iris, **h**eart defect, choanal **a**tresia, intrauterine growth **r**estriction, **g**enital anomalies, and **e**ar anomalies (see p. 376)

Limb–Body Wall Complex (see p. 361)

Megacystis-Microcolon-Intestinal Hypoperistalsis Syndrome: Autosomal recessive lethal condition caused by decreased muscle tone in the intestinal and urinary tracts, resulting in a markedly dilated urinary bladder and hypoperistalsis of the colon (occasional) (see p. 396)

Pentalogy of Cantrell: Combination of five anomalies: ectopia cordis, omphalocele, disruption of the distal sternum, anterior diaphragm, and diaphragmatic pericardium (see p. 405)

Sirenomelia (see p. 370)

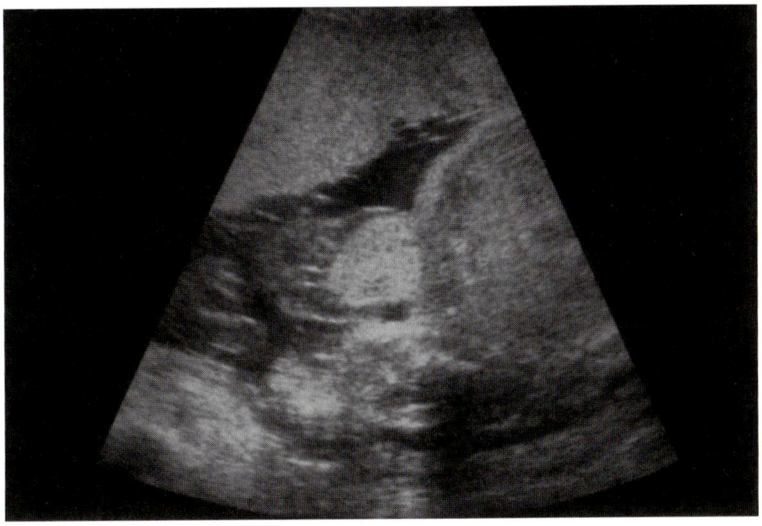

FIGURE 1-52 Transverse view through the insertion of the umbilical cord shows a small bowel-containing omphalocele.

ANTERIOR NECK MASS

Amniotic Band Syndrome: Condition caused by premature rupture of the amnion, resulting in an asymmetric, destructive fetal process whereby the fetus becomes adherent to, intertwined with, and tethered by the fibrous bands; associated with diverse anomalies (see p. 356)

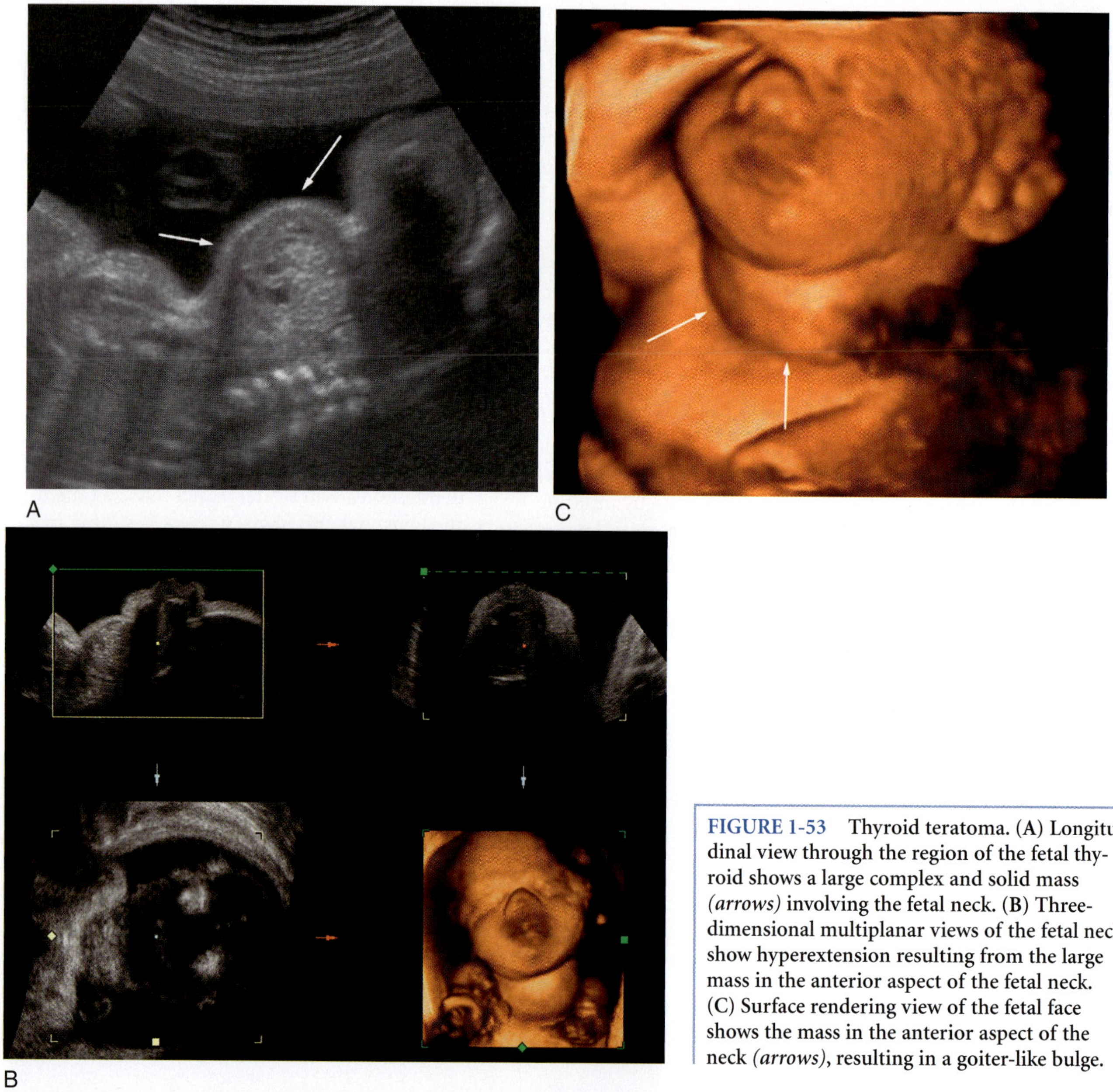

FIGURE 1-53 Thyroid teratoma. (**A**) Longitudinal view through the region of the fetal thyroid shows a large complex and solid mass *(arrows)* involving the fetal neck. (**B**) Three-dimensional multiplanar views of the fetal neck show hyperextension resulting from the large mass in the anterior aspect of the fetal neck. (**C**) Surface rendering view of the fetal face shows the mass in the anterior aspect of the neck *(arrows)*, resulting in a goiter-like bulge.

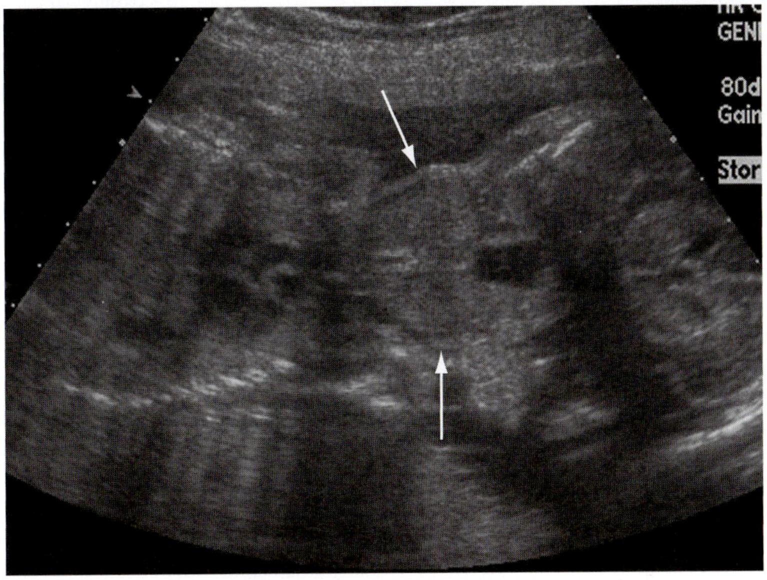

FIGURE 1-54 Coronal view through the fetal thyroid of a fetus with a goiter. Note the two enlarged lobes of the fetal thyroid *(arrows)* just below the level of the larynx.

Branchial Cleft Cyst

Cystic Hygroma (Lymphangioma) (see p. 515)

Goiter

Hemangioma (see p. 519)

Teratoma (see p. 525)

Thyroglossal Duct Cyst

ROTATION OF THE HEART

Absent Lung

Cardiosplenic Syndromes (Asplenia/ Polysplenia): Defects in lateralization of normal body asymmetry, including severe heart defects and anomalies of the intrathoracic and intraabdominal viscera (see p. 365)

Diaphragmatic Hernia

Goldenhar Syndrome: Asymmetry of the face and ears in conjunction with vertebral anomalies of the upper spine (occasional) (see p. 162)

Heart Anomaly (e.g., Conotruncal Anomalies or Ebstein Anomaly)

Intrathoracic Mass (see differential diagnosis for this condition) (see p. 61)

Pleural Effusion

Scimitar Syndrome: Dextroposition of the heart secondary to right pulmonary hypoplasia and anomalous pulmonary venous return (see p. 416)

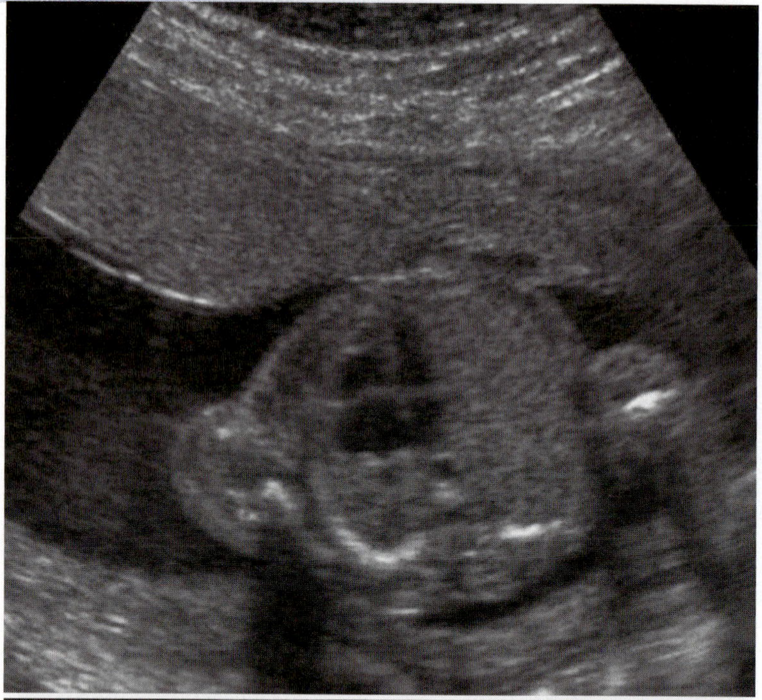

FIGURE 1-55 Transverse view through the fetal chest shows the heart is displaced into the right side of the thorax by a hypoplastic right lung.

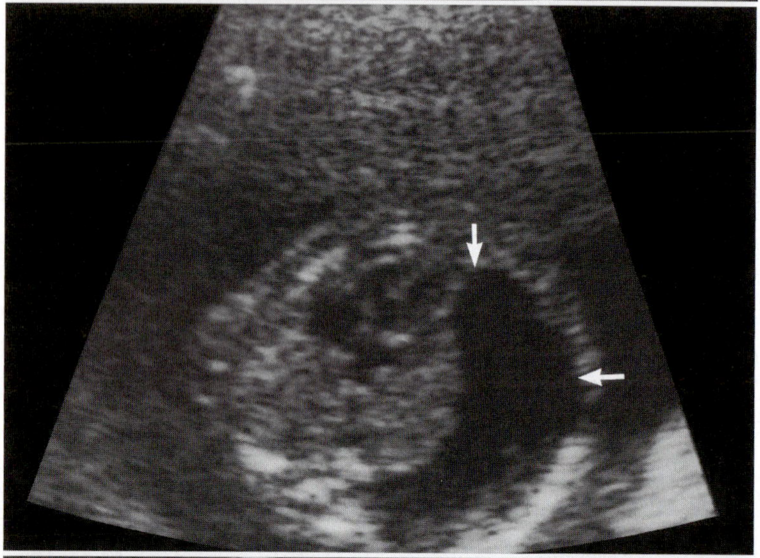

FIGURE 1-56 Transverse view through the fetal chest shows a large, unilateral, left pleural effusion *(arrows)*. The heart and mediastinum have been displaced into the right side of the chest.

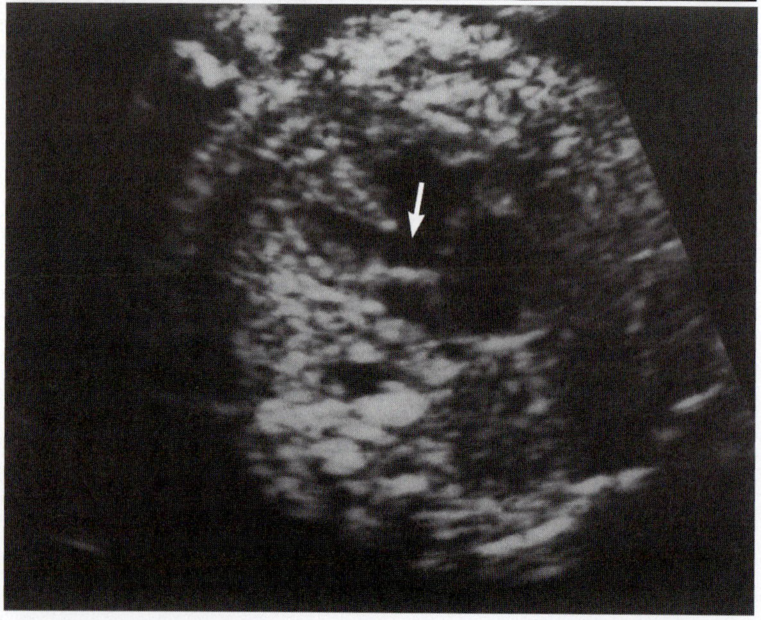

FIGURE 1-57 Heart anomaly. Transverse view through the chest of a fetus with a large ventricular septal defect *(arrow)*. The axis of the ventricular septum indicates that the heart is levorotated, almost to a 90-degree angle.

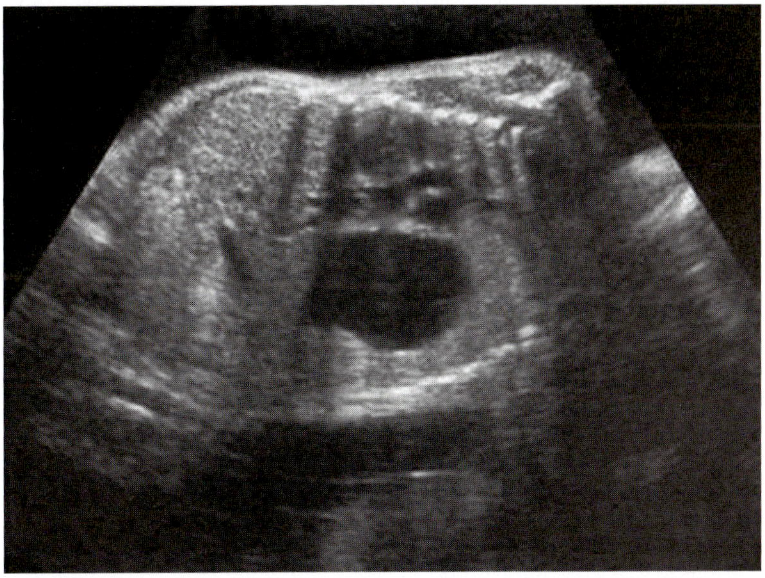
A

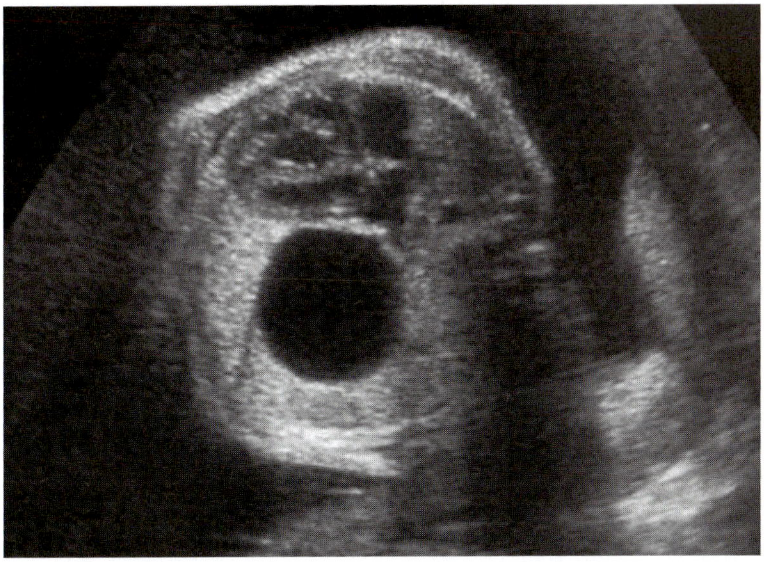
B

FIGURE 1-58 Type I congenital cystic adenomatoid malformation of the lung containing a large cyst. Longitudinal (A) and transverse (B) views of intrathoracic mass displacing the heart and mediastinum to the right.

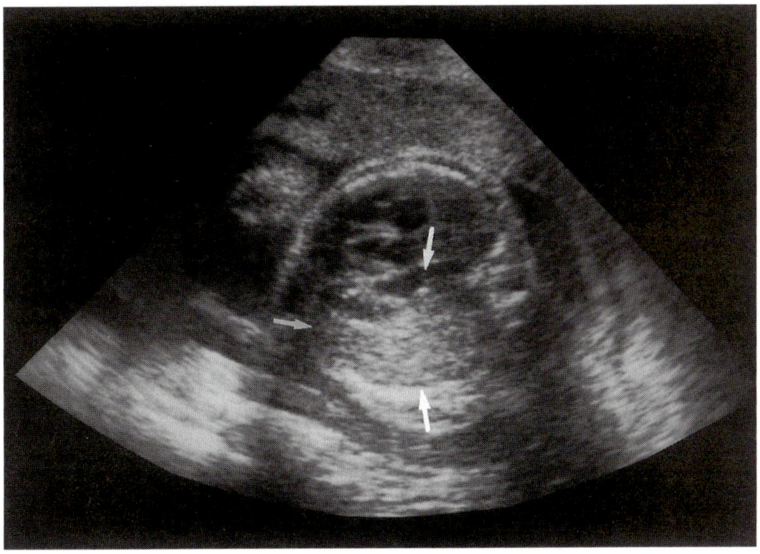

FIGURE 1-59 Diaphragmatic hernia. Transverse view through the chest of a third-trimester fetus with a left-sided diaphragmatic hernia. Note that the heart is deviated into the right side of the chest by a large complex mass in the left side of the thorax *(arrows)*.

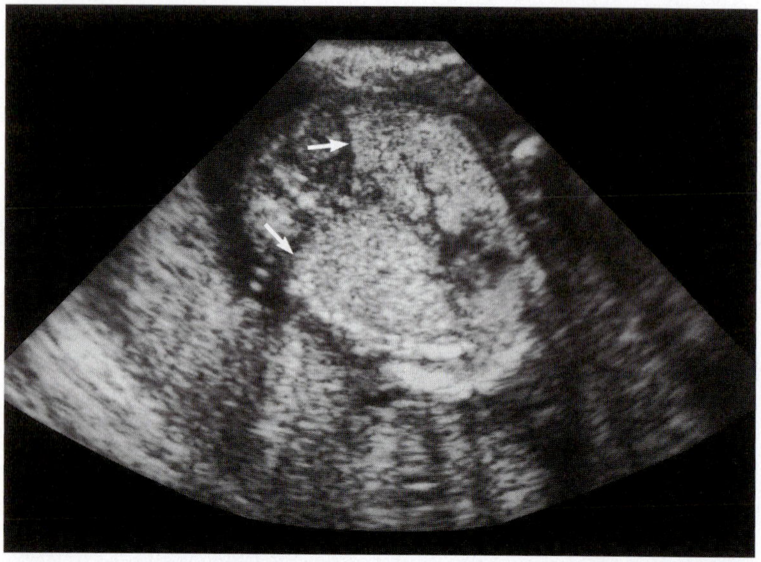

FIGURE 1-60 Laryngeal atresia. Longitudinal view of the chest of a fetus with complete obstruction of the larynx and trachea. Note the marked distention and increased echogenicity of the lungs, with inverted diaphragms *(arrows)*.

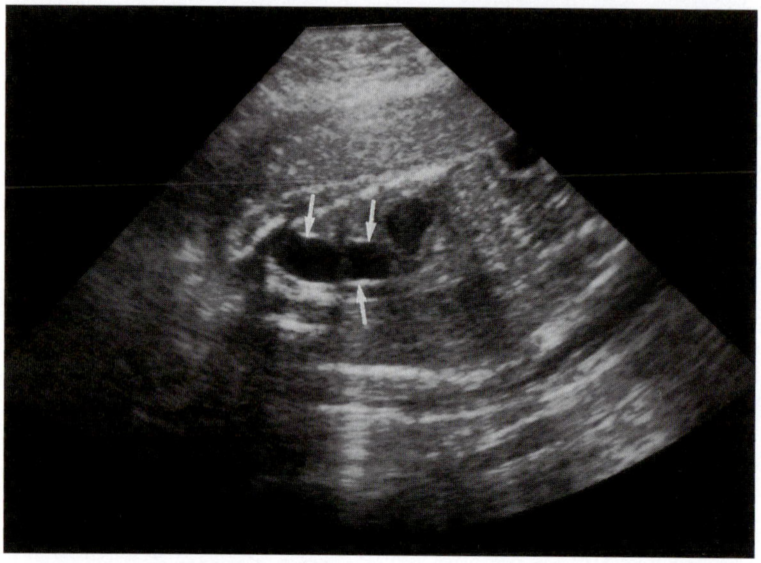

FIGURE 1-61 Esophageal duplication cyst. Longitudinal view of the fetal chest and abdomen reveals a tubular cystic mass *(arrows)* in the posterior aspect of the chest. Initially, the appearance of the mass suggested the possibility of an adenomatoid cystic malformation; however, it was found to be an esophageal duplication cyst at surgery.

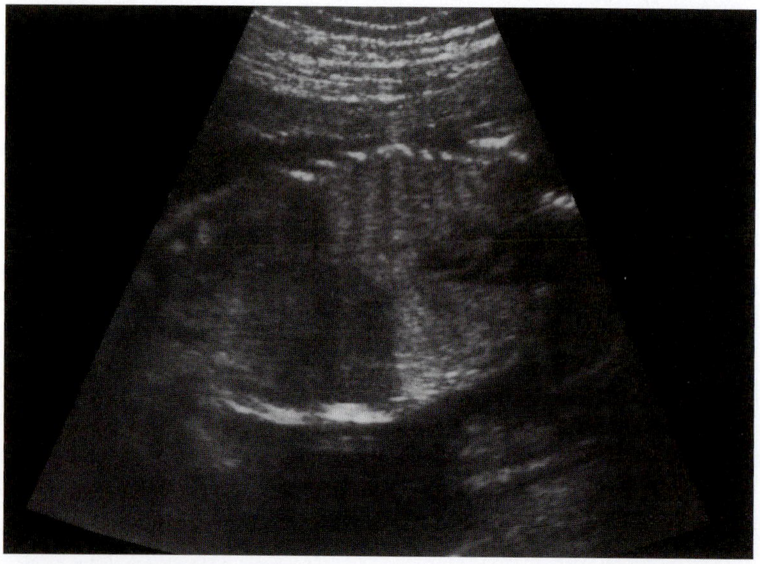

FIGURE 1-62 Tracheal stenosis. Longitudinal view of the chest of a third-trimester fetus shows mild distention of the lungs and hyperechogenicity. This neonate was diagnosed as having tracheal stenosis, which was repaired after birth.

INTRATHORACIC MASS

Bronchial Atresia (Solid or Cystic)

Congenital High Airway Obstruction Syndrome: Group of disorders characterized by complete obstruction of the upper airway, secondary to either laryngeal or glottic atresia and leading to massive enlargement of the lungs (see p. 380)

Cystic Adenomatoid Malformation

Cystic Hygroma (Cystic) (see p. 515)

Diaphragmatic Hernia (see differential diagnosis for this condition) (see p. 61)

Fraser Syndrome: Autosomal recessive syndrome featuring cryptothalmas; syndactyly; and genital, renal, and tracheal anomalies (see p. 160)

Fryns Syndrome: Autosomal recessive condition characterized by diaphragmatic defects, digital and facial abnormalities, and brain anomalies (see p. 325)

Marfan Syndrome: Autosomal dominant connective tissue disorder characterized by tall stature, long limbs, pectus deformities, congenital heart defects, and ocular anomalies (see p. 344)

Neuroblastoma (Cystic or Solid) (see p. 521)

Neurogenic or Bronchogenic Cyst (Cystic)

Sequestration (Solid)

Teratoma (Complex) (see p. 525)

Tracheal or Esophageal Duplication Cyst (Cystic)

CHROMOSOMAL ANOMALIES

Deletion 4p (Wolf-Hirschhorn Syndrome): Abnormality of chromosome 4 characterized by IUGR, facial dysmorphology, cardiac defects, and hypospadias (see p. 459)

Tetrasomy 12p (Pallister-Killian Syndrome): Mosaic aneuploidy characterized by multiple congenital abnormalities of the central nervous system, face, heart, and many other organs (see p. 471)

Trisomy 9: Occurring as a result of an extra chromosome 9, this is a severe abnormality characterized by multiple anomalies of practically all organ systems (see p. 478)

Trisomy 18 (Edwards Syndrome): Occurring as a result of an extra chromosome 18, this is a severe abnormality characterized by IUGR and multiple anomalies of the central nervous system, face, heart, and extremities (see p. 490)

DIAPHRAGMATIC HERNIA

SKELETAL DYSPLASIA

Apert Syndrome: Craniosynostosis, acrocephaly, and syndactyly (occasional) (see p. 304)

Chondrodysplasia Punctata: Heterogeneous group of bone dysplasias characterized by asymmetric limb shortening and abnormal early calcification of the proximal and distal epiphyses (occasional) (see p. 266)

OTHER SYNDROMES AND SEQUENCES

Fryns Syndrome: Autosomal recessive condition characterized by diaphragmatic defects, digital and facial abnormalities, and brain anomalies (see p. 325)

CHROMOSOMAL ABNORMALITIES

Deletion 4p (Wolf-Hirschhorn Syndrome): Abnormality of chromosome 4 characterized by IUGR, facial dysmorphology, cardiac defects, and hypospadias (see p. 459)

Tetrasomy 12p (Pallister-Killian Syndrome): Mosaic aneuploidy characterized by multiple congenital abnormalities of the central nervous system, face, heart, and many other organs (see p. 471)

Trisomy 9: Occurring as a result of an extra chromosome 9, this is a severe abnormality characterized by multiple anomalies of practically all organ systems (see p. 478)

Trisomy 18 (Edwards Syndrome): Occurring as a result of an extra chromosome 18, this is a severe abnormality characterized by IUGR and multiple anomalies of the central nervous system, face, heart, and extremities (see p. 490)

TERATOGEN

Imipramine (see p. 438)

NARROW CHEST

SKELETAL DYSPLASIA

Achondrogenesis: Lethal skeletal dysplasia characterized by extreme hypoplasia of the bones, micromelia, decreased ossification of the bones (particularly those of the skull and spine), and hydrops (see p. 253)

Achondroplasia, Homozygous: Autosomal dominant condition characterized by rhizomelic limb shortening (see p. 257)

Atelosteogenesis, Type I: Lethal skeletal dysplasia characterized by severe limb shortening and deficient ossification of the bones, resulting in micromelic dwarfism (see p. 260)

Camptomelic Dysplasia: Short-limbed skeletal dysplasia characterized by bowing of the long bones, particularly in the lower extremities; bell-shaped, narrow chest; and facial anomalies (see p. 262)

Ellis-van Creveld Syndrome: Autosomal recessive skeletal dysplasia characterized by disproportionately short extremities, narrow chest, polydactyly, and heart defects (see p. 272)

Jeune Thoracic Dystrophy (Asphyxiating Thoracic Dysplasia): Autosomal recessive skeletal dysplasia characterized by very narrow chest with short ribs, moderately short long-bones, and occasional polydactyly (see p. 278)

Majewski Syndrome (Short Rib–Polydactyly Syndrome, Type II): Autosomal recessive skeletal dysplasia characterized by short ribs, narrow thorax, polydactyly, and median facial cleft (see p. 283)

Metatropic Dysplasia: Short-limbed skeletal dysplasia characterized by progressive severe kyphoscoliosis, narrow chest, and metaphyseal flaring (see p. 285)

Osteogenesis Imperfecta: Heterogeneous group of conditions characterized by severe osseous fragility, decreased ossification, and multiple fractures (see p. 345)

Short Rib–Polydactyly Syndrome, Types I and III: Skeletal dysplasias characterized by short ribs, narrow chest, polydactyly, and short limbs (see p. 288)

Thanatophoric Dysplasia, Types I and II: Most common skeletal dysplasia; characterized by narrow chest; short ribs; short, bowed long bones; and flat vertebral bodies (see p. 294)

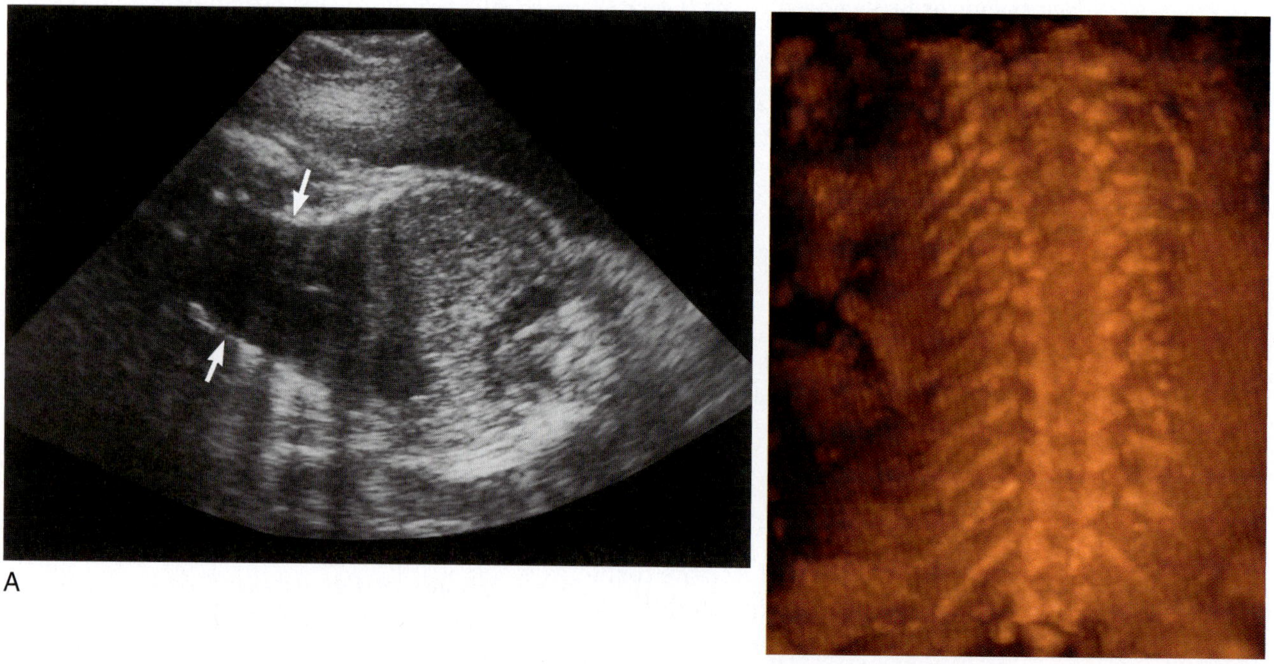

A

B

FIGURE 1-63 (A) Longitudinal view of the chest and abdomen of a fetus with severe skeletal dysplasia and short ribs. The width of the chest *(demarcated by the arrows)* is much smaller than that anticipated for the size of the fetal abdomen directly caudal to it. (B) Three-dimensional surface rendering of the skeleton of a fetus with Lejeune thoracic dystrophy shows the short fetal ribs.

NONSKELETAL DYSPLASIA

Caudal Regression Syndrome/Sirenomelia: Although of different etiologies, these two syndromes are similar; characterized by disruption of the caudal portion of the neural tube, absence or dysplasia of the sacrum, and renal and lower extremity anomalies (see p. 370)

Jarcho-Levin Syndrome (Spondylothoracic Dysplasia): Most common among Puerto Ricans; characterized by vertebral defects, resulting in a very short thorax and spine and a protuberant abdomen (see p. 332)

Multiple Pterygium Syndrome: Autosomal recessive condition characterized by multiple contractures and webbing across the joints, cystic hygromata, and facial defects (see p. 244)

Renal Agenesis and Syndromes Associated with Renal Agenesis (see p. 412)

ABDOMINAL FLUID COLLECTION OR CYST

Anterior Meningocele

Ascites

Bowel Obstruction (see differential diagnosis for this condition) (see p. 70)

Choledochal Cyst

Cloacal Abnormality (see p. 382)

Duplex Collecting System with Obstruction

Enlarged Bladder

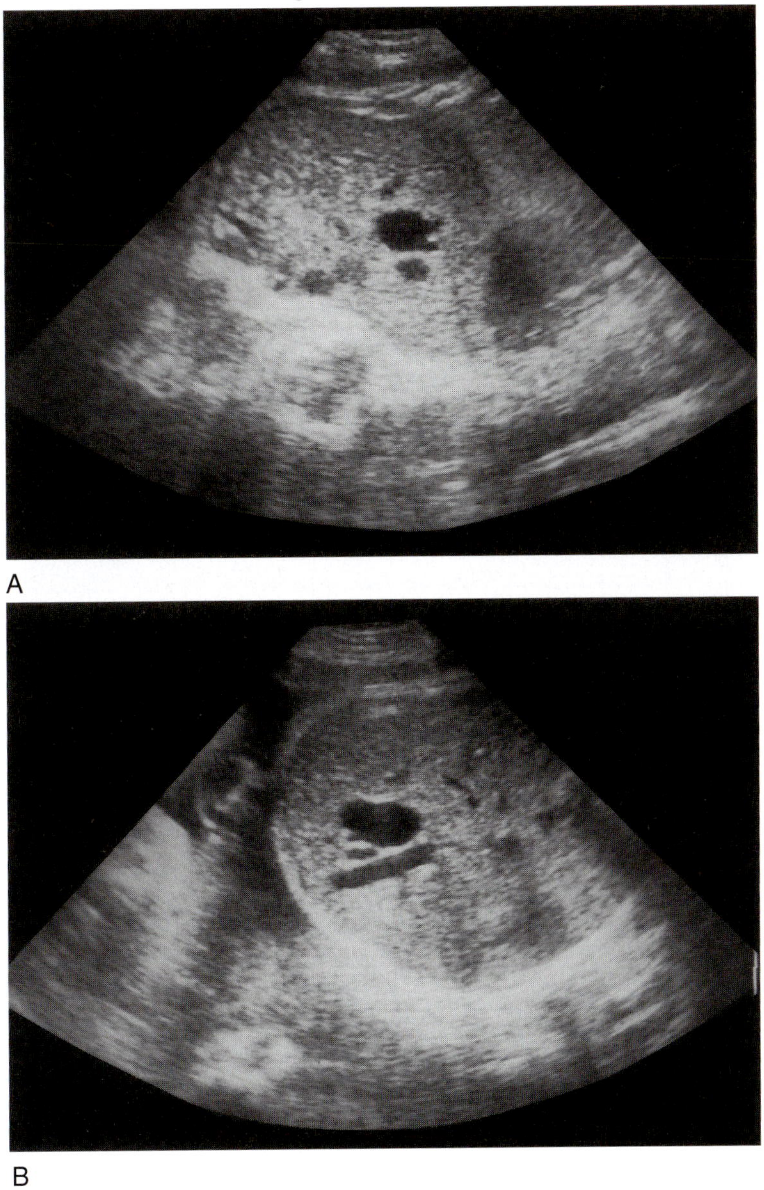

FIGURE 1-64 Longitudinal (A) and transverse (B) views through the fetal abdomen, at the level of the liver, reveal a cyst in the region of the gallbladder. This was diagnosed as a choledochal cyst.

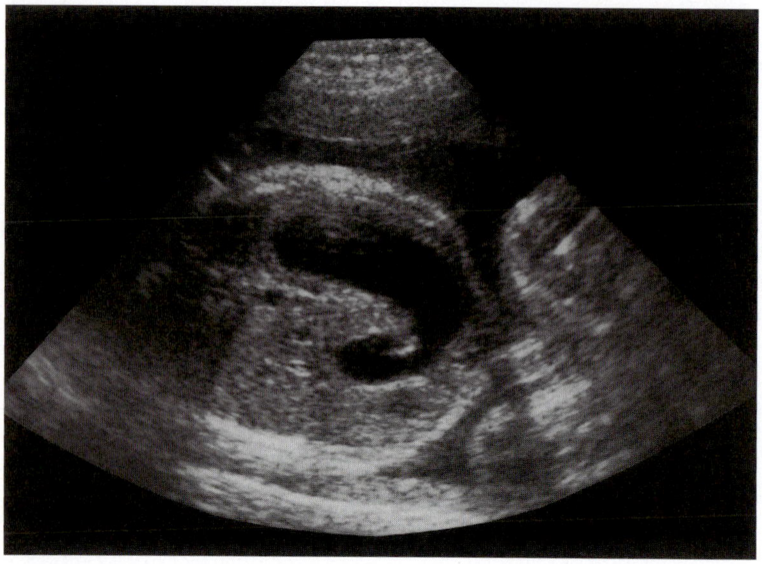

FIGURE 1-65 Duodenal atresia. Transverse view through the fetal abdomen, at the level of the stomach, shows a distended stomach and duodenum, consistent with duodenal atresia.

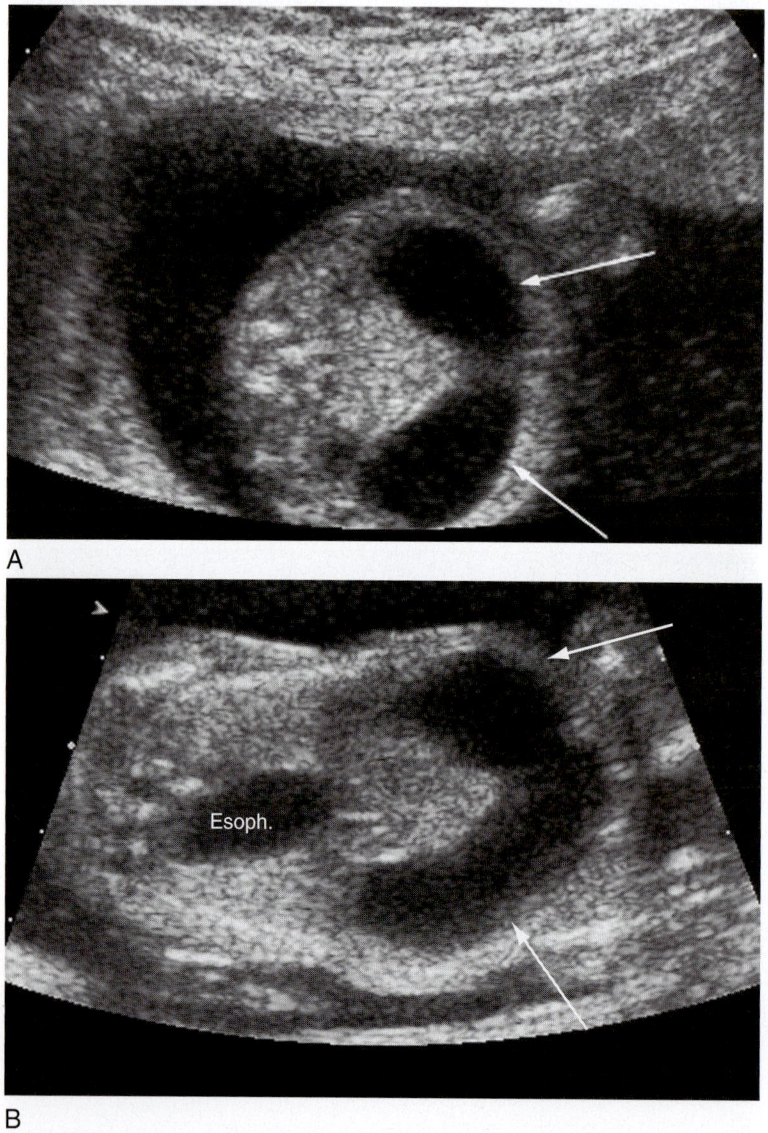

FIGURE 1-66 (A) C-shaped enlargement of the fetal stomach and duodenum *(arrows)*, typical of duodenal atresia with an esophageal atresia. (B) Longitudinal view shows a dilated esophagus *(Esoph.)* and the C-shaped distended stomach *(arrows)*.

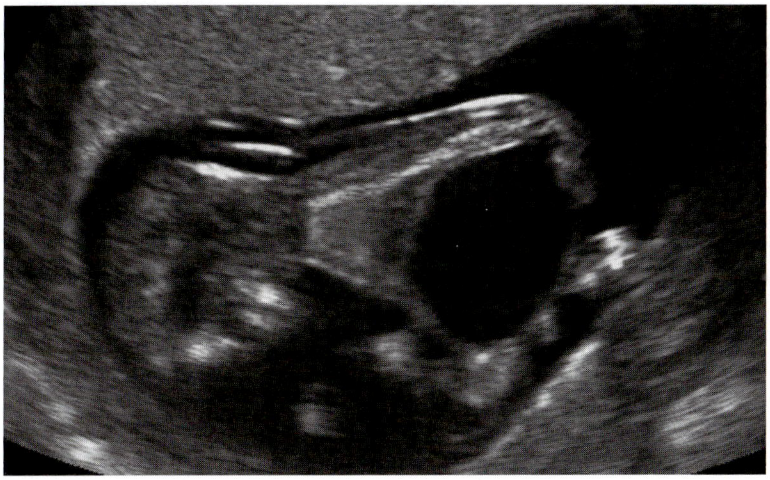

A

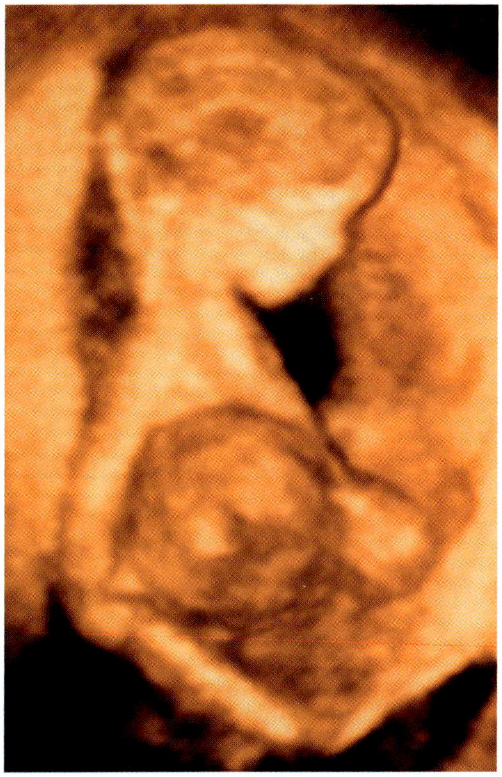

B

FIGURE 1-67 (**A**) Longitudinal view of late first-trimester fetus with complete bladder outlet obstruction resulting from posterior urethral valves. (**B**) Three-dimensional surface rendering of the same fetus shows severe distention of the fetal bladder.

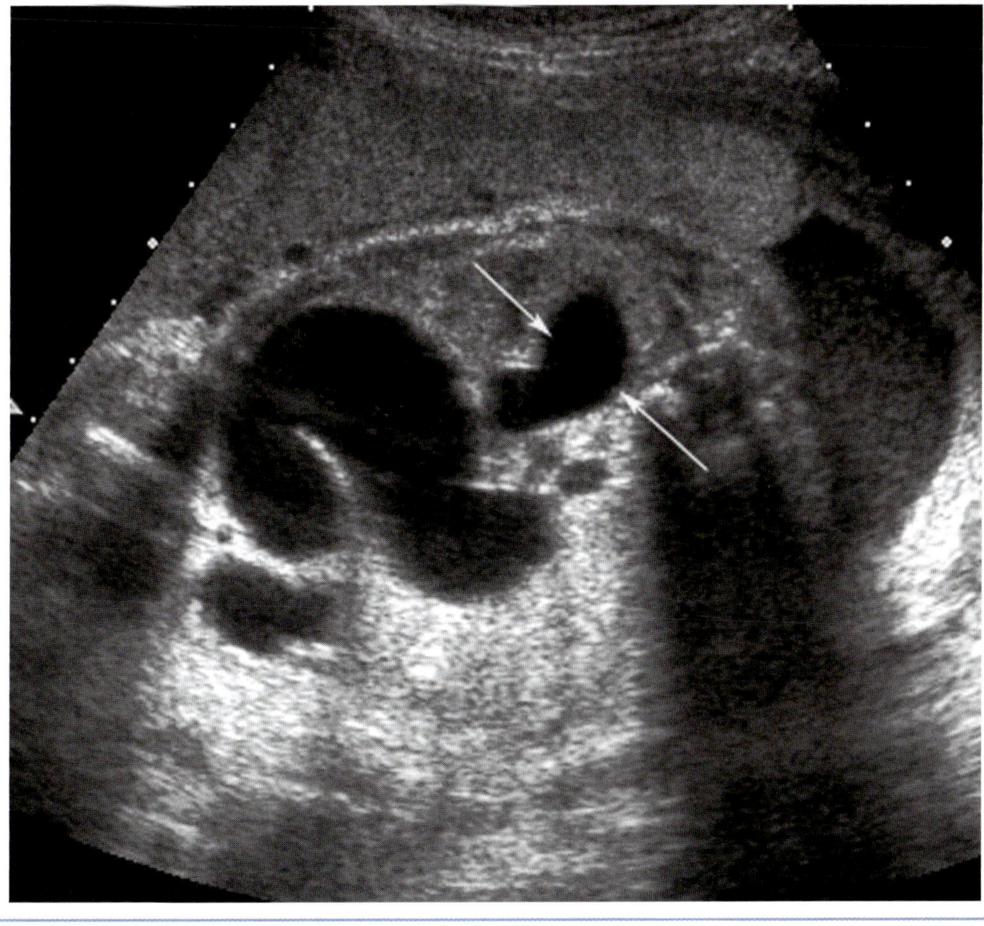

FIGURE 1-68 Third-trimester fetus with duplex collecting system shows dilation of the upper moiety *(arrows)* with a large serpiginous fluid collection denoting a dilated ureter.

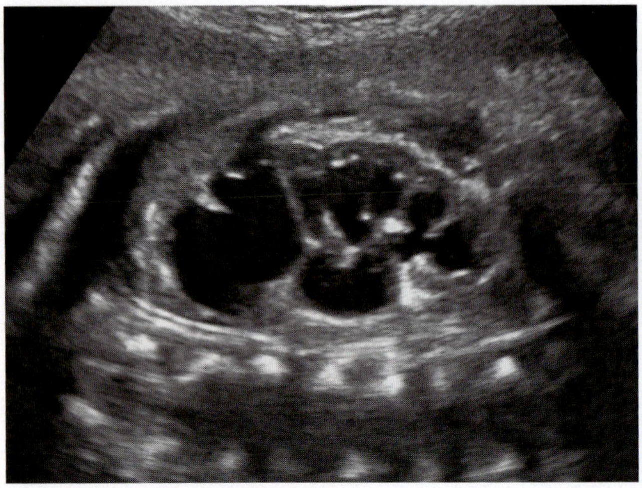

A

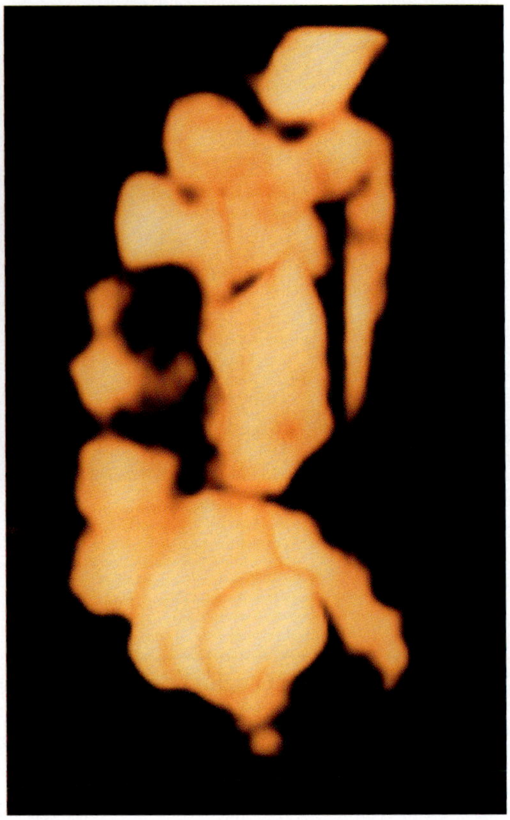

B

FIGURE 1-69 (A) Severely hydronephrotic fetal kidney in the third trimester with a duplex collecting system. (B) Inverse mode of three-dimensional volume data of the same hydronephrotic kidney shows the duplex collecting system with severe dilation.

Enteric Duplication Cyst

Hydrometrocolpos

Hydronephrosis (ureteropelvic junction obstruction or reflux) (see differential diagnosis for this condition) (see p. 75)

Hydroureter

Liver Cyst

Lymphangioma (see p. 515)

Meconium Cyst

Mesenteric Cyst

Multicystic Dysplastic Kidney

Neuroblastoma (see p. 521)

Ovarian Cyst

Perinephric Urinoma

Sacrococcygeal Teratoma

Umbilical Vein Varix

Urachal Cyst

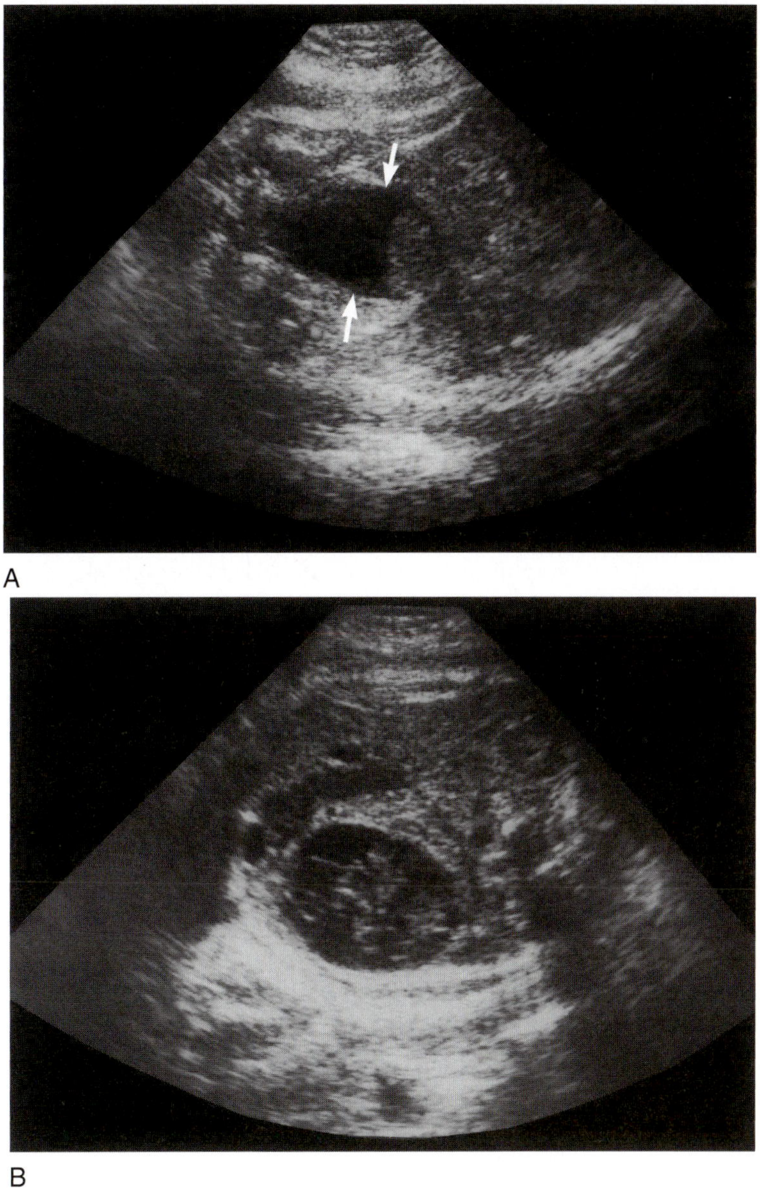

FIGURE 1-70 (A) Hydrometra/hematometra. Coronal view through the lower abdomen of a fetus with a cloacal abnormality. The cystic mass *(arrows)* is a hydrometrocolpos with some debris noted within the mass. (B) Fetal ovarian cyst. Transvaginal, transverse view through the fetal abdomen shows a cyst with internal echoes in a female fetus, consistent with a hemorrhagic ovarian cyst.

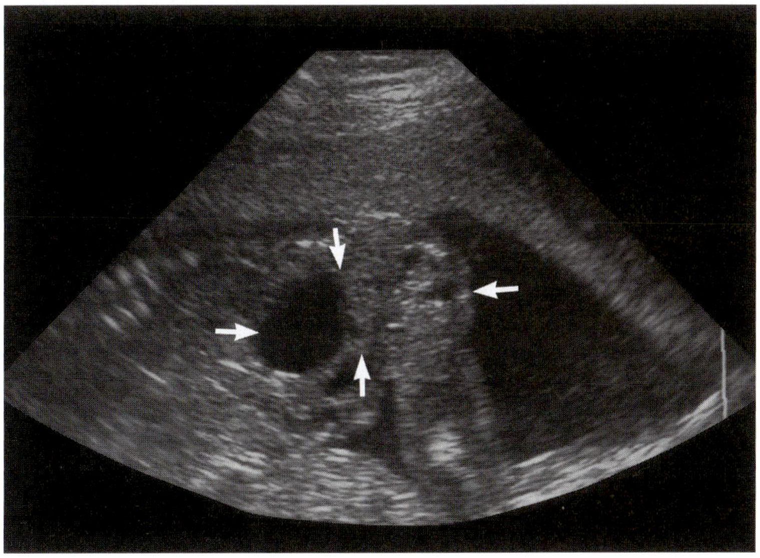

FIGURE 1-71 Sacrococcygeal teratoma. Longitudinal view of the lower abdomen and buttock of a fetus with a type IV sacrococcygeal teratoma *(arrows)*. The large cystic component of the mass is totally intraabdominal. In addition, a solid component extends to the level of the buttock.

HYPERECHOIC BOWEL

Ingestion of Blood by the Fetus

GROWTH ABNORMALITIES

IUGR (onset in early second trimester) (see p. 114)

CHROMOSOMAL ANOMALIES

Trisomy 21: Occurring as a result of an extra chromosome 21, this abnormality is characterized by nuchal fold thickening, short long-bones, abnormal nasal bone, heart defects, and other anomalies. Twenty-five percent of fetuses with Down syndrome do not display any sonographic abnormalities or markers (see p. 496)

OTHER SYNDROMES AND SEQUENCES

Alpha-Thalassemia (see p. 336)

Cystic Fibrosis: Autosomal recessive disorder characterized by chronic respiratory obstruction and infection, exocrine pancreatic insufficiency, and elevated sweat chlorine levels (see p. 322)

TERATOGENS

Cytomegalovirus (see p. 441)

Rubella (occasional) (see p. 449)

Varicella infection (see p. 456)

ECHOGENIC MASS IN ABDOMEN

SOLID OR COMPLEX

Adrenal Hemorrhage

Dermoid or Teratoma (see p. 525)

Dysplastic Kidney

Extralobar Sequestration

Hemangioma of the Liver (see p. 519)

Hemorrhagic Ovarian Cyst

Hepatoblastoma of the Liver

Meconium Cyst

Neuroblastoma (see p. 521)

Renal Mass (Wilms' tumor or hamartoma)

INTRAABDOMINAL CALCIFICATIONS

Adrenal Calcification (adrenal hemorrhage or neuroblastoma)

Gallstones

Idiopathic Arterial Calcification of Infancy: Rare autosomal recessive syndrome characterized by disruption and calcification of the internal elastic laminae of fetal arteries, with calcium

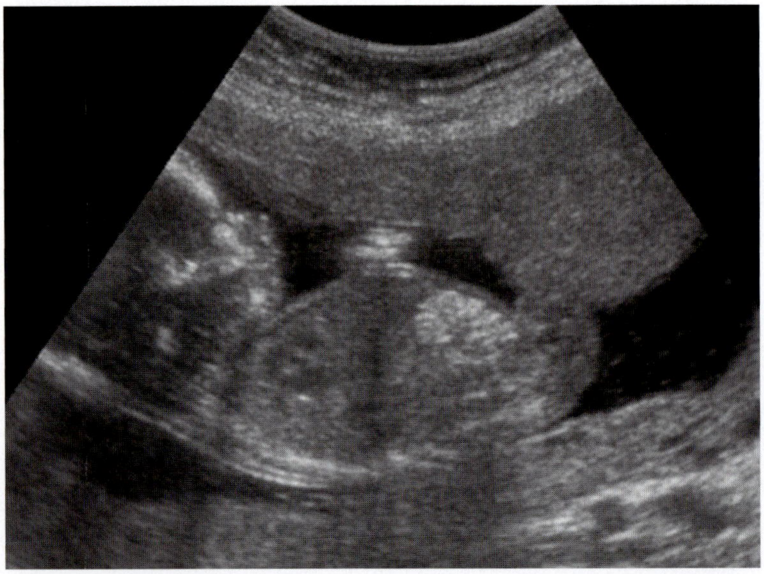

FIGURE 1-72 Longitudinal view of second-trimester fetus with hyperechoic bowel. Note that the echogenicity of the bowel is equal to that of bone.

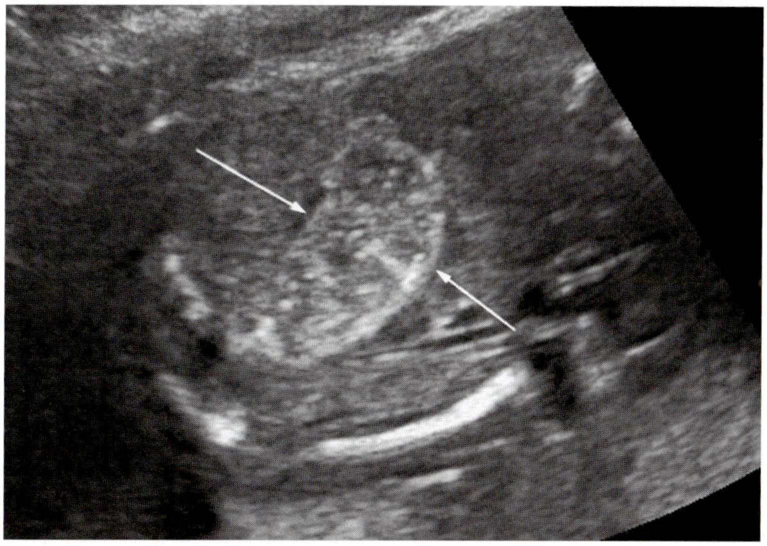

FIGURE 1-73 Second-trimester fetus with an intraabdominal dilated loop of bowel *(arrows)* containing increased echogenicity. Note the punctate calcifications in the lumen of the dilated loop of bowel, consistent with imperforate anus with a rectovesical fistula. The mixture of meconium and urine results in intraluminal calcifications.

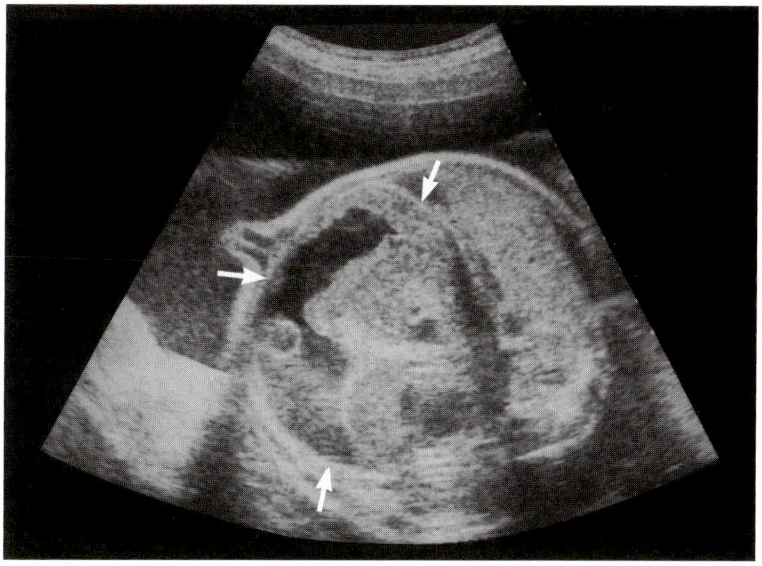

FIGURE 1-74 Intraabdominal teratoma. Transverse view through the fetal abdomen shows a large echogenic mass *(arrows)* that fills the entire intraabdominal cavity. This was found to be a well-differentiated, mature, totally internal, sacrococcygeal teratoma with features of fetus in fetu.

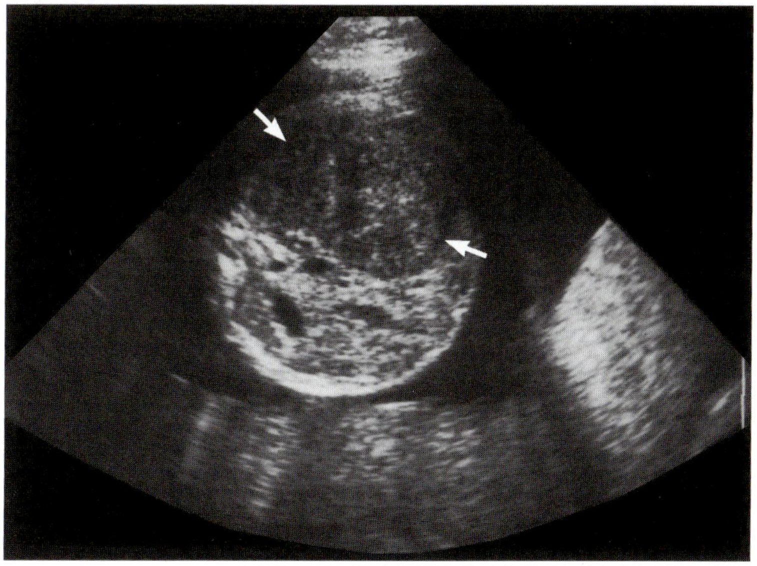

FIGURE 1-75 Transverse view through the fetal upper abdomen shows a solid mass *(arrows)* that was found, at birth, to be a mesoblastic nephroma.

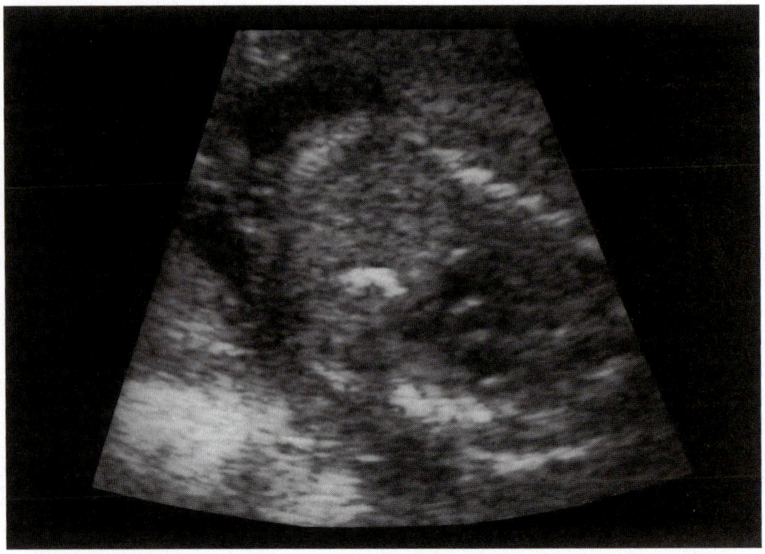

FIGURE 1-76 Liver calcifications. Oblique view through the fetal liver reveals a single, comma-shaped, hepatic calcification that is not associated with any other finding or mass. In most fetuses, this is a benign finding, although occasionally it indicates a TORCH infection.

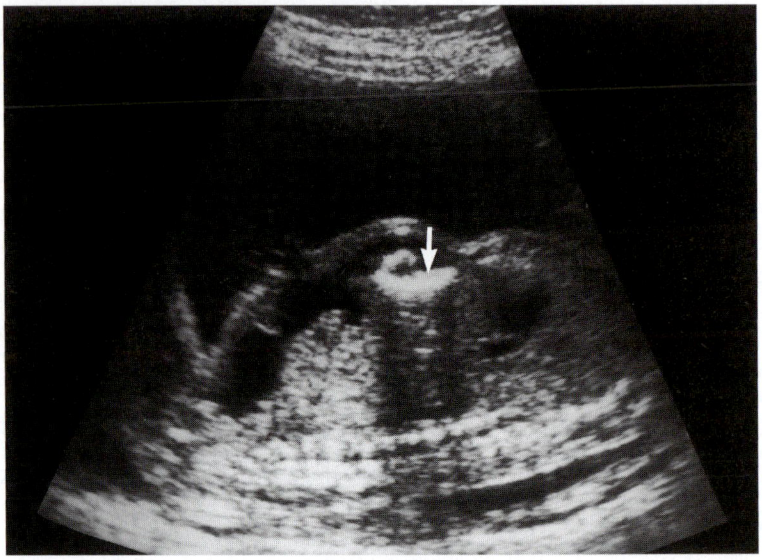

FIGURE 1-77 Meconium peritonitis. Longitudinal view of the abdomen of a fetus with meconium peritonitis reveals a moderate amount of ascites and an area of calcification *(arrow)*.

deposits leading to fibrosis and occlusion of the arteries, hydrops, and death (see p. 391)

Intraluminal Calcifications (imperforate anus with rectovesical fistula)

Isolated Liver Calcifications (normal variants)

Meconium Peritonitis (often associated with ascites)

TORCH Infections (see p. 441)

BOWEL OBSTRUCTION

FACIAL AND BRAIN ABNORMALITIES

Miller-Dieker Syndrome: Lissencephaly, type I; characterized by complete absence of gyri of the brain, microcephaly, and severe mental retardation (duodenal atresia) (see p. 208)

LIMB AND SKELETAL ABNORMALITIES

Fanconi Anemia: Autosomal recessive condition characterized by radial hypoplasia, absent thumbs, and tendency for leukemia (occasional) (see p. 229)

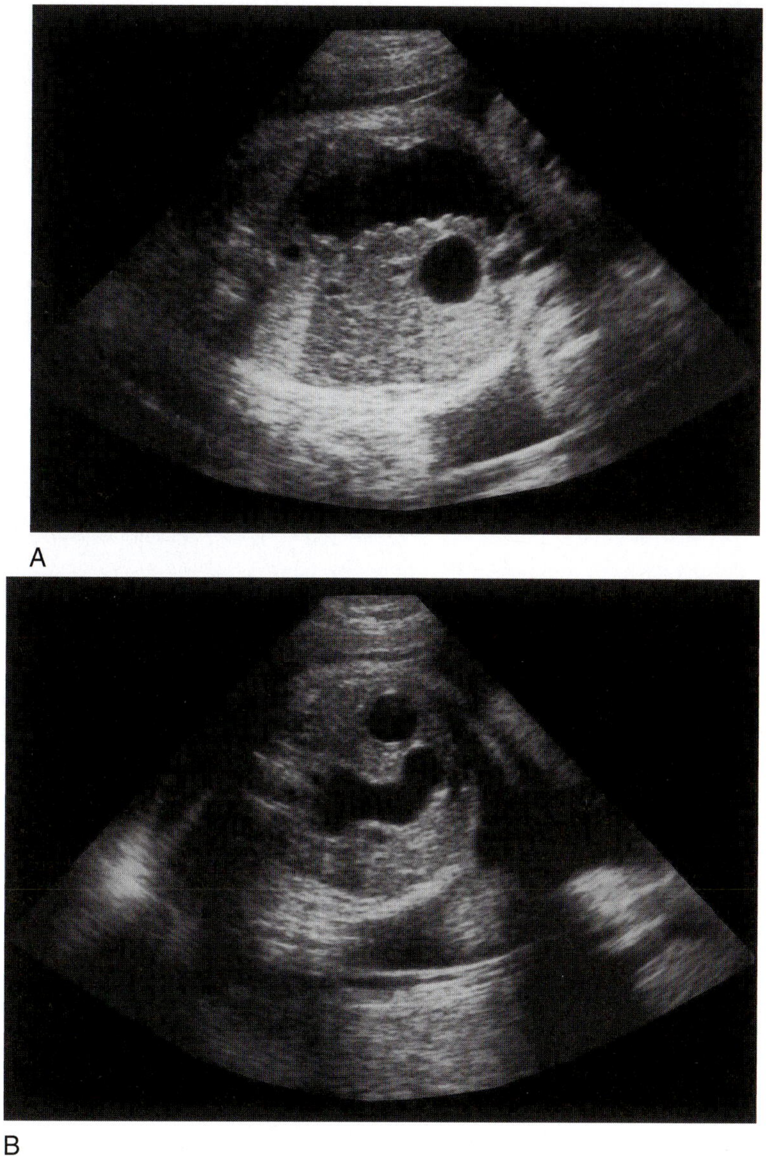

FIGURE 1-78 Transverse and oblique views through the abdomen of a fetus with proximal small bowel obstruction at the level of the duodenum. (A) In the transverse view, the classic double-bubble is seen. (B) In the oblique view, more of the duodenum is identified because of the slightly more distal obstruction.

Short Rib–Polydactyly Syndrome, Types I and III (imperforate anus and bowel atresia) (see p. 288)

CHROMOSOMAL ANOMALIES

Trisomy 21 (Down Syndrome): Occurring as a result of an extra chromosome 21, this abnormality is characterized by nuchal fold thickening, short long-bones, abnormal nasal bone, heart defects, and other anomalies. Twenty-five percent of fetuses with Down syndrome do not display any sonographic abnormalities or markers (duodenal atresia) (see p. 496)

Trisomy 22: Occurring as a result of an extra chromosome 22, this is a lethal abnormality characterized by multiple anomalies of the heart, face, extremities, and gastrointestinal and genitourinary systems (imperforate anus) (see p. 509)

OTHER SYNDROMES AND SEQUENCES

Alpha-Thalassemia (see p. 336)

Anterior Abdominal Wall Defect

Aplasia Cutis Congenita (ACC) (pyloric atresia) (see p. 338)

Bowel Atresia

Caudal Regression Syndrome/Sirenomelia: Although of different etiologies, these two syndromes are similar; characterized by disruption of the caudal portion of the neural tube, absence or dysplasia of the sacrum, and renal and lower extremity anomalies (imperforate anus) (see p. 370)

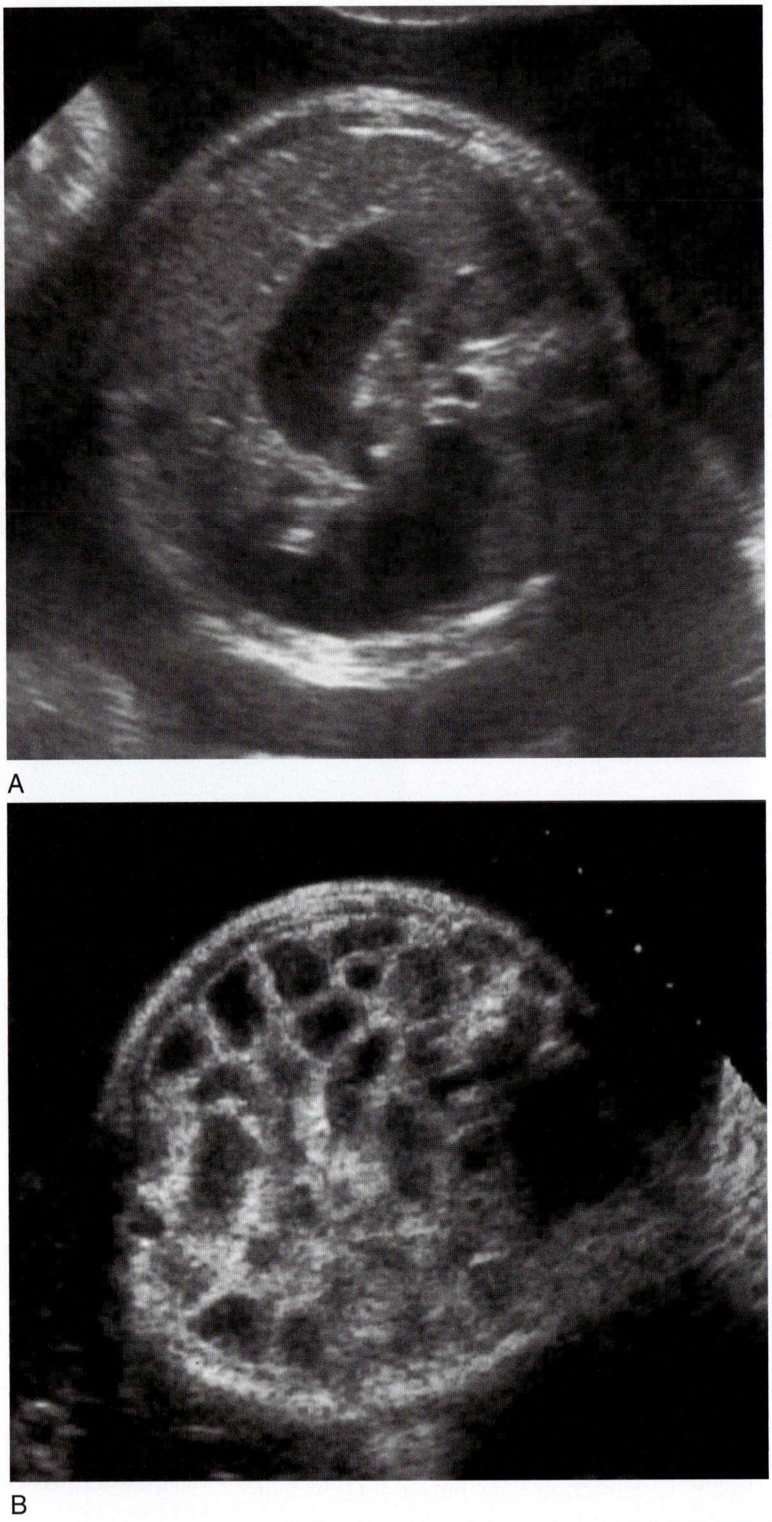

FIGURE 1-79 (A) Third-trimester fetus with duodenal atresia shows a dilated stomach and duodenum adjacent to the fetal liver. (B) Multiple loops of dilated bowel in third-trimester fetus with small bowel obstruction.

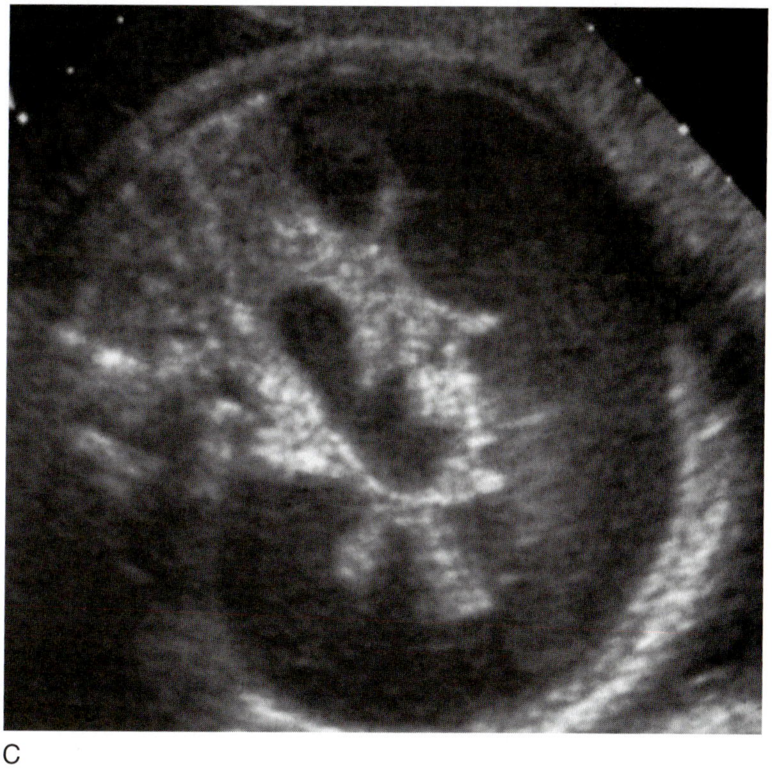

FIGURE 1-79, cont'd (C) Dilated single loop of colon shows typical markings of colonic haustra.

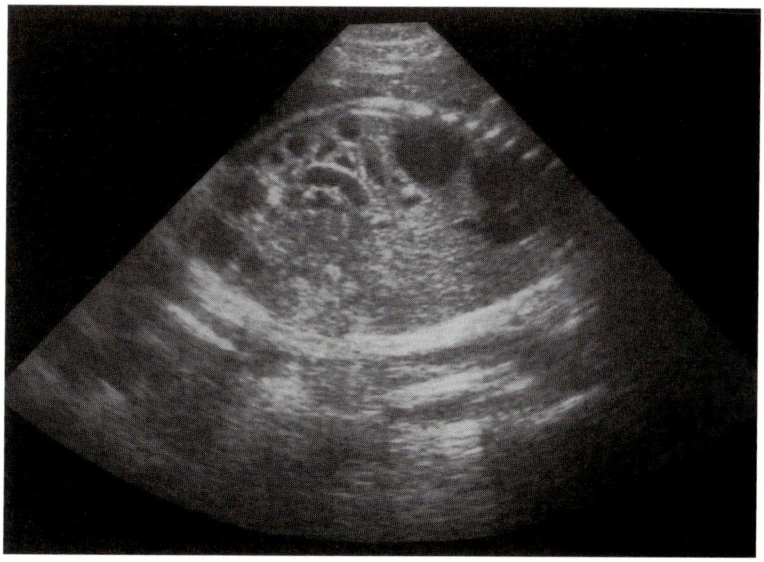

FIGURE 1-80 Longitudinal view of the abdomen of a fetus with cystic fibrosis. Note the multiple, slightly dilated loops of bowel and the dilated stomach secondary to meconium ileus.

CHARGE Association: Coloboma of the iris, **h**eart defect, choanal **a**tresia, intrauterine growth **r**estriction, **g**enital anomalies, and **e**ar anomalies (anal atresia and tracheoesophageal fistula) (see p. 376)

Cystic Fibrosis: Autosomal recessive disorder characterized by chronic obstruction and infection of the respiratory tract, exocrine pancreatic insufficiency, and elevated sweat chlorine levels (small bowel dilation) (see p. 322)

Fryns Syndrome: Autosomal recessive condition characterized by diaphragmatic defects, digital and facial abnormalities, and brain anomalies (malrotation) (see p. 325)

Imperforate Anus (occasional)

Malrotation of Bowel

Renal Agenesis (occasional) (see p. 412)

VATER Association: **V**ertebral defects, **a**nal atresia, **t**racheoesophageal fistula, **e**sophageal atresia, and **r**adial and renal dysplasias (anal atresia) (see p. 429)

Volvulus

TERATOGENS

Chlordiazepoxide (duodenal atresia) (see p. 437)

Clomiphene (esophageal atresia) (see p. 437)

Codeine (pyloric stenosis) (see p. 439)

Fluorouracil (esophageal and duodenal atresias) (see p. 435)

Oral contraceptives (anal and esophageal atresias) (see p. 437)

Syphilis (see p. 450)

Thalidomide (duodenal atresia) (see p. 437)

Trimethadione (esophageal atresia) (see p. 436)

ASCITES

GROWTH ABNORMALITIES

Perlman Syndrome: Autosomal recessive fetal overgrowth syndrome characterized by macrosomia, bilaterally enlarged kidneys, renal tumors, and other visceromegaly associated with polyhydramnios (see p. 147)

FACIAL AND BRAIN ABNORMALITIES

Fraser Syndrome: Autosomal recessive syndrome featuring cryptophthalmos; syndactyly; and genital, renal, and tracheal anomalies (occasional) (see p. 160)

CHROMOSOMAL ABNORMALITIES

Trisomy 21 (Down Syndrome): Occurring as a result of an extra chromosome 21, this abnormality is characterized by nuchal fold thickening, short long-bones, abnormal nasal bone, heart defects, and other anomalies. Twenty-five percent of fetuses with Down syndrome do not display any sonographic abnormalities or markers (see p. 496)

XO Syndrome (Turner Syndrome): Occurring as a result of a single X chromosome (XO), Turner syndrome is characterized primarily in early pregnancy by large cystic hygromata, lymphangiectasia, and heart defects. Affected infants who survive gestation may represent Turner mosaic individuals (see p. 510)

OTHER SYNDROMES AND SEQUENCES

Alpha-Thalassemia (see p. 336)

Cloacal Exstrophy Sequence: Complex disorder characterized by a combination of defects that include omphalocele, imperforate anus, cloacal exstrophy, spinal defects, and genital abnormalities (occasional) (see p. 382)

Congenital High Airway Obstruction Syndrome: Group of disorders characterized by

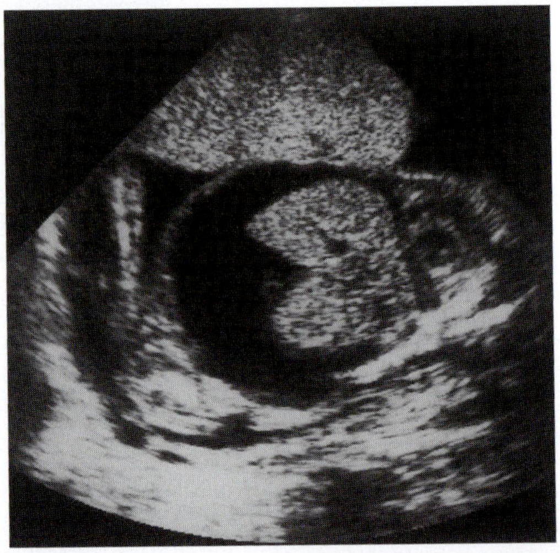

FIGURE 1-81 Longitudinal view of the abdomen of a fetus with ascites. This fetus did not have any evidence of skin edema or pleural effusions.

complete obstruction of the upper airway, secondary to either laryngeal or glottic atresia and leading to massive enlargement of the lungs (see p. 380)

Early Hydrops (see differential diagnosis for this condition) (see p. 111)

Meconium Peritonitis

Urinary Ascites Secondary to Genitourinary Obstruction

TERATOGENS

Cytomegalovirus (CMV) (see p. 441)

Parvovirus (see p. 446)

Syphilis (see p. 450)

Toxoplasmosis (see p. 452)

ABSENT STOMACH

Diaphragmatic Hernia

Normal Variant (warrants a repeat scan)

CHROMOSOMAL ANOMALIES

Deletion 4p (Wolf-Hirschhorn Syndrome): Abnormality of chromosome 4 characterized by IUGR, facial dysmorphology, cardiac defects, and hypospadias (diaphragmatic hernia) (see p. 459)

Tetrasomy 12p (Pallister-Killian Syndrome): Mosaic aneuploidy characterized by multiple congenital abnormalities of the central nervous system, face, heart, and many other organs (diaphragmatic hernia) (see p. 471)

Trisomy 9: Occurring as a result of an extra chromosome 9, this is a severe abnormality characterized by multiple anomalies of practically all organ systems (diaphragmatic hernia) (see p. 478)

Trisomy 18 (Edwards Syndrome): Occurring as a result of an extra chromosome 18, this is a severe abnormality characterized by IUGR and multiple anomalies of the central nervous system, face, heart, and extremities (tracheoesophageal fistula) (see p. 490)

OTHER SYNDROMES AND SEQUENCES

CHARGE Association: **C**oloboma of the iris, **h**eart defect, choanal **a**tresia, intrauterine growth **r**estriction, **g**enital anomalies, and **e**ar anomalies (tracheoesophageal fistula) (see p. 376)

CNS Anomalies Causing Inability to Swallow

Facial Anomalies, Such as Masses and Clefts, Causing Inability to Swallow

Fryns Syndrome: Autosomal recessive condition characterized by diaphragmatic defects, digital and facial abnormalities, and brain anomalies (diaphragmatic hernia) (see p. 325)

Marfan Syndrome: Autosomal dominant connective tissue disorder characterized by tall stature, long limbs, pectus deformities, congenital heart defects, and ocular anomalies (occasional diaphragmatic hernia) (see p. 344)

Renal Agenesis (Oligohydramnios) (see p. 412)

VATER Association: **V**ertebral defects, **a**nal atresia, **t**racheoesophageal fistula, **e**sophageal atresia, and **r**adial and renal dysplasias (tracheoesophageal fistula) (see p. 429)

HYDRONEPHROSIS

Duplex Collecting System

Ectopic Ureterocele

Intraabdominal Mass

Megacystis/Megaureter Posterior Urethral Valves

Ureteropelvic Junction Obstruction

Vesicoureteral Reflux (for specific syndrome, see differential diagnosis of syndromes associated with various renal anomalies) (see p. 79)

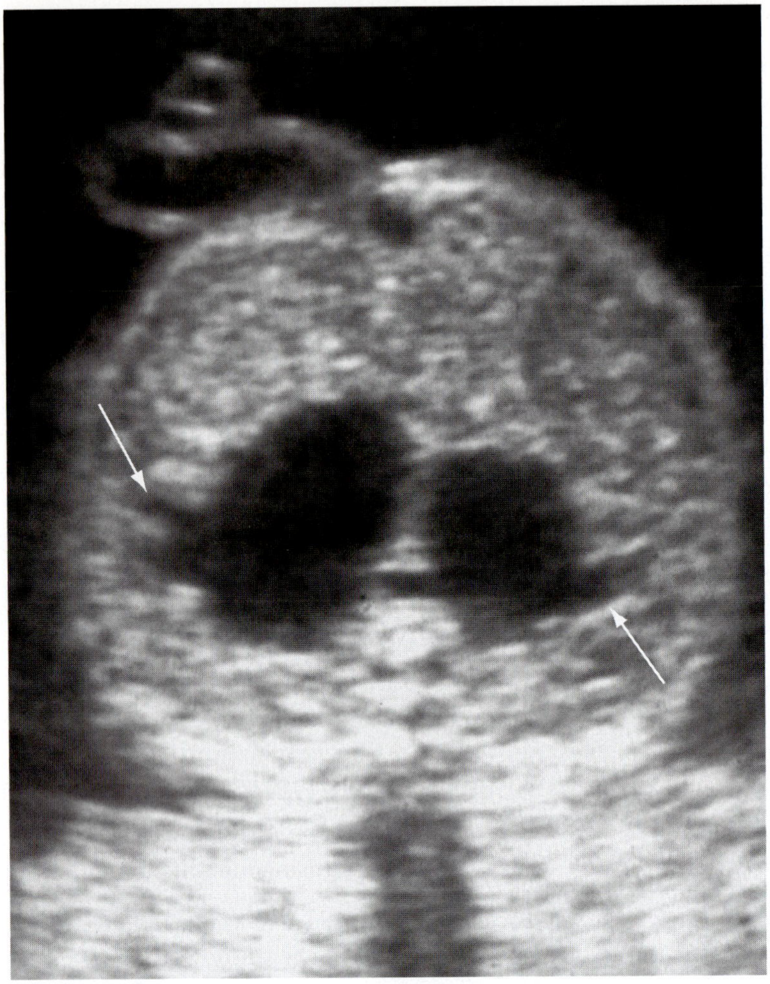

FIGURE 1-82 Early second-trimester fetus with severe bilateral hydronephrosis. Note bilateral caliectasis *(arrows)* and severe pyelectasis.

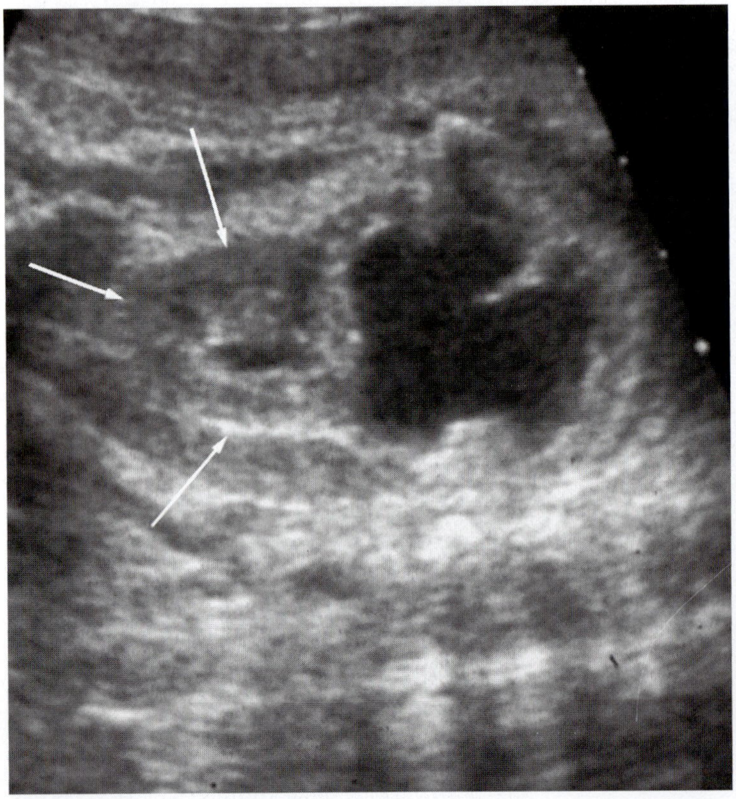

A

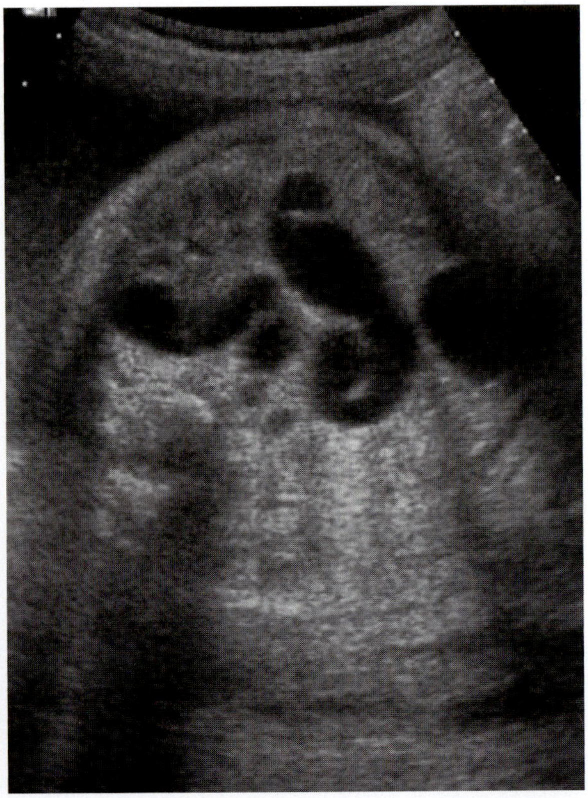

B

FIGURE 1-83 (**A**) Third-trimester fetus with hydronephrosis of the upper pole of a duplex collecting system. Arrows show the normal lower pole. (**B**) Multiple dilated loops of ureter in a third-trimester fetus with a duplex collecting system and dilation of both ureters.

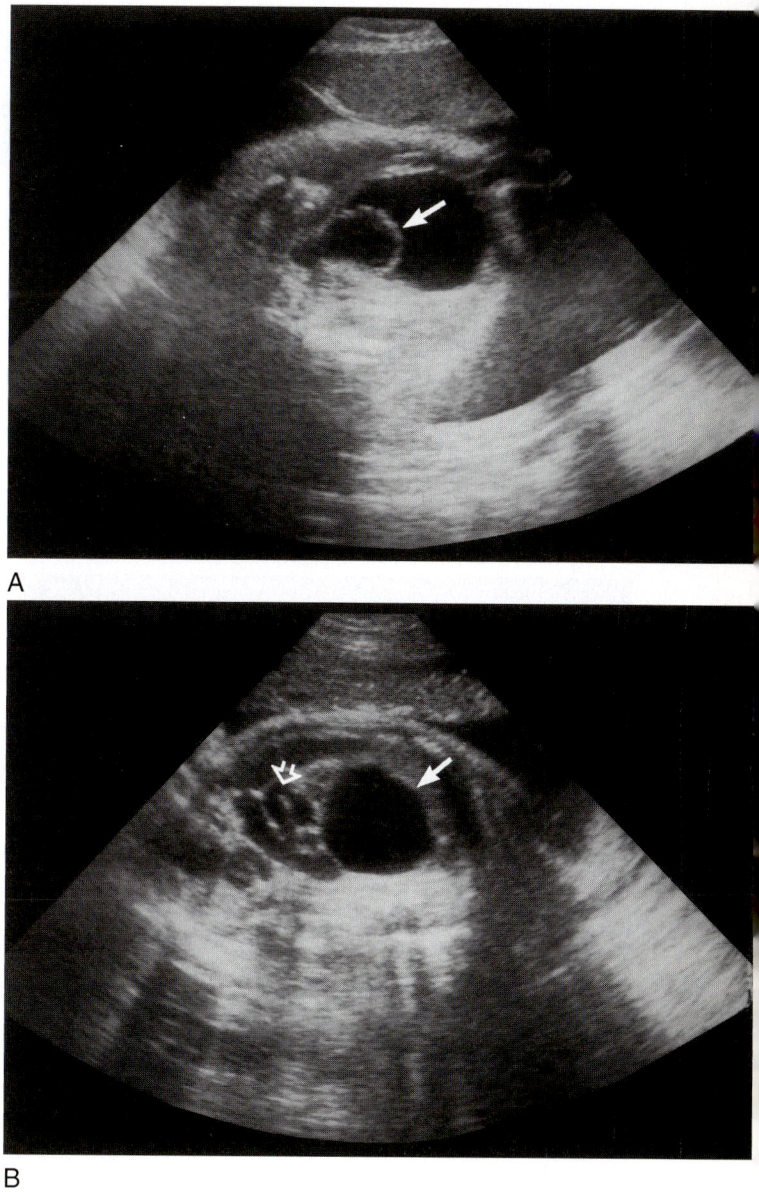

FIGURE 1-84 Longitudinal views of the fetal bladder and kidney showing (A) a ureterocele in the bladder *(arrow)* and (B) an obstructed, upper-pole moiety of a duplex collecting system *(solid arrow)* with a dilated ureter *(open arrow)*.

RENAL AGENESIS (Unilateral or Bilateral)

GROWTH ABNORMALITIES

Diabetic Embryopathy

Smith-Lemli-Opitz Syndrome: Autosomal recessive syndrome featuring microcephaly, mental retardation, and genital and renal anomalies (see p. 140)

FACIAL AND BRAIN ABNORMALITIES

Branchio-Oculo-Facial Syndrome: Autosomal dominant disorder characterized by mental retardation, growth deficiency, ocular defects, and clefting of the upper lip (occasional) (see p. 149)

Fraser Syndrome: Autosomal recessive syndrome featuring cryptophthalmos; syndactyly; and genital, renal, and tracheal anomalies (see p. 160)

Goldenhar Syndrome: Asymmetry of the face and ears in conjunction with vertebral anomalies of the upper spine (occasional) (see p. 162)

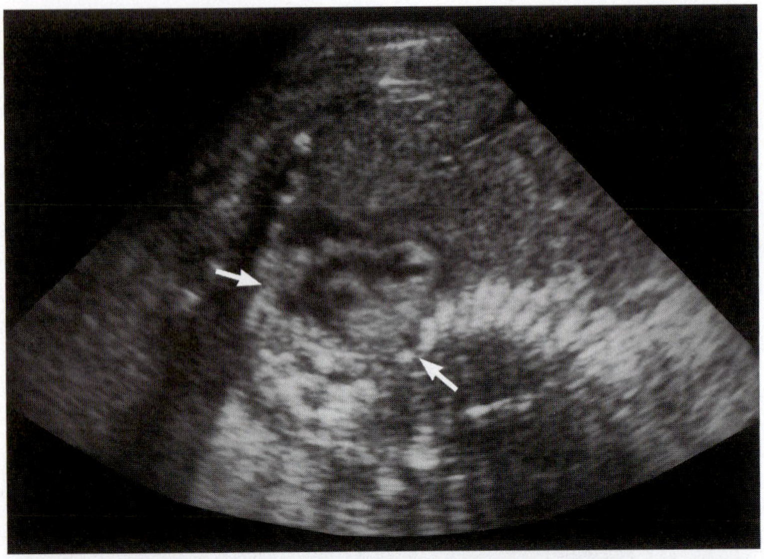

FIGURE 1-85 Longitudinal view of the chest of a fetus with renal agenesis in the second trimester. Note the complete absence of amniotic fluid. The chest *(arrows)* is extremely narrow, with space only for the heart. The lungs are not identified and probably are already hypoplastic.

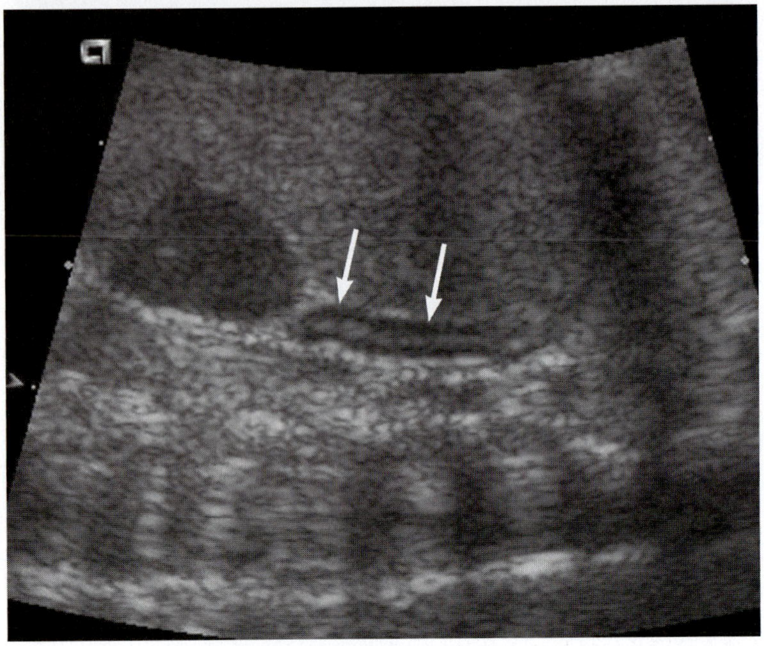

FIGURE 1-86 Absence of the fetal kidney demonstrated by the lying-down adrenal sign (arrows indicate adrenal).

LIMB AND SKELETAL ABNORMALITIES

Ectrodactyly–Ectodermal Dysplasia–Clefting (EEC) Syndrome: Autosomal dominant condition characterized by labial clefting, ectrodactyly (lobster-claw deformities of the limbs), and genitourinary tract anomalies (see p. 225)

Ellis-van Creveld Syndrome: Autosomal recessive skeletal dysplasia characterized by disproportionately short extremities, narrow chest, polydactyly, and heart defects (occasional) (see p. 272)

Short Rib–Polydactyly Syndrome, Types I and III: Skeletal dysplasias characterized by short ribs, narrow chest, polydactyly, and short limbs (see p. 288)

OTHER SYNDROMES AND SEQUENCES

Caudal Regression Syndrome/Sirenomelia: Although of different etiologies, these two syndromes are similar; characterized by disruption of the caudal portion of the neural tube, absence or dysplasia of the sacrum, and renal and lower extremity anomalies (see p. 370)

MURCS Association: Müllerian duct aplasia, **r**enal aplasia, **c**ervicothoracic **s**omite dysplasia (see p. 398)

Renal Agenesis (unilateral or bilateral) (see p. 412)

VATER Association: Vertebral defects, **a**nal atresia, **t**racheoesophageal fistula, **e**sophageal atresia, and **r**adial and renal dysplasias (see p. 429)

SYNDROMES ASSOCIATED WITH VARIOUS RENAL ANOMALIES

GROWTH ABNORMALITIES

Smith-Lemli-Opitz Syndrome: Autosomal recessive syndrome featuring microcephaly, mental retardation, and genital and renal anomalies (see p. 140)

FACIAL AND BRAIN ABNORMALITIES

Cerebrocostomandibular Syndrome: Autosomal recessive condition characterized by severe micrognathia, cleft palate, and vertebral body abnormalities associated with defective costal development (occasional) (see p. 152)

Fraser Syndrome: Autosomal recessive syndrome featuring cryptophthalmos; syndactyly; and genital, renal, and tracheal anomalies (see p. 160)

Goldenhar Syndrome: Asymmetry of the face and ears in conjunction with vertebral anomalies of the upper spine (occasional) (see p. 162)

Joubert Syndrome: Autosomal recessive syndrome characterized by dysmorphic facial features and agenesis of the cerebellar vermis (see p. 197)

Meckel-Gruber Syndrome: Autosomal recessive condition characterized by posterior encephalocele, postaxial polydactyly, and polycystic kidneys (see p. 199)

Miller-Dieker Syndrome: Lissencephaly, type I; characterized by complete absence of gyri of the brain, microcephaly, and severe mental retardation (see p. 208)

LIMB AND SKELETAL ABNORMALITIES

Camptomelic Dysplasia: Short-limbed skeletal dysplasia characterized by bowing of the long bones, particularly in the lower extremities; bell-shaped, narrow chest; and facial anomalies (occasional) (see p. 262)

Ectrodactyly–Ectodermal Dysplasia–Clefting (EEC) Syndrome: Autosomal dominant condition characterized by labial clefting, ectrodactyly (lobster-claw deformities of the limbs), and genitourinary tract anomalies (see p. 225)

Fanconi Anemia: Autosomal recessive condition characterized by radial hypoplasia, absent thumbs, and tendency for leukemia (see p. 229)

Femoral Hypoplasia–Unusual Facies Syndrome: Syndrome characterized by short lower limbs, especially hypoplastic femurs, and facial abnormalities; may be part of a spectrum of abnormalities that includes caudal regression syndrome (see p. 231)

Majewski Syndrome (Short Rib–Polydactyly Syndrome, Type II): Autosomal recessive

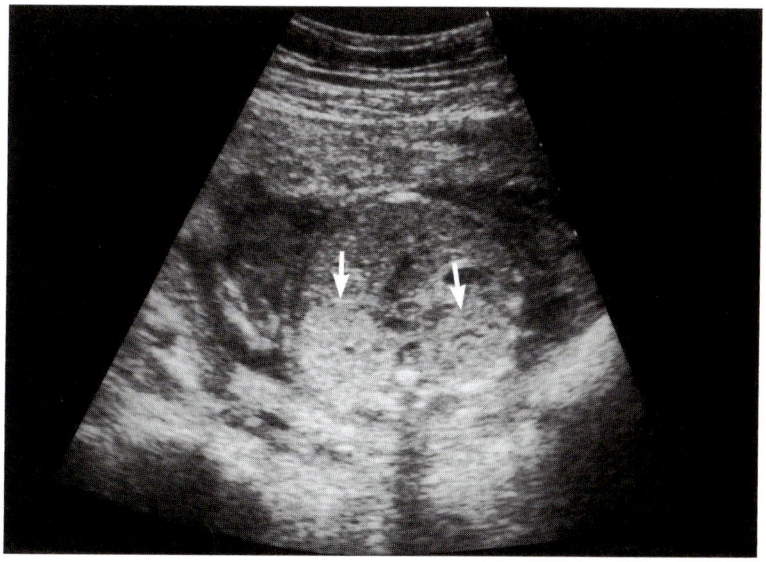

FIGURE 1-87 Transverse view through the abdomen of a fetus with bilateral, large, echogenic kidneys *(arrows)*. This fetus also had polydactyly, indicating Meckel-Gruber syndrome.

skeletal dysplasia characterized by short ribs, narrow thorax, polydactyly, and median facial cleft (occasional) (see p. 283)

Multiple Pterygium Syndrome: Autosomal recessive condition characterized by multiple contractures and webbing across the joints, cystic hygromata, and facial defects (occasional) (see p. 244)

Roberts Syndrome: Autosomal recessive condition characterized by severe shortening of the limbs (pseudothalidomide syndrome) and facial anomalies (occasional) (see p. 247)

Short Rib–Polydactyly Syndrome, Types I and III: Skeletal dysplasias characterized by short ribs, narrow chest, polydactyly, and short limbs (see p. 288)

Thanatophoric Dysplasia: Most common skeletal dysplasia; characterized by narrow chest; short ribs; short, bowed long bones; and flat vertebral bodies (see p. 294)

Thrombocytopenia–Absent Radius (TAR) Syndrome: Autosomal recessive syndrome characterized by radial aplasia and thrombocytopenia (occasional) (see p. 251)

CRANIOSYNOSTOSIS

Antley-Bixler Syndrome: Disorder characterized by craniosynostosis, resulting in severe brachycephaly, midfacial hypoplasia, multiple skeletal fusions, and contractures (occasional) (see p. 303)

Apert Syndrome: Craniosynostosis, acrocephaly, and syndactyly (occasional) (see p. 304)

CHROMOSOMAL ANOMALIES

Deletion 4p (Wolf-Hirschhorn Syndrome): Abnormality of chromosome 4 characterized by IUGR, facial dysmorphology, cardiac defects, and hypospadias (occasional) (see p. 459)

Deletion 11q (Jacobsen Syndrome): Deletion of the distal long arm of chromosome 11 characterized by multiple anomalies of practically all organ systems (occasional) (see p. 464)

Tetrasomy 12p (Pallister-Killian Syndrome): Mosaic aneuploidy characterized by multiple congenital abnormalities of the central nervous system, face, heart, and many other organs (see p. 471)

Triploidy: Occurring as a result of a complete extra set of chromosomes, this is a lethal abnormality characterized by severe early-onset IUGR and multiple anomalies of practically all organ systems (see p. 473)

Trisomy 9: Occurring as a result of an extra chromosome 9, this is a severe abnormality characterized by multiple anomalies of practically all organ systems (see p. 478)

Trisomy 13 (Patau Syndrome): Occurring as a result of an extra chromosome 13, this is a severe abnormality characterized by multiple anomalies of the central nervous system, face, heart, and extremities (see p. 483)

Trisomy 18 (Edwards Syndrome): Occurring as a result of an extra chromosome 18, this is a severe abnormality characterized by IUGR and multiple anomalies of the central nervous system, face, heart, and extremities (see p. 490)

Trisomy 21 (Down Syndrome): Occurring as a result of an extra chromosome 21, this abnormality is characterized by nuchal fold thickening, short long-bones, abnormal nasal bone, heart defects, and other anomalies. Twenty-five percent of fetuses with Down syndrome do not display any sonographic abnormalities or markers (see p. 496)

Trisomy 22: Occurring as a result of an extra chromosome 22, this is a lethal abnormality characterized by multiple anomalies of the heart, face, and extremities, gastrointestinal and genitourinary systems (see p. 509)

XO Syndrome (Turner Syndrome): Occurring as a result of a single X chromosome (XO), Turner syndrome is characterized primarily in early pregnancy by large cystic hygromata and lymphangiectasia, and heart defects. Affected infants who survive gestation may represent Turner mosaic individuals (see p. 510)

OTHER SYNDROMES AND SEQUENCES

Arthrogryposis: Sequence of neurologic, muscular, and connective tissue disorders leading to fetal joint contractures and rigidity, as well as decreased activity (occasional) (see p. 362)

Cardiosplenic Syndromes (Asplenia/Polysplenia): Defects in the lateralization of normal body asymmetry, including severe heart defects and anomalies of the intrathoracic and intraabdominal viscera (see p. 365)

Caudal Regression Syndrome/Sirenomelia: Although of different etiologies, these two syndromes are similar; characterized by disruption of the caudal portion of the neural tube, absence or dysplasia of the sacrum, and renal and lower extremity anomalies (see p. 370)

CHARGE Association: **C**oloboma of the iris, **h**eart defect, choanal **a**tresia, intrauterine growth **r**estriction, **g**enital anomalies, and **e**ar anomalies (occasional) (see p. 376)

Cloacal Exstrophy Sequence: Complex disorder characterized by a combination of defects that include omphalocele, imperforate anus, cloacal exstrophy, spinal defects, and genital abnormalities (occasional) (see p. 382)

Fryns Syndrome: Autosomal recessive condition characterized by diaphragmatic defects, digital and facial abnormalities, and brain anomalies (see p. 325)

Jarcho-Levin Syndrome (Spondylothoracic Dysplasia): Disorder occurring most commonly among Puerto Ricans; characterized by vertebral defects resulting in very short thorax and spine and protuberant abdomen (occasional) (see p. 332)

Klippel-Feil Syndrome: Abnormal cervical vertebrae, webbed neck, facial asymmetry (occasional) (see p. 394)

Megacystis–Microcolon–Intestinal Hypoperistalsis Syndrome: Autosomal recessive lethal condition caused by decreased muscle tone in the intestinal and urinary tracts, resulting in a markedly dilated urinary bladder and hypoperistalsis of the colon (see p. 396)

MURCS Association: **M**üllerian duct aplasia, **r**enal aplasia, **c**ervicothoracic **s**omite dysplasia (see p. 398)

Opitz Syndrome: Disorder characterized by ocular hypertelorism, micrognathia, and, in males, hypospadias (occasional) (see p. 399)

Proteus Syndrome: Asymmetric focal overgrowth, subcutaneous tumors, and hemihypertrophy (occasional) (see p. 352)

Prune-Belly Syndrome: Triad of abdominal wall distention, urinary tract obstruction, and cryptorchidism (see p. 408)

Renal Agenesis (Potter Syndrome) (see p. 412)

VATER Association: **V**ertebral defects, **a**nal atresia, **t**racheoesophageal fistula, **e**sophageal atresia, and **r**adial and renal dysplasias (see p. 429)

TERATOGENS

Cocaine (see p. 439)

Hydantoin (occasional) (see p. 436)

Imipramine (see p. 438)

Valproic acid (see p. 436)

ABSENT BLADDER

FACIAL AND BRAIN ABNORMALITIES

Meckel-Gruber Syndrome: Autosomal recessive condition characterized by posterior encephalocele, postaxial polydactyly, and polycystic kidneys (bilateral cystic kidneys) (see p. 199)

OTHER SYNDROMES AND SEQUENCES

Bilateral Cystic Dysplasia, Such as Multicystic Dysplastic Kidneys

Bladder Exstrophy (see p. 382)

Caudal Regression Syndrome/Sirenomelia: Although of different etiologies, these two syndromes are similar; characterized by disruption of the caudal portion of the neural tube, absence or dysplasia of the sacrum, and renal and lower extremity anomalies (see p. 370)

Cloacal Exstrophy Sequence: Complex disorder characterized by a combination of defects that include omphalocele, imperforate anus, cloacal exstrophy, spinal defects, and genital abnormalities (see p. 382)

Infantile Polycystic Kidney Disease (bilateral cystic kidneys) (see p. 329)

Intrauterine Growth Restriction (see differential diagnosis) (see p. 114)

MURCS Association: **M**üllerian duct aplasia, **r**enal aplasia, **c**ervicothoracic **s**omite dysplasia (renal agenesis) (see p. 398)

Normal Variant (warrants a repeat scan)

Renal Agenesis and Syndromes Featuring Renal Agenesis (see p. 412)

DISTENDED BLADDER

OTHER SYNDROMES AND SEQUENCES

Cloacal Exstrophy Sequence: Complex disorder characterized by a combination of defects that include omphalocele, imperforate anus, cloacal exstrophy, spinal defects, and genital abnormalities (see p. 382)

Megacystis–Microcolon–Intestinal Hypoperistalsis Syndrome: Autosomal recessive lethal condition caused by decreased muscle tone in the intestinal and urinary tracts, resulting in a markedly dilated urinary bladder and hypoperistalsis of the colon (see p. 396)

Posterior Urethral Valves and Other Form of Urethral Obstruction

Prune-Belly Syndrome: Triad of abdominal wall distention, urinary tract obstruction, and cryptorchidism (see p. 408)

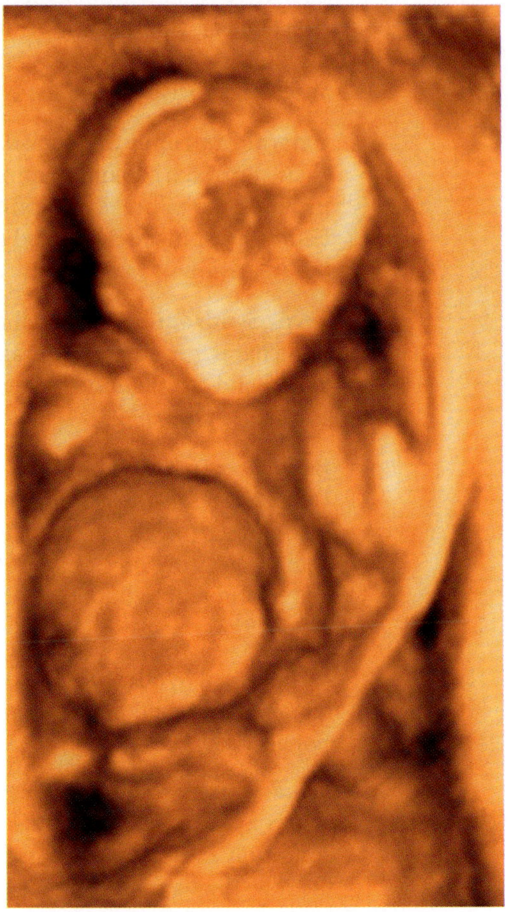

FIGURE 1-88 Three-dimensional surface rendering of the fetal bladder of an early second-trimester fetus with severe bladder outlet obstruction.

SUPRARENAL MASS

Duplex Collection System with Upper Pole Obstruction (Cystic)

Liver Cyst (Cystic)

Mass of Renal Origin (see Enlarged Kidneys, p. 84 in differential diagnosis)

Neuroblastoma (Cystic or Solid) (see p. 521)

Sequestration (Solid, Echogenic)

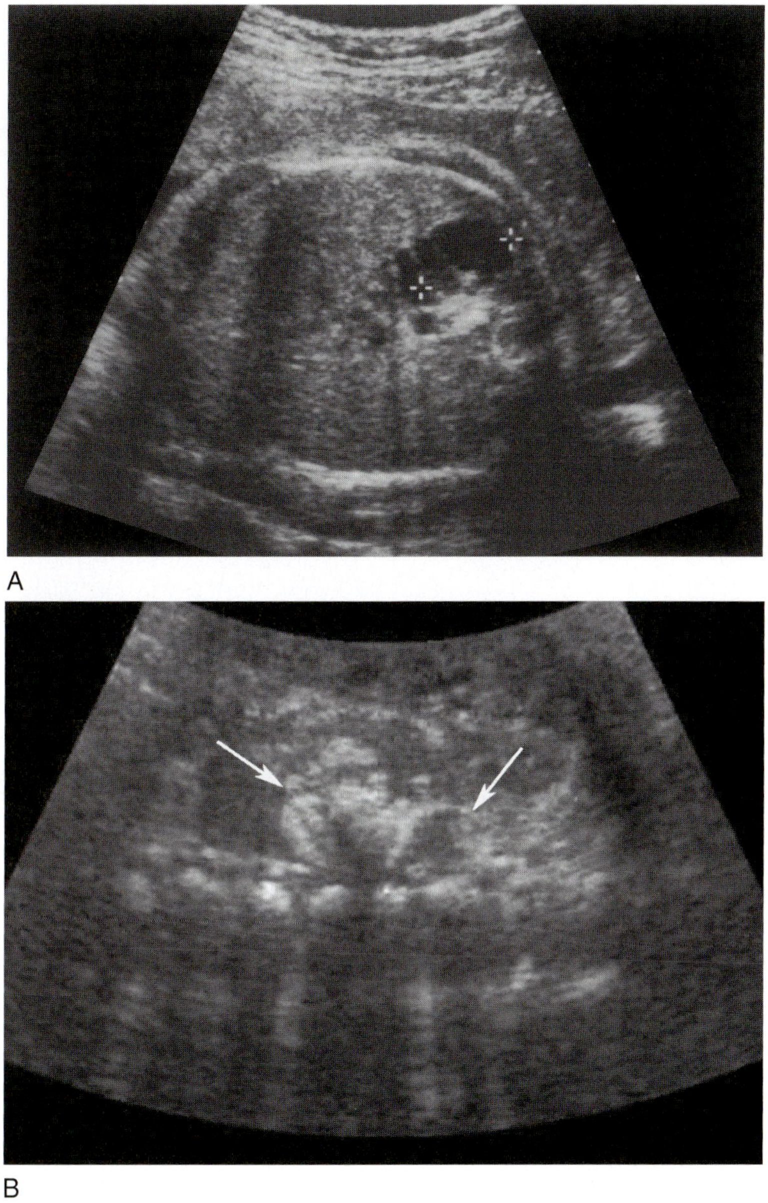

FIGURE 1-89 (A) Transverse view through the fetal abdomen reveals a cystic mass of the adrenal, which was consistent with a neuroblastoma (shown by calipers). (B) Echogenic mass *(arrows)* adjacent to the fetal spine of a different fetus, elevating the fetal kidney away from the spine. The mass is a neuroblastoma.

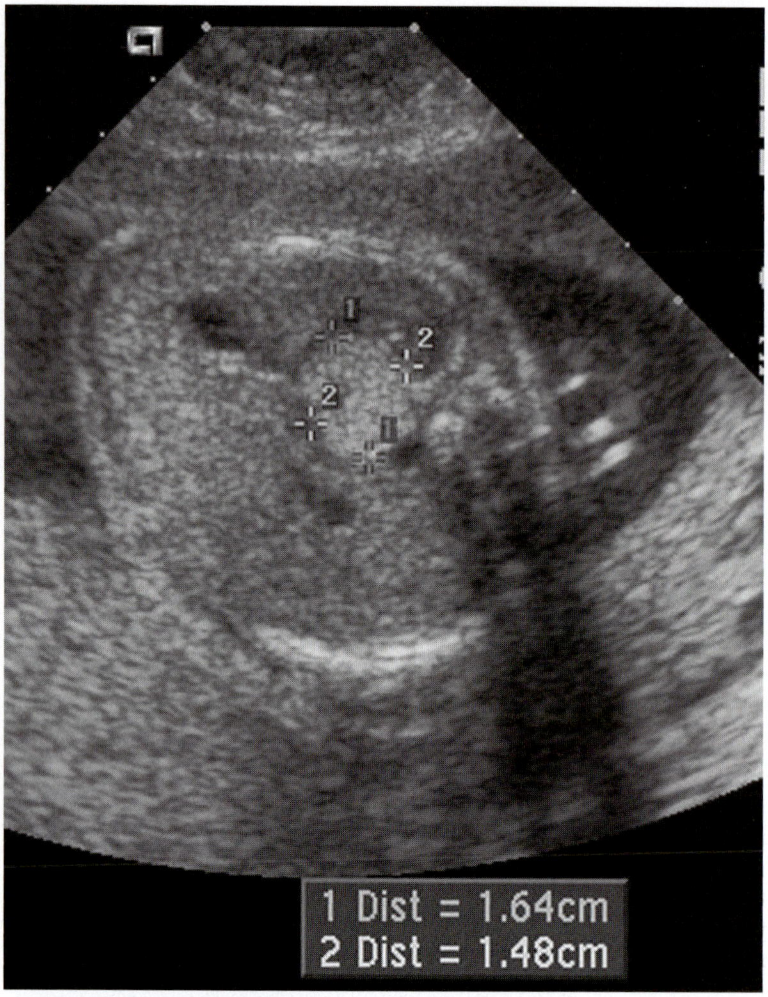

FIGURE 1-90 Echogenic mass *(calipers)* adjacent to the fetal spine in a cross-section through the abdomen. This is a subdiaphragmatic sequestration of the lung.

ENLARGED KIDNEYS

Adrenal Mass, Giving Impression of an Enlarged Kidney (neuroblastoma, hemorrhage)

Compensatory Hypertrophy with Absent Contralateral Kidney (unilateral)

Crossed-Fused Ectopia

Duplex Collecting System (with or without obstruction)

Hydronephrosis (including that associated with posterior urethral valves, megacystis/megaureter, prune-belly syndrome, and obstructive or reflux dilation of the collecting system)

Megacystis–Microcolon–Intestinal Hypoperistalsis Syndrome: Autosomal recessive lethal condition caused by decreased muscle tone in the intestinal and urinary tracts, resulting in a markedly dilated urinary bladder and hypoperistalsis of the colon (see p. 396)

Multicystic Dysplastic Kidney (usually unilateral)

Perinephric Urinoma (usually unilateral)

Tumor (Wilms' or hamartoma [mesoblastic nephroma], usually unilateral)

GROWTH ABNORMALITIES

Beckwith-Wiedemann Syndrome: Gigantism in utero in conjunction with macroglossia, omphalocele, and renal anomalies (see p. 142)

Perlman Syndrome: Autosomal recessive fetal overgrowth syndrome characterized by macrosomia, bilaterally enlarged kidneys, renal

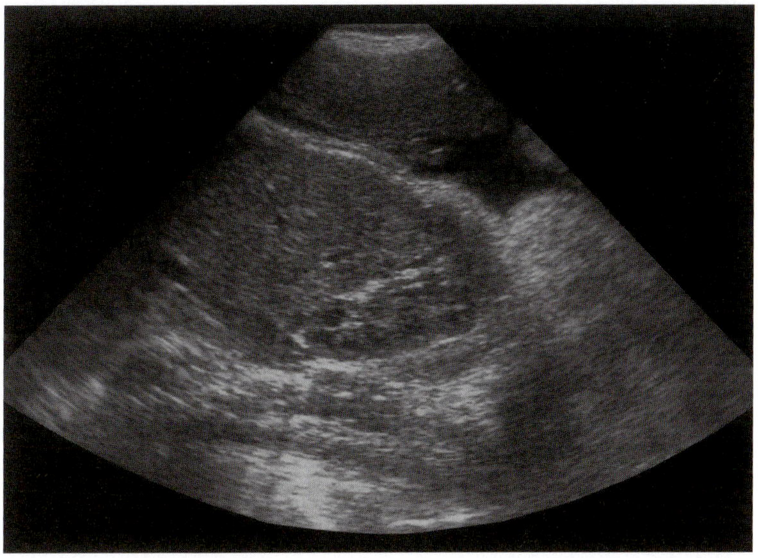

FIGURE 1-91 Crossed-fused ectopia. Longitudinal view of a fetal kidney shows its extended length and bilobed nature. The kidney extends downward, partly into the pelvis. The contralateral kidney was not identified, a finding consistent with crossed-fused ectopia.

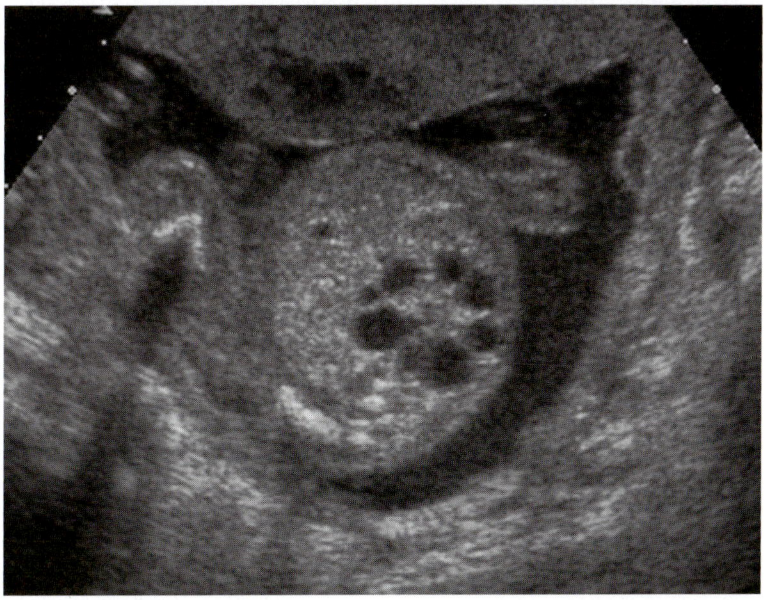

FIGURE 1-92 Transverse view through the fetal abdomen of a second-trimester fetus shows multiple cysts involving the fetal kidney consistent with a multicystic dysplastic kidney. The contralateral kidney was normal (not shown).

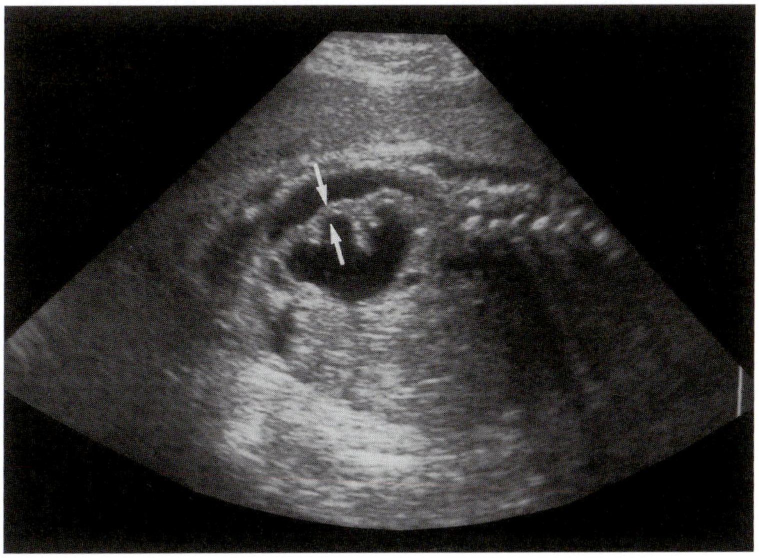

FIGURE 1-93 Longitudinal view of a fetal kidney with severe hydronephrosis. A urinoma around the outside of the renal cortex is visible. Note that the cortex *(arrows)* is thin as a result of pressure exerted from both sides.

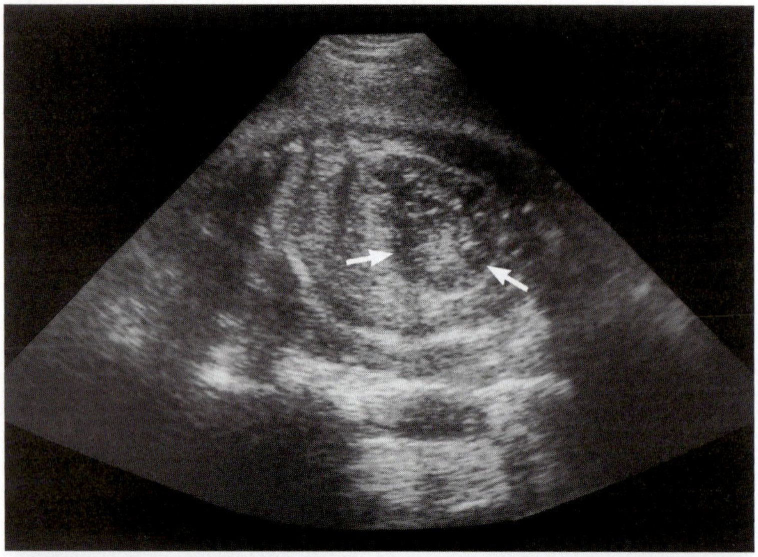

FIGURE 1-94 Longitudinal view of a fetal kidney shows an echogenic mass *(arrows)* involving the anterior surface of the lower pole of the kidney. This was diagnosed as a mesoblastic nephroma.

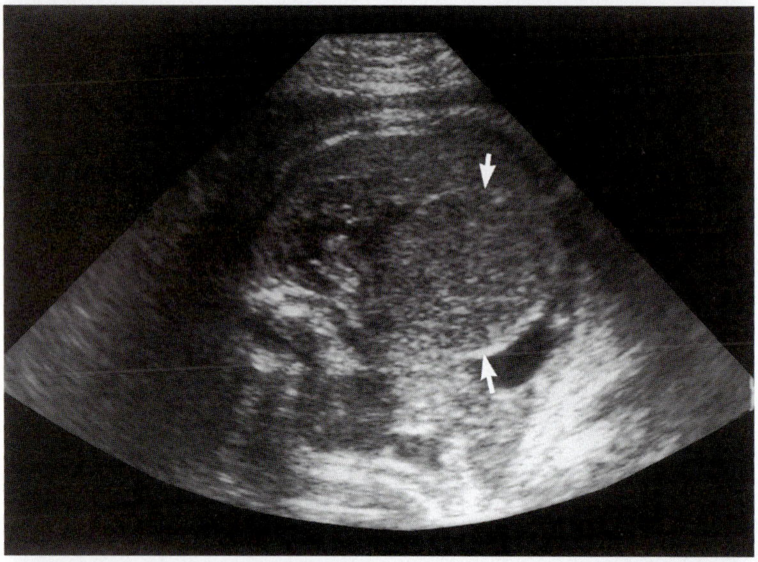

FIGURE 1-95 Longitudinal view through the fetal kidney shows a large solid mass *(arrows)* in the fetal kidney. This was shown at birth to be a Wilms' tumor.

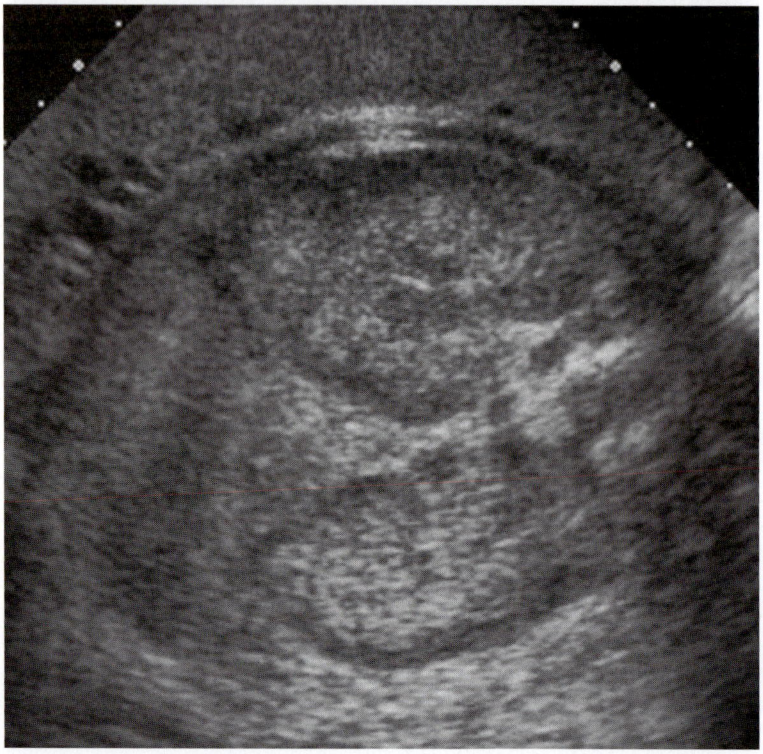

FIGURE 1-96 Bilaterally enlarged, abnormal-appearing kidneys in the third trimester associated with severe oligohydramnios. This fetus had autosomal recessive polycystic kidney disease. Note the lack of normal architecture of the kidneys.

tumors, and other visceromegaly associated with polyhydramnios (see p. 147)

FACIAL AND BRAIN ABNORMALITIES

Meckel-Gruber Syndrome: Autosomal recessive condition characterized by posterior encephalocele, postaxial polydactyly, and polycystic kidneys (bilateral) (see p. 199)

Oral-Facial-Digital Syndrome, Type I: X-linked dominant condition (lethal in males), OFD1 is one of nine syndromes (OFD1–OFD9) that include median cleft lip and palate, hypertelorism, micrognathia, and digital anomalies (adult-type polycystic kidney disease) (see p. 174)

CHROMOSOMAL ANOMALIES

Trisomy 13 (Patau Syndrome): Occurring as a result of an extra chromosome 13, this is a severe abnormality characterized by multiple anomalies of the central nervous system, face, heart, and extremities (bilateral) (see p. 483)

OTHER SYNDROMES AND SEQUENCES

Infantile Polycystic Kidney Disease (bilateral) (see p. 329)

Prune-Belly Syndrome: Triad of abdominal wall distention, urinary tract obstruction, and cryptorchidism (see p. 408)

GENITAL ANOMALIES

GROWTH ABNORMALITIES

Cornelia de Lange Syndrome: Facial/limb anomalies, growth restriction, and mental developmental delay (see p. 129)

Noonan Syndrome: Phenotypically, a Turner-like syndrome featuring short stature, webbed neck, cardiac abnormalities, and a normal karyotype (see p. 131)

Smith-Lemli-Opitz Syndrome: Autosomal recessive syndrome featuring microcephaly, mental retardation, and genital and renal anomalies (see p. 140)

FACIAL AND BRAIN ABNORMALITIES

Fraser Syndrome: Autosomal recessive syndrome featuring cryptophthalmos; syndactyly; and genital, renal, and tracheal anomalies (see p. 160)

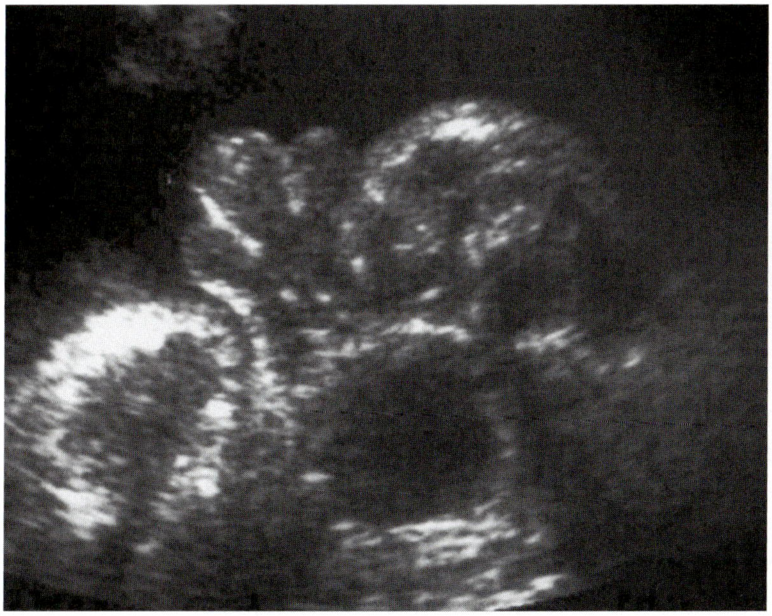

A

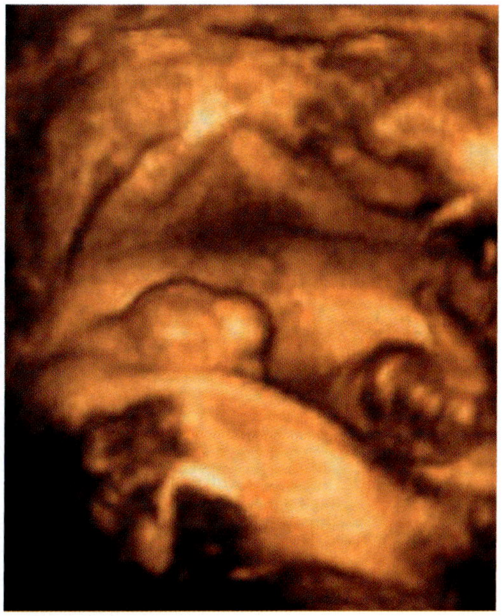

B

FIGURE 1-97 (A) Ambiguous genitalia in a karyotypically male fetus consistent with severe hypospadias (penile scrotal transposition). (B) Three-dimensional surface rendering of a fetus with severe hypospadias in the third trimester.

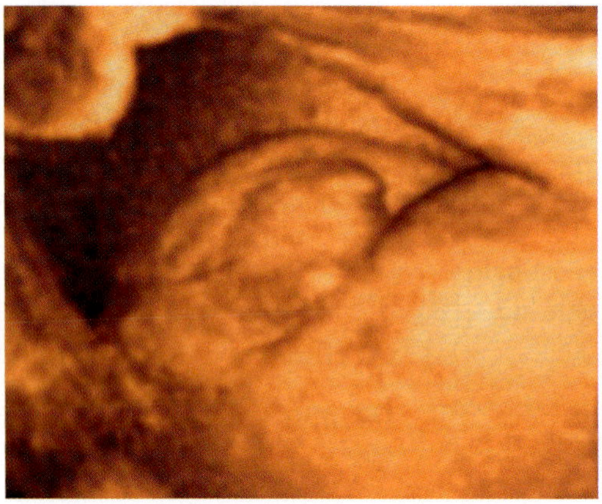

FIGURE 1-98 Third-trimester fetal genitals of a karyotypically female fetus with clitoral hypertrophy.

Hydrolethalus: Autosomal recessive disorder characterized by hydrocephalus, polydactyly, heart defects, and polyhydramnios (see p. 194)

Meckel-Gruber Syndrome: Autosomal recessive condition characterized by posterior encephalocele, postaxial polydactyly, and polycystic kidneys (see p. 199)

Miller-Dieker Syndrome: Lissencephaly, type I; characterized by complete absence of gyri of the brain, microcephaly, and severe mental retardation (see p. 208)

Neu-Laxova Syndrome: Autosomal recessive condition characterized by microcephaly, lissencephaly, exophthalmos, severe IUGR, swollen subcutaneous tissues, and ichthyosis (see p. 211)

Shprintzen Syndrome: Autosomal dominant syndrome characterized by short stature, mild mental retardation, micrognathia, and cardiac and limb abnormalities (occasional) (see p. 179)

Walker-Warburg Syndrome: Autosomal recessive condition characterized by severe, congenital, oculocerebral abnormalities, including lissencephaly, hydrocephalus, encephalocele, microcephaly, microphthalmia, and cataracts (occasional) (see p. 217)

LIMB AND SKELETAL ABNORMALITIES

Camptomelic Dysplasia: Short-limbed skeletal dysplasia characterized by bowing of the long bones, particularly in the lower extremities; bell-shaped, narrow chest; and facial anomalies (see p. 262)

Chondrodysplasia Punctata (Rhizomelic Type)**:** Heterogeneous group of bone dysplasias characterized by asymmetric limb shortening and abnormal early calcification of the proximal and distal epiphyses (occasional) (see p. 266)

Ectrodactyly–Ectodermal Dysplasia–Clefting (EEC) Syndrome: Autosomal dominant condition characterized by labial clefting, ectrodactyly (lobster-claw deformities of the limbs), and genitourinary tract anomalies (see p. 225)

Ellis-van Creveld Syndrome: Autosomal recessive skeletal dysplasia characterized by disproportionately short extremities, narrow chest,

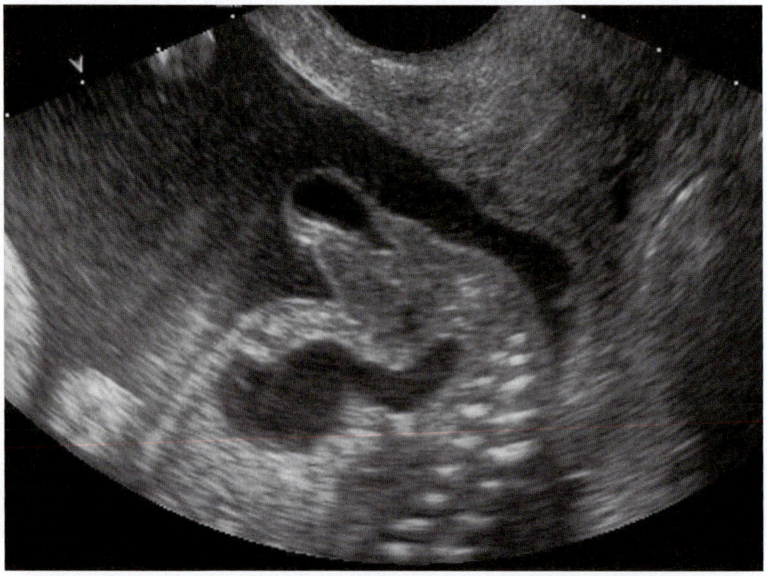

FIGURE 1-99 Lower body of a second-trimester fetus with prune-belly syndrome, scanned using the transvaginal approach. Note the distended fetal bladder and penile urethra consistent with megalourethra, both typical of this syndrome.

polydactyly, and heart defects (occasional) (see p. 272)

Fanconi Anemia: Autosomal recessive condition characterized by radial hypoplasia, absent thumbs, and tendency for leukemia (see p. 229)

Roberts Syndrome: Autosomal recessive condition characterized by severe shortening of the limbs (pseudothalidomide syndrome) and facial anomalies (see p. 247)

Short Rib–Polydactyly Syndrome, Types I and III: Skeletal dysplasias characterized by short ribs, narrow chest, polydactyly, and short limbs (see p. 288)

CRANIOSYNOSTOSIS

Antley-Bixler Syndrome: Disorder characterized by craniosynostosis, resulting in severe brachycephaly, midfacial hypoplasia, multiple skeletal fusions, and contractures (occasional) (see p. 303)

Apert Syndrome: Craniosynostosis/acrocephaly/syndactyly (occasional) (see p. 304)

Carpenter Syndrome: Autosomal recessive condition with acrocephaly, syndactyly, and preaxial polydactyly (see p. 310)

CHROMOSOMAL ANOMALIES

Deletion 4p (Wolf-Hirschhorn Syndrome): Abnormality of chromosome 4 characterized by IUGR, facial dysmorphology, cardiac defects, and hypospadias (see p. 459)

Deletion 11q (Jacobsen Syndrome): Deletion of the distal long arm of chromosome 11 characterized by multiple anomalies of practically all organ systems (see p. 464)

DiGeorge Syndrome: Also known as velocardiofacial syndrome or Shprintzen syndrome, this disorder results from a deletion of chromosome 22q11.2 and is characterized by cardiac abnormalities involving largely the great vessels, facial abnormalities, hypocalcemia, and hypoplasia of the thymus (occasional) (see p. 466)

Triploidy: Occurring as a result of a complete extra set of chromosomes, this is a lethal abnormality characterized by severe early-onset IUGR and multiple anomalies of practically all organ systems (see p. 473)

Trisomy 9: Occurring as a result of an extra chromosome 9, this is a severe abnormality characterized by multiple anomalies of practically all organ systems (see p. 478)

Trisomy 10: Rare abnormality with only those patients with mosaic trisomy 10 surviving to infancy. Abnormalities include IUGR and face, heart, hands, and feet anomalies (see p. 480)

Trisomy 18 (Edwards Syndrome): Occurring as a result of an extra chromosome 18, this is a severe abnormality characterized by IUGR and multiple anomalies of the central nervous system, face, heart, and extremities (see p. 490)

OTHER SYNDROMES AND SEQUENCES

Caudal Regression Syndrome/Sirenomelia: Although of different etiologies, these two syndromes are similar; characterized by disruption of the caudal portion of the neural tube, absence or dysplasia of the sacrum, and renal and lower extremity anomalies (see p. 370)

CHARGE Association: Coloboma of the iris, **h**eart defect, choanal **a**tresia, intrauterine growth **r**estriction, **g**enital anomalies, and **e**ar anomalies (see p. 376)

Cloacal Exstrophy Sequence: Complex disorder characterized by a combination of defects that include omphalocele, imperforate anus, cloacal exstrophy, spinal defects, and genital abnormalities (see p. 382)

Congenital Adrenal Hyperplasia: Characterized by a deficiency of one of the enzymes of cortisol biosynthesis (usually 21-hydroxylase deficiency), resulting in defective cortisol synthesis. Consequent overproduction and accumulation of cortisol precursors cause excessive production of androgens, leading to virilization of female fetuses (see p. 378)

Fryns Syndrome: Autosomal recessive condition characterized by diaphragmatic defects, digital and facial abnormalities, and brain anomalies (see p. 325)

Jarcho-Levin Syndrome (Spondylothoracic Dysplasia): Disorder occurring most commonly among Puerto Ricans; characterized by vertebral defects resulting in very short thorax and spine and protuberant abdomen (see p. 332)

MURCS Association: **Mü**llerian duct aplasia, **r**enal aplasia, **c**ervicothoracic **s**omite dysplasia (see p. 398)

Opitz Syndrome: Disorder characterized by ocular hypertelorism, micrognathia, and, in males, hypospadias (see p. 399)

Pena Shokeir Syndrome: Autosomal recessive condition characterized by IUGR, multiple joint contractures, facial anomalies, and pulmonary hypoplasia; also known as fetal akinesia/hypokinesia sequence or neurogenic arthrogryposis (see p. 402)

Prune-Belly Syndrome: Triad of abdominal wall distention, urinary tract obstruction, and cryptorchidism (see p. 408)

VATER Association: **V**ertebral defects, **a**nal atresia, **t**racheoesophageal fistula, **e**sophageal atresia, and **r**adial and renal dysplasias (see p. 429)

TERATOGENS

Azathioprine (see p. 435)

Carbamazepine (Tegretol) (see p. 436)

Chlorpheniramine (see p. 439)

Clomiphene (Clomid) (see p. 437)

Hydantoin (occasional) (see p. 436)

Oral contraceptives (see p. 437)

Progestin (females) (see p. 437)

Tetracycline (hypospadias) (see p. 434)

Valproic acid (see p. 436)

CONTRACTURES OF THE EXTREMITIES

GROWTH ABNORMALITIES

Cornelia de Lange Syndrome: Facial/limb anomalies, growth restriction, and mental developmental delay (see p. 129)

Seckel Syndrome: Autosomal recessive syndrome with severe IUGR, microcephaly, and severely abnormal profile (see p. 138)

Smith-Lemli-Opitz Syndrome: Autosomal recessive syndrome featuring microcephaly, mental retardation, and genital and renal anomalies (see p. 140)

FACIAL AND BRAIN ABNORMALITIES

Neu-Laxova Syndrome: Autosomal recessive condition characterized by microcephaly, lissencephaly, exophthalmos, severe IUGR, swollen subcutaneous tissues, and ichthyosis (see p. 211)

LIMB AND SKELETAL ABNORMALITIES

Freeman-Sheldon (Whistling Face) Syndrome: Autosomal dominant condition characterized by unusual facial features and skeletal anomalies, such as flexion deformities of the joints (see p. 237)

Larsen Syndrome: Condition characterized by abnormal facies and spine and limb abnormalities, including dislocations and hyperextensions at the joints (see p. 242)

Multiple Pterygium Syndrome: Autosomal recessive condition characterized by multiple contractures and webbing across the joints, cystic hygromata, and facial defects (see p. 244)

Roberts Syndrome: Autosomal recessive condition with severe shortening of the limbs (pseudothalidomide syndrome) and facial anomalies (see p. 247)

CRANIOSYNOSTOSIS

Antley-Bixler Syndrome: Disorder characterized by craniosynostosis, resulting in severe brachycephaly, midfacial hypoplasia, multiple skeletal fusions, and contractures (see p. 303)

CHROMOSOMAL ANOMALIES

Deletion 11q (Jacobsen Syndrome): Deletion of the distal long arm of chromosome 11 characterized by multiple anomalies of practically all organ systems (see p. 464)

Trisomy 9: Occurring as a result of an extra chromosome 9, this is a severe abnormality characterized by multiple anomalies of practically all organ systems (see p. 478)

Trisomy 18 (Edwards Syndrome): Occurring as a result of an extra chromosome 18, this is a severe abnormality characterized by IUGR and multiple anomalies of the central nervous system, face, heart, and extremities (see p. 490)

OTHER SYNDROMES AND SEQUENCES

Amniotic Band Syndrome: Condition caused by premature rupture of the amnion, resulting in an asymmetric, destructive fetal process whereby the fetus becomes adherent to, intertwined with, and tethered by the fibrous bands; associated with diverse anomalies (occasional) (see p. 356)

Arthrogryposis: Sequence of neurologic, muscular, and connective tissue disorders leading to fetal joint contractures and rigidity, as well as decreased activity (see p. 362)

Caudal Regression Syndrome/Sirenomelia: Although of different etiologies, these two syndromes are similar; characterized by disruption of the caudal portion of the neural tube, absence or dysplasia of the sacrum, and renal and lower extremity anomalies (see p. 370)

Cerebro-Oculo-Facio-Skeletal (COFS) Syndrome: Autosomal recessive condition characterized by joint contractures of all the extremities, with severe facial and brain abnormalities (see p. 374)

Pena Shokeir Syndrome: Autosomal recessive condition characterized by IUGR, multiple joint contractures, facial anomalies, and pulmonary hypoplasia; also known as fetal akinesia/hypokinesia sequence or neurogenic arthrogryposis (see p. 402)

CLENCHED HANDS

GROWTH ABNORMALITIES

Smith-Lemli-Opitz Syndrome: Autosomal recessive syndrome featuring microcephaly, mental retardation, and genital and renal anomalies (see p. 140)

FACIAL AND BRAIN ABNORMALITIES

Neu-Laxova Syndrome: Autosomal recessive condition characterized by microcephaly, lissencephaly, exophthalmos, severe IUGR, swollen subcutaneous tissues, and ichthyosis (see p. 211)

LIMB AND SKELETAL ABNORMALITIES

Freeman-Sheldon (Whistling Face) Syndrome: Autosomal dominant condition characterized by unusual facial features and skeletal anomalies, such as flexion deformities of the joints (see p. 237)

Multiple Pterygium Syndrome: Autosomal recessive condition characterized by multiple contractures and webbing across the joints, cystic hygromata, and facial defects (see p. 244)

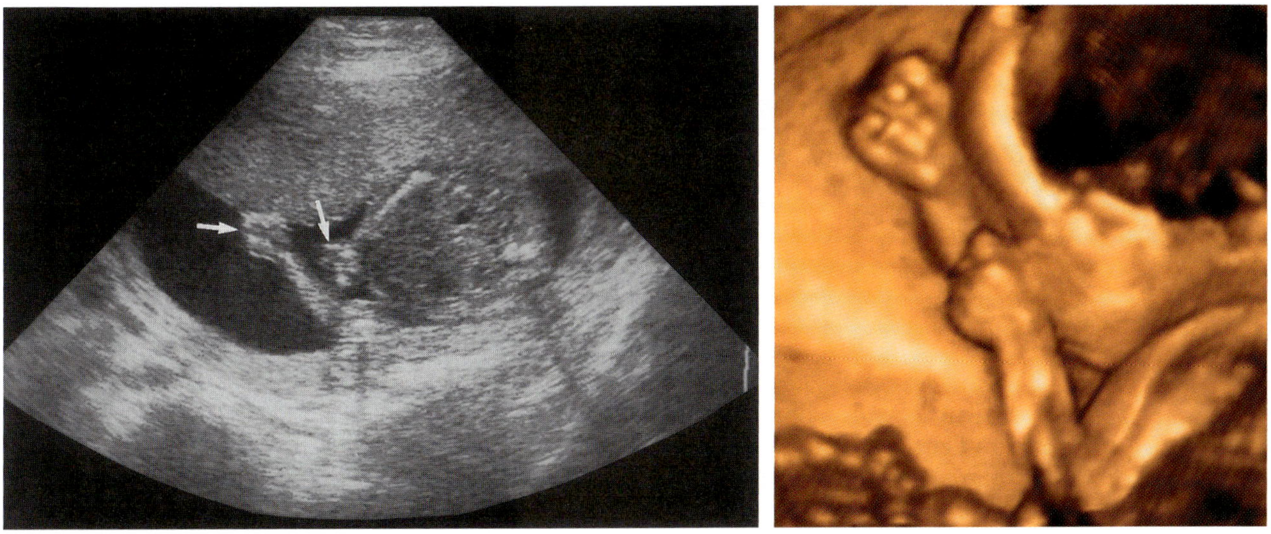

A B

FIGURE 1-100 (A) View of both forearms of a fetus with multiple contractures of all extremities. Note the clenched hands *(arrows)* in this fetus presumed to have Pena Shokeir syndrome. (B) Three-dimensional surface rendering shows bilateral clenched fists in a fetus with arthrogryposis. Note the overlapping digits.

CHROMOSOMAL ANOMALIES

Trisomy 9: Occurring as a result of an extra chromosome 9, this is a severe abnormality characterized by multiple anomalies of practically all organ systems (see p. 478)

Trisomy 13 (Patau Syndrome): Occurring as a result of an extra chromosome 13, this is a severe abnormality characterized by multiple anomalies of the central nervous system, face, heart, and extremities (occasional) (see p. 483)

Trisomy 18 (Edwards Syndrome): Occurring as a result of an extra chromosome 18, this is a severe abnormality characterized by IUGR and multiple anomalies of the central nervous system, face, heart, and extremities (see p. 490)

OTHER SYNDROMES AND SEQUENCES

Amniotic Band Syndrome: Condition caused by premature rupture of the amnion, resulting in an asymmetric destructive fetal process whereby the fetus becomes adherent to, intertwined with, and tethered by the fibrous bands; associated with diverse anomalies (occasional) (see p. 356)

Arthrogryposis: Sequence of neurologic, muscular, and connective tissue disorders leading to fetal joint contractures and rigidity, as well as decreased activity (see p. 362)

Cerebro-Oculo-Facio-Skeletal (COFS) Syndrome: Autosomal recessive condition characterized by joint contractures of all the extremities, with severe facial and brain abnormalities (see p. 374)

Pena Shokeir Syndrome: Autosomal recessive condition characterized by IUGR, multiple joint contractures, facial anomalies, and pulmonary hypoplasia; also known as fetal akinesia/hypokinesia sequence or neurogenic arthrogryposis (see p. 402)

POLYDACTYLY

GROWTH ABNORMALITIES

Smith-Lemli-Opitz Syndrome: Autosomal recessive syndrome featuring microcephaly, mental retardation, and genital and renal anomalies (see p. 140)

FACIAL AND BRAIN ABNORMALITIES

Branchio-Oculo-Facial Syndrome: Autosomal dominant disorder characterized by mental retardation, growth deficiency, ocular defects, and clefting of the upper lip (occasional) (see p. 149)

Hydrolethalus: Autosomal recessive disorder characterized by hydrocephalus, polydactyly, heart defects, and polyhydramnios (see p. 194)

Joubert Syndrome: Autosomal recessive syndrome characterized by dysmorphic facial features and agenesis of the cerebellar vermis (occasional) (see p. 197)

Meckel-Gruber Syndrome: Autosomal recessive condition characterized by posterior encephalocele, postaxial polydactyly, and polycystic kidneys (see p. 199)

Oral-Facial-Digital Syndrome, Type I: X-linked dominant condition (lethal in males), OFD1 is one of nine syndromes (OFD1–OFD9) that include median cleft lip and palate, hypertelorism, micrognathia, and digital anomalies (see p. 174)

Oral-Facial-Digital Syndrome, Type II (Mohr Syndrome): Autosomal recessive syndrome characterized by short stature; deafness; and facial, hand, and foot abnormalities (see p. 175)

LIMB AND SKELETAL ABNORMALITIES

Ellis-van Creveld Syndrome: Autosomal recessive skeletal dysplasia characterized by disproportionately short extremities, narrow chest, polydactyly, and heart defects (see p. 272)

Hypochondroplasia: Autosomal dominant skeletal dysplasia with moderate limb shortening; resembles achondroplasia but is less severe (occasional) (see p. 274)

Jeune Thoracic Dystrophy (Asphyxiating Thoracic Dysplasia): Autosomal recessive skeletal dysplasia characterized by very narrow chest with short ribs, moderately short long-bones, and occasional polydactyly (see p. 278)

Majewski Syndrome (Short Rib–Polydactyly Syndrome, Type II): Autosomal recessive skeletal dysplasia characterized by short ribs, narrow thorax, polydactyly, and median facial cleft (see p. 283)

Short Rib–Polydactyly Syndrome, Types I and III: Skeletal dysplasias characterized by short

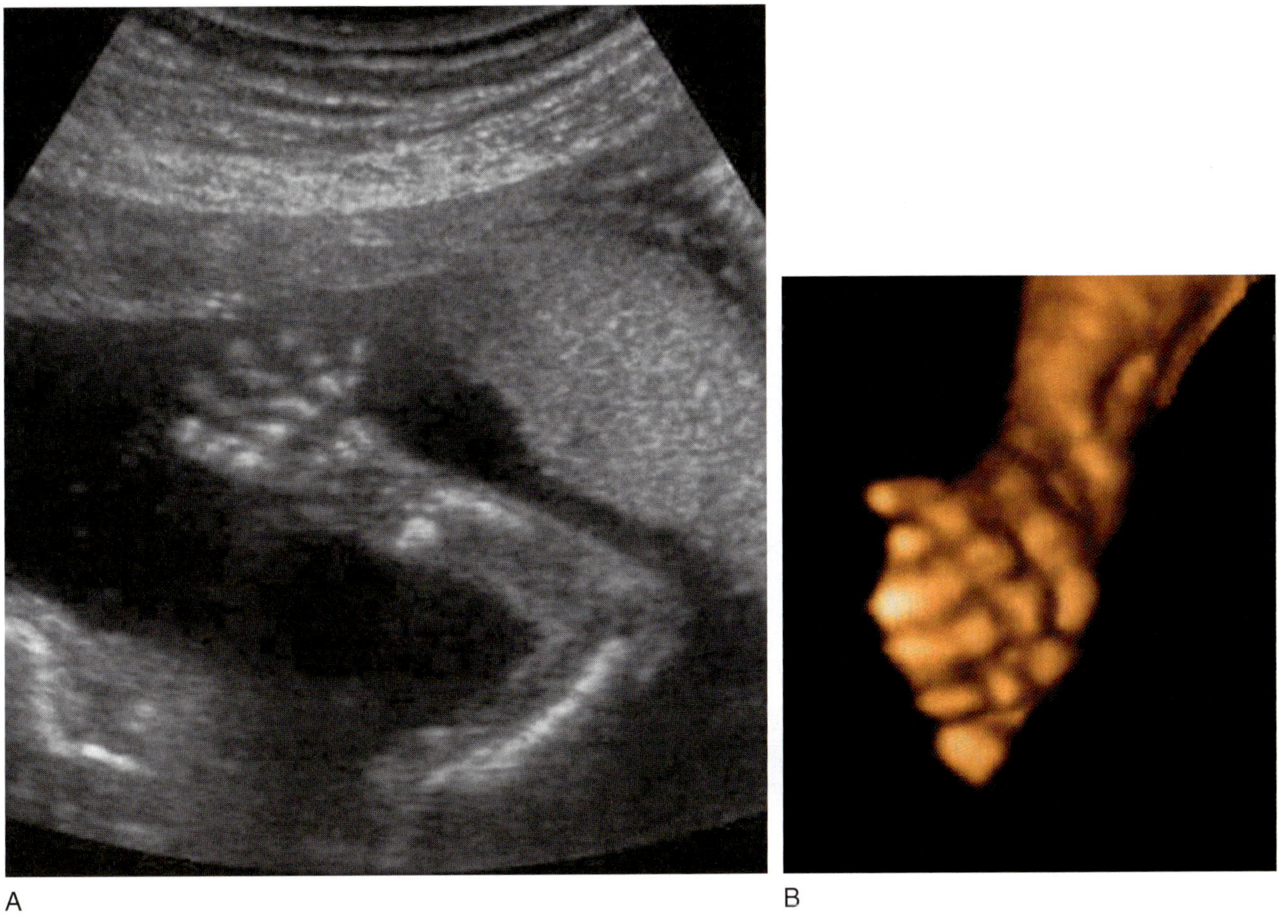

FIGURE 1-101 (A) Second-trimester fetus with polydactyly. (B) Three-dimensional surface rendering of a fetus with polydactyly.

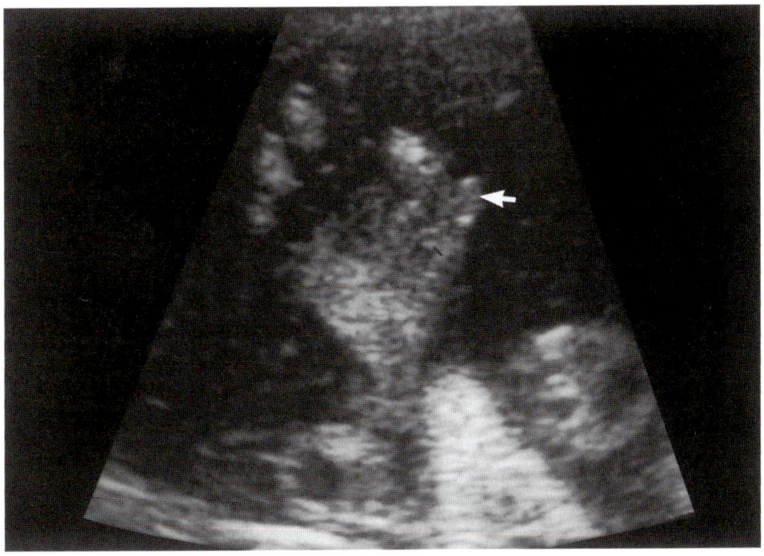

FIGURE 1-102 Preaxial polydactyly. View of the palm of the hand of a fetus with a duplicated thumb *(arrow)*.

ribs, narrow chest, polydactyly, and short limbs (see p. 288)

CRANIOSYNOSTOSIS

Saethre-Chotzen Syndrome: Autosomal dominant syndrome characterized by facial asymmetry, craniosynostosis of the coronal sutures, and digital abnormalities of the hands and feet (duplicated hallux, polysyndactyly) (see p. 320)

CHROMOSOMAL ANOMALIES

Deletion 4p (Wolf-Hirschhorn Syndrome): Abnormality of chromosome 4 characterized by IUGR, facial dysmorphology, cardiac defects, and hypospadias (see p. 459)

Trisomy 10: Rare abnormality with only those patients with mosaic trisomy 10 surviving to infancy. Abnormalities include IUGR and face, heart, hand, and feet anomalies (preaxial) (see p. 480)

Trisomy 13 (Patau Syndrome): Occurring as a result of an extra chromosome 13, this is a severe abnormality characterized by multiple anomalies of the central nervous system, face, heart, and extremities (see p. 483)

OTHER SYNDROMES AND SEQUENCES

Carpenter Syndrome: Autosomal recessive condition characterized by acrocephaly, syndactyly, and preaxial polydactyly (see p. 310)

CHARGE Association: **C**oloboma of the iris, **h**eart defect, choanal **a**tresia, intrauterine growth **r**estriction, **g**enital anomalies, and **e**ar anomalies (occasional) (see p. 376)

VATER Association: **V**ertebral defects, **a**nal atresia, **t**racheoesophageal fistula, **e**sophageal atresia, and **r**adial and renal dysplasias (occasional) (see p. 429)

TERATOGENS

Azathioprine (see p. 435)

Chlorpheniramine (see p. 439)

Clomiphene (see p. 437)

Phenylpropanolamine (see p. 439)

SYNDACTYLY

GROWTH ABNORMALITIES

Cornelia de Lange Syndrome: Facial/limb anomalies, growth restriction, and mental developmental delay (see p. 129)

Russell-Silver Syndrome: Asymmetric growth restriction of the skeleton in conjunction with a normal-size head and short stature (see p. 136)

Smith-Lemli-Opitz Syndrome: Autosomal recessive syndrome featuring microcephaly, mental retardation, and genital and renal anomalies (see p. 140)

FACIAL AND BRAIN ABNORMALITIES

Fraser Syndrome: Autosomal recessive syndrome featuring cryptophthalmos; syndactyly; and genital, renal, and tracheal anomalies (see p. 160)

Nager Syndrome: Acrofacial dysostosis syndrome similar to Treacher Collins syndrome, with mandibular hypoplasia, malformed ears, and abnormal radial ray (occasional) (see p. 171)

Neu-Laxova Syndrome: Autosomal recessive condition characterized by microcephaly, lissencephaly, exophthalmos, severe IUGR, swollen subcutaneous tissues, and ichthyosis (see p. 211)

Oral-Facial-Digital Syndrome, Type I: X-linked dominant condition (lethal in males), OFD1 is one of nine syndromes (OFD1–OFD9) that include median cleft lip and palate, hypertelorism, micrognathia, and digital anomalies (see p. 174)

Oral-Facial-Digital Syndrome, Type II (Mohr Syndrome): Autosomal recessive syndrome characterized by short stature; deafness; and facial, hand, and foot abnormalities (see p. 175)

LIMB AND SKELETAL ABNORMALITIES

Adams-Oliver Syndrome: Disorder characterized by terminal transverse defects of the upper and lower extremities, as well as denuded areas on the scalp with or without an underlying bony skull (bone) defect (occasional) (see p. 223)

Ectrodactyly–Ectodermal Dysplasia–Clefting (EEC) Syndrome: Autosomal dominant condition characterized by labial clefting, ectrodactyly (lobster-claw deformities of the limbs), and genitourinary tract anomalies (see p. 225)

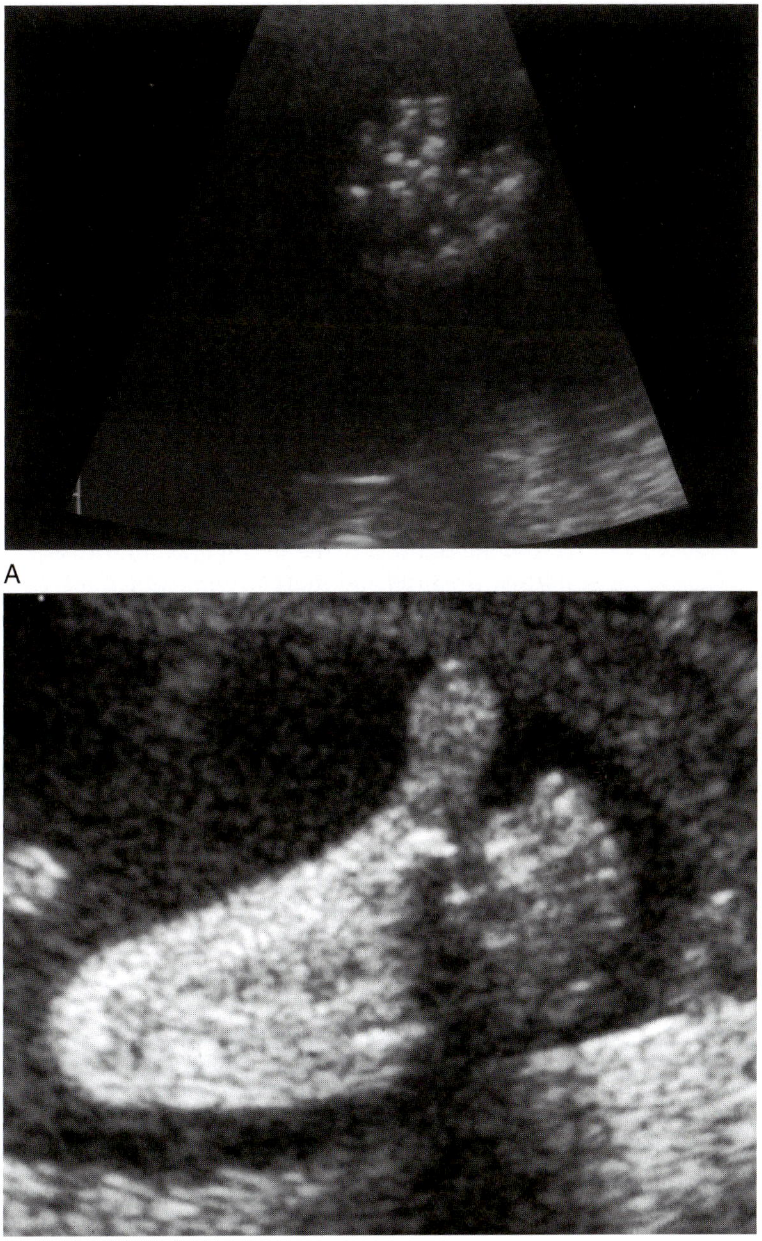

A

B

FIGURE 1-103 (A) Fingers of a fetus with syndactyly of fingers 3, 4, and 5, with bony fusion of the phalanges. (B) Plantar aspect of the foot of a fetus with polysyndactyly.

Holt-Oram Syndrome: Autosomal dominant condition characterized by upper extremity abnormalities, such as radial hypoplasia, and heart defects (see p. 238)

Roberts Syndrome: Autosomal recessive condition with severe shortening of the limbs (pseudothalidomide syndrome) and facial anomalies (see p. 247)

CRANIOSYNOSTOSIS

Apert Syndrome: Craniosynostosis, acrocephaly, and syndactyly (see p. 304)

Carpenter Syndrome: Autosomal recessive condition with acrocephaly, syndactyly, and preaxial polydactyly (see p. 310)

Pfeiffer Syndrome: Acrocephalic skull, craniosynostosis (particularly of the coronal and sagittal sutures), and syndactyly of hands and feet (occasional) (see p. 316)

CHROMOSOMAL ANOMALIES

Trisomy 10: Rare abnormality with only those patients with mosaic trisomy 10 surviving to infancy. Abnormalities include IUGR and face, heart, hand, and feet anomalies (see p. 480)

OTHER SYNDROMES AND SEQUENCES

VATER Association: **V**ertebral defects, **a**nal atresia, **t**racheoesophageal fistula, **e**sophageal atresia, **r**adial and renal dysplasias (occasional) (see p. 429)

TERATOGENS

Aminopterin (see p. 438)

Clomiphene (see p. 437)

Cyclophosphamide (see p. 435)

Cytarabine (see p. 435)

Methotrexate (see p. 435)

Phenothiazine (see p. 438)

Phenylephrine (see p. 439)

CLINODACTYLY

GROWTH ABNORMALITIES

Russell-Silver Syndrome: Asymmetric growth restriction of the skeleton in conjunction with a normal-size head and short stature (see p. 136)

LIMB AND SKELETAL ABNORMALITIES

Nager Syndrome: Acrofacial dysostosis syndrome similar to Treacher Collins syndrome; characterized primarily by mandibular hypoplasia, malformed ears, and abnormal radial ray (see p. 171)

Oral-Facial-Digital Syndrome, Type I: X-linked dominant condition (lethal in males), OFD1 is one of nine syndromes (OFD1-OFD9) that include median cleft lip and palate, hypertelorism, micrognathia, and digital anomalies (see p. 174)

Oral-Facial-Digital Syndrome, Type II (Mohr Syndrome): Autosomal recessive syndrome characterized by short stature; deafness; and facial, hand, and foot abnormalities (see p. 175)

CRANIOSYNOSTOSIS

Carpenter Syndrome: Autosomal recessive condition characterized by acrocephaly, syndactyly, and preaxial polydactyly (see p. 310)

CHROMOSOMAL ANOMALIES

Deletion 11q (Jacobsen Syndrome): Deletion of the distal long arm of chromosome 11

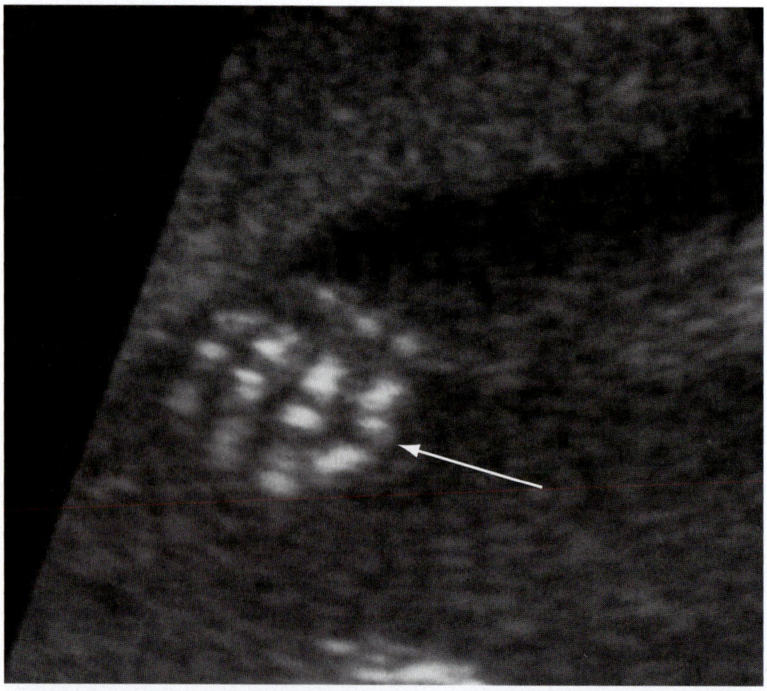

FIGURE 1-104 Second-trimester fetus with Down syndrome shows clinodactyly. Note hypoplasia of the phalanx of the fifth digit *(arrow)* with inward curvature of the fifth digit.

characterized by multiple anomalies of practically all organ systems (occasional) (see p. 464)

Tetrasomy 12p (Pallister-Killian Syndrome): Mosaic aneuploidy characterized by multiple congenital abnormalities of the central nervous system, face, heart, and many other organs (see p. 471)

Trisomy 21 (Down Syndrome): Occurring as a result of an extra chromosome 21, this abnormality is characterized by nuchal fold thickening, short long-bones, abnormal nasal bone, heart defects, and other anomalies. Twenty-five percent of fetuses with Down syndrome do not display any sonographic abnormalities or markers (see p. 496)

ASYMMETRIC LENGTHS OF EXTREMITIES

GROWTH ABNORMALITIES

Russell-Silver Syndrome: Asymmetric growth restriction of the skeleton in conjunction with a normal-size head and short stature (see p. 136)

LIMB AND SKELETAL ABNORMALITIES

Chondrodysplasia Punctata (Nonrhizomelic Type)**:** Heterogeneous group of bone dysplasias characterized by asymmetric limb shortening and abnormal early calcification of the proximal and distal epiphyses (see p. 266)

Femoral Hypoplasia–Unusual Facies Syndrome: Syndrome characterized by short lower limbs, especially hypoplastic femurs, and facial abnormalities; may be part of a spectrum of abnormalities that includes caudal regression syndrome (see p. 231)

Femur–Fibula–Ulna (FFU) Syndrome: Condition characterized by severe, asymmetric abnormalities of both upper and lower extremities (see p. 235)

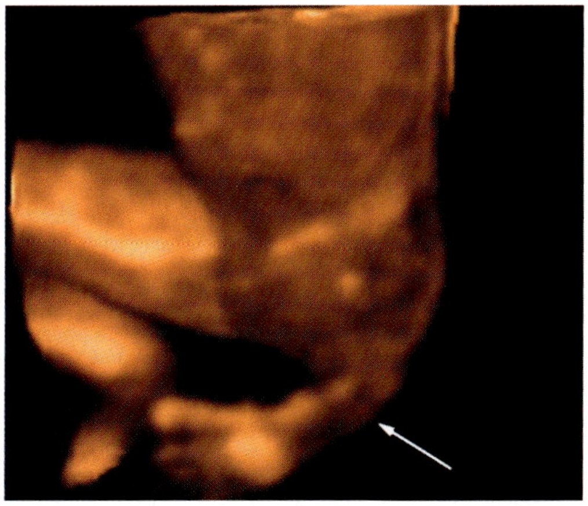

FIGURE 1-105 Three-dimensional surface rendering of an abnormal lower extremity. Note that the foot is almost directly attached to the hip *(arrow)*, with very little intervening leg present.

OTHER SYNDROMES AND SEQUENCES

Amniotic Band Syndrome: Condition caused by premature rupture of the amnion, resulting in an asymmetric, destructive fetal process whereby the fetus becomes adherent to, intertwined with, and tethered by the fibrous bands; associated with diverse anomalies (see p. 356)

Klippel-Trenaunay-Weber Syndrome: Large, cutaneous hemangiomata associated with hypertrophy of related bones and soft tissues (see p. 341)

Proteus Syndrome: Asymmetric focal overgrowth, subcutaneous tumors, and hemihypertrophy (see p. 352)

TERATOGENS

Amitriptyline (see p. 437)

Chlorpheniramine (see p. 439)

Cocaine (see p. 439)

Codeine (see p. 439)

Estrogen (see p. 437)

Fluorouracil (see p. 435)

Haloperidol (see p. 438)

Imipramine (see p. 438)

Indomethacin (see p. 439)

Meprobamate (see p. 438)

Nortriptyline (see p. 438)

Oral contraceptives (see p. 437)

Progestin (see p. 437)

Quinine (see p. 434)

Tetracycline (see p. 434)

Thalidomide (see p. 437)

Trimethadione (see p. 436)

Valproic acid (see p. 436)

SLIGHTLY SHORT FEMUR

GROWTH ABNORMALITIES

Early-Onset IUGR of All Types (including syndromes with early IUGR; see differential diagnosis) (see p. 114)

Russell-Silver Syndrome: Asymmetric growth restriction of the skeleton in conjunction with a normal-size head and short stature (see p. 136)

FACIAL AND BRAIN ABNORMALITIES

Neu-Laxova Syndrome: Autosomal recessive condition characterized by microcephaly, lissencephaly, exophthalmos, severe IUGR, swollen subcutaneous tissues, and ichthyosis (see p. 211)

Shprintzen Syndrome: Autosomal dominant syndrome characterized by short stature, mild mental retardation, micrognathia, and cardiac and limb abnormalities (see p. 179)

LIMB AND SKELETAL ABNORMALITIES

Achondroplasia (Heterozygous)**:** Autosomal dominant condition with rhizomelic limb shortening (nonlethal, heterozygous type usually is not apparent until late in the second trimester) (see p. 257)

Femoral Hypoplasia–Unusual Facies Syndrome: Syndrome with short lower limbs, hypoplastic femurs, and facial abnormalities; may be part of a spectrum of abnormalities that includes caudal regression syndrome (see p. 231)

Hypochondroplasia: Autosomal dominant skeletal dysplasia characterized by moderate limb shortening; resembles achondroplasia but is less severe (see p. 274)

Jeune Thoracic Dystrophy (Asphyxiating Thoracic Dysplasia): Autosomal recessive skeletal dysplasia characterized by very narrow chest with short ribs, moderately short long-bones, and occasional polydactyly (see p. 278)

Kniest Syndrome: Autosomal dominant condition characterized by kyphoscoliosis, platyspondyly, and shortened tubular long bones (occasional) (see p. 281)

Spondyloepiphyseal Dysplasia Congenita: Autosomal dominant, heterogeneous group of disorders, with a short spine with platyspondyly, which results in kyphoscoliosis and lordosis (see p. 291)

CHROMOSOMAL ANOMALIES

DiGeorge Syndrome: Also known as velocardiofacial syndrome or Shprintzen syndrome, this disorder results from a deletion of chromosome 22q11.2 and is characterized by cardiac abnormalities involving largely the great vessels, facial abnormalities, hypocalcemia, and hypoplasia of the thymus (see p. 466)

Tetrasomy 12p (Pallister-Killian Syndrome): Mosaic aneuploidy characterized by multiple congenital abnormalities of the central nervous system, face, heart, and many other organs (see p. 471)

Trisomy 21 (Down Syndrome): Occurring as a result of an extra chromosome 21, this abnormality is characterized by nuchal fold thickening, short long-bones, abnormal nasal bone, heart defects, and other anomalies. Twenty-five percent of fetuses with Down syndrome do not display any sonographic abnormalities or markers (see p. 496)

XO Syndrome (Turner Syndrome): Occurring as a result of a single X chromosome (XO), Turner syndrome is characterized primarily in early pregnancy by large cystic hygromata and lymphangiectasia, and heart defects. Affected infants who survive gestation may represent Turner mosaic individuals (see p. 510)

GENERALIZED SHORT AND BOWED LIMBS

FACIAL AND BRAIN ABNORMALITIES

Neu-Laxova Syndrome: Autosomal recessive condition characterized by microcephaly, lissencephaly, exophthalmos, severe IUGR, swollen subcutaneous tissues, and ichthyosis (see p. 211)

LIMB AND SKELETAL ABNORMALITIES

Achondrogenesis: Lethal skeletal dysplasia with extreme hypoplasia of the bones, micromelia, decreased ossification of the bones (particularly

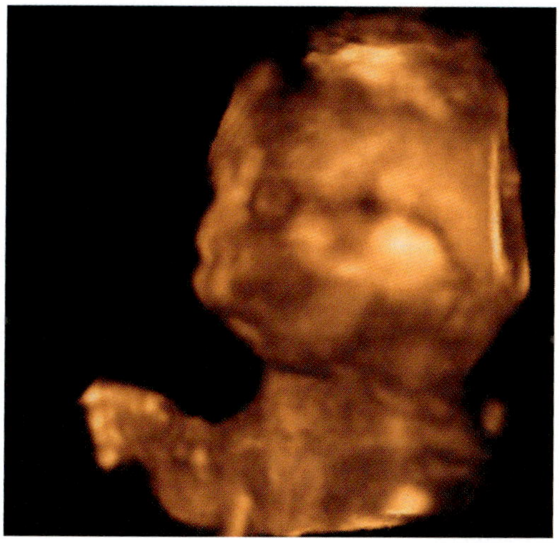

FIGURE 1-106 Markedly shortened extremity in a fetus with a skeletal dysplasia. Note the micrognathia.

those of the skull and spine), and hydrops (see p. 253)

Achondroplasia (Homozygous)**:** Autosomal dominant condition with rhizomelic limb shortening (nonlethal, heterozygous type usually is not apparent until late in the second trimester) (see p. 257)

Atelosteogenesis, Type I: Lethal skeletal dysplasia with severe limb shortening and deficient ossification of the bones, resulting in micromelic dwarfism (see p. 260)

Camptomelic Dysplasia: Short-limbed skeletal dysplasia characterized by bowing of the long bones, particularly in the lower extremities; bell-shaped, narrow chest; and facial anomalies (see p. 262)

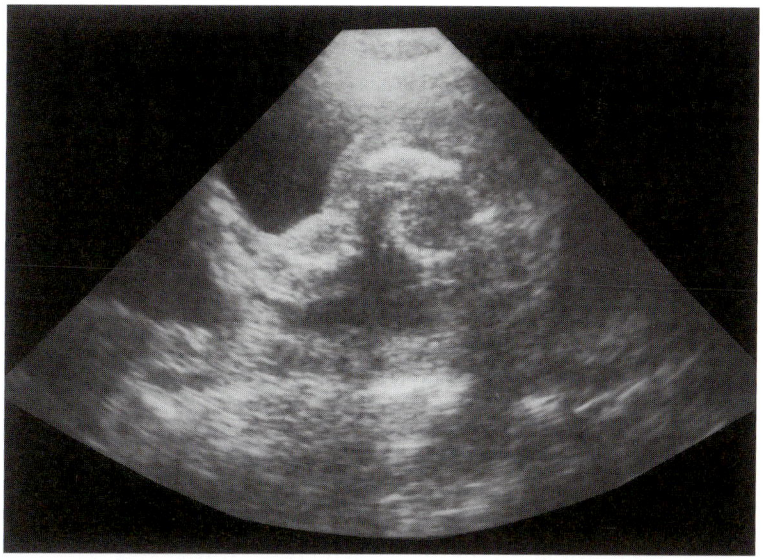

FIGURE 1-107 Longitudinal view of the lower extremity of a fetus with thanatophoric dysplasia. Note the bowed femur and tibia.

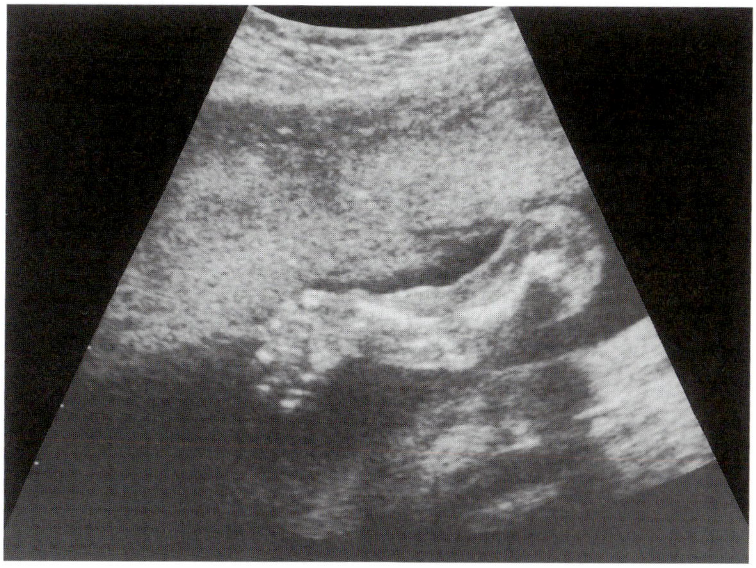

FIGURE 1-108 Longitudinal view of the upper extremity of a fetus with thanatophoric dysplasia.

Diastrophic Dysplasia: Skeletal dysplasia characterized by micromelia, club feet, hand abnormalities (hitchhiker thumb), and kyphoscoliosis (see p. 270)

Hypophosphatasia: Autosomal recessive condition characterized by severe demineralization of the bones and a congenital deficiency of alkaline phosphatase (see p. 275)

Majewski Syndrome (Short Rib–Polydactyly Syndrome, Type II): Autosomal recessive skeletal dysplasia characterized by short ribs, narrow thorax, polydactyly, and median facial cleft (see p. 283)

Metatropic Dysplasia: Short-limbed skeletal dysplasia characterized by progressive severe kyphoscoliosis, narrow chest, and metaphyseal flaring (see p. 285)

Roberts Syndrome: Autosomal recessive condition characterized by severe shortening of the limbs (pseudothalidomide syndrome) and facial anomalies (see p. 247)

Short Rib–Polydactyly Syndrome, Types I and III: Skeletal dysplasias characterized by short ribs, narrow chest, polydactyly, and short limbs (see p. 288)

Thanatophoric Dysplasia: Most common skeletal dysplasia characterized by narrow chest; short ribs; short, bowed long-bones; and flat vertebral bodies (see p. 294)

CRANIOSYNOSTOSIS

Antley-Bixler Syndrome: Disorder characterized by craniosynostosis, resulting in severe brachycephaly, midfacial hypoplasia, multiple skeletal fusions, and contractures (bowed bones, especially femur) (see p. 303)

OTHER SYNDROMES AND SEQUENCES

Osteogenesis Imperfecta: Heterogeneous group of conditions characterized by severe osseous fragility, decreased ossification, and multiple fractures (see p. 345)

ASYMMETRIC LIMB REDUCTION DEFECTS

GROWTH ABNORMALITIES

Cornelia de Lange Syndrome: Facial and limb malformations, growth restriction, and mental developmental delay (see p. 129)

Russell-Silver Syndrome: Asymmetric growth restriction of the skeleton in conjunction with a normal-size head and short stature (see p. 136)

FACIAL AND BRAIN ABNORMALITIES

Nager Syndrome: Acrofacial dysostosis syndrome similar to Treacher Collins syndrome; characterized primarily by mandibular hypoplasia, malformed ears, and abnormal radial ray (occasional) (see p. 171)

LIMB AND SKELETAL ABNORMALITIES

Adams-Oliver Syndrome: Disorder characterized by terminal transverse defects of the upper and lower extremities, as well as denuded areas on the scalp with or without an underlying bony skull (bone) defect (see p. 223)

Ectrodactyly–Ectodermal Dysplasia–Clefting (EEC) Syndrome: Autosomal dominant condition characterized by labial clefting and ectrodactyly (lobster-claw deformities of the limbs), as well as genitourinary tract anomalies (see p. 225)

Fanconi Anemia: Autosomal recessive condition characterized by radial hypoplasia, absent thumbs, and tendency for leukemia (see p. 229)

Femoral Hypoplasia–Unusual Facies Syndrome: Syndrome characterized by short lower limbs, especially hypoplastic femurs, and facial abnormalities; may be part of a spectrum of abnormalities that includes caudal regression syndrome (see p. 231)

Femur-Fibula-Ulna (FFU) Syndrome: Condition characterized by severe asymmetric abnormalities of both upper and lower extremities (see p. 235)

Holt-Oram Syndrome: Autosomal dominant condition characterized by upper extremity abnormalities, such as radial hypoplasia, and heart defects (see p. 238)

Roberts Syndrome: Autosomal recessive condition characterized by severe shortening of the limbs (pseudothalidomide syndrome) and facial anomalies (see p. 247)

Thrombocytopenia–Absent Radius (TAR) Syndrome: Autosomal recessive syndrome

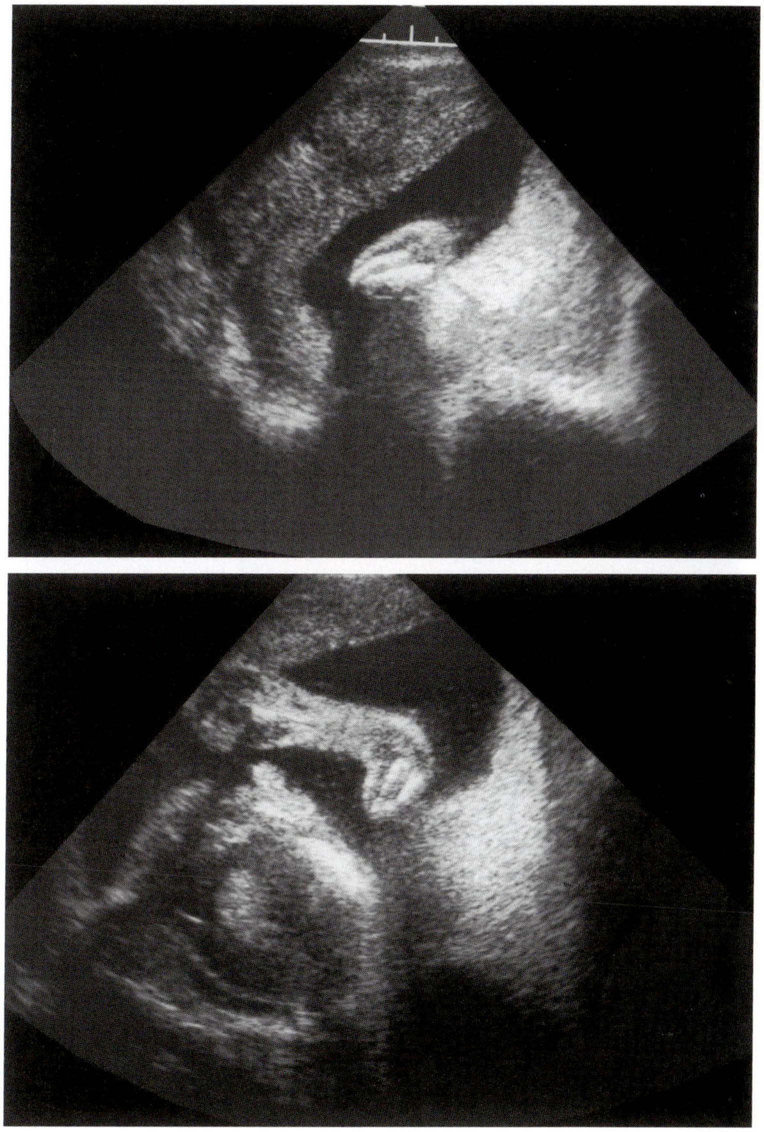

FIGURE 1-109 Two views of the forearm of a fetus with complete amputation at the midforearm level. Note that the lower portion of the forearm and hand are missing.

characterized by radial aplasia and thrombocytopenia (see p. 251)

CHROMOSOMAL ANOMALIES

Tetrasomy 12p (Pallister-Killian Syndrome): Mosaic aneuploidy characterized by multiple congenital abnormalities of the central nervous system, face, heart, and many other organs (see p. 471)

Trisomy 13 (Patau Syndrome): Occurring as a result of an extra chromosome 13, this is a severe abnormality characterized by multiple anomalies of the central nervous system, face, heart, and extremities (see p. 483)

Trisomy 18 (Edwards Syndrome): Occurring as a result of an extra chromosome 18, this is a severe abnormality characterized by IUGR and multiple anomalies of the central nervous system, face, heart, and extremities (see p. 490)

OTHER SYNDROMES AND SEQUENCES

Amniotic Band Syndrome: Condition caused by premature rupture of the amnion, resulting in an asymmetric, destructive fetal process whereby the fetus becomes adherent to, intertwined in, and tethered by the fibrous bands; associated with diverse anomalies (see p. 356)

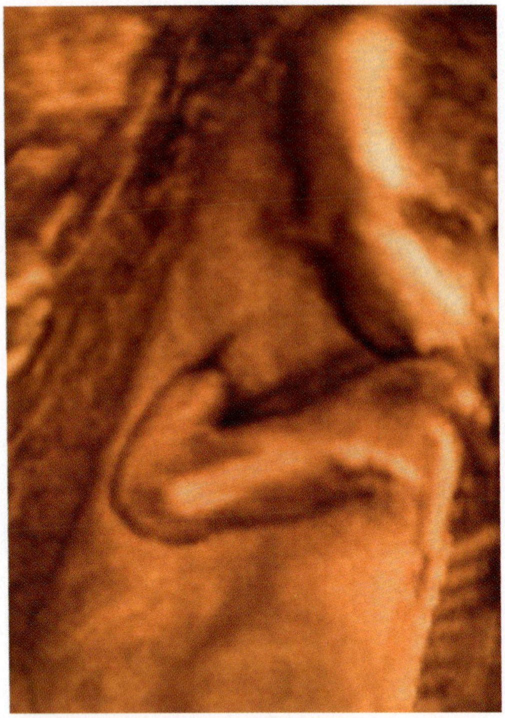

FIGURE 1-110 Surface rendering of a second-trimester fetal upper extremity showing transverse amputation below the elbow.

Caudal Regression Syndrome/Sirenomelia: Although of different etiologies, these two syndromes are similar; characterized by disruption of the caudal portion of the neural tube, absence or dysplasia of the sacrum, and renal and lower extremity anomalies (see p. 370)

MURCS Association: Müllerian duct aplasia, **r**enal aplasia, **c**ervicothoracic **s**omite dysplasia (occasional) (see p. 398)

Renal agenesis (occasional) (see p. 412)

VATER Association: Vertebral defects, **a**nal atresia, **t**racheoesophageal fistula, **e**sophageal atresia, and **r**adial and renal dysplasias (see p. 429)

TERATOGENS

Aminopterin (see p. 438)

Amitriptyline (see p. 437)

Cocaine (see p. 439)

Estrogen (see p. 437)

Fluorouracil (see p. 435)

Haloperidol (see p. 438)

Imipramine (see p. 438)

Progestin (see p. 437)

Tetracycline (see p. 434)

Thalidomide (see p. 437)

Valproic acid (see p. 436)

Warfarin (Coumadin) (see p. 435)

SHORT RADIAL RAY

GROWTH ABNORMALITIES

Cornelia de Lange Syndrome: Facial and limb malformations, growth restriction, and mental developmental delay (see p. 129)

FACIAL AND BRAIN ABNORMALITIES

Nager Syndrome: Acrofacial dysostosis syndrome similar to Treacher Collins syndrome; characterized primarily by mandibular hypoplasia, malformed ears, and abnormal radial ray (see p. 171)

LIMB AND SKELETAL ABNORMALITIES

Fanconi Anemia: Autosomal recessive condition characterized by radial hypoplasia, absent thumbs, and tendency for leukemia (see p. 229)

Holt-Oram Syndrome: Autosomal dominant condition characterized by upper extremity abnormalities, such as radial hypoplasia, and heart defects (see p. 238)

Roberts Syndrome: Autosomal recessive condition characterized by severe shortening of the limbs (pseudothalidomide syndrome) and facial anomalies (see p. 247)

Thrombocytopenia–Absent Radius (TAR) Syndrome: Autosomal recessive syndrome characterized by radial aplasia and thrombocytopenia (see p. 251)

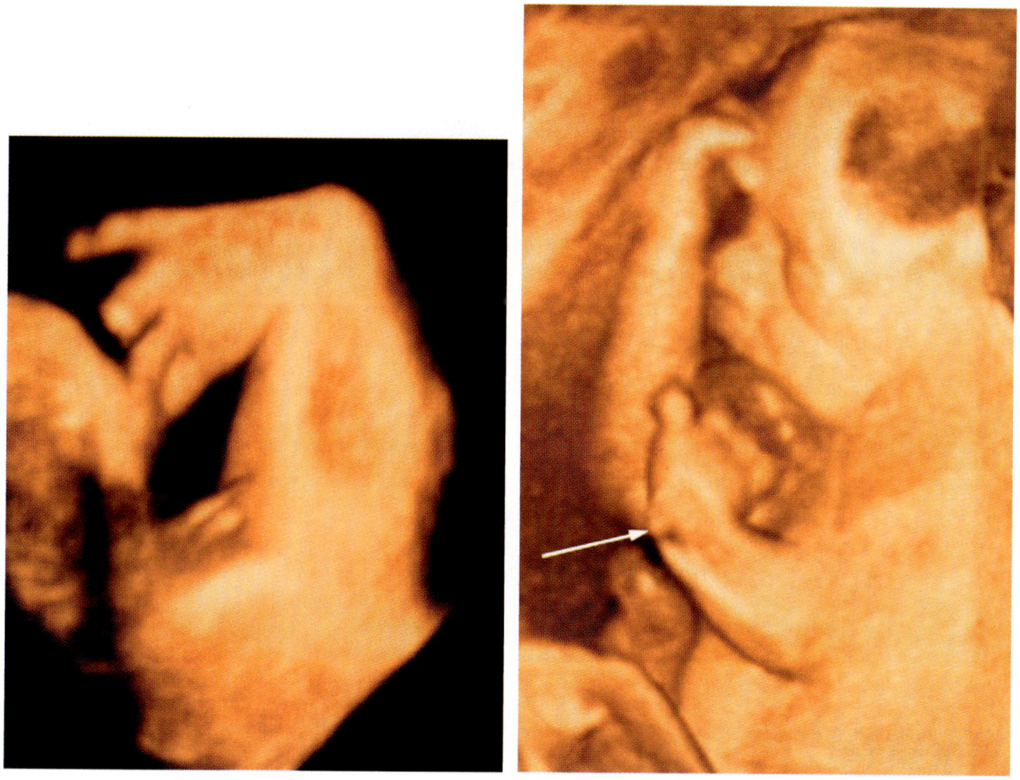

A B

FIGURE 1-111 (A) Surface rendering of third-trimester fetus with absent radius and thumb. Note acute angulation made by the hand and the forearm because of absence of thc radius. (B) Third-trimester fetus with short radial ray showing an abnormal angle *(arrow)* between the fetal hand and forearm resulting from the abnormal radius.

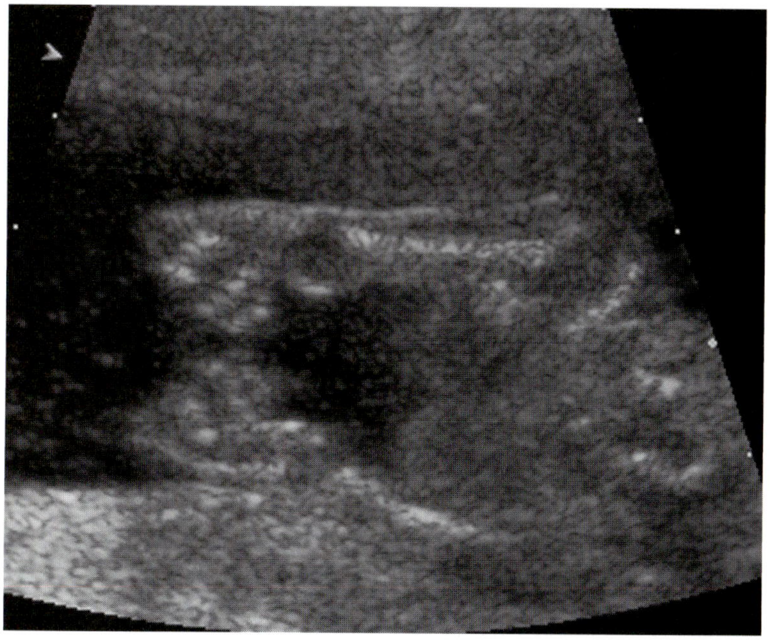

FIGURE 1-112 Bilateral radial ray abnormalities in a fetus with trisomy 18. Note symmetry of the abnormalities of the forearms with shortened ulna, absent radii, and club hands.

CHROMOSOMAL ANOMALIES

Trisomy 10: Rare abnormality with only those patients with mosaic trisomy 10 surviving to infancy. Abnormalities include IUGR and face, heart, hand, and feet anomalies (see p. 480)

Trisomy 13 (Patau Syndrome): Occurring as a result of an extra chromosome 13, this is a severe abnormality characterized by multiple anomalies of the central nervous system, face, heart, and extremities (see p. 483)

Trisomy 18 (Edwards Syndrome): Occurring as a result of an extra chromosome 18, this is a severe abnormality characterized by IUGR and multiple anomalies of the central nervous system, face, heart, and extremities (see p. 490)

OTHER SYNDROMES AND SEQUENCES

Amniotic Band Syndrome: Condition caused by premature rupture of the amnion, resulting in an asymmetric, destructive fetal process whereby the fetus becomes adherent to, intertwined in, and tethered by the fibrous bands; associated with diverse anomalies (see p. 356)

Renal Agenesis (occasional) (see p. 412)

VATER Association: **V**ertebral defects, **a**nal atresia, **t**racheoesophageal fistula, **e**sophageal atresia, **r**adial and renal dysplasias (see p. 429)

TERATOGENS

Fluorouracil (see p. 435)

Oral contraceptives (see p. 437)

Valproic acid (see p. 436)

CLUB FEET

FACIAL AND BRAIN ABNORMALITIES

Cerebrocostomandibular Syndrome: Autosomal recessive condition characterized by severe micrognathia, cleft palate, and vertebral body abnormalities associated with defective costal development (occasional) (see p. 152)

Hydrolethalus: Autosomal recessive disorder characterized by hydrocephalus, polydactyly, heart defects, and polyhydramnios (see p. 194)

Nager Syndrome: Acrofacial dysostosis syndrome similar to Treacher Collins syndrome; with mandibular hypoplasia, malformed ears, and abnormal radial ray (occasional) (see p. 171)

Stickler Syndrome: Autosomal dominant syndrome characterized by ocular defects, cleft palate, micrognathia/hypoplasia of the mandible, and early orthopedic degenerative abnormalities (see p. 181)

LIMB AND SKELETAL ABNORMALITIES

Adams-Oliver Syndrome: Disorder characterized by terminal transverse defects of the upper and lower extremities, as well as denuded areas on the scalp with or without an underlying bony skull (bone) defect (occasional) (see p. 223)

Atelosteogenesis, Type I: Lethal skeletal dysplasia with severe limb shortening and deficient ossification of bones, resulting in micromelic dwarfism (see p. 260)

Camptomelic Dysplasia: Short-limbed skeletal dysplasia characterized by bowing of the long bones, particularly in the lower extremities;

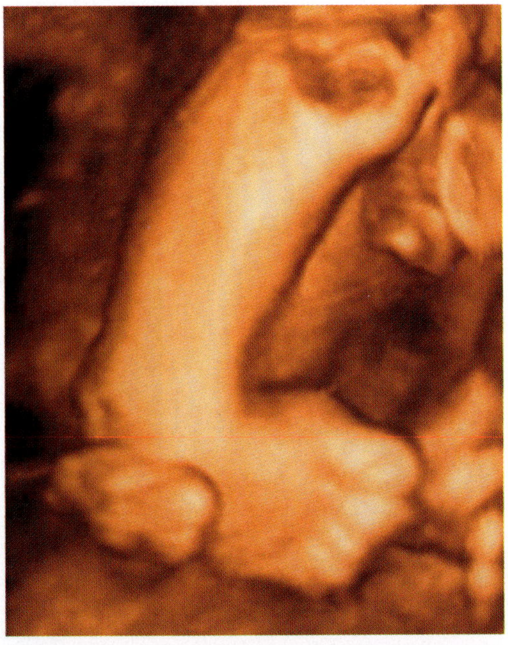

FIGURE 1-113 Surface rendering of third-trimester fetus with club foot.

bell-shaped, narrow chest; and facial anomalies (occasional) (see p. 262)

Diastrophic Dysplasia: Skeletal dysplasia characterized by micromelia, club feet, hand abnormalities (hitchhiker thumb), and kyphoscoliosis (see p. 270)

Ellis-van Creveld Syndrome: Autosomal recessive skeletal dysplasia characterized by disproportionately short extremities, narrow chest, polydactyly, and heart defects (see p. 272)

Femoral Hypoplasia–Unusual Facies Syndrome: Syndrome characterized by short lower limbs, especially hypoplastic femurs, and facial abnormalities; may be part of a spectrum of abnormalities that includes caudal regression syndrome (see p. 231)

Freeman-Sheldon (Whistling Face) Syndrome: Autosomal dominant condition characterized by unusual facial features and skeletal anomalies, such as flexion deformities of the joints (see p. 237)

Larsen Syndrome: Condition with abnormal facies and spine and limb abnormalities, including dislocations and hyperextensions at the joints (see p. 242)

Spondyloepiphyseal Dysplasia Congenita: Autosomal dominant, heterogeneous group of disorders with a short spine with platyspondyly, which results in kyphoscoliosis and lordosis (see p. 291)

CHROMOSOMAL ANOMALIES

Deletion 4p (Wolf-Hirschhorn Syndrome): Abnormality of chromosome 4 characterized by IUGR, facial dysmorphology, cardiac defects, and hypospadias (see p. 459)

Triploidy: Occurring as a result of a complete extra set of chromosomes, this is a lethal abnormality characterized by severe early-onset IUGR and multiple anomalies of practically all organ systems (see p. 473)

Trisomy 9: Occurring as a result of an extra chromosome 9, this is a severe abnormality characterized by multiple anomalies of practically all organ systems (see p. 478)

Trisomy 10: Rare abnormality with only those patients with mosaic trisomy 10 surviving to infancy. Abnormalities include IUGR and face, heart, hand, and feet anomalies (see p. 480)

Trisomy 18 (Edwards Syndrome): Occurring as a result of an extra chromosome 18, this is a severe abnormality characterized by IUGR and multiple anomalies of the central nervous system, face, heart, and extremities (see p. 490)

OTHER SYNDROMES AND SEQUENCES

Amniotic Band Syndrome: Condition caused by premature rupture of the amnion, resulting in an asymmetric, destructive fetal process whereby the fetus becomes adherent to, intertwined in, and tethered by the fibrous bands; associated with diverse anomalies (see p. 356)

Arthrogryposis: Sequence of neurologic, muscular, and connective tissue disorders leading to fetal joint contractures and rigidity, as well as decreased activity (see p. 362)

Caudal Regression Syndrome/Sirenomelia: Although of different etiologies, these two syndromes are similar; characterized by disruption of the caudal portion of the neural tube, absence or dysplasia of the sacrum, and renal and lower extremity anomalies (see p. 370)

Cerebro-Oculo-Facio-Skeletal (COFS) Syndrome: Autosomal recessive condition characterized by joint contractures of all the extremities, with severe facial and brain abnormalities (rockerbottom feet) (see p. 374)

Pena Shokeir Syndrome: Autosomal recessive condition characterized by IUGR, multiple joint contractures, facial anomalies, and pulmonary hypoplasia; also known as fetal akinesia/hypokinesia sequence or neurogenic arthrogryposis (see p. 402)

Pentalogy of Cantrell: Combination of five anomalies: ectopia cordis, omphalocele, disruption of distal sternum, anterior diaphragm, and diaphragmatic pericardium (occasional) (see p. 405)

Spinal Dysraphism (occasional) (see p. 418)

TERATOGENS

Carbamazepine (Tegretol) (see p. 436)

Aminopterin (see p. 438)

Clomiphene (see p. 437)

Cortisone (see p. 437)

Phenothiazine (see p. 438)

ROCKERBOTTOM FEET

LIMB AND SKELETAL ABNORMALITIES

Syndromes associated with lack of movement (see differential diagnosis of decreased activity) (see p. 113)

CRANIOSYNOSTOSIS

Antley-Bixler Syndrome: Disorder characterized by craniosynostosis, resulting in severe brachycephaly, midfacial hypoplasia, multiple skeletal fusions, and contractures (see p. 303)

CHROMOSOMAL ANOMALIES

Trisomy 18: Occurring as a result of an extra chromosome 18, this is a severe abnormality characterized by IUGR and multiple anomalies of the central nervous system, face, heart, and extremities (see p. 490)

OTHER SYNDROMES AND SEQUENCES

Cerebro-Oculo-Facio-Skeletal (COFS) Syndrome: Autosomal recessive condition characterized by joint contractures of all the extremities, with severe facial and brain abnormalities (see p. 374)

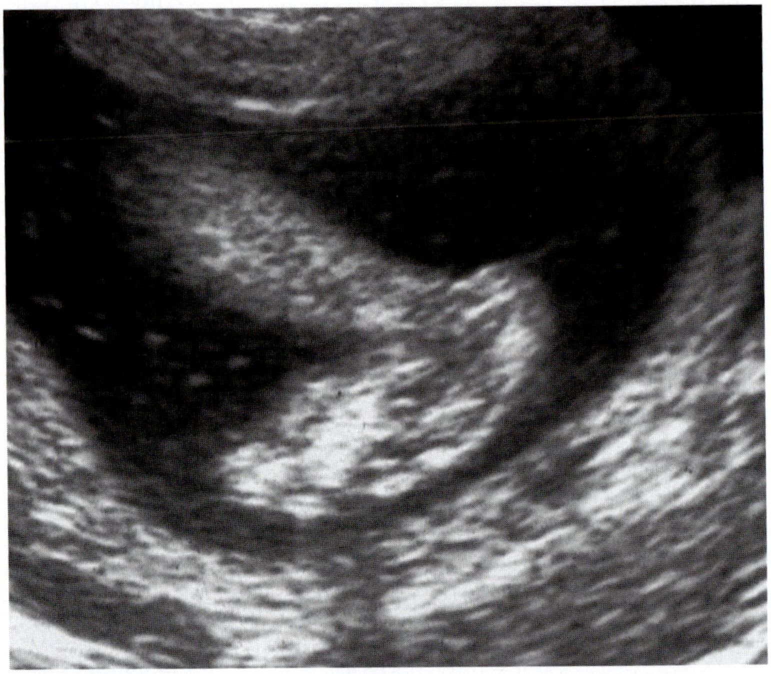

FIGURE 1-114 Longitudinal view of fetal foot with rockerbottom deformity.

FLARED METAPHYSES OR EPIPHYSES

LIMB AND SKELETAL ABNORMALITIES

Short Rib–Polydactyly Syndrome, Types I and III: Skeletal dysplasias characterized by short ribs, narrow chest, polydactyly, and short limbs (see p. 288)

Spondyloepiphyseal Dysplasia Congenita: Autosomal dominant, heterogeneous group of disorders characterized by a short spine with platyspondyly, which result in kyphoscoliosis and lordosis (see p. 291)

UNDEROSSIFICATION OF BONE

FACIAL AND BRAIN ABNORMALITIES

Cerebrocostomandibular Syndrome: Autosomal recessive condition characterized by severe micrognathia, cleft palate, and vertebral body abnormalities associated with defective costal development (ribs) (see p. 152)

LIMB AND SKELETAL ABNORMALITIES

Achondrogenesis: Lethal skeletal dysplasia characterized by extreme hypoplasia of the bones, micromelia, decreased ossification of the bones (particularly those of the skull and

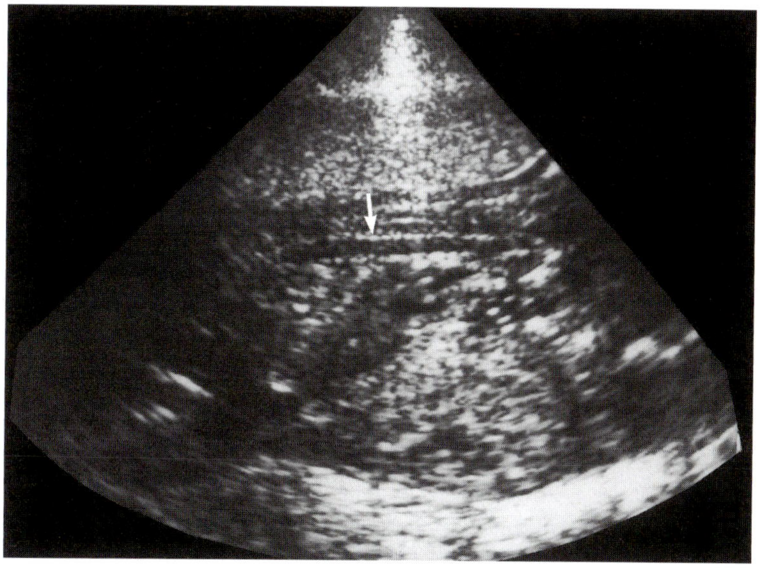

FIGURE 1-115 Longitudinal view of the spine of a fetus with achondrogenesis shows a remarkable lack of ossification of the spine *(arrow)*.

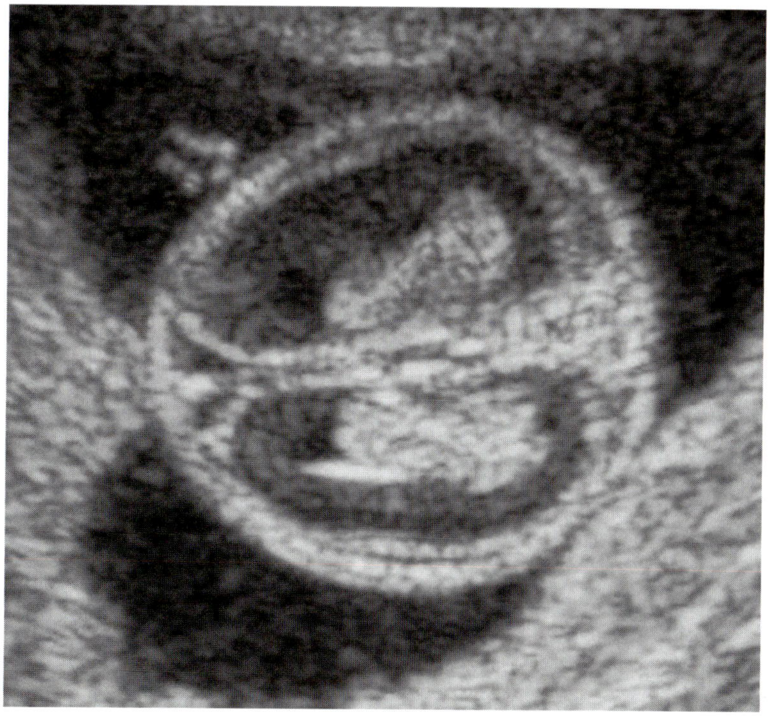

FIGURE 1-116 Early second-trimester fetus with osteogenesis imperfecta showing lack of ossification of the skull permitting excellent visualization of the brain.

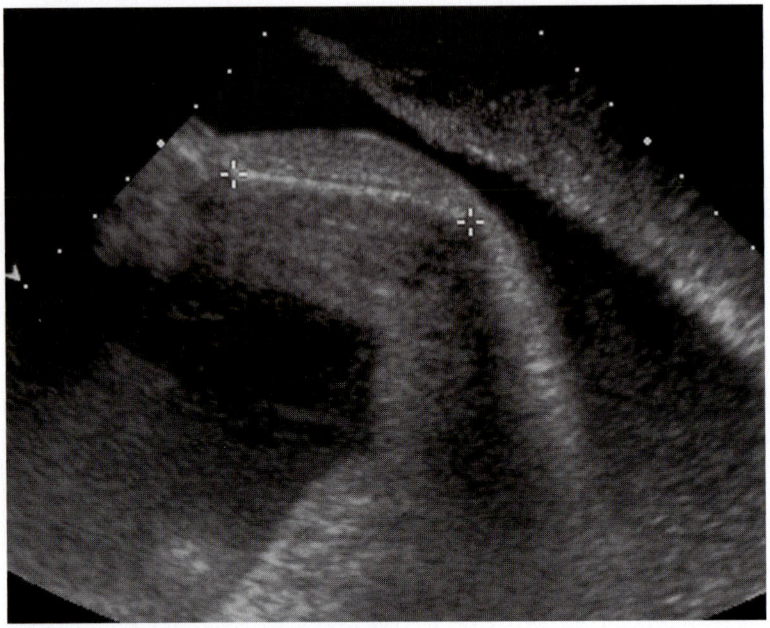

FIGURE 1-117 Third-trimester fetus with arthrogryposis with poor visualization of the long bones secondary to osteopenia.

spine), and hydrops (type I = skull; type II = spine) (see p. 253)

Adams-Oliver Syndrome: Disorder characterized by terminal transverse defects of the upper and lower extremities, as well as denuded areas on the scalp with or without an underlying bony skull (bone) defect (areas of skull) (see p. 223)

Arthrogryposis: Sequence of neurologic, muscular, and connective tissue disorders leading to fetal joint contractures and rigidity, as well as decreased activity (osteopenia) (see p. 362)

Atelosteogenesis, Type I: Lethal skeletal dysplasia characterized by severe limb shortening and deficient ossification of the bones, resulting in micromelic dwarfism (extremities) (see p. 260)

Hypophosphatasia: Autosomal recessive condition characterized by severe demineralization of the bones and congenital deficiency of alkaline phosphatase (skull) (see p. 275)

Osteogenesis Imperfecta: Heterogeneous group of conditions with severe osseous fragility, decreased ossification, and multiple fractures (skull) (see p. 345)

Short Rib–Polydactyly Syndrome, Types I and III: Skeletal dysplasias characterized by short ribs, narrow chest, polydactyly, and short limbs (spine) (see p. 288)

TERATOGENS

Aminopterin (see p. 438)

Carbamazepine (Tegretol) (see p. 436)

Fluphenazine (see p. 438)

CORD CYST/MASS

CHROMOSOMAL ANOMALIES

Trisomy 18 (Edwards Syndrome): Occurring as a result of an extra chromosome 18, this is a severe abnormality characterized by IUGR and multiple anomalies of the central nervous system, face, heart, and extremities (see p. 490)

OTHER

Allantoid Cyst

Aneurysm

Hemangioma (see p. 519)

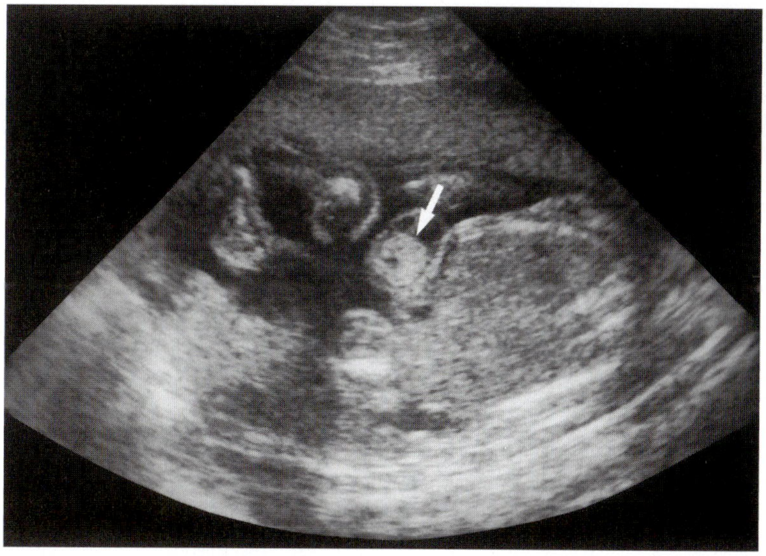

FIGURE 1-118 Cord hemangioma. Echogenic mass *(arrow)* is seen in the umbilical cord of a fetus who was otherwise normal. The mass was diagnosed as a hemangioma at birth.

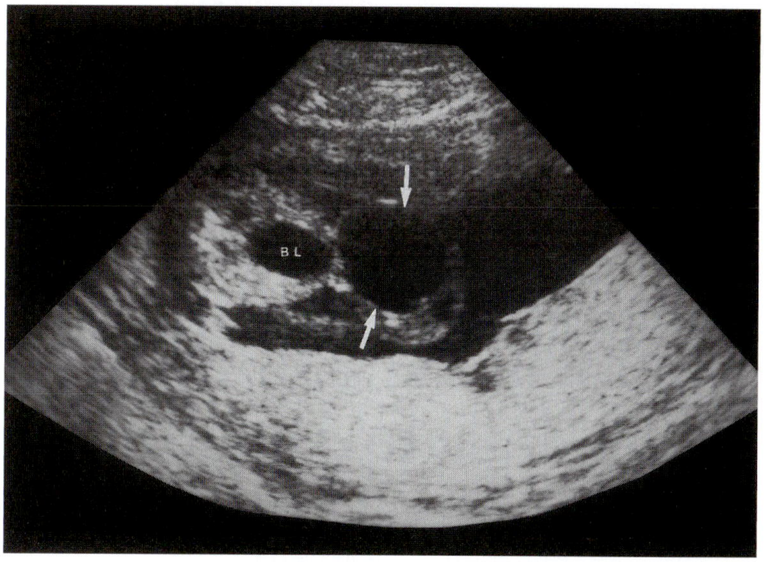

FIGURE 1-119 Longitudinal view of fetal bladder *(BL)* at the level of insertion of the cord. A large cyst *(arrows)* is located within the proximal portion of the cord. This was diagnosed at birth as a urachal cyst, which was successfully repaired.

Hematoma

Omphalomesenteric Cyst

Pseudocyst (Wharton Jelly Degeneration)

Teratoma (see p. 525)

Urachal Cyst

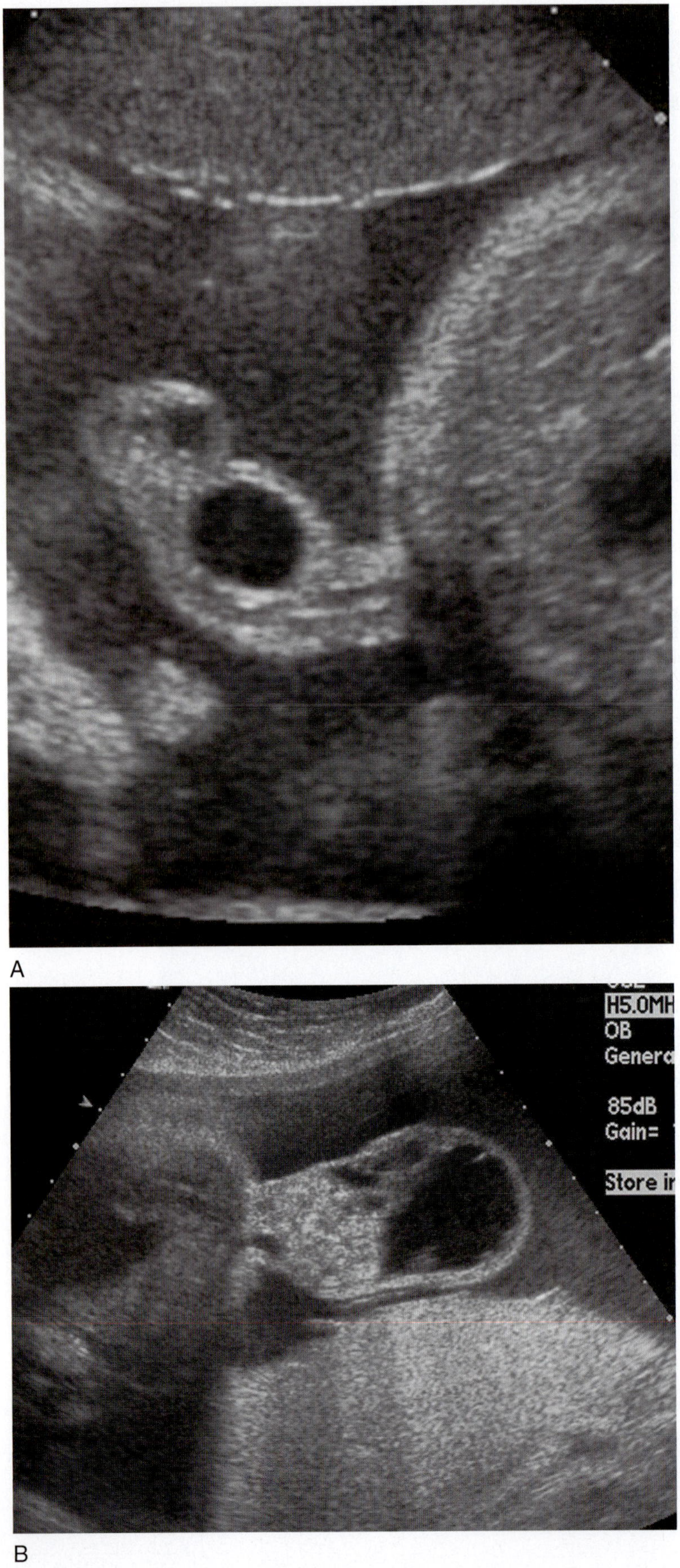

FIGURE 1-120 (**A**) Second-trimester fetus with small umbilical cord cyst. (**B**) Second-trimester fetus with a small bowel containing omphalocele and umbilical cord cyst.

HYDROPS

ANEMIA

Fetal–Maternal Hemorrhage

Isoimmune Parvovirus

Twin-to-Twin Transfusion Syndrome

CARDIOVASCULAR ANOMALIES

Arteriovenous Shunt (Aneurysm of Vein of Galen)

Bradycardia

Cardiomyopathy

Heart Defect

Tachycardia

Idiopathic Arterial Calcification of Infancy: Rare autosomal recessive syndrome characterized by disruption and calcification of the internal elastic laminae of fetal arteries, with calcium deposits leading to fibrosis and occlusion of the arteries, hydrops, and death (see p. 391)

CHROMOSOMAL ANOMALIES

Deletion 5p (Cri du Chat Syndrome): Abnormality of chromosome 5 characterized by microcephaly, hypertelorism, micrognathia, hydrops, and growth delay (see p. 457)

Tetrasomy 12p (Pallister-Killian Syndrome): Mosaic aneuploidy characterized by multiple congenital abnormalities of the central nervous system, face, heart, and many other organs (see p. 471)

Trisomy 21 (Down Syndrome): Occurring as a result of an extra chromosome 21, this abnor-

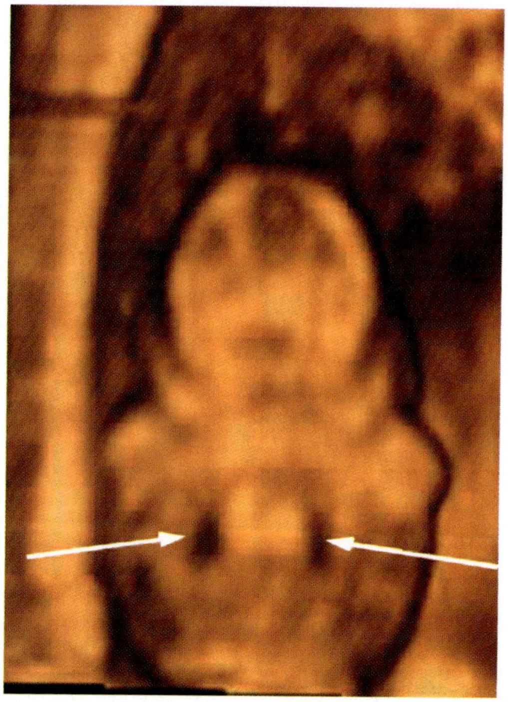

FIGURE 1-121 Three-dimensional surface rendering of a 8.5-week fetus with fetal hydrops and cystic hygromas. Note the bilateral pleural effusions *(arrows)*.

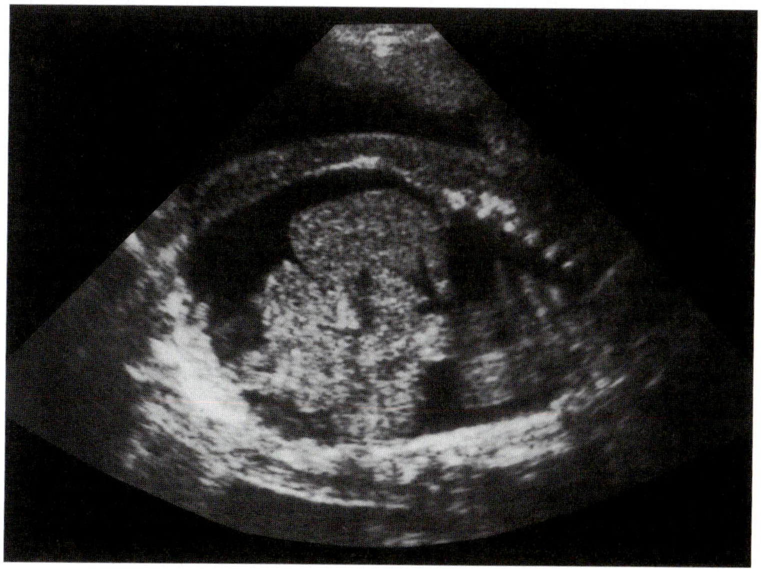

FIGURE 1-122 Longitudinal view of the chest and abdomen of a fetus with nonimmune hydrops. Evidence of ascites, pleural effusions, and skin edema is seen.

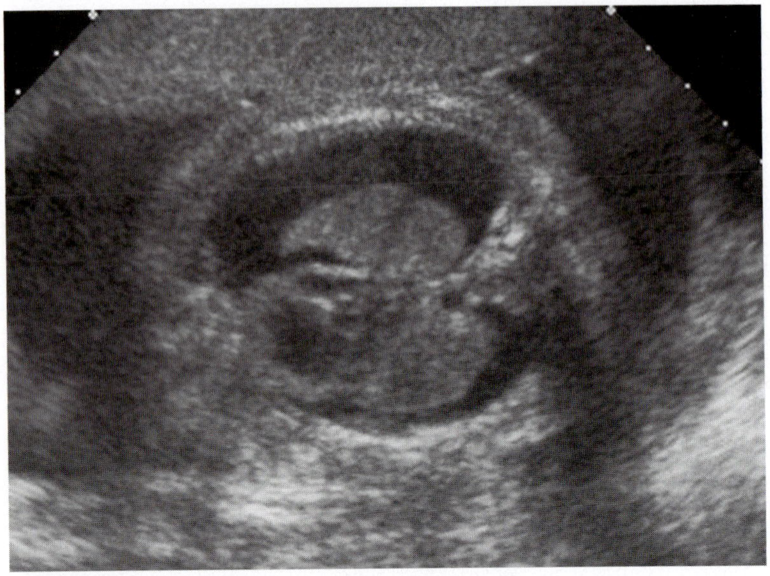

FIGURE 1-123 Transverse view through the fetal chest of a fetus with hydrops showing bilateral pleural effusions.

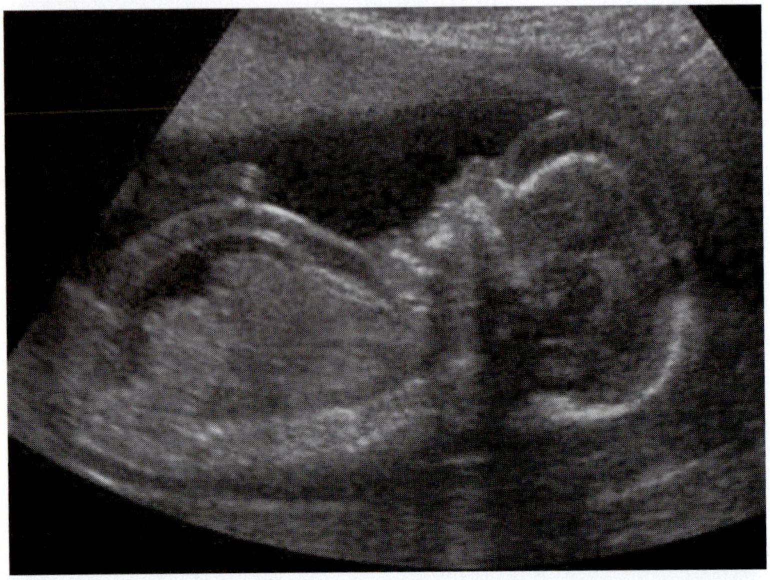

FIGURE 1-124 Second-trimester fetus with Down syndrome and fetal hydrops. Note severe scalp and skin edema, as well as ascites.

mality is characterized by nuchal fold thickening, short long-bones, abnormal nasal bone, heart defects, and other anomalies. Twenty-five percent of fetuses with Down syndrome do not display any sonographic abnormalities or markers (occasional) (see p. 496)

XO Syndrome (Turner Syndrome): Occurring as a result of a single X chromosome (XO), Turner syndrome is characterized primarily in early pregnancy by large cystic hygromata, lymphangiectasia, and heart defects. Affected infants who survive gestation may represent Turner mosaic individuals (see p. 510)

Other Chromosomal Abnormalities

TUMORS

Chest Masses (causing mediastinal compression) (see differential diagnosis for intrathoracic mass) (see p. 61)

Chorioangioma

Cystic Hygroma (see p. 515)

Gastrointestinal Obstructions

Hepatic Tumor (hemangioendothelioma)

Lymphangioma (see p. 515)

Teratoma (see p. 525)

MATERNAL INFECTION

Cytomegalovirus (see p. 441)

Parvovirus (see p. 446)

Syphilis (see p. 450)

Toxoplasmosis (see p. 452)

Varicella (see p. 456)

OTHER SYNDROMES

Achondrogenesis: Lethal skeletal dysplasia with extreme hypoplasia of the bones, micromelia, decreased ossification of the bones (particularly those of the skull and spine), and hydrops (see p. 253)

Alpha-Thalassemia (see p. 336)

Congenital High Airway Obstruction Syndrome: Group of disorders characterized by complete obstruction of the upper airway, secondary to either laryngeal or glottic atresia and leading to massive enlargement of the lungs (see p. 380)

Fryns Syndrome: Autosomal recessive condition with diaphragmatic defects, digital and facial abnormalities, and brain anomalies (occasional) (see p. 325)

Glycogen Storage Diseases

Multiple Pterygium Syndrome: Autosomal recessive condition with multiple contractures and webbing across joints, cystic hygromata, and facial defects (see p. 244)

Neu-Laxova Syndrome: Autosomal recessive condition with microcephaly, lissencephaly, exophthalmos, severe IUGR, swollen subcutaneous tissues, and ichthyosis (see p. 211)

Noonan Syndrome: Phenotypically, a Turner-like syndrome featuring short stature, webbed neck, cardiac abnormalities, and normal karyotype (see p. 131)

Osteogenesis Imperfecta: Heterogeneous group of conditions characterized by severe osseous fragility, decreased ossification, and multiple fractures (see p. 345)

DECREASED ACTIVITY

FACIAL AND BRAIN ABNORMALITIES

Neural Tube Defects (see p. 418)

LIMB AND SKELETAL ABNORMALITIES

Arthrogryposis: Sequence of neurologic, muscular, and connective tissue disorders leading to fetal joint contractures, rigidity, decreased activity (see p. 362)

Multiple Pterygium Syndrome: Autosomal recessive condition characterized by multiple contractures and webbing across the joints, cystic hygromata, and facial defects (see p. 244)

CRANIOSYNOSTOSIS

Antley-Bixler Syndrome: Disorder characterized by craniosynostosis, resulting in severe brachycephaly, midfacial hypoplasia, multiple skeletal fusions, and contractures (see p. 303)

OTHER SYNDROMES AND SEQUENCES

Caudal Regression Syndrome/Sirenomelia: Although of different etiologies, these two syndromes are similar; characterized by disruption of the caudal portion of the neural tube, absence or dysplasia of the sacrum, and renal and lower extremity anomalies (see p. 370)

Harlequin Syndrome and Other Restrictive Fetal Skin Diseases: Harlequin Syndrome: Autosomal recessive condition characterized by massive overgrowth of the keratin layers of skin, resulting in parchment appearance and clown-like face (see p. 339)

Pena Shokeir Syndrome: Autosomal recessive condition characterized by IUGR, multiple joint contractures, facial anomalies, and pulmonary hypoplasia; also known as fetal akinesia/hypokinesia sequence or neurogenic arthrogryposis (see p. 402)

INTRAUTERINE GROWTH RESTRICTION

GROWTH ABNORMALITIES

Cornelia de Lange Syndrome: Facial and limb malformations, growth restriction, and mental developmental delay (see p. 129)

Russell-Silver Syndrome: Asymmetric growth restriction of the skeleton in conjunction with a normal-size head and short stature (see p. 136)

Seckel Syndrome: Autosomal recessive syndrome characterized by severe IUGR with microcephaly and a severely abnormal profile (see p. 138)

Smith-Lemli-Opitz Syndrome: Autosomal recessive syndrome featuring microcephaly, mental retardation, and genital and renal anomalies (late onset) (see p. 140)

FACIAL AND BRAIN ABNORMALITIES

Branchio-Oculo-Facial Syndrome: Autosomal dominant disorder characterized by mental retardation, growth deficiency, ocular defects, and clefting of the upper lip (see p. 149)

Miller-Dieker Syndrome: Lissencephaly, type I; characterized by complete absence of gyri of the brain, microcephaly, and severe mental retardation (see p. 208)

Neu-Laxova Syndrome: Autosomal recessive condition characterized by microcephaly, lissencephaly, exophthalmos, severe IUGR, swollen subcutaneous tissues, and ichthyosis (see p. 211)

LIMB AND SKELETAL ABNORMALITIES

Adams-Oliver Syndrome: Disorder characterized by terminal transverse defects of the upper and lower extremities, as well as denuded areas on the scalp with or without an underlying bony skull (bone) defect (see p. 223)

Freeman-Sheldon (Whistling Face) Syndrome: Autosomal dominant condition characterized by unusual facial features and skeletal anomalies, such as flexion deformities of the joints (see p. 237)

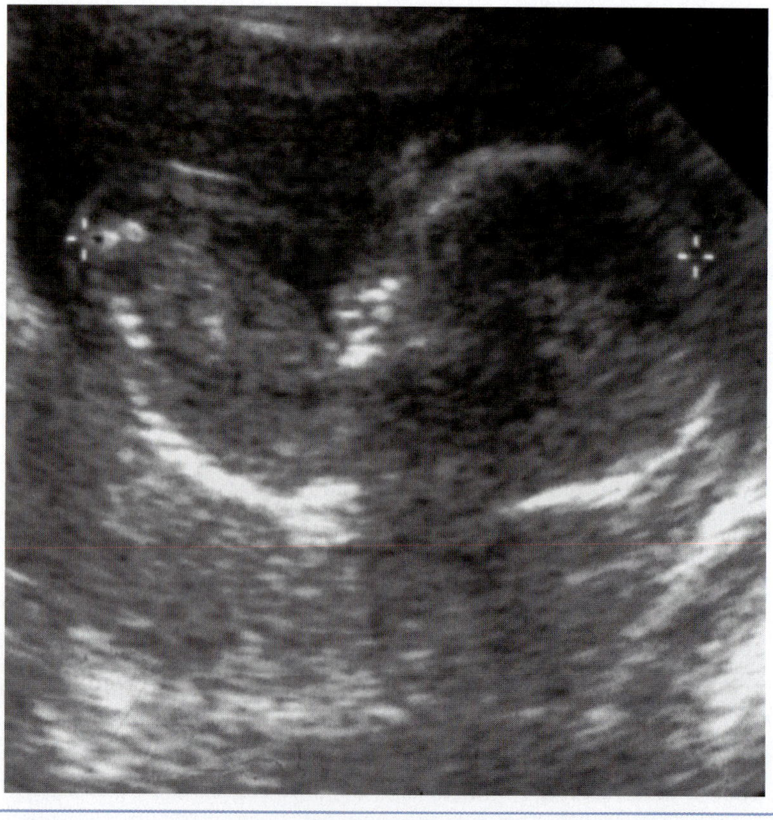

FIGURE 1-125 First-trimester fetus with triploidy and early-onset intrauterine growth restriction. Note that the body is small for the size of the head, characteristic of this condition.

Osteopetrosis: Autosomal recessive condition characterized by diffuse skeletal sclerosis and resulting in increased bone density, fractures, ventriculomegaly, and shortened long bones (see p. 287)

Roberts Syndrome: Autosomal recessive condition characterized by severe shortening of the limbs (pseudothalidomide syndrome) and facial anomalies (see p. 247)

CHROMOSOMAL ANOMALIES

Deletion 4p (Wolf-Hirschhorn Syndrome): Abnormality of chromosome 4 characterized by IUGR, facial dysmorphology, cardiac defects, and hypospadias (see p. 457)

Deletion 5p (Cri du Chat Syndrome): Abnormality of chromosome 5 characterized by microcephaly, hypertelorism, micrognathia, hydrops, and growth delay (see p. 459)

Deletion 11q (Jacobsen Syndrome): Deletion of the distal long arm of chromosome 11 characterized by multiple anomalies of practically all organ systems (see p. 464)

Triploidy: Occurring as a result of a complete extra set of chromosomes, this is a lethal abnormality characterized by severe early-onset IUGR and multiple anomalies of practically all organ systems (most severe) (see p. 473)

Trisomy 9: Occurring as a result of an extra chromosome 9, this is a severe abnormality characterized by multiple anomalies of practically all organ systems (see p. 478)

Trisomy 10: Rare abnormality with only those patients with mosaic trisomy 10 surviving to infancy. Abnormalities include IUGR and face, heart, hand, and feet anomalies (see p. 480)

Trisomy 18 (Edwards Syndrome): Occurring as a result of an extra chromosome 18, this is a severe abnormality characterized by IUGR and multiple anomalies of the central nervous system, face, heart, and extremities (see p. 490)

OTHER SYNDROMES AND SEQUENCES

Harlequin Syndrome: Autosomal recessive condition characterized by a massive overgrowth of the keratin layers of skin, resulting in parchment appearance and clown-like face (see p. 339)

TERATOGENS

Acetazolamide (see p. 438)

Alcohol (see p. 438)

Aminopterin (see p. 438)

Aspirin (occasional) (see p. 435)

Azathioprine (see p. 435)

Cocaine (see p. 439)

Cortisone (see p. 437)

Cytarabine (see p. 435)

Cytomegalovirus (see p. 441)

Hydantoin (see p. 436)

Hyperthermia (see p. 439)

Methotrexate (see p. 435)

Phenantoin (see p. 436)

Propranolol (see p. 439)

Radiation (see p. 439)

Rubella (see p. 449)

Smoking (see p. 440)

Toxoplasmosis (see p. 452)

Trimethadione (see p. 436)

Valproic acid (see p. 436)

Warfarin (Coumadin) (see p. 435)

ENLARGED PLACENTA

GROWTH ABNORMALITIES

Beckwith-Wiedemann Syndrome: Gigantism in utero in conjunction with macroglossia, omphalocele, and renal anomalies (see p. 142)

CHROMOSOMAL ANOMALIES

Triploidy: Occurring as a result of a complete extra set of chromosomes, this is a lethal abnormality characterized by severe early-onset IUGR and multiple anomalies of practically all organ systems (see p. 473)

TERATOGENS

Cytomegalovirus (CMV) (see p. 441)

Syphilis (see p. 450)

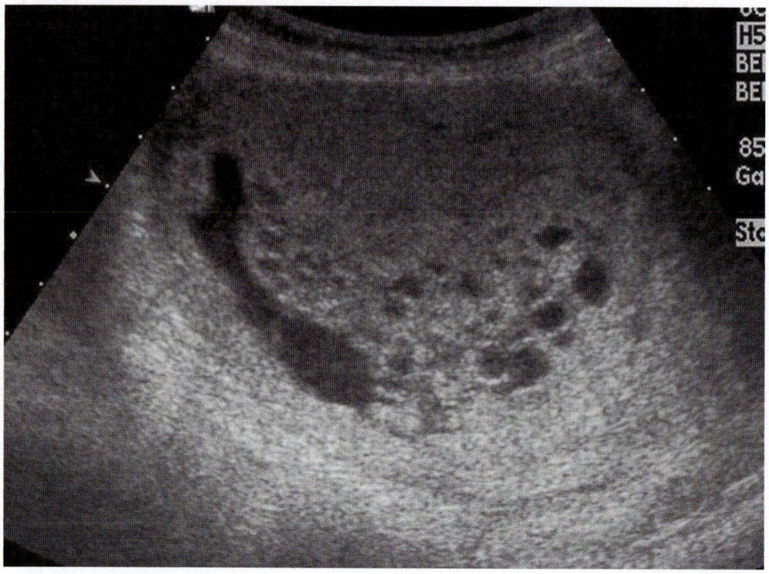

FIGURE 1-126 Enlarged placenta with multiple echolucencies consistent with molar pregnancy. This is often associated with triploidy.

POLYHYDRAMNIOS

GROWTH ABNORMALITIES

Beckwith-Wiedemann Syndrome: Gigantism in utero in conjunction with macroglossia, omphalocele, and renal anomalies (see p. 142)

Perlman Syndrome: Autosomal recessive fetal overgrowth syndrome characterized by macrosomia, bilaterally enlarged kidneys, renal tumors, and other visceromegaly associated with polyhydramnios (see p. 147)

FACIAL AND BRAIN ABNORMALITIES

Fraser Syndrome: Autosomal recessive syndrome featuring cryptophthalmos; syndactyly; and genital, renal, and tracheal anomalies (occasional) (see p. 160)

Goldenhar Syndrome: Asymmetry of the face and ears in conjunction with vertebral anomalies of the upper spine (see p. 162)

Hydrolethalus: Autosomal recessive disorder characterized by hydrocephalus, polydactyly, heart defects, and polyhydramnios (see p. 194)

Miller-Dieker Syndrome: Lissencephaly, type I; characterized by complete absence of gyri of the brain, microcephaly, and severe mental retardation (see p. 208)

Nager Syndrome: Acrofacial dysostosis syndrome similar to Treacher Collins syndrome; characterized primarily by mandibular hypoplasia, malformed ears, and abnormal radial ray (occasional) (see p. 171)

Neu-Laxova Syndrome: Autosomal recessive condition characterized by microcephaly, lissencephaly, exophthalmos, severe IUGR, swollen subcutaneous tissues, and ichthyosis (see p. 211)

Oral-Facial-Digital Syndrome, Type II (Mohr Syndrome): Autosomal recessive syndrome characterized by short stature, deafness, and facial, hand, and foot abnormalities (see p. 175)

Pierre Robin Syndrome: Hypoplasia of the mandible and cleft palate (see p. 177)

Stickler Syndrome: Autosomal dominant syndrome characterized by ocular defects, cleft palate, micrognathia/hypoplasia of the mandible, and early orthopedic degenerative abnormalities (see p. 181)

LIMB AND SKELETAL ABNORMALITIES

Achondrogenesis: Lethal skeletal dysplasia with extreme hypoplasia of the bones, micromelia, decreased ossification of the bones (particularly those of the skull and spine), and hydrops (see p. 253)

Arthrogryposis: Sequence of neurologic, muscular, and connective tissue disorders leading to fetal joint contractures and rigidity, as well as decreased activity (see p. 362)

Atelosteogenesis, Type I: Lethal skeletal dysplasia characterized by severe limb shortening and deficient ossification of the bones, resulting in micromelic dwarfism (see p. 260)

Cerebrocostomandibular Syndrome: Autosomal recessive condition characterized by severe micrognathia, cleft palate, and vertebral body abnormalities associated with defective costal development (see p. 152)

Diastrophic Dysplasia: Skeletal dysplasia characterized by micromelia, club feet, hand abnormalities (hitchhiker thumb), and kyphoscoliosis (see p. 270)

Jeune Thoracic Dystrophy (Asphyxiating Thoracic Dysplasia): Autosomal recessive skeletal dysplasia characterized by very narrow chest with short ribs, moderately short long-bones, and occasional polydactyly (see p. 278)

Kniest Syndrome: Autosomal dominant condition characterized by kyphoscoliosis, platyspondyly, and shortened tubular long bones (see p. 281)

Majewski Syndrome (Short Rib–Polydactyly Syndrome, Type II): Autosomal recessive skeletal dysplasia characterized by short ribs, narrow thorax, polydactyly, and median facial cleft (see p. 283)

Multiple Pterygium Syndrome: Autosomal recessive condition characterized by multiple contractures and webbing across the joints, cystic hygromata, and facial defects (see p. 244)

Roberts Syndrome: Autosomal recessive condition characterized by severe shortening of the limbs (pseudothalidomide syndrome) and facial anomalies (occasional) (see p. 247)

Short Rib–Polydactyly Syndrome, Types I and III: Skeletal dysplasias characterized by short ribs, narrow chest, polydactyly, and short limbs (see p. 288)

Thanatophoric Dysplasia: Most common skeletal dysplasia; narrow chest; short ribs; short, bowed long bones; flat vertebral bodies (see p. 294)

CRANIOSYNOSTOSIS

Antley-Bixler Syndrome: Disorder characterized by craniosynostosis, resulting in severe brachycephaly, midfacial hypoplasia, multiple skeletal fusions, and contractures (see p. 303)

CHROMOSOMAL ANOMALIES

Tetrasomy 12p (Pallister-Killian Syndrome): Mosaic aneuploidy characterized by multiple congenital abnormalities of the central nervous system, face, heart, and many other organs (see p. 471)

Trisomy 18: Occurring as a result of an extra chromosome 18, this is a severe abnormality characterized by IUGR and multiple anomalies of the central nervous system, face, heart, and extremities (see p. 490)

OTHER SYNDROMES AND SEQUENCES

Alpha-Thalassemia (see p. 336)

CHARGE Association: **C**oloboma of the iris, **h**eart defect, choanal **a**tresia, intrauterine growth **r**estriction, **g**enital anomalies, and **e**ar anomalies (see p. 376)

Cystic Fibrosis: Autosomal recessive disorder characterized by chronic respiratory obstruction and infection, exocrine pancreatic insufficiency, and elevated sweat chlorine levels (see p. 322)

Diabetes (see p. 146)

Fryns Syndrome: Autosomal recessive condition characterized by diaphragmatic defects, digital and facial abnormalities, and brain anomalies (see p. 325)

Idiopathic Arterial Calcification of Infancy: Rare autosomal recessive syndrome characterized by disruption and calcification of the internal elastic laminae of fetal arteries, with calcium deposits leading to fibrosis and occlusion of the arteries, hydrops, and death (see p. 391)

Maternal Diabetes (see p. 146)

Megacystis-Microcolon-Intestinal Hypoperistalsis Syndrome: Autosomal recessive lethal condition caused by decreased muscle tone in the intestinal and urinary tracts, resulting in markedly dilated urinary bladder and hypoperistalsis of the colon (occasional) (see p. 396)

Pena Shokeir Syndrome: Autosomal recessive condition characterized by IUGR, multiple joint contractures, facial anomalies, and pulmonary hypoplasia; also known as fetal akinesia/hypokinesia sequence or neurogenic arthrogryposis (see p. 402)

Tumors (see p. 515)

VATER Association: **V**ertebral defects, **a**nal atresia, **t**racheoesophageal fistula, **e**sophageal atresia, and **r**adial and renal dysplasias (see p. 429)

TERATOGENS

Cytomegalovirus (CMV) (see p. 441)

Parvovirus (see p. 446)

Varicella (see p. 456)

OLIGOHYDRAMNIOS

FACIAL AND BRAIN ABNORMALITIES

Fraser Syndrome: Autosomal recessive syndrome featuring cryptophthalmos, syndactyly, and genital, renal, and tracheal anomalies (occasional) (see p. 160)

Meckel-Gruber Syndrome: Autosomal recessive condition characterized by posterior encephalocele, postaxial polydactyly, and polycystic kidneys (see p. 199)

OTHER SYNDROMES AND SEQUENCES

Caudal Regression Syndrome/Sirenomelia: Although of different etiologies, these two syndromes are similar; characterized by disruption of the caudal portion of the neural tube, absence or dysplasia of the sacrum, and renal and lower extremity anomalies (see p. 370)

Cloacal Exstrophy Sequence: Complex disorder characterized by a combination of defects that include omphalocele, imperforate anus, cloacal exstrophy, spinal defects, and genital abnormalities (see p. 382)

Congenital High Airway Obstruction Syndrome: Group of disorders characterized by complete obstruction of the upper airway, secondary to either laryngeal or glottic atresia and leading to massive enlargement of the lungs (see p. 380)

Infantile Polycystic Kidney Disease (see p. 329)

Megacystis-Microcolon-Intestinal Hypoperistalsis Syndrome: Autosomal recessive lethal condition caused by decreased muscle tone in the intestinal and urinary tracts, resulting in markedly dilated urinary bladder and hypoperistalsis of the colon (see p. 396)

Prune-Belly Syndrome: Triad of abdominal wall distention, urinary tract obstruction, and cryptorchidism (see p. 408)

Renal Agenesis and Syndromes Featuring Renal Agenesis (see p. 412)

TERATOGEN

Cytomegalovirus (CMV) (see p. 441)

HEART DEFECTS

GROWTH ABNORMALITIES

Cornelia de Lange Syndrome: Facial and limb malformations, growth restriction, and mental developmental delay (see p. 129)

Noonan Syndrome: Phenotypically, a Turner-like syndrome featuring short stature, webbed neck, cardiac abnormalities, and normal karyotype (see p. 131)

Perlman Syndrome: Autosomal recessive fetal overgrowth syndrome characterized by macrosomia, bilaterally enlarged kidneys, renal tumors, and other visceromegaly associated with polyhydramnios (see p. 147)

Smith-Lemli-Opitz Syndrome: Autosomal recessive syndrome featuring microcephaly, mental retardation, and genital and renal anomalies (see p. 140)

FACIAL AND BRAIN ABNORMALITIES

Cerebrocostomandibular Syndrome: Autosomal recessive condition characterized by severe micrognathia, cleft palate, and vertebral body abnormalities associated with defective costal development (occasional ventriculoseptal defect) (see p. 152)

Goldenhar Syndrome: Asymmetry of the face and ears in conjunction with vertebral anomalies of the upper spine (occasional) (see p. 162)

Hydrolethalus: Autosomal recessive disorder characterized by hydrocephalus, polydactyly, heart defects, and polyhydramnios (see p. 194)

Meckel-Gruber Syndrome: Autosomal recessive condition characterized by posterior encephalocele, postaxial polydactyly, and polycystic kidneys (see p. 199)

Median Cleft Face: Midline facial defects resulting in hypertelorism and bifid or broad nasal bridge (occasional) (see p. 165), (occasional tetralogy of Fallot) (see p. 165)

Miller-Dieker Syndrome: Lissencephaly, type I; characterized by complete absence of gyri of the brain, microcephaly, and severe mental retardation (see p. 208)

Neu-Laxova Syndrome: Autosomal recessive condition characterized by microcephaly, lissencephaly, exophthalmos, severe IUGR, swollen subcutaneous tissues, and ichthyosis (occasional) (see p. 211)

Shprintzen Syndrome: Autosomal dominant syndrome characterized by short stature, mild mental retardation, micrognathia, and cardiac and limb abnormalities (see p. 179)

LIMB AND SKELETAL ABNORMALITIES

Adams-Oliver Syndrome: Disorder characterized by terminal transverse defects of the upper and lower extremities, as well as denuded areas on the scalp with or without an underlying bony skull (bone) defect (occasional) (see p. 223)

Camptomelic Dysplasia: Short-limbed skeletal dysplasia characterized by bowing of the long bones, particularly in the lower extremities; bell-shaped, narrow chest; and facial anomalies (occasional) (see p. 262)

Chondrodysplasia Punctata (Nonrhizomelic Type)**:** Heterogeneous group of bone dysplasias characterized by asymmetric limb shortening and abnormal early calcification of the proximal and distal epiphyses (occasional) (see p. 266)

Ellis-van Creveld Syndrome: Autosomal recessive skeletal dysplasia characterized by disproportionately short extremities, narrow chest, polydactyly, and heart defects (see p. 272)

Fanconi Anemia: Autosomal recessive condition characterized by radial hypoplasia, absent thumbs, and tendency for leukemia (occasional) (see p. 229)

Holt-Oram Syndrome: Autosomal dominant condition characterized by upper extremity abnormalities, such as radial hypoplasia, and heart defects (see p. 238)

Larsen Syndrome: Condition characterized by abnormal facies and spine and limb abnormalities, including dislocations and hyperextensions at the joints (occasional) (see p. 242)

Multiple Pterygium Syndrome: Autosomal recessive condition characterized by multiple contractures and webbing across the joints, cystic hygromata, and facial defects (occasional) (see p. 244)

Roberts Syndrome: Autosomal recessive condition characterized by severe shortening of the limbs (pseudothalidomide syndrome) and facial anomalies (occasional) (see p. 247)

Short Rib–Polydactyly Syndrome, Types I and III: Skeletal dysplasias characterized by short ribs, narrow chest, polydactyly, and short limbs (see p. 288)

Thanatophoric Dysplasia: Most common skeletal dysplasia; characterized by narrow chest; short ribs; short, bowed long bones; and flat vertebral bodies (occasional) (see p. 294)

Thrombocytopenia–Absent Radius (TAR) Syndrome: Autosomal recessive syndrome characterized by radial aplasia and thrombocytopenia (occasional) (see p. 251)

CRANIOSYNOSTOSIS

Antley-Bixler Syndrome: Disorder characterized by craniosynostosis, resulting in severe brachycephaly, midfacial hypoplasia, multiple skeletal fusions, and contractures (occasional) (see p. 303)

Apert Syndrome: Craniosynostosis, acrocephaly, and syndactyly (occasional) (see p. 304)

Carpenter Syndrome: Autosomal recessive condition characterized by acrocephaly, syndactyly, and preaxial polydactyly (see p. 310)

Pfeiffer Syndrome: Acrocephalic skull, craniosynostosis (particularly of the coronal and sagittal sutures), and syndactyly of hands and feet (occasional) (see p. 316)

CHROMOSOMAL ANOMALIES

Deletion 4p (Wolf-Hirschhorn Syndrome): Abnormality of chromosome 4 characterized by IUGR, facial dysmorphology, cardiac defects, and hypospadias (see p. 457)

Deletion 5p (Cri du Chat Syndrome): Abnormality of chromosome 5 characterized by microcephaly, hypertelorism, micrognathia, hydrops, and growth delay (see p. 459)

Deletion 11q (Jacobsen Syndrome): Deletion of the distal long arm of chromosome 11 characterized by multiple anomalies of practically all organ systems (see p. 464)

DiGeorge Syndrome: Also known as velocardiofacial syndrome or Shprintzen syndrome, this disorder results from a deletion of chromosome 22q11.2 and is characterized by cardiac abnormalities involving largely the great vessels, facial abnormalities, hypocalcemia, and hypoplasia of the thymus (see p. 466)

Tetrasomy 12p (Pallister-Killian Syndrome): Mosaic aneuploidy characterized by multiple congenital abnormalities of the central nervous system, face, heart, and many other organs (see p. 471)

Triploidy: Occurring as a result of a complete extra set of chromosomes, this is a lethal abnormality characterized by severe early-onset IUGR and multiple anomalies of practically all organ systems (see p. 473)

Trisomy 9: Occurring as a result of an extra chromosome 9, this is a severe abnormality characterized by multiple anomalies of practically all organ systems (see p. 478)

Trisomy 10: Rare abnormality with only those patients with mosaic trisomy 10 surviving to infancy. Abnormalities include IUGR and face, heart, hand, and feet anomalies (see p. 480)

Trisomy 13 (Patau Syndrome): Occurring as a result of an extra chromosome 13, this is a severe abnormality characterized by multiple anomalies of the central nervous system, face, heart, and extremities (see p. 483)

Trisomy 18 (Edwards Syndrome): Occurring as a result of an extra chromosome 18, this is a severe abnormality characterized by IUGR and multiple anomalies of the central nervous system, face, heart, and extremities (see p. 490)

Trisomy 21 (Down Syndrome): Occurring as a result of an extra chromosome 21, this abnormality is characterized by nuchal fold thickening, short long-bones, abnormal nasal bone, heart defects, other anomalies. Twenty-five percent of fetuses with Down syndrome do not display any sonographic abnormalities or markers (see p. 496)

Trisomy 22: Occurring as a result of an extra chromosome 22, this is a lethal abnormality characterized by multiple anomalies of the heart, face, extremities, and gastrointestinal and genitourinary systems (see p. 509)

XO Syndrome (Turner Syndrome): Occurring as a result of a single X chromosome (XO), Turner syndrome is characterized primarily in early pregnancy by large cystic hygromata, lymphangiectasia, and heart defects. Affected infants who survive gestation may represent Turner mosaic individuals (see p. 510)

OTHER SYNDROMES AND SEQUENCES

Cardiosplenic Syndromes (Asplenia/Polysplenia): Defects in lateralization of normal body asymmetry, including severe heart defects and anomalies of intrathoracic and intra-abdominal viscera (see p. 365)

Caudal Regression Syndrome/Sirenomelia: Although of different etiologies, these two syndromes are similar; characterized by disruption of the caudal portion of the neural tube, absence or dysplasia of the sacrum, and renal and lower extremity anomalies (occasional) (see p. 370)

CHARGE Association: **C**oloboma of the iris, **h**eart defect, choanal **a**tresia, intrauterine growth **r**estriction, **g**enital anomalies, and **e**ar anomalies (see p. 376)

Fryns Syndrome: Autosomal recessive condition characterized by diaphragmatic defects, digital and facial abnormalities, and brain anomalies (occasional) (see p. 325)

Infantile Polycystic Kidney Disease (see p. 329)

Klippel-Feil Syndrome: Abnormal cervical vertebrae, webbed neck, and facial asymmetry (occasional) (see p. 394)

Marfan Syndrome: Autosomal dominant connective tissue disorder characterized by tall stature, long limbs, pectus deformities, congenital heart defects, and ocular anomalies (see p. 344)

Opitz Syndrome: Disorder characterized by ocular hypertelorism, micrognathia, and, in males, hypospadias (occasional) (see p. 399)

Pena Shokeir Syndrome: Autosomal recessive condition characterized by IUGR, multiple joint contractures, facial anomalies, and pulmonary hypoplasia; also known as fetal akinesia/hypokinesia sequence or neurogenic arthrogryposis (occasional) (see p. 402)

Pentalogy of Cantrell: Combination of five anomalies: ectopia cordis, omphalocele, disruption of distal sternum, anterior diaphragm, and diaphragmatic pericardium (see p. 405)

Renal Agenesis (occasional) (see p. 412)

Scimitar Syndrome: Dextroposition of the heart secondary to right pulmonary hypoplasia and anomalous pulmonary venous return (see p. 416)

Tuberous Sclerosis: Autosomal dominant condition characterized by hamartomatous lesions throughout many tissues, including the brain, skin, heart, and kidneys (see p. 353)

VATER Association: **V**ertebral defects, **a**nal atresia, **t**racheoesophageal fistula, **e**sophageal atresia, and **r**adial and renal dysplasias (occasional) (see p. 429)

TERATOGENS

Alcohol (see p. 438)

Azathioprine (see p. 435)

Carbamazepine (see p. 436)

Chlordiazepoxide (see p. 437)

Clomiphene (Clomid) (see p. 437)

Cocaine (see p. 439)

Codeine (see p. 439)

Cortisone (see p. 437)

Cyclophosphamide (see p. 435)

Cytarabine (see p. 435)

Dextroamphetamine (see p. 439)

Estrogen (see p. 437)

Hydantoin (occasional) (see p. 436)

Indomethacin (see p. 439)

Meclizine (see p. 436)

Meprobamate (see p. 438)

Methotrexate (see p. 435)

Oral contraceptives (see p. 437)

Parvovirus (see p. 446)

Phenantoin (see p. 436)

Phenylketonuria (see p. 439)

Progestin (see p. 437)

Quinine (see p. 434)

Rubella (see p. 449)

Smoking (see p. 440)

Thalidomide (see p. 437)

Trimethadione (see p. 436)

Valproic acid (see p. 436)

Warfarin (Coumadin) (see p. 435)

ECHOGENIC INTRACARDIAC FOCUS

Cardiac tumors (e.g., rhabdomyoma, myxoma)

Normal variant

Tuberous sclerosis (rhabdomyoma) (see p. 353)

CHROMOSOMAL ANOMALIES

Trisomy 13 (Patau Syndrome): Occurring as a result of an extra chromosome 13, this is a

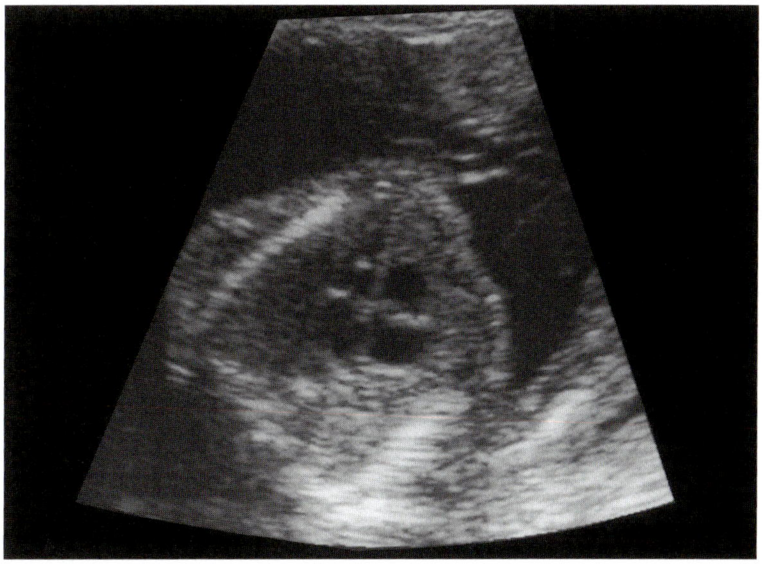

FIGURE 1-127 Four-chamber view of the heart shows an echogenic focus within the left ventricle. In 90% of fetuses with this finding, the echogenic focus is in the left ventricle. When the focus occurs in both ventricles, the risk of chromosomal abnormalities is greater than when it occurs in only one ventricle.

severe abnormality characterized by multiple anomalies of the central nervous system, face, heart, and extremities (see p. 483)

Trisomy 21 (Down Syndrome): Occurring as a result of an extra chromosome 21, this abnormality is characterized by nuchal fold thickening, short long-bones, abnormal nasal bone, heart defects, and other anomalies. Twenty-five percent of fetuses with Down syndrome do not display any sonographic abnormalities or markers (see p. 496)

ABNORMAL HEART APPEARANCE

ENLARGED HEART

Cardiac Tumor

Cardiomyopathy

Ebstein Anomaly

PARALLEL GREAT VESSELS

Double-Outlet Right Ventricle

Transposition of the Great Vessels

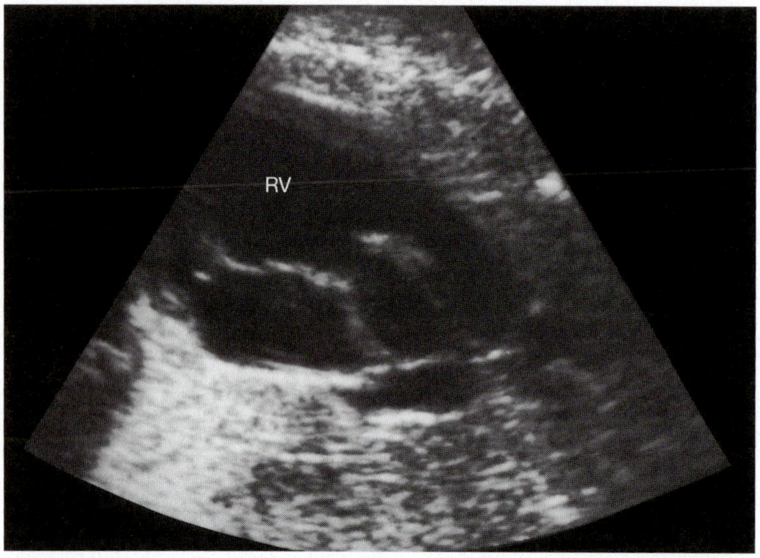

FIGURE 1-128 Double-outlet right ventricle. Short-axis view of the fetal heart shows that the right ventricle *(RV)* gives rise to two parallel great vessels.

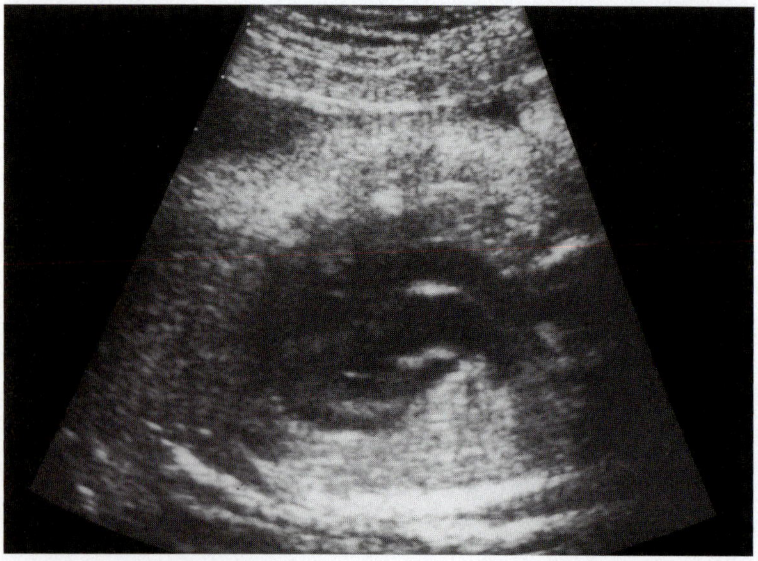

FIGURE 1-129 Transposition of the great arteries. Short-axis view of the fetal heart shows that each ventricle gives rise to a great vessel, in a parallel configuration.

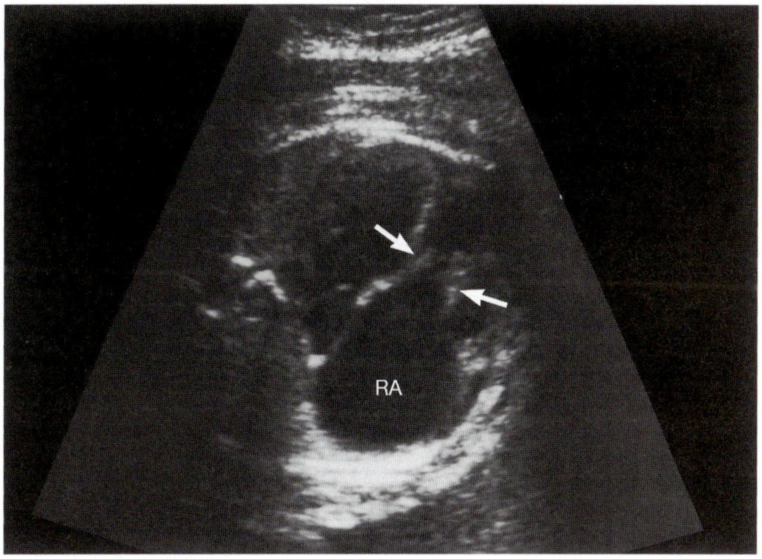

FIGURE 1-130 Ebstein anomaly. Four-chamber view of the fetal heart reveals markedly enlarged right atrium *(RA)* secondary to tricuspid valve *(arrows)* displaced into the right ventricle.

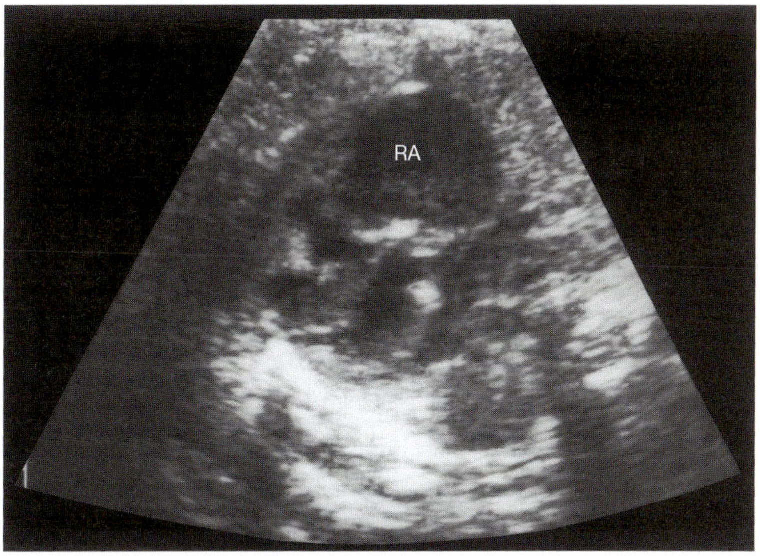

FIGURE 1-131 Pulmonic stenosis. Four-chamber view of the fetal heart shows markedly enlarged right atrium *(RA)*. The valves are normally placed in this fetus; however, outlet obstruction (secondary to pulmonic stenosis) resulted in marked tricuspid regurgitation.

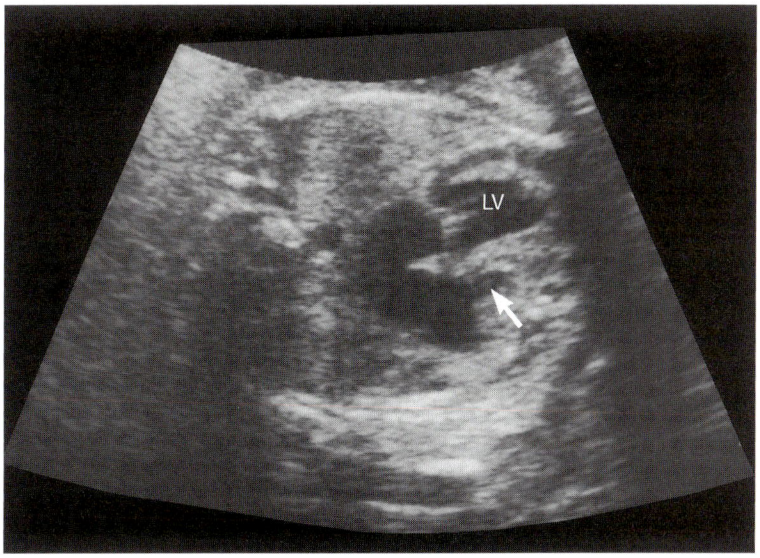

FIGURE 1-132 Four-chamber view of the heart shows a normal-size left ventricle *(LV)* and tiny right ventricle *(arrow)* in this fetus with tricuspid atresia.

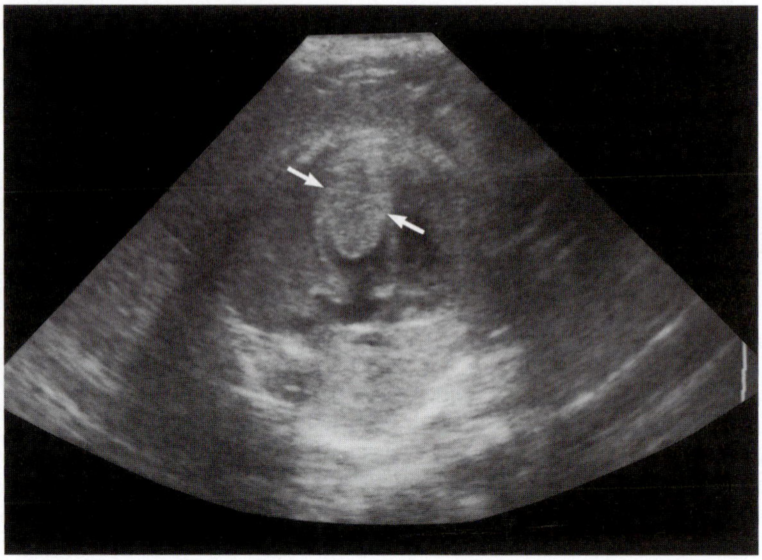

FIGURE 1-133 Cardiac tumor. Four-chamber view of the fetal heart shows that the left ventricle is practically filled by a large echogenic mass, which is consistent with a cardiac tumor *(arrows)*.

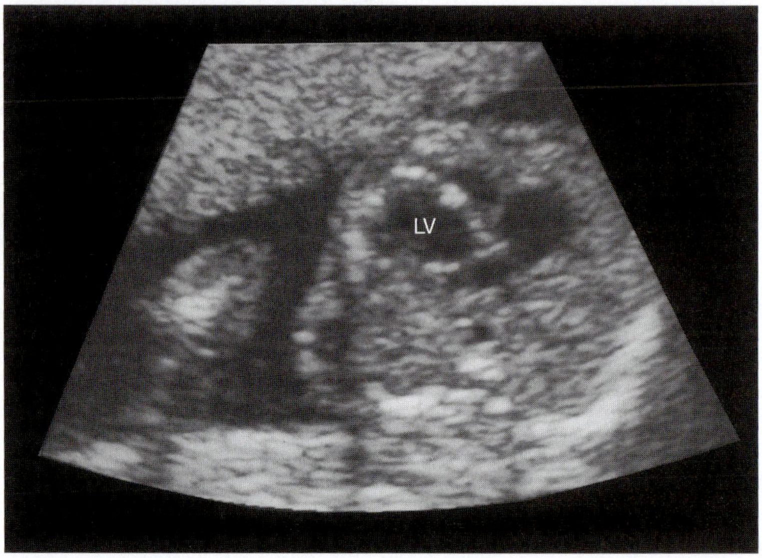

FIGURE 1-134 Four-chamber view of the fetal heart shows that the left ventricle *(LV)* is enlarged and has an echogenic rim. On real-time scanning, the ventricle was practically noncontractile, a finding consistent with severe fibroelastosis secondary to critical aortic stenosis.

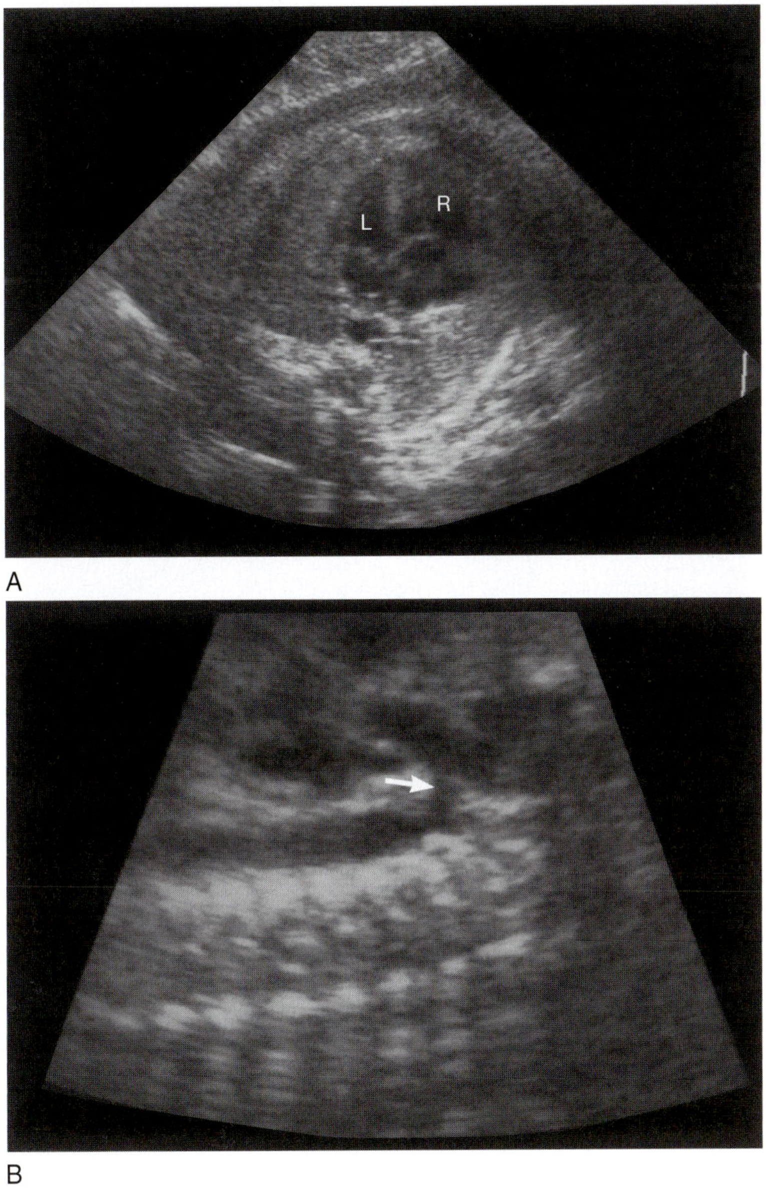

FIGURE 1-135 Coarctation of the aorta. (A) Four-chamber view of the fetal heart shows that the left side *(L)* is smaller than the right side *(R)* of the heart. This is an indirect sign of coarctation of the aorta. (B) View showing the aortic arch. Arrow indicates the area of narrowing.

ENLARGED RIGHT SIDE OF THE HEART (COMPARED WITH THE LEFT)

Ebstein Anomaly

Premature Closure of the Ductus Arteriosis

Pulmonic Stenosis

Tricuspid Regurgitation

SMALLER RIGHT SIDE OF THE HEART (COMPARED WITH THE LEFT)

Pulmonic Atresia

Tricuspid Atresia

ENLARGED LEFT SIDE OF THE HEART (COMPARED WITH THE RIGHT)

Cardiac Tumor

Critical Aortic Stenosis

Endocardial Fibroelastosis

Tricuspid Atresia

SMALLER LEFT SIDE OF THE HEART (COMPARED WITH THE RIGHT)

Coarctation of the Aorta

Hypoplastic Left Heart Syndrome

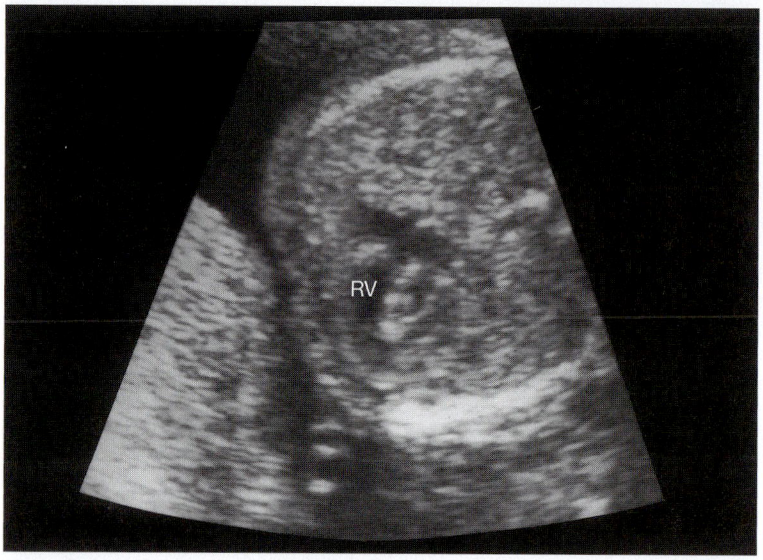

FIGURE 1-136 Four-chamber view of the fetal heart shows a normal-appearing right ventricle *(RV)*. The left ventricle is very small and echogenic, with no obvious blood flow through it, a finding consistent with hypoplastic left heart.

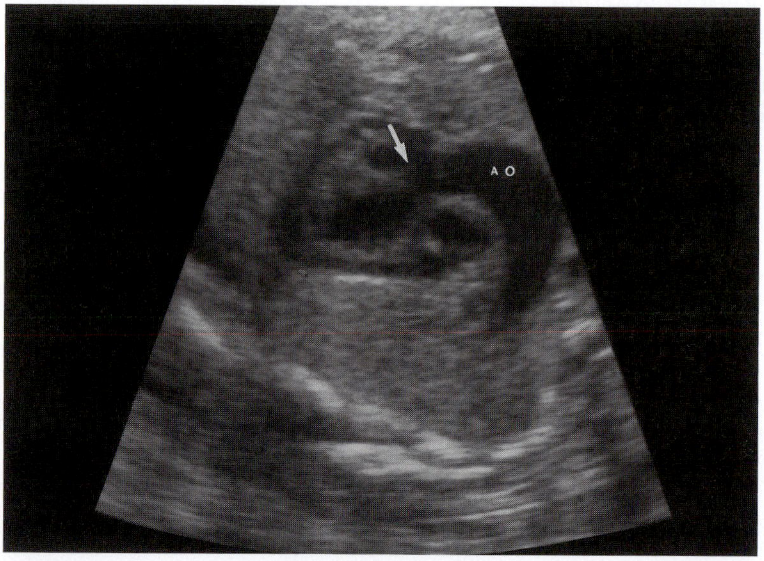

FIGURE 1-137 Short-axis view of the fetal heart reveals an enlarged aorta *(AO)* overriding a ventricular septal defect *(arrow)*. This fetus had severe tetralogy of Fallot.

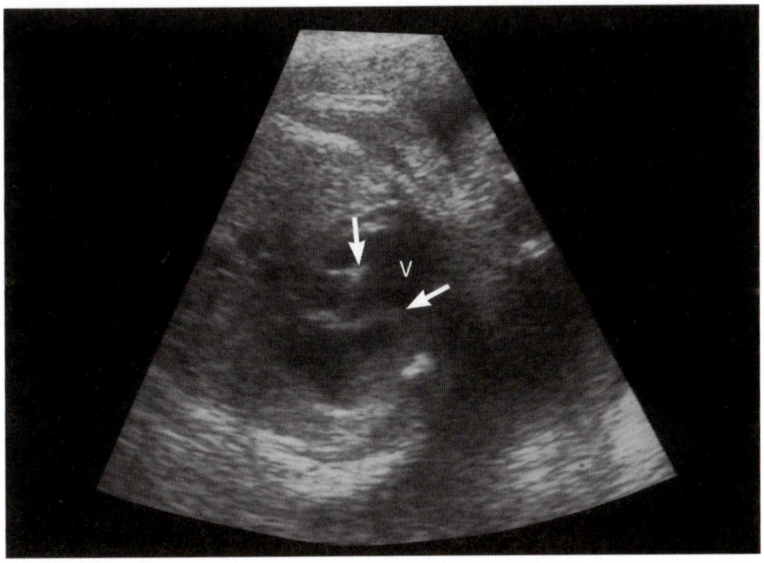

FIGURE 1-138 Four-chamber view of the fetal heart shows that only one ventricle *(V)* is identified. This case of double-inlet left ventricle shows that both atrioventricular valves *(arrows)* are leading into a single ventricle.

SINGLE GREAT VESSEL

Tetralogy of Fallot

Truncus Arteriosus

SINGLE VENTRICLE

Complete Atrioventricular Canal (illusion of single ventricle)

Double-Inlet Left Ventricle

Double-Outlet Right Ventricle

Hypoplastic Left Heart Syndrome

Tricuspid Atresia

2 Syndromes

Syndromes Featuring Growth Restriction

CORNELIA DE LANGE SYNDROME

DESCRIPTION AND DEFINITION

Synonym: Brachmann-de Lange syndrome

Described by Brachmann in 1916 and by de Lange in 1933, this syndrome is of unknown etiology but is recognizable by characteristic facial and limb malformations, as well as prenatal and postnatal growth restriction and mental developmental delay.

ABNORMALITIES DETECTABLE BY ULTRASOUND

Intrauterine growth restriction (IUGR) with biometry demonstrating poor growth; onset at 20 to 25 weeks' gestation

Brachycephaly

Microcephaly

Micrognathia

Micromelia, syndactyly, and ulnar dysplasia with abnormal contractures of the upper extremities

Micromelia and syndactyly of the lower extremities

Oligodactyly

Nuchal lucency thickening (first trimester)

Cystic hygroma

Cardiac defects, including ventricular septal defect and atrial septal defect

Undescended testicles and hypospadias

MAJOR DIFFERENTIAL DIAGNOSES

Apert syndrome (nuchal lucency and limb anomalies)

Chromosomal abnormalities (nuchal lucency and limb anomalies)

DiGeorge syndrome (nuchal lucency, micrognathia, short bones)

Fanconi anemia (short radial ray)

Holt-Oram syndrome (short radial ray and heart defect)

Multiple pterygium syndrome (nuchal lucency and limb anomalies)

Roberts' syndrome (nuchal lucency and limb anomalies)

Smith-Lemli-Opitz syndrome (nuchal lucency and limb anomalies)

Thrombocytopenia with absent radius syndrome (short radial ray)

ULTRASOUND DIAGNOSIS

An ultrasound diagnosis has been established prenatally as early as 12 weeks' gestation, based on the observation of nuchal lucency and generalized skin edema. A persistently flexed fore-

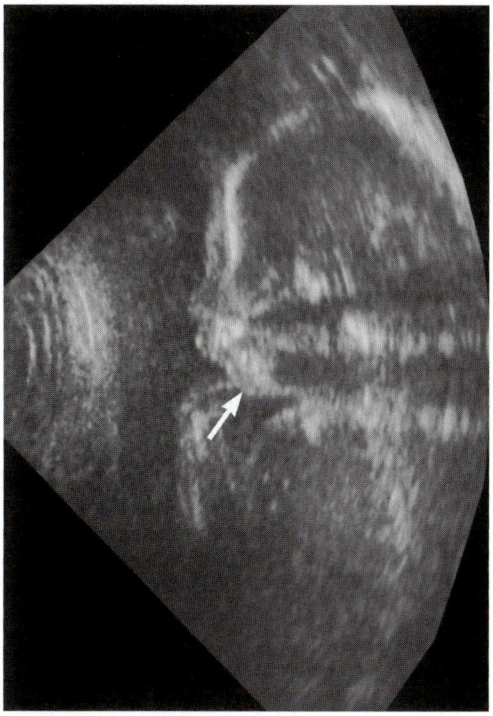

FIGURE 2-1 Sagittal view of the profile of fetus with Cornelia de Lange syndrome shows micrognathia. Arrow indicates chin of fetus.

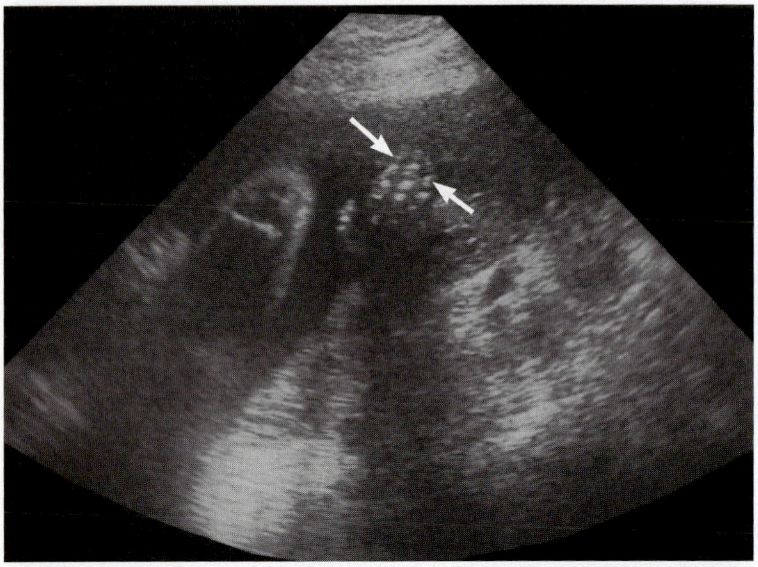

A

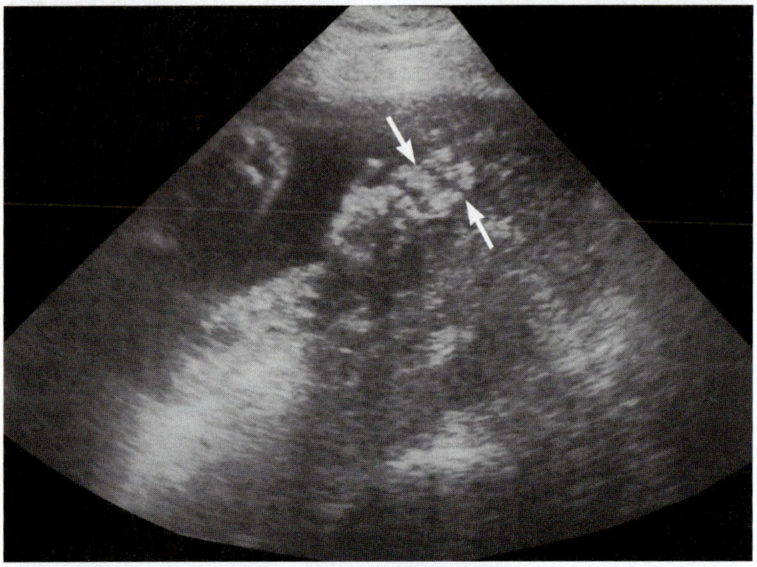

B

FIGURE 2-2 (**A, B**) Views of both hands of the fetus shown in Figure 2-1. The digits *(arrows)* are fused, which is consistent with syndactyly of the fingers of both hands.

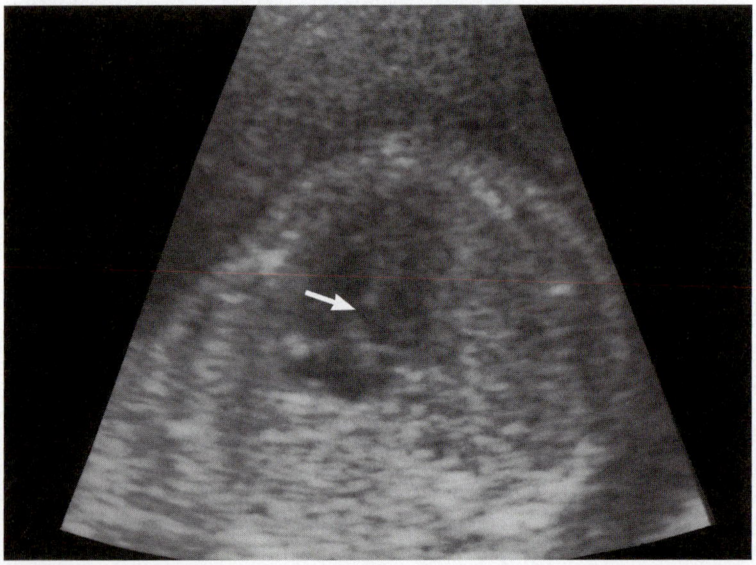

FIGURE 2-3 Four-chamber view of the heart of the fetus shown in Figures 2-1 and 2-2 reveals a ventricular septal defect *(arrow)* and levorotation of the heart, which are signs consistent with congenital heart disease.

arm has been observed in a fetus as early as 14 weeks. Cystic hygromas and early-onset growth restriction have been noted at 15 weeks. Growth restriction has been described between 20 and 25 weeks.

HEREDITY

Features of Cornelia de Lange syndrome have been observed to occur with partial trisomy of the distal portion of chromosome 3. Another locus associated with this syndrome has been reported at 5p13. This may account for some, but not all, cases of the so-called familial Cornelia de Lange syndrome.

Etiology is unknown. However, there has been a suggestion of autosomal dominance, with sporadic reports of mildly affected mothers giving birth to severely affected children. For unaffected parents, the syndrome is thought to have a sporadic hereditary pattern, with no increased recurrence rate.

NATURAL HISTORY AND OUTCOME

Children with this syndrome are severely retarded and growth restricted. Survivors are severely mentally impaired and have hearing loss, speech delay, failure to thrive, feeding difficulties, vomiting, swallowing problems, and behavioral difficulties.

Suggested Reading

Allderdice PW, Browne N, Murphy DP: Chromosome 3 duplication q21-qter deletion p25-pter syndrome in children of carriers of a pericentric inversion inv(3)(p25q21). *Am J Hum Genet* 27:699–718, 1975.

Brachmann W: Ein fall von symmetrischer monodaktylie durch Ulnadefekt, mit symmetrischer flughautbildung in den ellenbeugen, sowie anderen abnormitaten (zwerghaftogkeit, halsrippen, behaarung). *Jarb Kinder Phys Erzie* 84:225–235, 1916.

Bruner JP, Hsia YE: Prenatal findings in Brachmann-de Lange syndrome. *Obstet Gynecol* 76:966–968, 1990.

de Lange C: Sur un type nouveau de degenerescence (typus Amstelodamensis). *Arch Med Enfants* 36:713–719, 1933.

Drolshagen LF, Durmon G, Berumen M, Burks DD: Prenatal ultrasonographic appearance of "Cornelia de Lange" syndrome. *J Clin Ultrasound* 20:470–474, 1992.

Huang WH, Porto M: Abnormal first-trimester fetal nuchal translucency and Cornelia De Lange syndrome. *Obstet Gynecol* 99:956–958, 2002.

Jones KL: *Smith's recognizable patterns of human malformations.* Philadelphia, 2006, Elsevier.

Kliewer MA, Kahler SG, Hertzberg BS, Bowie JD: Fetal biometry in the Brachmann-de Lange syndrome. *Am J Med Genet* 47:1035–1041, 1993.

Manouvrier S, Espinasse M, Vaast P, et al: Brachmann-de Lange syndrome: pre- and postnatal findings. *Am J Med Genet* 62:268–273, 1996.

Marino T, Wheeler PG, Simpson LL, Craigo SD, Bianchi DW: Fetal diaphragmatic hernia and upper limb anomalies suggest Brachmann-de Lange syndrome. *Prenat Diagn* 22:144–147, 2002.

Ranzini AC, Day-Salvatore D, Farren-Chavez D, McLean DA, Greco R: Prenatal diagnosis of de Lange syndrome. *J Ultrasound Med* 16:755–758, 1997.

Robinson LK, Wolfsberg E, Jones KL: Brachmann-de Lange syndrome: evidence for autosomal dominant inheritance. *Am J Med Genet* 22:109–115, 1985.

Sekimoto H, Osada H, Kimura H, Kamiyama M, Arai K, Sekiya S: Prenatal findings in Brachmann-de Lange syndrome. *Arch Gynecol Obstet* 263:182–184, 2002.

Wilson GN, Hieber VC, Schmickel RD: The association of chromosome 3 duplication and the Cornelia de Lange syndrome. *J Pediatr* 93:783–788, 1978.

NOONAN SYNDROME

DESCRIPTION AND DEFINITION

This is a "Turner-like syndrome" featuring short stature, short neck with webbing, cardiac anomalies, and a phenotype similar to that of Turner syndrome but with normal karyotype.

ABNORMALITIES DETECTABLE BY ULTRASOUND

Common Findings:

Thickened nuchal lucency in the late first trimester; small, lateral, cystic hygromata in the second trimester

Right heart defects, particularly pulmonic stenosis and septal defects

Hypertelorism

Low-set ears

Hemivertebrae

Cryptorchidism

Micropenis

Occasional Findings:

Full-blown hydrops

Pleural effusions

Skin edema

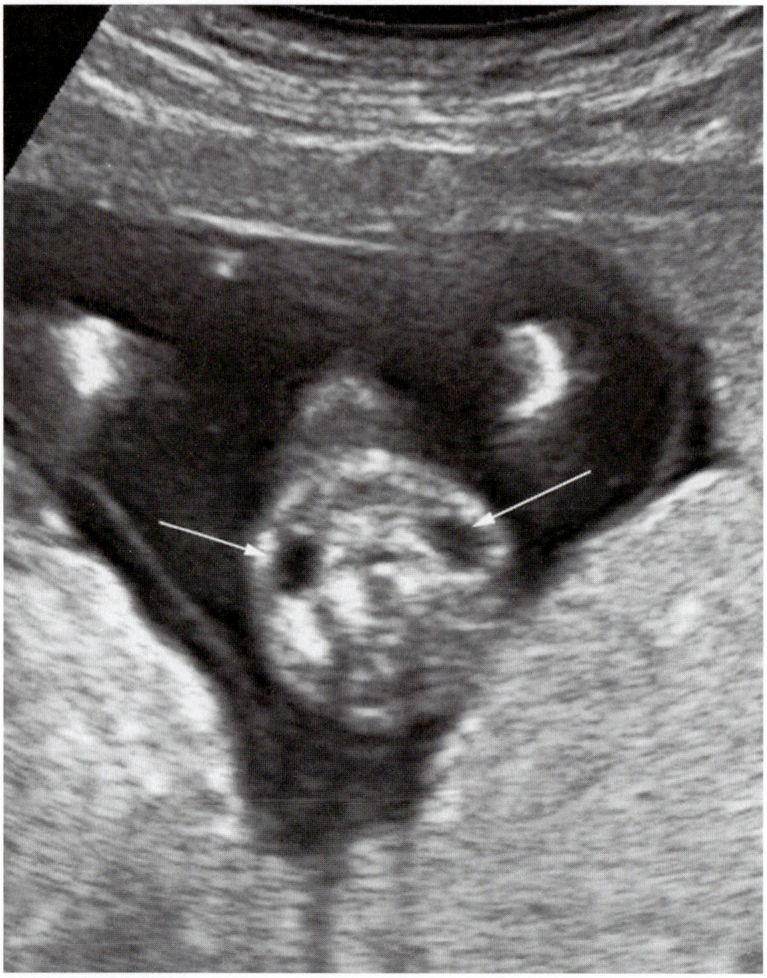

A

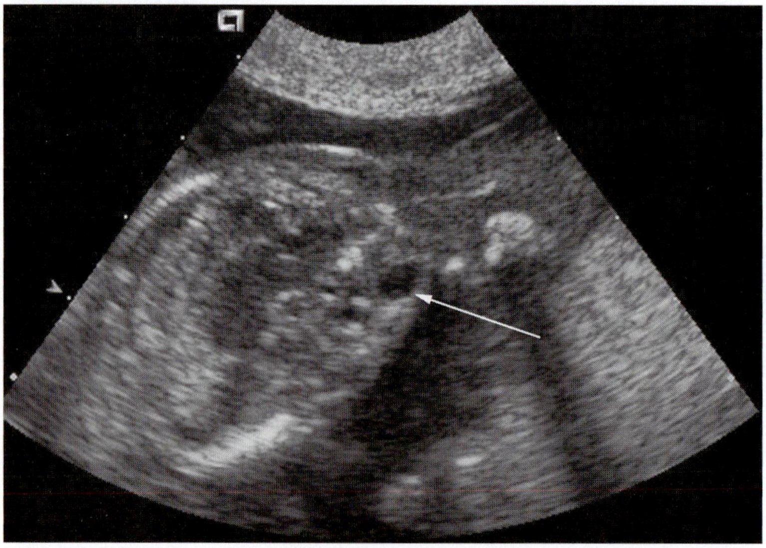

B

FIGURE 2-4 Late first-trimester fetus with Noonan syndrome. (**A, B**) Transverse and oblique views of the fetal neck show bilateral paired small cystic hygromas in the jugular region of the fetal neck *(arrows)*.

Continued

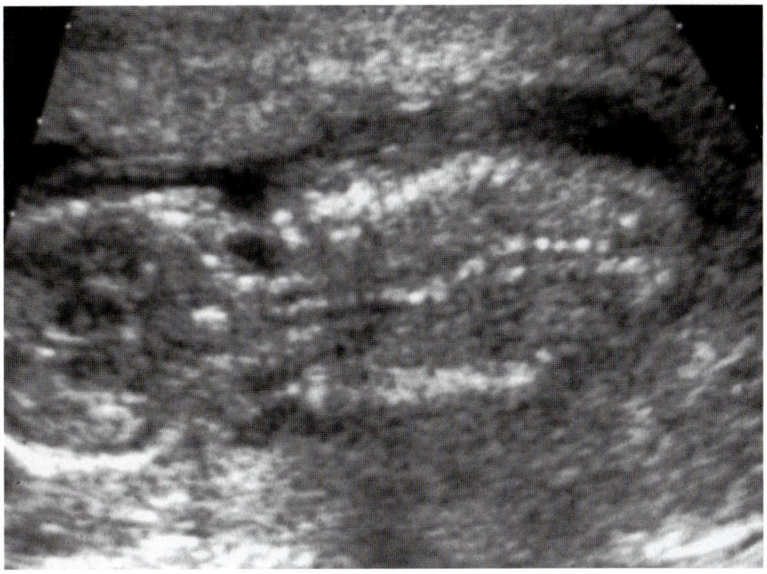

C

FIGURE 2-4, cont'd (C) Longitudinal view through the fetal body shows two hemivertebra (midthoracic and upper lumbar) and two small, paired cystic hygromas at the lateral aspects of the neck, typical of fetuses with Noonan syndrome.

MAJOR DIFFERENTIAL DIAGNOSES

Many other syndromes feature nuchal lucency in the first trimester, including thc following:

- Achondrogenesis
- Achondroplasia
- Apert syndrome (craniosynostosis, acrocephaly, and syndactyly)
- Arthrogryposis
- Cardiosplenic syndromes
- Caudal regression syndrome/sirenomelia
- Cerebrocostomandibular syndrome
- CHARGE association
- Congenital adrenal hyperplasia
- Congenital high airway obstruction syndrome
- Cornelia de Lange syndrome
- Cri du chat syndrome (5p deletion)
- Deletion 11q (Jacobsen syndrome)
- DiGeorge syndrome
- Ectrodactyly–ectodermal dysplasia–clefting (EEC) syndrome
- Ellis-van Creveld syndrome
- Fanconi anemia
- Fryns syndrome
- Holoprosencephaly sequence
- Holt-Oram syndrome
- Hydrolethalus
- Hypophosphatasia
- Jarcho-Levin syndrome
- Jeune thoracic dystrophy
- Joubert syndrome
- Multiple pterygium syndrome
- Noonan syndrome
- Osteogenesis imperfecta
- Parvovirus
- Pentalogy of Cantrell
- Perlman syndrome
- Roberts' syndrome
- Smith-Lemli-Opitz syndrome
- Tetrasomy 12p (Pallister-Killian syndrome)
- Thanatophoric dysplasia
- Triploidy
- Trisomy 9
- Trisomy 10
- Trisomy 13 (Patau syndrome)
- Trisomy 18 (Edwards' syndrome)
- Trisomy 21 (Down syndrome)
- Trisomy 22 (occasional)
- XO syndrome (Turner syndrome)

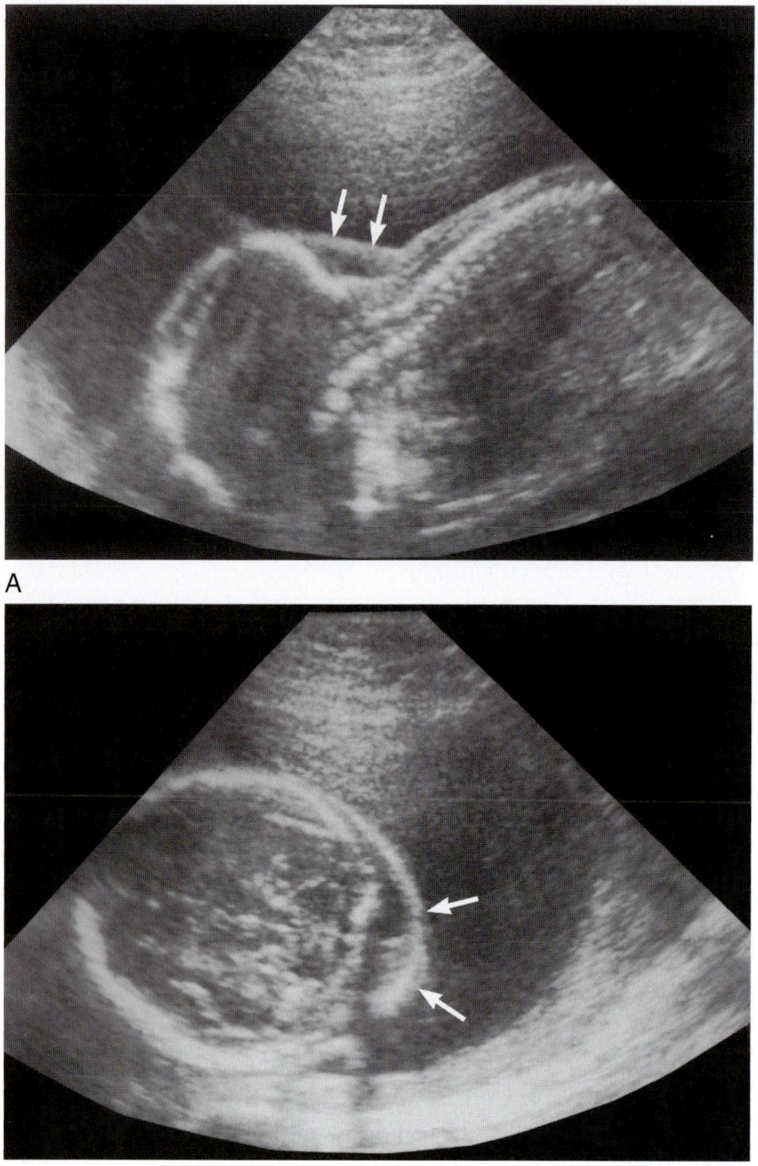

A

B

FIGURE 2-5 Longitudinal (A) and transverse (B) views of the back of the head and neck of a fetus with Noonan syndrome. A thickened, nuchal fold *(arrows)* is visible, as is a small cystic hygroma within the fold.

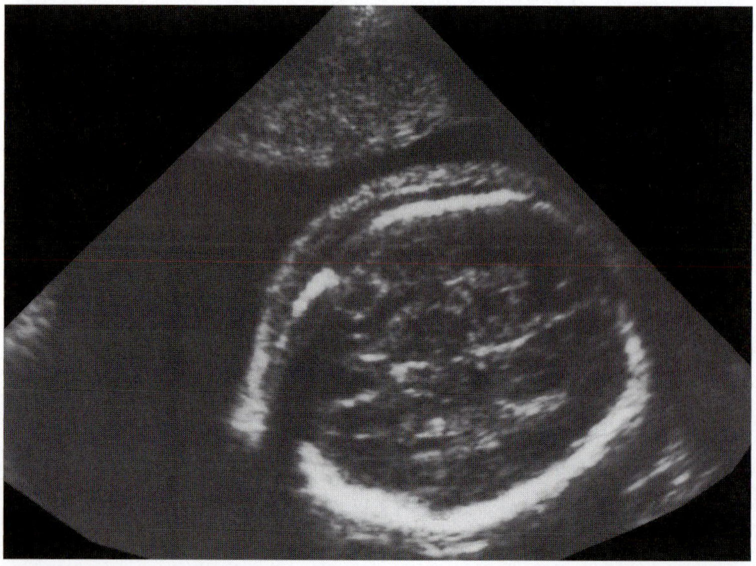

FIGURE 2-6 Third-trimester sonographic image of a fetus with Noonan syndrome shows the development of hydrops and skin edema. The transverse view of the fetal head shows significant scalp edema.

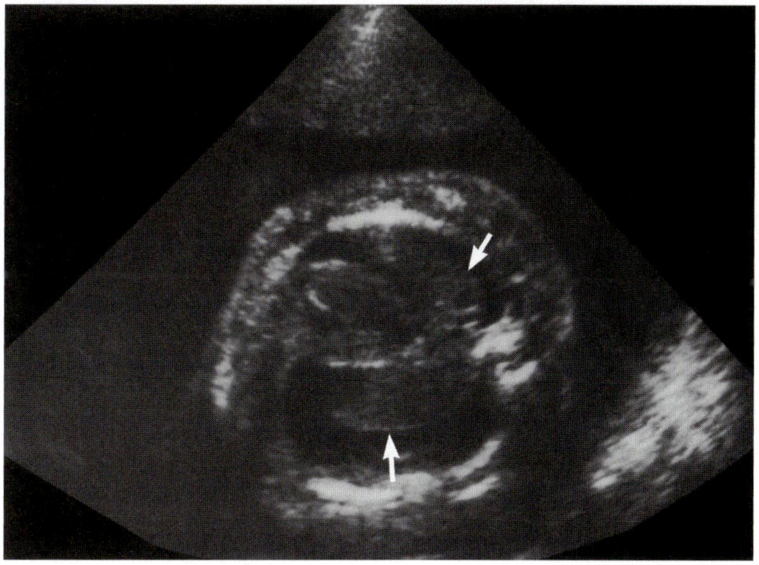

FIGURE 2-7 Transverse view of the thorax of the fetus shown in Figure 2-5 with hydrops reveals pleural effusions (arrows point to the lungs), as well as skin edema of the thorax.

ULTRASOUND DIAGNOSIS

A careful echocardiogram in the second trimester may reveal right heart abnormalities. The genitals should be evaluated to rule out gonadal hypoplasia in males. Noonan syndrome is most often identified in the late first trimester, recognized by a thickened nuchal lucency or cystic hygroma. When a fetus presents with cystic hygromata and a normal karyotype, Noonan syndrome is the most likely diagnosis. Nuchal thickening may continue into the second trimester when small, lateral, cystic hygromata can persist, accompanied by nuchal swelling similar to that seen in Down syndrome. Progression of these findings occasionally leads to full-blown hydrops, pleural effusions, and skin edema, placing the fetus at risk for intrauterine death.

HEREDITY

Noonan syndrome is considered an autosomal dominant condition. Several reports have shown the disorder in a parent and child. However, in more than 50% of cases it is a sporadic anomaly, occurring in families with no prior history. Mutations at the 12q24.1 locus (a gene coding for the nonreceptor protein tyrosine phosphate [SHP-2]) have been implicated in some cases.

NATURAL HISTORY AND OUTCOME

Diffuse lymphedema can develop, placing affected fetuses at risk for hydrops and intrauterine death.

Children with Noonan syndrome can develop peripheral edema and often are left with a webbed neck from the original cystic hygroma present during early gestation. The timing of these manifestations may vary among infants, occurring either in utero or in childhood. Affected children have short stature, and 25% have mental retardation (seldom severe). There is a tendency toward coagulation and bleeding abnormalities, including thrombocytopenia, von Willebrand disease, and factor XI deficiency. Other symptoms include gastrointestinal dysfunction, pulmonic stenosis, cardiomyopathy, and genital abnormalities such as cryptorchidism.

It is sometimes difficult to recognize individuals with Noonan syndrome until they themselves have affected children. A neonate with Noonan syndrome should trigger further evaluation of the family.

Suggested Reading

Achiron R, Heggesh J, Grisaru D, et al: Noonan syndrome: a cryptic condition in early gestation. *Am J Med Genet* 92:159–165, 2000.

Allanson JE: Syndrome of the month: Noonan syndrome. *J Med Genet* 24:9–13, 1987.

Allanson JE, Hall JG, Hughes HE, Preus M, Witt RD: Noonan syndrome: the changing phenotype. *Am J Med Genet* 21:507–514, 1985.

Baird PA, De Jong BP: Noonan's syndrome (XX and XY Turner phenotype) in three generations of a family. *J Pediatr* 80:110–114, 1972.

Benacerraf BR, Greene MF, Holmes LB: The prenatal sonographic features of Noonan's syndrome. *J Ultrasound Med* 8:59–63, 1989.
Celermajer JM, Bowdler JD, Cohen DH: Pulmonary stenosis in patients with the Turner phenotype in the male. *Am J Dis Child* 116:351–358, 1968.
Char F, Rodriquez-Fernandez HL, Scott CI Jr, et al: The Noonan syndrome—a clinical study of forty-five cases. *Birth Defects Orig Art Ser* 8:110–118, 1972.
deHaan M, van de Kamp JJP, Briet E, Dubbeldam J: Noonan syndrome: partial factor XI deficiency. *Am J Med Genet* 29:277–282, 1988.
Donnenfeld AE, Nazir MA, Sindoni F, Librizzi RJ: Prenatal sonographic documentation of cystic hygroma regression in Noonan syndrome. *Am J Med Genet* 39:461–465, 1991.
Kalousek DK, Seller MJ: Differential diagnosis of posterior cervical hygroma in previable fetuses. *Am J Med Genet Suppl* 3:83–92, 1987.
Jones, KL: *Smith's recognizable patterns of human malformations.* Philadelphia, 2006, Elsevier.
Menashe M, Arbel R, Raveh D, Achiron R, Yagel S: Poor prenatal detection rate of cardiac anomalies in Noonan syndrome. *Ultrasound Obstet Gynecol* 19:51–55, 2002.
Mendez HMM, Opitz JM: Noonan syndrome: a review. *Am J Med Genet* 21:493–506, 1985.
Nisbet DL, Griffin DR, Chitty LS: Prenatal features of Noonan syndrome. *Prenat Diagn* 19:642–647, 1999.
Noonan JA: Hypertelorism with Turner phenotype. A new syndrome with associated congenital heart disease. *Am J Dis Child* 116:373–380, 1968.
Nora JJ, Nora AH, Sinha AK, Spangler RD, Lubs HA Jr: The Ullrich-Noonan syndrome (Turner phenotype). *Am J Dis Child* 127:48–55, 1974.
Opitz JM: The Noonan syndrome. *Am J Med Genet* 21:515–518, 1985 (editorial).
Ragavan M, Vause S: Prenatal diagnosis of Noonan's syndrome: a case report. *J Obstet Gynaecol* 25:305–306, 2005.
Schluter G, Steckel M, Schiffmann H, et al: Prenatal DNA diagnosis of Noonan syndrome in a fetus with massive hygroma colli, pleural effusion and ascites. *Prenat Diagn* 25:574–576, 2005.
Sharland M, Patton MA, Talbot S, Chitolie A, Bevan DH: Coagulation-factor deficiencies and abnormal bleeding in Noonan's syndrome. *Lancet* 339:19–21, 1992.
Witt DR, Hoyme E, Zonana J, et al: Lymphedema in Noonan syndrome: clues to pathogenesis and prenatal diagnosis and review of the literature. *Am J Med Genet* 27:841–856, 1987.
Witt DR, McGillivray BC, Allanson JE, et al: Bleeding diathesis in Noonan syndrome: a common association. *Am J Med Genet* 31:305–317, 1988.
Zarabi M, Mieckowski GC, Mazer J: Cystic hygroma associated with Noonan's syndrome. *J Clin Ultrasound* 11:398–400, 1983.

RUSSELL-SILVER SYNDROME

DESCRIPTION AND DEFINITION

Synonym: Russell-Silver dwarfism

The main feature of this syndrome is asymmetric growth restriction of the skeleton, often occurring with a normal-size head and short stature.

ABNORMALITIES DETECTABLE BY ULTRASOUND

Limb asymmetry

Short long-bones (asymmetric, when comparing sides)

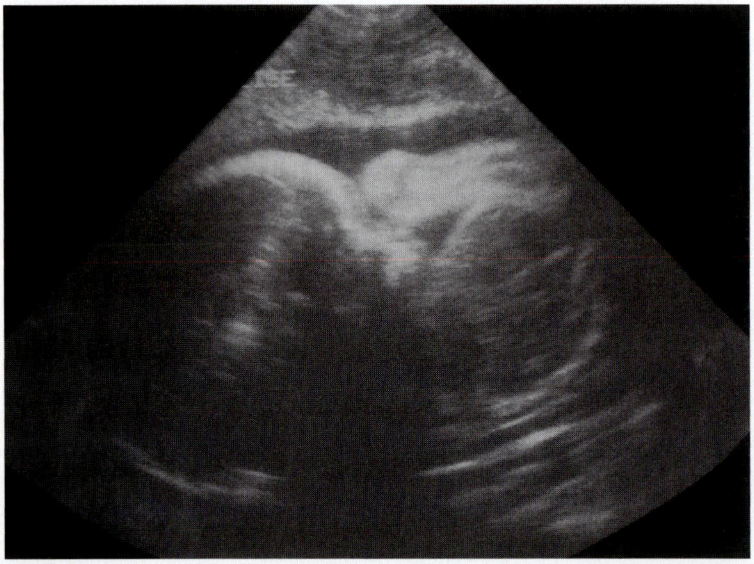

FIGURE 2-8 Longitudinal view of a third-trimester fetus with Russell-Silver syndrome shows an unusually small body and leg compared with the fetal head, which is normal size for gestational age. There is severe growth restriction of the fetal body and extremities.

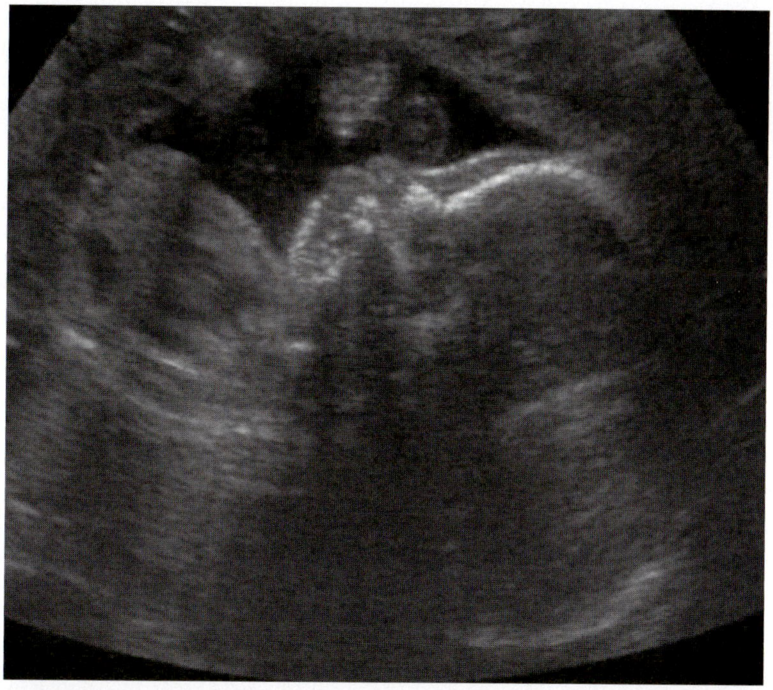

A

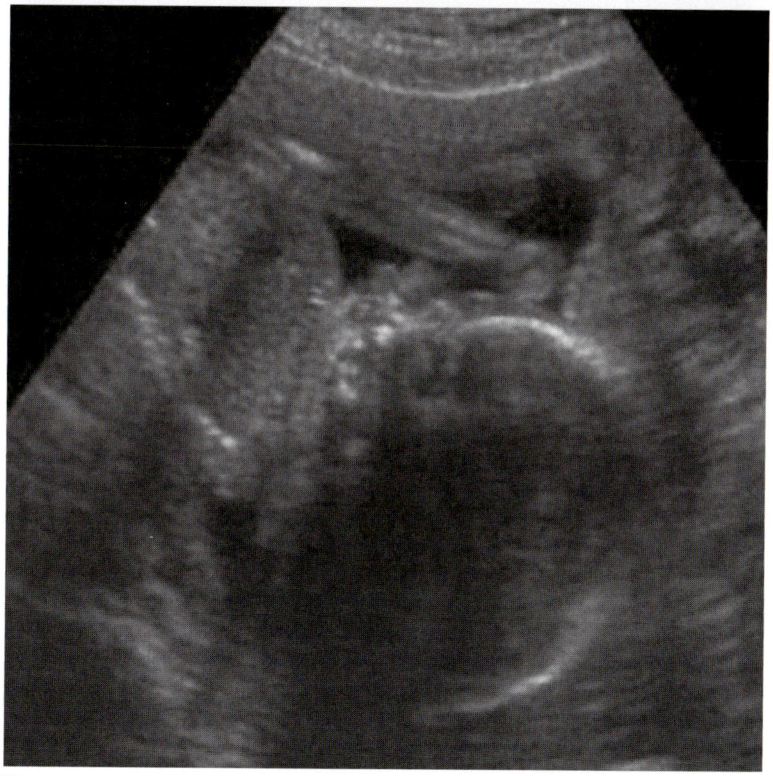

B

FIGURE 2-9 (**A, B**) Two longitudinal views of an early third-trimester fetus with severe asymmetric growth restriction. Note the large head compared to the small body, typical of Russell-Silver syndrome.

Fifth-finger clinodactyly

Syndactyly of the second and third toes

Prominent forehead

Micrognathia

IUGR (onset in second trimester)

MAJOR DIFFERENTIAL DIAGNOSES

Other causes of IUGR should be considered (see differential diagnosis, Chapter 1). However, the hallmark for diagnosis of Russell-Silver syndrome is the demonstration of limb-length asymmetry, which would be unusual in other forms of growth restriction.

Chromosomal anomalies associated with pronounced IUGR (e.g., triploidy and trisomy 18) can be confused with this syndrome.

Teratogens such as alcohol, infection (cytomegalovirus [CMV], rubella and toxoplasmosis) can cause early IUGR and are included in the differential diagnosis.

ULTRASOUND DIAGNOSIS

Prenatal ultrasound diagnosis is determined on the basis of abnormal biometry and short femurs (with asymmetry, when comparing the two femurs). In some cases, prenatal features include a two-vessel cord and a thickened placenta. At 18 and 23 weeks' gestation, femur length measures below the 5th percentile, and follow-up scans show femoral asymmetry and growth restriction. The earliest detection of long bone below the 5th percentile was at 18 weeks; however, it is more likely that Russell-Silver syndrome may not be easily detected until the late second trimester, when limb growth abnormalities are more recognizable.

HEREDITY

The etiology and, therefore, the heredity of this syndrome are unknown. Evidence suggests that this syndrome represents a new dominant mutation. Chromosomal rearrangements that may be associated with forms of this syndrome include a mutation at 17q25 and maternal uniparental disomy for chromosome 7, although this mutation accounts for only 10% of affected cases.

NATURAL HISTORY AND OUTCOME

Affected children tend to be small, but they have normal intelligence. Psychomotor development and final height are variable, but children can grow up to 5 feet.

Suggested Reading

Duncan PA, Hall JG, Shapiro LR, Vibert BK: Three-generation dominant transmission of the Silver-Russell syndrome. *Am J Med Genet* 35:245–250, 1990.

Falkert A, Dittmann K, Seelbach-Gobel B: Silver-Russell syndrome as a cause for early intrauterine growth restriction. *Prenat Diagn* 25:497–501, 2005.

Jones KL: *Smith's recognizable patterns of human malformations.* Philadelphia, 2006, Elsevier.

Kozot D, Schmitt S, Bernasconi F, et al: Uniparental disomy 7 in Silver-Russell syndrome and primordial growth retardation. *Hum Mol Genet* 4:583–587, 1995.

Midro AT, Debek K, Sawicka A, Marcinkiewicz D, Rogowska M: Second observation of Silver-Rusel [sic] syndrome in a carrier of a reciprocal translocation with one breakpoint at site 17q25. *Clin Genet* 44:53–55, 1993 (letter).

Patton MA: Russell-Silver syndrome. *J Med Genet* 25:557–560, 1988.

Silver HK: Asymmetry, short stature, and variations in sexual development: a syndrome of congenital malformations. *Am J Dis Child* 107:495–515, 1964.

Tanner JM, Lejarraga H, Cameron N: The natural history of the Silver-Russell syndrome: a longitudinal study of thirty-nine cases. *Pediatr Res* 9:611–623, 1975.

Wax JR, Burroughs R, Wright MS: Prenatal sonographic features of Russell-Silver syndrome. *J Ultrasound Med* 16:253–255, 1996.

SECKEL SYNDROME

DESCRIPTION AND DEFINITION

Synonym: Bird-like dwarfism

This syndrome is characterized by severe IUGR, prominent nose, microcephaly, micrognathia, and mental deficiency.

ABNORMALITIES DETECTABLE BY ULTRASOUND

Early-onset IUGR

Microcephaly

Severe micrognathia

Abnormal facial profile with prominent nose

Dislocated joints (particularly at the radial head)

Flexion deformities at the hips and knees

MAJOR DIFFERENTIAL DIAGNOSIS

Other syndromes featuring microcephaly and abnormal facies:

Adams-Oliver syndrome

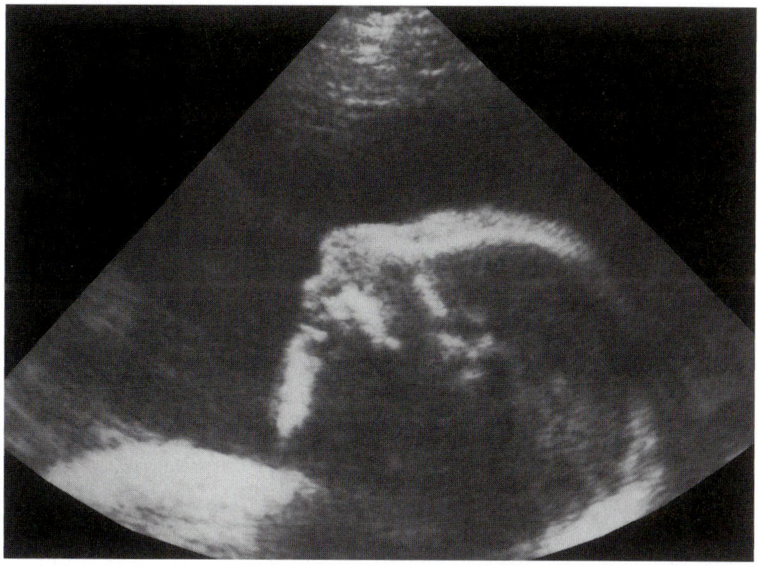

FIGURE 2-10 Longitudinal view of the head of a fetus with an abnormal facial profile suggestive of Seckel syndrome. Note the beak-like appearance of the nose, small forehead with microcephaly, and micrognathia.

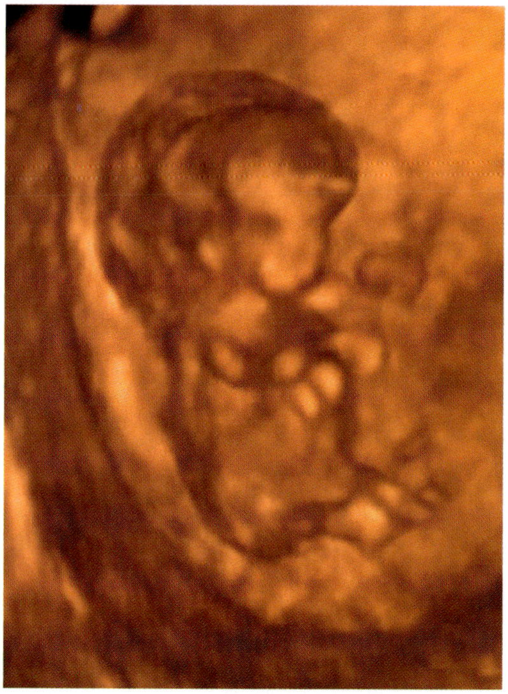

FIGURE 2-11 Three-dimensional image of a first-trimester fetus with cystic hygromas and lymphatic enlargement of the neck and body.

Branchio-oculo-facial syndrome

Cerebrocostomandibular syndrome

Cerebro-oculo-facio-skeletal (COFS) syndrome

Chromosomal abnormalities (e.g., trisomies 5p [cri du chat], 9, and 13)

Cornelia de Lange syndrome

DiGeorge syndrome

Dubowitz syndrome

Freeman-Sheldon syndrome

Neu-Laxova syndrome

Teratogen exposure (e.g., fetal alcohol syndrome)

ULTRASOUND DIAGNOSIS

Two reports on prenatal ultrasound diagnosis of Seckel syndrome cite the detection of severe growth restriction and microcephaly as early as 17 weeks, accompanied by the abnormal facial features consistent with the syndrome. At 30 weeks' gestation, a cystic abnormality of the posterior fossa has been described, along with beak-like facies, abnormal binocular and ocular measurements, and IUGR.

HEREDITY

This is an autosomal recessive syndrome with clinical and genetic heterogeneity. Two different loci have been mapped to this disorder: 3q22.1-q24 and 18p11.31-q11.2

NATURAL HISTORY AND OUTCOME

The syndrome is characterized by moderate-to-severe mental deficiency, abnormal joints with a characteristic stance secondary to flexion of the hips and knees, very short stature, increased risk for development of myelodysplasia, and other hematologic abnormalities.

Suggested Reading

Borglum AD, Balslev T, Haagerup A, et al: A new locus for Seckel syndrome on chromosome 18p11.31-q11.2. *Eur J Hum Genet* 9:753–757, 2001.

Faivre L, Le Merrer M, Lyonnet S, et al: Clinical and genetic heterogeneity of Seckel syndrome. *Am J Med Genet* 112:379–383, 2002.

Featherstone LS, Sherman SJ, Quigg MH: Prenatal diagnosis of Seckel syndrome. *J Ultrasound Med* 15:85–88, 1996.

Goodship J, Gill H, Carter J, Jackson A, Splitt M, Wright M: Autozygosity mapping of a seckel syndrome locus to chromosome 3q22.1-q24. *Am J Hum Genet* 67:498–503, 2000.

Mann TP, Russell A: A study of a microcephalic midget of extreme type. *Proc R Soc Med* 52:1024, 1959.

Seckel HPG: *Bird-headed dwarfs: studies in developmental anthropology including human proportions.* Springfield, Ill, 1960, Charles C Thomas.

SMITH-LEMLI-OPITZ SYNDROME

DESCRIPTION AND DEFINITION

First described by Smith in 1964, this syndrome consists of microcephaly, mental retardation, and genital abnormalities.

ABNORMALITIES DETECTABLE BY ULTRASOUND

Common Findings:

Microcephaly

Heart defects

Abnormal genitals:

- Hypospadias
- Cryptorchidism
- Micropenis
- Ambiguous genitalia

Female-appearing genitals with a male karyotype (in severely affected fetuses—type II or severe lethal form)

Limb abnormalities:

- Syndactyly of the second and third toes
- Postaxial polydactyly
- Clenched hands
- Valgus deformity of the feet

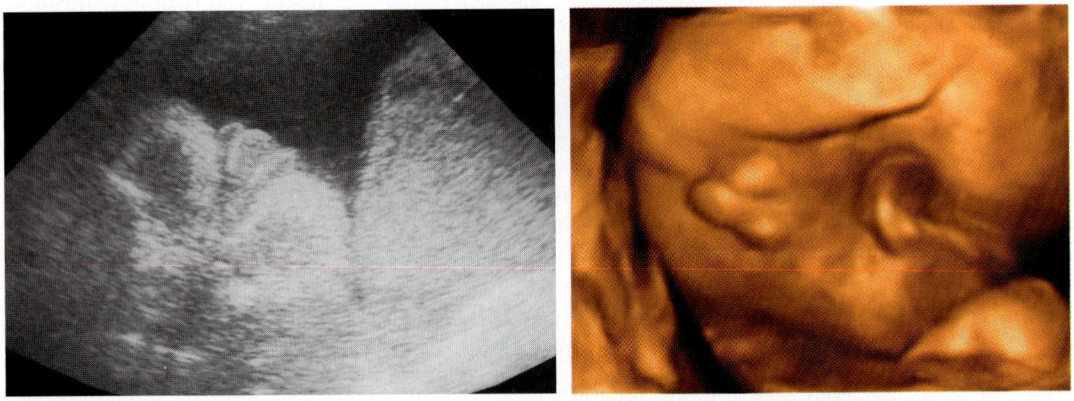

A B

FIGURE 2-12 (A) View of the genitals of a karyotypically male fetus with ambiguous genitalia, sonographically suggestive of a female phenotype, which is a feature of fetuses with Smith-Lemli-Opitz syndrome. (B) Three-dimensional image of a different second-trimester fetus with ambiguous genitalia consistent with a severe form of hypospadias called penile scrotal transposition.

Renal anomalies:

- Hydronephrosis
- Cystic kidneys
- Hypoplastic kidneys

Nuchal lucency in first trimester

IUGR (late onset)

Occasional Findings:

Cerebellar hypoplasia

Ventriculomegaly

Agenesis of the corpus callosum

Holoprosencephaly

Hypertelorism

Cataracts

Micrognathia

Cleft palate

MAJOR DIFFERENTIAL DIAGNOSES

Other syndromes featuring postaxial polydactyly, including the following:

- Ellis-van Creveld syndrome (skeletal dysplasia)
- Joubert syndrome
- Meckel Gruber syndrome
- Mohr syndrome
- Oral-facial-digital syndromes
- Short rib–polydactyly syndromes (skeletal dysplasia)
- Trisomy 13

Other syndromes featuring genital anomalies, including the following:

- Carpenter syndrome (also associated with brachycephaly, cranial synostosis, and polydactyly)
- CHARGE association
- Cloacal exstrophy
- Congenital adrenal hyperplasia
- Cornelia de Lange syndrome
- MURCS (müllerian duct aplasia, renal aplasia, cervicothoracic somite dysplasia) association
- Opitz G/BBB syndrome

Other syndromes featuring syndactyly of the second and third toes and genital anomalies:

- Cornelia de Lange syndrome

See Chapter 1 for information on the differential diagnosis of microcephaly and first-trimester nuchal lucency, as well as complete differential diagnoses for the features mentioned.

ULTRASOUND DIAGNOSIS

The ultrasound diagnosis of this syndrome has frequently been established in the first trimester, as early as 11 weeks' gestation when fetuses with this syndrome have a nuchal lucency similar to that seen in fetuses with chromosomal abnormalities. Although the nuchal lucency tends to resolve with time, karyotyping is helpful, particularly when a male karyotype is present and the genital anatomy of a female is visualized sonographically. Abnormalities of the limbs (e.g., polydactyly) have been detected by ultrasound as early as 12 weeks.

The demonstration of genital and limb defects has been the hallmark of sonographic diagnosis of this syndrome later in gestation, particularly in patients at increased risk. The finding of female genitalia with a male karyotype is highly suggestive of Smith-Lemli-Opitz syndrome.

The biochemical prenatal diagnosis is based on elevated 7-dehydrocholesterol in the amniotic fluid and using chorionic villus sampling.

HEREDITY

The syndrome has an autosomal recessive pattern of inheritance.

The etiology is a metabolic defect that leads to multiple congenital malformations. It results from a deficiency of 7-dehydrocholesterol reductase (DHCR7) that leads to a surplus of 7-dehydrocholesterol (a cholesterol precursor). The DHCR7 gene is located at 11q12-13. The deficiency of cholesterol has facilitated prenatal diagnosis, using elevated amniotic fluid 7-dehydrocholesterol and undetectable amniotic fluid unconjugated estriol.

NATURAL HISTORY AND OUTCOME

The syndrome is thought to be caused, in part, by a deficiency of DHCR7, thus making this syndrome a metabolic defect that leads to multiple congenital malformations. The deficiency of cholesterol, confirmed by reduced levels of amniotic fluid cholesterol, has facilitated prenatal diagnosis. The defect in DHCR7 may lend itself to treatment through gene therapy in the future.

Two types of Smith-Lemli-Opitz syndrome are reported: type I and type II. Type II is considered the more severe or lethal form. However, both types have similar features and appear to be associated with the same defect in cholesterol biosynthesis. The two types are believed to represent a spectrum of the same disorder. Fetuses with type II likely have a more severe mutation (i.e., homozygotes) with no DHCR7 activity compared with fetuses with type I who have some residual enzyme activity.

Neonatal death is common with the more severe form of the syndrome. Affected children have failure to thrive, gastrointestinal difficulties, moderate-to-severe mental deficiency, and behavioral problems. Twenty percent of survivors die in the first year of life.

Suggested Reading

Bick DP, McCorkle D, Stanley WS, et al: Prenatal diagnosis of Smith-Lemli-Opitz syndrome in a pregnancy with low maternal serum oestriol and a sex-reversed fetus. *Prenat Diagn* 19:68–71, 1999.

Blair HR, Martin JK: A syndrome characterized by mental retardation, short stature, craniofacial dysplasia, and genital anomalies occurring in siblings. *J Pediatr* 69:457–459, 1966.

Cotlier E, Rice P: Cataracts in the Smith-Lemli-Opitz syndrome. *Am J Ophthalmol* 72:955–959, 1971.

Dallaire L, Mitchell G, Giguere R, et al: Prenatal diagnosis of Smith-Lemli-Opitz syndrome is possible by measurement of 7-dehydrocholesterol in amniotic fluid. *Prenat Diagn* 15:855–858, 1995.

Degenhardt F, Muhlhaus K: Delayed bone growth as a sonographic sign in the early detection of Smith-Lemli-Opitz syndrome (German). *Z Geburtshilfe Perinatol* 192:169–172, 1988.

Goldenberg A, Wolf C, Chevy F, et al: Antenatal manifestations of Smith-Lemli-Opitz (RSH) syndrome: a retrospective survey of 30 cases. *Am J Med Genet* 124:423–426, 2004.

Hobbins JC, Jones OW, Gottesfeld S, Persutte W: Transvaginal ultrasonography and transabdominal embryoscopy in the first-trimester diagnosis of Smith-Lemli-Opitz syndrome, type II. *Am J Obstet Gynecol* 171:546–549, 1994.

Hyett JA, Clayton PT, Moscoso G, Nicolaides KH: Increased first trimester nuchal translucency as a prenatal manifestation of Smith-Lemli-Opitz syndrome. *Am J Med Genet* 58:374–376, 1995.

Irons M, Elias ER, Tint GS, et al: Abnormal cholesterol metabolism in the Smith-Lemli-Opitz syndrome: report of clinical and biochemical findings in four patients and treatment in one patient. *Am J Med Genet* 50:347–352, 1994.

Irons MB, Tint GS: Prenatal diagnosis of Smith-Lemli-Opitz syndrome. *Prenat Diagn* 18:369–372, 1998.

Loeffler J, Utermann G, Witsch-Baumgartner M: Molecular prenatal diagnosis of Smith-Lemli-Opitz syndrome is reliable and efficient. *Prenat Diagn* 22:827–830, 2002.

Maymon R, Ogle RF, Chitty LS: Smith-Lemli-Opitz syndrome presenting with persisting nuchal oedema and non-immune hydrops. *Prenat Diagn* 19:105–107, 1999.

Smith DW, Lemli L, Opitz JM: A newly recognized syndrome of multiple congenital anomalies. *J Pediatr* 64:210–217, 1964.

Tint GS, Abuelo D, Till M, et al: Fetal Smith-Lemli-Opitz syndrome can be detected accurately and reliably by measuring amniotic fluid dehydrocholesterols. *Prenat Diagn* 18:651–658, 1998.

Tint GS, Irons M, Elias ER, et al: Defective cholesterol biosynthesis associated with the Smith-Lemli-Opitz syndrome. *N Engl J Med* 330:107–113, 1994.

Syndromes Featuring Fetal Overgrowth

BECKWITH-WIEDEMANN SYNDROME

DESCRIPTION AND DEFINITION

This syndrome, initially described by Beckwith and Wiedemann in the mid-1960s, is characterized by gigantism in utero, macroglossia, omphalocele, and renal abnormalities.

ABNORMALITIES DETECTABLE BY ULTRASOUND

Common Findings:

Organ hypertrophy, particularly the following:

- Enlargement and echogenicity of the kidneys
- Overall macrosomia
- Macroglossia, with protrusion of the tongue through an open mouth

Omphalocele

Polyhydramnios

Occasional Findings:

Cryptorchidism

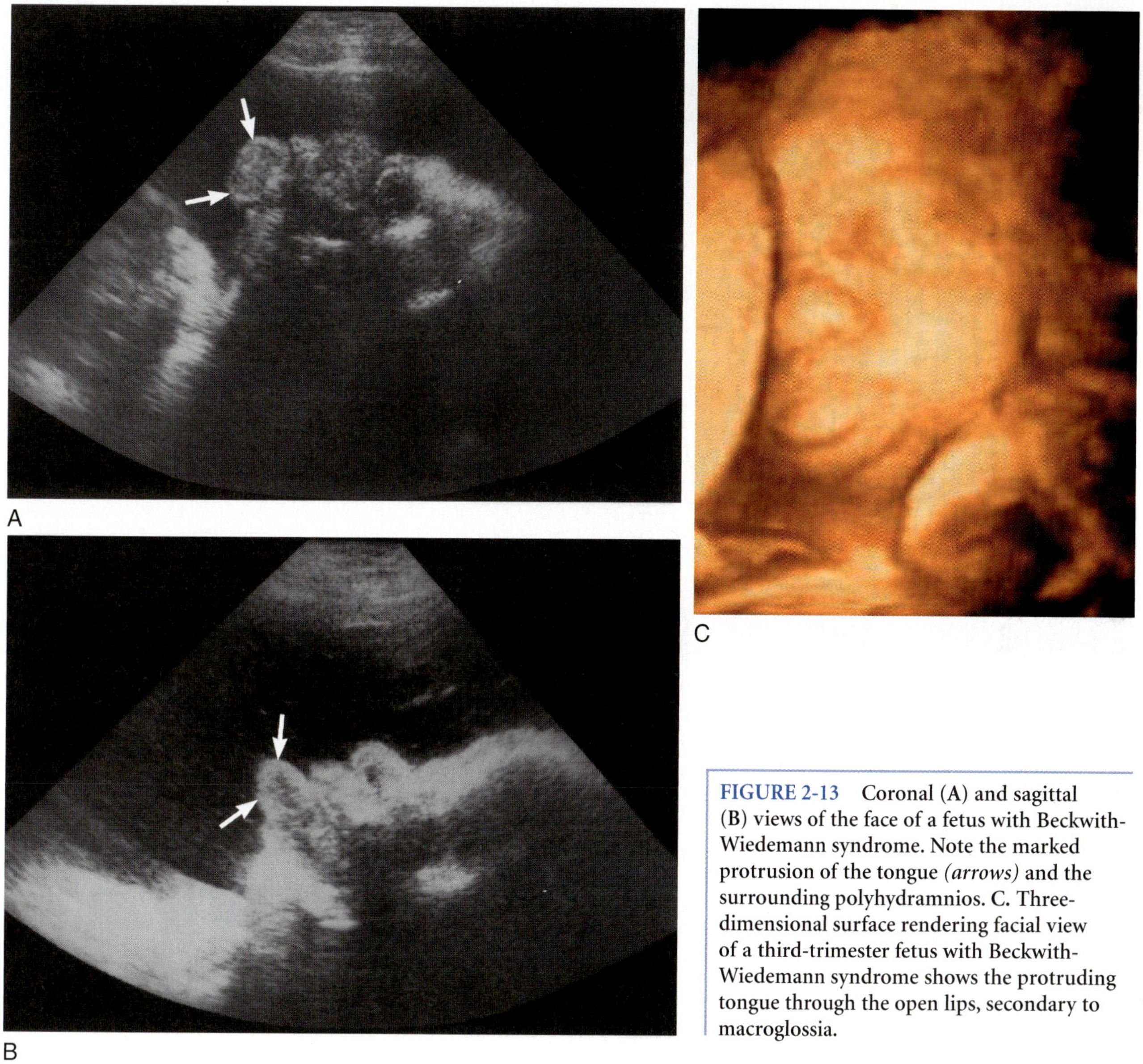

FIGURE 2-13 Coronal (A) and sagittal (B) views of the face of a fetus with Beckwith-Wiedemann syndrome. Note the marked protrusion of the tongue *(arrows)* and the surrounding polyhydramnios. C. Three-dimensional surface rendering facial view of a third-trimester fetus with Beckwith-Wiedemann syndrome shows the protruding tongue through the open lips, secondary to macroglossia.

Hypospadias

Cardiomyopathy with cardiomegaly

Enlarged pancreas

Placental abnormalities suggesting a partial mole, similar to triploidy

MAJOR DIFFERENTIAL DIAGNOSES

Other syndromes associated with macrosomia:

- Marshall-Smith syndrome
- Maternal diabetes
- Perlman syndrome
- Sotos' syndrome
- Weaver syndrome

Beckwith-Wiedemann syndrome should be suspected if macrosomia is associated with an omphalocele.

ULTRASOUND DIAGNOSIS

Since the first reported ultrasound diagnosis of this syndrome in 1980, there have been many reports of associated sonographic findings. They include the development of macrosomia (usually in the late second or third trimester), enlargement of the kidneys, omphalocele, and macroglossia. Usually, polyhydramnios is present. One report describes an enlarged pancreas in the second trimester.

There are some reports of associated placental enlargement, with villus hydrops. The diagnosis can be established as early as 12 weeks'

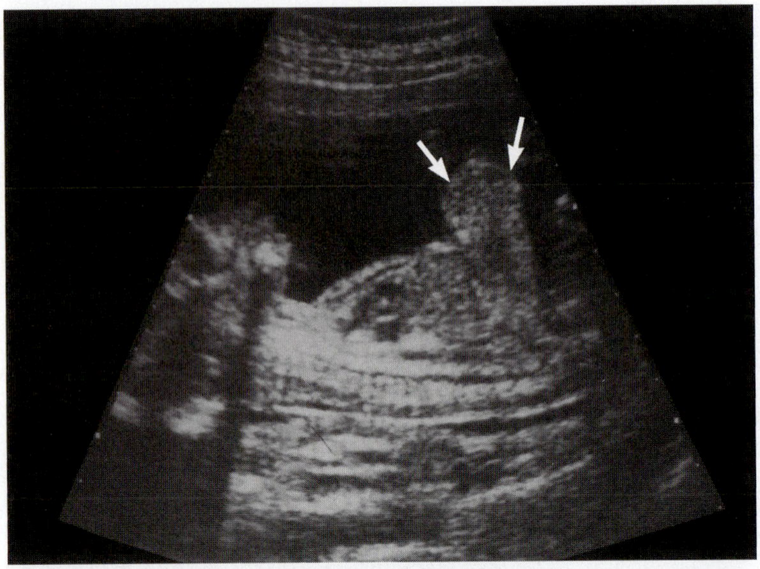

A

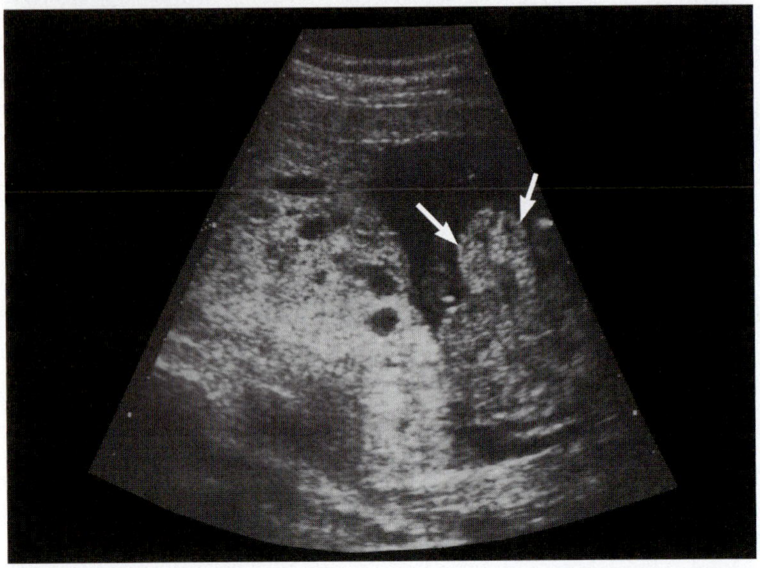

B

FIGURE 2-14 (A) Longitudinal view of an early second-trimester fetus with Beckwith-Wiedemann syndrome and an omphalocele *(arrows)*. (B) Transverse view of the same fetus with omphalocele *(arrows)*. Note that the placenta has multiple echolucencies, a sign consistent with hydropic changes of the placenta, as is seen in partial moles.

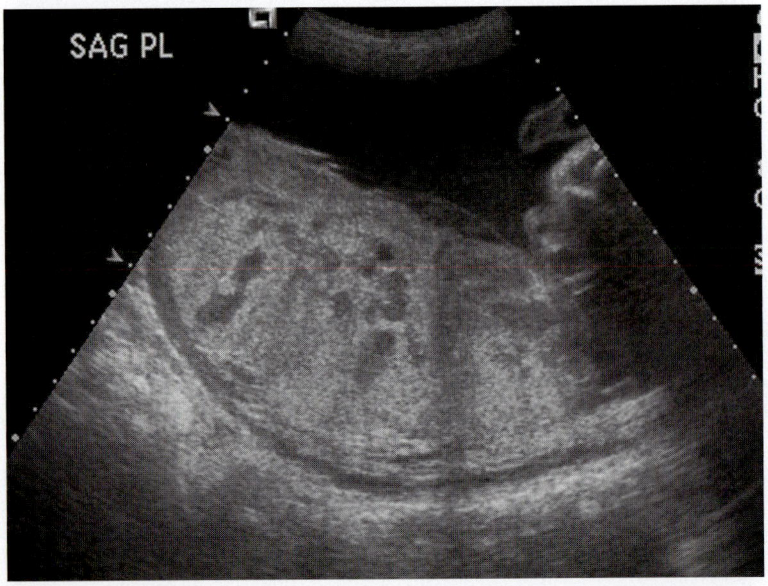

FIGURE 2-15 Second-trimester fetus with Beckwith-Wiedemann syndrome shows multiple echolucencies within the placenta mimicking a partial mole.

gestation, particularly when an omphalocele is present. In cases without an omphalocele, gigantism may not be detectable until later, making the diagnosis difficult, if not impossible, in early gestation.

HEREDITY

Although most often sporadic, there is evidence that a minority of cases are autosomal dominant, with an excess of transmitting females. The genetics of this syndrome are complex and beyond the scope of this book. The genes responsible for this syndrome are polymorphic loci located at 11p15.5. Defective, inverted, or deleted maternal genes at that locus (and the paternal duplications) and uniparental disomy are responsible for the syndrome in many of affected individuals.

NATURAL HISTORY AND OUTCOME

Fetuses with Beckwith-Wiedemann syndrome have a tendency to be born prematurely because of polyhydramnios and preterm enlargement of the uterus. Neonates can develop hypoglycemia and hyperviscosity syndrome. Macroglossia can lead to swallowing and respiratory difficulties. The 20% infant mortality rate can be attributed to dystocia, neonatal hypoglycemia, seizures, and cardiac failure. Other risks include childhood neoplasms, such as Wilms' tumor, hepatoblastoma, and other neoplasias. Close monitoring for tumor development is warranted. Survivors tend to be generally healthy.

Suggested Reading

Carseldine DB, Crocker EF, Walker AG, et al: The pre- and postnatal appearance of the kidneys in Beckwith-Wiedemann syndrome. *Australas Radiol* 27:30–32, 1983.

Cobellis G, Iannoto P, Stabile M, et al: Prenatal ultrasound diagnosis of macroglossia in the Wiedemann-Beckwith syndrome. *Prenat Diagn* 8:79–81, 1988.

Grundy H, Walton S, Burlbaw J, et al: Beckwith-Wiedemann syndrome: prenatal ultrasound diagnosis using standard kidney to abdominal circumference ratio. *Am J Perinatol* 2:236–239, 1985.

Harker CP, Winter T III, Mack L: Prenatal diagnosis of Beckwith-Wiedemann syndrome. *AJR Am J Roentgenol* 168:520–522, 1997.

Hillstrom MM, Brown DL, Wilkins-Haug L, Genest DR: Sonographic appearance of placenta villous hydrops associated with Beckwith-Wiedemann syndrome. *J Ultrasound Med* 14:61–64, 1995.

Jones KL: *Smith's recognizable patterns of human malformations.* Philadelphia, 2006, Elsevier.

Koontz WL, Shaw LA, Lavery JP: Antenatal sonographic appearance of Beckwith-Wiedemann syndrome. *J Clin Ultrasound* 14:57–59, 1986.

Lage JM: Placentomegaly with massive hydrops of the placental stem villi, diploid DNA content, and fetal omphaloceles: possible association with Beckwith-Wiedemann syndrome. *Hum Pathol* 22:591, 1991.

Lodeiro JG, Byers JW, Chuipek S, et al: Prenatal diagnosis and perinatal management of the Beckwith-Wiedemann syndrome: a case and review. *Am J Perinatol* 6:446, 1989.

Meizner I, Carmi R, Katz M, et al: In utero prenatal diagnosis of Beckwith-Wiedemann syndrome: a case report. *Eur J Obstet Gynecol Reprod Biol* 32:259, 1989.

Moutou C, Junien C, Henry I, Bonaiti-Pellie CJ: Beckwith-Wiedemann syndrome: a demonstration of the mechanisms responsible for the excess of transmitting females. *Med Genet* 29:217–220, 1992.

Mulik V, Wellesley D, Sawdy R, Howe DT: Unusual prenatal presentation of Beckwith-Wiedemann syndrome. *Prenat Diagn* 24:501–503, 2004.

O'Grady JP, Tunney C, Pflueger SMV, et al: Beckwith-Wiedemann syndrome: prenatal ultrasonic diagnosis and clinical implications. *J Matern Fetal Med* 1:70–74, 1992.

Pelizzo G, Conoscenti G, Kalache KD, Vesce F, Guerrini P, Cavazzini L: Antenatal manifestation of congenital pancreatoblastoma in a fetus with Beckwith-Wiedemann syndrome. *Prenat Diagn* 23:292–294, 2003.

Ranzini AC, Day-Salvatore D, Turner T, Smulian JC, Vintzileos AM: Intrauterine growth and ultrasound findings in fetuses with Beckwith-Wiedemann syndrome. *Obstet Gynecol* 89:538–542, 1997.

Reish O, Lerer I, Amiel A, et al: Wiedemann-Beckwith syndrome: further prenatal characterization of the condition. *Am J Med Genet* 107:209–213, 2002.

Shah YG, Metlay L: Prenatal ultrasound diagnosis of Beckwith-Wiedemann syndrome. *J Clin Ultrasound* 18:597–600, 1990.

Shapiro LR, Duncan PA, Davidian MM, et al: The placenta in familial Beckwith-Wiedemann syndrome. *Birth Defects* 18:203, 1982.

Takayama M, Soma H, Yaguchi S, et al: Abnormally large placenta associated with Beckwith-Wiedemann syndrome. *Gynecol Obstet Invest* 22:165, 1986.

Viljoen DL, Jaquire Z, Woods DL: Prenatal diagnosis in autosomal dominant Beckwith-Wiedemann syndrome. *Prenat Diagn* 11:167–175, 1991.

Weinstein L, Anderson C: In utero diagnosis of Beckwith-Wiedemann syndrome by ultrasound. *Radiology* 134:474, 1990.

Weissman A, Mashiach S, Achiron R: Macroglossia: prenatal ultrasonographic diagnosis and proposed management. *Prenat Diagn* 15:66–69, 1995 (short communication).

Wieacker P, Wilhelm C, Greiner P, et al: Prenatal diagnosis of Wiedemann-Beckwith syndrome. *J Perinat Med* 17:351, 1989.

Williams DH, Gauthier DW, Maizels M: Prenatal diagnosis of Beckwith-Wiedemann syndrome. *Prenat Diagn* 25:879–884, 2005.

Winter SC, Curry CJR, Smith JC, et al: Prenatal diagnosis of the Beckwith-Wiedemann syndrome. *Am J Med Genet* 24:137, 1986.

MATERNAL DIABETES

DESCRIPTION AND DEFINITION

Fetuses of diabetic mothers tend to be macrosomic and are at increased risk for developing major malformations, particularly if the mother's diabetes was not effectively managed during organogenesis in the early first trimester.

ABNORMALITIES DETECTABLE BY ULTRASOUND

Fetal overgrowth is the most common finding, with routine biometry demonstrating growth acceleration by the end of the second trimester.

Malformations associated with maternal diabetes include the following:

- Anencephaly, holoprosencephaly, and neural tube defects
- Caudal regression syndrome
- Cardiac abnormalities, including transposition of the great arteries, ventricular septal defects, and tetralogy of Fallot
- Renal anomalies, including renal hypoplasia (unilateral or bilateral) and hydronephrosis
- Polyhydramnios

MAJOR DIFFERENTIAL DIAGNOSES

Other syndromes associated with macrosomia:

- Beckwith-Wiedemann syndrome
- Marshall-Smith syndrome
- Perlman syndrome
- Sotos' syndrome
- Weaver syndrome

ULTRASOUND DIAGNOSIS

The diagnosis of macrosomia can be made in the late second trimester and in the third trimester, using biometry to demonstrate pronounced enlargement in abdominal circumference, head circumference, and thickness of the echogenic fat stripe around the abdomen and head. This stripe of soft tissue or fat can sometimes be mistaken for skin edema, as seen in hydrops. The lengths of the long bones tend to be normal, with the pattern of macrosomia focused on the abdominal circumference, shoulder width, and soft tissues rather than on the skeleton. Polyhydramnios often is associated with pregnancy in diabetic women, but it does not develop until the third trimester.

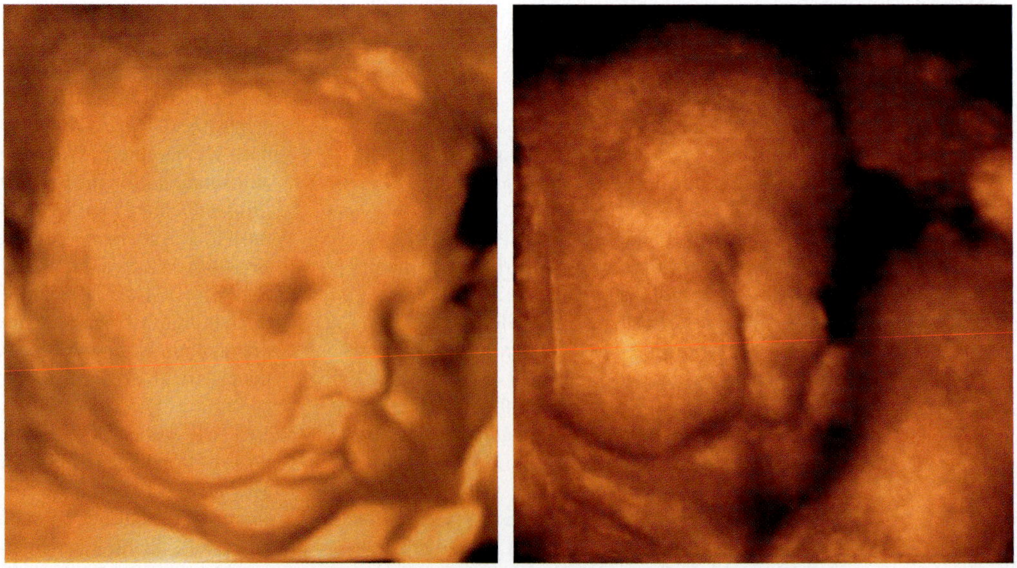
A B

FIGURE 2-16 (A, B) Three-dimensional surface rendering of two different fetuses with severe macrosomia. Note the large cheeks of both fetuses, a facial feature typical of fetuses with macrosomia.

Structural abnormalities (e.g., anencephaly and neural tube defects) can be diagnosed early in gestation, often by the late first trimester. They are most common in diabetic women who did not have good glycemic control during organogenesis. Eighteen weeks' gestation is considered an ideal time for evaluating the fetus of a diabetic mother, including examination of the heart, kidneys, brain, spine, and extremities. Major neural tube defects, however, have been diagnosed as early as 12 weeks.

HEREDITY

Consideration of a hereditary pattern is not applicable to this syndrome.

NATURAL HISTORY AND OUTCOME

During pregnancy, diabetic women may encounter complications related to structural abnormalities of their fetuses. Other complications include those associated with macrosomia, dystocia, and polyhydramnios. Fetuses of diabetic mothers tend to have delayed lung development, which must be factored into obstetric management when contemplating early delivery. There is an increased fetal death rate, particularly in late pregnancy, and a risk of fetal growth restriction in diabetic mothers with vasculopathies.

Suggested Reading

Albert TJ, Landon MB, Wheller JJ, et al: Prenatal detection of fetal anomalies in pregnancies complicated by insulin-dependent diabetes mellitus. *Am J Obstet Gynecol* 174:1424–1428, 1996.

Cousins L: Congenital anomalies among infants of diabetic mothers. *Am J Obstet Gynecol* 147:333–338, 1983.

Greene M, Hare J, Cloherty J, Benacerraf B, Soeldner JS: First trimester hemoglobin Al and risk for major malformation and spontaneous abortion in diabetic pregnancy. *Teratology* 39:225–231, 1989.

Greene MF, Benacerraf BR: Prenatal diagnosis in diabetic gravidas: utility of ultrasound and maternal serum alpha-fetoprotein screening. *Obstet Gynecol* 77:520–524, 1991.

Landon MB: Prenatal diagnosis of macrosomia in pregnancy complicated by diabetes mellitus. *J Matern Fetal Med* 9:52–54, 2000.

PERLMAN SYNDROME

DESCRIPTION AND DEFINITION

Perlman syndrome is a fetal overgrowth syndrome characterized by macrosomia, bilaterally enlarged kidneys, renal tumors, and other visceromegaly associated with polyhydramnios.

ABNORMALITIES DETECTABLE BY ULTRASOUND

Common Findings:

First trimester:

- Cystic hygroma
- Thickened nuchal lucency

Second and third trimesters:

- Macrosomia
- Enlarged kidneys
- Renal tumors (hamartoma, Wilms' tumor)
- Cardiac abnormalities
- Visceromegaly
- Ascites
- Polyhydramnios

MAJOR DIFFERENTIAL DIAGNOSES

Beckwith-Wiedemann syndrome

Simpson-Golabi-Behmel syndrome

Other syndromes associated with enlarged kidneys (but *not* associated with macrosomia):

- Meckel-Gruber syndrome
- Polycystic kidney syndromes

ULTRASOUND DIAGNOSIS

Perlman syndrome has been detected at 18 weeks, with cystic hygromata, cardiac defect, enlarged echogenic kidneys, hepatomegaly, polyhydramnios, and macrosomia or overgrowth. This syndrome has manifested in the first trimester as a thickened nuchal translucency or cystic hygroma.

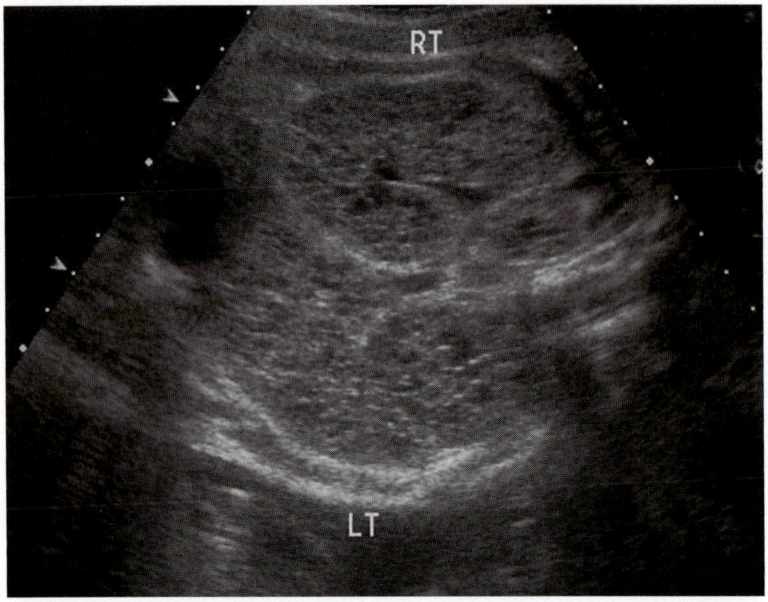

A

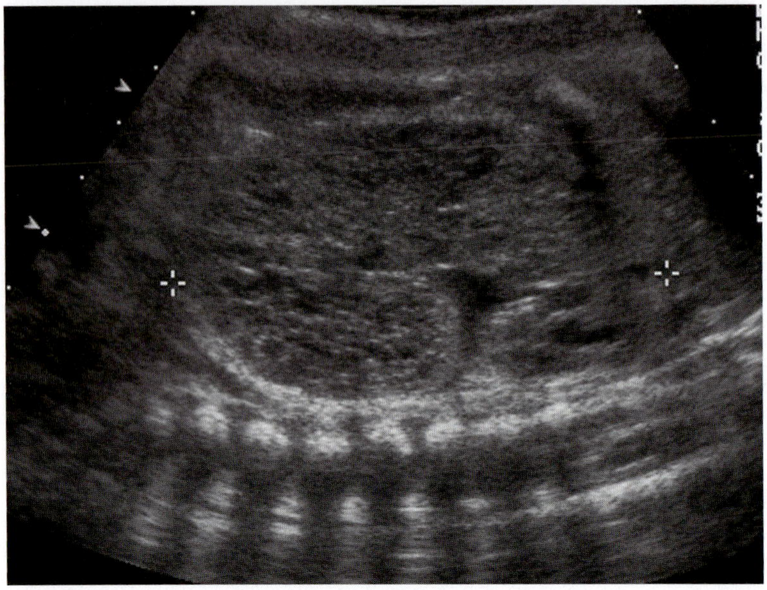

B

FIGURE 2-17 **(A, B) Coronal and longitudinal views of enlarged kidneys in a fetus that was very large. These large echogenic kidneys can be seen in fetuses with Perlman syndrome.**

HEREDITY

This syndrome is thought to be an autosomal recessive syndrome.

NATURAL HISTORY AND OUTCOME

There are severe neurodevelopmental deficits and a downhill course. The prognosis is dismal, with death usually occurring within the first year of life.

Suggested Reading

Chitty LS, Clark T, Maxwell D: Perlman syndrome—a cause of enlarged, hyperechogenic kidneys. *Prenat Diagn* 18:1163–1168, 1998 (short communication).

DeRoche ME, Craffey A, Greenstein R, Borgida AF: Antenatal sonographic features of Perlman syndrome. *J Ultrasound Med* 23:561–564, 2004.

Henneveld HT, van Lingen RA, Hamel BCJ, Stolte-Dijkstra I, van Essen AJ: Perlman syndrome: four additional cases and review. *Am J Med Genet* 86:439–446, 1999.

Perlman M, Levin M, Wittels B: Syndrome of fetal gigantism, renal hamartomas and nephroblastomatosis with Wilms' tumour. *Cancer* 35:1212–1217, 1975.

Perlman M, Goldberg GM, Bar-Ziv J, Danovitch G: Renal hamartomas and nephroblastomatosis with fetal gigantism: a familial syndrome. *J Pediatr* 83:414–418, 1973.

Schilke K, Schaefer F, Waldherr R, et al: A case of Perlman syndrome: fetal gigantism, renal dysplasia, and severe neurological deficits. *Am J Med Genet* 91:29–33, 2000.

Syndromes Featuring Primarily Facial Anomalies

BRANCHIO-OCULO-FACIAL SYNDROME

DESCRIPTION AND DEFINITION

This syndrome is characterized by mental retardation, growth deficiency, ocular defects, and clefting of the upper lip.

ABNORMALITIES DETECTABLE BY ULTRASOUND

Common Findings:

Pseudo-cleft lip, which is characterized by incomplete bilateral clefts

Microphthalmia or anophthalmia

Prenatal growth deficiency

Occasional Findings:

Microcephaly

Orbital cyst

Cataract

Cleft palate

Ear abnormalities

Renal agenesis

Polydactyly

MAJOR DIFFERENTIAL DIAGNOSES

Cerebro-oculo-facio-skeletal (COFS) syndrome

Goldenhar syndrome

Median cleft face

Oral-facial-digital syndromes

Trisomy 13

Van der Woude syndrome

Walker-Warburg syndrome

ULTRASOUND DIAGNOSIS

Prenatal detection of this syndrome in a patient was accomplished at 27 weeks, with sonographic diagnosis of bilateral incomplete cleft lip and anophthalmia. An earlier scan at 15 weeks in this patient was reported as unremarkable, although limited.

HEREDITY

This is an autosomal dominant disorder.

NATURAL HISTORY AND OUTCOME

Most individuals with this condition have normal intelligence, although 25% have mild mental retardation. Additional abnormalities noted after birth are low-set ears with some conductive hearing loss and supra-auricular sinuses. Affected individuals have dental abnormalities, micrognathia, and premature graying of the scalp hair.

Suggested Reading

Bromley B, Miller WA, Mansour R, Benacerraf B: Prenatal findings of branchio-oculo-facial syndrome. *J Ultrasound Med* 17:475–477, 1998.

Jones KL: *Smith's recognizable patterns of human malformations.* Philadelphia, 2006, Elsevier.

Lin AE, Gorlin RJ, Lurie IW, et al: Further delineation of the branchio-oculo-facial syndrome. *Am J Med Genet* 56:42–59, 1995.

McCool M, Weaver DD: Branchio-oculo-facial syndrome: broadening the spectrum. *Am J Med Genet* 49:414–421, 1994.

Richardson E, Davison C, Moore AT: Colobomatous microphthalmia with midfacial clefting: part of the spectrum of branchio-oculo-facial syndrome? *Ophthalmol Genet* 17:59–65, 1996.

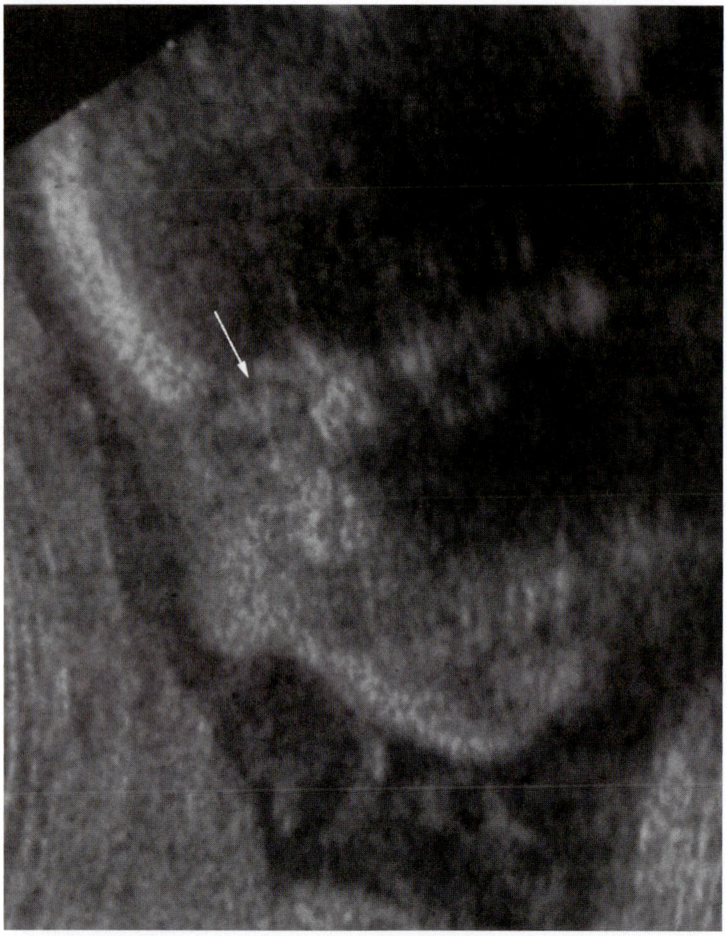

A

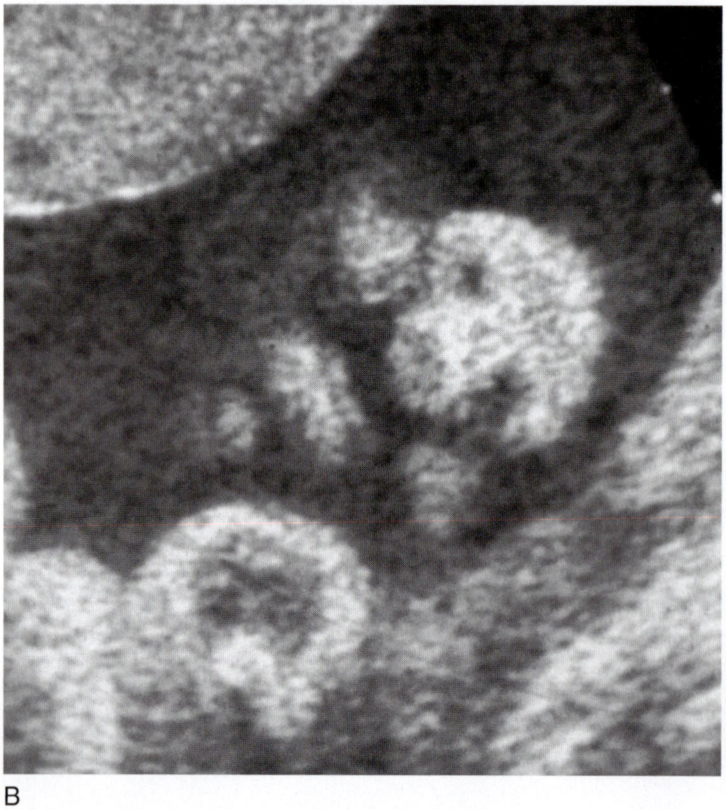

B

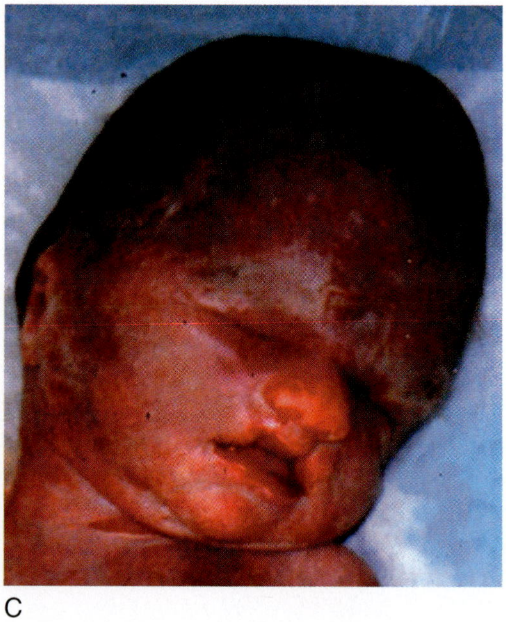

C

FIGURE 2-18 (A) Third-trimester fetus with branchio-oculo-facial syndrome shows absence of the orbit *(arrow)*. (B) Coronal view through the fetal mouth of the same third-trimester fetus shows bilateral incomplete cleft lip not involving the nose. (C) Same third-trimester fetus with anophthalmia and incomplete cleft, both features typical of branchio-oculo-facial syndrome. (Panels B and C from Bromley B, Miller WA, Mansour R, Benacerraf B: Prenatal findings of branchio-oculo-facial syndrome. *J Ultrasound Med* 17:475–477, 1998.)

CATARACTS

DESCRIPTION AND DEFINITION

Congenital cataracts can be part of many different syndromes, although they also can be an isolated finding, inherited as an autosomal dominant condition.

ABNORMALITIES DETECTABLE BY ULTRASOUND

Dense, echogenic lenses of the eyes are best seen using high-frequency (e.g., 7-MHz) transducers and even a transvaginal approach.

Associated abnormalities depend on whether the presence of these cataracts is part of a syndrome (see next section) or an isolated occurrence.

MAJOR DIFFERENTIAL DIAGNOSES

Arthrogryposis

Branchio-oculo-facial syndrome

Cerebro-oculo-facio-skeletal (COFS) syndrome

Chondrodysplasia punctata

Coloboma

Congenital aniridia

Congenital infections

Down syndrome

Enzymatic disorders

Glucose-6-phosphate dehydrogenase (G6PD) deficiency

Hallermann-Streiff syndrome

Homocystinuria

Hypochondroplasia

Kniest syndrome

Marfan syndrome

Microphthalmia

Multiple pterygium syndrome

Neu-Laxova syndrome

Roberts' syndrome

Smith-Lemli-Opitz syndrome

Stickler syndrome

Teratogens (see list in Chapter 1)

Walker-Warburg syndrome

ULTRASOUND DIAGNOSIS

Prenatal sonographic diagnosis of congenital cataracts has been established in patients at risk for autosomal dominant transmission of the condition. In several cases, ultrasound studies have established a prenatal diagnosis of cataracts, sometimes as early as 15 weeks' gestation, using a high-frequency transducer (6.5–7 MHz, transvaginally) to demonstrate an opaque fetal lens in the anterior aspect of the orbit. However, the threshold for diagnosis of cataracts remains uncertain, and mild forms of cataracts may not be detectable early.

HEREDITY

Both autosomal dominant and autosomal recessive inheritance have been reported. The inheritance of certain syndromes associated with cataracts is dependent on the syndrome itself.

NATURAL HISTORY AND OUTCOME

The outcome for fetuses with cataracts depends on the underlying associated syndrome. Isolated cataracts are treatable by surgery in infancy.

Suggested Reading

Bronshtein M, Zimmer EZ, Gershoni-Baruch R, et al: First and second trimester diagnosis of fetal ocular defects and associated anomalies: report of eight cases. *Obstet Gynecol* 7:443–449, 1991.

Cengiz B, Baxi L: Congenital cataract in triplet pregnancy after IVF with frozen embryos: prenatal diagnosis and management. *Fetal Diagn Ther* 16:234–236, 2001.

Drysdale K, Kyle PM, Sepulveda W: Prenatal detection of congenital inherited cataracts. *Ultrasound Obstet Gynecol* 9:62–63, 1997.

Gaary EA, Rawnsley E, Marin-Padilla JM, Morse CL, Crow HC: In utero detection of fetal cataracts. *J Ultrasound Med* 4:234–236, 1993.

Mashiach R, Vardimon D, Kaplan B, Shalev J, Meizner I: Early sonographic detection of recurrent fetal eye anomalies. *Ultrasound Obstet Gynecol* 24:640–643, 2004.

Monteagudo A, Timor-Tritsch IE, Friedman AH, Santos R: Autosomal dominant cataracts of the fetus: early detection by transvaginal ultrasound. *Ultrasound Obstet Gynecol* 8:104–108, 1996.

Pedreira DA, Diniz EM, Schultz R, Faro LB, Zugaib M: Fetal cataract in congenital toxoplasmosis. *Ultrasound Obstet Gynecol* 13:266–267, 1999.

Romain M, Awoust J, Dugauquier C, Van Maldergem L: Prenatal ultrasound detection of congenital cataract in trisomy 21. *Prenat Diagn* 19:780–782, 1999.

Zimmer EZ, Bronshtein M, Ophir E, et al: Sonographic diagnosis of fetal congenital cataracts. *Prenat Diagn* 13:503–511, 1993.

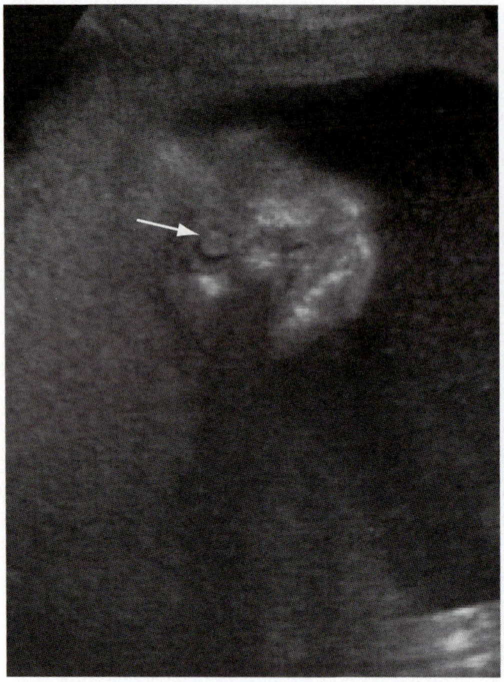

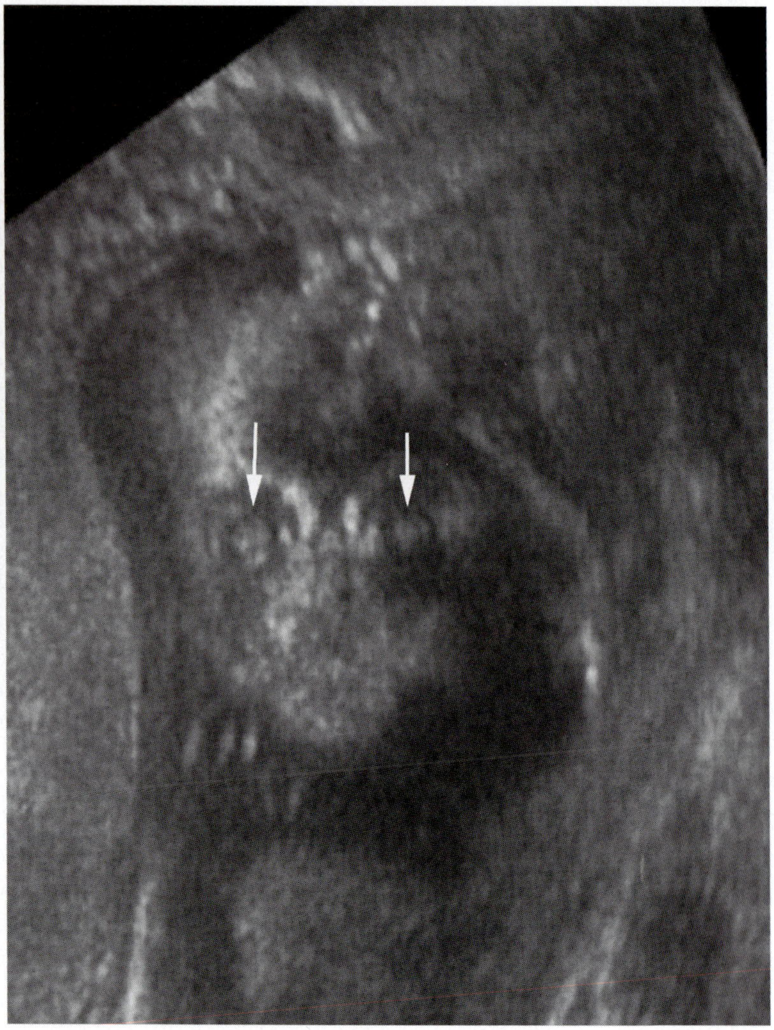

FIGURE 2-19 (A) Coronal view through a second-trimester fetal face shows echogenic opacity of the fetal lens *(arrow)* consistent with a cataract. Note that this fetus also has a facial cleft. (B) Fetus with trisomy 13 who has bilateral cataracts. Note the increased opacification of the lenses *(arrows)*.

CEREBROCOSTOMANDIBULAR SYNDROME

DESCRIPTION AND DEFINITION

Synonym: Rib gap defects with micrognathia

This is an autosomal recessive condition, characterized by severe micrognathia, cleft palate, and vertebral body abnormalities associated with defective costal development.

ABNORMALITIES DETECTABLE BY ULTRASOUND

Common Findings:

Micrognathia

Hemivertebrae

Narrow chest

Rib deformities

Decreased ossification of the ribs, particularly posteriorly

Cystic hygroma/nuchal thickening

Polyhydramnios

Occasional Findings:

Microcephaly

Choanal atresia

Hypoplasia of the bones of the upper extremities

Renal anomalies

Club feet

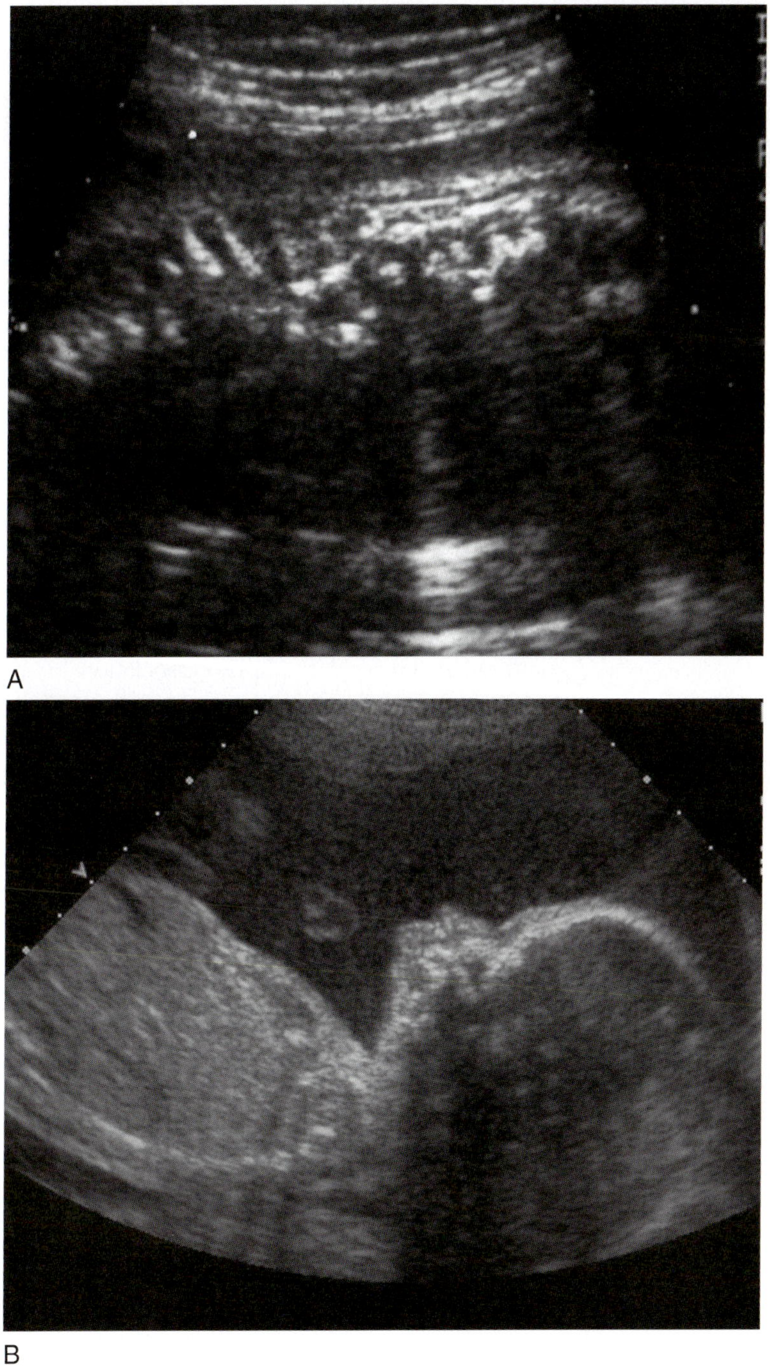

FIGURE 2-20 (A) Coronal view through the fetal spine shows multiple vertebral body abnormalities of the thoracic and lumbar spine. These findings are seen in fetuses with cerebrocostomandibular syndrome. (B) Profile view of a second-trimester fetus with severe micrognathia, a finding that can be seen in fetuses with cerebrocostomandibular syndrome.

Scoliosis

Ventricular septal defect

Intracranial abnormalities (e.g., ventriculomegaly and agenesis of the corpus callosum)

Meningomyelocele

Omphalocele

MAJOR DIFFERENTIAL DIAGNOSES

Other syndromes associated with micrognathia:

- Cornelia De Lange syndrome
- Goldenhar syndrome
- Joubert syndrome
- Nager syndrome
- Neu-Laxova syndrome
- Oral-facial-digital syndromes
- Pena Shokeir syndrome
- Pierre Robin syndrome
- Seckel syndrome
- Shprintzen syndrome

Smith-Lemli-Opitz syndrome

Stickler syndrome

Treacher Collins syndrome

Other syndromes and associations with rib abnormalities:

Jarcho-Levin syndrome

Klippel Feil syndrome

MURCS (**mü**llerian duct aplasia, **r**enal aplasia, **c**ervicothoracic **s**omite dysplasia) association

Spondylocostal dysplasia

Spondylothoracic dysplasia

VATER (**v**ertebral defects, **a**nal atresia, **t**racheoesophageal fistula, **e**sophageal atresia, and **r**adial and renal dysplasias) association

ULTRASOUND DIAGNOSIS

There are several reports of prenatal diagnosis of this syndrome, starting at 12 weeks' gestation with thickened nuchal translucency and at 16 weeks' gestation with an essentially absent mandible. Other findings include polyhydramnios, mild pyelectasis, lack of visible ossification of the ribs, severe micrognathia, and IUGR.

HEREDITY

This is an autosomal recessive condition, although there have been occasional reports of autosomal dominant transmission.

NATURAL HISTORY AND OUTCOME

The outcome of affected newborns varies, depending on the degree of abnormality. Severe micrognathia and cleft palate in an infant with serious respiratory difficulty may indicate cerebrocostomandibular syndrome. The manifestations of the disorder are extremely variable in severity and expression. Approximately half of affected infants die by the end of the first year, usually as a result of severe respiratory problems. One third of survivors have mental deficiency.

Suggested Reading

Jones KL: *Smith's recognizable patterns of human malformations.* Philadelphia, 2006, Elsevier.

Ibba RM, Corda A, Zoppi MA, Floris M, Todde P, Monni G: Cerebro-costo-mandibular syndrome: early sonographic prenatal diagnosis. *Ultrasound Obstet Gynecol* 10:142–144, 1997.

Kirk EP, Arbuckle S, Ramm PL, Ades LC: Severe micrognathia, cleft palate, absent olfactory tract, and abnormal rib development: cerebro-costo-mandibular syndrome or a new syndrome? *Am J Med Genet* 84:120–124, 1999.

Lee W, McNie B, Chaiworapongsa T, et al: Three-dimensional ultrasonographic presentation of micrognathia. *J Ultrasound Med* 21:775–781, 2002.

Megier P, Ayeva-Derman M, Esperandieu O, Aubry MC, Couly G, Deroches A: Prenatal ultrasonographic diagnosis of the cerebro-costo-mandibular syndrome: case report and review of the literature. *Prenat Diagn* 12:1294–1299, 1998.

Merlob P, Schonfeld A, Grunebaum M, Mor N, Reisner SH: Autosomal dominant cerebro-costo-mandibular syndrome: ultrasonographic and clinical findings. *Am J Med Genet* 26:195–202, 1987.

Morin G, Gekas J, Naepels P, et al: Cerebro-costo-mandibular syndrome in a father and a female fetus: early prenatal ultrasonographic diagnosis and autosomal dominant transmission. *Prenat Diagn* 10:890–893, 2001.

CLEFT LIP AND PALATE

DESCRIPTION AND DEFINITION

Paramedian cleft lip and palate occur when the inner maxillary segment and lateral maxillary prominences fail to close by approximately 8 to 9 weeks' gestation. The condition can occur as a unilateral or bilateral defect.

ABNORMALITIES DETECTABLE BY ULTRASOUND

Bilateral complete cleft lip and palate, in which the inner maxillary segment (just under the nose) forms a flap that protrudes anteriorly and can easily be seen in both coronal and sagittal views

Complete cleft lip and palate (unilateral or bilateral), in which the defect extends into the nasal region and the anterior third of the palate, causing widening and flattening of the nostril

Incomplete cleft lip, which involves only the lip and generally produces more subtle sonographic findings (e.g., minimal distortion of the nose)

Hypertelorism

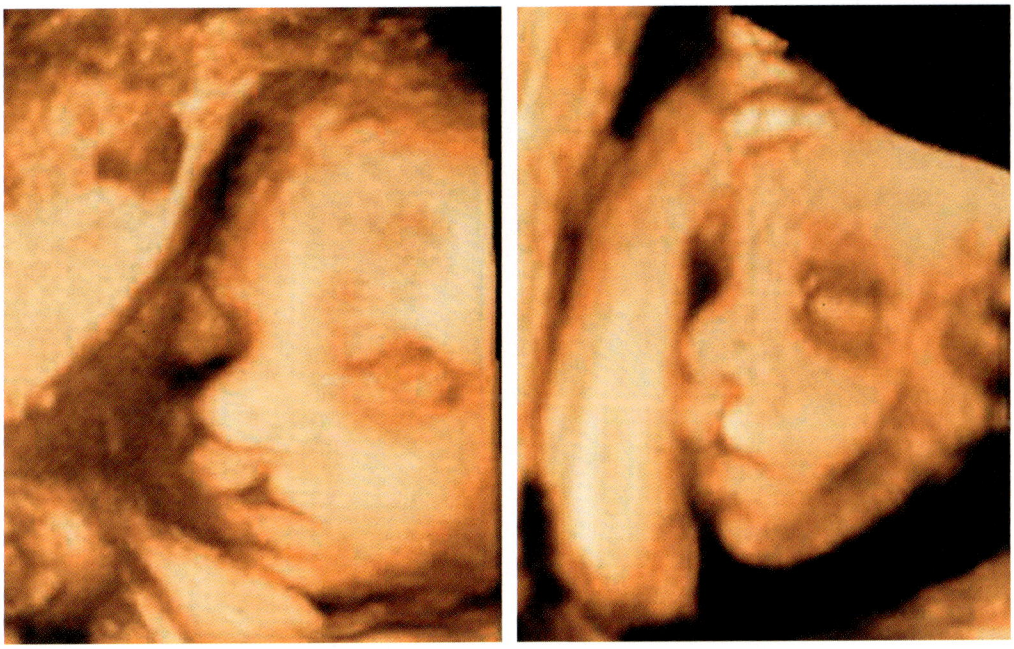

A B

FIGURE 2-21 (A, B) Incomplete cleft lip only seen on three-dimensional surface reconstruction at 29 weeks. Note the limited distortion of the nose and the rest of the face.

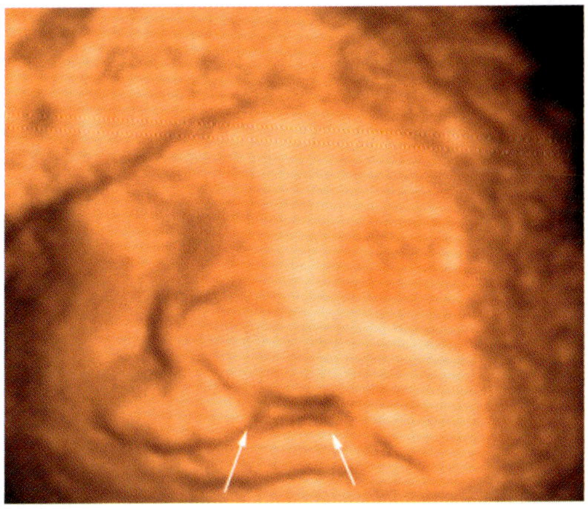

FIGURE 2-22 Third-trimester fetus with a unilateral complete cleft lip and palate seen using three-dimensional surface reconstruction. Note that the cleft is wide *(arrows)*, causing a large gap between the portions of the upper lip and flattening of the nose on one side.

Abnormalities of the nose

Range of clinical manifestations depends on the etiology of the cleft lip and palate in any given fetus, as well as any associated syndromes that may be present.

Midline clefts are associated with the most severe syndromes and anomalies affecting other organ systems. Midline cleft lip and palate is characterized by maxillary hypoplasia or absence of the premaxilla and hypotelorism.

MAJOR DIFFERENTIAL DIAGNOSES

Van der Woude syndrome, which has an autosomal dominant pattern of inheritance, is a labial cleft syndrome associated with small pits on the lower lip and variable clefting of the upper lip and palate.

Although most *children* with cleft lip and palate have isolated lesions that can successfully be repaired with plastic surgery, most *fetuses* with cleft lip and palate have multiple severe abnormalities associated with the defect and a high incidence of chromosomal anomalies. Less than 50% of fetuses with cleft lip and palate diagnosed in utero have this abnormality as an isolated lesion.

Associated congenital syndromes:

- Adams-Oliver syndrome
- Amniotic band syndrome
- Arthrogryposis
- Branchio-oculo-facial syndrome
- Camptomelic dysplasia
- Caudal regression syndrome/sirenomelia

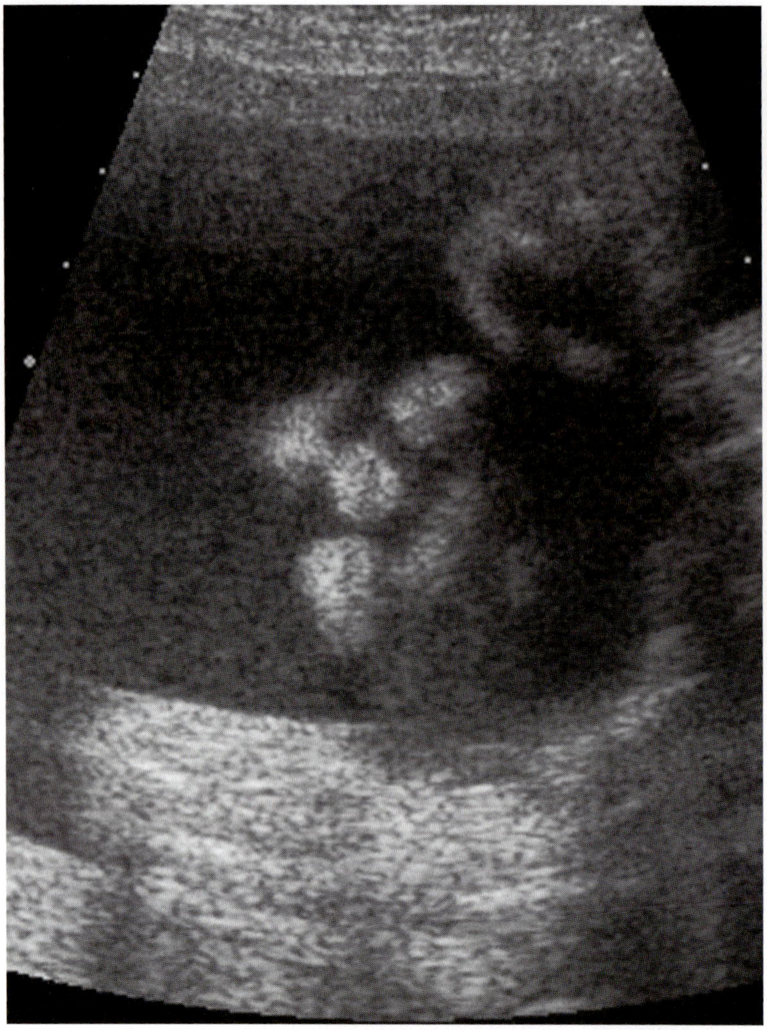

A

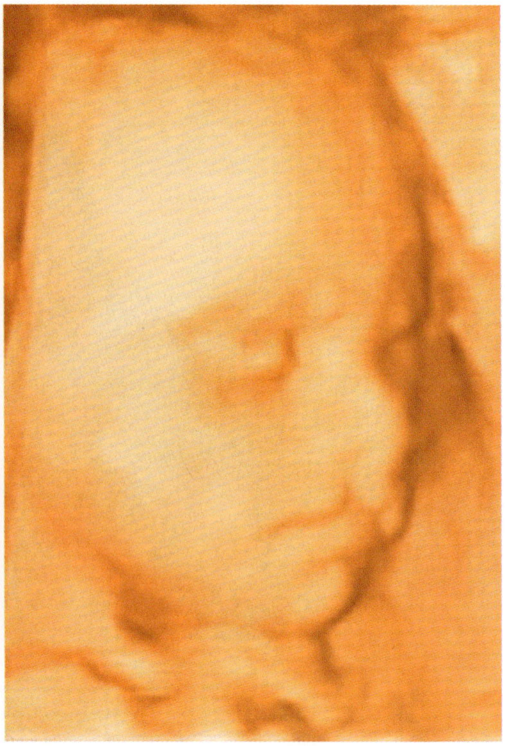

B

FIGURE 2-23 (A) Bilateral cleft lip seen coronally in two dimensions shows that the cleft is symmetric on either side of the inner maxillary segment. (B) Third-trimester fetus with bilateral cleft lip without cleft palate seen with three-dimensional surface reconstruction. Note the intactness of the nose and the relatively narrow cleft compared to fetus shown in Figure 2-22.

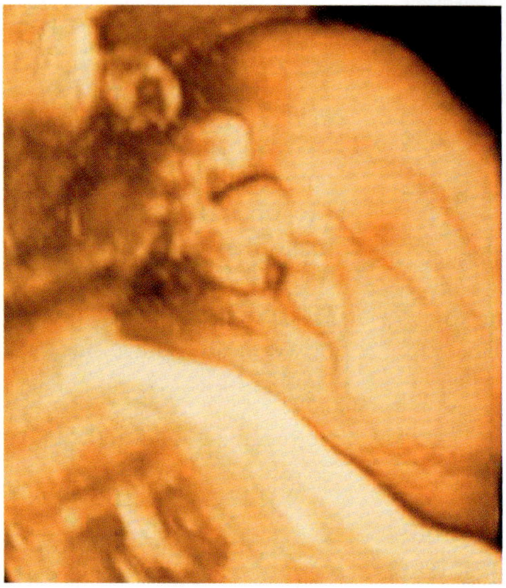

FIGURE 2-24 Bilateral complete cleft lip and palate in third trimester fetus seen using three-dimensional surface reconstruction. Note that the cleft is best seen on one side involving the base of the nostril.

Cerebro-oculo-facio-skeletal (COFS) syndrome

CHARGE association

Chromosomal anomalies

Crouzon syndrome

Diastrophic dysplasia

DiGeorge syndrome

Ectrodactyly–ectodermal dysplasia–clefting (EEC) syndrome

Fraser syndrome

Fryns syndrome

Goldenhar syndrome

Gorlin syndrome

Holoprosencephaly

Hydrolethalus

Larsen syndrome

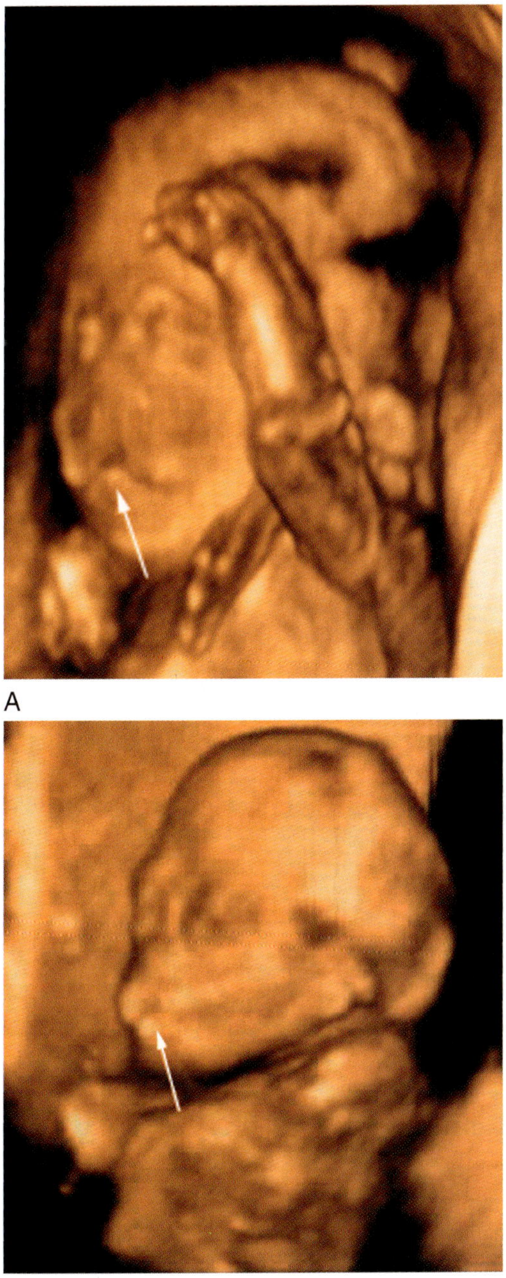

A

B

FIGURE 2-25 (A, B) Two different fetuses with median cleft lip and palate at 17 and 18 weeks. Both fetuses have trisomy 13 and holoprosencephaly. A large central cleft *(arrows)* is midline and is associated with a hypoplastic nose and hypotelorism.

Majewski syndrome (short rib–polydactyly syndrome, type II)

Meckel-Gruber syndrome

MURCS (**mü**llerian duct aplasia, **r**enal aplasia, **c**ervicothoracic **s**omite dysplasia) association

Nager syndrome

Neu-Laxova syndrome

Opitz syndrome

Oral-facial-digital syndrome, type I

Oral-facial-digital syndrome, type II (Mohr syndrome)

Pena Shokeir syndrome

Pierre Robin syndrome

Roberts' syndrome

Septo-optic dysplasia

Shprintzen syndrome

Smith-Lemli-Opitz syndrome

Stickler syndrome

Van der Woude syndrome

Walker-Warburg syndrome

Associated teratogens:

Alcohol

Carbamazepine (Tegretol)

Codeine

Cortisone

Ethosuximide

Fluphenazine

Hydantoin

Hyperthermia

Imipramine

Metronidazole (Flagyl)

Phenantoin

Quinine

Radiation

Trimethadione

Valproic acid

Abnormalities associated with midline cleft lip and palate:

Holoprosencephaly

Mohr syndrome

Oral-facial-digital syndrome

Short rib–polydactyly of the Majewski type

Trisomy 13

ULTRASOUND DIAGNOSIS

Cleft lip and palate can be diagnosed by sonography as early as 14 or 15 weeks' gestation and by embryoscopy as early as 11 weeks.

Bilateral complete cleft lip and palate is the form that is most easily diagnosed because of the free inner maxillary segment under the nose. This segment protrudes anteriorly like a mass and can easily be seen, both coronally and sagittally, in the early second trimester. Unilateral complete cleft lip and palate also is detectable early because of disruption of the inner maxillary segment and nose complex. Incomplete cleft lip (involving only the lip), produces far more subtle sonographic signs.

Midline clefts often involve hypotelorism and absence of the nose. Usually, they are seen in conjunction with syndromes featuring other, multiple, severe abnormalities, such as holoprosencephaly.

HEREDITY

Van der Woude syndrome, an autosomal dominant condition, is associated with up to a 50% risk of facial clefting in the offspring of affected parents. Although the sole manifestation of this syndrome may be symmetric pits or eminences of the lower lip, as many as 50% of gene carriers have cleft lip, cleft palate, or both. Approximately 2% of all cases of cleft lip and palate may be due to Van der Woude syndrome.

In general, for patients who have had one affected child with neither parent affected, the risk of recurrence of labial clefting in future pregnancies is 4%; if two affected children are born to unaffected parents, the risk rises to 10%. In families with one parent and one child with a cleft lip and palate, the risk of clefting in future pregnancies is 14%. Because more than half of the cases of cleft lip and palate occurring in fetuses are associated with broad patterns of dysmorphology, the recurrence risk for those families may be different and is based on the other abnormalities present.

NATURAL HISTORY AND OUTCOME

Isolated cleft lip and palate is treatable with plastic surgery, usually with an excellent outcome. However, because of the widely differing types of abnormalities associated with cleft lip and palate, the prognosis varies greatly depending on the underlying abnormality.

Suggested Reading

Baraitser M, Winter RM: *Color atlas of congenital malformation syndromes.* London, 1996, Mosby-Wolfe.

Benacerraf BR, Frigoletto FD, Bieber FR: The fetal face: ultrasound examination. *Radiology* 153:495–497, 1984.

Benacerraf BR, Frigoletto FD, Greene MF: Abnormal facial features and extremities in human trisomy syndromes: prenatal ultrasound appearance. *Radiology* 159:243–246, 1986.

Benacerraf BR, Mulliken JB: Fetal cleft lip/palate: sonographic diagnosis and postnatal outcome. *Plast Reconstr Surg* 92:1045–1051, 1993.

Berge SJ, Plath H, Van de Vondel PT, et al: Fetal cleft lip and palate: sonographic diagnosis, chromosomal abnormalities, associated anomalies and postnatal outcome in 70 fetuses. *Ultrasound Obstet Gynecol* 18:422–431, 2001.

Campbell S, Lees C, Moscoso G, Hall P: Ultrasound antenatal diagnosis of cleft palate by a new technique: the 3D "reverse face" view. *Ultrasound Obstet Gynecol* 25:12–18, 2005.

Cash C, Set P, Coleman N: The accuracy of antenatal ultrasound in the detection of facial clefts in a low-risk screening population. *Ultrasound Obstet Gynecol* 18:432–436, 2001.

Chmait R, Pretorius D, Jones M, et al: Prenatal evaluation of facial clefts with two-dimensional and adjunctive three-dimensional ultrasonography: a prospective trial. *Am J Obstet Gynecol* 187:946–949, 2002.

Chmait R, Pretorius D, Moore T, et al: Prenatal detection of associated anomalies in fetuses diagnosed with cleft lip with or without cleft palate in utero. *Ultrasound Obstet Gynecol* 27:173–176, 2006.

Ghi T, Tani G, Savelli L, Colleoni GG, Pilu G, Bovicelli L: Prenatal imaging of facial clefts by magnetic resonance imaging with emphasis on the posterior palate. *Prenat Diagn* 23:970–975, 2003.

Hegge FN, Prescott GH, Watson PT: Fetal facial abnormalities identified during obstetric sonography. *J Ultrasound Med* 5:679–684, 1986.

Jones KL: *Smith's recognizable patterns of human malformations.* Philadelphia, 2006, Elsevier.

Jones MC: Prenatal diagnosis of cleft lip and palate: detection rates, accuracy of ultrasonography, associated anomalies, and strategies for counseling. *Cleft Palate Craniofac J* 39:169–173, 2002.

Kraus BS, Kitamura H, Ooe T: Malformations associated with cleft lip and palate in human embryos and fetuses. *Am J Obstet Gynecol* 86:321–328, 1963.

Meizner I, Katz M, Bar-Ziv J, Insler V: Prenatal sonographic detection of fetal facial malformations. *Isr J Med Sci* 23:881–885, 1987.

Robinson JN, McElrath TF, Benson CB, et al: Prenatal ultrasonography and the diagnosis of fetal cleft lip. *J Ultrasound Med* 20:1165–1170, 2001.

Rotten D, Levaillant JM: Two- and three-dimensional sonographic assessment of the fetal face. 2. Analysis of cleft lip, alveolus and palate. *Ultrasound Obstet Gynecol* 24:402–411, 2004.

Saltzman DH, Benacerraf BR, Frigoletto FD: Diagnosis and management of fetal facial clefts. *Am J Obstet Gynecol* 155:377–379, 1986.

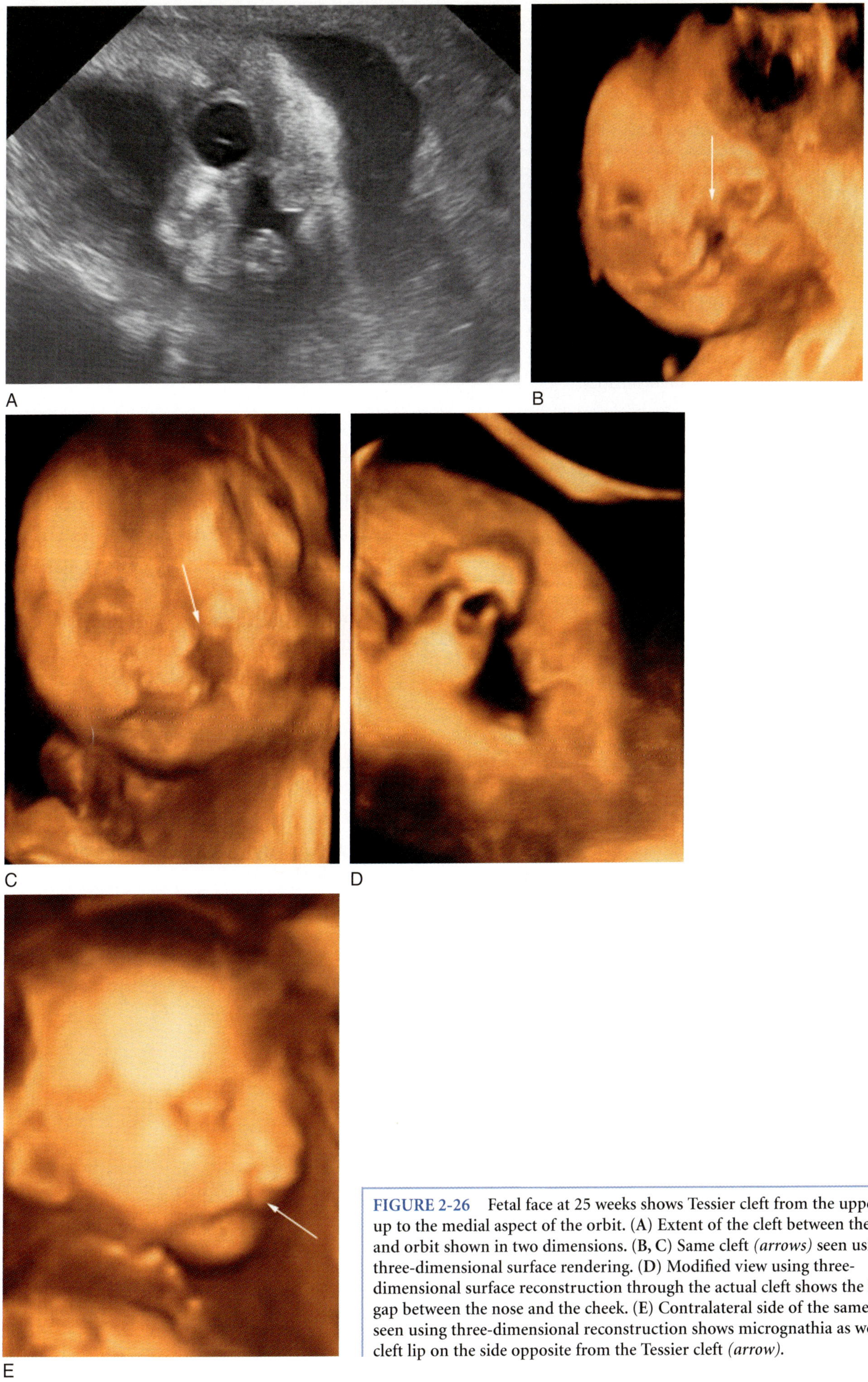

FIGURE 2-26 Fetal face at 25 weeks shows Tessier cleft from the upper lip up to the medial aspect of the orbit. (A) Extent of the cleft between the lip and orbit shown in two dimensions. (B, C) Same cleft *(arrows)* seen using three-dimensional surface rendering. (D) Modified view using three-dimensional surface reconstruction through the actual cleft shows the large gap between the nose and the cheek. (E) Contralateral side of the same fetus seen using three-dimensional reconstruction shows micrognathia as well as a cleft lip on the side opposite from the Tessier cleft *(arrow)*.

Savoldelli G, Schmid W, Schinzel A: Prenatal diagnosis of cleft lip and palate by ultrasound. *Prenat Diagn* 2:313–317, 1982.

Van der Woude A: Fistula labii inferioris congenita and its association with cleft lip and palate. *Am J Hum Genet* 6:244, 1954.

Wayne C, Cook K, Sairam S, Hollis B, Thilaganathan B: Sensitivity and accuracy of routine antenatal ultrasound screening for isolated facial clefts. *Br J Radiol* 75:584–589, 2002.

FRASER SYNDROME

DESCRIPTION AND DEFINITION

Fraser syndrome is a disorder characterized by cryptophthalmos; syndactyly; and genital, renal, and tracheal abnormalities.

ABNORMALITIES DETECTABLE BY ULTRASOUND

Common Abnormalities:

Cryptophthalmos* (93%)

Syndactyly (57%)

Genital abnormalities (49%)

Abnormalities of the ears (44%)

Nose abnormalities (37%)

Urinary tract hypoplasia or agenesis† (37%)

Laryngeal stenosis or atresia‡ (21%)

*Cryptophthalmos is not a prerequisite for establishing the diagnosis of Fraser syndrome, but it is the most common anomaly in this syndrome and often is associated with a broad, depressed nasal bridge.

†Oligohydramnios may be associated with renal agenesis.

‡Polyhydramnios occasionally is associated with laryngeal atresia, with markedly hyperextended and echogenic lungs.

Occasional Anomalies:

Microcephaly, hydrocephalus, and neural tube defect

Facial cleft

Hypertelorism

Ascites

MAJOR DIFFERENTIAL DIAGNOSES

Branchio-oculo-facial syndrome (eye and facial)

Cerebro-oculo-facio-skeletal (COFS) syndrome (eye and facial)

CHARGE association (facial and genital abnormalities)

Fryns syndrome (facial and genital abnormalities)

Goldenhar syndrome (facial anomalies)

Opitz syndrome (facial and genital abnormalities)

Potter sequence

Smith-Lemli-Opitz syndrome (genitourinary anomalies)

Trisomy 13

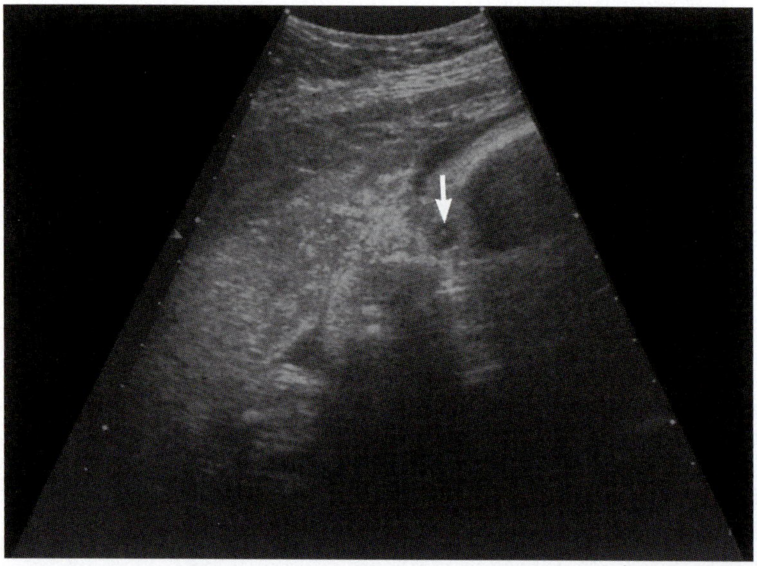

FIGURE 2-27 Coronal view of the fetal face shows microphthalmia, a feature commonly associated with Fraser syndrome. The orbit *(arrow)* is much smaller than normal for this third-trimester gestational age.

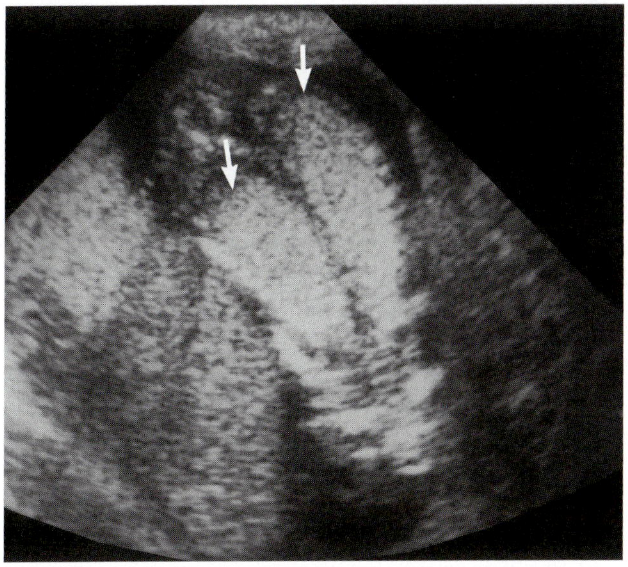

FIGURE 2-28 Longitudinal view of an early second-trimester fetus with tracheal atresia, a feature associated with Fraser syndrome. Note hyperexpansion of the lungs, inverted hemidiaphragms *(arrows)*, and marked hyperechoic lungs.

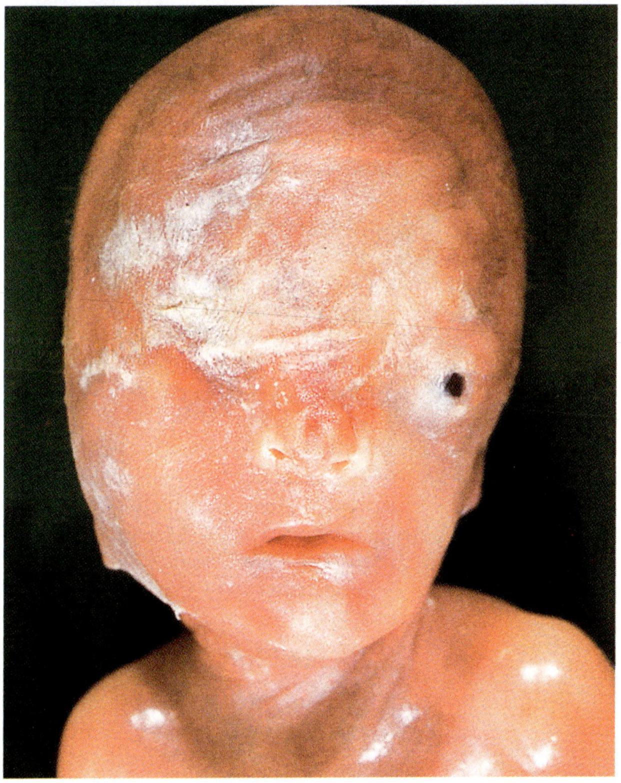

FIGURE 2-29 Eye anomalies in a neonate with Fraser syndrome. (From Keeling JW: *Fetal pathology.* London, 1994, Churchill Livingstone.)

Because of the number of different malformations associated with Fraser syndrome (not all of which are manifested in any one case), the differential diagnosis is broad and varies according to the presentation of each individual case.

ULTRASOUND DIAGNOSIS

In several cases occurring in families with an affected older sibling, prenatal diagnosis of Fraser syndrome has been established as early as 16–18 weeks' gestation. Sonographic diagnosis is based on the presence of highly variable anomalies, which can range from complete renal agenesis, associated with oligohydramnios; to complete tracheal agenesis, leading to huge hyperechoic lungs; to nonlethal sonographically subtle malformations, such as cryptophthalmos, facial asymmetry, and unilateral renal agenesis. Prenatal detection of cryptophthalmos was made at 26 weeks in a fetus with unilateral microphthalmos, unilateral renal agenesis, and syndactyly. The large echogenic lungs seen in this syndrome can mimic cystic adenomatoid malformations.

HEREDITY

Fraser syndrome has an autosomal recessive pattern of inheritance.

NATURAL HISTORY AND OUTCOME

Neonates having this disorder with associated renal agenesis or tracheal atresia will be stillborn. Eye anomalies and resultant impaired visual perception are frequent problems.

Suggested Reading

Balci S, Altinok G, Ozaltin F, Aktas D, Niron EA, Onol B: Laryngeal atresia presenting as fetal ascites, oligohydramnios and lung appearance mimicking cystic adenomatoid malformation in a 25-week-old fetus with Fraser syndrome. *Prenat Diagn* 19:856–858, 1999.

Berg C, Geipel A, Germer U, Pertersen-Hansen A, Koch-Dorfler M, Gembruch U: Prenatal detection of Fraser syndrome without cryptophthalmos: case report and review of the literature. *Ultrasound Obstet Gynecol* 18:76–80, 2001.

Boyd PA, Keeling JW, Lindenbaum RH: Fraser syndrome (cryptophthalmos-syndactyly syndrome): a review of eleven cases with postmortem findings. *Am J Med Genet* 31:159–168, 1988.

Bronshtein M, Zimmer E, Gershoni-Baruch R, et al: First and second trimester diagnosis of fetal ocular defects and associated anomalies: report of eight cases. *Obstet Gynecol* 77:443–449, 1991.

Burn J, Marwood RP: Fraser syndrome presenting as bilateral renal agenesis in three sibs. *J Med Genet* 19:360–361, 1982.

Feldman E, Shalev E, Weiner E, Cohen H, Zuckerman H: Microphthalmia—prenatal ultrasonic diagnosis: a case report. *Prenat Diagn* 5:205–207, 1985.

Francannet C, Lefrancois P, Dechelotte P, et al: Fraser syndrome with renal agenesis in two consanguineous Turkish families. *Am J Med Genet* 36:477–479, 1990.

Fraser GR: Our genetical "load": a review of some aspects of genetical variation. *Ann Hum Genet* 25:387–415, 1962.

Gattuso J, Patton MA, Baraitser M: The clinical spectrum of the Fraser syndrome: report of three new cases and review. *J Med Genet* 24:549–555, 1987.

Jones KL: *Smith's recognizable patterns of human malformations.* Philadelphia, 2006, Elsevier.

Karas DE, Respler DS: Fraser syndrome: a case report and review of the otolaryngologic manifestations. *Int J Pediatr Otorhinolaryngol* 31:85–90, 1995.

Kohl T, Hering R, Bauriedel G, et al: Fetoscopic and ultrasound-guided decompression of the fetal trachea in a human fetus with Fraser syndrome and congenital high airway obstruction syndrome (CHAOS) from laryngeal atresia. *Ultrasound Obstet Gynecol* 27:84–88, 2006.

Lane MA, Harman CR, Pelech AN, et al: Antenatal diagnosis, perinatal management, and pulmonary complications as a result of laryngeal compromise in Fraser syndrome. *J Matern Fetal Med* 4:280–284, 1995.

Levine RS, Powers T, Rosenberg HK, et al: The cryptophthalmos syndrome. *AJR Am J Roentgenol* 143:375–376, 1984.

Lurie IW, Cherstvoy ED: Renal agenesis as a diagnostic feature of the cryptophthalmos-syndactyly syndrome. *Clin Genet* 25:528–532, 1984.

Philip N, Gamberelli D, Guys JM, Camboulives J, Ayme S: Epidemiological study of congenital diaphragmatic defects with special reference to aetiology. *Eur J Pediatr* 150:726–729, 1991.

Pilu G, Reece EA, Romero R, et al: Prenatal diagnosis of craniofacial malformations with ultrasonography. *Am J Obstet Gynecol* 155:45–50, 1986.

Ramsing M, Rehder H, Holzgreve W, Meinecke P, Lenz W: Fraser syndrome (cryptophthalmos with syndactyly) in the fetus and newborn. *Clin Genet* 37:84–96, 1990.

Rousseau T, Laurent N, Thauvin-Robinet C, et al: Prenatal diagnosis and intrafamilial clinical heterogeneity of Fraser syndrome. *Prenat Diagn* 22:692–696, 2002.

Schauer GM, Dunn LK, Godmilow L, Eagle RC Jr, Knisely AS: Prenatal diagnosis of Fraser syndrome at 18.5 weeks gestation, with autopsy findings at 19 weeks. *Am J Med Genet* 37:583–591, 1990.

Serville F, Carles D, Boussin B: Fraser syndrome: prenatal ultrasonic detection. *Am J Med Genet* 32:561–563, 1989 (letter).

Vijayaraghavan SB, Suma N, Lata S, Kamakshi K: Prenatal sonographic appearance of cryptophthalmos in Fraser syndrome. *Ultrasound Obstet Gynecol* 25:629–630, 2005.

GOLDENHAR SYNDROME

DESCRIPTION AND DEFINITION

Synonyms: Hemifacial microsomia, oculoauriculovertebral spectrum, first and second branchial arch syndrome

The primary feature of this syndrome is asymmetry of the face and ears, which may occur with vertebral abnormalities. Goldenhar syndrome is the result of abnormalities of the first and second branchial arches.

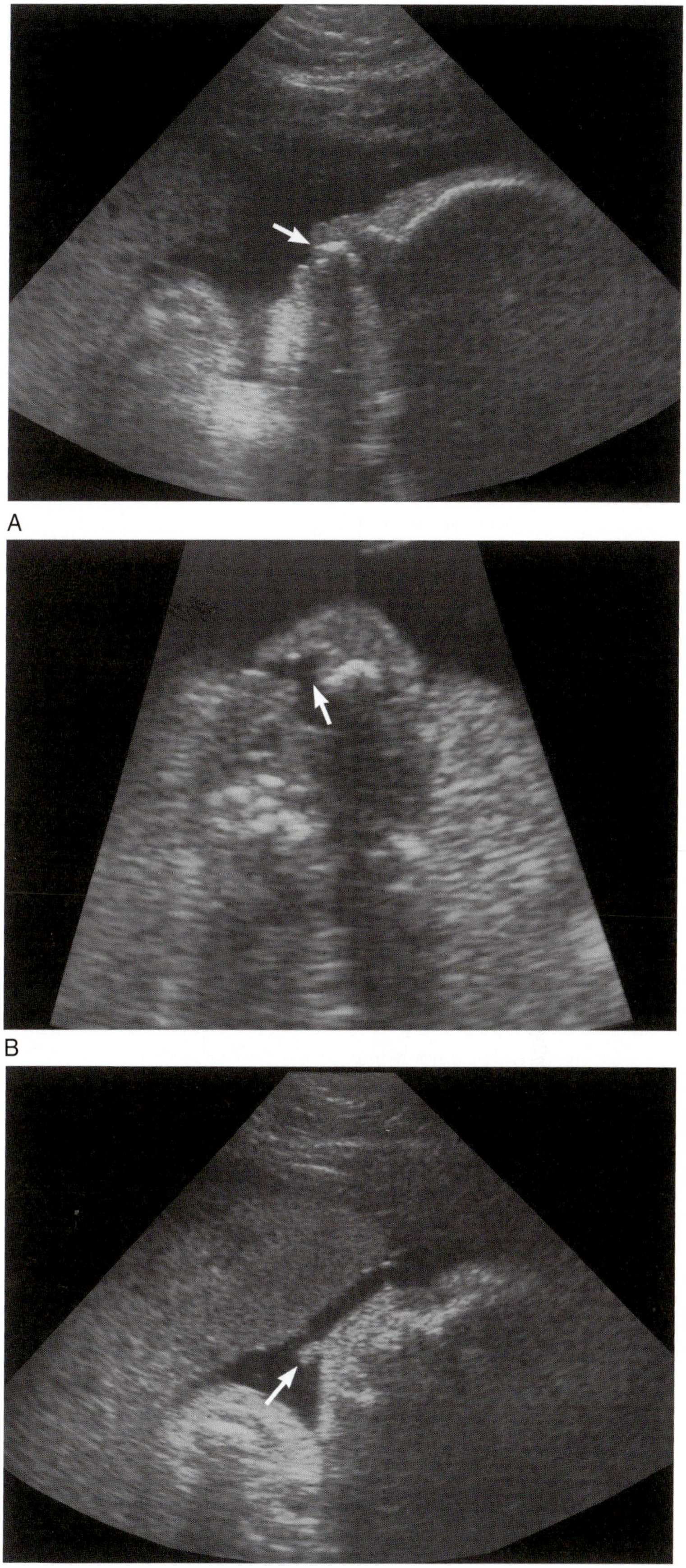

A

B

C

FIGURE 2-30 Multiple views of the fetal face and head of a third-trimester fetus with Goldenhar syndrome (hemifacial microsomia). (A) Paramedian sagittal view through the fetal face shows the cleft, which involves the upper lip and nose *(arrow)*. (B) Coronal view through the upper lip reveals a cleft lip and palate, involving one side more than the other, with a clear cleft connecting the nostril to the roof of the mouth *(arrow)*. (C) View of the lower face and neck of this fetus reveals a skin tag, low set and anterior, which is consistent with a malformed ear *(arrow)*.

ABNORMALITIES DETECTABLE BY ULTRASOUND

Common Findings:

Hypoplasia of the mandible, usually unilateral, involving the temporomandibular joint and malformations of the ear, in addition to multiple skin tags around the ear area and proximal mandibular region

Marked asymmetry of the soft tissues of the jaw

Microphthalmia

Hemivertebrae along the cervical and, occasionally, the thoracic regions

Polyhydramnios

Occasional Findings:

Cardiac defect (e.g., ventricular septal defect)

Cleft lip and palate

Unilateral renal and lung abnormalities

Ventriculomegaly

MAJOR DIFFERENTIAL DIAGNOSES

Branchio-oculo-facial syndrome

Cerebro-oculo-facio-skeletal (COFS) syndrome

Fraser syndrome

Fryns syndrome

Klippel-Feil sequence

Nager syndrome

Opitz syndrome

Stickler syndrome

Shprintzen syndrome

Treacher Collins syndrome

Trisomy 13

Trisomy 18

ULTRASOUND DIAGNOSIS

Goldenhar syndrome has been detected sonographically in several cases. The diagnosis is based on identification of facial abnormalities, such as clefts, micrognathia, other malformations that are asymmetric and unilateral (e.g., hydronephrosis, absence of a lung, vertebral abnormalities, ventriculomegaly), and polyhydramnios.

HEREDITY

The pattern of inheritance for Goldenhar syndrome is unknown. The syndrome occurs sporadically.

NATURAL HISTORY AND OUTCOME

Cosmetic surgery is the main treatment modality for this syndrome. Children with this syndrome have normal intelligence. Handicaps are related to the degree of deafness and microphthalmia associated with the syndrome. Early intervention is helpful.

Suggested Reading

Benacerraf BR, Frigoletto FD: Prenatal ultrasonographic recognition of Goldenhar's syndrome. *Am J Obstet Gynecol* 159:950–952, 1988.

De Catte L, Laubach M, Legein J, Goossens A: Early prenatal diagnosis of oculoauriculovertebral dysplasia or the Goldenhar syndrome. *Ultrasound Obstet Gynecol* 8:422–424, 1996.

Jones KL: *Smith's recognizable patterns of human malformations.* Philadelphia, 2006, Elsevier.

Martinelli P, Maruotti GM, Agangi A, Mazzarelli LL, Bifulco G, Paladini D: Prenatal diagnosis of hemifacial microsomia and ipsilateral cerebellar hypoplasia in a fetus with oculoauriculovertebral spectrum. *Ultrasound Obstet Gynecol* 24:199–201, 2004.

Tamas DE, Mahony BS, Bowie JD, Woodruff WW III, Kay HH: Prenatal sonographic diagnosis of hemifacial microsomia (Goldenhar-Gorlin syndrome). *J Ultrasound Med* 5:461–463, 1986.

Thomas P: Goldenhar syndrome and hemifacial microsomia: observations on three patients. *Eur J Pediatr* 133:287–292, 1980.

Volpe P, Gentile M: Three-dimensional diagnosis of Goldenhar syndrome. *Ultrasound Obstet Gynecol* 24:798–800, 2004.

Witters I, Schreurs J, Van Wing J, Wouters W, Fryns JP: Prenatal diagnosis of facial clefting as part of the oculo-auriculo-vertebral spectrum. *Prenat Diagn* 21:62–64, 2001.

MEDIAN CLEFT FACE SYNDROME

DESCRIPTION AND DEFINITION

Synonym: Frontonasal dysplasia sequence

This is a syndrome of midline facial defects involving the eyes, nose, and forehead. Hypertelorism, bifid nose, and broad nasal bridge are the major features of this abnormality, first described by DeMyer and Sedano in 1967 and 1970.

ABNORMALITIES DETECTABLE BY ULTRASOUND

Common Findings:

Hypertelorism

Malformations of the nose, visible in both coronal and sagittal views, ranging from a notched, slightly broadened nasal tip to a completely divided nose with absence of the premaxilla and nasal tip and a median cleft lip

Occasional Findings:

Microphthalmia

Agenesis of the corpus callosum

Lipoma of the corpus callosum

Frontal encephalocele

Tetralogy of Fallot

MAJOR DIFFERENTIAL DIAGNOSES

Branchio-oculo-facial syndrome

Chromosomal abnormalities (e.g., triploidy and trisomy 13)

Craniosynostosis syndromes (e.g., Pfeiffer syndrome and Apert syndrome)

Fetal drug effects (i.e., from aminopterin or methotrexate)

Frontal encephalocele

Mohr syndrome

Opitz syndrome

Oral-facial-digital syndrome, type I

Other causes of hypertelorism, such as cleft lip/palate and Pena Shokeir syndrome (see differential diagnosis of hypertelorism, p. 5)

Shprintzen syndrome

Van der Woude syndrome

ULTRASOUND DIAGNOSIS

The diagnosis of frontonasal dysplasia has been established by ultrasound studies as early as 21 weeks' gestation, based on detection of abnormal midface and encephalocele.

HEREDITY

The pattern of inheritance for median cleft face syndrome is unknown. This syndrome is considered to be sporadic, although there are rare reports of familial recurrence.

NATURAL HISTORY AND OUTCOME

The outcome depends on the severity of the defect and associated anomalies. Major cosmetic surgery may be necessary. Although most children have normal intelligence, mild mental delays have been reported in 8%–12%.

Suggested Reading

Chervanak FA, Tortora M, Mayden K, et al: Antenatal diagnosis of median cleft face syndrome: sonographic demonstration of cleft lip and hypertelorism. *Am J Obstet Gynecol* 149:94–97, 1984.

DeMyer W: The median cleft face syndrome: differential diagnosis of cranium bifidum occultum, hypertelorism, and median cleft nose, lip and palate. *Neurology* 17:961, 1967.

Frattarelli JL, Boley TJ, Miller RA: Prenatal diagnosis of frontonasal dysplasia (median cleft syndrome). *J Ultrasound Med* 15:81–83, 1996.

Fryburg JS, Persing JA, Lin KY: Frontal dysplasia in two consecutive generations. *Am J Med Genet* 46:712–714, 1993.

Guion-Almeida ML, Richieri-Costa A, Saavedra D, Cohen MM: Fronto-nasal dysplasia: analysis of 21 cases and literature review. *Int J Oral Maxifac Surg* 25:91–97, 1996.

Johnson JM, Benoit B, Pierre-Louis J, Keating S, Chitayat D: Early prenatal diagnosis of oculoauriculofrontonasal syndrome by three-dimensional ultrasound. *Ultrasound Obstet Gynecol* 25:184–186, 2005.

Lees MM, Hodgkins P, Reardon W, et al: Frontonasal dysplasia with optic disc anomalies and other midline craniofacial defects: a report of six cases. *Clin Dysmorphol* 7:157–162, 1998.

Martinelli P, Russo R, Agangi A, Paladini D: Prenatal ultrasound diagnosis of frontonasal dysplasia. *Prenat Diagn*. 22:375–379, 2002.

Sedano HO, Cohen MM, Jirasek J, Gorlin RJ: Frontonasal dysplasia. *J Pedriatr* 76:906–913, 1970.

Selano HO, Gorlin RJ: Frontonasal malformation as a field defect and in syndromal associations. *Oral Surg* 65:704–710, 1988.

Shipp TD, Mulliken JB, Bromley B, Benacerraf B: Three-dimensional diagnosis of frontonasal malformation and unilateral cleft lip/palate. *Ultrasound Obstet Gynecol* 20:290–293, 2002.

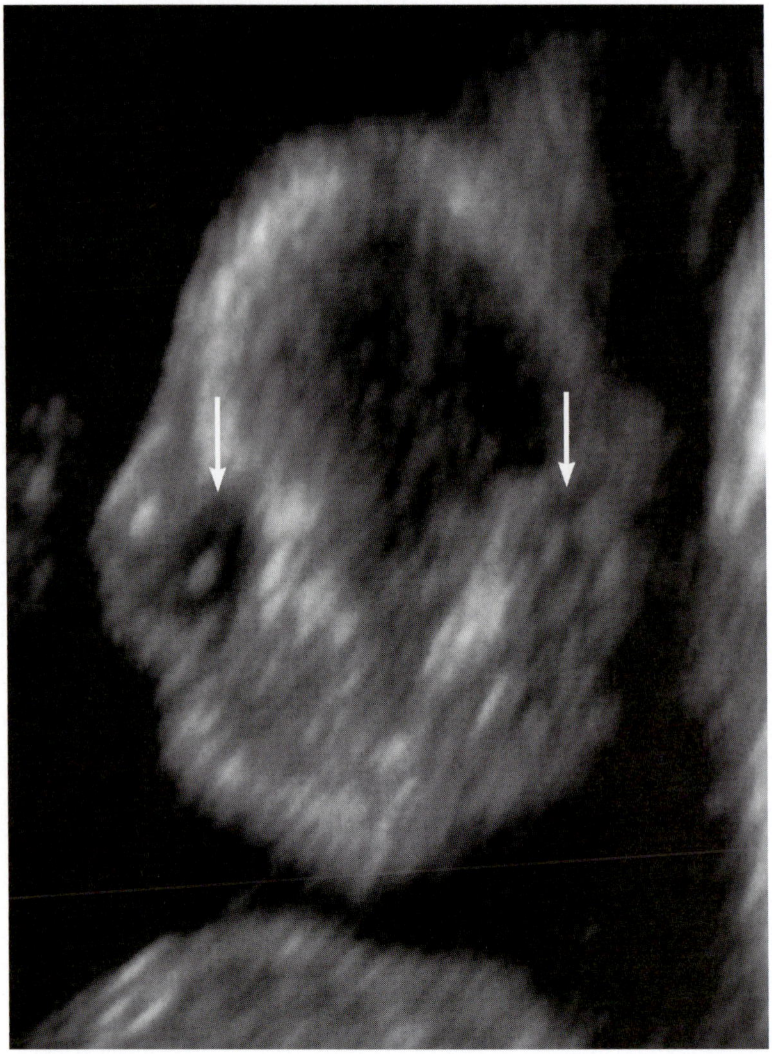

A

FIGURE 2-31 Median cleft face syndrome. (A) Two-dimensional coronal view through second-trimester fetal face with median cleft face syndrome shows severe hypertelorism caused by a midline facial cleft. *Arrows,* orbits.

Continued

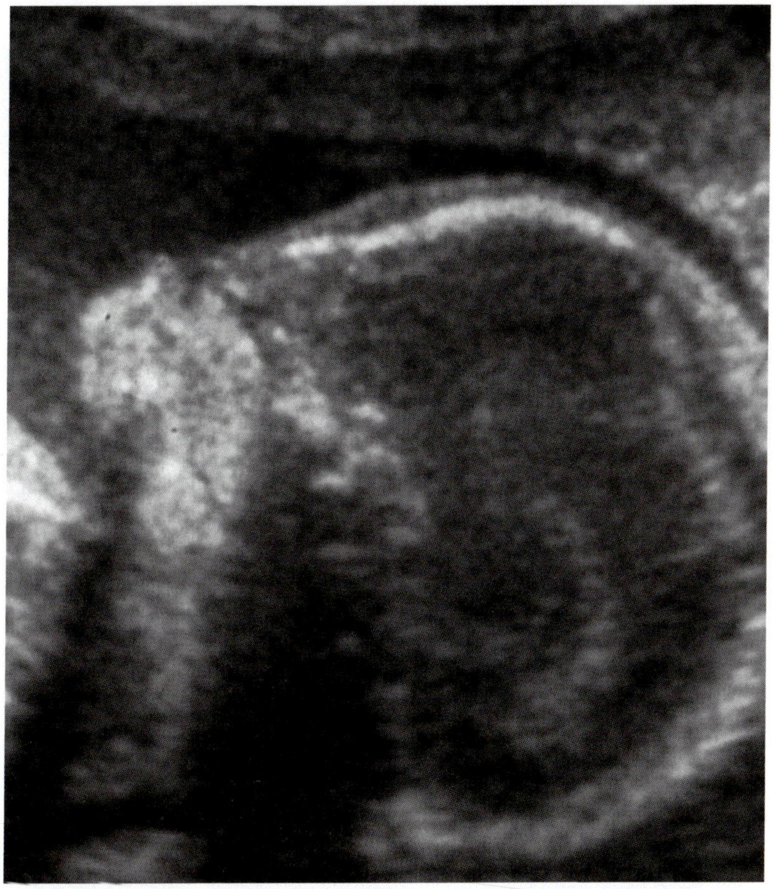

B

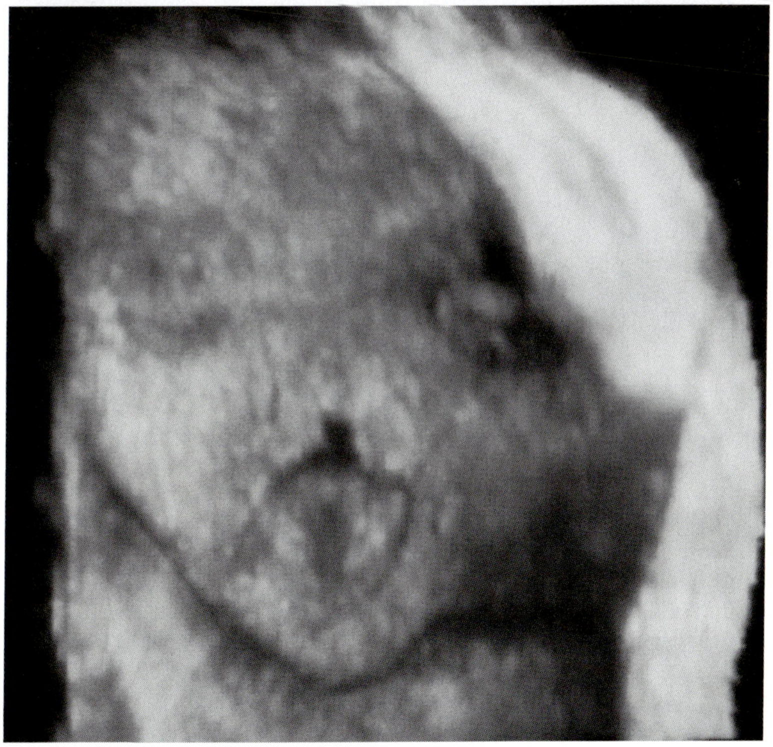

C

FIGURE 2-31, cont'd Median cleft face syndrome. (B) Profile of the same fetus with absence of the nose and completely flat facial profile. (C, D) Three-dimensional views of the same fetus with a flat fetal face attributable to a severe midline cleft, resulting in absence of the nose, hypertelorism, and frontal bossing. These findings are typical of median cleft face or frontal nasal dysplasia.

Continued

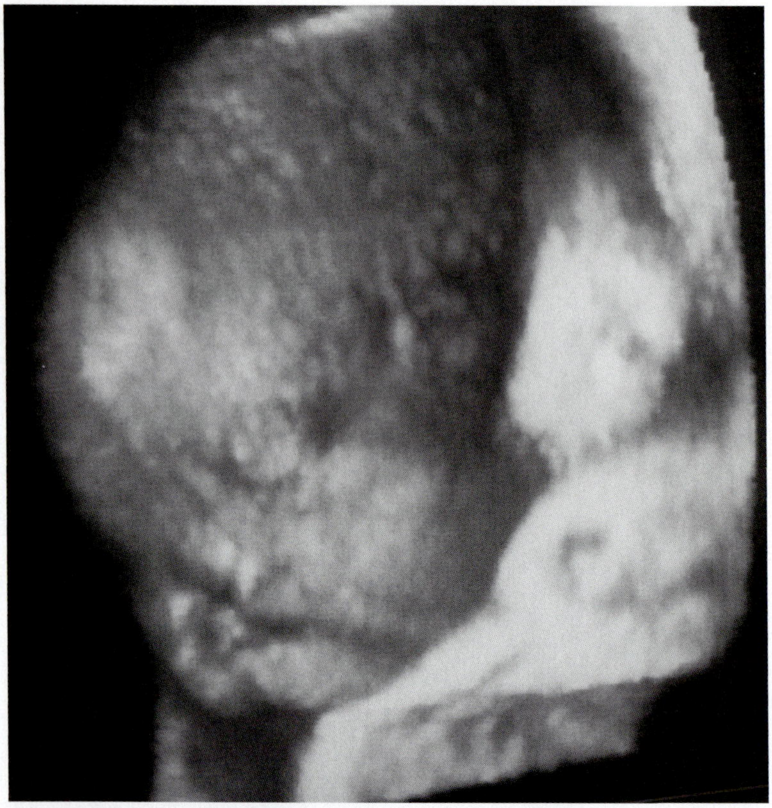

D

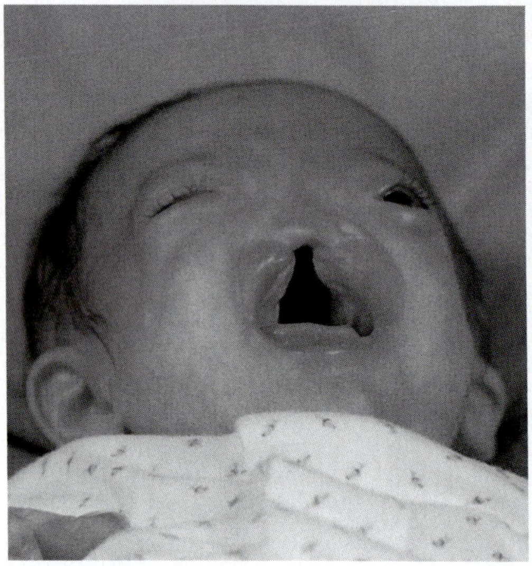

E

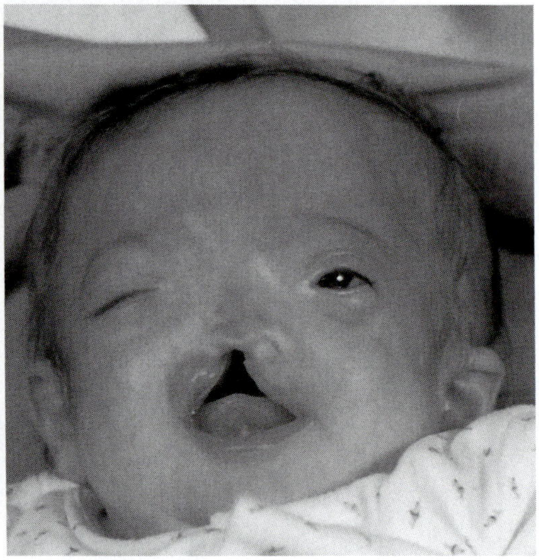

F

FIGURE 2-31, cont'd Median cleft face syndrome. (**C, D**) Three-dimensional views of the same fetus with a flat fetal face attributable to a severe midline cleft, resulting in absence of the nose, hypertelorism, and frontal bossing. These findings are typical of median cleft face or frontal nasal dysplasia. (**E, F**) Photographs of the child postnatally showing these malformations prior to surgery. (E and F from Shipp TD, Mulliken JB, Bromley B, Benacerraf B: *Ultrasound Obstet Gynecol* 20:290–293, 2002.)

MICROPHTHALMIA/ANOPHTHALMIA

DESCRIPTION AND DEFINITION

Microphthalmia (microphthalmos) is a disorder characterized by decreased size of the eyeball and orbit and is generally associated with other abnormalities/syndromes. It can be unilateral or bilateral and is responsible for a small percentage of congenital heritable blindness.

Anophthalmia, which represents the most severe form of the microphthalmic spectrum, refers to complete absence of the ocular primordia.

ABNORMALITIES DETECTABLE BY ULTRASOUND

Small orbits

Extremely small ocular primordia or absent primordia

Syndromes associated with microphthalmia and anophthalmia have different, distinguishing sonographic features that should be sought when evaluating a fetus with small orbits.

MAJOR DIFFERENTIAL DIAGNOSES

Alcohol syndrome (fetal)

Branchio-oculo-facial syndrome

Cerebro-oculo-facio-skeletal (COFS) syndrome

CHARGE association

Deletion 4p syndrome (Wolf-Hirschhorn syndrome)

Fanconi anemia

Fraser syndrome

Fryns syndrome

Goldenhar syndrome

Meckel-Gruber syndrome

Neu-Laxova syndrome

Proteus syndrome

Roberts' syndrome

TORCH (**t**oxoplasmosis, **o**ther infections, **r**ubella, **c**ytomegalovirus infection, and **h**erpes simplex) infection

Triploidy

Trisomy 9

Trisomy 13 (Patau syndrome)

Walker-Warburg syndrome

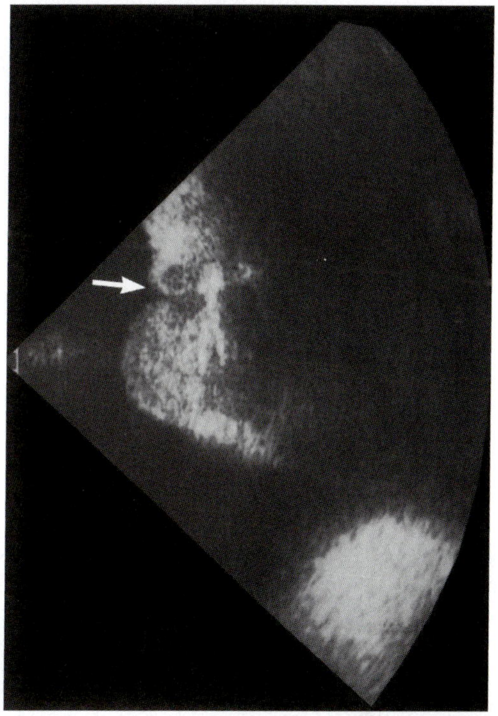

FIGURE 2-32 Coronal view of the facial soft tissues of a fetus with anophthalmia. Note that no orbit is visible at an orbit's usual location *(arrow)*.

ULTRASOUND DIAGNOSIS

Ultrasound studies can be used to demonstrate the size of the orbits. Coronal and transverse views of the orbit are the most useful for measuring the size of the orbits and evaluating their symmetry. Prenatal diagnosis of isolated microphthalmia has been established as early as 16 weeks' gestation in a patient with a family history of the anomaly.

The presence of an echogenic round lens in the anterior portion of the orbit is helpful in assessing the presence and size of the primordia.

HEREDITY

Both microphthalmia and anophthalmia may occur in the same family. Although isolated microphthalmia usually occurs sporadically, it may be inherited as an autosomal dominant, recessive, or X-linked pattern. Lenz microphthalmia is X-linked and associated with microcephaly, syndactyly, and kyphoscoliosis. The etiology and inheritance depend on the underlying syndrome.

NATURAL HISTORY AND OUTCOME

Microphthalmia can occur as one of a number of different disorders (see Chapter 1, p. 2). Some of these disorders, such as chromosomal abnormalities, are severe and lethal. Alternatively, microphthalmia can be an isolated finding and can even be unilateral, which generally is associated with a good prognosis. The prognosis depends on the associated anomalies.

Suggested Reading

Chen CP, Wang KG, Huang JK, et al: Prenatal diagnosis of otocephaly with microphthalmia/anophthalmia using ultrasound and magnetic resonance imaging. *Ultrasound Obstet Gynecol* 22:214–215, 2003.

Feldman E, Shalev E, Weiner E, Cohen H, Zuckerman H: Microphthalmia—prenatal ultrasonic diagnosis: a case report. *Prenat Diagn* 5:205–207, 1985.

Fryns JP, Kleczkowska A, Moerman P, van den Berghe K, van den Berghe H: Double autosomal trisomy (lq21.2-qter and 14 pter-ql3) in a female fetus with nuchal oedema. *Ann Genet* 30:240–242, 1987.

Jones KL: *Smith's recognizable patterns of human malformations*. Philadelphia, 2006, WB Saunders.

Shulman LP, Gordon PL, Emerson DS, Wilroy RS, Elias S: Prenatal diagnosis of isolated bilateral microphthalmia with confirmation by evaluation of products of conception obtained by dilation and evacuation. *Prenat Diagn* 13:403–409, 1993.

Warburg M: The heterogeneity of microphthalmos. *Int Ophthalmol* 4:45–65, 1981.

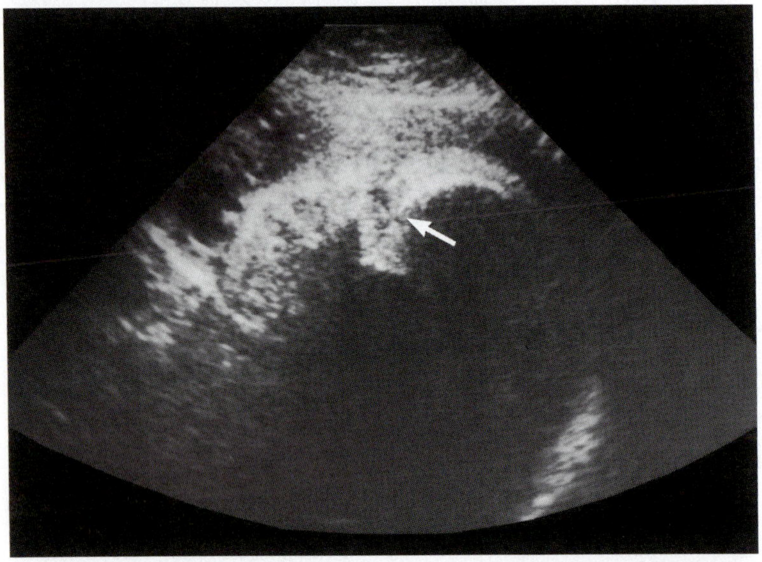

A

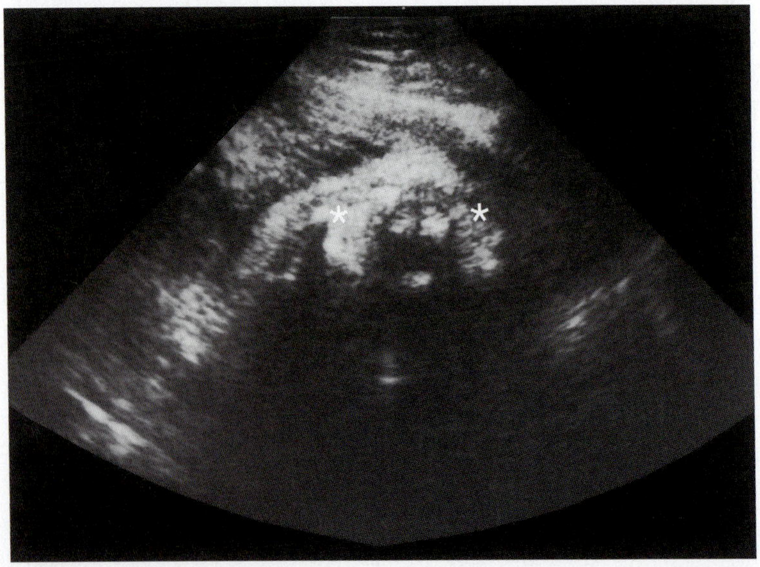

B

FIGURE 2-33 **(A)** Parasagittal view of the facial profile of a fetus with anophthalmia shows absence of the orbit *(arrow)*. **(B)** Transverse view of the same fetus at the level of the orbits. Asterisk marks the location where the orbits normally would be found. An echogenic mass of bone is seen instead.

NAGER SYNDROME

DESCRIPTION AND DEFINITION

Synonym: Acrofacial dysostosis

Nager syndrome (acrofacial dysostosis) is similar to Treacher Collins syndrome. It is primarily an abnormality manifested by mandibular hypoplasia; malformed, low-set ears; and an abnormal radial aspect of the hand and forearm.

ABNORMALITIES DETECTABLE BY ULTRASOUND

Common Findings:

Severe micrognathia and mandibular hypoplasia

Cleft palate

Malformed, low-set ears

Hypoplasia of the thumbs

Abnormalities of other digits

Short radial ray (to some degree)

Short forearms

Occasional Findings:

Cleft lip

Syndactyly, clinodactyly, and other anomalies of the fingers and toes

Club feet

Limb reduction defects

Polyhydramnios

MAJOR DIFFERENTIAL DIAGNOSES

Other syndromes involving facial and/or forearm anomalies:

Cornelia de Lange syndrome

Ectrodactyly–ectodermal dysplasia–clefting (EEC) syndrome

Fanconi anemia

Femur-fibula-ulna (FFU) syndrome

Holt-Oram syndrome

Multiple pterygium syndrome

Oral-facial-digital syndrome, type I

Oral-facial-digital syndrome, type II (Mohr syndrome)

Pena Shokeir syndrome

Pierre Robin syndrome

Roberts' syndrome

Thrombocytopenia–absent radius (TAR) syndrome

Treacher Collins syndrome

Trisomy 18 (Edwards' syndrome)

ULTRASOUND DIAGNOSIS

Nager syndrome has been detected sonographically as early as 16 weeks on the basis of severe micrognathia. Nager syndrome also has been diagnosed prenatally at 23 weeks and in a different case at 30 weeks, when a severe mandibular abnormality, malformed ears, malformed upper extremities, and polyhydramnios were noted.

HEREDITY

The etiology of this syndrome is unknown, so its pattern of inheritance is undetermined. Evidence of both autosomal dominant and autosomal recessive inheritance has been noted in several families.

NATURAL HISTORY AND OUTCOME

Early intervention, involving plastic surgery for mandibular abnormalities and early hearing aid intervention for deafness, has been found to be beneficial. Perinatal mortality in these cases is related to respiratory distress, and management is similar to that for Pierre-Robin syndrome.

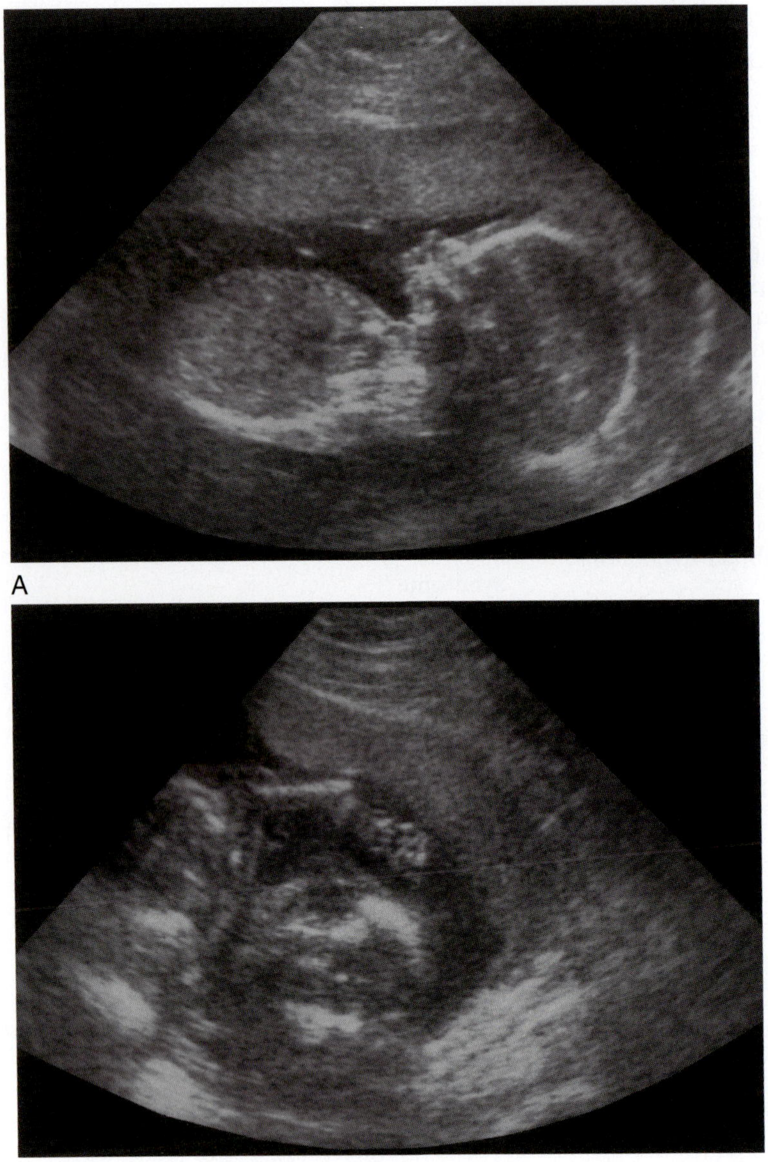

A

B

FIGURE 2-34 (A) Sagittal view of the face of a second-trimester fetus, presumed to have Nager syndrome, shows severe micrognathia. (B) View of the forearm of the same fetus reveals a deformity involving the lower arm and hand.

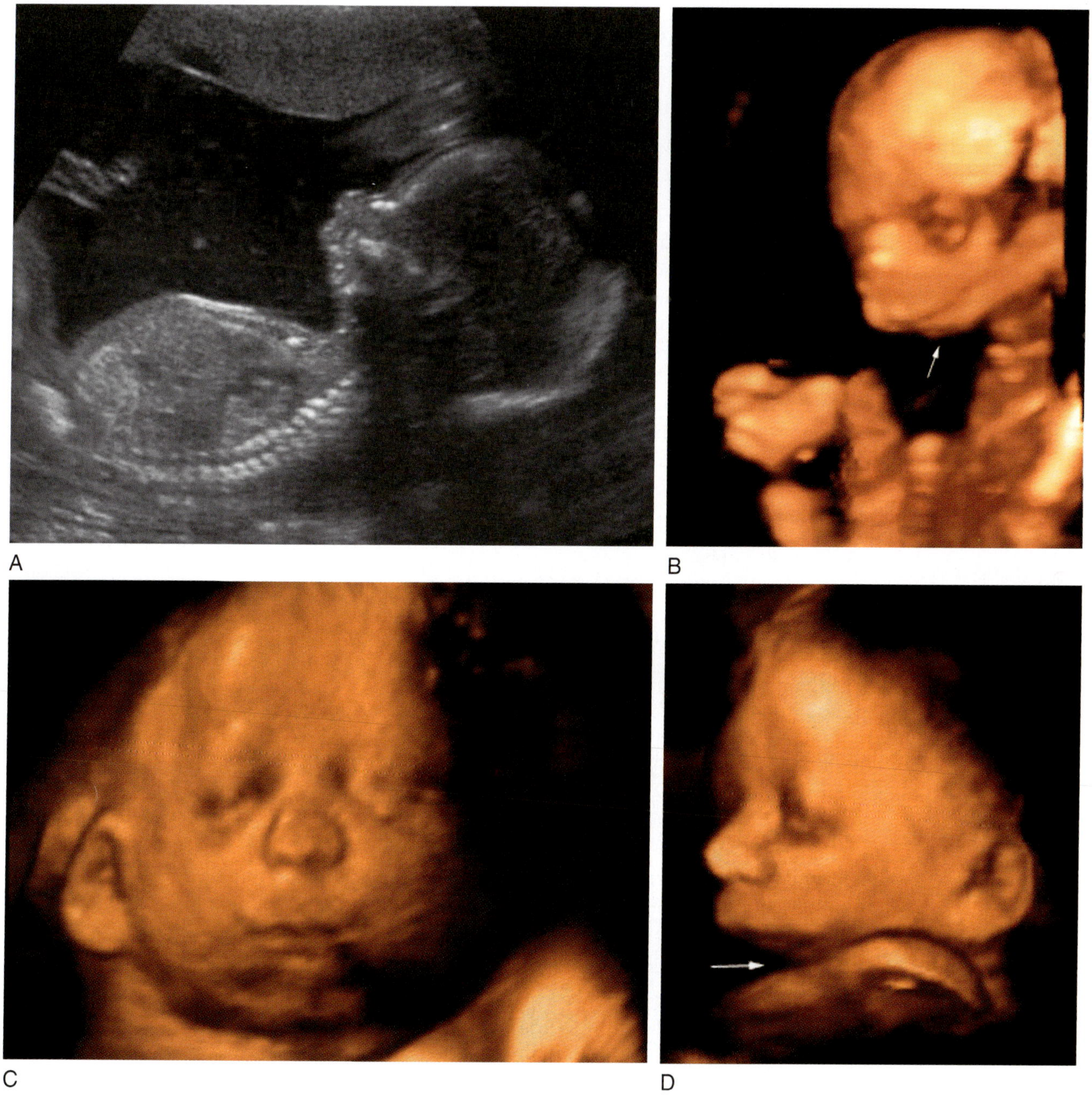

FIGURE 2-35 (**A**) Profile view of a second-trimester fetus with Nager syndrome shows severe micrognathia. (**B**) Three-dimensional surface rendering of the same fetus shows extreme micrognathia *(arrow)*. (**C, D**) Surface rendering of the same fetus in the third trimester shows extreme micrognathia *(arrow)*, almost giving the impression of an absent jaw.

Suggested Reading

Benson CB, Pober BR, Hirsh MP, Doubilet PM: Sonography of Nager acrofacial dysostosis syndrome in utero. *J Ultrasound Med* 7:163–167, 1988.

Hecht JT, Immken LL, Harris LF, Malini S, Scott CI Jr: The Nager syndrome. *Am J Med Genet* 27:965–969, 1987.

Jones KL: *Smith's recognizable patterns of human malformations.* Philadelphia, 2006, Elsevier.

Paladini D, Tartaglione A, Lamberti A, Lapadula C, Martinelli P: Prenatal ultrasound diagnosis of Nager syndrome. *Ultrasound Obstet Gynecol* 21:195–197, 2003.

Zori RT, Grat BA, Bent-Williams A, et al: Preaxial acrofacial dysostosis (Nager syndrome) associated with an inherited and apparently balanced X;9 translocation: prenatal and postnatal late replication studies. *Am J Med Genet* 46:379–383, 1993.

ORAL-FACIAL-DIGITAL SYNDROME, TYPE I (OFD1)

DESCRIPTION AND DEFINITION

Synonyms: OFD syndrome 1, oral-facial-digital syndrome, Papillon-Leage Psaume syndrome

Papillon-Leage and Psaume first described this syndrome in 1954. It is characterized by facial and digital abnormalities, as well as anomalies of the oral cavity. OFD1 is one of nine syndromes (OFD1–OFD9) with similarities that include median cleft lip and palate, hypertelorism, micrognathia, and digital anomalies. Associated polycystic kidney disease seems to be specific to OFD1.

ABNORMALITIES DETECTABLE BY ULTRASOUND

Common Findings:

Median cleft lip and cleft palate

Shortening of the digits

Clinodactyly

Polydactyly

Syndactyly

Adult-type polycystic kidney disease

Brain abnormalities (e.g., vermian hypoplasia, agenesis of the corpus callosum, porencephaly)

Occasional Findings:

Facial asymmetry

MAJOR DIFFERENTIAL DIAGNOSES

Hydrolethalus (central nervous system [CNS] and polydactyly)

Majewski syndrome (midline facial cleft and polydactyly)

Meckel-Gruber syndrome (CNS and polydactyly)

Median cleft lip syndrome (broad nasal bridge/ bifid nasal tip)

Other types of oral-facial-digital syndrome (heterogeneous group of defects involving face and limbs)

Smith-Lemli-Opitz syndrome (facial and renal anomalies, polydactyly)

ULTRASOUND DIAGNOSIS

Prenatal diagnosis of OFD1 based on micrognathia, cleft palate, limb abnormalities, and hydrocephalus has been reported. Brain malformations are present in only 20% of affected fetuses and therefore may not always be detectable sonographically.

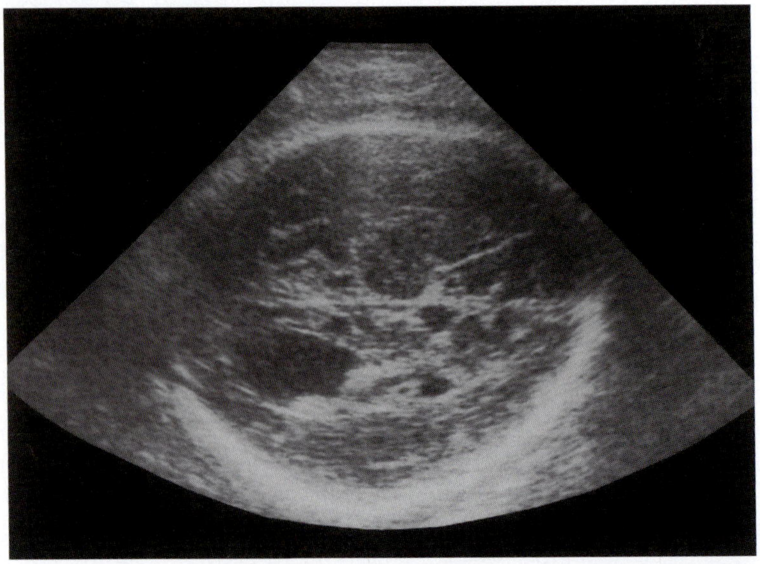

FIGURE 2-36 Transverse view though the fetal head during the third trimester shows teardrop-shaped dilation of the occipital horn of the lateral ventricles. This fetus had agenesis of the corpus callosum and oral-facial-digital syndrome, type I.

HEREDITY

OFD1 is transmitted as an X-linked dominant condition and is lethal in males. The mutation in OFD1 has been localized to the Xp22.2-Xp22.3 locus.

NATURAL HISTORY AND OUTCOME

The prognosis is poor. One third of affected fetuses die in infancy, and approximately 50% of survivors have mental deficiency. In survivors, treatment focuses on plastic surgery for correction of oral and facial abnormalities.

Suggested Reading

Feather SA, Woolf AS, Donnai D, et al: The oral-facial-digital syndrome type I (OFD1): a cause of polycystic kidney disease and associated malformations, maps to Xp22.2-Xp22.3. *Hum Mol Genet* 6:1163–1167, 1997.

Gillerot Y, Heimann M, Fourneau C, et al: Oral-facial-digital syndrome type I in a newborn male. *Am J Med Genet* 46:335–338, 1993.

Jones KL: *Smith's recognizable patterns of human malformation,* ed 6. Philadelphia, 2006, Elsevier.

Larralde de Luna M, Raspa ML, Ibargoyen J: Oral-facial-digital type I syndrome of Papillon-Leage and Psaume. *Pediatr Dermatol* 9:52–56, 1992.

Shipp TD, Chu GC, Benacerraf B: Prenatal diagnosis of oral-facial-digital syndrome, type 1. *J Ultrasound Med* 19:491–494, 2000.

Thauvin-Robinet C, Rousseau T, Durand C, et al: Familial orofaciodigital syndrome type I revealed by ultrasound prenatal diagnosis of porencephaly. *Prenat Diagn* 21:466–470, 2001.

ORAL-FACIAL-DIGITAL SYNDROME, TYPE II (MOHR SYNDROME)

DESCRIPTION AND DEFINITION

Synonym: Mohr syndrome

There are nine types of OFD syndrome; Mohr syndrome is type II. As described in 1941 by Mohr, the syndrome is characterized by short stature; deafness; and abnormalities of the nose, lips, tongue, and mandible, as well as of the hands and feet.

ABNORMALITIES DETECTABLE BY ULTRASOUND

Common Findings:

Facial clefts

Broad nasal bridge

Bifid nasal tip

Micrognathia

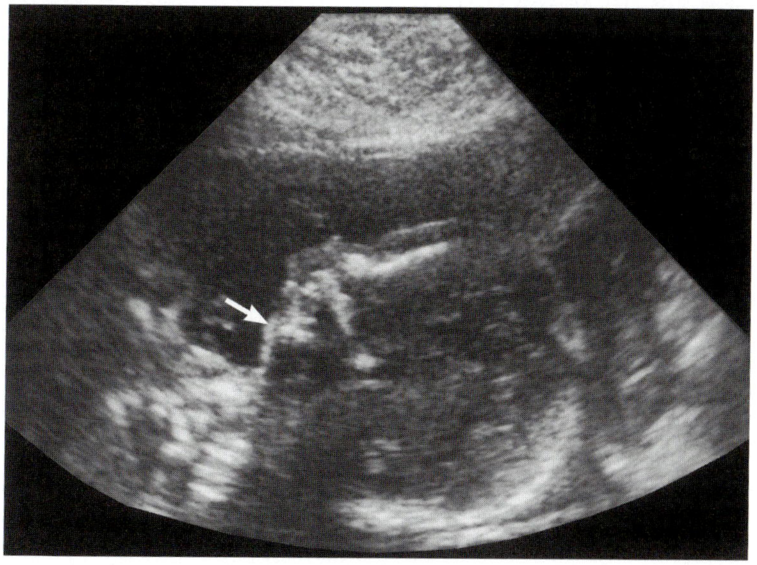

FIGURE 2-37 Longitudinal view of a second-trimester fetus with severe micrognathia, as can be seen in fetuses with Mohr syndrome. Arrow points to the chin.

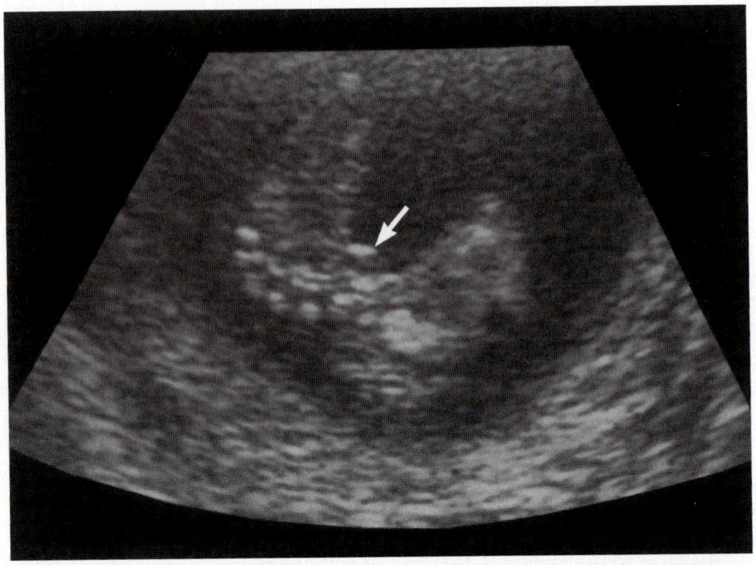

FIGURE 2-38 Preaxial polydactyly *(arrow)* in a second-trimester fetus, which is consistent with the features of Mohr syndrome.

Multiple tumors of the tongue

Digital abnormalities (e.g., polysyndactyly)

Clinodactyly of the fifth digit

Bifid hallux

Occasional Findings:

Intracranial anomalies (agenesis of the corpus callosum, arachnoid cyst, cerebellar abnormalities, microcephaly, porencephaly, ventriculomegaly)

MAJOR DIFFERENTIAL DIAGNOSES

Carpenter syndrome (bifid hallux)

Hydrolethalus (CNS and preaxial polydactyly)

Majewski syndrome (facial cleft and polydactyly)

Meckel-Gruber syndrome (CNS and polydactyly)

Median cleft lip syndrome (bifid nasal tip)

Oral-facial-digital syndrome, types I and III–IX (heterogeneous group of defects involving the face and limbs, as well as other associated malformations)

Saethre-Chotzen syndrome (duplicated hallux)

Smith-Lemli-Opitz syndrome (facial, polydactyly, renal anomalies)

ULTRASOUND DIAGNOSIS

Prenatal diagnosis of oral-facial-digital syndrome, type II (Mohr syndrome) has been established at 20 weeks' gestation. Findings have included a cystic mass in the posterior fossa, ventriculomegaly, small occipital encephalocele, polyhydramnios, micrognathia, polydactyly, and clubbed feet.

HEREDITY

This syndrome has an autosomal recessive pattern of inheritance.

NATURAL HISTORY AND OUTCOME

Survival is dependent on the severity of abnormalities. Those who do survive tend to have less severe anomalies and have normal intelligence.

Suggested Reading

Mohr OL: A hereditary sublethal syndrome in man. *Skr Norske Vidensk Akad, I Mat Naturv Klasse* 14:1–18, 1941.

Prpic I, Cekada S, Franulovic J: Mohr syndrome (oro-facial-digital syndrome II): a familial case with different phenotype findings. *Clin Genet* 48:304–307, 1995.

Reardon W, Harbord MG, Hall-Craggs MA, et al: Central nervous system malformations in Mohr's syndrome. *J Med Genet* 26:659–663, 1989.

Rimoin DL, Edgerton MT: Genetic and clinical heterogeneity in the oral-facial-digital syndromes. *J Pediatr* 71:94–102, 1967.

Suresh S, Rajesh K, Suresh I, et al: Prenatal diagnosis of orofaciodigital syndrome: Mohr type. *J Ultrasound Med* 14:863–866, 1995.

PIERRE ROBIN SYNDROME

DESCRIPTION AND DEFINITION

Pierre Robin syndrome is thought to occur secondary to hypoplasia of the mandible early in gestation, leading to retrognathia and a high potential for airway obstruction. The primary defect is hypoplasia of the mandible, with the tongue falling more posteriorly than normal, resulting in interference of normal closure of the posterior soft palate.

ABNORMALITIES DETECTABLE BY ULTRASOUND

Micrognathia

Cleft palate

Polyhydramnios

MAJOR DIFFERENTIAL DIAGNOSES

Although the Pierre Robin syndrome occurs as an isolated finding in otherwise normal individuals who outgrow this condition, the differential diagnosis for the finding of micrognathia includes the following:

- Achondrogenesis
- Aicardi syndrome
- Amniotic band syndrome
- Antley-Bixler syndrome
- Atelosteogenesis
- Camptomelic dysplasia
- Carpenter syndrome
- Cerebrocostomandibular syndrome
- Cerebro-oculo-facio-skeletal (COFS) syndrome
- CHARGE association
- Chromosomal anomalies
- Cleidocranial dysostosis
- Cornelia de Lange syndrome
- Cri du chat syndrome (5p deletion)
- Crouzon syndrome
- Diastrophic dysplasia
- DiGeorge syndrome
- Ectrodactyly–ectodermal dysplasia–clefting (EEC) syndrome
- Femoral hypoplasia–unusual facies syndrome
- Fryns syndrome
- Goldenhar syndrome
- Hydrolethalus
- Infantile polycystic kidney disease
- Joubert syndrome
- Meckel-Gruber syndrome
- Multiple pterygium
- MURCS (**mü**llerian duct aplasia, **r**enal aplasia, **c**ervicothoracic **s**omite dysplasia) association
- Nager syndrome
- Neu-Laxova syndrome
- Opitz syndrome
- Oral-facial-digital syndrome, type I
- Oral-facial-digital syndrome, type II (Mohr syndrome)
- Pena Shokeir syndrome
- Roberts' syndrome
- Russell-Silver syndrome
- Seckel syndrome
- Shprintzen syndrome
- Smith-Lemli-Opitz syndrome
- Stickler syndrome
- Thrombocytopenia–absent radius (TAR) syndrome
- Treacher Collins syndrome

Teratogens

Alcohol

Amitriptyline

Methotrexate

Valproic acid

ULTRASOUND DIAGNOSIS

Prenatal diagnosis of Robin anomalad has occurred at 13 weeks, although most affected cases reportedly are detected in the middle of the second trimester, seen as micrognathia on a sagittal

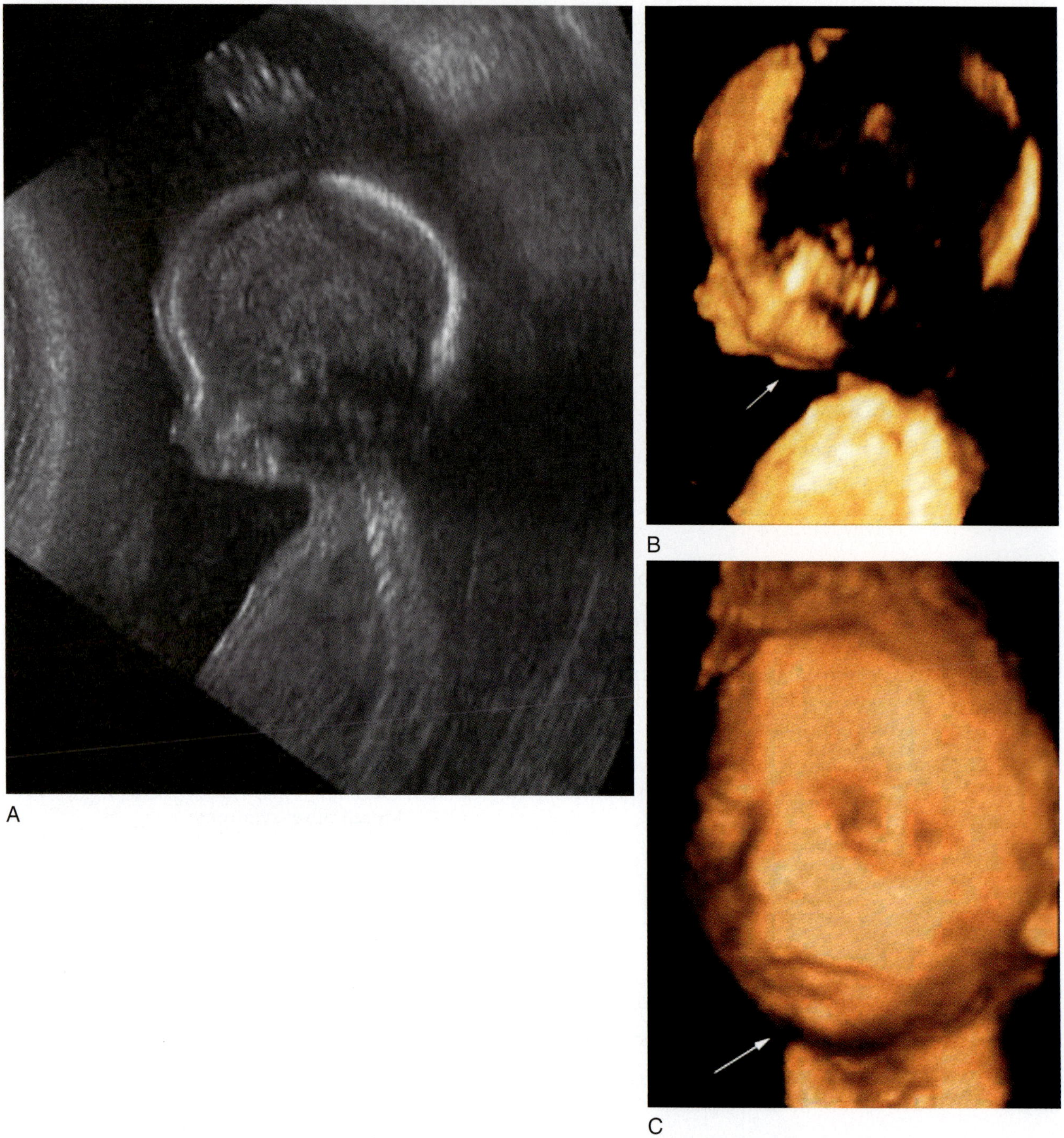

FIGURE 2-39 (A) Two-dimensional profile view of a second-trimester fetus with micrognathia, typical of Pierre Robin syndrome. (B) Three-dimensional surface rendering of the same fetus shows the small jaw *(arrow)*. (C) Early third-trimester fetus with micrognathia, typical of Pierre Robin syndrome. *Arrow* = jaw.

view of the fetal face. The posteriorly displaced tongue that never reaches the alveolar ridge (glossoptosis) is another helpful sonographic feature of this syndrome.

Robin anomalad may be associated with polyhydramnios, particularly in the third trimester. The cleft palate defect usually is not detectable sonographically because it affects the posterior aspect of the palate. A careful survey of the rest of the fetal anatomy is recommended because micrognathia is a feature of all the syndromes listed, each with its own sonographic features and pattern of inheritance.

HEREDITY

Pierre Robin syndrome is generally considered to be a sporadic abnormality, although there are reports of both autosomal recessive and autosomal dominant patterns of inheritance. Robin anomalad may be a feature of other syndromes, such as trisomy 18, Stickler syndrome, and others. In those cases, the etiology and heredity depend on the associated syndrome.

NATURAL HISTORY AND OUTCOME

Pierre Robin syndrome may lead to emergent airway obstruction, necessitating intubation or tracheotomy to prevent sudden death. Chronic airway obstruction may lead to hypoxia, cor pulmonale, failure to thrive, and mental retardation. Over time and with proper management, mandibular growth will take place, and the prognosis often is excellent for those who survive the early period of respiratory compromise. However, when this abnormality occurs as part of a syndrome, the prognosis depends on the severity of the syndrome and its associated anomalies.

Suggested Reading

Bixler D, Christian JC: Pierre-Robin syndrome occurring in two related sibships. *Birth Defects* 7:67–71, 1971.

Bromley B, Benacerraf BR: Fetal micrognathia: associated anomalies and outcome. *J Ultrasound Med* 13:529–533, 1994.

Bronshtein M, Blazer S, Zalel Y, Zimmer EZ: Ultrasonographic diagnosis of glossoptosis in fetuses with Pierre Robin sequence in early and mid pregnancy. *Am J Obstet Gynecol* 193:1561–1564, 2005.

Hsieh YY, Chang CC, Tsai HD, Yang TC, Lee CC, Tsai CH: The prenatal diagnosis of Pierre-Robin sequence. *Prenat Diagn* 19:567–569, 1999.

Jones KL: *Smith's recognizable patterns of human malformations*. Philadelphia, 2006, WB Saunders.

Lee W, McNie B, Chaiworapongsa T, et al: Three-dimensional ultrasonographic presentation of micrognathia. *J Ultrasound Med* 21:775–781, 2002.

Megier P, Ayeva-Derman M, Esperandieu O, Aubry MC, Couly G, Desroches A: Prenatal ultrasonographic diagnosis of the cerebro-costo-mandibular syndrome: case report and review of the literature. *Prenat Diagn* 18:1294–1299, 1998.

Meizner I, Katz M, Bar-Ziv J, Insler V: Prenatal sonographic detection of fetal facial malformations. *Isr J Med Sci* 23:881–885, 1987.

Morin G, Gekas J, Naepels P, et al: Cerebro-costo-mandibular syndrome in a father and a female fetus: early prenatal ultrasonographic diagnosis and autosomal dominant transmission. *Prenat Diagn* 21:890–893, 2001.

Pilu G, Romero R, Reece A, Jeanty P, Hobbins JC: The prenatal diagnosis of Robin anomalad. *Am J Obstet Gynecol* 154:630–632, 1986.

Shechter SA, Sherer DM, Geilfuss CJ, Metlay LA, Woods JR Jr: Prenatal sonographic appearance and subsequent management of a fetus with otomandibular limb hypogenesis syndrome associated with pulmonary hypoplasia. *J Clin Ultrasound* 18:661–665, 1990.

Soulier M, Sigaudy S, Chau C, Philip N: Prenatal diagnosis of Pierre-Robin sequence as part of Stickler syndrome. *Prenat Diagn* 22:567–568, 2002.

Teoh M, Meagher S: First-trimester diagnosis of micrognathia as a presentation of Pierre Robin syndrome. *Ultrasound Obstet Gynecol* 21:616–618, 2003.

SHPRINTZEN SYNDROME

DESCRIPTION AND DEFINITION

Synonym: Velocardiofacial syndrome, DiGeorge syndrome, CATCH 22 (**c**ardiac defect, **a**bnormal facies, **t**hymic hypoplasia, **c**left palate, **h**ypocalcemia), 22q11 deletion syndrome

Described in 1978, this syndrome includes short stature, mild mental retardation, ear and hearing abnormalities, micrognathia, and cardiac and limb defects. In 1965, DiGeorge described this syndrome as DiGeorge syndrome (primarily cardiac anomalies), and in 1978, Shprintzen reported a group of patients with cleft palate and prominent nose, calling it Shprintzen syndrome. It was determined that both of these syndromes actually are manifestations of a deletion of chromosome 22q11.2 (see DiGeorge Syndrome).

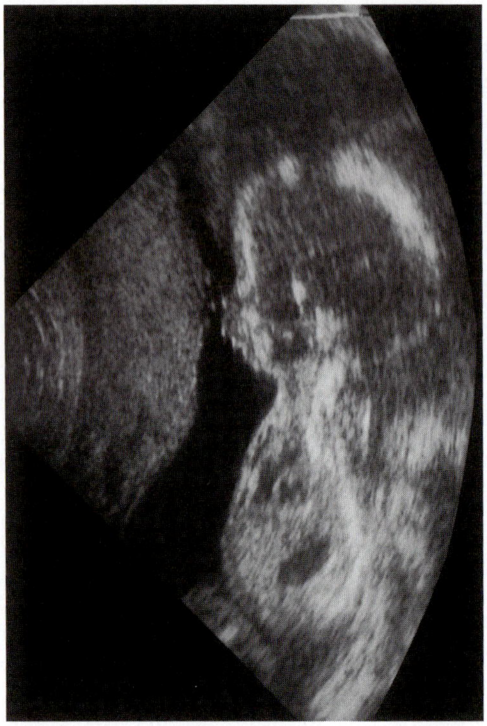

FIGURE 2-40 Longitudinal view of a second-trimester fetus with Shprintzen syndrome. Note the small chin, which is consistent with micrognathia.

ABNORMALITIES DETECTABLE BY ULTRASOUND

Common Findings:

Microcephaly

Micrognathia

Facial cleft

Short long-bones

Cardiac defects

Occasional Findings:

Pierre Robin syndrome

Holoprosencephaly

Umbilical hernia

Cryptorchidism

Hypospadias

MAJOR DIFFERENTIAL DIAGNOSES

Disorders associated with the findings of micrognathia and slightly short limbs:

- Branchio-oculo-facial syndrome
- Cerebro-oculo-facio-skeletal (COFS) syndrome
- Chromosomal abnormalities (e.g., triploidy, trisomy 18 [Edwards' syndrome])
- Cornelia de Lange syndrome
- Ectrodactyly–ectodermal dysplasia–clefting (EEC) syndrome
- Fanconi anemia
- Femoral hypoplasia–unusual facies syndrome
- Femur-fibula-ulna syndrome
- Holt-Oram syndrome
- Multiple pterygium syndrome
- Neu-Laxova syndrome
- Oral-facial-digital syndrome, type II (Mohr syndrome)
- Roberts' syndrome
- Russell-Silver syndrome
- Seckel syndrome
- Skeletal dysplasias (camptomelic syndrome, diastrophic dysplasia)
- Stickler syndrome
- Thrombocytopenia–absent radius (TAR) syndrome

ULTRASOUND DIAGNOSIS

The author had an opportunity to perform sonographic studies on a patient carrying a fetus with Shprintzen syndrome. The patient previously had a child with Pierre Robin syndrome.

At 16 weeks' gestation, mild micrognathia and a slightly short femur were noted in this fetus, although amniocentesis revealed a normal karyotype. The patient returned for follow-up scans, which confirmed the micrognathia, as well as the reduced femoral and humeral lengths (particularly the radial and ulnar lengths). By 27.5 weeks' gestation, the ulnar and radial lengths were equivalent to those expected at 21 to 22 weeks' gestation. There was some discrepancy between the long bone measurements when comparing sides, with the radius and ulna on one side being 5 mm longer than those on the contralateral side.

After birth, a ventricular septal defect was identified, as well as features consistent with Shprintzen syndrome.

HEREDITY

The syndrome has an autosomal dominant pattern of inheritance and is caused by the interstitial deletion of chromosome 22q11.21-q11.23. This defect is thought to be related to DiGeorge syndrome and likely is part of the same genetic defect.

NATURAL HISTORY AND OUTCOME

Hypotonia, mental retardation, and language and hearing problems are among the findings in affected individuals. Occasional abnormalities include absent T-cell function and absent thymic tissue.

Suggested Reading

(Also see DiGeorge syndrome)

Driscoll DA, Spinner NB, Budarf ML, et al: Deletions and microdeletions of 22q11.2 in velocardio-facial syndrome. *Am J Med Genet* 44:261–268, 1992.

Jones KL: *Smith's recognizable patterns of human malformations.* Philadelphia, 2006, Elsevier.

Ryan AK, Goodship JA, Wilson DI, et al: Spectrum of clinical features associated with interstitial chromosome 22q11 deletions: a European collaborative study. *J Med Genet* 34:798–804, 1997.

Shprintzen RJ, Goldberg RB, Lewin ML, et al: A new syndrome involving cleft palate, cardiac anomalies, typical facies, and learning disabilities; velo-cardio-facial syndrome. *Cleft Palate J* 15:56–62, 1978.

STICKLER SYNDROME

DESCRIPTION AND DEFINITION

Synonym: Hereditary arthroophthalmopathy

This syndrome was introduced by Stickler in 1965 as an autosomal dominant syndrome characterized by ocular defects, cleft palate, micrognathia/ hypoplasia of the mandible, and orthopedic abnormalities, including mild spondyloepiphyseal dysplasia unrelated to trauma.

ABNORMALITIES DETECTABLE BY ULTRASOUND

Mandibular hypoplasia (micrognathia)

Cleft palate

Cataracts

Clubbed foot

Polyhydramnios

Major Differential Diagnoses

Syndromes featuring micrognathia:

- Achondrogenesis
- Aicardi syndrome
- Amniotic band syndrome
- Atelosteogenesis
- Camptomelic dysplasia

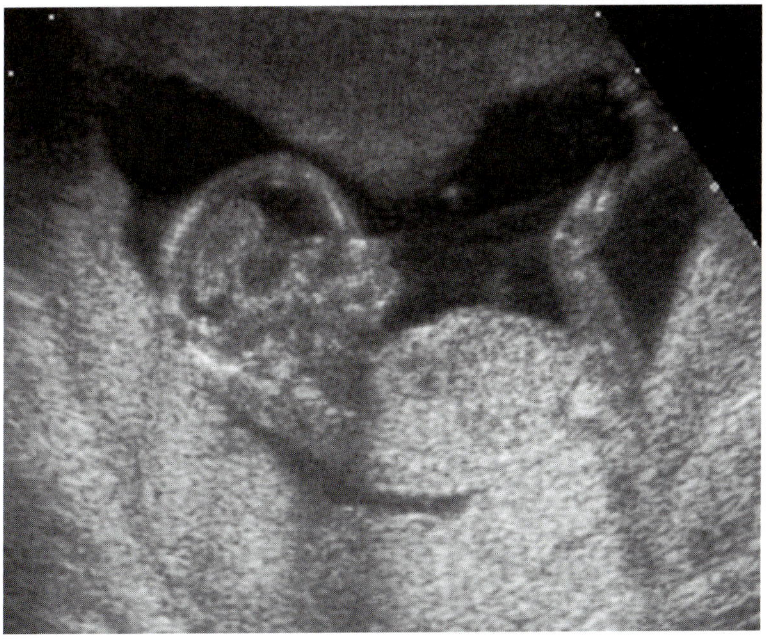
A

FIGURE 2-41 Stickler syndrome. (A) Longitudinal view of an early second-trimester fetus with Stickler syndrome.

Continued

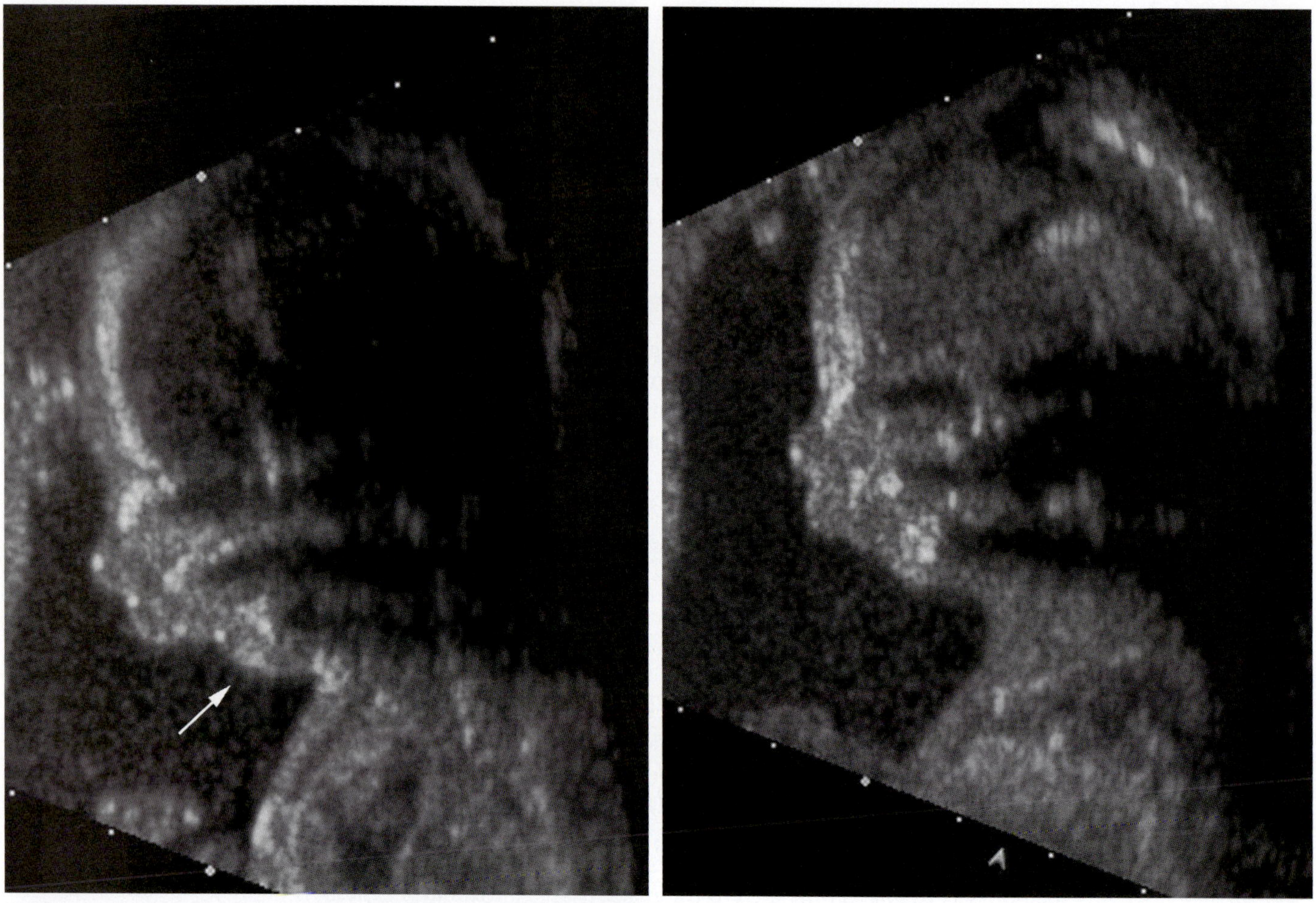

B C

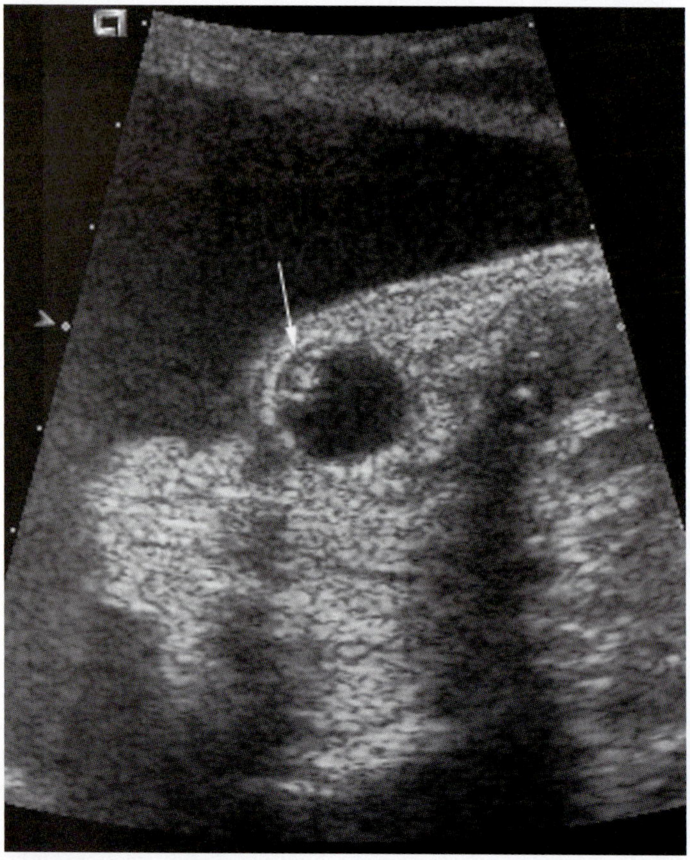

D

FIGURE 2-41, cont'd Stickler syndrome. (B, C) Magnified views of the same fetus showing a small chin *(arrow)*. (D) Magnified view of the fetal eye with a cataract. Note opacification of the center of the lens *(arrow)*. Cataracts can be a feature of Stickler syndrome.

Carpenter syndrome

Cerebrocostomandibular syndrome

CHARGE association

Chromosomal anomalies

Cornelia de Lange syndrome

Crouzon syndrome

Diastrophic dysplasia

Ectrodactyly–ectodermal dysplasia–clefting (EEC) syndrome

Femoral hypoplasia–unusual facies syndrome

Fryns syndrome

Goldenhar syndrome

Hydrolethalus

Infantile polycystic kidney disease

Joubert syndrome

Meckel-Gruber syndrome

Multiple pterygium

MURCS (**mü**llerian duct aplasia, **r**enal aplasia, **c**ervicothoracic **s**omite dysplasia) association

Nager syndrome

Neu-Laxova syndrome

Oral-facial-digital syndrome, type I

Oral-facial-digital syndrome, type II (Mohr syndrome)

Pena Shokeir syndrome

Pierre Robin syndrome

Roberts' syndrome

Seckel syndrome

Shprintzen syndrome

Smith-Lemli-Opitz syndrome

Thrombocytopenia–absent radius (TAR) syndrome

Treacher Collins syndrome

Teratogens

Alcohol

Amitriptyline

Methotrexate

Valproic acid

ULTRASOUND DIAGNOSIS

This syndrome can be detected sonographically by isolated polyhydramnios in a patient at risk for this familial autosomal dominant disorder. Polyhydramnios occurs as a result of abnormal swallowing of amniotic fluid. This syndrome also has been diagnosed prenatally by detection of micrognathia.

HEREDITY

The pattern of inheritance for this syndrome is autosomal dominant. Most cases are associated with the gene that encodes for type II collagen (COL2A1) on chromosome 12q13, although other, less common mutations exist (COL11A1 and COL11A2).

NATURAL HISTORY AND OUTCOME

Progressive myopia may lead to retinal detachment and result in blindness. Skeletal abnormalities often result in premature degenerative changes in the joints of young adults. Affected individuals have mitral valve prolapse and should use preoperative antibiotics for dental procedures.

Suggested Reading

Ahmad N, Richards AJ, Murfett HC, et al: Prevalence of mitral valve prolapse in Stickler syndrome. *Am J Med Genet* A 116:234–237, 2003.

Liberfarb R, Goldblatt A: Prevalence of mitral-valve prolapse in the Stickler syndrome. *Am J Med Genet* 24:387–392, 1986.

Opitz JM: Ocular anomalies in malformation syndromes. *Trans Am Acad Ophthalmol Otolaryngol* 76:1193–1202, 1972.

Snead MP, Yates JR: Clinical and molecular genetics of Stickler syndrome. *J Med Genet* 36:353–359, 1999.

Soulier M, Sigaudy S, Chau C, Philip N: Prenatal diagnosis of Pierre-Robin sequence as part of Stickler syndrome. *Prenat Diagn* 22:567–568, 2002.

Stickler GB, Belau PG, Raffell FJ, et al: Hereditary progressive arthro-ophthalmopathy. *Mayo Clin Proc* 40:433–455, 1965.

Stickler GB, Hughes W, Houchin P: Clinical features of hereditary progressive arthroophthalmopathy (Stickler syndrome): a survey. *Genet Med* 3:192–196, 2001.

Vuoristo MM, Pappas JG, Jansen V, Ala-Kokko L: A stop codon mutation in COL11A2 induces exon skipping and leads to non-ocular Stickler syndrome (review). *Am J Med Genet A* 130:160–164, 2004.

TREACHER COLLINS SYNDROME

DESCRIPTION AND DEFINITION

Synonym: Mandibulofacial dysostosis

Characterized by abnormalities involving the first branchial arch, Treacher Collins syndrome features malformations of the lower eyelids; palpebral fissures; hypoplasia of the malar bone and mandible; anomalies of the auricles and external auditory meatus; a high arched or cleft palate, or both; and deafness.

ABNORMALITIES DETECTABLE BY ULTRASOUND

Micrognathia

Abnormal orbits with ocular fissures slanted downward

Hypoplastic zygomata

Malformed ears, with either absent auricles or floppy, hypoplastic auricles that are low set and associated with skin tags

Choanal atresia

Cleft palate

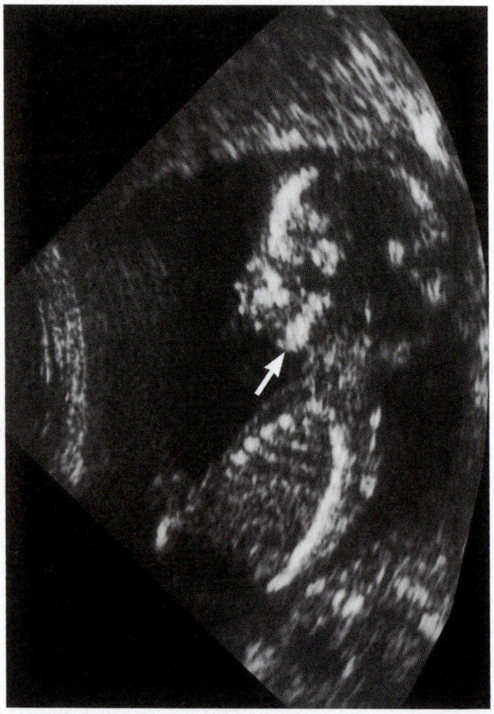

FIGURE 2-42 Longitudinal view of a second-trimester fetus with Treacher Collins syndrome shows severe micrognathia *(arrow)*.

MAJOR DIFFERENTIAL DIAGNOSES

Cerebrocostomandibular syndrome

Chromosomal anomalies

- Triploidy
- Trisomy 13 (Patau syndrome)
- Trisomy 18 (Edwards' syndrome)

Cornelia de Lange syndrome

Femoral hypoplasia–unusual facies syndrome

Fraser syndrome

Fryns syndrome

Goldenhar syndrome (hemifacial microsomia)

Joubert syndrome

Klippel-Feil sequence

Multiple pterygium syndrome

Nager (acrofacial dysostosis) syndrome

Neu-Laxova syndrome

Oral-facial-digital syndrome, type I

Oral-facial-digital syndrome, type II (Mohr syndrome)

Pena Shokeir syndrome

Pierre Robin syndrome

Seckel syndrome

Shprintzen syndrome

Stickler syndrome

ULTRASOUND DIAGNOSIS

Early sonographic diagnosis at 15 weeks' gestation has been reported in several cases, based on detection of micrognathia and other abnormalities of the face, such as abnormal positioning of the eyes and choanal atresia. Ear abnormalities are visible sonographically, particularly when the external ear is malformed and displaced downward.

HEREDITY

The syndrome has an autosomal dominant pattern of inheritance. However, as many as 60% of cases are new mutations, occurring in previously unaffected families. Mutations of the gene at locus 5q32-33.1 are thought to be responsible for some cases of this syndrome.

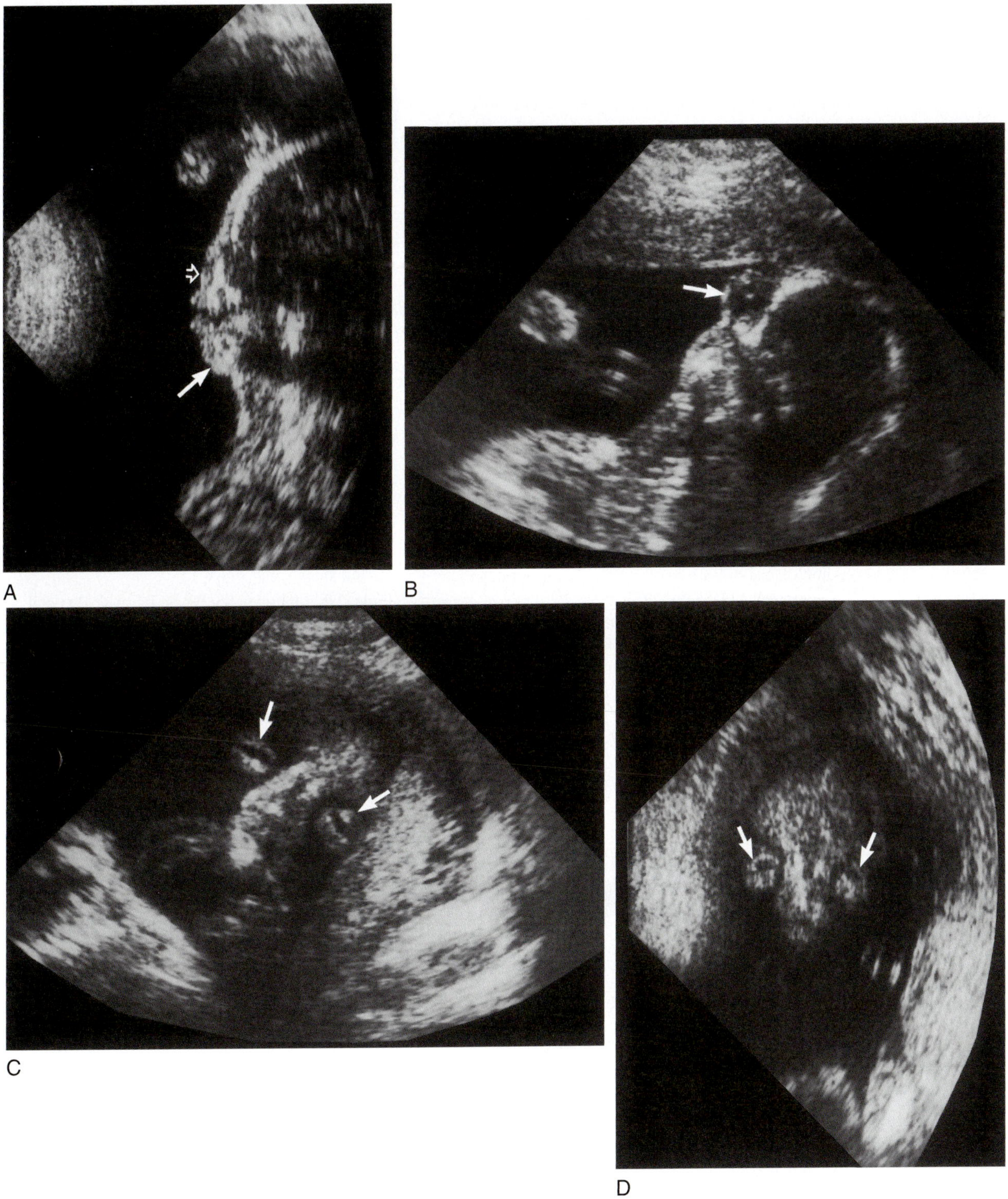

FIGURE 2-43 (A) Sagittal view of the fetal profile in Treacher Collins syndrome. Note complete absence of the nose *(open arrow)*, choanal atresia, severe micrognathia, and very small mandible *(solid arrow)*. (B) Oblique view of the fetal face shows proptosis of the eye *(arrow)*. (C, D) Coronal views of the soft tissues of the face in the same fetus. Note hypertelorism, severe orbital proptosis, and downslanting palpebral fissures. Arrows indicate locations of the eyes.

NATURAL HISTORY AND OUTCOME

There is marked variability in the expression of this syndrome, even within a given family. The spectrum ranges from fetuses with very mild features to severely affected fetuses with significant handicaps. Therefore the outcome also varies, ranging from a normal outcome to severe physical handicaps resulting from abnormalities such as arrhinia (absence of the nose), choanal atresia, hypoplastic orbits, corneal exposure, and need for a tracheotomy. Most affected individuals have normal intelligence.

Because mildly affected individuals have a 50% chance of having an affected fetus, many of these individuals seek prenatal diagnostic services.

Suggested Reading

Behrents RG, McNamara JA, Avery JK: Prenatal mandibulofacial dysostosis (Treacher Collins syndrome). *Cleft Palate J* 14:13–34, 1977.

Cohen J, Ghezi F, Goncalves L, et al: Prenatal sonographic diagnosis of Treacher Collins syndrome: a case and review of the literature. *Am J Perinatol* 12:416–419, 1995.

Crane JP, Beaver HA: Midtrimester sonographic diagnosis of mandibulofacial dysostosis. *Am J Med Genet* 25:251–255, 1986.

Hansen M, Lucarelli MJ, Whiteman DAH, Mulliken JB: Treacher Collins syndrome: phenotypic variability in a family, including an infant with arhinia and uveal colobomas. *Am J Med Genet* 61:71–74, 1996.

Hsu TY, Hsu JJ, Chang SY, Chang MS: Prenatal three-dimensional sonographic images associated with Treacher Collins syndrome. *Ultrasound Obstet Gynecol* 19:413–422, 2002.

Jones KL: *Smith's recognizable patterns of human malformations.* Philadelphia, 2006, Elsevier.

Meizner I, Carmi R, Katz M: Prenatal ultrasonic diagnosis of mandibulofacial dysostosis (Treacher Collins syndrome). *J Clin Ultrasound* 19:124–127, 1991.

Milligan DA, Harlass FE, Duff P, Kopelman JN: Recurrence of Treacher Collins' syndrome with sonographic findings. *Milit Med* 159:250–252, 1994.

Nicolaides KH, Johansson D, Donnai D, Rodeck CH: Prenatal diagnosis of mandibulofacial dysostosis. *Prenat Diagn* 4:201–205, 1984.

Ochi H, Matsubara K, Ito M, Kusanagi Y: Prenatal sonographic diagnosis of Treacher Collins syndrome. *Obstet Gynecol* 91:862, 1998.

Ruangvutilert P, Sutantawibul A, Sunsaneevithayakul P, Limwongse C: Ultrasonographic prenatal diagnosis of Treacher Collins syndrome: a case report. *J Med Assoc Thai* 86:482–488, 2003.

Tamas DE, Mahoney BS, Bowie JD, et al: Prenatal sonographic diagnosis of hemifacial microsomia (Goldenhar-Gorlin syndrome). *J Ultrasound Med* 5:461–463, 1986.

Tanaka Y, Kanenishi K, Tanaka H, Yanagihara T, Hata T: Antenatal three-dimensional sonographic features of Treacher Collins syndrome. *Ultrasound Obstet Gynecol* 19:414–415, 2002.

VAN DER WOUDE SYNDROME

DESCRIPTION AND DEFINITION

Synonym: Lip-pit syndrome

Autosomal dominant labial clefting syndrome characterized by pits in the lower lip and variable cleft lip and palate.

ABNORMALITIES DETECTABLE BY ULTRASOUND

The lower lip pits are not detectable sonographically, but cleft lip and palate involving the upper lip are visible in the early second trimester using both two-dimensional and three-dimensional ultrasound. Appearance of the cleft associated with this syndrome is similar to the paramedian cleft lip and palate that occur from lack of closure of the inner maxillary segment and the lateral maxillary prominences around weeks 8 to 9 (see Cleft Lip and Palate, p. 14).

MAJOR DIFFERENTIAL DIAGNOSES

Fetuses identified in utero with cleft lip and palate have high incidences of chromosomal abnormality and other syndromes (see differential diagnosis of cleft lip and palate, p. 14). Fewer than half of the fetuses with cleft lip and palate seen in utero have labial clefting as an isolated lesion, and only a small proportion of those are due to Van der Woude syndrome.

ULTRASOUND DIAGNOSIS

Cleft lip and palate can be diagnosed by sonography as early as 14 or 15 weeks. Van der Woude syndrome has been diagnosed by embryoscopy as early as 11 weeks.

Complete cleft lip and palate is easily diagnosed using either two-dimensional or three-dimensional ultrasound by observing the defect

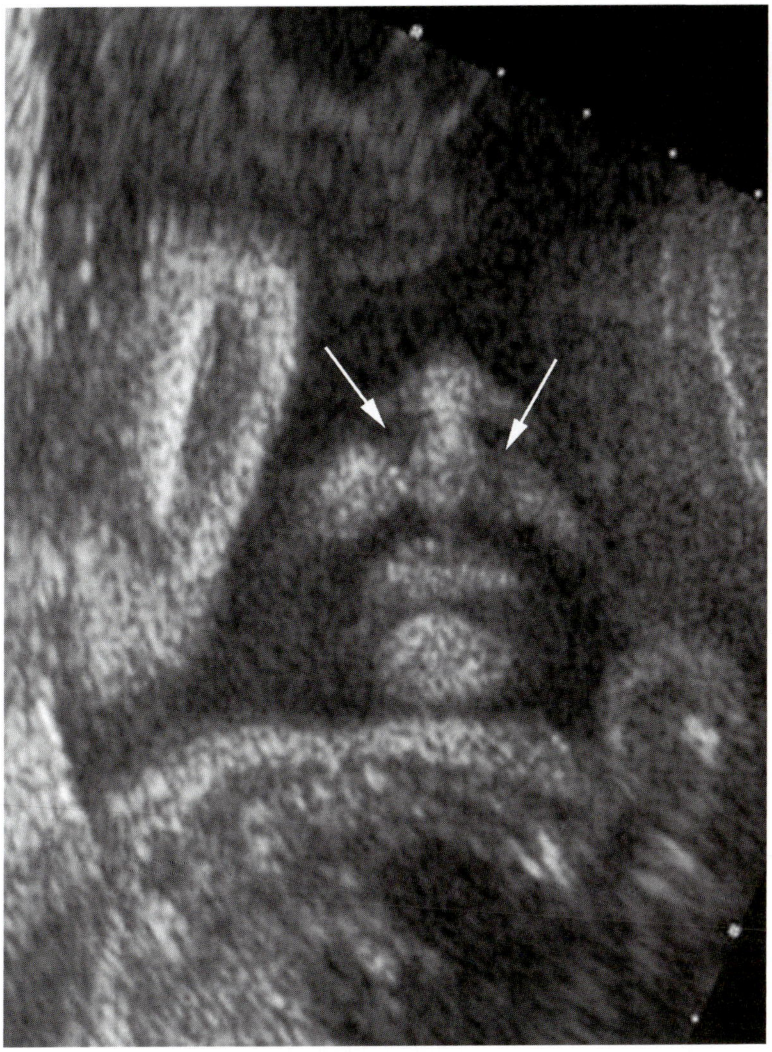

A

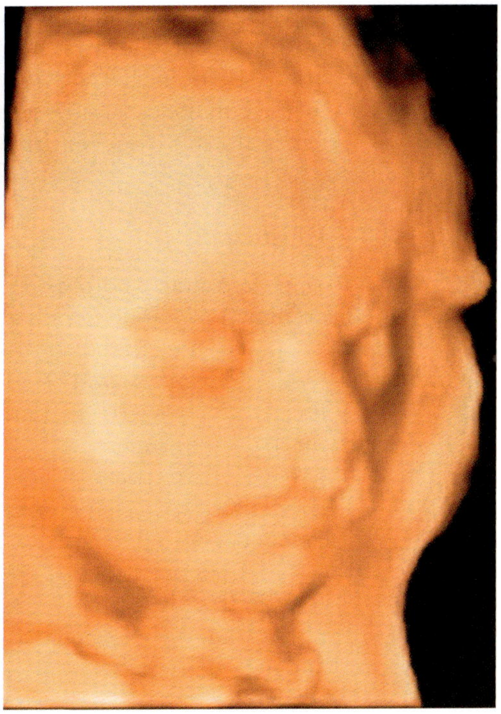

B

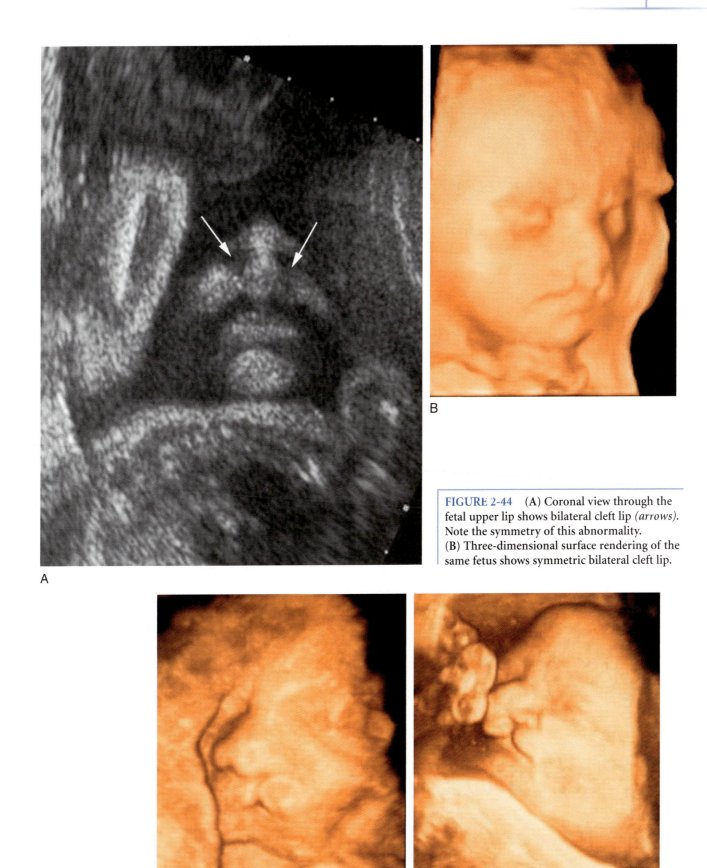

FIGURE 2-44 (A) Coronal view through the fetal upper lip shows bilateral cleft lip *(arrows)*. Note the symmetry of this abnormality. (B) Three-dimensional surface rendering of the same fetus shows symmetric bilateral cleft lip.

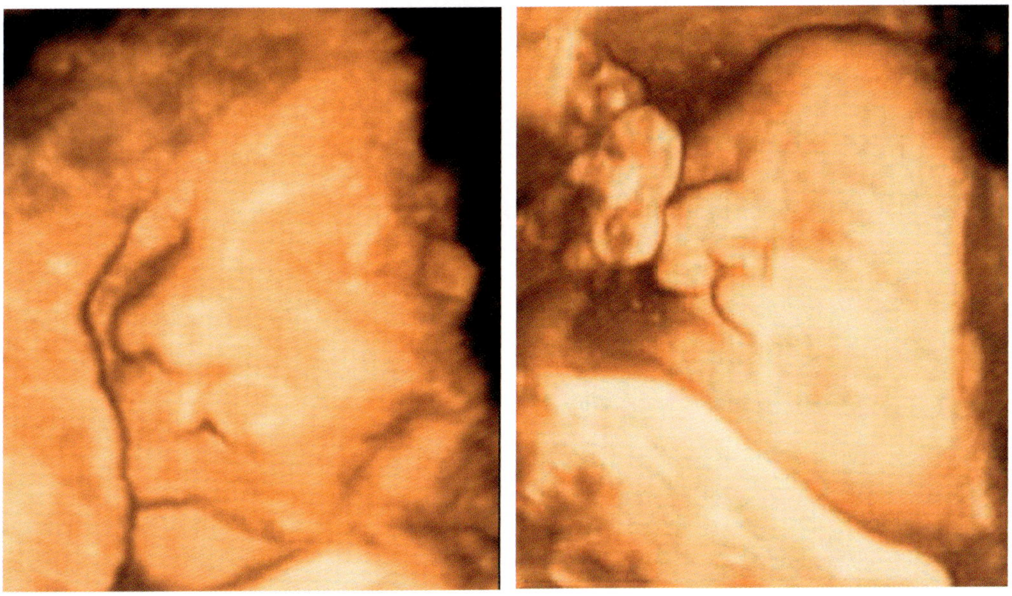

A B

FIGURE 2-45 (A) Thirty-week-old fetus with unilateral cleft lip. (B) Surface rendering of a cleft lip in a different fetus at 37 weeks shows both cleft lip and palate.

in the fetal maxilla and protrusion of the intermaxillary segment forward. Incomplete cleft lip (involving only the lip) is more subtle because of the lack of maxillary defect. Imaging must be focused on the facial surface to visualize the defect in the soft tissues of the lip.

HEREDITY

Van der Woude syndrome is an autosomal dominant condition, resulting in up to 50% risk of facial clefting in the offspring of affected parents. Although this syndrome may be manifested only by symmetric pits or eminencies of the lower lip, as many as 50% of gene carriers have cleft lip or palate or both. Approximately 2% of all cases of cleft lip and palate may be due to Van der Woude syndrome. The gene for this disorder has been mapped to 1q32-41. Mutations in this locus (interferon-inhibiting factor-6) can lead to popliteal pterygium syndrome, and both of these syndromes have occurred in the same family.

NATURAL HISTORY AND OUTCOME

Individuals with Van der Woude syndrome have isolated facial clefts that are reparable with plastic surgery, resulting in good outcomes.

Suggested Reading

Benacerraf BR, Mulliken JB: Fetal cleft lip/palate: sonographic diagnosis and postnatal outcome. *Plast Reconstr Surg* 92:1045–1051, 1993.

Dommergues M, Lemerrer M, Couly G, Delezoide AL, Dumez Y: Prenatal diagnosis of cleft lip at 11 menstrual weeks using embryoscopy in the Van der Woude syndrome. *Prenat Diagn* 15:378–381, 1995.

Jones KL: *Smith's recognizable patterns of human malformations*. Philadelphia, 2006, WB Saunders.

Kondo S, Schutte BC, Richardson RJ, et al: Mutations in IRF6 cause Van der Woude and popliteal pterygium syndromes. *Nat Genet* 32:285–289, 2002.

Lipson A: Van der Woude syndrome and limb defects: the chance of recurrence. *J Med Genet* 26:347–348, 1989.

Van der Woude A: Fistula labii inferioris congenita and its association with cleft lip and palate. *Am J Hum Genet* 6:244, 1954.

Syndromes Featuring Primarily Brain Anomalies

AICARDI SYNDROME

DESCRIPTION AND DEFINITION

Synonym: Agenesis of the corpus callosum with chorioretinal abnormality

This syndrome, first described by Aicardi in 1969, is a rare X-linked syndrome characterized by agenesis of the corpus callosum, chorioretinal abnormalities, and infantile seizures.

ABNORMALITIES DETECTABLE BY ULTRASOUND

Common Findings:

Ventriculomegaly

Agenesis of the corpus callosum

Interhemispheric cyst

Asymmetric orbits

Occasional Findings:

Dandy-Walker abnormality

Cortical heterotopia

Hemivertebrae

MAJOR DIFFERENTIAL DIAGNOSES

Other syndromes primarily affecting the brain and associated with agenesis of the corpus callosum:

- Miller-Dieker syndrome
- Neu-Laxova syndrome
- Walker-Warburg syndrome

Syndromes associated with lissencephaly:

- Miller-Dieker syndrome
- Walker-Warburg syndrome

Trisomy 18

Brain injuries (e.g., schizencephaly, porencephalic cyst)

Dandy-Walker cyst

Lobar and semilobar holoprosencephaly

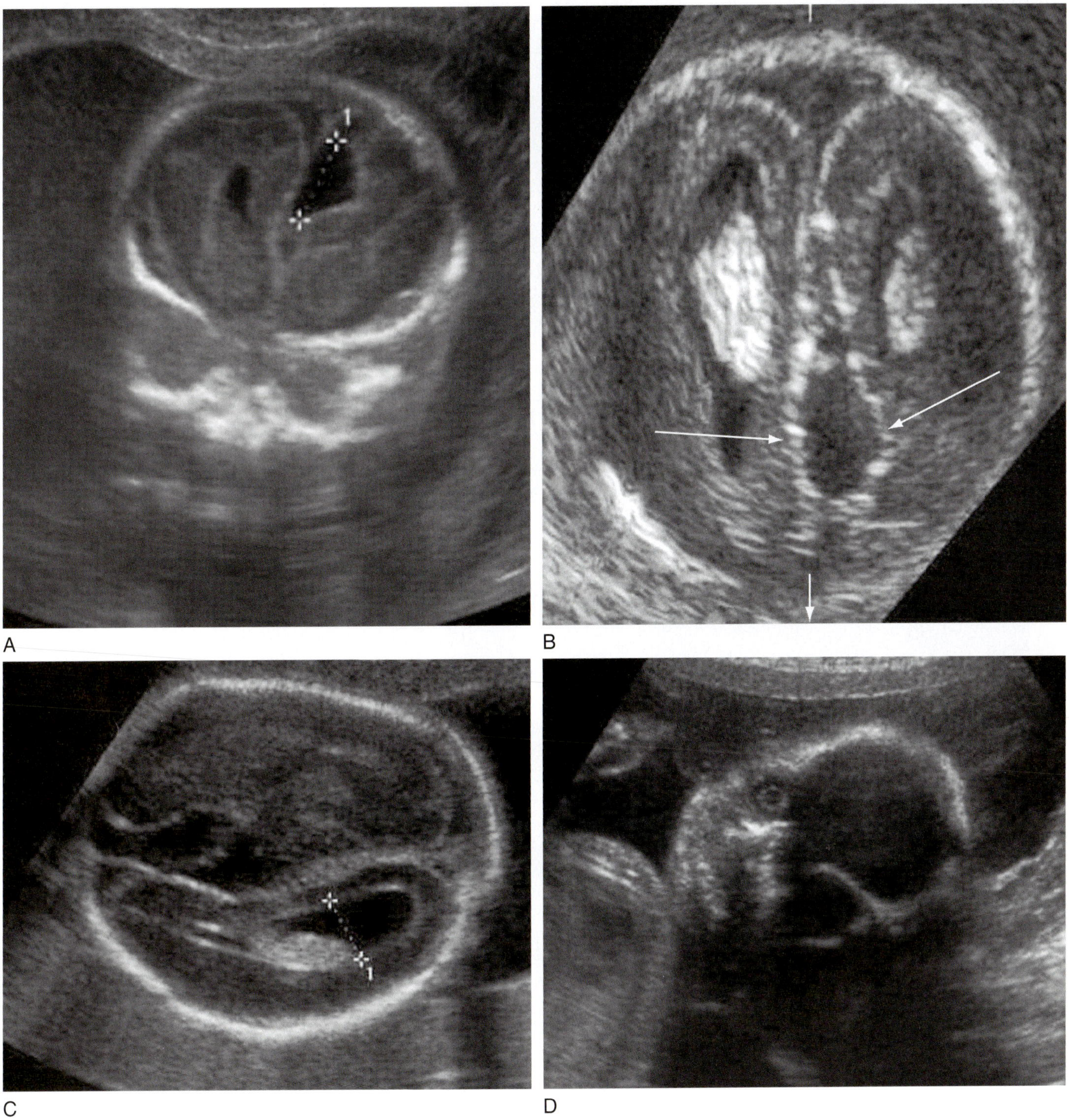

FIGURE 2-46 (A) Coronal view of the fetal brain shows an inner hemispheric cyst *(calipers)*. This fetus also had agenesis of the corpus callosum, both of which are features of Aicardi syndrome. (B) Reconstructed axial view of the same fetus shows the inner hemispheric cyst *(arrows)*. Note parallel orientation of the lateral ventricles, typical of agenesis of the corpus callosum. (C) Axial view of a fetus thought to have Aicardi syndrome shows the typical teardrop-shaped occipital horn of the lateral ventricle *(calipers)*, typical of agenesis of the corpus callosum and colpocephaly. In the midline is a cystic area representing the inner hemispheric cyst. (D) Same fetus thought to have Aicardi syndrome shows asymmetry of the size of the orbits.

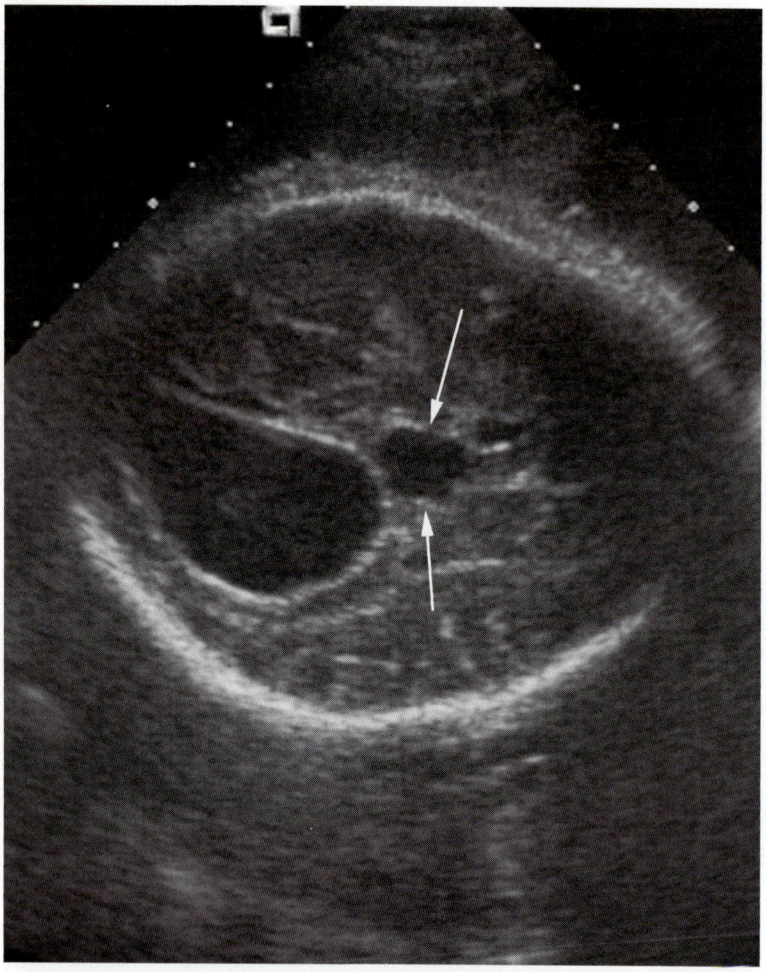

FIGURE 2-47 Third-trimester fetus with Aicardi syndrome has a high-riding third ventricle *(arrows)*. Note associated arachnoid cyst posteriorly in a fetus who also had agenesis of the corpus callosum.

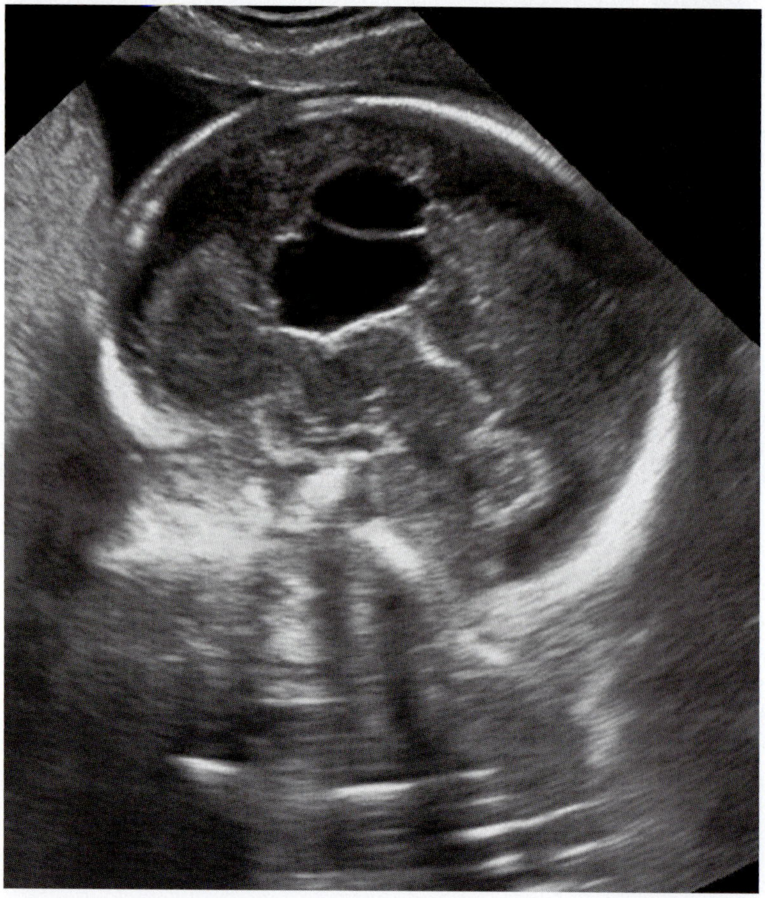

A

FIGURE 2-48 Complex inner hemispheric cyst in a female fetus that also had agenesis of the corpus callosum. (A) Midline sagittal view with the septate inner hemispheric cyst.

Continued

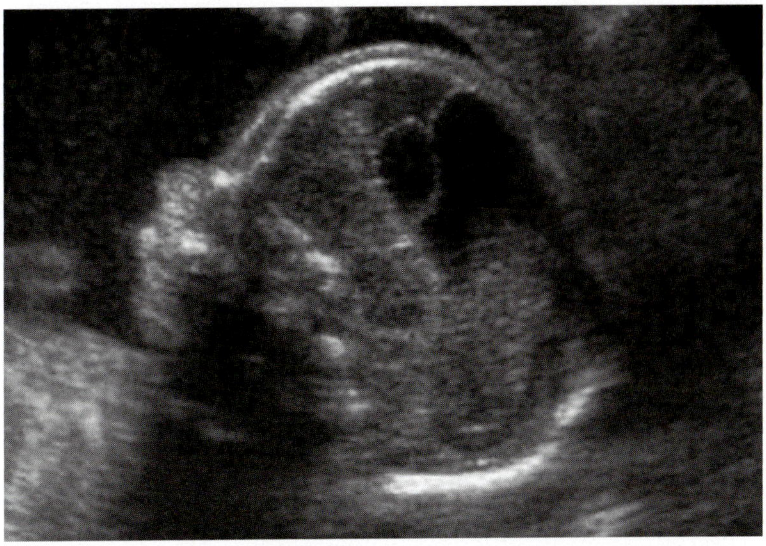

B

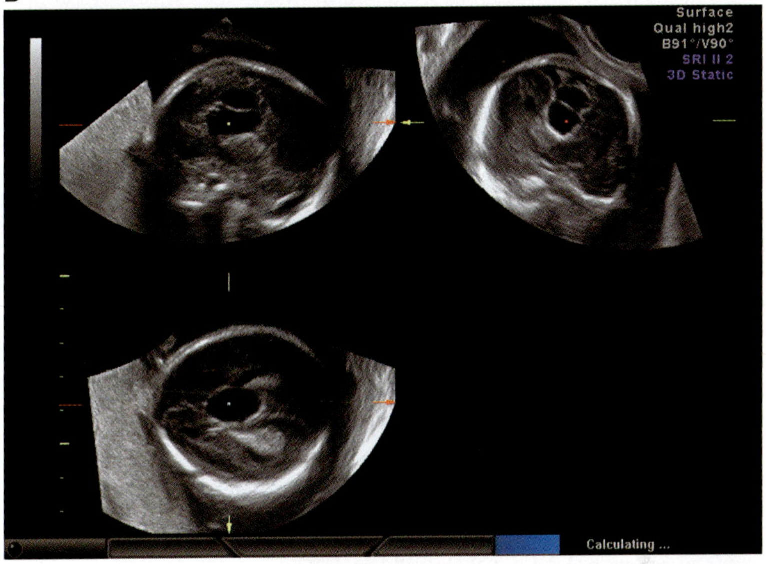

C

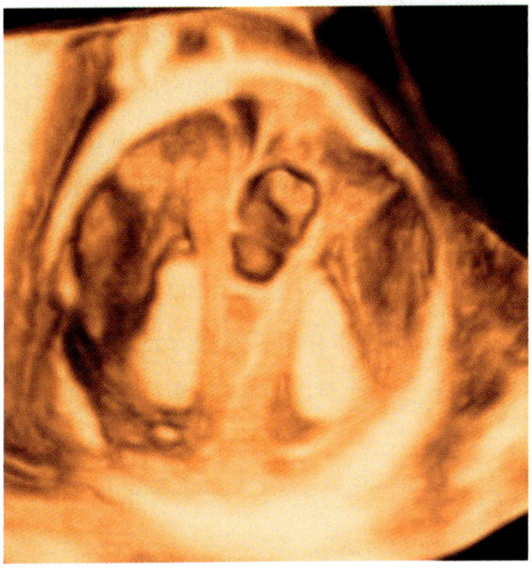

D

FIGURE 2-48, cont'd Complex inner hemispheric cyst in a female fetus that also had agenesis of the corpus callosum. (B) Profile of fetus with mild micrognathia. (C) Multiplanar three-dimensional display of the septate inner hemispheric cyst shown in three planes, with the reconstructed C plane demonstrating the parallel orientation of the lateral ventricles. (D) Surface rendering view of the inside of the fetal brain shows the parallel orientation of the choroid plexuses as well as the cavity of the inner hemispheric cyst.

ULTRASOUND DIAGNOSIS

The diagnosis of Aicardi syndrome has been made in the third trimester by detection of an interhemispheric cyst and mild ventriculomegaly in a female fetus. One of the reported cases had a normal 18-week scan, which indicates that agenesis of the corpus callosum may not always be detectable on a routine scan until after 18 weeks. The combination of an interhemispheric cyst with a high-riding third ventricle in a female fetus should raise the suspicion of Aicardi syndrome.

HEREDITY

Aicardi syndrome is a rare X-linked syndrome that is lethal in males. Only female fetuses are known to have Aicardi syndrome; therefore, this syndrome should be considered only if the fetus is female. This syndrome is considered to be a new mutation because affected individuals have not been known to reproduce.

NATURAL HISTORY AND OUTCOME

Aicardi syndrome has an extremely poor prognosis, with severe psychomotor retardation and severe seizure disorders. Some of the orbital abnormalities, particularly optic atrophy and chorioretinal abnormality, typically are not identified sonographically.

Suggested Reading

Aicardi J, Lefebvre J, Lerique-Koechlin A: A new syndrome: spasms in flexion, callosal agenesis, ocular abnormalities. *Electroencephalogr Clin Neurophysiol* 19:609–610, 1965.

Bromley B, Krishnamoorthy KS, Benacerraf BR: Aicardi syndrome: prenatal sonographic findings. A report of two cases. *Prenat Diag* 20:344–346, 2000.

Donnenfeld AE, Packer RJ, Zackai EH, Chee CM, Sellinger B, Emanuel BS: Clinical, cytogenetic, and pedigree findings in 18 cases of Aicardi syndrome. *Am J Med Genet* 32:461–467, 1989.

Pilu G, Sandri F, Perolo A, et al: Sonography of fetal agenesis of the corpus callosum: a survey of 35 cases. *Ultrasound Obstet Gynecol* 3:318–329, 1993.

GORLIN SYNDROME

DESCRIPTION AND DEFINITION

Gorlin syndrome is characterized by macrocephaly, cysts of the jaw, basal cell carcinomas and nevi, and other tumors.

ABNORMALITIES DETECTABLE BY ULTRASOUND

Common Findings:

Ventriculomegaly

Macrocephaly with frontal bossing

Calcification of the falx

Prognathism

Cleft lip and palate

Short fourth metacarpal

Misshapen ribs

Scoliosis

Vertebral abnormalities

Occasional Findings:

Agenesis of the corpus callosum

Hypertelorism

MAJOR DIFFERENTIAL DIAGNOSES

The most obvious prenatal sonographic feature of this syndrome reportedly is mild ventriculomegaly, a nonspecific finding that can be present in many different syndromes, including chromosomal anomalies and infections.

Syndromes and Conditions Associated with Ventriculomegaly and Cleft Lip and Palate:

Camptomelic dysplasia

Chromosomal anomalies

Crouzon syndrome

Fryns syndrome

Goldenhar syndrome

Hydrolethalus

Meckel-Gruber syndrome

Multiple pterygium syndrome

Neu-Laxova syndrome

Oral-facial-digital syndrome, type I

Oral-facial-digital syndrome, type II (Mohr syndrome)

Walker-Warburg syndrome

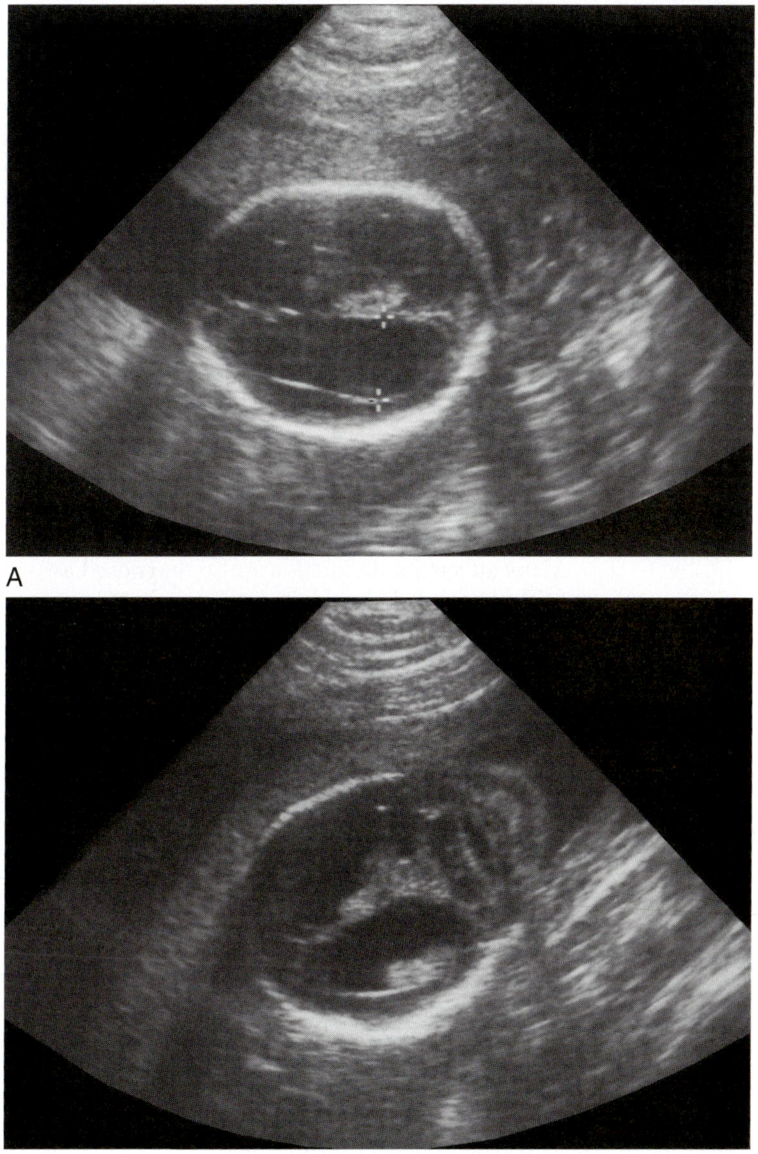

A

B

FIGURE 2-49 Transverse (A) and coronal (B) views through the fetal head in the second trimester show moderate ventriculomegaly, as can be seen in fetuses with Gorlin syndrome.

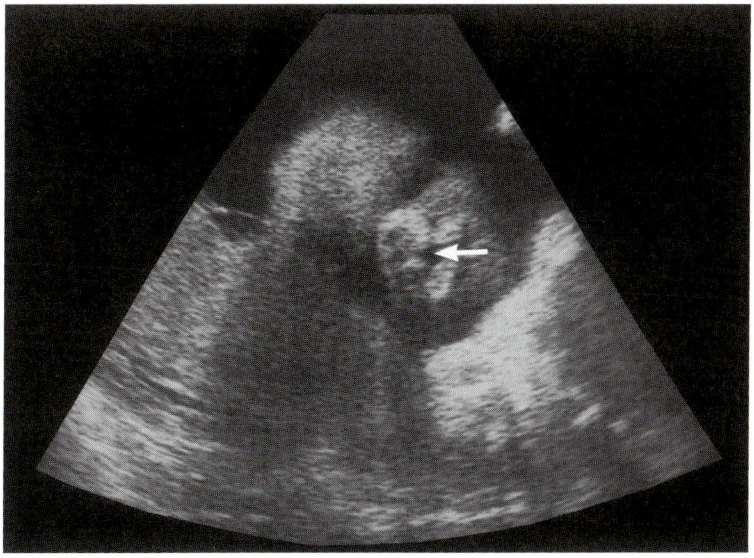

FIGURE 2-50 Coronal view through the fetal face shows a cleft lip and palate *(arrow)*, as can be seen in fetuses with Gorlin syndrome.

ULTRASOUND DIAGNOSIS

In three instances, the prenatal ultrasound diagnosis of Gorlin syndrome has been established as early as 19 weeks' gestation. Features identified included cleft lip and palate and mild ventriculomegaly with macrocephaly.

HEREDITY

Gorlin syndrome has an autosomal dominant pattern of inheritance. The gene responsible for this syndrome has been mapped to 9;22.3-q31.

NATURAL HISTORY AND OUTCOME

Tumors are a common feature of this syndrome, and vigilance is required for their detection. Many affected individuals are also diagnosed as having medulloblastomas, meningiomas, fibromas, lipomas, neurofibromas, ovarian tumors, leukemias, or other cancers. Some patients are mentally deficient.

Suggested Reading

Bialer MG, Gailani MR, McLaughlin JA, Petrikovsky B, Bale AE: Prenatal diagnosis of Gorlin syndrome. *Lancet* 344:477, 1994.

Gorlin JR, Goltz RW: Multiple nevoid basal cell epithelioma, jaw cysts, and bifid ribs: a syndrome. *N Engl J Med* 262:908, 1960.

Hogge WA, Blank C, Roochvarg LB, et al: Gorlin syndrome (naevoid basal cell carcinoma syndrome): prenatal detection in a fetus with macrocephaly and ventriculomegaly. *Prenat Diagn* 14:725–727, 1994.

Jones KL: *Smith's recognizable patterns of human malformations.* Philadelphia, 2006, WB Saunders.

Petrikovsky BM, Bialer MG, McLaughlin JA, Bale AE: Sonographic and DNA-based prenatal detection of Gorlin syndrome. *J Ultrasound Med* 15:493–495, 1996.

HYDROLETHALUS

DESCRIPTION AND DEFINITION

Hydrolethalus was first described in 1981 in Finland, based on 28 cases. It is a lethal malformation, features of which include ventriculomegaly, small occipital encephalocele, micrognathia, polydactyly, cardiac defects, and polyhydramnios.

ABNORMALITIES DETECTABLE BY ULTRASOUND

Thickened nuchal translucency

Ventriculomegaly

Micrognathia

Microphthalmia

Cleft lip and palate

Low-set ears

Neural tube defects

Cardiac defects (e.g., ventricular septal defect, endocardial cushion defect)

Postaxial polydactyly of the hands

Preaxial polydactyly of the feet (hallux duplication)

Clubbed feet

Hypospadias

Polyhydramnios

MAJOR DIFFERENTIAL DIAGNOSES

Syndromes and conditions associated with multiple anomalies, including ventriculomegaly and limb anomalies:

Apert syndrome

Chromosomal abnormalities

Fanconi anemia

Fryns syndrome

Meckel-Gruber syndrome

Oral-facial-digital syndrome, type I

Oral-facial-digital syndrome, type II (Mohr syndrome)

Pfeiffer syndrome

Syndromes and Conditions Associated with Ventriculomegaly and Cleft Lip and Palate:

Camptomelic dysplasia

Chromosomal anomalies

Crouzon syndrome

Fryns syndrome

Goldenhar syndrome

Gorlin syndrome

Meckel-Gruber syndrome

Multiple pterygium syndrome

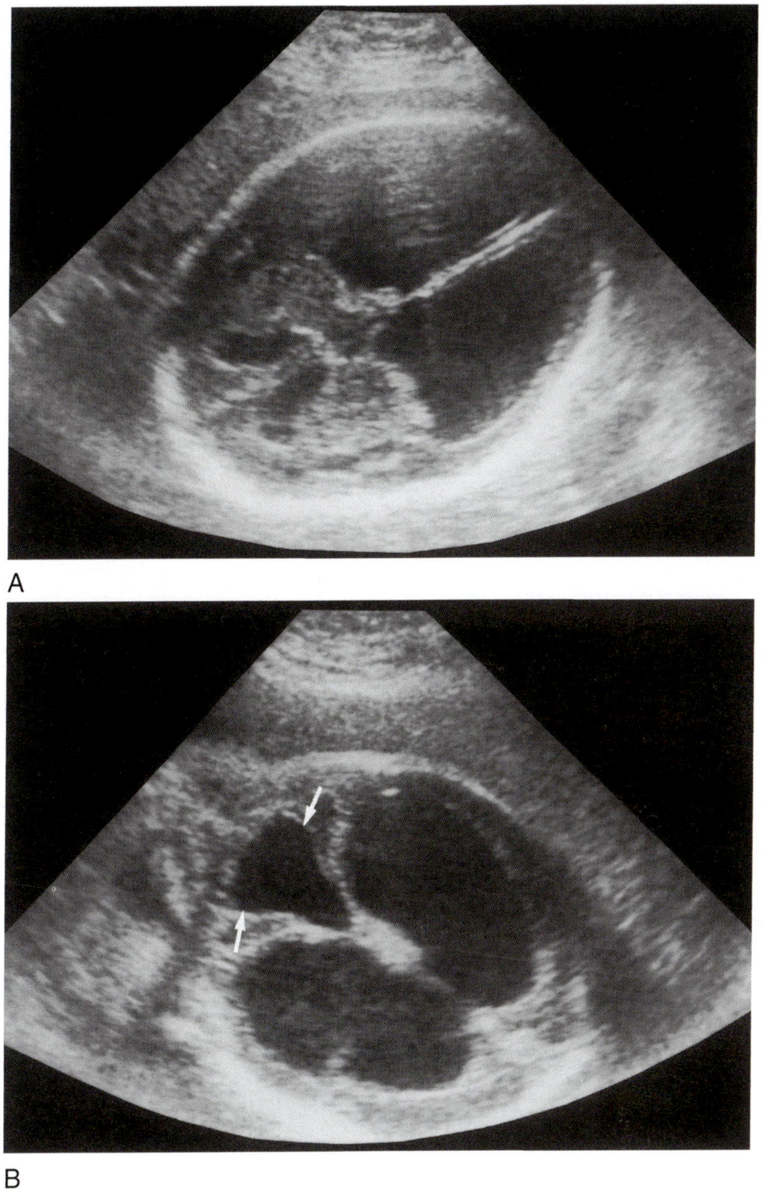

FIGURE 2-51 Transverse (A) and coronal (B) views of the fetal head show severe ventriculomegaly and a Dandy-Walker cyst *(arrows)*, as can be seen in fetuses with hydrolethalus.

Neu-Laxova syndrome

Oral-facial-digital syndrome, type I

Oral-facial-digital syndrome, type II (Mohr syndrome)

Roberts' syndrome

Walker-Warburg syndrome

ULTRASOUND DIAGNOSIS

The ultrasound diagnosis of this syndrome has been made several times, including as early as 12 weeks in two different reports, based on a thickened nuchal translucency and other anomalies, such as encephalocele, limb abnormalities, omphalocele, and cardiac defect. The diagnosis usually depends on intracranial abnormalities, such as ventriculomegaly and neural tube defects with limb abnormalities. The reported cases in the third trimester show sonographic evidence of severe ventriculomegaly and polyhydramnios.

HEREDITY

The pattern of inheritance for hydrolethalus is autosomal recessive. Locus is reportedly at 11p23-25.

NATURAL HISTORY AND OUTCOME

As the name suggests, hydrolethalus is a lethal syndrome. Affected fetuses usually exhibit severe IUGR. Most affected individuals are stillborn; the rest die shortly after birth.

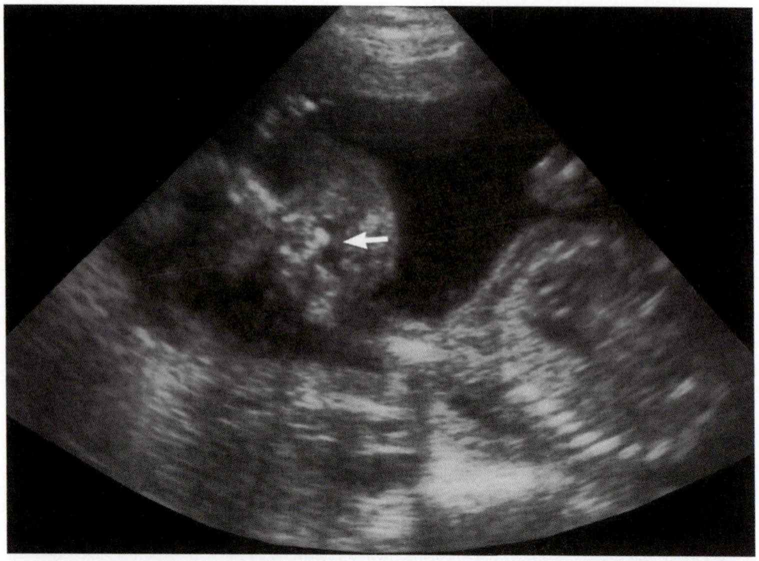

A

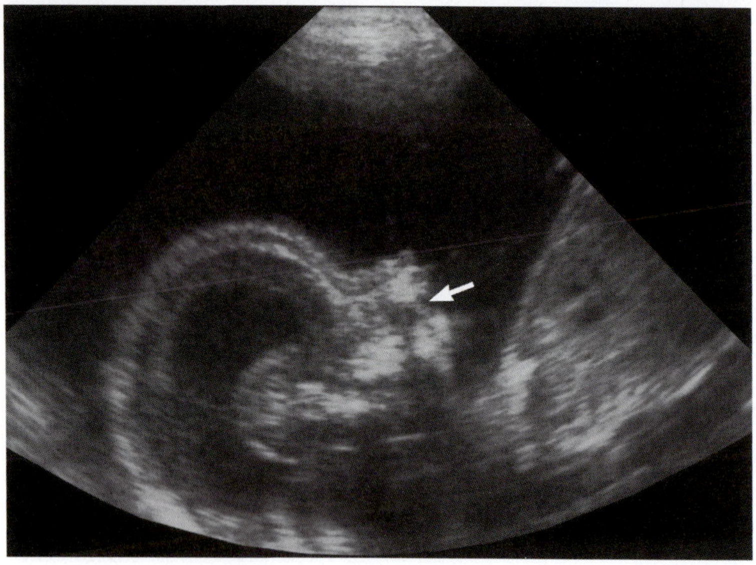

B

FIGURE 2-52 **(A)** Coronal view through the fetal face shows bilateral cleft lip and palate *(arrow),* a characteristic feature of fetuses with hydrolethalus syndrome. **(B)** Longitudinal view of the same fetus as in panel A shows disruption of the midface by cleft lip and palate *(arrow),* as can be seen in fetuses with hydrolethalus syndrome. Note ventriculomegaly.

Suggested Reading

Ammala P, Salonen R: First-trimester diagnosis of hydrolethalus syndrome. *Ultrasound Obstet Gynecol* 5:60–62, 1995.

Anyane-Yeboa K, Collins M, Kupsky W, et al: Hydrolethalus (Salonen-Herva-Norio) syndrome: further clinicopathological delineation. *Am J Med Genet* 26:899–907, 1987.

Authton DJ, Cassidy SB: Hydrolethalus syndrome: report of apparent mild case, literature review and differential diagnosis. *Am J Med Genet* 27:935–942, 1987.

Camera G, Carbone LD, Centa A, et al: Prenatal diagnosis of hydrolethalus (Salonen-Herva-Norio syndrome) in a woman with unknown risk: presentation of a case with long survival. *Pathologica* 83:359–364, 1991.

Chan BC, Shek TW, Lee CP: First-trimester diagnosis of hydrolethalus syndrome in a Chinese family. *Prenat Diagn* 24:587–590, 2004.

de Ravel TJ, van der Griendt MC, Evan P, Wright CA: Hydrolethalus syndrome in a non-Finnish family: confirmation of the entity and early prenatal diagnosis. *Prenat Diagn* 19:279–281, 1999.

Hartikainen-Sorri A, Kirkinen P, Herva R: Prenatal detection of hydrolethalus syndrome. *Prenat Diagn* 3:219–224, 1983.

Herva R, Seppanen U: Roentgenologic findings of the hydrolethalus syndrome. *Pediatr Radiol* 14:41–43, 1984.

Norgard M, Yankowitz J, Rhead W, Kanis AB, Hall BD: Prenatal ultrasound findings in hydrolethalus: continuing difficulties in diagnosis. *Prenat Diagn* 16:173–179, 1996.

Pryde PG, Qureshi F, Hallak M, et al: Two consecutive hydrolethalus syndrome-affected pregnancies in a nonconsanguineous black couple: discussion of problems in prenatal differential diagnosis of midline malformation syndromes. *Am J Med Genet* 46:537–541, 1993.

Salonen R, Herva R: Hydrolethalus syndrome. *J Med Genet* 27:756–759, 1990.

Salonen R, Herva R, Norio R: The hydrolethalus syndrome: delineation of a "new" lethal malformation syndrome based on 28 patients. *Clin Genet* 19:321–330, 1981.

Siffring PA, Forrest TS, Frick MP: Sonographic detection of hydrolethalus syndrome. *J Clin Ultrasound* 19:43–47, 1991.

JOUBERT SYNDROME

DESCRIPTION AND DEFINITION

First described by Marie Joubert in 1968, Joubert syndrome is a condition characterized by dysmorphic facial features and cerebellar vermis agenesis.

ABNORMALITIES DETECTABLE BY ULTRASOUND

Dandy-Walker variant

Occipital encephalocele

Ventriculomegaly

Micrognathia

Multicystic kidneys

Polydactyly

Thickened nuchal fold

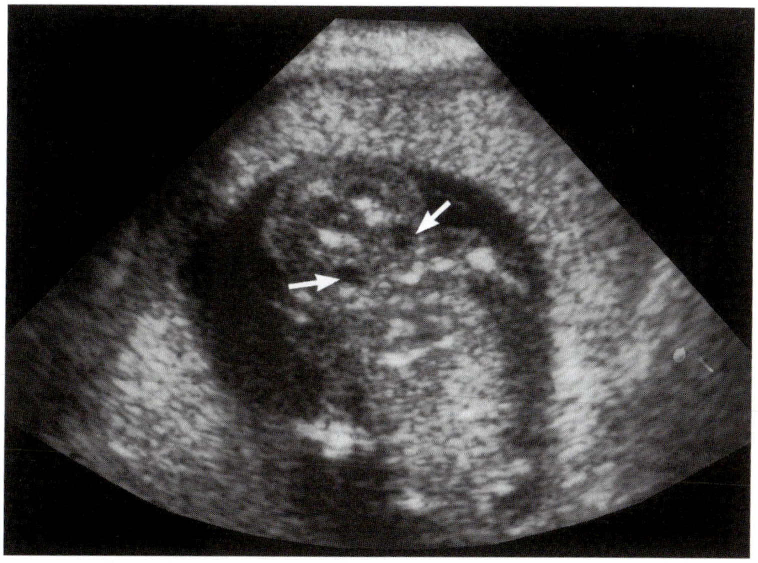

FIGURE 2-53 Longitudinal view of a late first-trimester fetus with Joubert syndrome. Note bilateral nuchal cystic hygroma *(arrows)* accompanied by thickened nuchal fold.

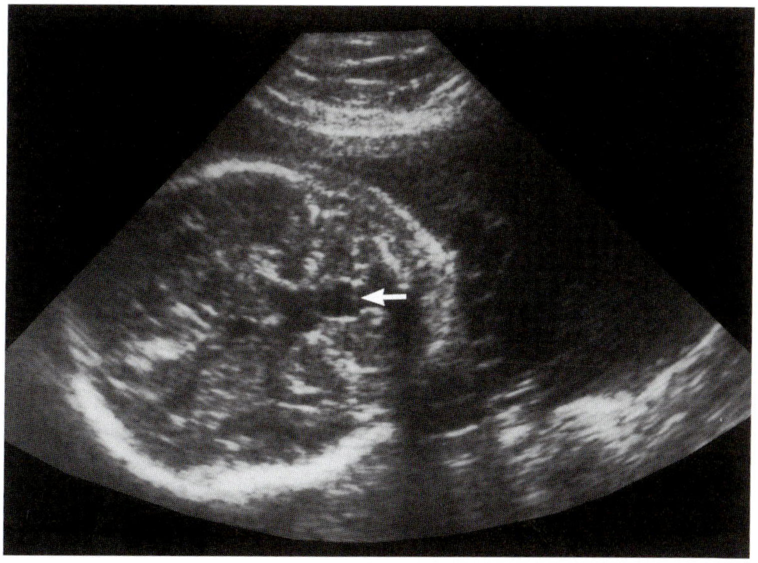

FIGURE 2-54 Modified transverse view through fetal posterior fossa shows Dandy-Walker variant. Arrow points to communication between fourth ventricle and cisterna magna, a feature of Joubert syndrome.

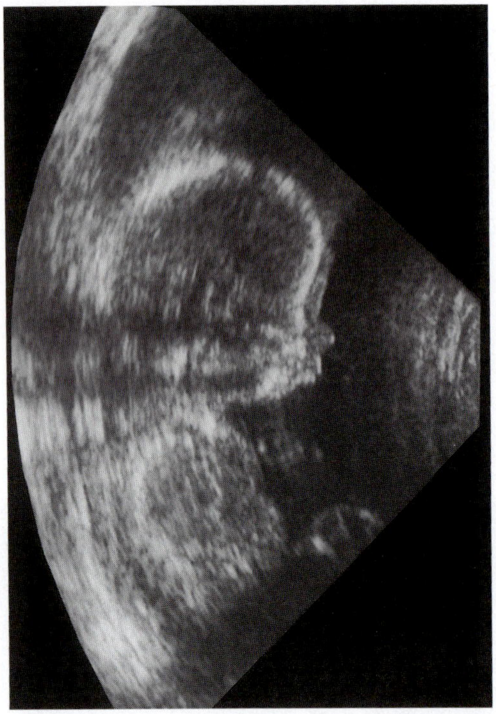

FIGURE 2-55 Longitudinal view of a fetus with Joubert syndrome reveals micrognathia.

MAJOR DIFFERENTIAL DIAGNOSES

Syndromes and Conditions Associated with Vermian Agenesis:

- Aicardi syndrome
- Arthrogryposis
- CHARGE association
- Chromosomal abnormalities
  - Triploidy
  - Trisomy 9
  - Tetrasomy 12p (Pallister-Killian syndrome)
  - Trisomy 18 (Edwards' syndrome)
- Fryns syndrome
- Meckel-Gruber syndrome
- MURCS (**m**üllerian duct aplasia, **r**enal aplasia, **c**ervicothoracic **s**omite dysplasia) association
- Neu-Laxova syndrome
- Opitz syndrome
- Oral-facial-digital syndrome, type I
- Oral-facial-digital syndrome, type II (Mohr syndrome)
- Smith-Lemli-Opitz syndrome
- Walker-Warburg syndrome

ULTRASOUND DIAGNOSIS

The diagnosis of Joubert syndrome has been possible after 17 weeks. Prenatal diagnosis of this syndrome has been reported in at least 11 fetuses, 6 of which had vermian hypoplasia, 4 enlarged cisterna magna, 4 occipital encephalocele, 2 thickened nuchal translucency, and 1 each with polydactyly, ventriculomegaly, renal cysts, and genital abnormality. The author has detected Joubert syndrome in the first trimester, based on a thickened nuchal lucency. Later in the second trimester, Dandy-Walker variant (vermian agenesis) and micrognathia were demonstrated, establishing the prenatal diagnosis of Joubert syndrome in a family with a previously affected child.

HEREDITY

The pattern of inheritance for this syndrome is autosomal recessive.

NATURAL HISTORY AND OUTCOME

The outcome of patients with Joubert syndrome is variable, depending on the degree of severity and number of associated malformations. Postnatal life is characterized by episodes of apnea, abnormal eye movements, ataxia, and psychomotor retardation.

Suggested Reading

Aslan H, Ulker V, Gulcan EM, et al: Prenatal diagnosis of Joubert syndrome: a case report. *Prenat Diagn* 22:13–16, 2002.

Cantani A, Lucenti P, Ranzani GA, Santoro C: Joubert syndrome: review of the fifty-three cases so far published. *Ann Genet* 33:96–98, 1990.

Doherty D, Glass IA, Siebert JR, Strouse PJ, et al: Prenatal diagnosis in pregnancies at risk for Joubert syndrome by ultrasound and MRI. *Prenat Diagn* 25:442–447, 2005.

Joubert M, Eiserung JJ, Preston RJ, Anderman F: Familial agenesis of the cerebellar vermis. *Neurology* 19:813–825, 1969.

Kroes HY, Nievelstein RJ, Barth PG, et al: Cerebral, cerebellar, and colobomatous anomalies in three related males: sex-linked inheritance in a newly recognized syndrome with features overlapping with Joubert syndrome. *Am J Med Genet A* 135:297–301, 2005.

Ni Scanaill S, Crowley P, Hogan M, Stuart B: Abnormal prenatal sonographic findings in the posterior cranial fossa: a case of Joubert's syndrome. *Ultrasound Obstet Gynecol* 13:71–74, 1999.

Squires LA, Raymond G, Neumeyer AM, Krishnamoorthy KS, Buyse ML: Dysmorphic features of Joubert syndrome. *Dysmorphol Clin Genet* 5:72–77, 1991.

Wang P, Chang FM, Chang CH, Yu CH, Jung YC, Huang CC: Prenatal diagnosis of Joubert syndrome complicated with encephalocele using two-dimensional and three-dimensional ultrasound. *Ultrasound Obstet Gynecol* 14:360–362, 1999.

MECKEL-GRUBER SYNDROME

DESCRIPTION AND DEFINITION

Synonym: Dysencephalia splanchnocystica

Meckel-Gruber syndrome is characterized by a posterior encephalocele, postaxial polydactyly, and cystic kidneys.

ABNORMALITIES DETECTABLE BY ULTRASOUND

Posterior encephalocele (80%)

Polydactyly (75%)

Cystic dysplasia of the kidneys (95%)

Microcephaly

Cerebellar hypoplasia

Dandy-Walker abnormalities

Ventriculomegaly

Arnold-Chiari malformation

Agenesis of the corpus callosum

Microphthalmia

Micrognathia

Cleft palate

Cardiac defects

Cryptorchidism

Oligohydramnios is often associated with this syndrome, secondary to renal dysplasia. Hepatic fibrosis also may be a feature, but it has not been detectable on prenatal sonograms.

MAJOR DIFFERENTIAL DIAGNOSES

Autosomal recessive polycystic kidney disease (infantile)

Hydrolethalus syndrome

Joubert syndrome

Oral-facial-digital syndrome, type I

Oral-facial-digital syndrome, type II (Mohr syndrome)

Short rib–polydactyly syndromes

Smith-Lemli-Opitz syndrome

Trisomy 13 (Patau syndrome, which can mimic Meckel-Gruber syndrome)

ULTRASOUND DIAGNOSIS

Ultrasound diagnosis of Meckel-Gruber syndrome has been established as early as the first trimester, at 10 to 11 weeks' gestation, with demonstration of polydactyly and an encephalocele. Although oligohydramnios (secondary to renal abnormalities) may complicate the diagnosis in many cases, prenatal diagnosis of this condition has been reported at all gestational ages.

HEREDITY

This syndrome has an autosomal recessive pattern of inheritance.

NATURAL HISTORY AND OUTCOME

Meckel-Gruber syndrome is a lethal malformation. Affected infants die within the first few days of life.

Suggested Reading

Braithwaite JM, Economides DL: First-trimester diagnosis of Meckel-Gruber syndrome by transabdominal sonography in a low-risk case (Short Communication). *Prenat Diagn* 15:1168–1170, 1995.

Budorick NE, Pretorius DH, McGahan JP, et al: Cephalocele detection in utero: sonographic and clinical features. *Ultrasound Obstet Gynecol* 5:77–85, 1995.

Dumez Y, Dommergues M, Gubler M, et al: Meckel-Gruber syndrome: prenatal diagnosis at 10 menstrual weeks using embryoscopy (short communication). *Prenat Diagn* 14:141–144, 1994.

Gallimore AP, Davies PF: Meckel syndrome: prenatal ultrasonographic diagnosis in two cases showing marked differences in phenotypic expression. *Australas Radiol* 36:62–64, 1992.

Gruber GB: Beitraege zur Frag 'gekoppelter' missbildungen (akrocephalo-syndactylie und dysencephalia splanchnocystica). *Beitr Pathol Anat* 93:459–476, 1934.

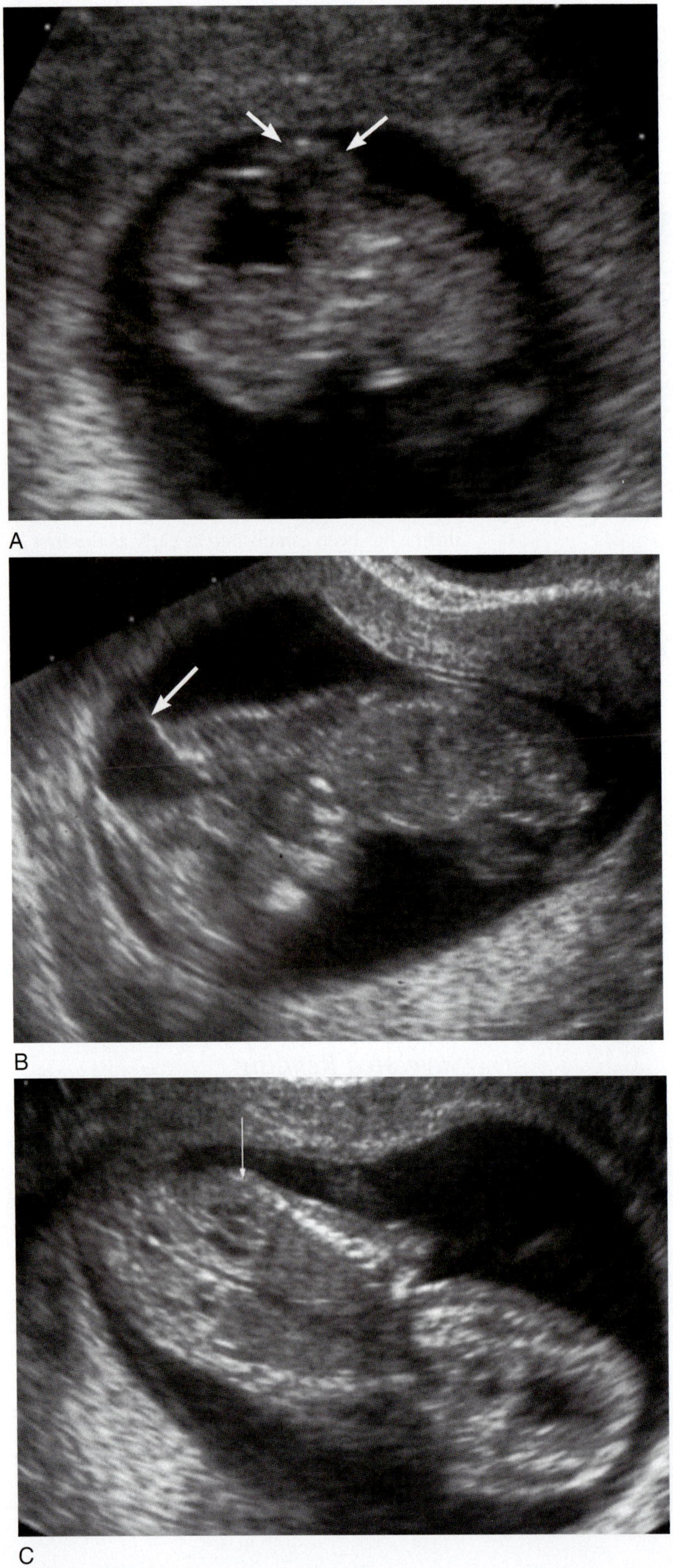

FIGURE 2-56 (**A**) An 8.5-week fetus with Meckel-Gruber syndrome. Note the larger than normal posterior cystic area accompanied by an irregularity in the occipital region of the fetal head *(arrows)*. **B–E:** Same fetus with Meckel-Gruber syndrome at 12 weeks. (**B**) Posterior view shows posterior encephalocele *(arrow)*. (**C**) Coronal view through the fetal head and body shows a cystic kidney *(arrow)*.

Continued

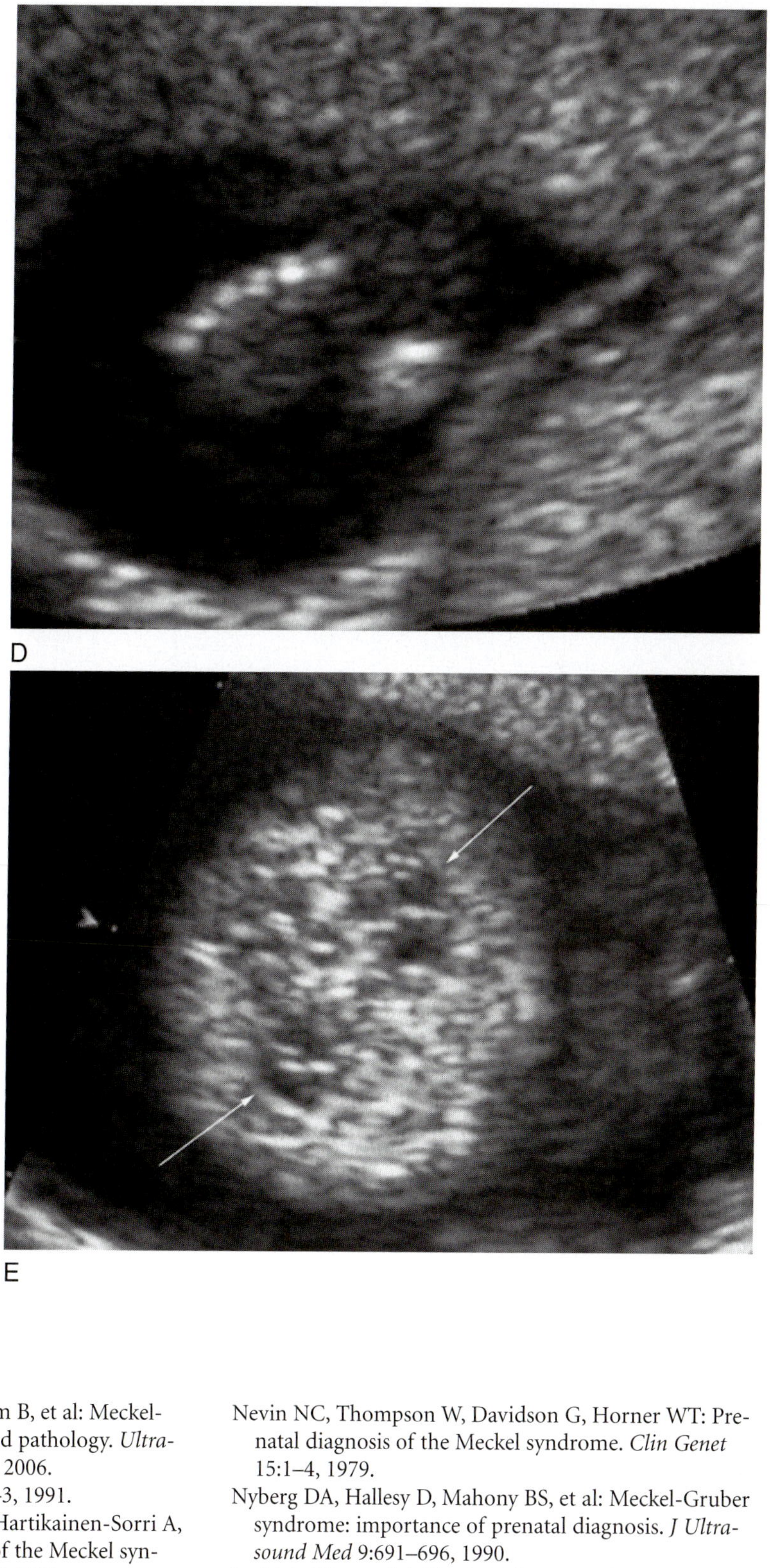

FIGURE 2-56, cont'd (D) Evidence of polydactyly. (E) Transverse view through both kidneys shows that both kidneys are cystic *(arrows)*.

Ickowicz V, Eurin D, Maugey-Laulom B, et al: Meckel-Gruber syndrome: sonography and pathology. *Ultrasound Obstet Gynecol* 27:296–300, 2006.

Jaffe R: Meckel syndrome. *Fetus* 1:1–3, 1991.

Karjalainen O, Pertti A, Seppala M, Hartikainen-Sorri A, Ryynanen M: Prenatal diagnosis of the Meckel syndrome. *Obstet Gynecol* 57:13S–15S, 1981.

Mecke S, Passarge E: Encephalocele, polycystic kidneys and polydactyly as an autosomal recessive trait simulating certain other disorders. *Ann Genet (Paris)* 14:97–103, 1971.

Meckel JF: Beschreibung zweier, durch sehr aehnliche Bildungsabweichungen entstellter geschwister. *Dtsch Arch Physiol* 7:99–172, 1822.

Nevin NC, Thompson W, Davidson G, Horner WT: Prenatal diagnosis of the Meckel syndrome. *Clin Genet* 15:1–4, 1979.

Nyberg DA, Hallesy D, Mahony BS, et al: Meckel-Gruber syndrome: importance of prenatal diagnosis. *J Ultrasound Med* 9:691–696, 1990.

Pachi A, Giancotti A, Torcia F, de Prosperi V, Maggi E: Meckel-Gruber syndrome: ultrasonographic diagnosis at 13 weeks' gestational age in an at-risk case. *Prenatal Diagn* 9:187–190, 1989.

Pardes JG, Engel IA, Blomquist K, Magid MS, Kazam E: Ultrasonography of intrauterine Meckel's syndrome. *J Ultrasound Med* 3:33–35, 1984.

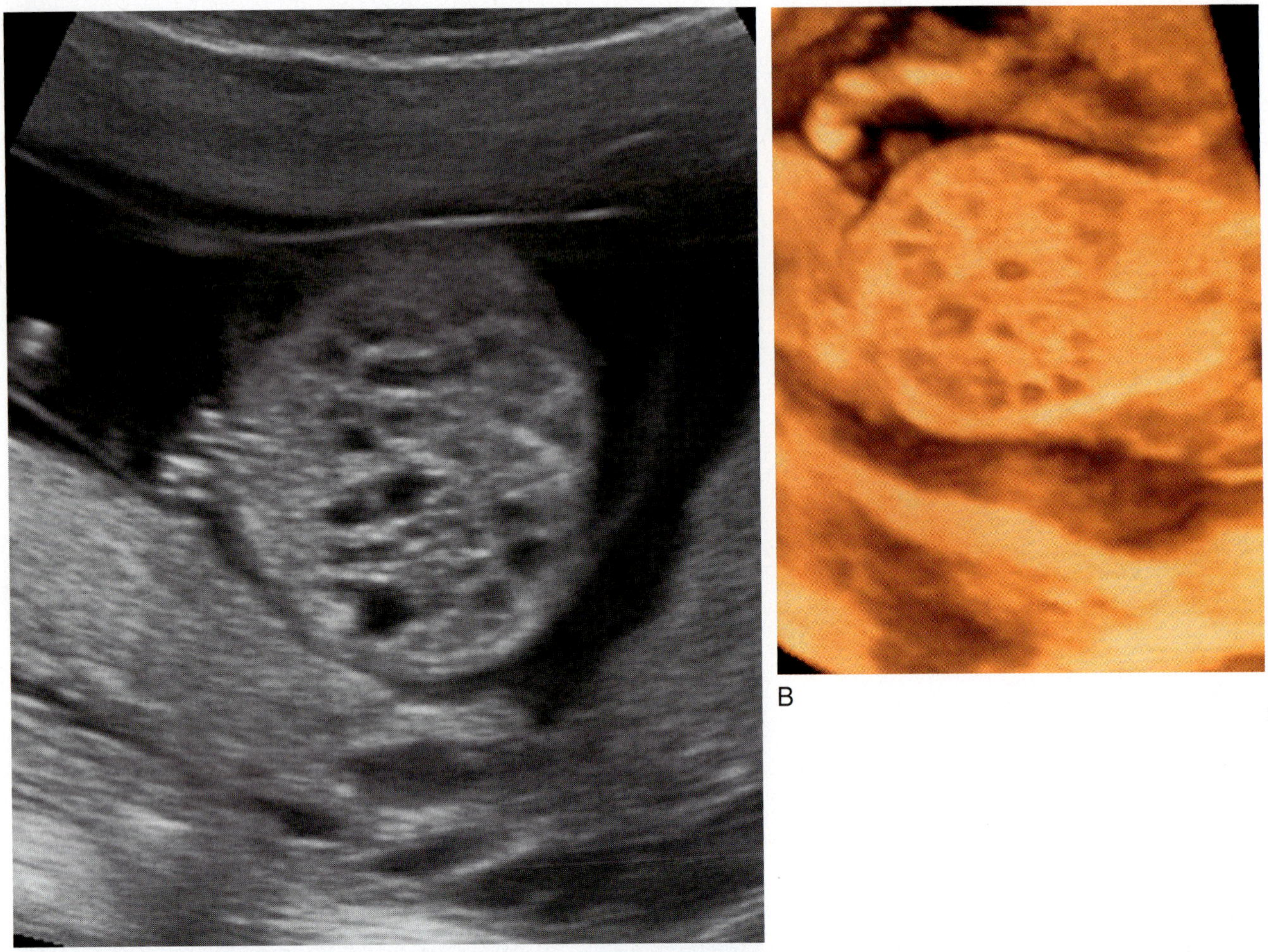

A B

FIGURE 2-57 A 14-week fetus with Meckel-Gruber syndrome. (**A**) Transverse view through the fetal kidneys shows that both kidneys are cystic, consistent with Meckel-Gruber syndrome. (**B**) Three-dimensional rendering of the cystic kidneys taken coronally.

Ramadani HM, Nasrat HA: Prenatal diagnosis of recurrent Meckel syndrome. *Int J Gynecol Obstet* 39:327–332, 1992.

Scully RE, Mark EJ, McNeely BU: Case records of the Massachusetts General Hospital: case 11-1983. *N Engl J Med* 308:642–648, 1983.

Sepulveda W, Sebier NJ, Souka A, Snijders RJM, Nicolaides KH: Diagnosis of the Meckel-Gruber syndrome at eleven to fourteen weeks' gestation. *Am J Obstet Gynecol* 176:316–319, 1997.

Simpson JL, Mills J, Rhoads GG, et al: Genetic heterogeneity in neural tube defects. *Ann Genet (Paris)* 34:279–286, 1991.

Su SL, Liu CM, Lee JN: Prenatal diagnosis of Meckel-Gruber syndrome: case reports. *Kaohsiung J Med Sci* 11:127–132, 1995.

Tanriverdi HA, Hendrik HJ, Ertan K, Schmidt W: Meckel Gruber syndrome: a first trimester diagnosis of a recurrent case. *Eur J Ultrasound* 15:69–72, 2002.

Weinstein BJ, Benacerraf BR: Meckel syndrome, first trimester diagnosis. *Fetus* 4:4–5, 1994.

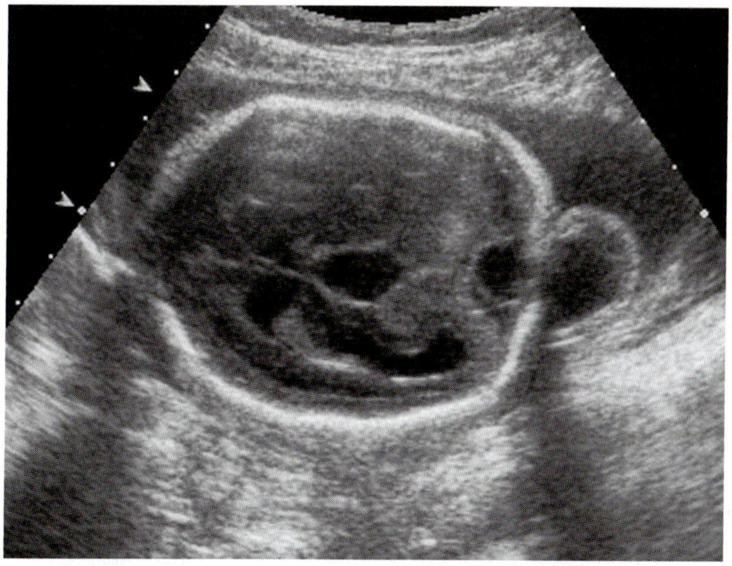

A

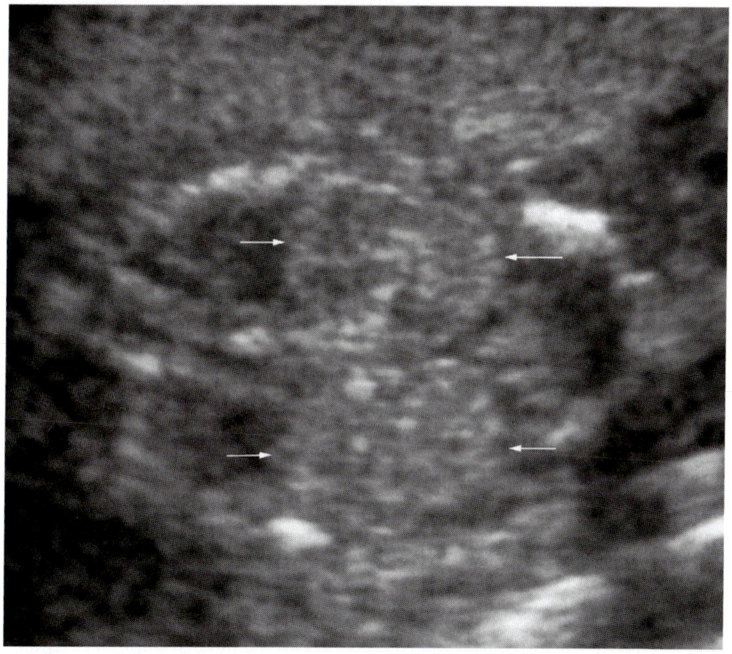

B

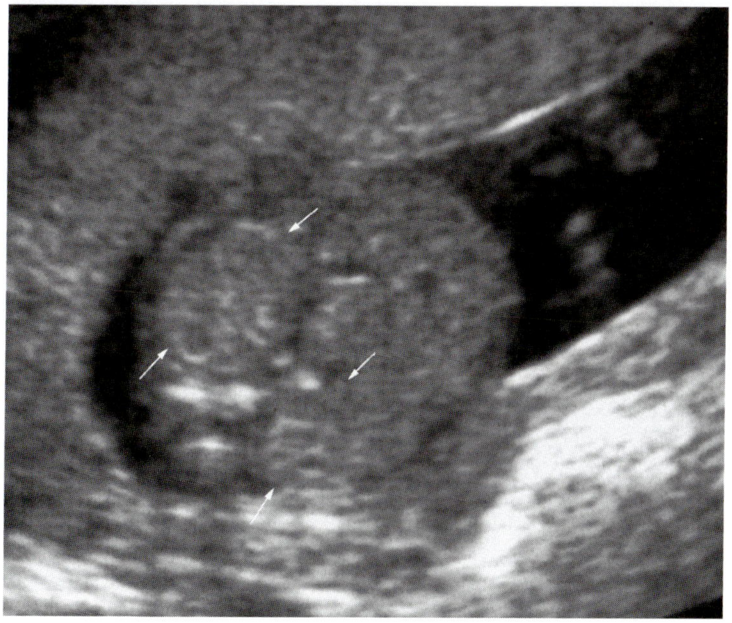

C

FIGURE 2-58 Second-trimester fetus with Meckel-Gruber syndrome. (**A**) Transverse view through the fetal head shows posterior encephalocele and small cyst in the posterior fossa. Note ventriculomegaly and enlarged third ventricle, suggesting agenesis of corpus callosum. (**B, C**) Longitudinal and transverse views of the fetal abdomen of the same fetus show large echogenic kidneys consistent with cystic kidneys *(arrows)*.

Continued

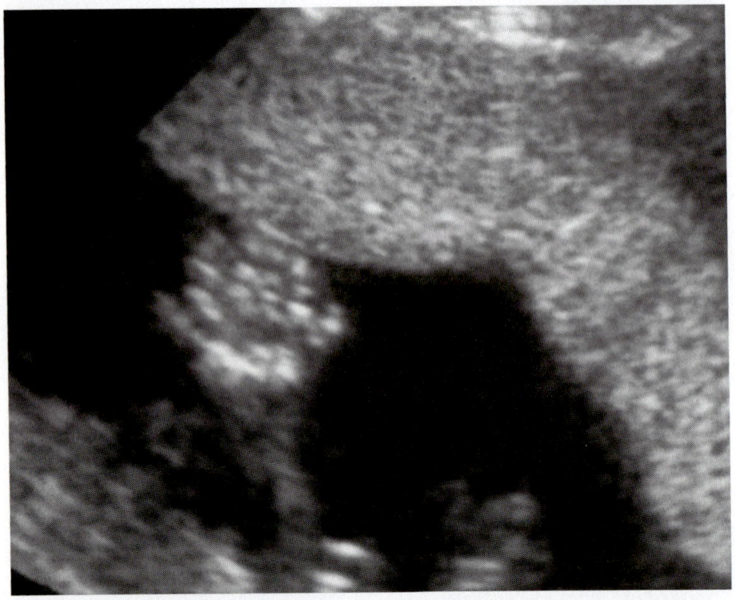
D

FIGURE 2-58, cont'd Second-trimester fetus with Meckel-Gruber syndrome. (D) View of the hand of the same fetus shows polydactyly.

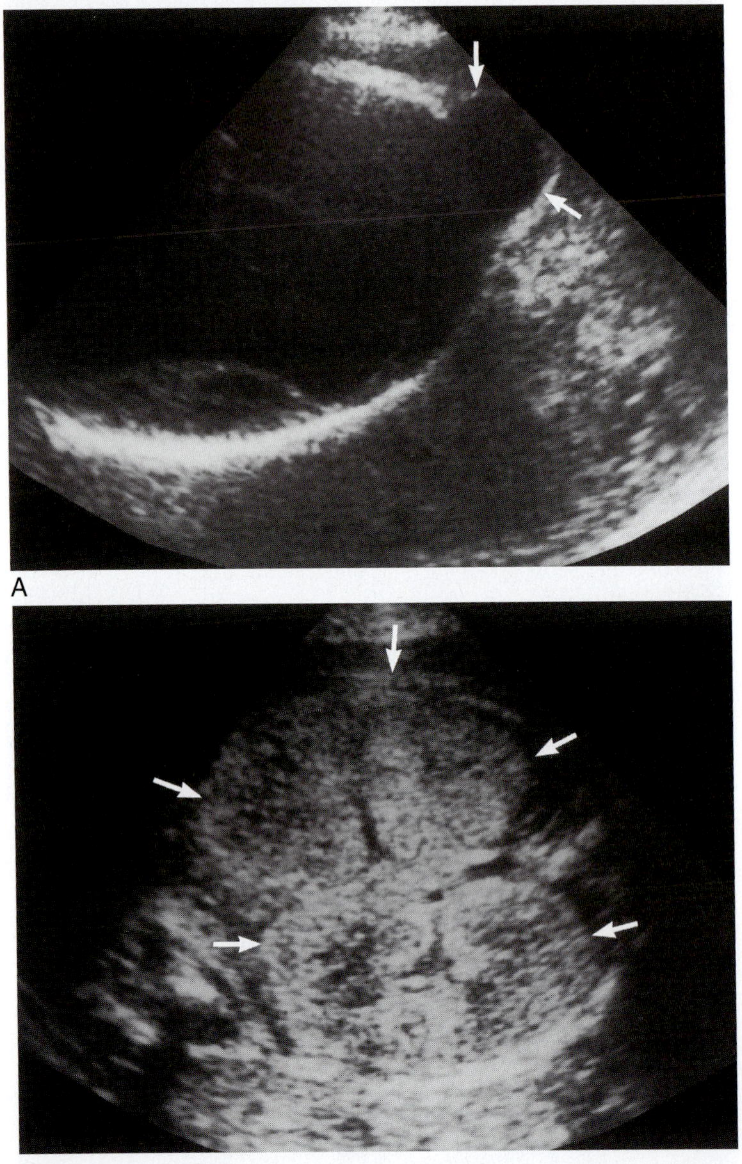
A

B

FIGURE 2-59 (A) Transverse view through the head of a fetus with Meckel-Gruber syndrome shows not only ventriculomegaly but also a posterior encephalocele *(arrows)*. (B) Coronal view through the fetal kidneys of the same fetus shows bilateral, large, echogenic kidneys *(arrows)*.

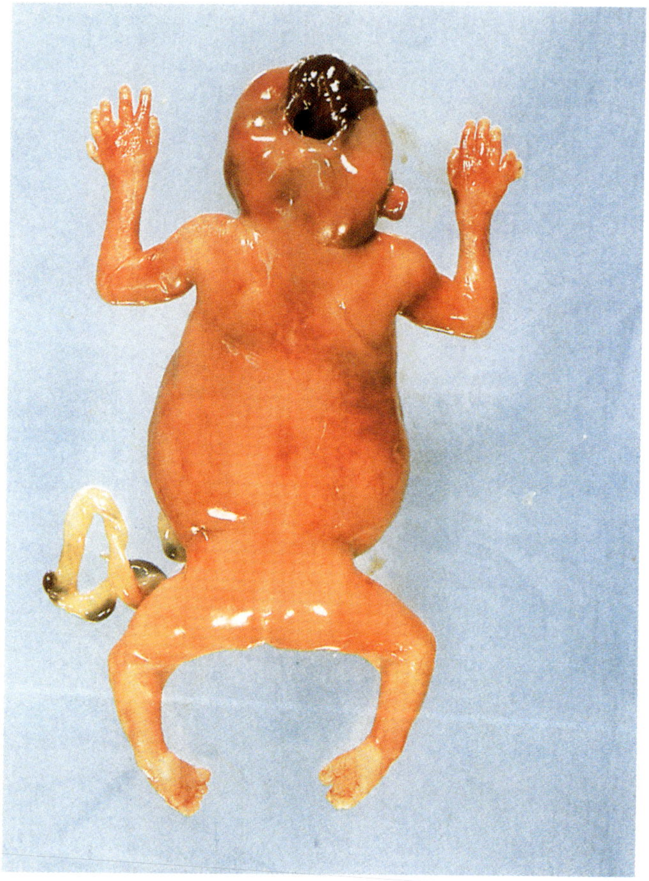

FIGURE 2-60 Postmortem examination of a fetus with Meckel-Gruber syndrome reveals the typical features of the syndrome: encephalocele, polydactyly, and enlarged kidneys (as evidenced by bulging flanks). (From Keeling JW: *Fetal pathology.* London, 1994, Churchill Livingstone.)

MICROCEPHALY

DESCRIPTION AND DEFINITION

Microcephaly represents a group of disorders characterized by a small head and associated with abnormal neurologic findings and mental retardation.

ABNORMALITIES DETECTABLE BY ULTRASOUND

Head circumference >3 standard deviations below the mean for gestational age

Associated brain abnormalities

Holoprosencephaly

Intracranial calcifications

Ventriculomegaly (as may occur in fetuses with neural tube defects)

Lissencephaly

Neural tube defects

Associated ultrasound findings depend on the etiologic factors underlying the microcephaly. If it is one feature of a syndrome, the associated abnormalities will depend on the characteristics of the syndrome present.

MAJOR DIFFERENTIAL DIAGNOSES

Adams-Oliver syndrome

Branchio-oculo-facial syndrome

Cerebrocostomandibular syndrome

Cerebro-oculo-facio-skeletal (COFS) syndrome

Chondrodysplasia punctata (rhizomelic type)

Cornelia de Lange syndrome

Cri du chat syndrome

Deletion 4p (Wolf-Hirschhorn syndrome)

Deletion 5p (cri du chat syndrome)

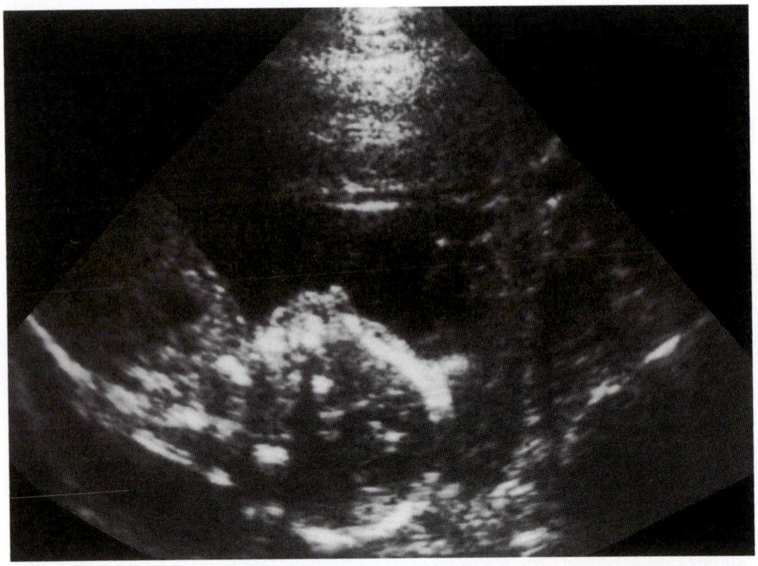

FIGURE 2-61 Longitudinal view of the face of a second-trimester fetus with microcephaly. Note the prominence of the face, which is secondary to the small size of the head.

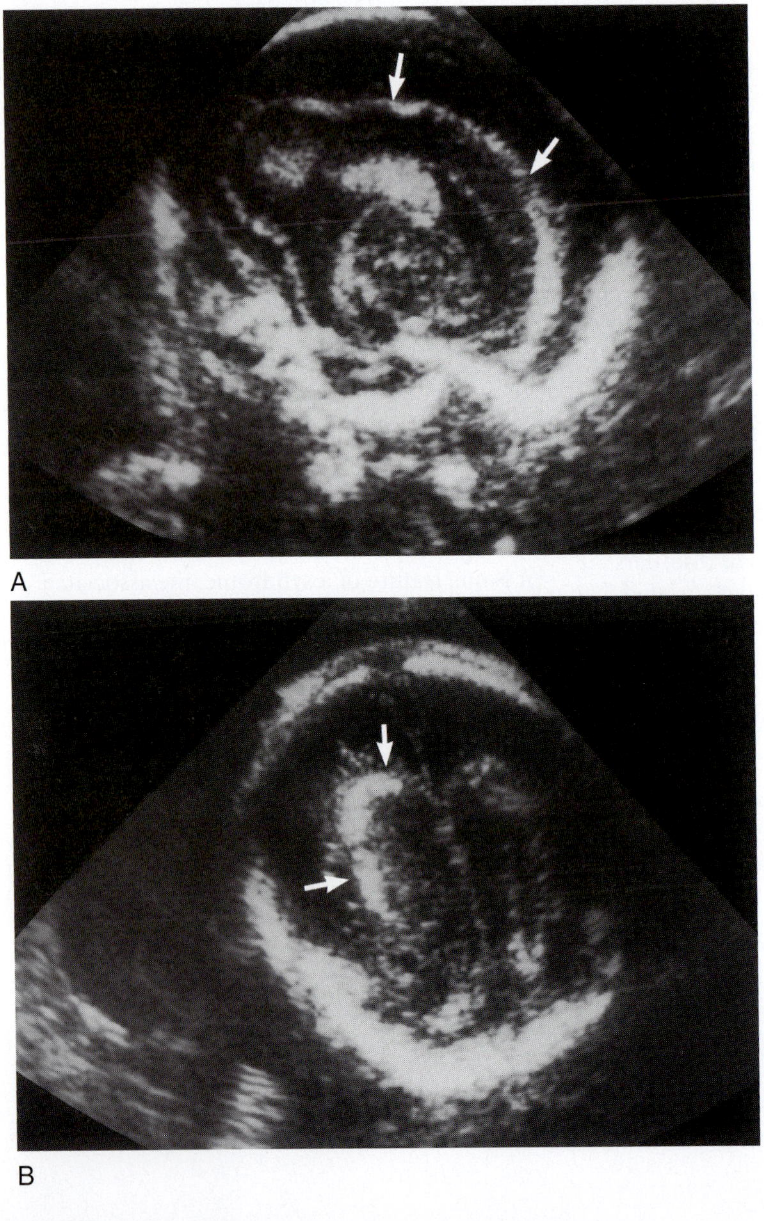

FIGURE 2-62 (**A, B**) Transvaginal views through the fetal head show calcifications along the junction of the gray and white matter *(arrows)*. These extensive calcifications are secondary to intrauterine infection. This fetus had severe microcephaly at birth.

Deletion 11q (Jacobsen syndrome)

DiGeorge syndrome

Fanconi anemia

Fraser syndrome

Freeman-Sheldon (whistling face) syndrome

Holoprosencephaly

Lissencephaly

Meckel-Gruber syndrome

Miller-Dieker syndrome

Multiple pterygium syndrome

Neu-Laxova syndrome

Neural tube defects (associated with Arnold-Chiari type II malformations)

Oral-facial-digital syndrome, type II (Mohr syndrome)

Roberts' syndrome

Seckel syndrome

Shprintzen syndrome

Smith-Lemli-Opitz syndrome

Triploidy

Trisomy 9

Trisomy 13 (Patau syndrome)

Walker-Warburg syndrome

Teratogens

Alcohol

Aminopterin

Chlordiazepoxide (Librium)

Chlorpropamide

Clomiphene

Cytomegalovirus (CMV)

Folic acid metabolism disorders

Hydantoin (occasional)

Hyperthermia

Methotrexate

Phenantoin

Phenothiazine

Phenylketonuria (PKU)

Radiation

Rubella

Toxoplasmosis

Trimethadione

Valproic acid

Varicella

ULTRASOUND DIAGNOSIS

The prenatal sonographic diagnosis of microcephaly is quite variable and depends on the onset of growth restriction of the fetal head. Although certain abnormalities (e.g., Neu-Laxova syndrome) have early-onset growth restriction of the head, there are many cases of microcephaly in which fetal head growth remains normal until 22 weeks' gestation. Therefore, microcephaly often is *not* detectable at 16 weeks' gestational age, when sonograms usually are performed. For example, a patient with PKU may have an affected fetus whose head circumference does not meet the criterion of 3 standard deviations below the mean until late in the second trimester.

Intracranial abnormalities, such as periventricular calcifications, present clues to the diagnosis of microcephaly and, in cases of intrauterine infection, usually predate the lag in fetal head growth by several weeks.

HEREDITY

There are some cases of autosomal recessive microcephaly syndromes. However, in most cases, the pattern of inheritance is dependent on the particular syndrome present.

NATURAL HISTORY AND OUTCOME

Because of the heterogeneity of microcephaly, the prognosis is dependent on associated anomalies and the particular syndrome present. In the absence of associated anomalies, the affected child is likely to have significant mental and physical developmental deficits.

Suggested Reading

Bromley B, Benacerraf BR: Difficulties in the prenatal diagnosis of microcephaly. *J Ultrasound Med* 14:303–305, 1995.

Chervenak FA, Jeanty P, Cantraine F, et al: The diagnosis of fetal microcephaly. *Am J Obstet Gynecol* 149:512–517, 1984.

Chervenak FA, Rosenberg J, Brightman RC, et al: A prospective study of the accuracy of ultrasound in predicting fetal microcephaly. *Obstet Gynecol* 69:908–910, 1987.

Kurtz AB, Wapner RJ, Rubin CS, et al: Ultrasound criteria for in utero diagnosis of microcephaly. *J Clin Ultrasound* 8:11–16, 1980.

Romero, R: Prenatal diagnosis of congenital anomalies. East Norwalk, CT, 1988, Appleton & Lange.

Schwarzler P, Homfray T, Bernard JP, Bland JM, Ville Y: Late onset microcephaly: failure of prenatal diagnosis. *Ultrasound Obstet Gynecol* 22:640–642, 2003.

MILLER-DIEKER SYNDROME (LISSENCEPHALY, TYPE I)

DESCRIPTION AND DEFINITION

Miller-Dieker syndrome (lissencephaly, type I) is characterized by complete absence of gyri and sulci in the brain, resulting in severe mental retardation and poor survival.

ABNORMALITIES DETECTABLE BY ULTRASOUND

Lack of normally developing gyri in the brain (seen sonographically after 24 weeks)

Mild ventriculomegaly

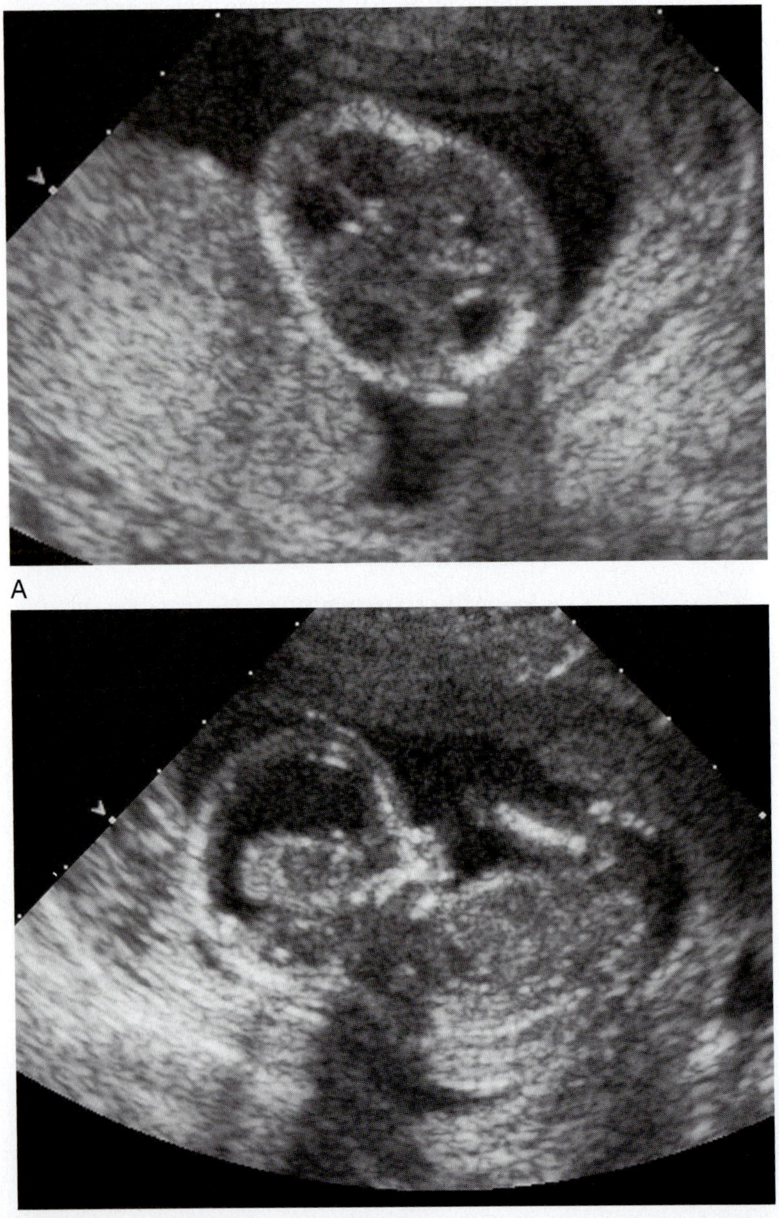

A

B

FIGURE 2-63 Early second-trimester fetus with Miller-Dieker syndrome. (A) Transverse view through the fetal head shows a Dandy-Walker abnormality. (B) Longitudinal view through the same fetus shows enlarged lateral ventricles. This fetus was proved by amniocentesis to have Miller-Dieker syndrome.

Prominent sylvian fissure

Underdeveloped corpus callosum

Microcephaly (late-developing)

IUGR

Cardiac defects

Renal dysplasia

Duodenal atresia

Cryptorchidism

Polyhydramnios

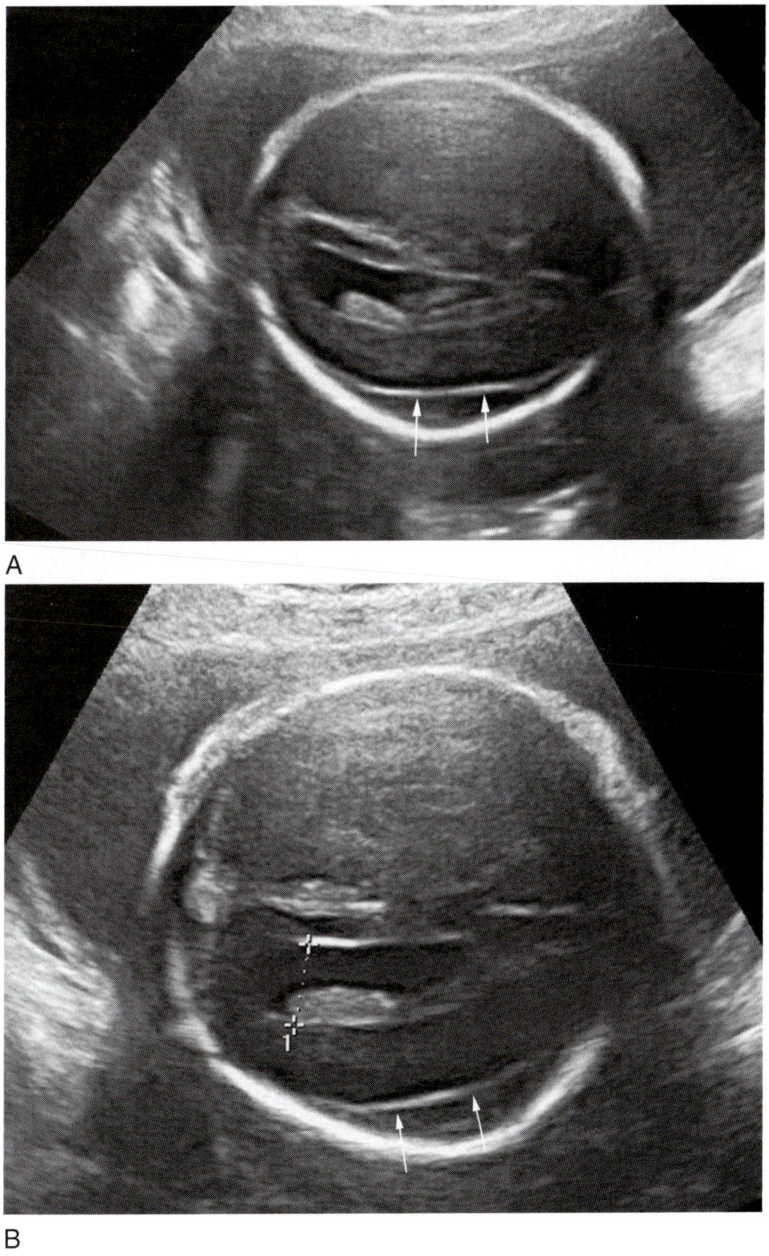

FIGURE 2-64 (A, B) A 30-week fetus with mild ventriculomegaly and evidence of a smooth brain. Note the smooth nature of the sylvian fissure *(arrows)*, which appears abnormal at 30 weeks.

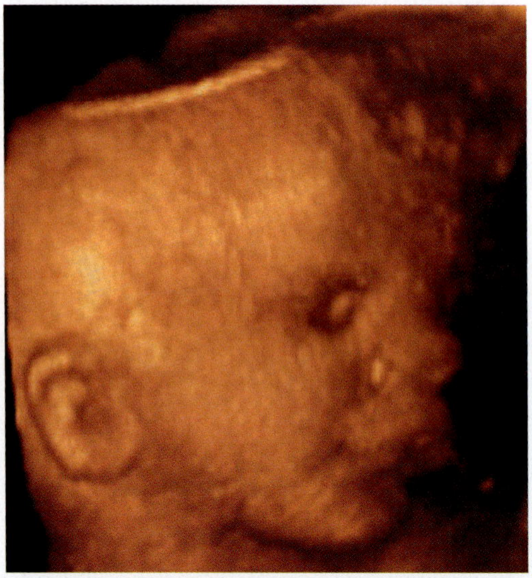

FIGURE 2-65 Surface rendering of a third-trimester fetal face with Miller-Dieker syndrome. Note low-set rotated ear and micrognathia.

MAJOR DIFFERENTIAL DIAGNOSES

Other Forms of Lissencephaly:

Walker-Warburg syndrome (lissencephaly, type II)

Neu-Laxova syndrome

Syndromes and Conditions Associated with Microcephaly:

Adams-Oliver syndrome

Agenesis of the corpus callosum

Branchio-oculo-facial syndrome

Cerebrocostomandibular syndrome

Cerebro-oculo-facio-skeletal (COFS) syndrome

Chondrodysplasia punctata (rhizomelic type)

Cornelia de Lange syndrome

Cri du chat syndrome

Deletion 4p (Wolf-Hirschhorn syndrome)

Deletion 5p (cri du chat syndrome)

Deletion 11q (Jacobsen syndrome)

DiGeorge syndrome

Fanconi anemia

Fraser syndrome

Freeman-Sheldon (whistling face) syndrome

Meckel-Gruber syndrome

Multiple pterygium syndrome

Neu-Laxova syndrome

Neural tube defects (associated with Arnold-Chiari type II malformations)

Oral-facial-digital syndrome, type II (Mohr syndrome)

Roberts' syndrome

Seckel syndrome

Shprintzen syndrome

Smith-Lemli-Opitz syndrome

Triploidy

Trisomy 9

Trisomy 13 (Patau syndrome)

Walker-Warburg syndrome

Teratogens

Alcohol

Aminopterin

Chlordiazepoxide (Librium)

Chlorpropamide

Clomiphene

Cytomegalovirus (CMV)

Folic acid metabolism disorders

Hydantoin (occasional)

Hyperthermia

Phenantoin

Phenothiazine

Phenylketonuria (PKU)

Radiation

Rubella

Toxoplasmosis

Trimethadione

Valproic acid

ULTRASOUND DIAGNOSIS

The ultrasound diagnosis of Miller-Dieker syndrome has been established prenatally as early as 23 weeks' gestation, based on the findings of progressive microcephaly and lack of progression of sulci and gyri formation. Because the brain of a typical fetus usually is smooth during the first half of pregnancy, sonography often is not a useful diagnostic study before the late second or early third trimester. In patients known to be at increased risk because of parental translocations, the diagnosis of 17p13 can be made by karyotyping. By the third trimester, most patients have polyhydramnios and IUGR, an unusual combination that should prompt an amniocentesis. The sonographic diagnosis of this disorder remains elusive at less than 23 weeks because of the normally smooth brain appearance at earlier gestational ages.

HEREDITY

Miller-Dieker syndrome is associated with a deletion at the 17p13.3 locus. Patients who have balanced translocations may be at risk for bearing offspring with this disorder.

NATURAL HISTORY AND OUTCOME

Neonates with Miller-Dieker syndrome have very severe mental retardation, failure to thrive, and seizures. Profoundly retarded, affected individuals usually die within the first 2 years of life.

Suggested Reading

Alvarez LA, Yamamoto T, Wong B, et al: Miller-Dieker syndrome: a disorder affecting specific pathways of neuronal migration. *Neurology* 36:489–493, 1986.

Blaas H, Eik-Nex SH, Kiserud T, van der Hagen CB, Smedvig E: Lissencephaly, type I. *Fetus* 2:1–4, 1992.

Dieker H, Edwards RH, ZuRhein G, et al: The lissencephaly syndrome. *Birth Defects* 5:53, 1969.

Dobyns WB, Kirkpatrick JB, Hittner HM, et al: Syndromes with lissencephaly II: Walker-Warburg and cerebro-oculomuscular syndromes and a new type I lissencephaly. *Am J Med Genet* 22:157–195, 1985.

Dobyns WB, Stratton RF, Greenberg F: Syndromes with lissencephaly I: Miller-Dieker and Norman-Roberts syndrome and isolated lissencephaly. *Am J Med Genet* 18:509–526, 1984.

Dobyns WB, Stratton RF, Parke JT, et al: Miller-Dieker syndrome: lissencephaly and monosomy 17p. *J Pediatr* 102:552–558, 1983.

Fong KW, Ghai S, Toi A, Blaser S, Winsor EJ, Chitayat D: Prenatal ultrasound findings of lissencephaly associated with Miller-Dieker syndrome and comparison with pre- and postnatal magnetic resonance imaging. *Ultrasound Obstet Gynecol* 24:716–723, 2004.

Greenberg F, Courtney KB, Wessels RA, et al: Prenatal diagnosis of deletion 17p13 associated with DiGeorge anomaly. *Am J Med Genet* 31:1–4, 1988.

Greenberg F, Stratton RF, Lockhart LH, et al: Familial Miller-Dieker syndrome associated with pericentric inversion of chromosome 17. *Am J Med Genet* 23:853–859, 1986.

Holzgreve W, Feil R, Louwen FR, Miny P: Prenatal diagnosis and management of fetal hydrocephaly and lissencephaly. *Childs Nerv Sys* 9:408–412, 1993.

Jones KL: *Smith's recognizable patterns of human malformation,* ed 6. Philadelphia, 2006, Elsevier.

McGahan JP, Grix A, Gerscovich O: Prenatal diagnosis of lissencephaly: Miller-Dieker syndrome. *J Clin Ultrasound* 22:560–563, 1994.

Miller JQ: Lissencephaly in two siblings. *Neurology* 13:841, 1963.

Okamura K, Murotsuki J, Sakai T, et al: Prenatal diagnosis of lissencephaly by magnetic resonance image. *Fetal Diagn Ther* 8:56–59, 1993.

Saltzman DH, Krauss CM, Goldman JM, Benacerraf BR: Prenatal diagnosis of lissencephaly. *Prenat Diagn* 11:139–143, 1991.

Stratton RF, Dobyns WB, Airhart SD, Ledbetter DH: New chromosomal syndrome: Miller-Dieker syndrome and monosomy 17p13. *Hum Genet* 67:193–200, 1984.

van Allen M, Clarren SK: A spectrum of gyral anomalies in Miller-Dieker (lissencephaly) syndrome. *J Pediatr* 102:559–564, 1983.

NEU-LAXOVA SYNDROME

DESCRIPTION AND DEFINITION

Neu-Laxova syndrome is characterized by microcephaly, lissencephaly, exophthalmos, severe IUGR, and subcutaneous edema.

ABNORMALITIES DETECTABLE BY ULTRASOUND

Common Findings:

Severe, early-onset IUGR

Microcephaly

Lissencephaly

Absence of the corpus callosum

Hypoplasia of the cerebellum and cerebrum

Ocular hypertelorism with protruding eyes and absent lids

Cataracts

Microphthalmia

Micrognathia

Short neck

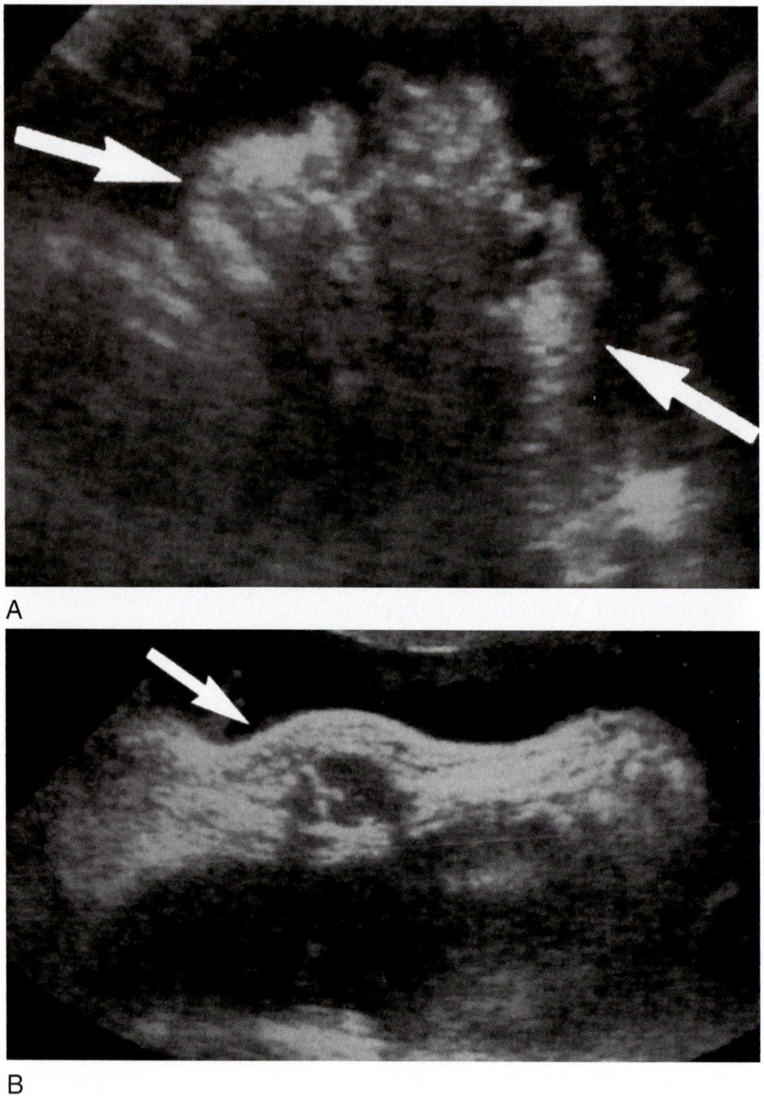

FIGURE 2-66 (A) Profile *(arrows)* of a fetus with Neu-Laxova syndrome shows extreme microcephaly. (B) Longitudinal view of the lower extremity of the same fetus reveals a joint contracture *(arrow),* resulting in hyperextension at the knee. (From Gulmezoglu AM, Ekiei E: *J Clin Ultrasound* 22:48–51, 1994.)

Abnormal skin, with swollen subcutaneous tissue and ichthyosis

Short limbs

Syndactyly of the fingers

Edema of the hands and feet

Flexion contractures

Hypoplastic genitals

Small placenta

Polyhydramnios

Occasional Findings:

Cardiac defects

Facial clefting

Dandy-Walker malformation

Ventriculomegaly

Hydranencephaly

Spina bifida

MAJOR DIFFERENTIAL DIAGNOSES

Other Forms of Lissencephaly:

Miller-Dieker syndrome

Walker-Warburg syndrome (lissencephaly, type II)

Anomalies Associated with Dyskinesia/Akinesia:

Arthrogryposis

Multiple pterygium syndrome

Pena Shokeir syndrome

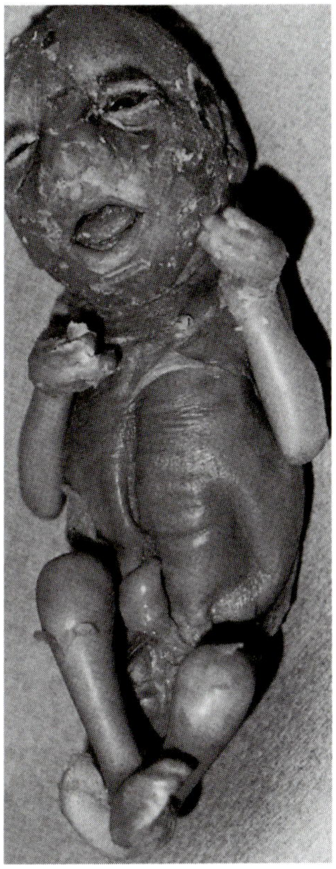

FIGURE 2-67 Neonate with Neu-Laxova syndrome. Note protruding eyeballs, micrognathia, limb contractures, skin edema, and ichthyosis. (From Bronshtein M, Blumenfeld I, Cohen I, Blumenfeld Z: *J Clin Ultrasound* 21:648–650, 1993.)

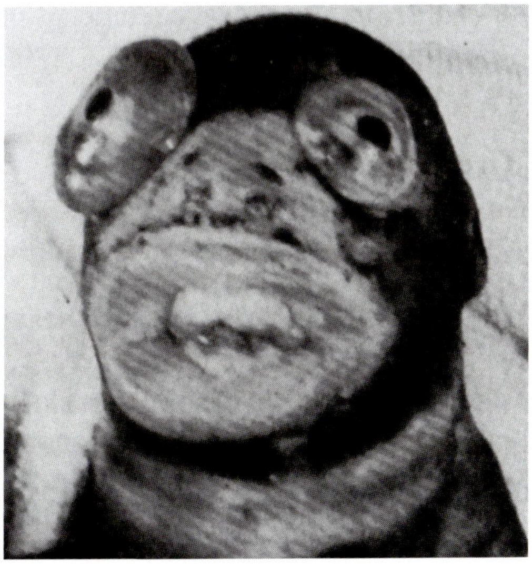

FIGURE 2-68 Frontal view of an infant with Neu-Laxova syndrome shows the externalized eyes and overall marked edema of soft tissues. (From Broderick K, Oyer R, Chatwani A: *Am J Obstet Gynecol* 158:574–575, 1988.)

Syndromes and Conditions Associated with Microcephaly and IUGR*:

Cerebro-oculo-facio-skeletal (COFS) syndrome

Chromosomal abnormalities

Cornelia de Lange syndrome

Freeman-Sheldon syndrome

Miller-Dieker syndrome

Rubella

Seckel syndrome

Smith-Lemli-Opitz syndrome

Toxoplasmosis

ULTRASOUND DIAGNOSIS

The diagnosis of this condition has been made in the mid-second trimester (19–21 weeks), using sonographic features such as intrauterine growth retardation, microcephaly, polyhydramnios, exophthalmos, cataracts, cystic hygromata, syndactyly, clubbed foot, joint contractures, and abnormal facies. There is one reported diagnosis of this condition at 17 weeks in a family with two prior affected pregnancies. The diagnosis at 17 weeks was based on family history along with growth restriction, microcephaly, thickened nuchal fold, and abnormal posturing of the extremities.

HEREDITY

The pattern of inheritance for Neu-Laxova syndrome is autosomal recessive.

NATURAL HISTORY AND OUTCOME

This is a lethal syndrome. Most infants are stillborn or die in the early neonatal period.

Suggested Reading

Allias F, Buenerd A, Bouvier R, et al: The spectrum of type III lissencephaly: a clinicopathological update. *Fetal Pediatr Pathol* 23:305–317, 2004.

Broderick K, Oyer R, Chatwani A: Neu-Laxova syndrome: a case report. *Am J Obstet Gynecol* 158:574–575, 1988.

Bronshtein M, Blumenfeld I, Cohen I, Blumenfeld Z: Fetal ultrasonographic detection of hypodontia in the Neu-Laxova syndrome. *J Clin Ultrasound* 21:648–650, 1993.

Driggers RW, Isbister S, McShane C, Stone K, Blakemore K: Early second trimester prenatal diagnosis of Neu-Laxova syndrome. *Prenat Diagn* 22:118–120, 2002.

*See Appendixes and p. 30 of Chapter 1 for microcephaly.

Durr-e-Sabih, Khan AN, Sabih Z: Prenatal sonographic diagnosis of Neu-Laxova syndrome. *J Clin Ultrasound* 29:531–534, 2001.

Gulmezoglu AM, Ekici E: Sonographic diagnosis of Neu-Laxova syndrome. *J Clin Ultrasound* 22:48–51, 1994.

Jones KL: *Smith's recognizable patterns of human malformations,* ed 6. Philadelphia, 2006, Elsevier.

Kainer F, Prechtl FR, Dudenhausen JW, Ungers M: Qualitative analysis of fetal movement patterns in the Neu-Laxova syndrome. *Prenat Diagn* 16:667–669, 1996.

Manning MA, Cunniff CM, Colby CE, El-Sayed YY, Hoyme HE: Neu-Laxova syndrome: detailed prenatal diagnostic and post-mortem findings and literature review. *Am J Med Genet* 125:240–249, 2004.

Mihci E, Simsek M, Mendilcioglu I, Tacoy S, Karaveli S: Evaluation of a fetus with Neu-Laxova syndrome through prenatal, clinical, and pathological findings. *Fetal Diagn Ther* 20:167–170, 2005.

Muller LM, de Jong G, Mouton SC, et al: A case of the Neu-Laxova syndrome: prenatal ultrasonographic monitoring in the third trimester and the histopathological findings. *Am J Med Genet* 26:421–429, 1987.

Rode ME, Mennuti MT, Giardine RM, Zackai EH, Driscoll DA: Early ultrasound diagnosis of Neu-Laxova syndrome. *Prenat Diagn* 21:575–580, 2001.

Shapiro I, Borochowitz Z, Degani S, et al: Neu-Laxova syndrome: prenatal ultrasonographic diagnosis, clinical and pathological studies, and new manifestations. *Am J Med Genet* 43:602–605, 1992.

Shivarajan MA, Suresh S, Jagadeesh S, Lata S, Bhat L: Second trimester diagnosis of Neu Laxova syndrome. *Prenat Diagn* 23:21–24, 2003.

Tolmie JL, Mortimer G, Doyle D, et al: The Neu-Laxova syndrome in female sibs: clinical and pathological features with prenatal diagnosis in the second sib. *Am J Med Genet* 27:175–182, 1987.

SEPTO-OPTIC DYSPLASIA

DESCRIPTION AND DEFINITION

Synonym: De Morsier syndrome

This is a syndrome characterized by absence of the septum pellucidum and hypoplasia of the optic nerves, commonly associated with agenesis of the corpus callosum.

ABNORMALITIES DETECTABLE BY ULTRASOUND

Common Findings:

Absent cavum septi pellucidi, with communication between the frontal horns across the midline

Ventriculomegaly

Agenesis of (or thinned) corpus callosum (may not be detected until after 20 weeks)

Occasional Findings:

Craniofacial abnormalities, such as clefting and hypotelorism

Schizencephaly

MAJOR DIFFERENTIAL DIAGNOSES

Holoprosencephaly (lobar or alobar)

Syndromes associated with agenesis of the corpus callosum and brain abnormalities (see differential diagnosis section for complete list).

- Aicardi syndrome
- Apert syndrome
- Fryns syndrome
- Meckel-Gruber syndrome
- Miller-Dieker syndrome
- Neu-Laxova syndrome
- Oral-facial-digital syndrome, type I
- Walker-Warburg syndrome

ULTRASOUND DIAGNOSIS

Because the prenatal diagnosis of septo-optic dysplasia is dependent on *not* visualizing the cavum septum pellucidum, the diagnosis is easy to miss in the second trimester. Agenesis of the corpus callosum may not be detected until after 20 weeks. Therefore, it is not surprising that the diagnosis of this entity is generally made in the third trimester and overlooked in many cases in the second trimester. Reported diagnoses have occurred at 29 and 30 weeks' gestation.

HEREDITY

This syndrome is sporadic, with several different etiologies reported, including autosomal recessive inheritance, infectious etiology, teratogens, and vascular disruptions.

NATURAL HISTORY AND OUTCOME

This syndrome is associated with visual impairment, hypoplastic optic disks, and hypopituitarism. The developmental outcome is controversial because this syndrome has been

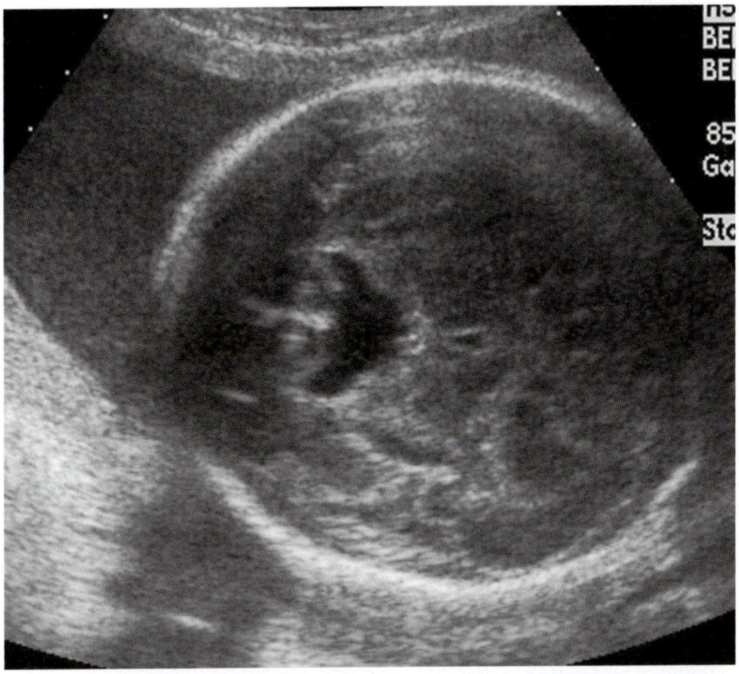

A

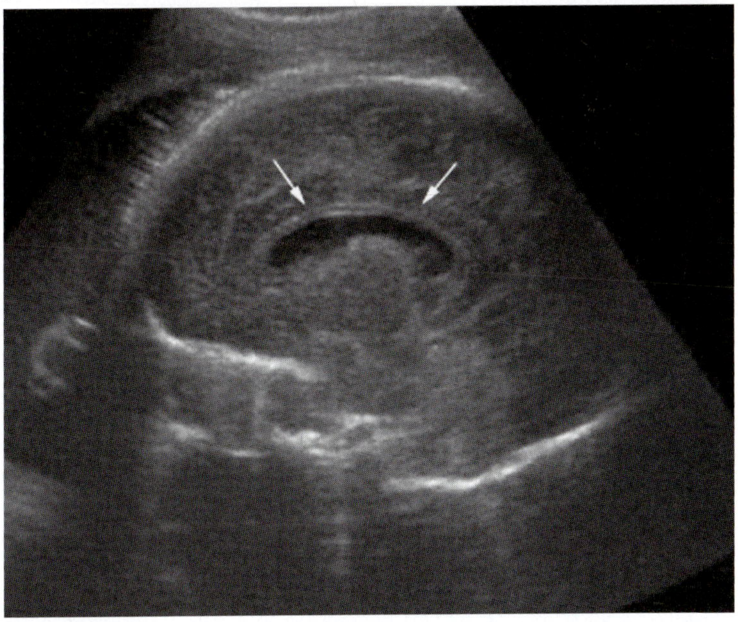

B

FIGURE 2-69 (A) Transverse view through the fetal head of a third-trimester fetus with septo-optic dysplasia. Note direct communication between the two frontal horns. (B) Sagittal view through the midline of the brain of the same fetus shows that the corpus callosum is present but thinned *(arrows)*.

associated with an excess of cerebral palsy, mental retardation, and seizures. In fetuses with other abnormalities such as schizencephaly, the prognosis of intellectual performance is poor. In those with uncomplicated absence of the cavum septi pellucidi and hypoplasia of the optic nerve, the cognitive outcome is good.

Suggested Reading

Jones KL: *Smith's recognizable patterns of human malformation,* ed 6. Philadelphia, 2006, Elsevier.

Lepinard C, Coutant R, Boussion F, et al: Prenatal diagnosis of absence of the septum pellucidum associated with septo-optic dysplasia. *Ultrasound Obstet Gynedol* 25:73–75, 2005.

Malinger G, Lev D, Kidron D, Heredia F, Hershkovitz R, Lerman-Sagie T: Differential diagnosis in fetuses with absent septum pellucidum. *Ultrasound Obstet Gynecol* 25:42–49, 2005.

Nyberg, DA, McGahan JP, Pretorius DH, Pilu G: *Diagnostic imaging of fetal anomalies.* Philadelphia, 2003, Lippincott Williams & Wilkins.

Pilu G, Tani G, Carletti A, Malaigia S, Ghi T, Rizzo N: Difficult early sonographic diagnosis of absence of the fetal septum pellucidum. *Ultrasound Obstet Gynecol* 25:70–72, 2005.

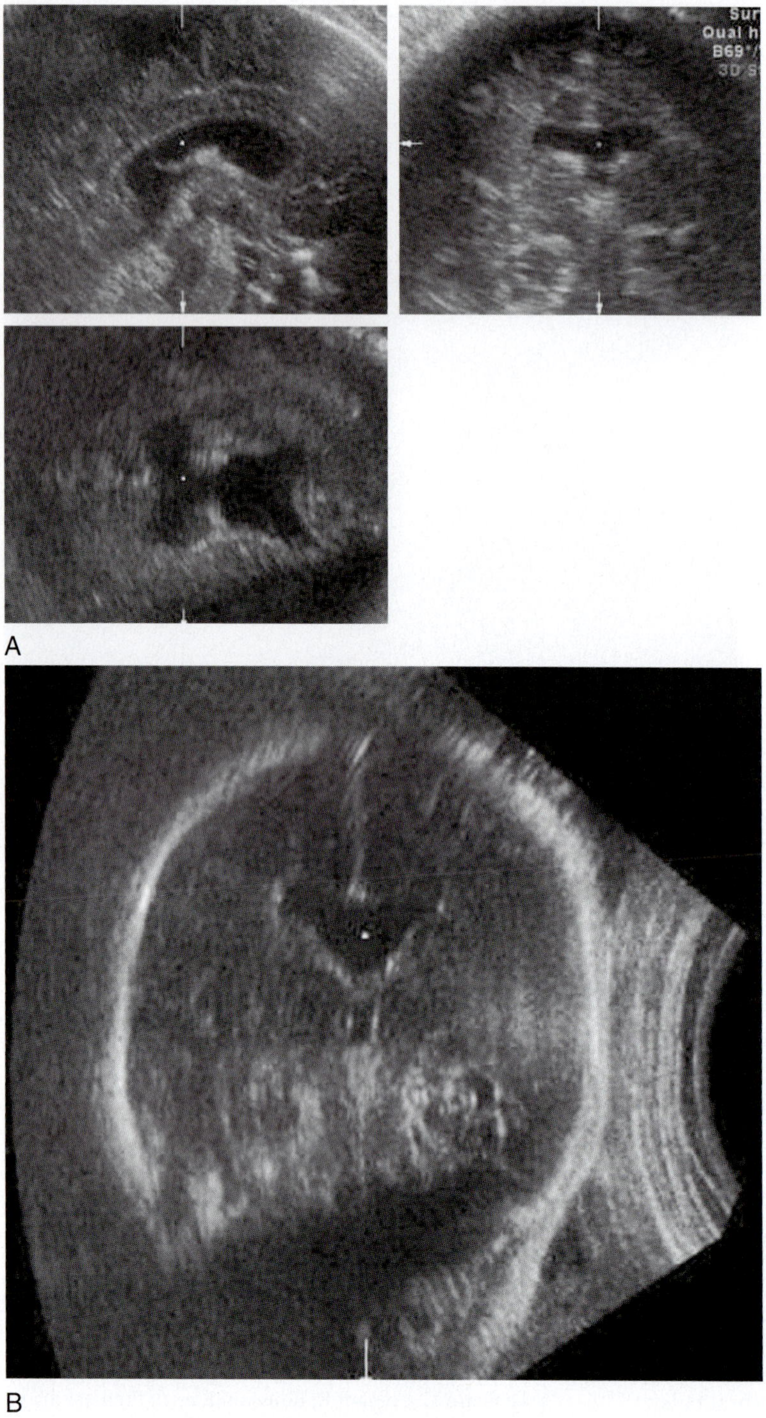

FIGURE 2-70 Three-dimensional reconstruction of brain images of a third-trimester fetus with septo-optic dysplasia. (A) Three orthogonal views show the communication between left and right ventricular systems. (B) Reconstructed coronal view shows the triangular-shaped connection between the frontal horns and lack of cavum septum pellucidum.

WALKER-WARBURG SYNDROME

DESCRIPTION AND DEFINITION

Synonym: Lissencephaly, type II

First reported by Walker in 1942 and further described by Warburg in 1971, this syndrome is characterized by severe congenital oculocerebral abnormalities, including lissencephaly and ventriculomegaly. The acronym associated with this syndrome is HARD(E): **h**ydrocephalus, **a**gyria, **r**etinal **d**ysplasia, and (sometimes) **e**ncephalocele.

ABNORMALITIES DETECTABLE BY ULTRASOUND

Common Findings:

Widespread agyria or lissencephaly

Ventriculomegaly (in nearly 100% of cases)

Occipital encephalocele (25%)

Dandy-Walker malformation (50%)

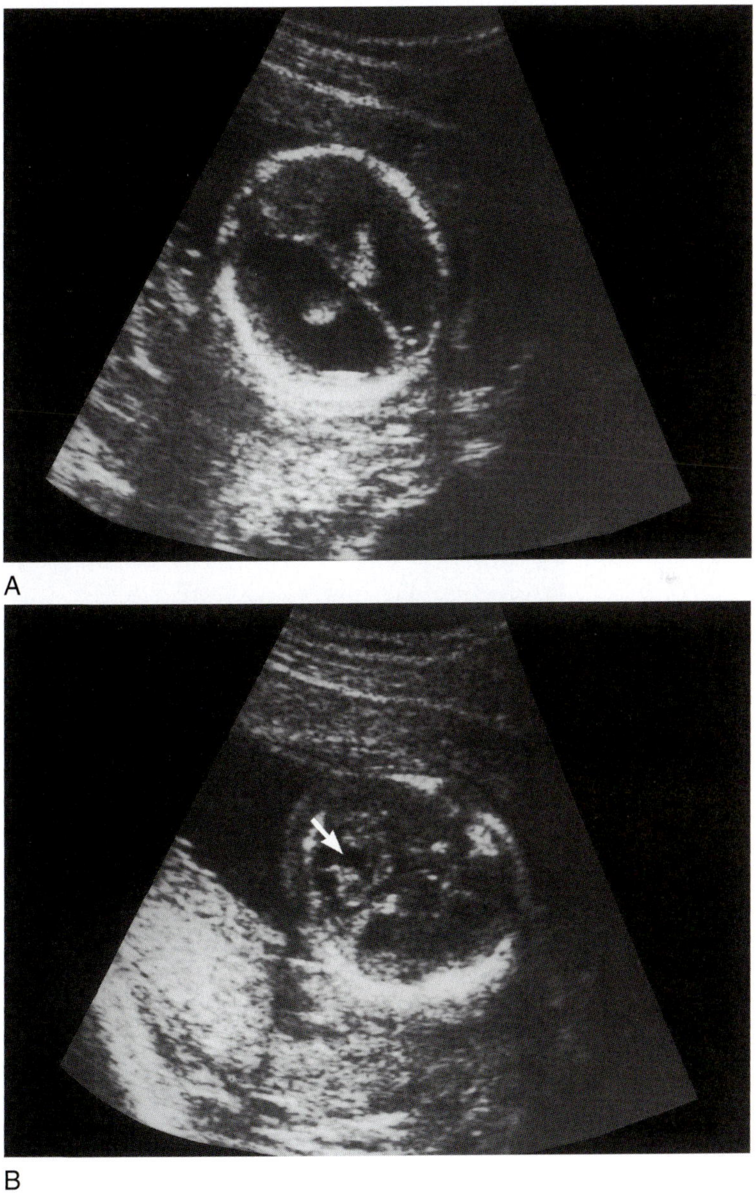

A

B

FIGURE 2-71 Views of the head of a fetus with Walker-Warburg syndrome show marked ventriculomegaly. (A) Choroid plexus are free floating in the large lateral ventricles. (B) Posterior fossa and Dandy-Walker variant *(arrow)* are seen in this view.

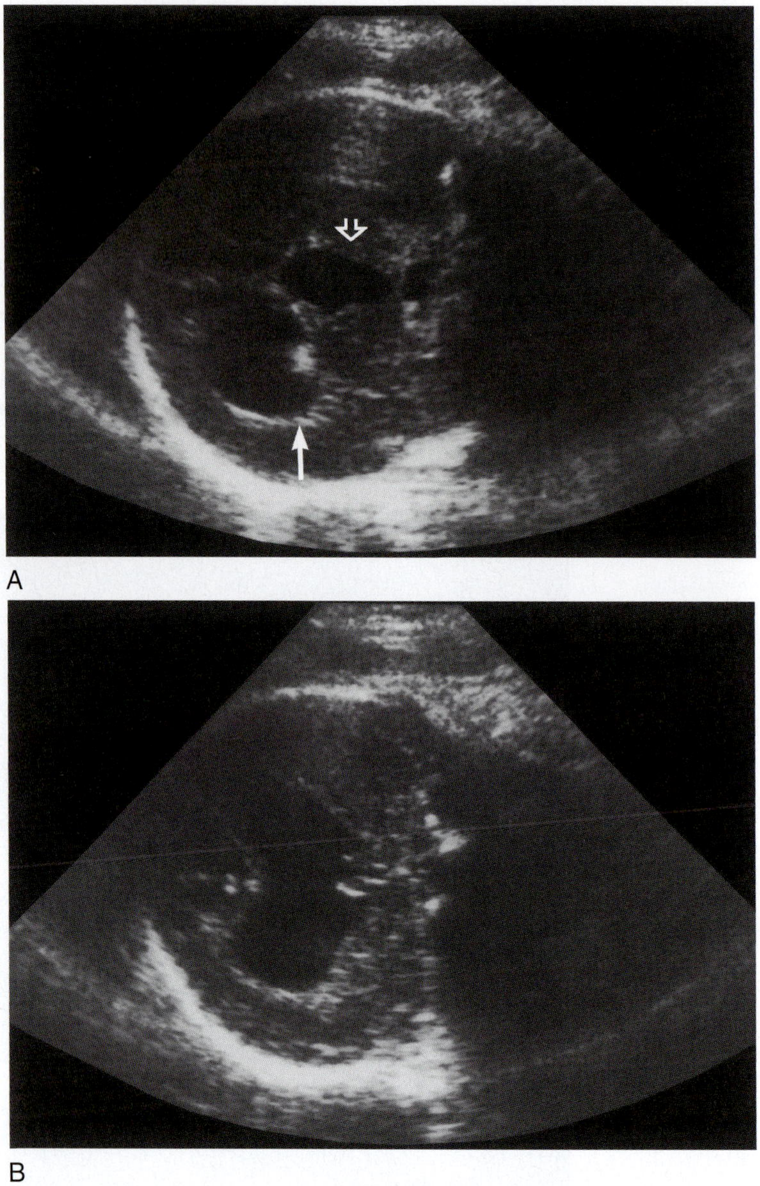

FIGURE 2-72 (A, B) Coronal views of the head of a third-trimester fetus with Walker-Warburg syndrome. Note ventriculomegaly (solid arrow indicates lateral ventricle) and dilated third ventricle *(open arrow)*, features consistent with agenesis of the corpus callosum.

Microcephaly (16%)

Agenesis of the corpus callosum

Eye abnormalities (almost 100%) including:

- Microphthalmia (50%)
- Congenital cataracts (35%)
- Retinal detachment
- Retinal dysplasia

Occasional Findings:

Cleft lip

Genital abnormalities

MAJOR DIFFERENTIAL DIAGNOSES

Other Syndromes and Conditions Associated with Microcephaly, Ventriculomegaly, Dandy-Walker Malformation, and/or Encephalocele:

Cerebro-oculo-facio-skeletal (COFS) syndrome

Cri du chat syndrome

Fryns syndrome

Meckel-Gruber syndrome

Miller-Dieker syndrome

Neu-Laxova syndrome

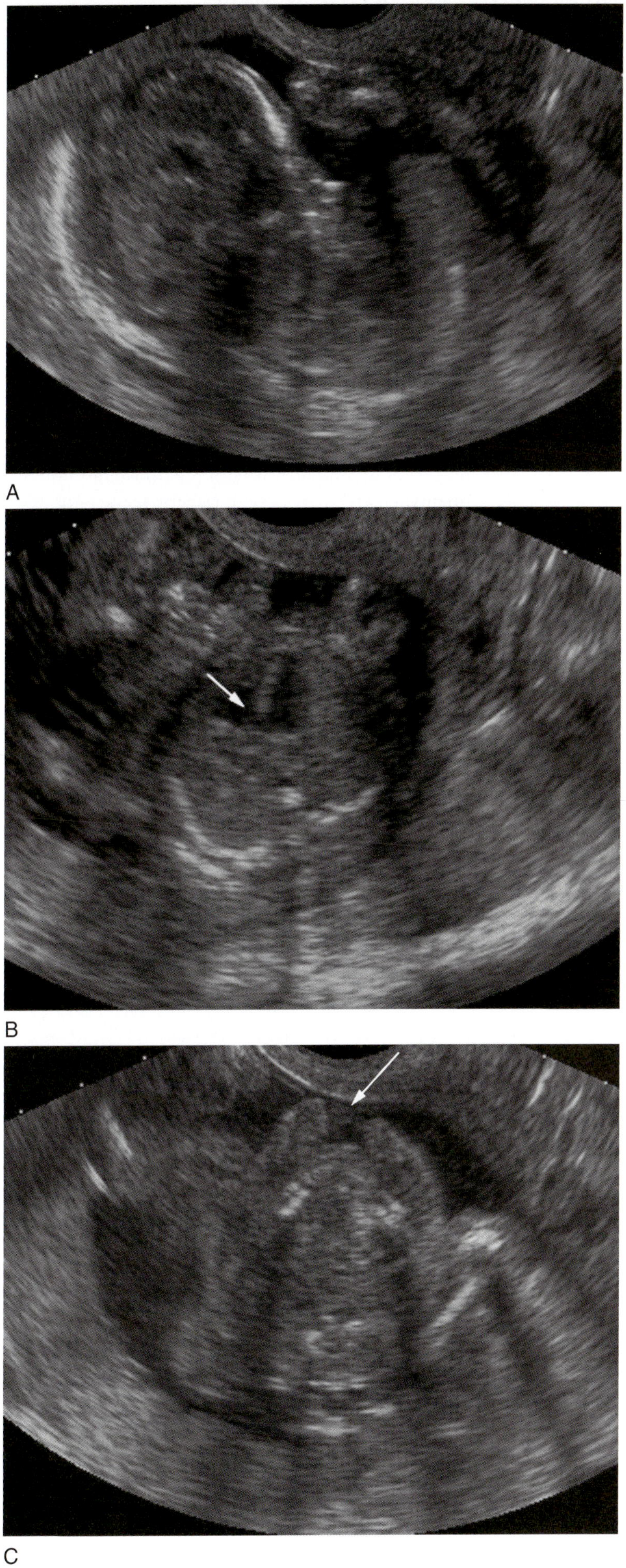

FIGURE 2-73 Second-trimester fetus with Walker-Warburg syndrome. (**A**) Fetus with oligohydramnios and obvious asymmetric intrauterine growth restriction (small body for size of head). (**B**) Four-chamber view of the heart with a ventricular septal defect *(arrow)*. (**C**) Axial view through the fetal upper lip shows a large cleft *(arrow)*.

TORCH (**t**oxoplasmosis, **o**ther infections, **r**ubella, **c**ytomegalovirus infection, and **h**erpes simplex) infections

Trisomy 13 (Patau syndrome)

Trisomy 18 (Edwards' syndrome)

ULTRASOUND DIAGNOSIS

There are several reports of the prenatal sonographic diagnosis of Walker-Warburg syndrome as early as the first trimester, particularly in cases of severe intracranial anomalies such as encephalocele. These are best seen endovaginally. Most of the early diagnoses of Walker-Warburg syndrome have been made in the second trimester in patients with previous affected pregnancies who are at high risk for recurrence. Detection is based on ventriculomegaly with associated posterior fossa abnormalities in a family at genetic risk for the syndrome.

Later in gestation, the ocular abnormalities associated with Walker-Warburg syndrome may be evident on ultrasound studies. These abnormalities include conical opacities within the globe between the lens and the retina.

HEREDITY

The pattern of inheritance for this syndrome is autosomal recessive.

NATURAL HISTORY AND OUTCOME

Walker-Warburg syndrome has a dismal prognosis and usually is lethal within the first year of life.

Suggested Reading

Beinder EJ, Pfeiffer RA, Bornemann A, Wenkel H: Second-trimester diagnosis of fetal cataract in a fetus with Walker-Warburg syndrome. *Fetal Diagn Ther* 12:197–199, 1997.

Blin G, Rabbe A, Ansquer Y, Meghdiche S, Floch-Tudal C, Mandelbrot L: First-trimester ultrasound diagnosis in a recurrent case of Walker-Warburg syndrome. *Ultrasound Obstet Gynecol* 26:297–299, 2005.

Chitayat D, Toi A, Babul R, et al: Prenatal diagnosis of retinal nonattachment in the Walker-Warburg syndrome. *Am J Med Genet* 56:351–358, 1995.

Crowe C, Jassani M, Dickerman L: The prenatal diagnosis of the Walker-Warburg syndrome. *Prenat Diagn* 6:177–185, 1986.

Dobyns WB, Pagon RA, Armstrong D, et al: Diagnostic criteria for Walker-Warburg syndrome. *Am J Med Genet* 32:195–210, 1989.

Donnai D, Farndon PA: Walker-Warburg syndrome (Warburg syndrome, HARD +/E syndrome). *J Med Genet* 23:200–203, 1986.

Farrell SA, Toi A, Leadman ML, Davidson RG, Caco C: Prenatal diagnosis of retinal detachment in Walker-Warburg syndrome. *Am J Med Genet* 28:619–624, 1987.

Gasser B, Lindner V, Dreyfus M, et al: Prenatal diagnosis of Walker-Warburg syndrome in three sibs. *Am J Med Genet* 76:107–110, 1998.

Holzgreve W, Feil R, Louwen F, Miny P: Prenatal diagnosis and management of fetal hydrocephaly and lissencephaly. *Childs Nerv Syst* 9:408–412, 1993.

Jones KL: *Smith's recognizable patterns of human malformations,* ed 6. Philadelphia, 2006, Elsevier.

Maynor CH, Hertzberg BS, Ellington KS: Antenatal sonographic features of Walker-Warburg syndrome: value of endovaginal sonography. *J Ultrasound Med* 11:301–303, 1992.

Miller G, Ladda RL, Towfighi J: Cerebro-ocular dysplasia-muscular dystrophy (Walker-Warburg) syndrome: findings in a 20-week old fetus. *Acta Neuropathol* 82:234–238, 1991.

Monteagudo A, Alayon A, Mayberry P: Walker-Warburg syndrome: case report and review of the literature. *J Ultrasound Med* 20:419–426, 2001.

Murphy KJ, PeBenito R, Storm RL, Ferrerti C, Liu DP: Walker-Warburg syndrome: case report and literature review. *Ophthalmic Paediatr Genet* 11:103–108, 1990.

Rodgers BL, Vanner LV, Pai GS, Sens MA: Walker-Warburg syndrome: report of three affected sibs. *Am J Med Genet* 49:198–201, 1994.

van Zalen-Sprock PM, van Vugt JM, van Geijn HP: First-trimester sonographic detection of neurodevelopmental abnormalities in some singlegene disorders. *Prenat Diagn* 16:199–202, 1996.

Vohra N, Ghidini A, Alvarez M, Lockwood C: Walker-Warburg syndrome: prenatal ultrasound findings. *Prenat Diagn* 13:575–579, 1993.

Walker AE: Lissencephaly. *Arch Neurol Psychiatry* 48:13–29, 1942.

Warburg M: The heterogeneity of microphthalmia in the mentally retarded. *Birth Defects* 7:136–154, 1971.

X-LINKED HYDROCEPHALUS SYNDROME

DESCRIPTION AND DEFINITION

Synonym: X-linked aqueductal stenosis

First described in 1949 by Bickers and Adams, X-linked hydrocephalus syndrome was further delineated by Bianchine and Lewis as a syndrome characterized by conditions having the acronym of MASA (**m**ental retardation, **a**dducted thumbs, **s**huffling gait, and **a**phasia).

ABNORMALITIES DETECTABLE BY ULTRASOUND

Ventriculomegaly of the lateral ventricles, with a normal fourth ventricle

Thumbs flexed over the palms in an adducted position

MAJOR DIFFERENTIAL DIAGNOSES

Syndromes and Conditions Associated with Ventriculomegaly*:

Abnormalities of the neural tube

Chromosomal anomalies

Genetic syndromes

Gorlin syndrome

Hydrolethalus syndrome

Intracranial cysts

Intracranial hemorrhage

In utero infections

Meckel-Gruber syndrome

Miller-Dieker syndrome

Walker-Warburg syndrome (lissencephaly, type II)

ULTRASOUND DIAGNOSIS

Hydrocephalus is detectable early and can be very severe; alternatively, it may not manifest until the third trimester. If hydrocephalus is present, prenatal sonographic detection of this syndrome is possible as early as 16 weeks' gestation. Second-trimester detection is limited, however, because of late development of hydrocephalus in some cases. The adducted thumbs that are often a feature of this syndrome are detectable in the second trimester.

HEREDITY

This syndrome has an X-linked recessive pattern of inheritance. There are many other causes of aqueductal stenosis, and X-linked hydrocephalus represents only a small fraction of all cases. Among males with aqueductal stenosis, 25% are thought to exhibit an X-linked mode of inheritance.

Other causes of hydrocephalus are genetic, infectious (including toxoplasmosis and cytomegalovirus in utero), teratogenic, and neoplastic (including pinealomas) in origin.

NATURAL HISTORY AND OUTCOME

Outcomes are variable, depending on the severity of the hydrocephalus.

Suggested Reading

Bickers DS, Adams RD: Hereditary stenosis of the aqueduct of Sylvius as a cause of congenital hydrocephalus. *Brain* 72:246–262, 1949.

Brocard O, Ragage C, Vibert M, et al: Prenatal diagnosis of X-linked hydrocephalus. *J Clin Ultrasound* 21:211–214, 1993.

Edwards JH: The syndrome of sex-linked hydrocephalus. *Arch Dis Child* 36:486–493, 1961.

Jones KL: *Smith's recognizable patterns of human malformation,* ed 6. Philadelphia, 2006, Elsevier.

Ko TM, Hwa HL, Tseng LH, et al: Prenatal diagnosis of X-linked hydrocephalus in a Chinese family with four successive affected pregnancies. *Prenat Diagn* 14:57–60, 1994.

Pomili G, Venti Donti G, Alunni Carrozza L, et al: MASA syndrome: ultrasonographic evidence in a male fetus. *Prenat Diagn* 20:1012–1014, 2000.

Renier D, Sainte-Rose C, Pierre-Kahn A, Hirsch JF: Prenatal hydrocephalus: outcome and prognosis. *Childs Nerv Syst* 4:213–222, 1988.

Zlotogora J, Sagi M, Cohen T: Familial hydrocephalus of prenatal onset. *Am J Med Genet* 49:202–204, 1994.

*See Appendixes and p. 27 for a complete list of syndromes associated with ventriculomegaly.

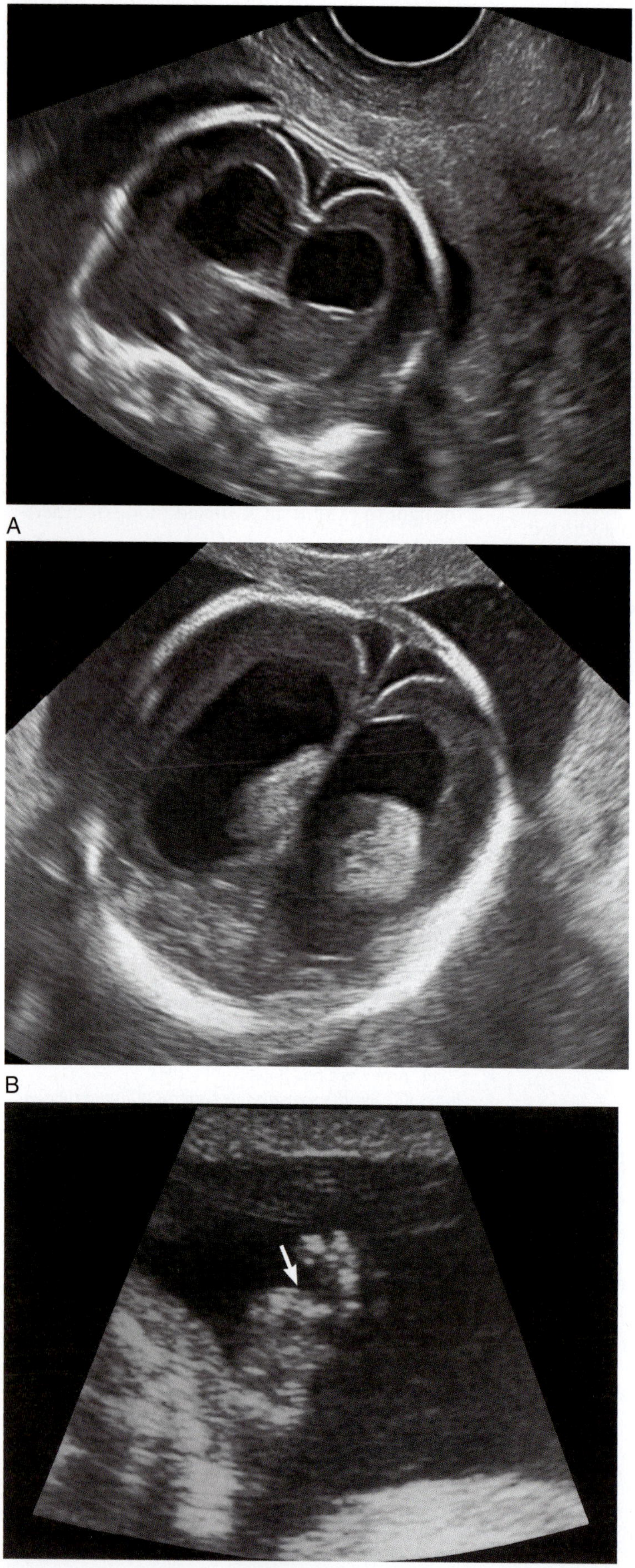

FIGURE 2-74 (**A, B**) Hydrocephalus. Coronal and modified transverse views through the ventricular system of a 20-week fetus with ventriculomegaly. Note that the choroids are asymmetric and do not fill the ventricle. (**C**) Hand of a fetus with aqueductal stenosis shows adduction of the fetal thumb *(arrow)* across the palm, characteristic of this disorder.

Limb Abnormalities

ADAMS-OLIVER SYNDROME

DESCRIPTION AND DEFINITION

This syndrome, first described by Adams and Oliver in 1945, is characterized by terminal transverse defects of the upper and lower extremities as well as denuded areas on the scalp, with or without an underlying bony skull defect.

ABNORMALITIES DETECTABLE BY ULTRASOUND

Common Findings:

Limb abnormalities, characterized by variable degrees of transverse limb defects (lower and upper extremities)

IUGR

Decreased ossification of some areas of the skull

Occasional Findings:

Encephalocele

Acrania

Microcephaly

Facial cleft

Cardiac defects

Clubbed feet

Syndactyly

MAJOR DIFFERENTIAL DIAGNOSES

Amniotic band syndrome

Ectrodactyly-ectodermal dysplasia-clefting (EEC) syndrome

Femoral hypoplasia–unusual facies syndrome

Limb–body wall defect

Oral-mandibular-limb defect

Roberts' syndrome

Sirenomelia

ULTRASOUND DIAGNOSIS

The detection of a fetus with Adams-Oliver syndrome was accomplished at 26 weeks. The same patient, with a known family history, had a second affected fetus detected at 22 weeks. The diagnosis was based on transverse limb defects and scalp abnormalities, with swelling of the scalp and decreased ossification of the skull.

HEREDITY

There have been reports of both an autosomal dominant and an autosomal recessive form of inheritance. There is a large amount of variability in the phenotype of this syndrome, with transverse defects ranging from just the distal toes to entire distal limbs.

NATURAL HISTORY AND OUTCOME

The prognosis is excellent, although surgical intervention often is required to close the skull or scalp defects that may expose the brain. The etiology of this syndrome is thought to be related to vascular disruption sequences, which result in interruption of the distal aspects of the affected extremities and other organs. This may explain the occasional association with acrania and Poland anomalad.

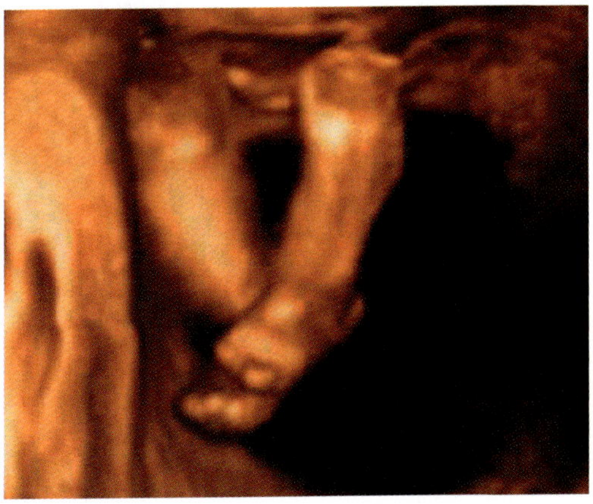

FIGURE 2-75 Three-dimensional surface-rendered image of second-trimester fetal feet shows absence of the first three toes of one foot.

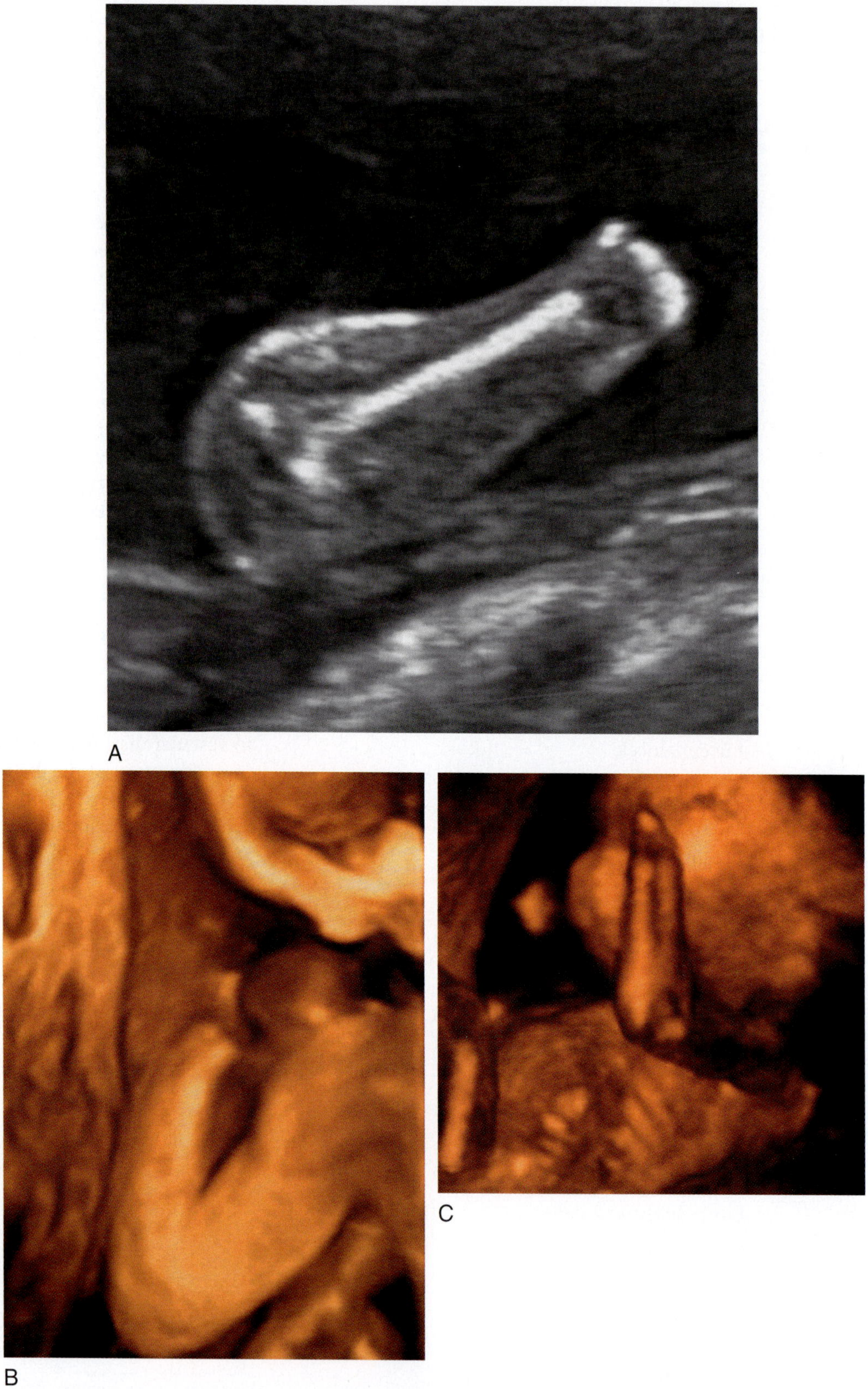

FIGURE 2-76 Two different fetuses in the second trimester with absence of the hand, as can be seen in fetuses with Adams-Oliver syndrome. (A, B) Two-dimensional and three-dimensional images of the same second-trimester fetus with a missing hand. (C) Missing hand on a different second-trimester fetus.

Suggested Reading

Adams FH, Oliver CP: Hereditary deformities in man due to arrested development. *J Hered* 36:2–7, 1945.

Becker R, Kunze J, Horn D, et al: Autosomal recessive type of Adams-Oliver syndrome: prenatal diagnosis. *Ultrasound Obstet Gynecol* 20:506–510, 2002.

Hoyme HE, Der Kaloustian VM, Hoff H, Entin MA, Guttmacher AE: Possible common pathogenetic mechanisms for Poland sequence and Adams-Oliver syndrome: an additional clinical observation. *Am J Med Genet* 42:398–399, 1992.

Jones KL: *Smith's recognizable patterns of human malformation,* ed 6. Philadelphia, 2006, Elsevier.

Kuster W, Lenz W, Kaariaiinen H, Majewski F: Congenital scalp defects with distal limb anomalies (Adams-Oliver syndrome): report of ten cases and review of the literature. *Am J Med Genet* 31:99–115, 1988.

Pereira-Da-Silva L, Leal F, Cassiano Santos G, Videira Amaral JM, Feijoo MJ: Clinical evidence of vascular abnormalities at birth in Adams-Oliver syndrome: report of two further cases. *Am J Med Genet* 94:75–76, 2000.

ECTRODACTYLY–ECTODERMAL DYSPLASIA–CLEFTING (EEC) SYNDROME

DESCRIPTION AND DEFINITION

Ectrodactyly–ectodermal dysplasia–clefting (EEC) syndrome is an inherited malformation characterized by labial clefting and ectrodactyly (lobster-claw deformity of the limbs).

ABNORMALITIES DETECTABLE BY ULTRASOUND

Common Findings:

Cleft lip, with or without cleft palate (72%)

Abnormalities of the hands and feet, including syndactyly and ectrodactyly (84%)

Urinary tract abnormalities, including megaureter, hydronephrosis, ureterocele, renal aplasia, and genital abnormalities (52%)

Occasional Findings:

Semilobar holoprosencephaly

Choanal atresia

Malformed ears

Micrognathia

Cystic hygroma

MAJOR DIFFERENTIAL DIAGNOSES

Syndromes and Conditions Associated with Facial Clefts and Abnormal Extremities:

Adams-Oliver syndrome

Amniotic band syndrome

Nager syndrome

Oral-facial-digital syndromes

Roberts' syndrome

Stickler syndrome

Triploidy

Trisomy 13 (Patau syndrome)

Trisomy 18 (Edwards' syndrome)

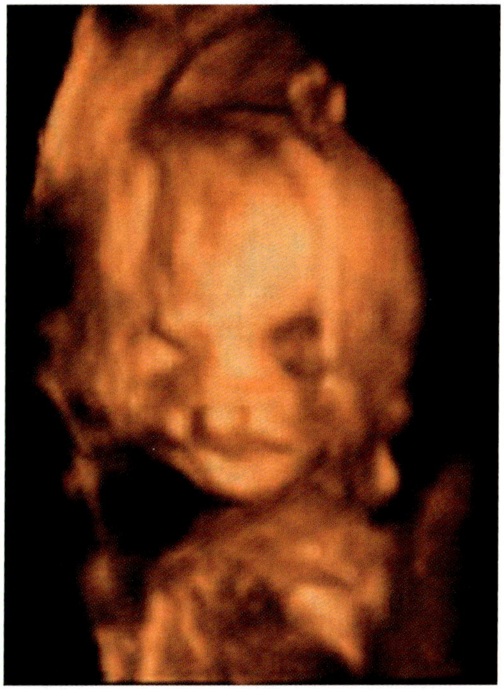

FIGURE 2-77 Surface rendering of a second-trimester fetus with bilateral complete cleft lip and palate, as can be seen in fetuses with ectrodactyly–ectodermal dysplasia–clefting (EEC) syndrome.

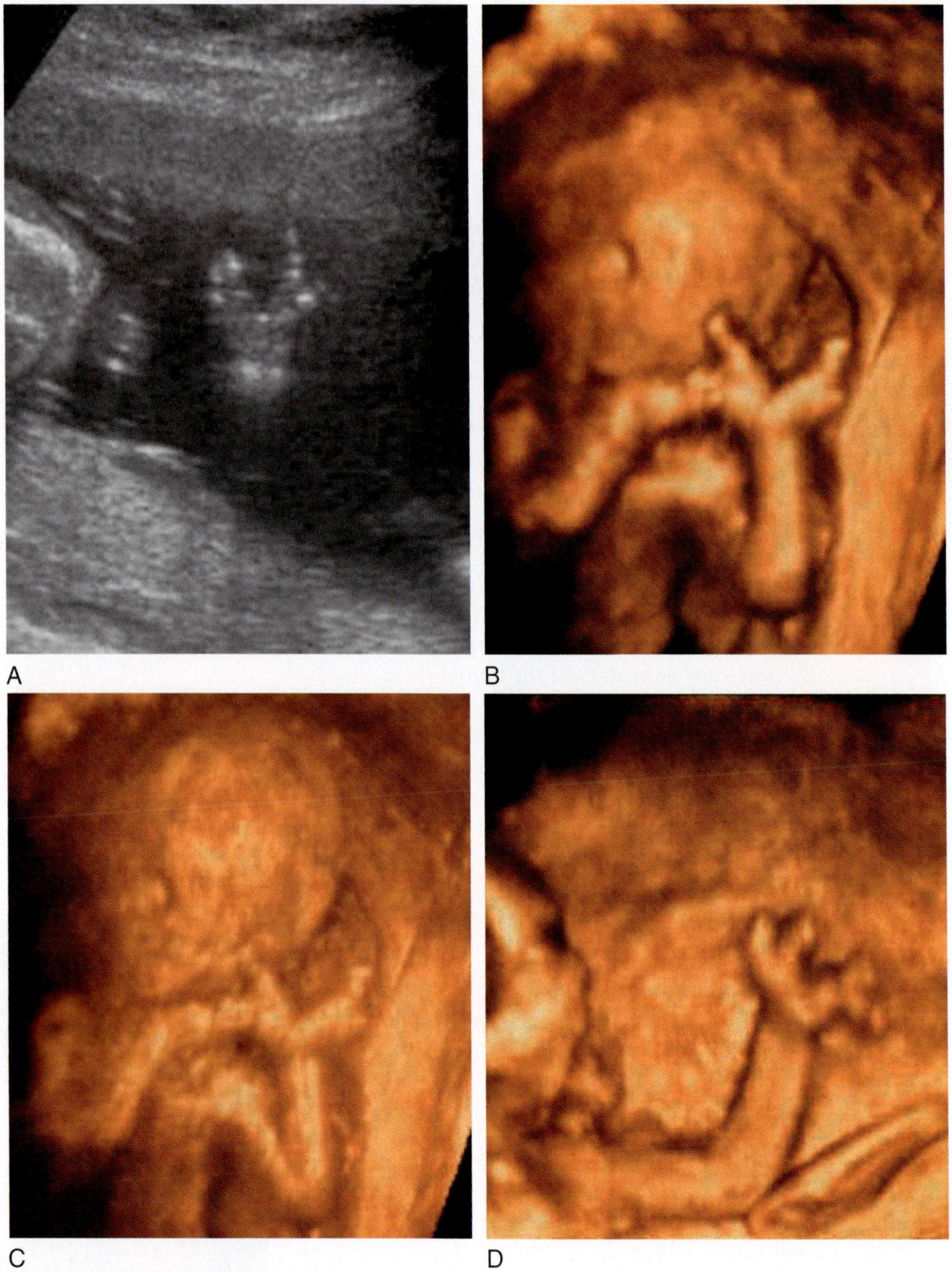

FIGURE 2-78 Second-trimester fetus with lobster-claw hands. (**A**) Two-dimensional image of a lobster-claw abnormality shows a split between the middle and ring fingers and syndactyly. (**B–D**) Three-dimensional surface rendering of the same fetus shows the hand deformity in both soft tissue and bony settings.

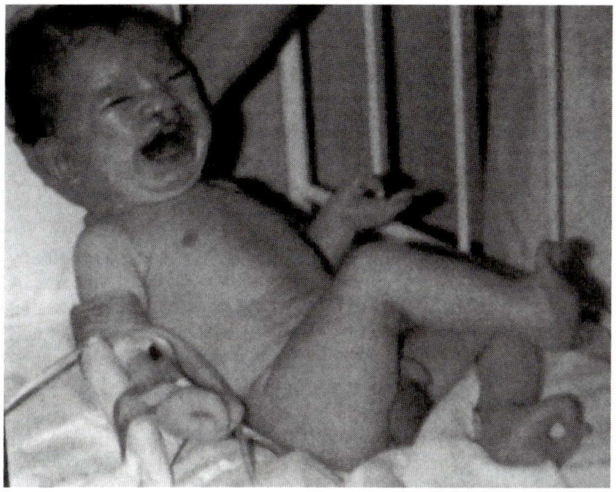

FIGURE 2-79 Postnatal appearance of the face and extremities of an infant with ectrodactyly–ectodermal dysplasia–clefting (EEC) syndrome. (From Kohler R, Sousa P, Jorge CS: *J Ultrasound Med* 8:337, 1989.)

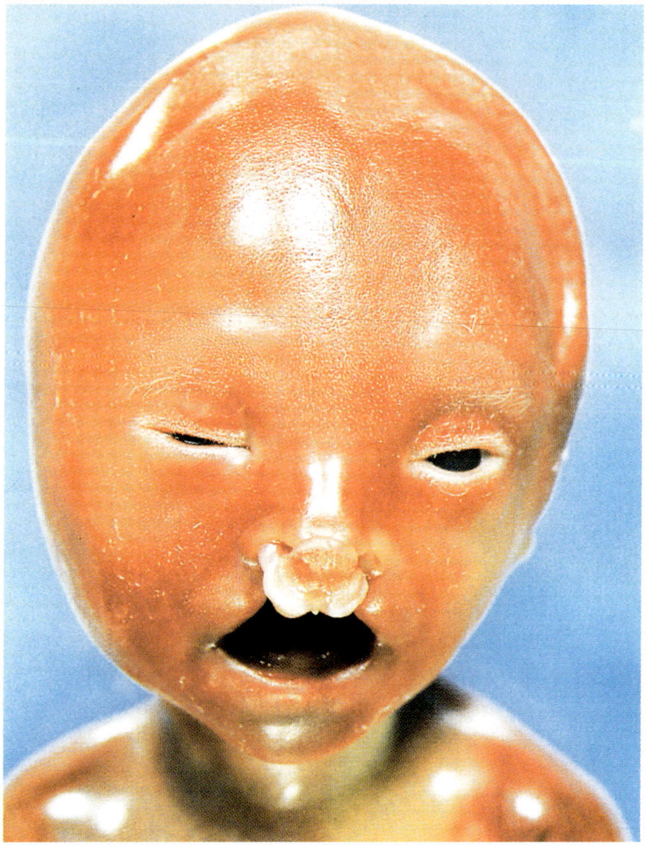

FIGURE 2-80 Frontal view of a fetus with ectrodactyly–ectodermal dysplasia–clefting (EEC) syndrome shows the facial cleft. (From Keeling JW: *Fetal pathology.* London, 1994, Churchill Livingstone.)

ULTRASOUND DIAGNOSIS

The ultrasound diagnosis of EEC syndrome has been established as early as 14 weeks' gestational age, as well as at 16 and 30 weeks. Findings include facial clefting and abnormalities of the hands. Early abnormalities also include first-trimester nuchal fold thickness and a cystic mass involving the umbilical cord (close to the fetal insertion). There is one reported case with associated large nephritic cyst and severe oligohydramnios.

HEREDITY

EEC syndrome has an autosomal dominant pattern of inheritance, with variable expression. There are reports of abnormalities of the long arm of chromosome 7, suggesting that this syndrome may be related to the split hand/split

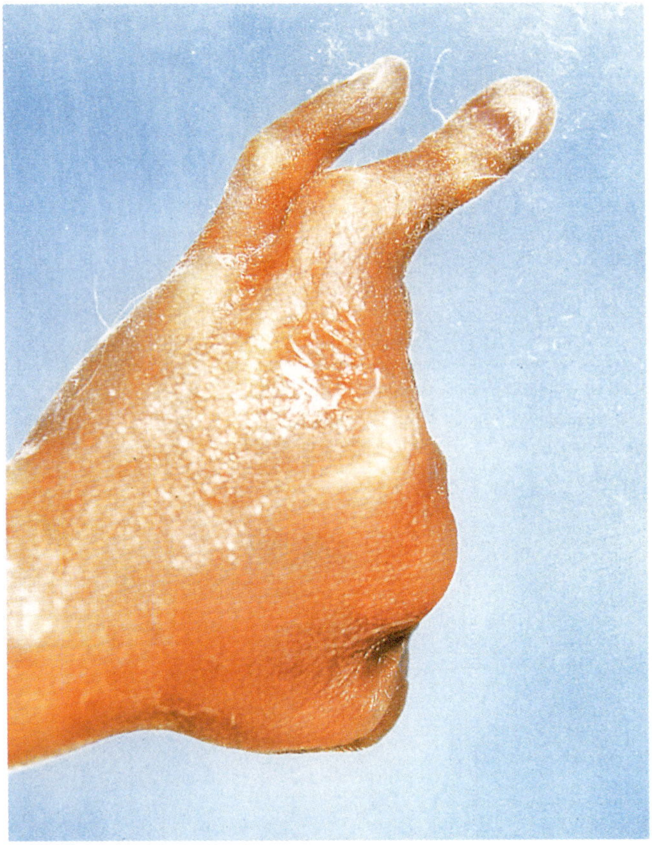

FIGURE 2-81 Severe malformation of the hand in a fetus with ectrodactyly–ectodermal dysplasia–clefting (EEC) syndrome. (From Keeling JW: *Fetal pathology.* London, 1994, Churchill Livingstone.)

foot malformation that has been mapped to 7q21-q22.

NATURAL HISTORY AND OUTCOME

Children with this disorder have normal intelligence. Treatment is focused on surgical correction of facial and limb deformities. Postnatal problems may involve abnormalities of the tear duct, which can cause corneal damage, as well as anomalies of the hair, teeth, skin, and nails.

Suggested Reading

Anneren G, Andersson T, Lindgren PG, Kjartansson S: Ectrodactyly–ectodermal dysplasia–clefting syndrome (EEC): the clinical variation and prenatal diagnosis. *Clin Genet* 40:257–262, 1991.

Brill CB, Hsu LYF, Hirschhorn K: The syndrome of ectrodactyly, ectodermal dysplasia and cleft lip and palate: report of a family demonstrating dominant inheritance pattern. *Clin Genet* 3:295–302, 1972.

Bronshtein M, Gershoni-Baruch R: Prenatal transvaginal diagnosis of the ectrodactyly, ectodermal dysplasia, cleft palate (EEC) syndrome. *Prenat Diagn* 13:519–522, 1993.

Chuangsuwanich T, Sunsaneevithayakul P, Muangsomboon K, Limwongse C: Ectrodactyly-ectodermal dysplasia-clefting (EEC) syndrome presenting with a large nephrogenic cyst, severe oligohydramnios and hydrops fetalis: a case report and review of the literature. *Prenat Diagn* 25:210–215, 2005.

Henrion R, Oury JF, Aubry JP, Aubry MC: Prenatal diagnosis of ectrodactyly. *Lancet* 2:319, 1980.

Jones KL: *Smith's recognizable patterns of human malformations,* ed 6. Philadelphia, 2006, Elsevier.

Kohler R, Sousa P, Jorge CS: Prenatal diagnosis of the ectrodactyly, ectodermal dysplasia, cleft palate (EEC) syndrome. *J Ultrasound Med* 8:337–339, 1989.

Lacombe D, Serville F, Marchand D, Battin J: Split hand/split foot deformity and LADD syndrome in a family: overlap between the EEC and LADD syndromes. *J Med Genet* 30:700–730, 1993.

Leung KY, MacLachaln NA, Sepulveda W: Prenatal diagnosis of ectrodactyly: the "lobster claw" anomaly. *Ultrasound Obstet Gynecol* 6:443–446, 1995.

Maas SM, de Jong TPVM, Buss P, Hennekam RCM: ECC syndrome and genitourinary anomalies: an update. *Am J Med Genet* 63:472–478, 1996.

Penchaszadeh VB, De Negrotti TC: Ectrodactyly–ectodermal dysplasia–clefting (EEC) syndrome: dominant inheritance and variable expression. *J Med Genet* 13:281–284, 1976.

Scherer SW, Poorkaj P, Massa H, et al: Physical mapping of the split hand/split foot locus on chromosome 7 and implication in syndromic ectrodactyly. *Hum Mol Genet* 3:1345–1354, 1994.

FANCONI ANEMIA

DESCRIPTION AND DEFINITION

Fanconi pancytopenia syndrome is an autosomal recessive condition characterized by radial hypoplasia and pancytopenia with a tendency for leukemia.

ABNORMALITIES DETECTABLE BY ULTRASOUND

Common Findings:

Short radial ray; abnormalities of the thumb and digits

Short stature

Genitourinary abnormalities, including abnormalities of the kidneys, ureters, and genitals

Abnormal nuchal translucency—first trimester

Occasional Findings:

Ventriculomegaly

Absence of the corpus callosum

Gastrointestinal obstruction

Cardiac defects

Microcephaly

Microphthalmos

MAJOR DIFFERENTIAL DIAGNOSES

Cornelia de Lange syndrome

Holt-Oram syndrome

Nager syndrome

Roberts' syndrome

Thrombocytopenia–absent radius (TAR) syndrome

Trisomy 13 (Patau syndrome)

Trisomy 18 (Edwards' syndrome)

VATER (**v**ertebral defects, **a**nal atresia, **t**racheo-esophageal fistula, **e**sophageal atresia, and **r**adial and renal dysplasias) association

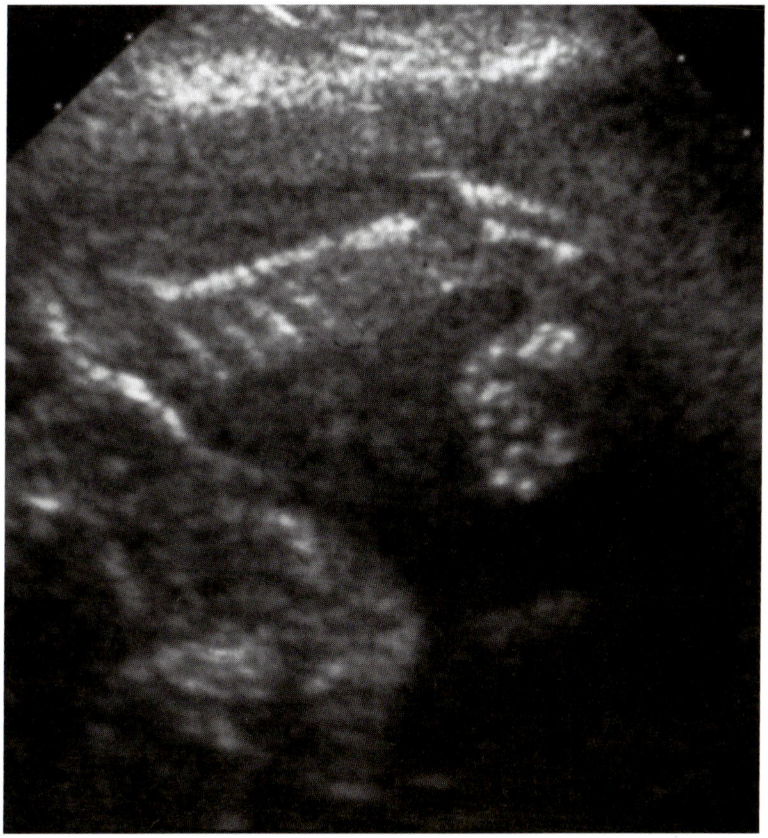

FIGURE 2-82 Two-dimensional image of second-trimester fetus with a short radial ray characteristic of Fanconi syndrome. Note that the hand is at a right angle to the lower arm because of deformity of the forearm.

ULTRASOUND DIAGNOSIS

Prenatal ultrasound detection is contingent on finding abnormalities of the radial ray and thumb. There is also a report of abnormal motor behavior, in the form of excessive bursts of fetal kicking, in an affected second-trimester fetus.

The most successful means of establishing a prenatal diagnosis for affected families involves DNA evaluation of fetal blood or cultured amniotic fluid cells, rather than ultrasound findings. Using DNA analysis in a family previously affected by this condition, the diagnosis of Fanconi anemia has been made at 14 weeks' gestation.

HEREDITY

The pattern of inheritance for Fanconi anemia is autosomal recessive. At least eight different complementation groups are recognized, although the phenotypes are not specific to the groups.

NATURAL HISTORY AND OUTCOME

Not all affected infants have skeletal or dysmorphic findings. In some children, the onset of hematologic abnormalities several years after birth may be the first manifestation of the disorder. Hematologic abnormalities, as well as progression to myelodysplastic disorders, and malignant tumors can lead to death in some affected individuals.

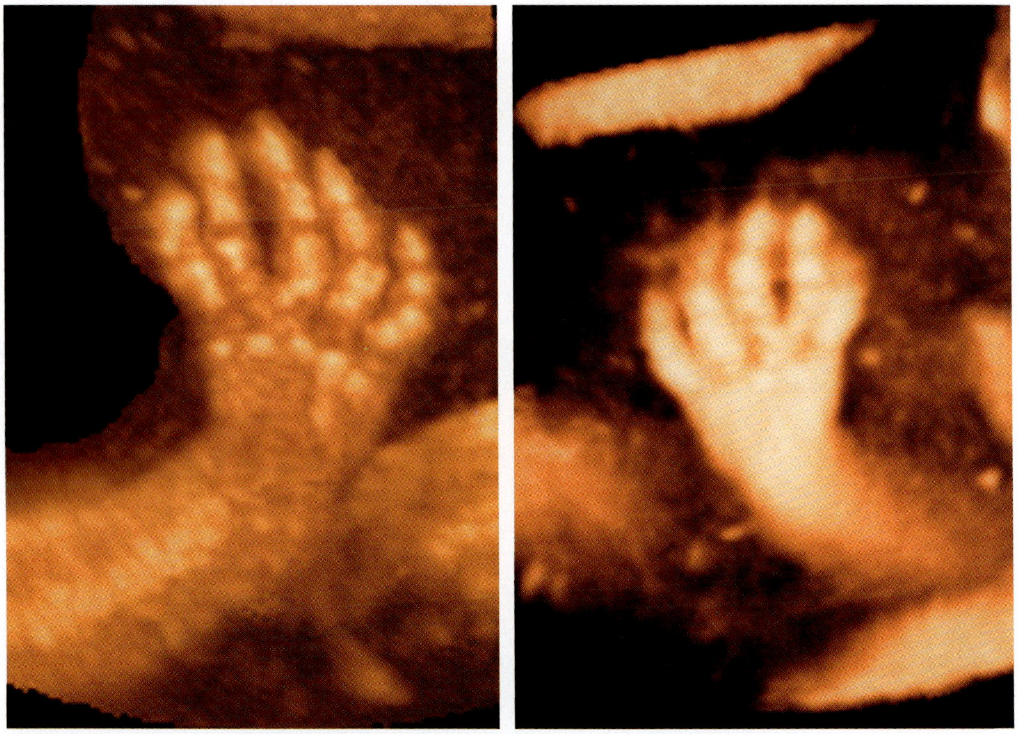

A B

FIGURE 2-83 (A, B) Three-dimensional surface rendering shows both soft tissues and bony features of a fetus with a radial ray abnormality and digitalization of the thumb. These findings are features of fetuses with Fanconi syndrome. Note that the hand is at an angle with respect to the forearm because of the radial abnormality.

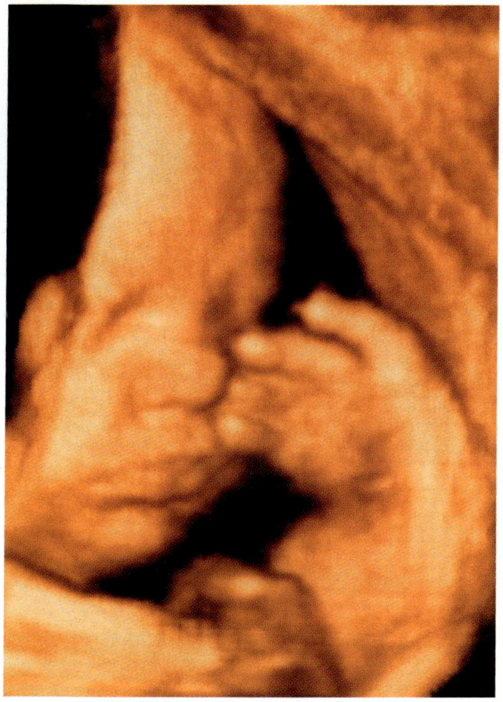

FIGURE 2-84 Severe radial ray abnormality of a third-trimester fetus. Note that the surface rendering image of the arm and the hand shows that the hand is at a right angle to the forearm because of the radial ray abnormality. The thumb could not be identified sonographically.

Suggested Reading

Auerbach AD: Umbilical cord blood transplants for genetic disease: diagnostic and ethical issues in fetal studies. *Blood Cells* 20:303–309, 1994.

de Vries JI, Laurini RN, Visser GH: Abnormal motor behaviour and developmental postmortem findings in a fetus with Fanconi anaemia. *Early Hum Dev* 36:137–142, 1994.

Jones KL: *Smith's recognizable patterns of human malformations,* ed 6. Philadelphia, 2006, Elsevier.

Kwee ML, Lo TF Jr, Arwert F, et al: Early prenatal diagnosis of Fanconi anaemia in a twin pregnancy, using DNA analysis. *Prenat Diagn* 16:345–348, 1996.

Merrill A, Rosenblum-Vos L, Driscoll DA, Daley K, Treat K: Prenatal diagnosis of Fanconi anemia (Group C) subsequent to abnormal sonographic findings. *Prenat Diagn* 25:20–22, 2005.

Tercanli S, Miny P, Siebert MS, Hosli I, Surbek DV, Holzgreve W: Fanconi anemia associated with increased nuchal translucency detected by first-trimester ultrasound. *Ultrasound Obstet Gynecol* 17:160–162, 2001.

FEMORAL HYPOPLASIA–UNUSUAL FACIES SYNDROME

DESCRIPTION AND DEFINITION

Characterized by short lower limbs, resulting from bilateral or unilateral hypoplastic femurs, this syndrome may be found in infants of diabetic mothers. It is thought to fall within a spectrum of abnormalities ranging from the milder form of proximal femoral deficiency syndrome to caudal regression syndrome, in which the deficiency involves the sacrum and fetal pelvis. The only difference between femoral hypoplasia–unusual facies syndrome and proximal femoral deficiency syndrome may be the presence of facial anomalies in the former.

ABNORMALITIES DETECTABLE BY ULTRASOUND

Cleft palate

Micrognathia

Low-set ears

Vertebral abnormalities

Dysplasia of the sacrum

Short and bowed femurs, either bilateral or unilateral

Variable hypoplasia of the humeri

Clubfoot

Urinary tract abnormalities

MAJOR DIFFERENTIAL DIAGNOSES

Amniotic band syndrome

Camptomelic dysplasia

Caudal regression syndrome

Exposure to drugs (thalidomide)

Femur–fibula–ulna (FFU) syndrome

Osteogenesis imperfecta

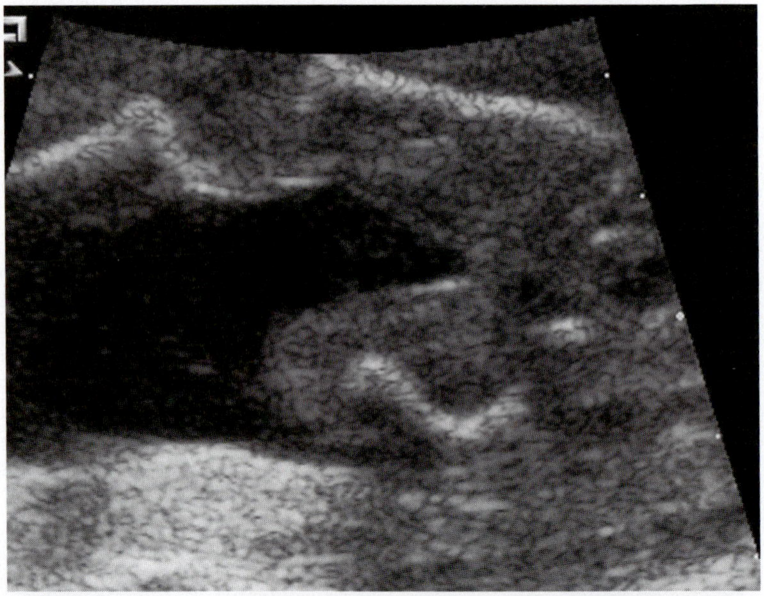

A

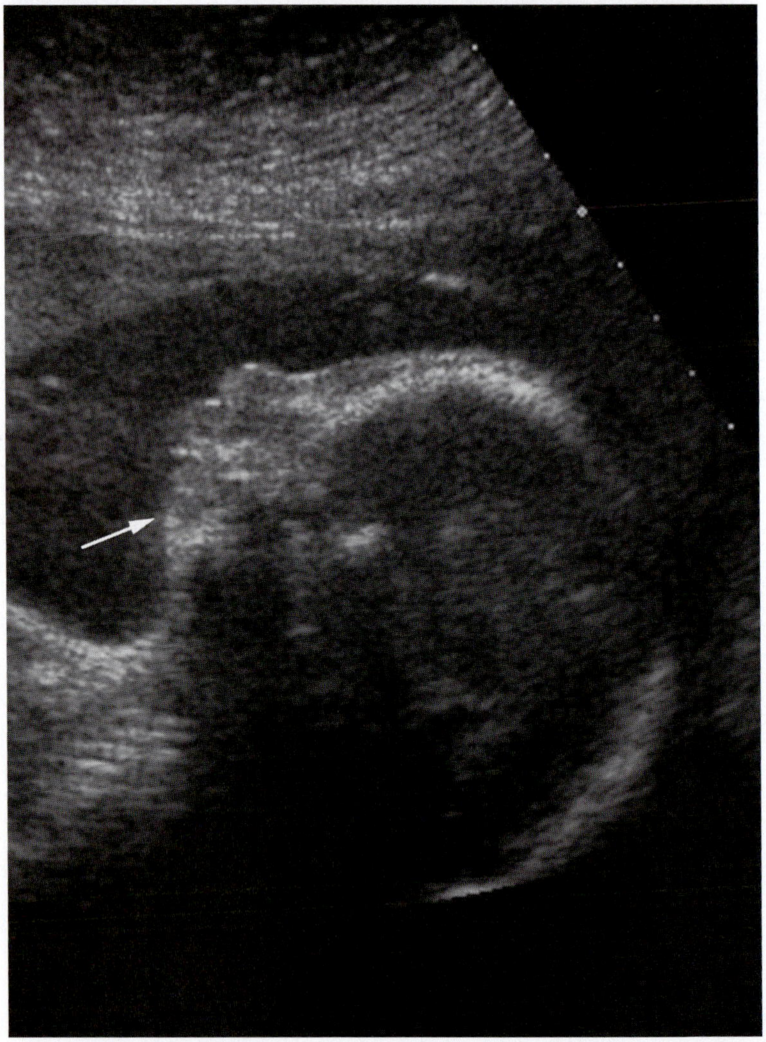

B

FIGURE 2-85 Second-trimester fetus with femoral hypoplasia unusual facies. (A) View through both femurs shows that one femur appears normal and the other is foreshortened and bowed. (B) Fetal face of the same fetus with femoral abnormality shows micrognathia *(arrow)*.

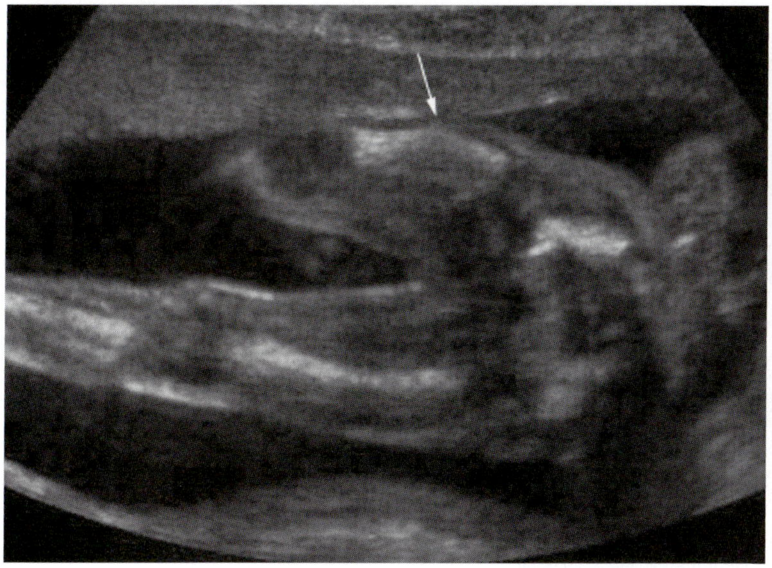
A

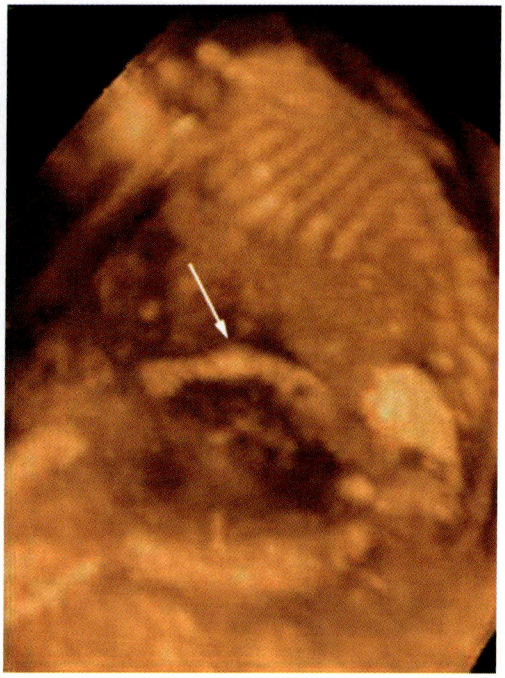
B

FIGURE 2-86 (A) Unilateral bowed femur *(arrow)* shown in two dimensions. (B) Unilateral bowed femur *(arrow)* shown in three dimensions.

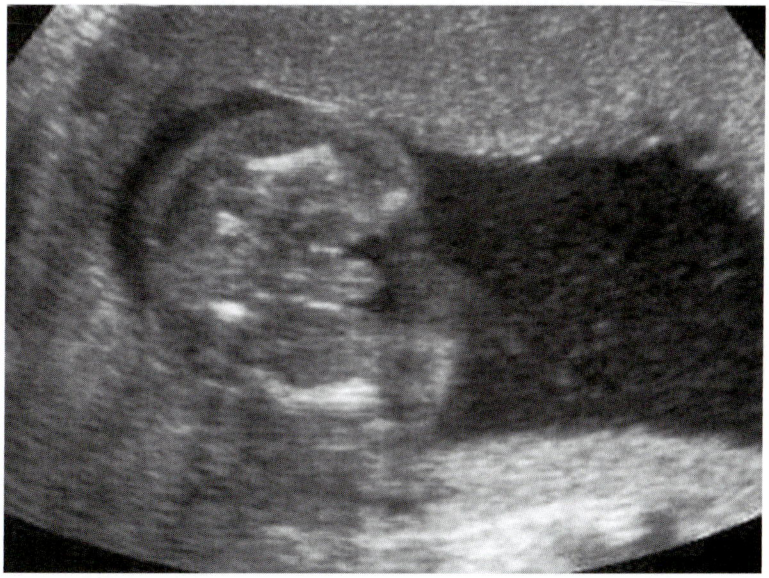
A

FIGURE 2-87 (A) Second-trimester fetus with femoral hypoplasia–unusual facies syndrome shows that both femurs are symmetrically short.

Continued

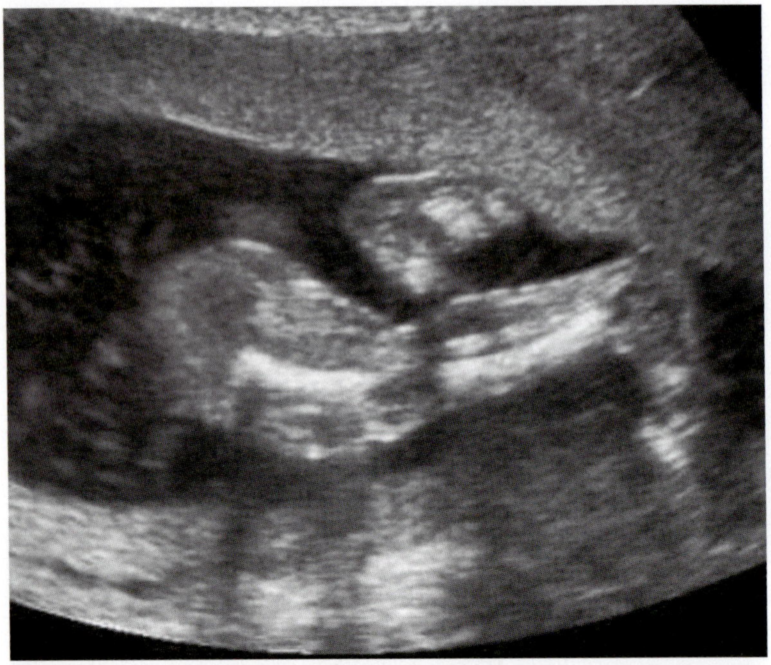

B

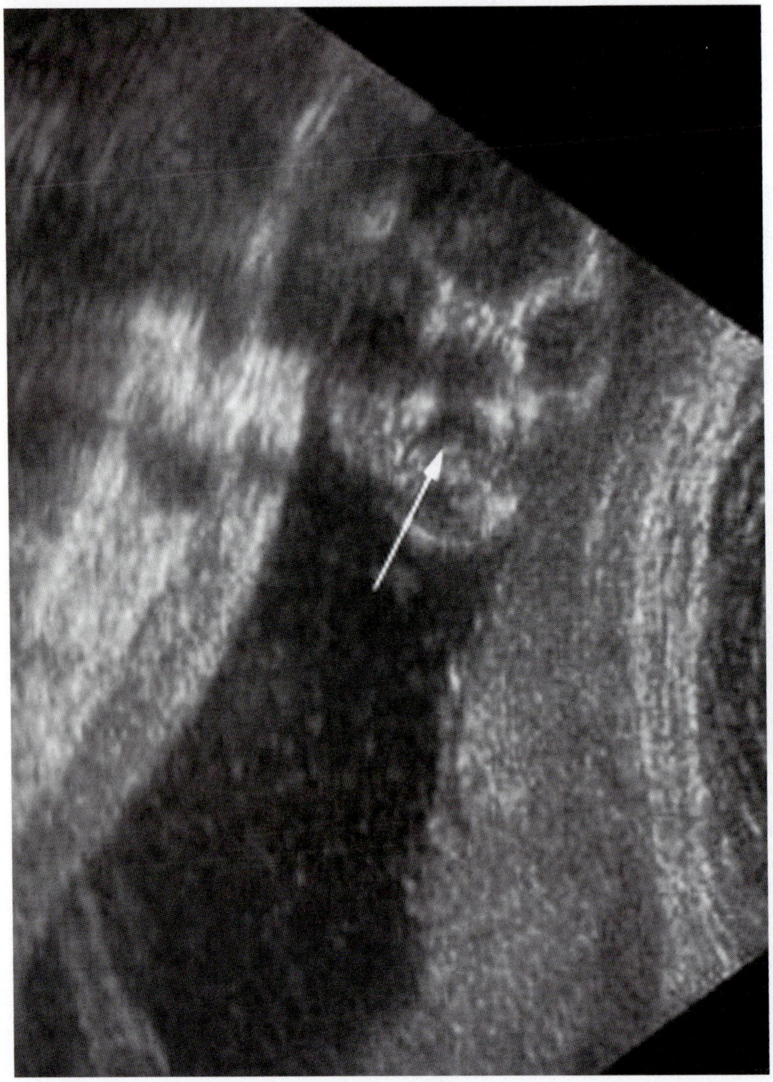

C

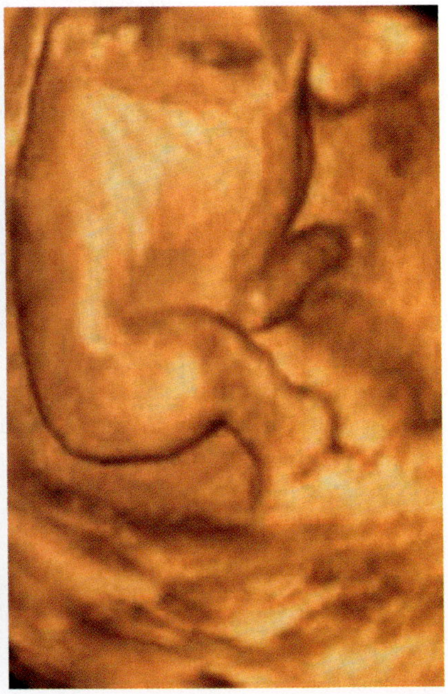

D

FIGURE 2-87, cont'd (B) Second-trimester fetus with femoral hypoplasia–unusual facies syndrome shows a short femur. (C) Cleft lip and palate *(arrow)* seen on a coronal view of the face. (D) Three-dimensional surface rendering of the lower extremity of the same fetus shows the short thigh as a result of the very short femur.

ULTRASOUND DIAGNOSIS

Prenatal diagnosis of this syndrome has been established by transvaginal ultrasound as early as 14 weeks' gestation. The unilateral form is easily diagnosed on the basis of a discrepancy between the measurements of the femora. Other findings may include facial defects, hypoplastic humeri, fibular hypoplasia, and renal abnormalities.

HEREDITY

The etiology of this syndrome is unknown, and the majority of cases are sporadic. There may be an association with diabetic mothers, and familial cases have been reported occasionally.

NATURAL HISTORY AND OUTCOME

Individuals with this disorder have normal intelligence. Treatment includes orthopedic procedures to correct the femoral abnormalities.

Suggested Reading

Ashkenazy M, Lurie S, Ben-Itzhak I, Appleman Z, Caspi B: Unilateral congenital short femur: a case report. *Prenat Diagn* 10:67–70, 1990.

Bau CH, Ribeiro CA, Ribeiro SA, Flores RZ: Bilateral femoral hypoplasia associated with Rokitansky sequence: another example of a mesodermal malformation spectrum? *Am J Med Genet* 49:205–206, 1994.

Bronshtein M, Deitsch M: Early diagnosis of proximal femoral deficiency. *Gynecol Obstet Invest* 34:246–248, 1992.

Bronshtein M, Keret D, Deutsch M, Liberson A, Bar Chava I: Transvaginal sonographic detection of skeletal anomalies in the first and early second trimesters. *Prenat Diagn* 13:597–601, 1993.

Camera G, Dodero D, Parodi M, Zucchinetti P, Camera A: Antenatal ultrasonographic diagnosis of a proximal femoral focal deficiency. *J Clin Ultrasound* 21:475–479, 1993.

Crum A: Femoral hypoplasia-unusual facies syndrome. *Fetus* 4:5–8, 1994.

Filly AL, Robnett-Filly B, Filly RA: Syndromes with focal femoral deficiency: strengths and weaknesses of prenatal sonography. *J Ultrasound Med* 23:1511–1516, 2004.

Goncalves LF, De Luca GR, Vitorello DA, et al: Prenatal diagnosis of bilateral proximal femoral hypoplasia. *Ultrasound Obstet Gynecol* 8:127–130, 1996.

Goncalves LF, Piper JM, Jeanty P: The accuracy of prenatal ultrasonography in detecting congenital anomalies. *Am J Obstet Gynecol* 171:1606–1612, 1994.

Graham M: Congenital short femur: prenatal sonographic diagnosis. *J Ultrasound Med* 4:361–363, 1985.

Hadi HA, Wade A: Prenatal diagnosis of unilateral proximal femoral focal deficiency in diabetic pregnancy: a case report. *Am J Perinatal* 10:285–287, 1993.

Hinson RM, Miller RC, Macri CJ: Femoral hypoplasia and maternal diabetes: consider femoral hypoplasia/unusual facies syndrome. *Am J Perinatol* 13:433–436, 1996.

Jeanty P, Kleinman G: Proximal femoral focal deficiency. *J Ultrasound Med* 8:639–642, 1989.

Jones KL: *Smith's recognizable patterns of human malformations,* ed 6. Philadelphia, 2006, Elsevier.

Kelly TE: Proximal focal femoral deficiency (familial). *Birth Defects* 10:508–509, 1974.

Keret D, Timor IE: Familial congenital short femur: intrauterine detection and follow-up by ultrasound. *Orthop Rev* 27:500–504, 1988.

Robinow M, Sonek J, Buttino L, Veghte A: Femoral–facial syndrome: prenatal diagnosis, autosomal dominant inheritance. *Am J Med Genet* 57:397–399, 1995.

Sen Gupta DK, Gupta SK: Familiar bilateral proximal femoral focal deficiency: report of a kindred. *J Bone Joint Surg* 66:1470–1472, 1984.

Tadmor OP, Hammerman C, Rabinowitz R, et al: Femoral hypoplasia, unusual facies syndrome: prenatal ultrasonographic observations. *Fetal Diagn Ther* 8:279–284, 1993.

FEMUR–FIBULA–ULNA (FFU) SYNDROME

DESCRIPTION AND DEFINITION

This syndrome of unknown etiology is characterized by severe, asymmetric abnormalities of both upper and lower limbs.

ABNORMALITIES DETECTABLE BY ULTRASOUND

Severe abnormalities of the limbs

Hypoplasia or aplasia of the femur and fibula

Abnormalities of the arm, ranging from absence of the arm to absence of the fingers

Para-axial hemimelia of the ulna and fibula, with lesser involvement of the humerus

MAJOR DIFFERENTIAL DIAGNOSES

Syndromes and Conditions Associated with Asymmetric Abnormalities of the Extremities:

Amniotic band syndrome

Caudal regression syndrome

Cornelia de Lange syndrome

Ectrodactyly–ectodermal dysplasia–clefting (EEC) syndrome

Fanconi anemia

Femoral hypoplasia–unusual facies

Holt–Oram syndrome

MURCS (**mü**llerian duct aplasia, **r**enal aplasia, **c**ervicothoracic **s**omite dysplasia) association

Nager syndrome

Oral-facial-digital (Mohr) syndrome

Roberts' syndrome

Russell-Silver syndrome

Thrombocytopenia–absent radius (TAR) syndrome

VATER (**v**ertebral defects, **a**nal atresia, **t**racheo-esophageal fistula, **e**sophageal atresia, and **r**adial and renal dysplasias) association

ULTRASOUND DIAGNOSIS

The prenatal diagnosis of this condition was first established in 1988 at 28 weeks' gestation, when an ultrasonogram revealed asymmetric limb abnormalities. More recently, prenatal diagnosis has been made at 19 weeks, seen as asymmetric shortening of both femora, bilateral hypoplastic tibiae, and absent fibulae. One of the hands was also abnormal. The diagnosis is based on three affected limbs.

HEREDITY

The etiology of this syndrome is unknown but has a 2:1 male/female predominance.

NATURAL HISTORY AND OUTCOME

Physical disabilities can be extensive. However, there is no evidence of mental retardation or reduced life expectancy associated with FFU syndrome.

Suggested Reading

Capece G, Fasolino A, Della Monica M, et al: Prenatal diagnosis of femur-fibula-ulna complex by ultrasonography in a male fetus at 24 weeks of gestation. *Prenat Diagn* 14:502–505, 1994.

Florio I, Wisser J, Huch R, Huch A: Prenatal ultrasound diagnosis of a femur-fibula-ulna complex during the first half of pregnancy. *Fetal Diagn Ther* 14:310–312, 1999.

Geipel A, Berg C, Germer U, Krokowski M, Smrcek J, Gembruch U: Prenatal diagnosis of femur-fibula-ulna complex by ultrasound examination at 20 weeks of gestation. *Ultrasound Obstet Gynecol* 22:79–81, 2003.

Hirose K, Koyanagi T, Hara K, Inoue M, Nakano H: Antenatal ultrasound diagnosis of the femur-fibula-ulna syndrome. *J Clin Ultrasound* 16:199–203, 1988.

Lenz W, Zygulska M, Horst J: FFU complex: an analysis of 491 cases. *Hum Genet* 91:347–356, 1993.

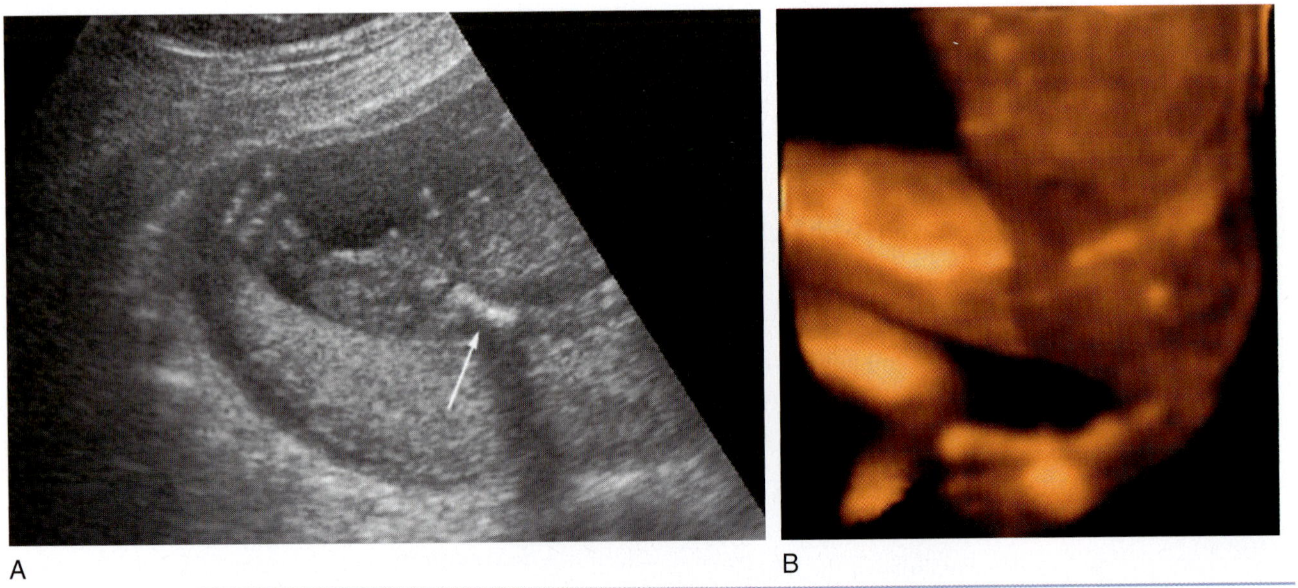

FIGURE 2-88 Second-trimester fetus with unilateral lower limb abnormality. **(A)** Two-dimensional image shows the iliac crest *(arrow)*. Note that the foot is almost directly attached to the hip in this case, with almost complete absence of the intervening leg. **(B)** Same deformity shown with three-dimensional surface rendering.

FREEMAN-SHELDON (WHISTLING FACE) SYNDROME

DESCRIPTION AND DEFINITION

Synonym: Whistling face syndrome

Described by Freeman and Sheldon in 1938, this rare disorder is characterized by unusual facial features and skeletal abnormalities similar to arthrogryposis.

ABNORMALITIES DETECTABLE BY ULTRASOUND

Abnormal facies

Sloping forehead

Deep-set eyes

Small nose

Long philtrum, giving the appearance of a "whistling face"

Microcephaly

Kyphoscoliosis

Ulnar deviation of the hands, with flexion deformity of the fingers

Clubbed feet

Contractures of the hips and knees

IUGR

Incomplete descent of testes

MAJOR DIFFERENTIAL DIAGNOSES

Amniotic band syndrome

Antley-Bixler syndrome

Arthrogryposis multiplex

Cerebro-oculo-facio-skeletal (COFS) syndrome

Cornelia de Lange syndrome

Multiple pterygium syndrome

Pena Shokeir syndrome

Seckel syndrome

Smith-Lemli-Opitz syndrome

Trisomy 18 (Edwards' syndrome)

ULTRASOUND DIAGNOSIS

This condition has been diagnosed prenatally by ultrasound at 20 weeks' gestational age in a family with an affected father, presuming autosomal dominance of the syndrome. The sonographic features leading to the diagnosis included clubbed foot and abnormal facial features.

I also examined a fetus with this disorder in the third trimester. Sonographic findings included an abnormal facial profile and contractures of the extremities.

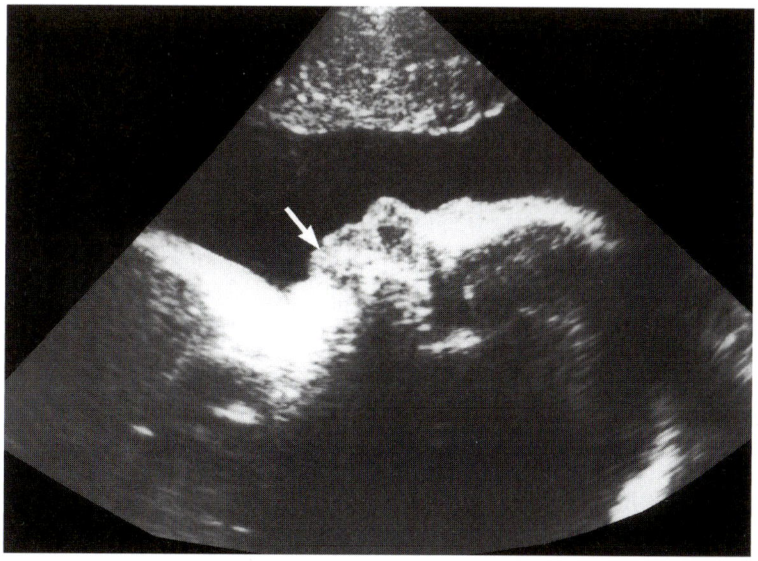

FIGURE 2-89 Profile of a fetus with whistling face syndrome. Note the unusually pursed configuration of the lips *(arrow)*.

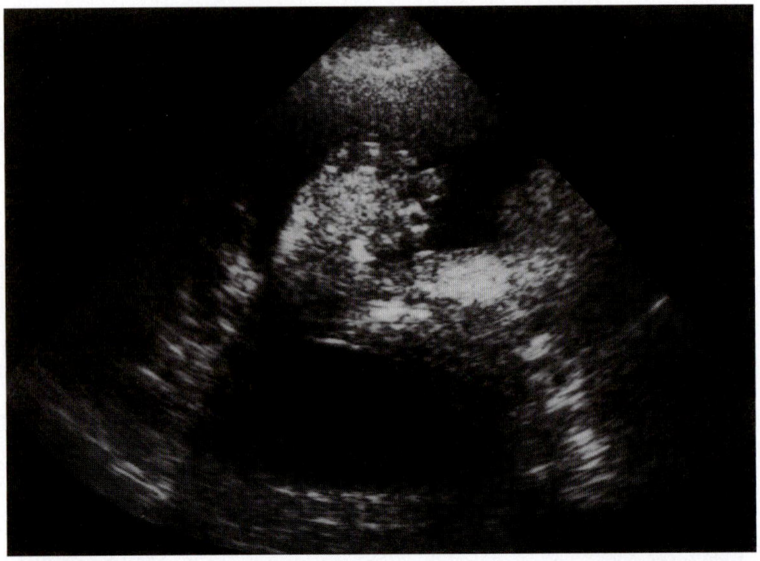

FIGURE 2-90 Lower extremity and foot of the same fetus shown in Figure 2-89. Note severe clubbing of the foot.

HEREDITY

The syndrome has an autosomal dominant inheritance pattern, but most cases are sporadic.

NATURAL HISTORY AND OUTCOME

Most individuals with this disorder have normal intelligence, although mental deficiency and seizures have been reported as part of the syndrome. In most cases, treatment focuses on corrective orthopedic surgery for an arthrogryposis-like disorder, as well as treatment for strabismus and/or blepharoptosis.

Suggested Reading

Baty BJ, Cubberley D, Morris C, et al: Prenatal diagnosis of distal arthrogryposis. *Am J Med Genet* 29:501–510, 1988.

Jones KL: *Smith's recognizable patterns of human malformations,* ed 6. Philadelphia, 2006, Elsevier.

O'Keefe M, Crawford J, Young J, Macrae W: Ocular abnormalities in the Freeman-Sheldon syndrome. *Am J Ophthalmol* 102:346–348, 1986.

Robbins-Furman P, Hecht JT, Rocklin M, et al: Prenatal diagnosis of Freeman-Sheldon syndrome (whistling face) (short communication). *Prenat Diagn* 15:179–182, 1995.

Vanek J, Janda J, Amblerova V, Losan F: Freeman-Sheldon syndrome: a disorder of congenital myopathic origin? *J Med Genet* 23:231–236, 1986.

HOLT-ORAM SYNDROME

DESCRIPTION AND DEFINITION

Described by Holt and Oram in 1960, this condition is characterized by skeletal malformations, particularly involving the upper extremities, and cardiac defects.

ABNORMALITIES DETECTABLE BY ULTRASOUND

Abnormal upper extremities with left side predominance in severity

Absent thumbs

Syndactyly

Phocomelia

Radial hypoplasia

Ulnar abnormalities

Clavicular abnormalities

Humeral abnormalities

Cardiac defects, primarily atrial and ventricular septal defects, affecting 85% of individuals with this abnormality

Abnormal nuchal translucency—first trimester

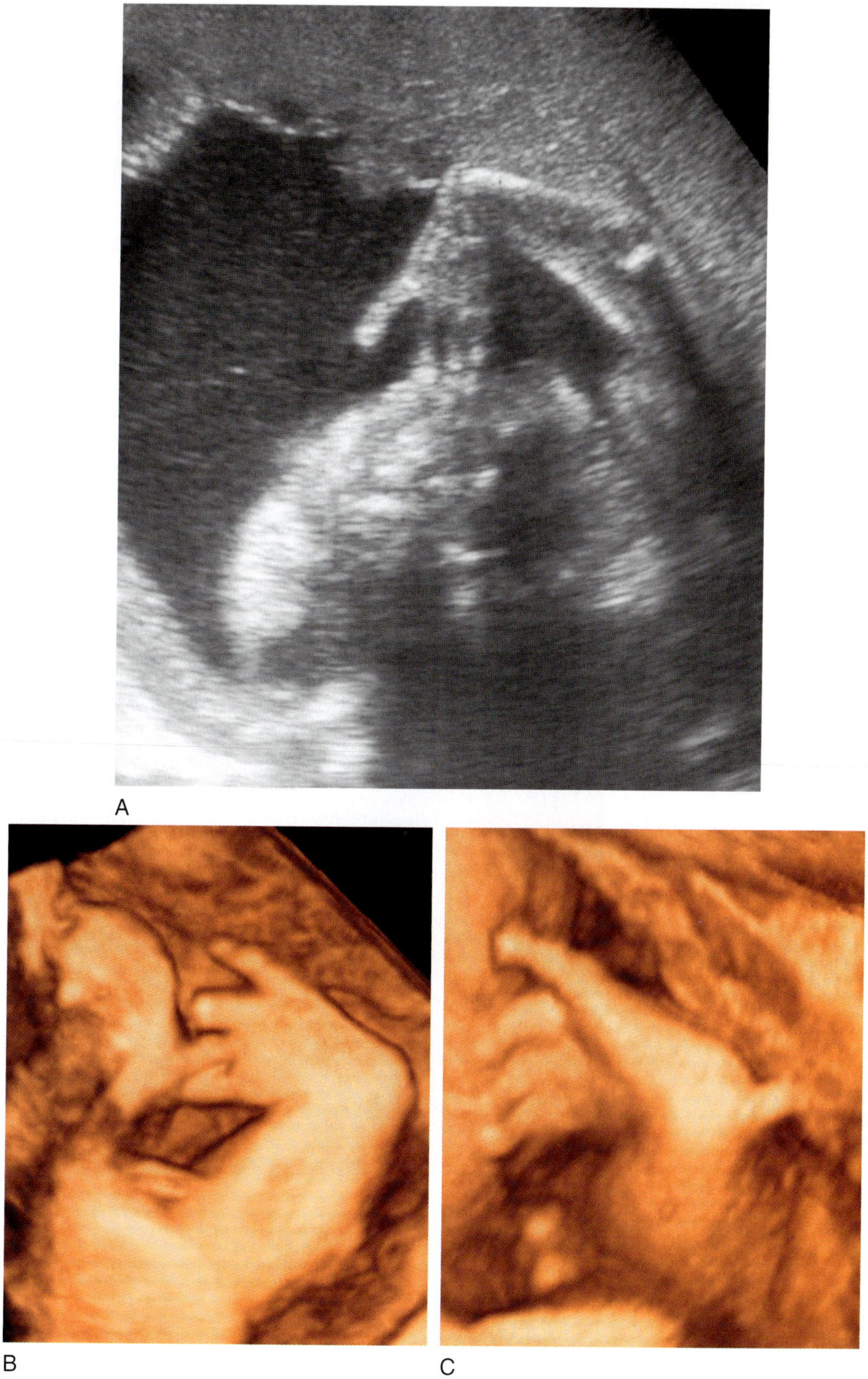

FIGURE 2-91 Second-trimester fetus with Holt-Oram syndrome. (A) Absent radial ray and thumb in a late second-trimester fetus with Holt-Oram syndrome. (B, C) Surface rendering of one of the arms of the same fetus shows abnormal angulation of the hand with respect to the forearm as a result of the absent radius and thumb.

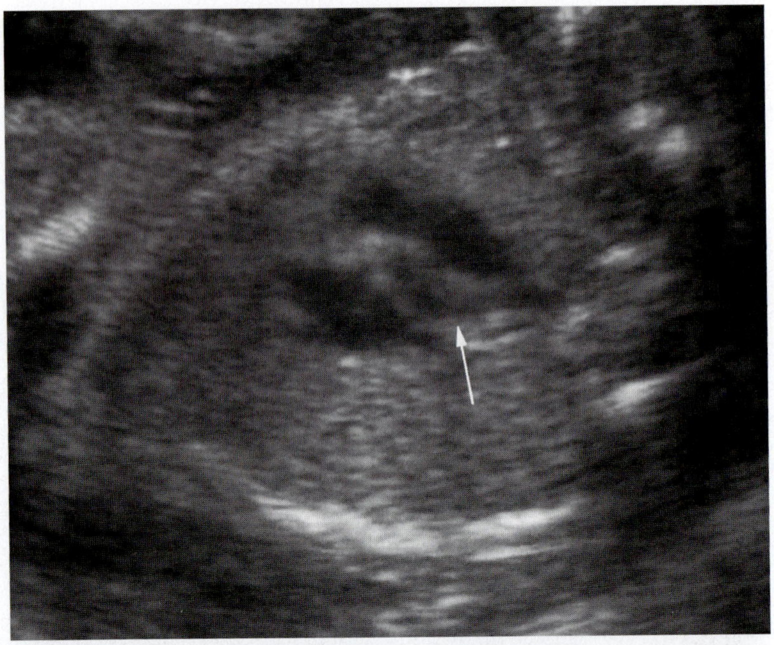

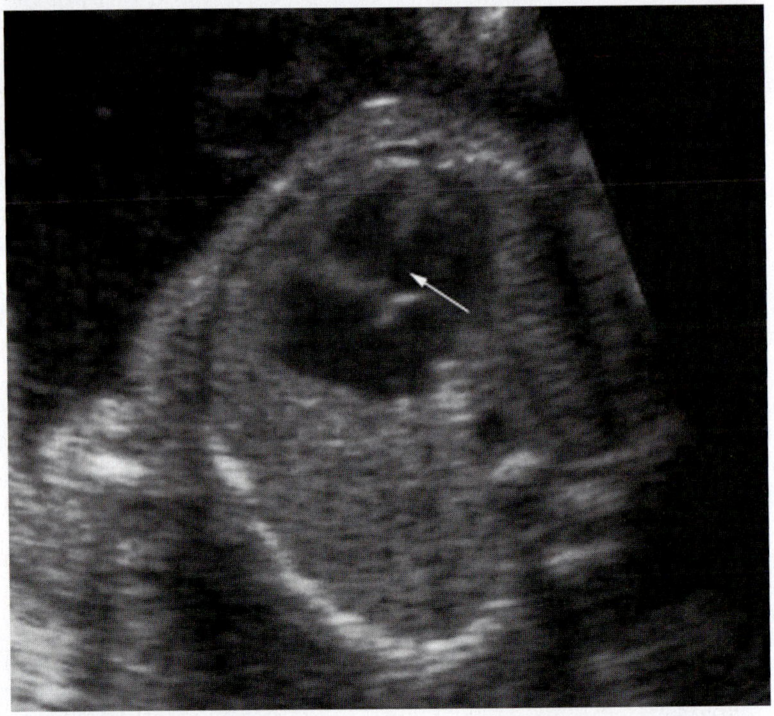

FIGURE 2-92 Second-trimester fetus with Holt-Oram syndrome. A, B. Abnormal heart. (A) Small aortic root *(arrow)*. (B) Four-chamber view of the heart with a large ventricular septal defect *(arrow)*.

Continued

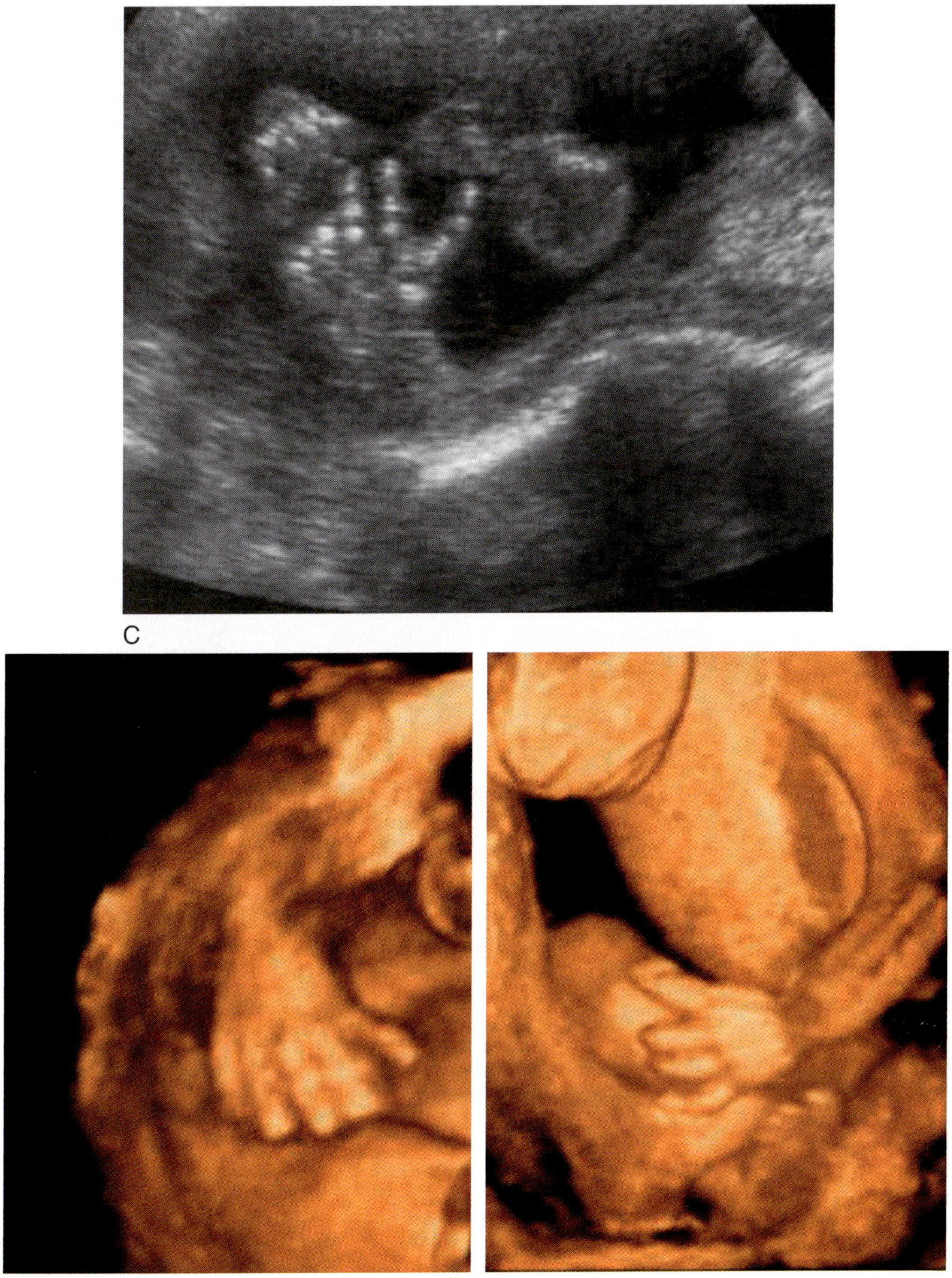

C

D

E

FIGURE 2-92, cont'd Second-trimester fetus with Holt-Oram syndrome. (C) Two-dimensional image of the abnormal hand with digitalization of the thumb. (D) Same hand with three-dimensional surface reconstruction shows that the thumb is digitalized in the same plane of the other four fingers. (E) Contralateral hand shows fusion of the thumb and first digit, consistent with syndactyly of a digitalized thumb and index finger.

MAJOR DIFFERENTIAL DIAGNOSES

Cornelia de Lange syndrome

Fanconi anemia

Nager syndrome (acrofacial dysostosis)

Roberts' syndrome

Thrombocytopenia–absent radius (TAR) syndrome

Trisomy 13 (Patau syndrome)

Trisomy 18 (Edwards' syndrome)

VATER (**v**ertebral defects, **a**nal atresia, **t**racheoesophageal fistula, **e**sophageal atresia, and **r**adial and renal dysplasias) association

ULTRASOUND DIAGNOSIS

The prenatal sonographic diagnosis of this malformation can be established as early as the second trimester if the abnormalities involving the forearm and thumb are sought specifically. This is most often the case in families known to be at increased risk.

HEREDITY

Holt-Oram syndrome has an autosomal dominant inheritance pattern with variable expression. Although it does not account for all affected individuals, the gene most often responsible for this disorder is located on the long arm of chromosome 12 (12q24.1) in the TBX5 of T-box 5 gene.

NATURAL HISTORY AND OUTCOME

Because of the autosomal dominant nature of this syndrome, families with an affected parent generally seek prenatal diagnosis of the offspring. Cardiac abnormalities may require surgical correction after birth, and some affected individuals have cardiac conduction disease and arrhythmias. Orthopedic procedures may be necessary for limb abnormalities.

Suggested Reading

Basson CT, Cowley GS, Solomon SD, et al: The clinical and genetic spectrum of the Holt-Oram syndrome (heart-hand syndrome). *N Engl J Med* 330:885–891, 1994.

Brons JTJ, Van Geijn HP, Wladimiroff JW, et al: Prenatal ultrasound diagnosis of the Holt-Oram syndrome. *Prenat Diagn* 8:175–181, 1988.

Holt M, Oram S: Familial heart disease with skeletal malformations. *Br Heart J* 22:236–242, 1960.

Hurst JA, Hall CM, Baraitser M: The Holt-Oram syndrome. *J Med Genet* 28:406–410, 1991.

Jones KL: *Smith's recognizable patterns of human malformations,* ed 6. Philadelphia, 2006, Elsevier.

Newbury-Ecob RA, Leanage R, Raeburn JA, Young ID: Holt-Oram syndrome: a clinical genetic study. *J Med Genet* 33:300–307, 1996.

Poznanski AK, Gall JC Jr, Stern AM: Skeletal manifestations of the Holt-Oram syndrome. *Radiology* 94:45–54, 1970.

Sepulveda W, Enriquez G, Martinez JL, Mejia R: Holt-Oram syndrome: contribution of prenatal 3-dimensional sonography in an index case. *J Ultrasound Med* 23:983–987, 2004.

Terrett JA, Newbury-Ecob R, Cross GS, et al: Holt-Oram syndrome is a genetically heterogeneous disease with one locus mapping to human chromosome 12q. *Nat Genet* 6:401–404, 1994.

Tongsong T, Chanprapaph P: Prenatal sonographic diagnosis of Holt-Oram syndrome. *J Clin Ultrasound* 28:98–100, 2000.

LARSEN SYNDROME

DESCRIPTION AND DEFINITION

First described by Larsen in 1950, this syndrome is an inherited disorder of collagen formation that leads to multiple joint dislocations, abnormal facies, spinal abnormalities, and neck instability.

ABNORMALITIES DETECTABLE BY ULTRASOUND

Common Findings:

Hypertelorism

Depressed nasal bridge

Cleft palate

Spinal abnormalities

Dysraphia

Scoliosis

Vertebral abnormalities

Dislocations at the elbows, hips, and knees

Hyperextension at the knees

Club feet

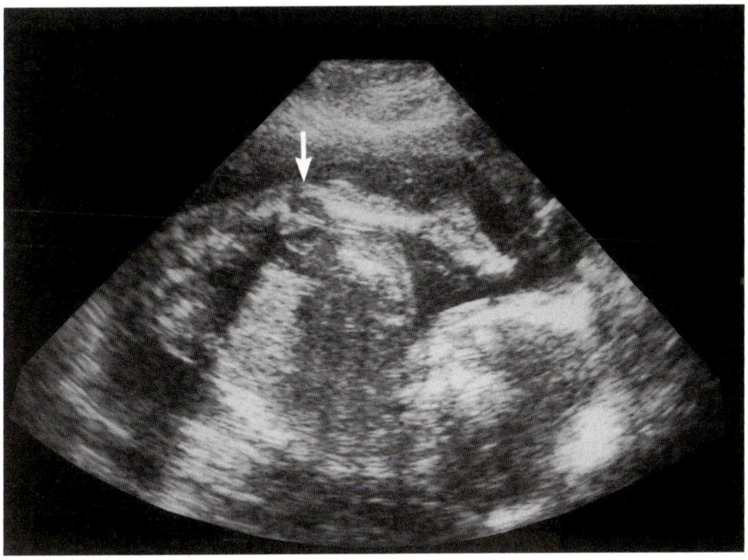

FIGURE 2-93 Longitudinal view of a second-trimester fetus with a deformity of the lower extremity typical of fetuses with Larsen syndrome. Note hyperextension of the fetal lower extremities, with dislocation at the knee *(arrow)*. The fetal feet are in close proximity to the fetal head.

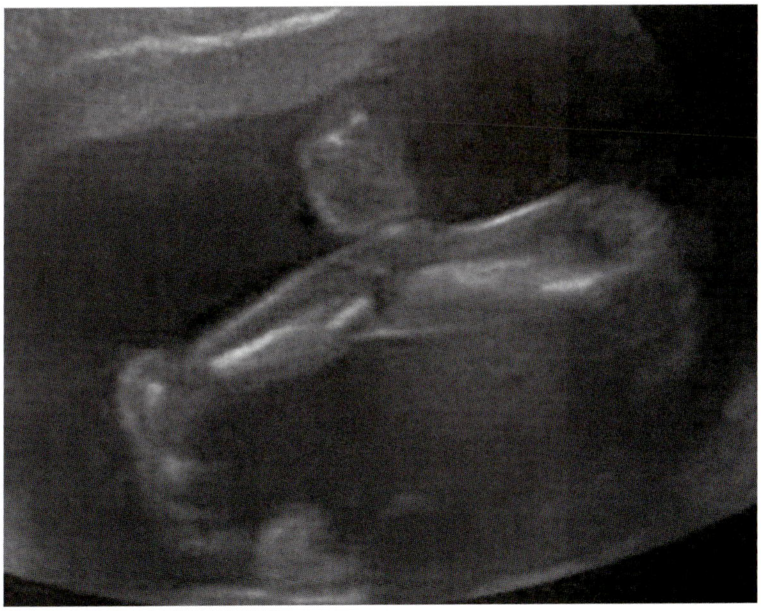

FIGURE 2-94 Longitudinal two-dimensional view of a fetal leg shows hyperextension of the leg at the knee.

Occasional Findings:

Cleft lip

Tracheomalacia

Cardiac defects

MAJOR DIFFERENTIAL DIAGNOSES

Other Syndromes and Conditions Associated with Dislocations and Hyperextensions:

Arthrogryposis multiplex

Pena Shokeir syndrome

Trisomy 18 (Edwards' syndrome)

Other Conditions Associated with Decreased Mobility of the Lower Extremities:

Muscle anomalies

Neurologic anomalies

ULTRASOUND DIAGNOSIS

The diagnosis of Larsen syndrome has been established by transvaginal sonography in a fetus as young as 15 weeks' gestation. Features have included hyperextension of the legs at the knees, moderate micrognathia, right pelvic kidney, single umbilical artery, clinodactyly of the fifth digit, and clubbed feet. Other episodes of prenatal diagnosis include detection of lower limb abnormalities at 20 and 21 weeks in families with previously affected infants. The diagnosis has been made at 28 weeks in a fetus without a family history.

HEREDITY

The origin of Larsen syndrome is unknown, but its pattern of inheritance is autosomal dominant in most cases. However, autosomal recessive inheritance has been suggested in a minority of cases.

NATURAL HISTORY AND OUTCOME

Aggressive orthopedic management and treatment of cervical spine instability and tracheomalacia are often required for individuals with this syndrome.

A rare lethal form of Larsen syndrome also exists. This form of the disorder may be autosomal recessive and includes more severe joint and spinal abnormalities (shortening of the upper limbs, hypoplastic vertebral bodies, multiple joint dislocation, and redundant neck skin). Death occurs as a result of pulmonary hypoplasia.

Suggested Reading

Jones KL: *Smith's recognizable patterns of human malformations,* ed 6. Philadelphia, 2006, Elsevier.

Larsen W, Schottstaedt ER, Bose FC: Multiple congenital dislocation associated with characteristic facial abnormality. *J Pediatr* 37:574, 1950.

Lewit N, Batino S, Groisman GM, Stark H, Bronshtein M: Early prenatal diagnosis of Larsen's syndrome by transvaginal sonography. *J Ultrasound Med* 14:627–629, 1995.

Mostello D, Hoechstetter L, Bendon RW, et al: Prenatal diagnosis of recurrent Larsen syndrome: further definition of a lethal variant. *Prenat Diagn* 11:215–225, 1991.

Rochelson B, Petrikovsky B, Shmoys S: Prenatal diagnosis and obstetric management of Larsen syndrome. *Obstet Gynecol* 81:845–847, 1993.

Shih JC, Peng SS, Hsiao SM, et al: Three-dimensional ultrasound diagnosis of Larsen syndrome with further characterization of neurological sequelae. *Ultrasound Obstet Gynecol* 24:89–93, 2004.

Tongsong T, Wanapirak C, Pongsatha S, Sudasana J: Prenatal sonographic diagnosis of Larsen syndrome. *J Ultrasound Med* 19:419–421, 2000.

MULTIPLE PTERYGIUM SYNDROME (LETHAL TYPE)

DESCRIPTION AND DEFINITION

This condition is characterized by multiple contractures and pterygium (or webbing) across joints, cystic hygromata, and hypoplastic lungs. Some investigators have postulated that the syndrome is caused by abnormalities involving collagen, connective tissue function, lymphatics, and muscle development. Other investigators suggest that it is related to decreased intrauterine movement in early gestation, the cause of which is unknown.

ABNORMALITIES DETECTABLE BY ULTRASOUND

Common Findings:

Flexion contractures of the limbs at all joints

Pterygia involving the cervical, chin area, axillary, antecubital, popliteal, and ankle joints

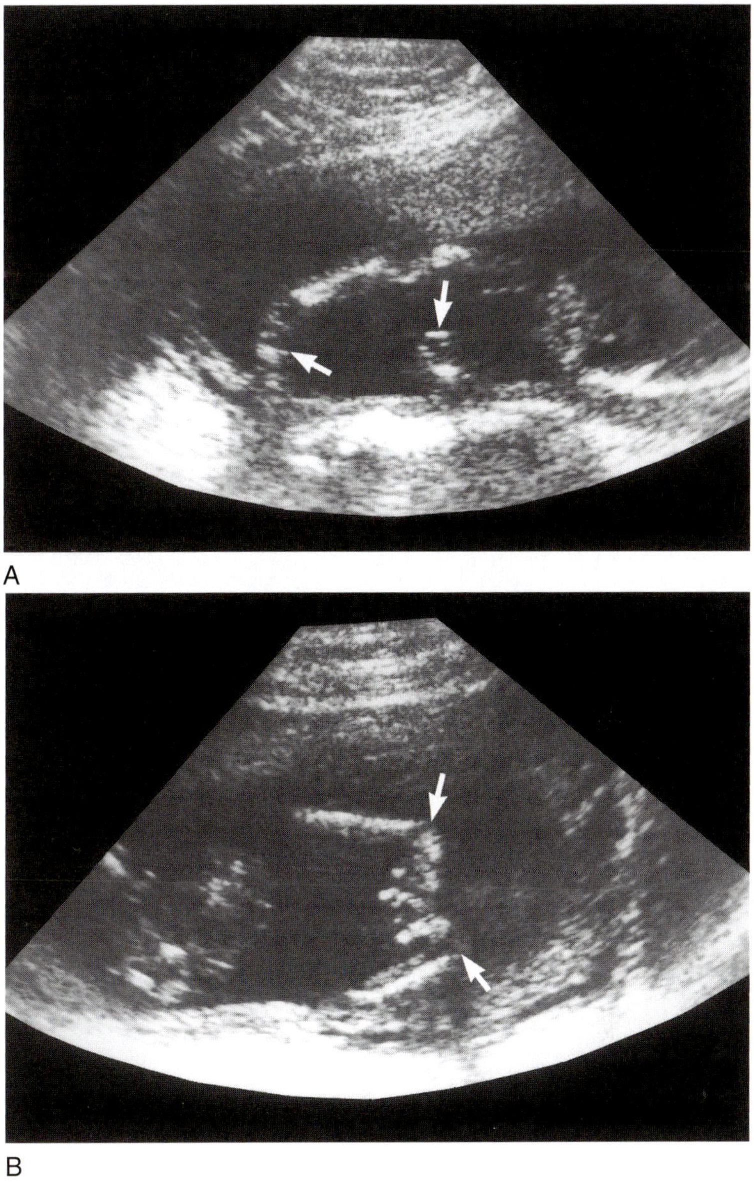

FIGURE 2-95 (**A**) Long-axis view of one of the lower extremities of a second-trimester fetus with multiple pterygium syndrome. Note the clubbed feet *(arrows)*. (**B**) Coronal view through the upper extremities of the same fetus shows marked contractures of the upper extremities at the elbows and wrists *(arrows)*.

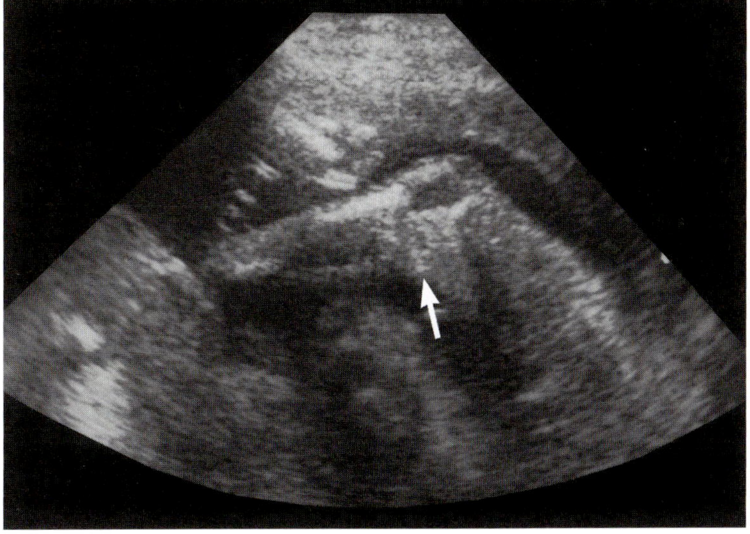

FIGURE 2-96 Long-axis view of a fetal leg shows a contracture at the knee *(arrow)*, as seen in fetuses with multiple pterygium syndrome.

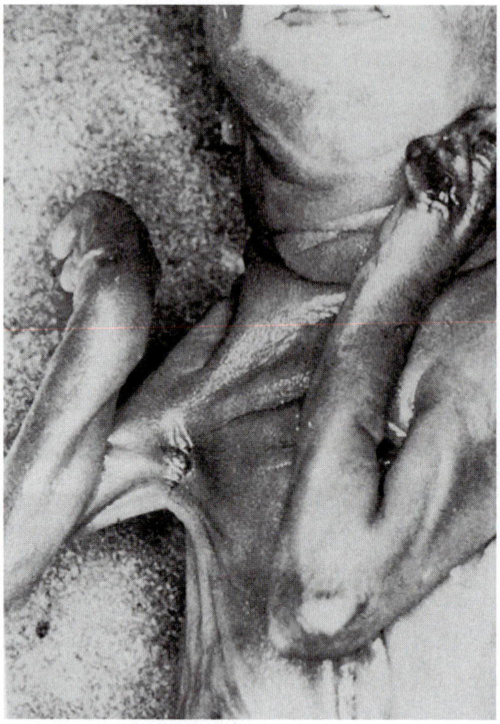

FIGURE 2-97 Axillary pterygia and contractures of the extremities typical of multiple pterygium syndrome. (From Anthony J, Mascarenhas L, O'Brien J, Battachargee AK, Gould S: *Ultrasound Obstet Gynecol* 3:212–216, 1993.)

Neck edema, consistent with cystic hygroma

Micrognathia

Cleft palate

Hypertelorism

Small chest

Polyhydramnios

Hydrops

Occasional Findings:

Cardiac defects

Hydronephrosis

Microcephaly

Ventriculomegaly

Vertebral body abnormalities

MAJOR DIFFERENTIAL DIAGNOSES

Other Syndromes and Conditions Associated with Flexion Contractures of the Extremities:

Amniotic band sequence

Antley-Bixler syndrome

Arthrogryposis multiplex

Caudal regression syndrome

Cerebro-oculo-facio-skeletal (COFS) syndrome

Cornelia de Lange syndrome

Freeman-Sheldon (whistling face) syndrome

Neu-Laxova syndrome

Pena Shokeir syndrome

Roberts' syndrome

Seckel syndrome

Other Conditions Associated with Decreased Mobility of the Lower Extremities:

Muscle anomalies

Neurologic anomalies

Chromosomal Abnormalities:

Triploidy

Trisomy 18 (Edwards' syndrome)

ULTRASOUND DIAGNOSIS

Prenatal ultrasound diagnosis of this syndrome has been established as early as 12 and 16 weeks' gestation, based on the findings of abnormal fetal positioning, particularly of the limbs, and thickened nuchal lucency. Frank cystic hygromata, as well as hydrops, have been seen sonographically starting at 13 weeks in fetuses with this syndrome. Hydrops is commonly seen in affected fetuses.

HEREDITY

The pattern of inheritance for this syndrome is autosomal recessive in most cases, although there have been occasional reports of X-linked inheritance.

NATURAL HISTORY AND OUTCOME

All infants with this disorder die in the neonatal period as a result of pulmonary hypoplasia.

Many fetuses develop hydrops and polyhydramnios. Some fetuses die early in utero, whereas others survive into the third trimester without hydrops, then die at birth.

Suggested Reading

Anthony J, Mascarenhas L, O'Brien J, Battachargee AK, Gould S: Lethal multiple pterygium syndrome. The importance of fetal posture in mid-trimester diagnosis by ultrasound: discussion and case report. *Ultrasound Obstet Gynecol* 3:212–216, 1993.

Chen M, Chan GS, Lee CP, Tang MH: Sonographic features of lethal multiple pterygium syndrome at 14 weeks. *Prenat Diagn* 25:475–478, 2005.

Hartwig NG, Vermeij-Keers C, Bruijn JA, et al: Case of lethal multiple pterygium syndrome with special reference to the origin of pterygia. *Am J Med Genet* 33:537–541, 1989.

Hertzberg BS, Kliewer MA, Paulyson-Nunez K: Lethal multiple pterygium syndrome: antenatal ultrasonographic diagnosis. *J Ultrasound Med* 19:657–660, 2000.

Isaacson G, Gargus JJ, Mahoney MJ: Lethal multiple pterygium syndrome in an 18 week fetus with hydrops. *Am J Med Genet* 17:835–839, 1984.

Izquierdo LA, Castellano TM, Clericuzio CL, et al: Pterygium syndrome, multiple lethal. *Fetus* 3:9–11, 1993.

Lockwood C, Irons M, Troiani J, et al: The prenatal sonographic diagnosis of lethal multiple pterygium syndrome: a heritable cause of recurrent abortion. *Am J Obstet Gynecol* 159:474–476, 1988.

Martin NJ, Hill JB, Cooper DH, O'Brien GD, Masel JP: Lethal multiple pterygium syndrome: three consecutive cases in one family. *Am J Med Genet* 24:295–304, 1986.

Moerman P, Fryns JP, Cornelis A, et al: Pathogenesis of the lethal multiple pterygium syndrome. *Am J Med Genet* 35:415–421, 1990.

Suma V, Marini A, Bellitti F, Serpotta G, Saia R: Pterygium syndrome, multiple lethal. *Fetus* 4:13–16, 1994.

van Regemorter N, Wilkin P, Englert Y, et al: Lethal multiple pterygium syndrome. *Am J Med Genet* 17:827–834, 1984.

Zeitune M, Fejgin MD, Abramowicz J, Ben Aderet N, Goodman RM: Short communication: prenatal diagnosis of the pterygium syndrome. *Prenat Diagn* 8:145–149, 1988.

ROBERTS' SYNDROME

DESCRIPTION AND DEFINITION

Synonym: Pseudothalidomide syndrome

This disorder, which is thought to be the same syndrome as SC phocomelia, is characterized by severe shortening of the limbs and facial anomalies.

ABNORMALITIES DETECTABLE BY ULTRASOUND

Common Findings:

Cleft lip with or without cleft palate

Hypertelorism

Micrognathia

Microcephaly

Severe hypomelia of the limbs (more severe in the upper limbs) with varying degrees of limb reduction involving the humerus, radius, and ulna

Absence or hypoplasia of the humerus, femur, tibia, and fibula

Oligodactyly, syndactyly

Flexion contractures of all the joints of the extremities

IUGR

Cryptorchidism

Occasional Findings:

Encephalocele

Ventriculomegaly

Craniosynostosis

Microphthalmia

Cataract

Cardiac abnormality

Renal abnormality

Abnormal genitalia

Cystic hygromata

Polyhydramnios

MAJOR DIFFERENTIAL DIAGNOSES

Amniotic band sequence

Ectrodactyly–ectodermal dysplasia–clefting (EEC) syndrome

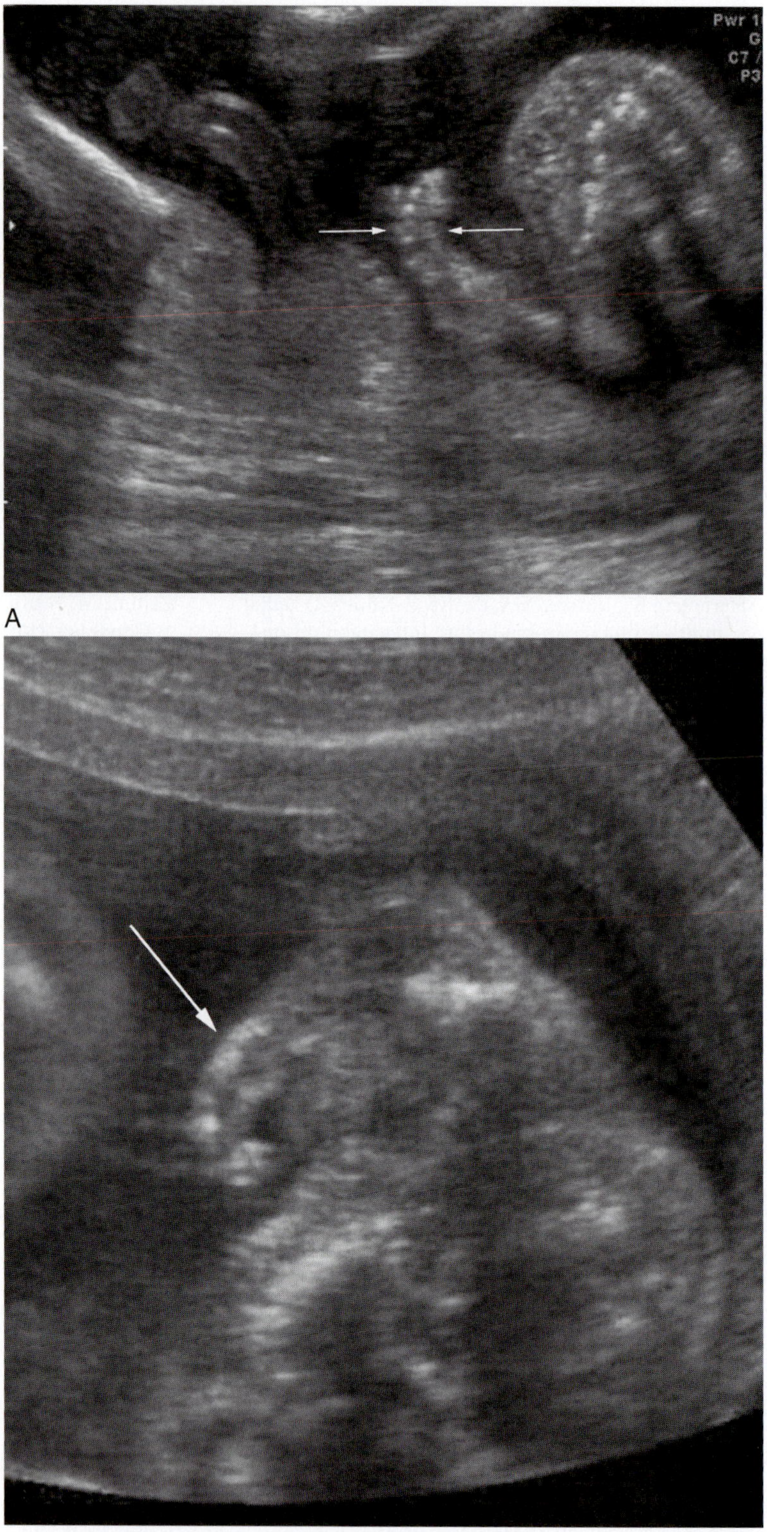

FIGURE 2-98 (A) Longitudinal view of the fetal arm showing marked shortening of the entire arm and a few digits on the end of a very short upper extremity *(arrows)*. (B) Same upper extremity shows the hand *(arrow)* essentially attached to the fetal shoulder. This type of deformity is common in fetuses with Roberts' syndrome.

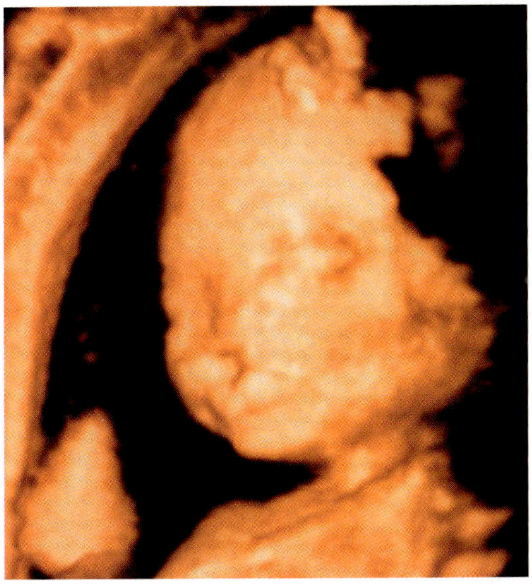

FIGURE 2-99 Surface rendering of the fetal face of a second-trimester fetus with a severe facial cleft.

Fanconi anemia

Femoral hypoplasia–unusual facies syndrome

Femur–fibula–ulna (FFU) syndrome

Holt-Oram syndrome

Nager syndrome

Oral-facial-digital (Mohr) syndrome

Thrombocytopenia–absent radius (TAR) syndrome

VATER (**v**ertebral defects, **a**nal atresia, **t**racheoesophageal fistula, **e**sophageal atresia, and **r**adial and renal dysplasias) association

ULTRASOUND DIAGNOSIS

This syndrome is associated with multiple congenital abnormalities that are detectable sonographically beginning in the late first trimester. On the basis of limb and facial abnormalities demonstrated by transvaginal sonography, a prenatal sonographic diagnosis has been established in several cases as early as 12 weeks' gestation. Cystic hygromata and polyhydramnios are among the sonographically detectable features of this syndrome.

The diagnosis also can be established by chorionic villus sampling or amniocentesis based on premature separation of the centromeric heterochromatin of some chromosomes. Such DNA evaluation is useful in families known to be at risk for this disorder.

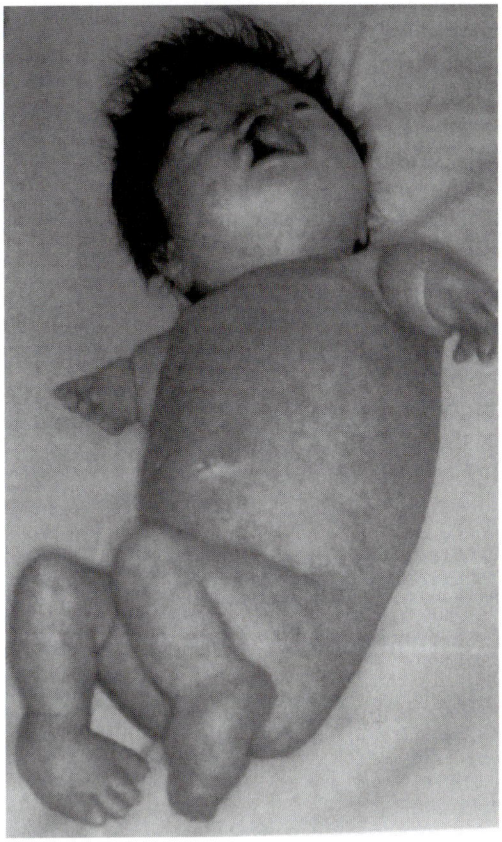

FIGURE 2-100 Postnatal photograph of a neonate with the typical features of Roberts' syndrome, including tetraphocomelia with absence of the forearms, club foot, microcephaly, hypertelorism, and facial cleft. (From Benzacken B, Savary JB, Manouvrier S, Bucourt M, Gonzales J: *Prenat Diagn* 16:125–130, 1996.)

HEREDITY

This syndrome has an autosomal recessive inheritance pattern with variable penetrance. Roberts' syndrome and SC phocomelia are most likely part of a spectrum, representing variable severities of the same disorder.

NATURAL HISTORY AND OUTCOME

Many individuals with this syndrome are stillborn or die in infancy. Those who survive have severe mental retardation and growth deficiency.

Suggested Reading

Benzacken B, Savary JB, Manouvrier S, Bucourt M, Gonzales J: Prenatal diagnosis of Roberts syndrome: two new cases. *Prenat Diagn* 16:125–130, 1996.

Freeman MVR, Williams DW, Schimke RN, Temtamy SA: The Roberts syndrome. *Clin Genet* 5:1–16, 1974.

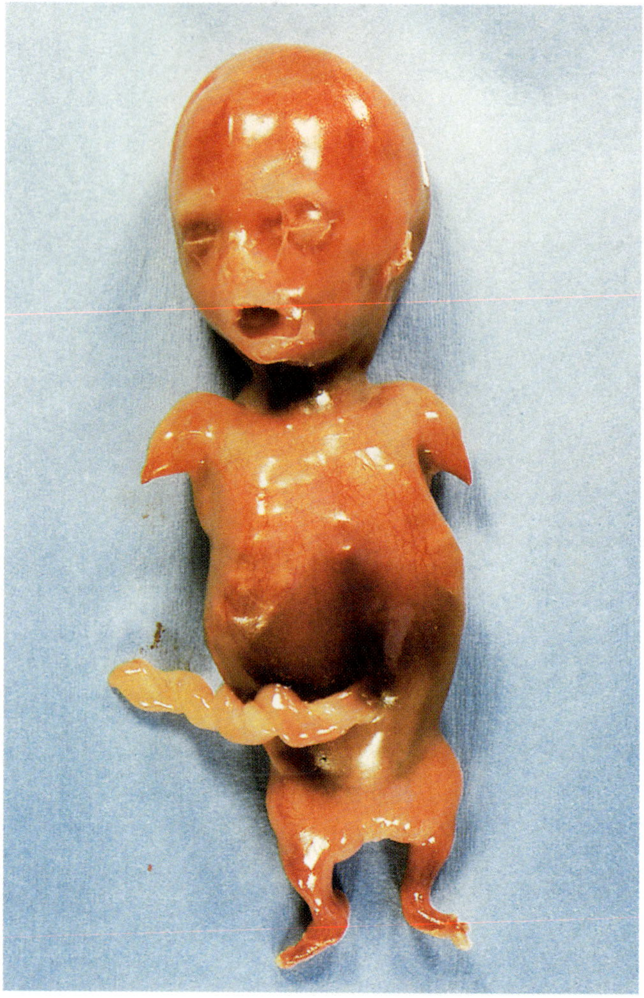

FIGURE 2-101 Pathology specimen of a fetus with Roberts' syndrome shows severe limb defects. (From Keeling JW: *Fetal pathology*. London, 1994, Churchill Livingstone.)

Herrmann J, Feingold M, Tuffli GA, Opitz JM: A familial dysmorphogenetic syndrome of limb deformities, characteristic facial appearance and associated anomalies: the "pseudothalidomide" or "SC syndrome." *Birth Defects Orig Art Series* 5:81–89, 1969.

Jones KL: *Smith's recognizable patterns of human malformations,* ed 6. Philadelphia, 2006, Elsevier.

Paladini D, Palmieri S, Lecora M, et al: Prenatal ultrasound diagnosis of Roberts syndrome in a family with negative history. *Ultrasound Gynecol* 7:208–210, 1996.

Roberts JB: A child with double cleft of lip and palate, protrusion of the intermaxillary portion of the upper jaw and imperfect development of the bones of the four extremities. *Ann Surg* 70:252–254, 1919.

Stioui S, Privitera O, Brambati B, et al: First-trimester prenatal diagnosis of Roberts syndrome (short communication). *Prenat Diagn* 12:145–149, 1992.

Trombly JF, Yeomans ER, Lester JW: Diagnosis of phocomelia by transvaginal sonography. *J Ultrasound Med* 11:309–311, 1992.

Van Den Berg DJ, Francke U: Roberts syndrome: a review of 100 cases and a new rating system for severity. *Am J Med Genet* 47:1104–1123, 1993.

Waldenmaier C, Aldenhoff P, Klemm T: Roberts syndrome. *Hum Genet* 40:345–349, 1978.

THROMBOCYTOPENIA–ABSENT RADIUS (TAR) SYNDROME

DESCRIPTION AND DEFINITION

This is an autosomal recessive syndrome characterized by radial aplasia and thrombocytopenia.

ABNORMALITIES DETECTABLE BY ULTRASOUND

Common Findings:

Bilateral absence of the radius, with hypoplasia or absence of the ulna

Thumbs present (invariably)

Abnormal humerus

Abnormalities of the lower extremities, including dislocations and absence of the fibulae (50%)

Occasional Findings:

Cleft palate

Micrognathia

Vermian hypoplasia

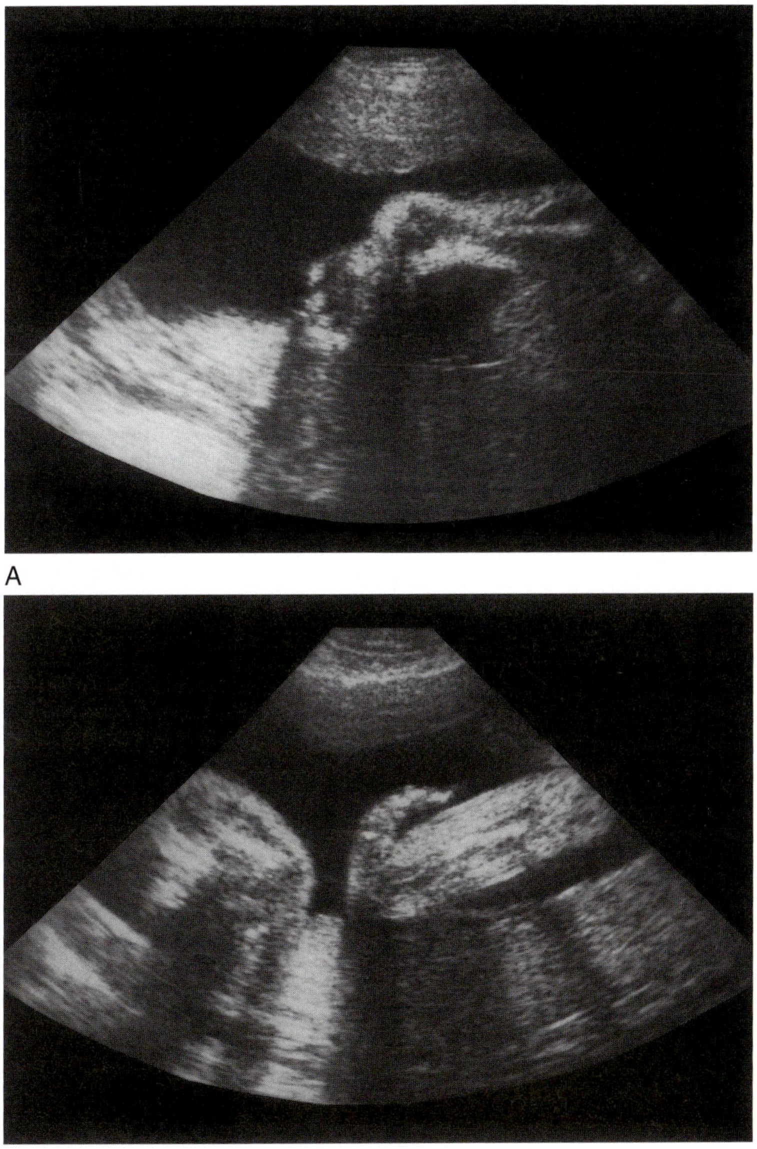

A

B

FIGURE 2-102 (A, B) Long-axis views of both extremities in a late second-trimester fetus with thrombocytopenia–absent radius (TAR) syndrome reveal a foreshortened lower arm. Note that the elbow and hand are in close proximity to each other.

Congenital cardiac defects, primarily tetralogy of Fallot and atrial septal defects

Renal anomalies

MAJOR DIFFERENTIAL DIAGNOSES

Cornelia de Lange syndrome

Fanconi anemia

Holt-Oram syndrome

Nager syndrome (acrofacial dysostosis)

Radial aplasia

Roberts' syndrome

Trisomy 13 (Patau syndrome)

Trisomy 18 (Edwards' syndrome)

VATER (**v**ertebral defects, **a**nal atresia, **t**racheo-esophageal fistula, **e**sophageal atresia, and **r**adial and renal dysplasias) association

ULTRASOUND DIAGNOSIS

The prenatal diagnosis of TAR syndrome has been established in many cases and is possible in the early second trimester. The diagnosis of this syndrome is based largely on the finding of upper extremity skeletal abnormalities.

The diagnosis of thrombocytopenia can be confirmed by umbilical blood sampling before delivery, in case a transfusion of platelets is necessary.

HEREDITY

The syndrome has an autosomal recessive pattern of inheritance.

NATURAL HISTORY AND OUTCOME

In the past, many affected individuals died from complications of thrombocytopenia and hemorrhage. Currently, however, particularly when a prenatal diagnosis is established, platelet transfusion is used to prevent perinatal hemorrhage, thus improving prognosis. Thrombocytopenia usually is present in early infancy and becomes less profound with age. Other abnormalities, such as orthopedic and cardiac anomalies, must be treated.

Suggested Reading

Bellver J, Lara C, Perez-Aytes A, Pellicer A, Remohi J, Serra V: First-trimester diagnosis of thrombocytopenia-absent radius (TAR) syndrome in a triplet pregnancy. *Prenat Diagn* 25:332–334, 2005.

Boute O, Depret-Mosser S, Vinatier D, et al: Prenatal diagnosis of thrombocytopenia–absent radius syndrome. *Fetal Diagn Ther* 11:224–230, 1996.

Donnenfeld AE, Wiseman B, Lavi E, Weiner S: Prenatal diagnosis of thrombocytopenia–absent radius syndrome by ultrasound and cordocentesis. *Prenat Diagn* 10:29–35, 1990.

Filkins K, Russo J: Prenatal diagnosis of thrombocytopenia–absent radius syndrome using ultrasound and fetoscopy. *Prenat Diagn* 4:139–142, 1984.

Hedberg VA, Lipton JM: Thrombocytopenia with absent radii: a review of 100 cases. *Am J Pediatr Hematol Oncol* 10:51–64, 1988.

Homans AC, Cohen JL, Mazur EM: Defective megakaryocytopoiesis in the syndrome of thrombocytopenia with absent radii. *Br J Haematol* 70:205–210, 1988.

Jones KL: *Smith's recognizable patterns of human malformations,* ed 6. Philadelphia, 2006, Elsevier.

Labrune PH, Pons JC, Khalil M, et al: Antenatal thrombocytopenia in three patients with TAR (thrombocytopenia with absent radii) syndrome. *Prenat Diagn* 13:463–466, 1993.

Luthy DA, Hall JG, Graham CB: Prenatal diagnosis of thrombocytopenia with absent radii. *Clin Genet* 15:495–499, 1979.

Luthy DA, Mack L, Hirsch J, Cheng E: Prenatal ultrasound diagnosis of thrombocytopenia with absent radii. *Am J Obstet Gynecol* 141:350–351, 1981.

Ray R, Zorn E, Kelly T, Hall JG, Sommer A: Lower limb anomalies in the thrombocytopenia–absent radius (TAR) syndrome. *Am J Med Genet* 7:523–528, 1980.

Shelton SD, Paulyson K, Kay HH: Prenatal diagnosis of thrombocytopenia absent radius (TAR) syndrome and vaginal delivery. *Prenat Diagn* 19:54-57, 1999.

Tongsong T, Sirichotiyakul S, Chanprapaph P: Prenatal diagnosis of thrombocytopenia-absent-radius (TAR) syndrome. *Ultrasound Obstet Gynecol* 15:256–258, 2000.

Skeletal Dysplasias

ACHONDROGENESIS

DESCRIPTION AND DEFINITION

Achondrogenesis is a lethal skeletal dysplasia characterized by extreme hypoplasia of the bones, resulting in marked micromelia, disproportionately large calvaria, and decreased bone ossification. Types IA and IB are distinguished histopathologically and previously were known as the Parenti-Fraccaro type. Type II is the Langer-Saldino type and represents a spectrum of the disorder that now includes hypochondrogenesis and may have longer limbs.

ABNORMALITIES DETECTABLE BY ULTRASOUND

Type IA and IB Achondrogenesis:

Gross, severe shortening of the limbs

Short, flared ribs

Poorly ossified iliac bones, spine, and skull

Enlarged head

Micrognathia

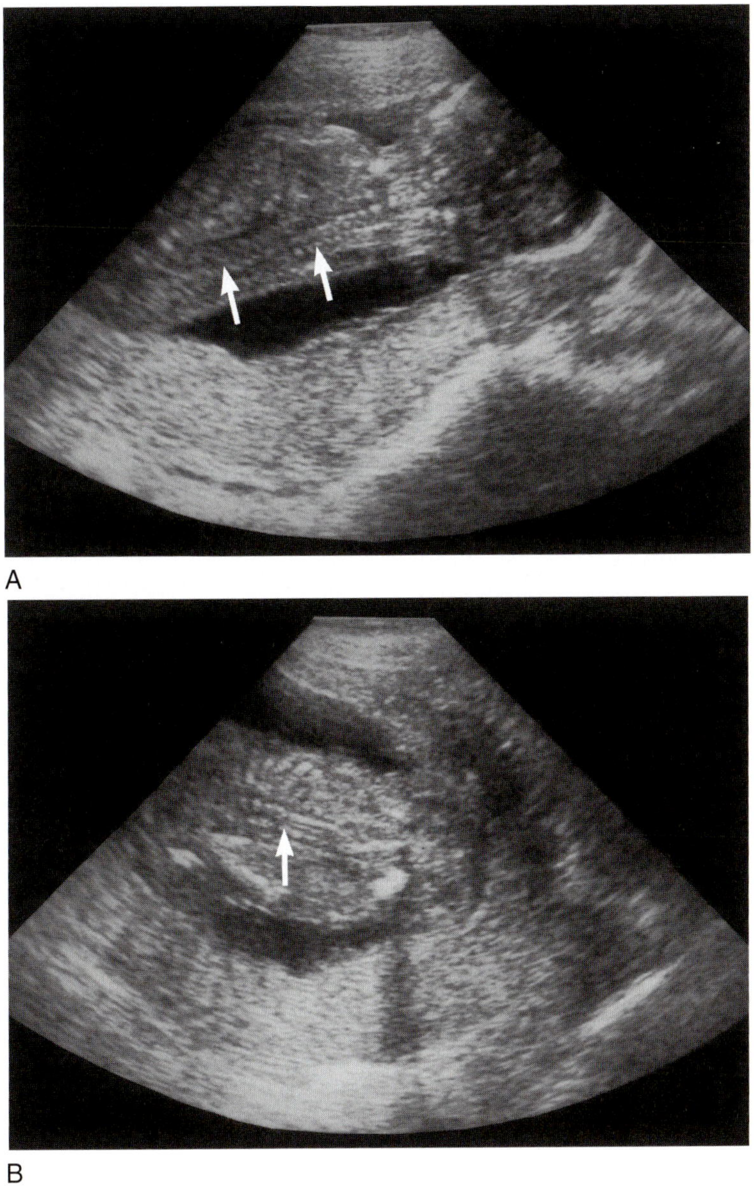

FIGURE 2-103 Longitudinal (A) and coronal (B) views of a fetus with achondrogenesis, type I. Note severe hypomineralization of the spine *(arrows)* and short limbs.

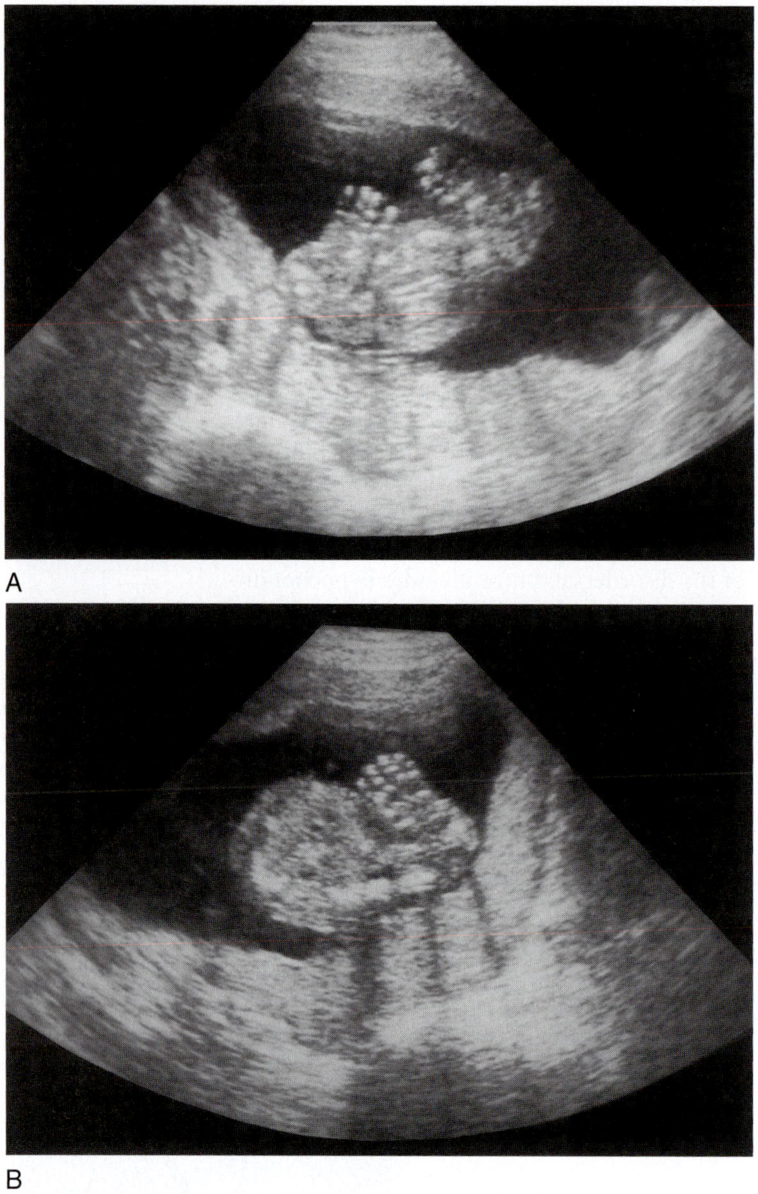

FIGURE 2-104 Long-axis (A) and short-axis (B) views of the upper extremities in the same fetus as in Figure 2-103 reveal marked foreshortening of the long bones with severe deformity of the bones.

Polyhydramnios

Hydrops

Type II (Langer-Saldino) Achondrogenesis (Features As Listed Above, with the Following Exceptions)

Relatively normal skull ossification

Enlarged head

More variable limb shortening from very short to near normal

Characteristic absence of spine ossification

MAJOR DIFFERENTIAL DIAGNOSES

Syndromes and Conditions Associated with Poorly Ossified Bones and Short Limbs:

Atelosteogenesis

Hypophosphatasia

Osteogenesis imperfecta

ULTRASOUND DIAGNOSIS

The diagnosis of this disorder has been established by several investigators at 12 to 14 weeks' gestation, based on thickened nuchal lucency

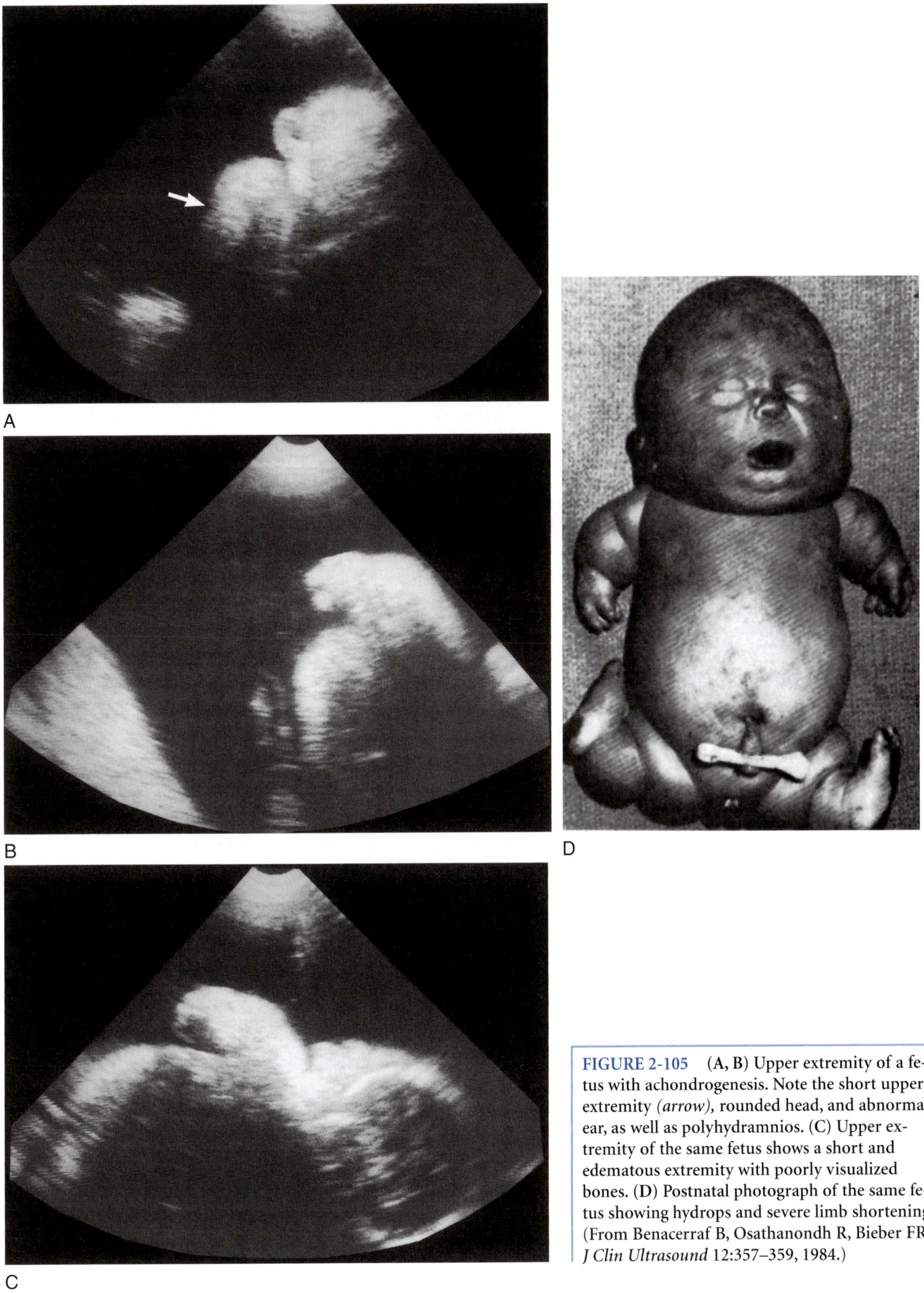

FIGURE 2-105 (**A, B**) Upper extremity of a fetus with achondrogenesis. Note the short upper extremity *(arrow)*, rounded head, and abnormal ear, as well as polyhydramnios. (**C**) Upper extremity of the same fetus shows a short and edematous extremity with poorly visualized bones. (**D**) Postnatal photograph of the same fetus showing hydrops and severe limb shortening. (From Benacerraf B, Osathanondh R, Bieber FR: *J Clin Ultrasound* 12:357–359, 1984.)

and early detection of abnormal limb formation and movement. Even early in development, the lack of ossification of the spine, severe shortening of the limbs, large skull, and occasional cystic hygroma with hydrops are recognizable characteristics.

HEREDITY

Type I achondrogenesis (A and B) has an autosomal recessive pattern of inheritance. Although the gene locus for type IA is unknown, the gene locus for type IB is the same (located on 5q) as for other forms of skeletal dysplasias, including diastrophic dysplasia, atelosteogenesis type II, and multiple epiphyseal dysplasia.

Achondrogenesis type II occurs sporadically and is thought to involve an abnormality in the gene that encodes type II collagen (COL2A1). This indicates a likely autosomal dominant inheritance for this disorder but with a new mutation, because affected individuals do not live to reproduce. Other conditions also thought to involve anomalies of the same gene include spondyloepimetaphyseal dysplasia, Kniest syndrome, spondyloepiphyseal dysplasia congenita, and Stickler syndrome.

NATURAL HISTORY AND OUTCOME

Achondrogenesis is characterized by lack of cartilaginous matrix formation. Achondrogenesis is a lethal condition. Infants with this disorder either are stillborn or die within 24 hours of birth as a result of pulmonary hypoplasia.

Suggested Reading

Benacerraf B, Osathanondh R, Bieber FR: Achondrogenesis type I: ultrasound diagnosis in utero. *J Clin Ultrasound* 12:357–359, 1984.

Fisk NM, Vaughan J, Smidt M, Wigglesworth J: Transvaginal ultrasound recognition of nuchal edema in the first-trimester diagnosis of achondrogenesis. *J Clin Ultrasound* 19:586–590, 1991.

Glenn LW, Teng SSK: In utero sonographic diagnosis of achondrogenesis. *J Clin Ultrasound* 13:195–198, 1985.

Goncalves L, Jeanty P: Fetal biometry of skeletal dysplasias: a multicentric study. *J Ultrasound Med* 13:767–775, 1994.

Gordienko IY, Grechanina EY, Sopko NI, Tarapurova EN, Mikchailets LP: Prenatal diagnosis of osteochondrodysplasias in high risk pregnancy. *Am J Med Genet* 63:90–97, 1996.

Graham D, Tracey J, Winn K, Corson V, Sanders RC: Early second trimester sonographic diagnosis of achondrogenesis. *J Clin Ultrasound* 11:336–338, 1983.

Jaeger HJ, Schmitz-Stolbrink A, Hulde J, et al: The boneless neonate: a severe form of achondrogenesis type I. *Pediatr Radiol* 24:319–321, 1994.

Johnson VP, Yiu-Chiu VS, Wierda DR, Holzwarth DR: Midtrimester prenatal diagnosis of achondrogenesis. *J Ultrasound Med* 3:223–226, 1984.

Jones KL: *Smith's recognizable patterns of human malformations,* ed 6. Philadelphia, Elsevier, 2006.

Knowlton S, Graves C, Tiller GE, Jeanty P: Achondrogenesis. *Fetus* 2:13–18, 1992.

Kocakoc E, Kiris A: Achondrogenesis type II with normally developed extremities: a case report. *Prenat Diagn* 22:594–597, 2002.

Krakow D, Williams J 3rd, Poehl M, Rimoin DL, Platt LD: Use of three-dimensional ultrasound imaging in the diagnosis of prenatal-onset skeletal dysplasias. *Ultrasound Obstet Gynecol* 21:467–472, 2003.

Mahony BS, Filly RA, Cooperberg PL: Antenatal sonographic diagnosis of achondrogenesis. *J Ultrasound Med* 3:333–335, 1984.

Meizner I, Barnhard Y: Achondrogenesis type I diagnosed by transvaginal ultrasonography at 13 weeks' gestation. *Am J Obstet Gynecol* 173:1620–1622, 1995.

Ozeren S, Yuksel A, Tukel T: Prenatal sonographic diagnosis of type I achondrogenesis with a large cystic hygroma. *Ultrasound Obstet Gynecol* 13:75–76, 1999.

Pretorius DH, Rumack CM, Manco-Johnson ML, et al: Specific skeletal dysplasias in utero: sonographic diagnosis. *Radiology* 159:237–242, 1986.

Seperti-Furga A, Hastbacka J, Wilcox WR, et al: Achondrogenesis type IB is caused by mutations in the diastrophic dysplasia sulfate transporter gene. *Nat Genet* 12:100–102, 1996.

Sharony R, Browne C, Lachman RS, Rimoin DL: Prenatal diagnosis of the skeletal dysplasias. *Am J Obstet Gynecol* 169:668–675, 1993.

Smith WL, Brettweiser D, Dinno N: In utero diagnosis of achondrogenesis, type I. *Clin Genet* 19:51–54, 1981.

Soothill PW, Vuthiwong C, Rees H: Achondrogenesis type 2 diagnosed by transvaginal ultrasound at 12 weeks' gestation. *Prenat Diagn* 13:523–528, 1993.

Tennstedt C, Bartho S, Bollmann R, et al: Osteochondrodysplasias. Prenatal diagnosis and pathological-anatomic findings. *Zentralbl Pathol* 139:71–80, 1993.

Wasant P, Waeteekul S, Rimoin DL, Lachman RS: Genetic skeletal dysplasia in Thailand: the Siriraj experience. *SE Asian J Trop Med Publ Health* 1:59–67, 1995.

Wladimiroff JW, Niermeijer MF, Laar J, Jahoda M, Stewart PA: Prenatal diagnosis of skeletal dysplasia by real-time ultrasound. *Obstet Gynecol* 63:360–364, 1984.

Won HS, Yoo HK, Lee PR, et al: A case of achondrogenesis type II associated with huge cystic hygroma: prenatal diagnosis by ultrasonography. *Ultrasound Obstet Gynecol* 14:288–290, 1999.

ACHONDROPLASIA

DESCRIPTION AND DEFINITION

This is the most common chondrodysplasia. Characterized by rhizomelic limb shortening, it is lethal when homozygous and nonlethal when heterozygous.

ABNORMALITIES DETECTABLE BY ULTRASOUND

Common Findings:

Homozygous achondroplasia: The more severe form of the disease resembles thanatophoric dysplasia; characterized by thoracic constriction and long-bone shortening in the early second trimester.

Heterozygous achondroplasia: Usually associated with normal sonograms until after the second trimester. Long-bone shortening becomes apparent after 22 to 24 weeks' gestation. Features of this disorder are most notable in the third trimester and include:

Megalocephaly

Low nasal bridge

Frontal bossing

Mildly to moderately shortened femur and humerus

Short, trident-like hand with fingers of similar lengths

Accentuated lumbar lordosis

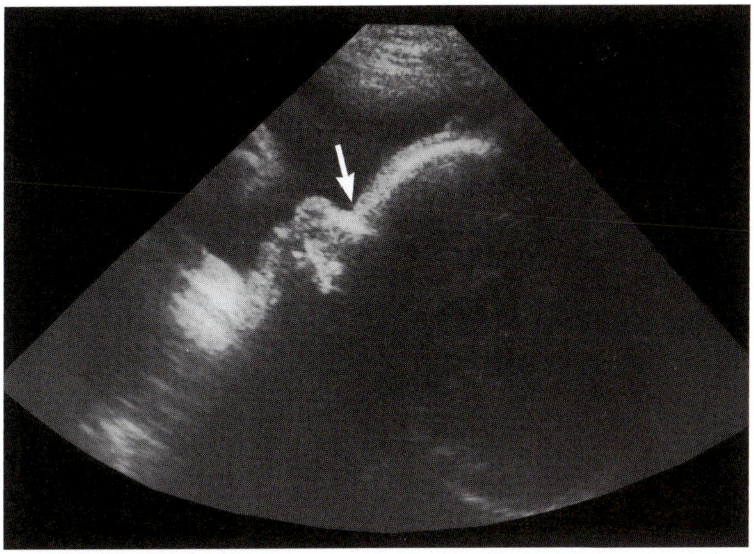

FIGURE 2-106 Profile view of a fetus with achondroplasia reveals marked frontal bossing and a depressed nasal bridge *(arrow)*.

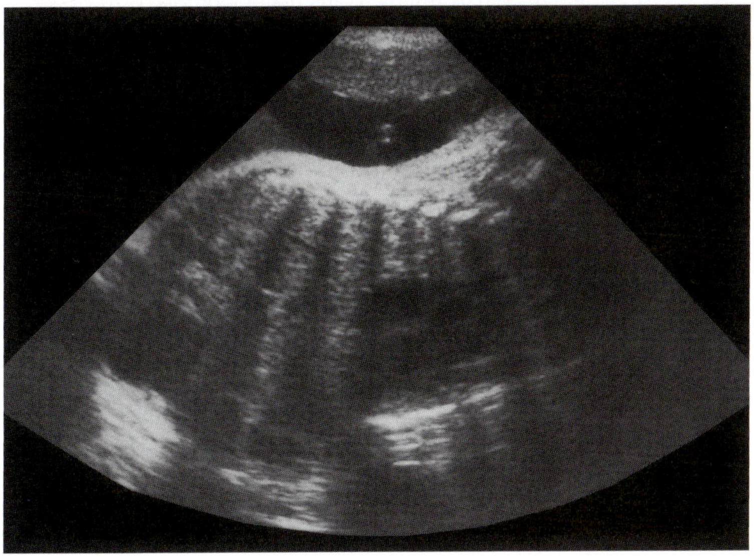

FIGURE 2-107 Coronal view of the fetal chest shows no evidence of thoracic narrowing in this fetus.

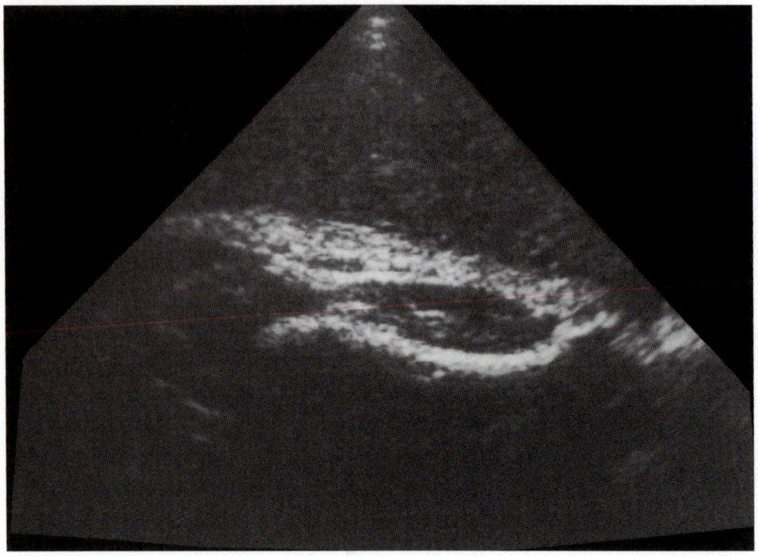

FIGURE 2-108 Long-axis view of the fetal femur shows an unusual configuration of the femur, with some bowing. The length of the femur lagged 6 weeks behind that expected for dates.

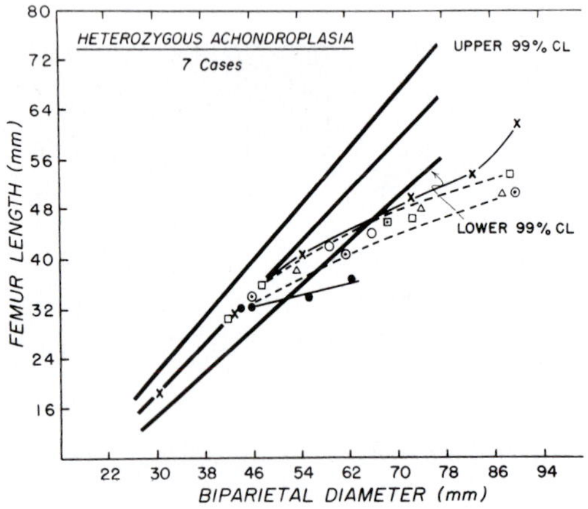

FIGURE 2-109 Length of the femora in seven fetuses with heterozygous achondroplasia, compared with the biparietal diameters and femur lengths in normal fetuses. Note that the femur length in fetuses with heterozygous achondroplasia is normal until the biparietal diameter has reached at least 54 mm, when the growth curves representing the femora flatten in affected cases. (From Kurtz AB, Filly RA, Wapner RJ: *J Ultrasound Med* 5:137–140, 1986.)

Occasional Findings:

Mild ventriculomegaly

Thickened nuchal translucency reported in first trimester (one report)

MAJOR DIFFERENTIAL DIAGNOSES

Other Skeletal Dysplasias with Late Sonographic Manifestations or Nonskeletal Dysplasias Associated with Mildly Short Femurs:

Asymmetric growth restriction

Down syndrome

Hypochondroplasia

Kniest syndrome

Russell-Silver syndrome

Shprintzen syndrome

Spondyloepiphyseal dysplasia

XO (Turner) syndrome

ULTRASOUND DIAGNOSIS

The earliest prenatal sonographic diagnosis of *homozygous achondroplasia* is at 13 weeks' gestation, although in most cases the diagnosis is easily established by 15 weeks' gestational age because of the discrepancy between biparietal diameter and femoral length.

Heterozygous achondroplasia usually is associated with a normal second-trimester ultrasound. Occasionally, biometry becomes abnormal as early as 20 weeks' gestation but in many cases not until after 22 weeks. Fetuses known to be at risk must be monitored by sonograms into the late second trimester before normalcy can be confirmed. Interval growth, measured between two scans, is helpful in evaluating skeletal growth in fetuses at risk. In seven cases of heterozygous achondroplasia reported by Kurtz et al., the gestational age at the time of sonographic diagnosis varied between 21 and 27 weeks.

Facial features of heterozygous achondroplasia are visible sonographically and include frontal bossing and an abnormally low nasal bridge. Some fetuses have mild ventriculomegaly and macrocephaly, with a biparietal diameter larger than expected for gestational age.

There is a single report of achondroplasia in which the first sonographic finding was a thickened nuchal translucency. A karyotype by chorionic villus sampling was normal, but follow-up ultrasound was suspicious for limb shortening below 2 standard deviations at 18 weeks. A G380R mutation was found in the locus gene encoding for the fibroblast growth factor receptor 3 (FGFR3) on chromosome 4p16.3 using villi obtained at chorionic villus sampling.

HEREDITY

The pattern of inheritance for achondroplasia is autosomal dominant, although a fresh mutation is suspected in 80% to 90% of cases. Older paternal age has been implicated in some cases. The gene responsible for the abnormality maps to 4p16.3 and represents a mutation in the FGFR3 gene.

Nonmutational homozygous achondroplasia usually arises in families in which both parents are heterozygous for the disorder.

NATURAL HISTORY AND OUTCOME

Homozygous achondroplasia is a lethal condition. Infants with heterozygous achondroplasia generally survive and exhibit normal intelligence. However, they tend to have health problems associated with stenosis of the spinal canal, kyphosis, spinal disk abnormalities, and occasional spinal cord compression. Orthopedic and neurosurgical intervention is sometimes required to treat these conditions.

Suggested Reading

Bellus GA, Escallon CS, Ortiz de Luna RO, et al: First-trimester prenatal diagnosis in a couple at risk for homozygous achondroplasia. *Lancet* 344:1511–1512, 1994.

Cordone M, Lituania M, Bocchino G, et al: Ultrasonographic features in a case of heterozygous achondroplasia at 25 weeks' gestation. *Prenat Diagn* 13:395–401, 1993.

Francomano CA, Ortiz de Luna RI, Hefferon TW, et al: Localization of the achondroplasia gene to the distal 2.5 Mb of human chromosome 4p. *Hum Mol Genet* 3:787–792, 1994.

Francomano CA, Pyeritz RE: Achondroplasia is not caused by mutation in the gene for type II collagen. *Am J Med Genet* 29:955–961, 1988.

Goncalves L, Jeanty P: Fetal biometry of skeletal dysplasias: a multicentric study. *J Ultrasound Med* 13:977–985, 1994.

Guzman ER, Day-Salvatore D, Westover T, et al: Prenatal ultrasonographic demonstration of the trident hand in heterozygous achondroplasia. *J Ultrasound Med* 13:63–66, 1994.

Hall JG: The natural history of achondroplasia. In Nicoletti B, Kopits SE, Ascani E, McKusick VA, editors: *Human achondroplasia: a multidisciplinary approach.* New York, Plenum Press, 1988.

Hall JG, Golbus MS, Graham CB, et al: Failure of early prenatal diagnosis in classic achondroplasia. *Am J Med Genet* 3:371–375, 1979.

Krakow D, Williams J 3rd, Poehl M, Rimoin DL, Platt LD: Use of three-dimensional ultrasound imaging in the diagnosis of prenatal-onset skeletal dysplasias. *Ultrasound Obstet Gynecol* 21:467–472, 2003.

Kurtz AB, Filly RA, Wapner RJ, et al: In utero analysis of heterozygous achondroplasia: variable time of onset as detected by femur length measurements. *J Ultrasound Med* 5:137–140, 1986.

Parilla BV, Leeth EA, Kambich MP, Chilis P, MacGregor SN: Antenatal detection of skeletal dysplasias. *J Ultrasound Med* 22:255–228, 2003.

Patel MD, Filly RA: Homozygous achondroplasia: US distinction between homozygous, heterozygous, and unaffected fetuses in the second trimester. *Radiology* 196:541–545, 1995.

Pretorius DH, Rumack CM, Manco-Johnson ML, et al: Specific skeletal dysplasias in utero: sonographic diagnosis. *Radiology* 159:237–242, 1986.

Rousseau F, Bonaventure J, Legeai-Mallet L, et al: Mutations in the gene encoding fibroblast growth factor receptor-3 in achondroplasia. *Nature* 371:252–254, 1994.

Ruano R, Molho M, Roume J, Ville Y: Prenatal diagnosis of fetal skeletal dysplasias by combining two-dimensional and three-dimensional ultrasound and intrauterine three-dimensional helical computer tomography. *Ultrasound Obstet Gynecol* 24:134–140, 2004.

Sharony R, Browne C, Lachman RS, Rimoin DL: Prenatal diagnosis of the skeletal dysplasias. *Am J Obstet Gynecol* 169:668–675, 1993.

Shiang R, Thompson LM, Zhu YZ, et al: Mutations in the transmembrane domain of FGFR3 cause the most common genetic form of dwarfism, achondroplasia. *Cell* 78:335–342, 1994.

Sukcharoen N: Sonographic prenatal diagnosis of heterozygous achondroplasia: a case report. *J Med Assoc Thailand* 77:549–553, 1994.

Tonni G, Ventura A, De Felice C: First trimester increased nuchal translucency associated with fetal achondroplasia. *Am J Perinatol* 22:145–148, 2005.

Wasant P, Waeteekul S, Rimoin DL, Lachman RS: Genetic skeletal dysplasia in Thailand: the Siriraj experience. *SE Asian J Trop Med Publ Health* 1:59–67, 1995.

ATELOSTEOGENESIS, TYPE I

DESCRIPTION AND DEFINITION

Synonym: Spondylohumerofemoral hypoplasia

This lethal chondrodysplasia is characterized by severe limb shortening and deficient ossification of bones, resulting in micromelic dwarfism.

ABNORMALITIES DETECTABLE BY ULTRASOUND

Depressed nasal bridge

Hypertelorism

Micrognathia

Abnormal vertebral bodies

Thoracic platyspondyly with coronal clefts

Narrow thoracic cage

Gross shortening of all limbs (deficient ossification)

Markedly foreshortened or absent humeri and femora

Proximal flaring of the humerus and femur

Bowed radius, ulna, and tibia

Absent fibula

Club feet

Polyhydramnios

MAJOR DIFFERENTIAL DIAGNOSES

Other Skeletal Dysplasias Associated with Micromelia and Reduced Ossification:

Achondrogenesis

Hypophosphatasia

Osteogenesis imperfecta

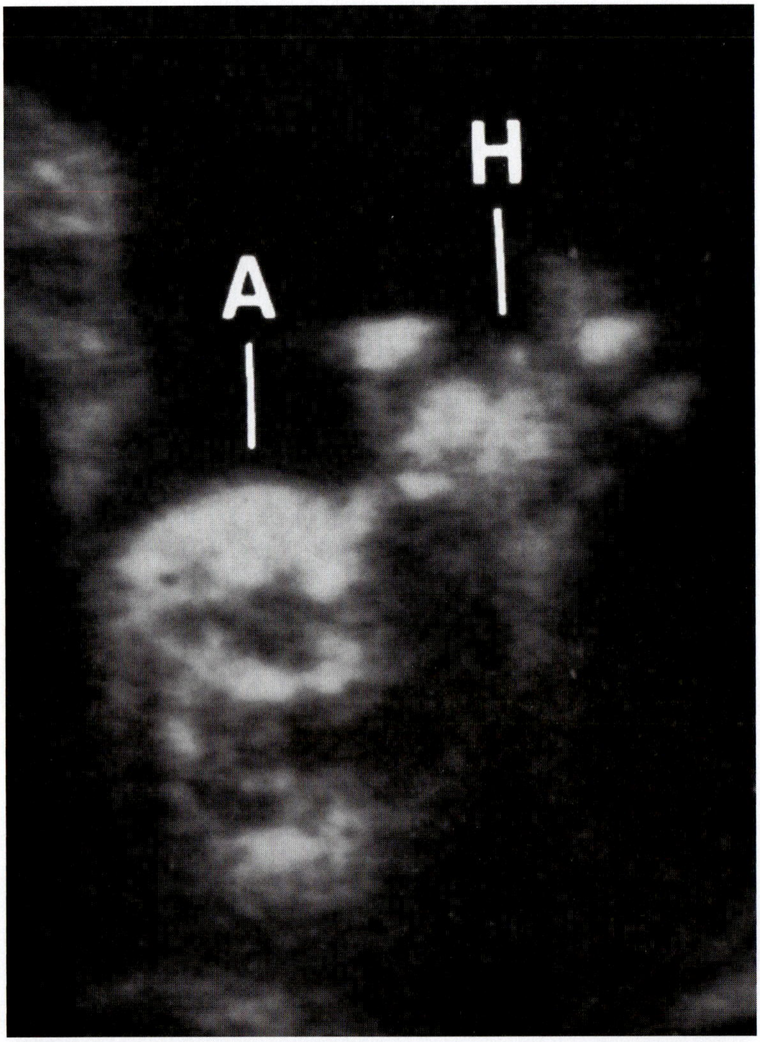

FIGURE 2-110 Upper extremity of a fetus with atelosteogenesis. *A*, Arm; *H*, hand. (From Chervenak FA, Isaacson G, Rosenberg JC, Kardon NB: *J Ultrasound Med* 5:111–113, 1986.)

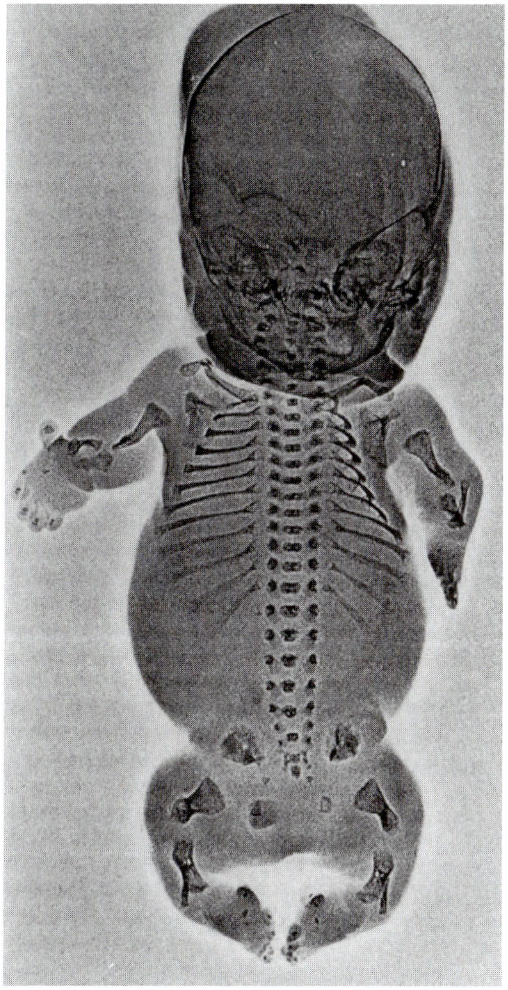

FIGURE 2-111 Xerogram shows the skeletal abnormalities associated with atelosteogenesis. Note flattening of the vertebral bodies, wide proximal metaphyses, distal hypoplasia of humeri, and bowed ulna and radius. The femora and tibiae are short, with rounded metaphyses. (From Nores JA, Rotmensch S, Romero R: *Prenat Diagn* 12:741–753, 1992.)

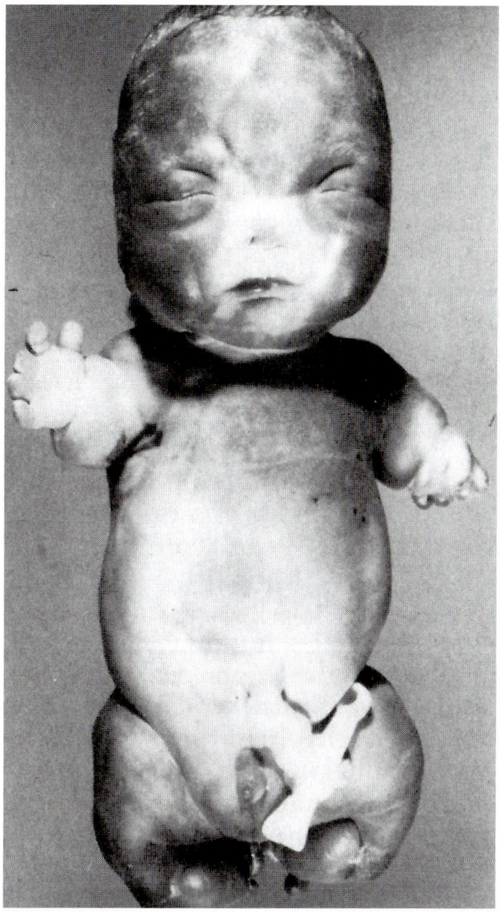

FIGURE 2-112 Postmortem photograph depicts hypertelorism and limb shortening in a fetus with atelosteogenesis. (From Chervenak FA, Isaacson G, Rosenberg JC, Kardon NB: *J Ultrasound Med* 5:111–113, 1986.)

Other Skeletal Dysplasias Associated with Similar Limb Shortening:

Camptomelic dysplasia

Ellis-van Creveld syndrome

Homozygous achondroplasia

Metatropic dysplasia

Roberts' syndrome

Short rib–polydactyly syndromes

Thanatophoric dysplasia

ULTRASOUND DIAGNOSIS

The diagnosis of this disorder is based on the identification of severely abnormal, tubular bones; underossification of posterior neural arches, humeri, radii, ulnae, and fibulae as well as other small tubular bones. Second- and third-trimester detection has been accomplished, starting at 15 weeks.

HEREDITY

The pattern of inheritance for this disorder is thought to be autosomal dominance, with all cases being a new mutation. The gene responsible for this disorder is filamin B (FLNB) located at 3p14. This gene has an impact on vertebral segmentation and formation of joints and cartilage.

NATURAL HISTORY AND OUTCOME

This form of atelosteogenesis is a lethal disorder. Fetuses with this syndrome either are stillborn or die shortly after birth.

Suggested Reading

Bejjani BA, Oberg KC, Wilkins I, et al: Prenatal ultrasonographic description and postnatal pathological findings in atelosteogenesis type 1. *Am J Med Genet* 79:392–395, 1998.

Chervenak FA, Isaacson G, Rosenberg JC, Kardon NB: Antenatal diagnosis of frontal cephalocele in a fetus with atelosteogenesis. *J Ultrasound Med* 5:111–113, 1986.

den Hollander NS, Stewart PA, Brandenburg H, van der Harten J, Gaillard HL: Atelosteogenesis, type I. *Fetus* 3;7564:23–26, 1993.

Greally MT, Jewett T, Smith WL Jr, Penick GD, Williamson RA: Lethal bone dysplasia in a fetus with manifestations of atelosteogenesis I and boomerang dysplasia. *Am J Med Genet* 47:1086–1091, 1993.

Nores JA, Rotmensch S, Romero R, et al: Atelosteogenesis type II: sonographic and radiological correlation. *Prenat Diagn* 12:741–753, 1992.

Sharony R, Browne C, Lachman RS, Rimoin DL: Prenatal diagnosis of the skeletal dysplasias. *Am J Obstet Gynecol* 169:668–675, 1993.

Tennstedt C, Bartho S, Bollmann R, et al: Osteochondrodysplasias. Prenatal diagnosis and pathological-anatomic findings. *Zentralbl Pathol* 139:71–80, 1993.

Ueno K, Tanaka M, Miyakoshi K, et al: Prenatal diagnosis of atelosteogenesis type I at 21 weeks' gestation. *Prenat Diagn* 22:1071–1075, 2002.

Wasant P, Waeteekul S, Rimoin DL, Lachman RS: Genetic skeletal dysplasia in Thailand: the Siriraj experience. *SE Asian J Trop Med Publ Health* 1:59–67, 1995.

CAMPTOMELIC DYSPLASIA

DESCRIPTION AND DEFINITION

Camptomelic dysplasia, which is usually lethal, is a short-limbed dysplasia characterized by bowing of the long bones, particularly of the lower extremities.

ABNORMALITIES DETECTABLE BY ULTRASOUND

Common Findings:

Hypertelorism

Cleft palate

Micrognathia

Ventriculomegaly

Marked bowing of the femur and tibia that may mimic a fracture

Hypoplastic fibula

Hypoplastic scapulae

Bell-shaped, narrow chest

Ambiguous genitalia in males

Occasional Findings:

Nuchal translucency abnormality

Cardiac defects

Large biparietal diameter

Flattened nose

Renal anomalies

Large kidneys

Hydronephrosis

Clubfeet

MAJOR DIFFERENTIAL DIAGNOSES

Other Skeletal Dysplasias Associated with Similar Limb Shortening:

Diastrophic dysplasia

Femur-fibula-ulna (FFU) syndrome

Hypophosphatasia

Osteogenesis imperfecta, with fractures of the long bones of the lower extremities

Roberts' syndrome

Thanatophoric dysplasia

ULTRASOUND DIAGNOSIS

The prenatal diagnosis of this condition has been established in the early- to mid-second trimester (17–18 weeks' gestation), based on short long-bone measurements with marked bowing. In addition to the bowing of the femur and tibia and the partial absence of the fibula, other sonographic findings may include short ribs, large biparietal diameter, flattened nose, clubfeet, bell-shaped chest, micrognathia, polyhydramnios or oligohydramnios, and large kidneys.

HEREDITY

The pattern of inheritance is thought to be autosomal dominant, with most cases being a new mutation. The gene involved with this disorder is SOX9, located on the 17q chromosome. SOX9 regulates the expression of COL2A1 and is involved with bone, cartilage, and testicular development.

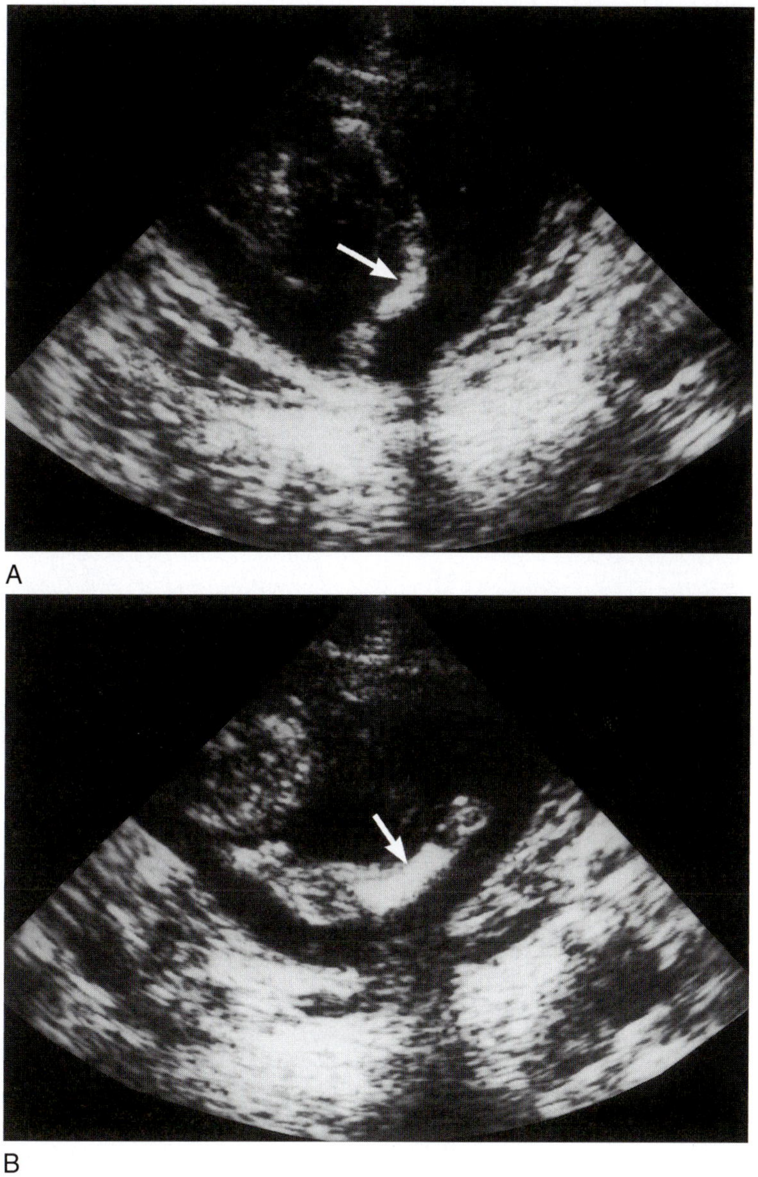

FIGURE 2-113 (A, B) Long-axis views of both lower extremities of a fetus with camptomelic dysplasia. Note bowing of the long bones in both lower extremities *(arrows)* and absence of the fibula bilaterally.

NATURAL HISTORY AND OUTCOME

Most affected infants die of respiratory insufficiency during the neonatal period. The remainder have failure to thrive and usually die within the first year of life.

Suggested Reading

Balcar I, Bieber FR: Sonographic and radiological findings in camptomelic dysplasia. *AJR Am J Roentgenol* 141:481–482, 1983.

Cordone M, Lituania M, Zampatti C, et al: In utero ultrasonographic features of camptomelic dysplasia. *Prenat Diagn* 9:745–750, 1989.

Cumming WA, Ohison A, Ali A: Brief clinical report: camptomelia, cervical lymphocele, polycystic dysplasia, short gut, polysplenia. *Am J Med Genet* 25:783–790, 1986.

Foster JW, Dominguez-Steglich MA, Guioli S, et al: Camptomelic dysplasia and autosomal sex reversal caused by mutations in an SRY-related gene. *Nature* 372:525–530, 1994.

Fryns JP, van den Berghe K, van Assche A, van den Berghe H: Prenatal diagnosis of camptomelic dwarfism. *Clin Genet* 19:199–201, 1981.

Gillerot Y, Vanheck CA, Foulon M, et al: Camptomelic syndrome: manifestations in a 20-week fetus and case history of a 5-year-old child. *Am J Med Genet* 34:589–592, 1989.

Goncalves L, Jeanty P: Fetal biometry of skeletal dysplasias: a multicentric study. *J Ultrasound Med* 13:767–775, 1994.

Jones KL: *Smith's recognizable patterns of human malformations,* ed 6. Philadelphia, Elsevier, 2006.

Michel-Calemard L, Lesca G, Morel Y, Boggio D, Plauchu H, Attia-Sobol J: Campomelic acampomelic dysplasia presenting with increased nuchal translucency in the first trimester. *Prenat Diagn* 2004;24:519–523.

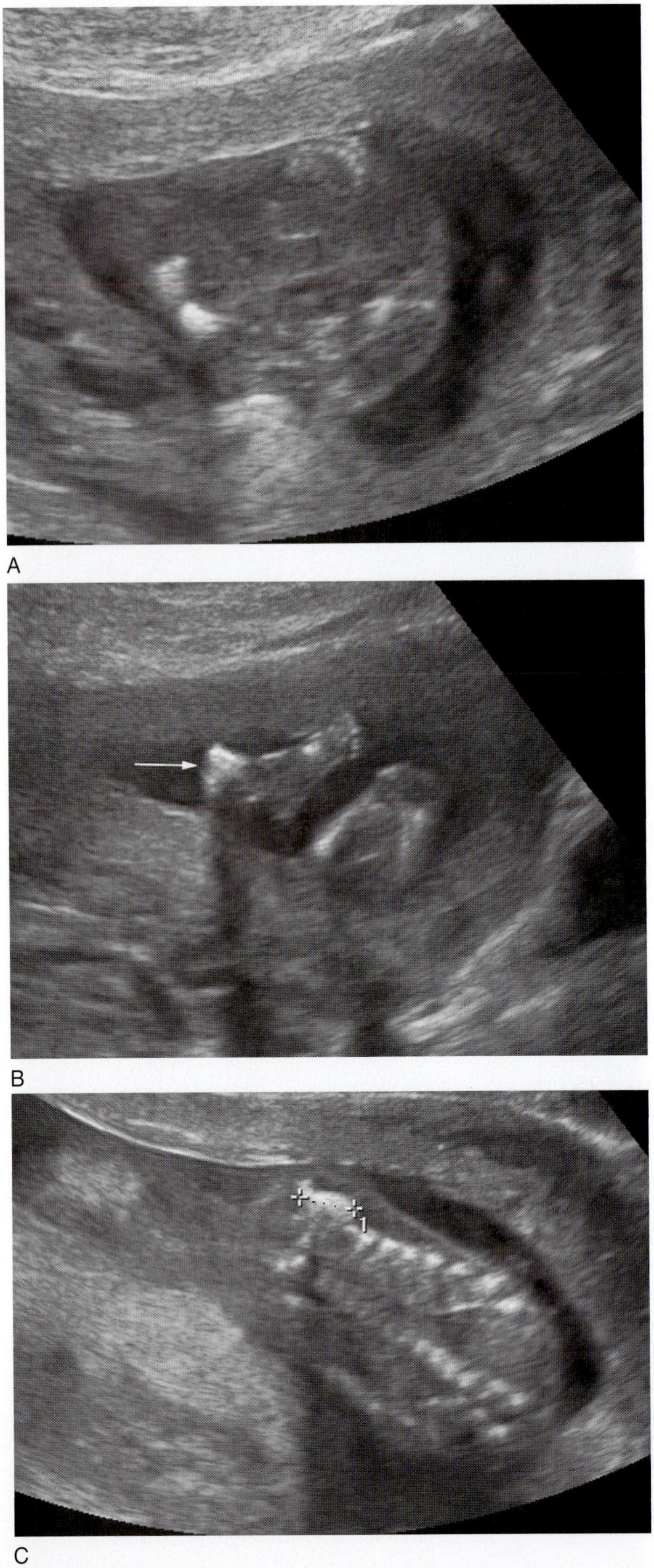

FIGURE 2-114 Early second-trimester fetus with camptomelic dysplasia. (**A, B**) Fetal lower extremity which shows bowed short femur (**A**) and acute bowing of the tibia (**B**, *arrow*). (**C**) Hypoplastic scapula indicated by calipers.

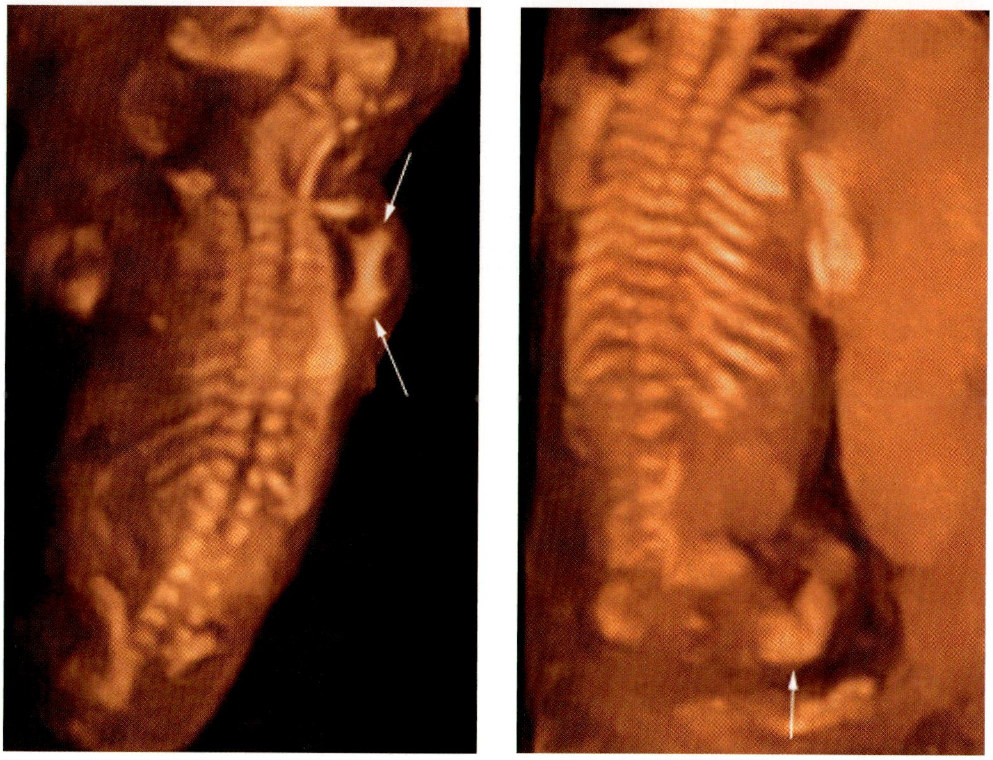

D E

FIGURE 2-114, cont'd (D, E) Three-dimensional surface rendering in skeletal mode of the same fetus shows hypoplastic scapula (D, *arrows*) and marked bowed shortening of the femur (E, *arrow*).

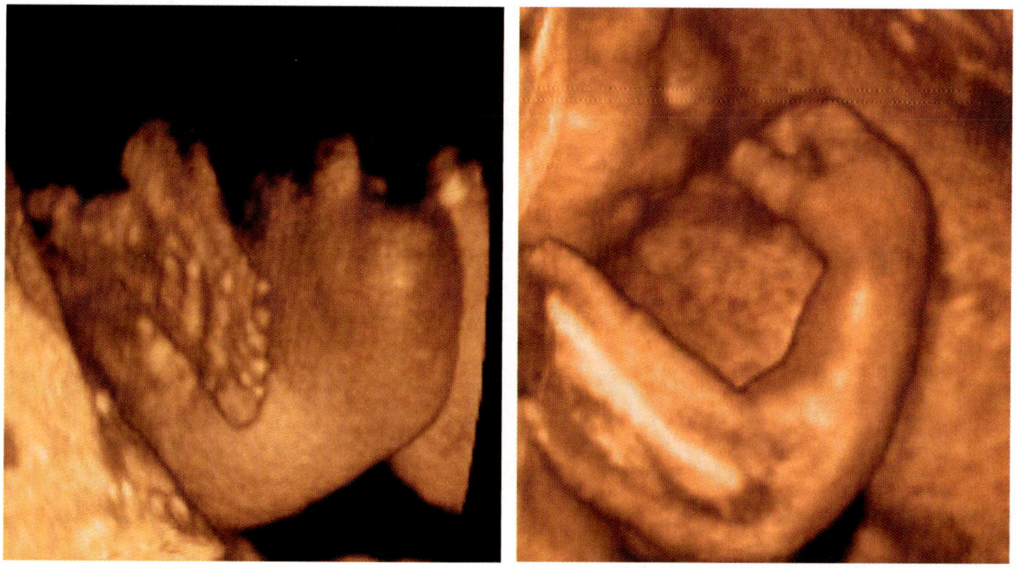

A B

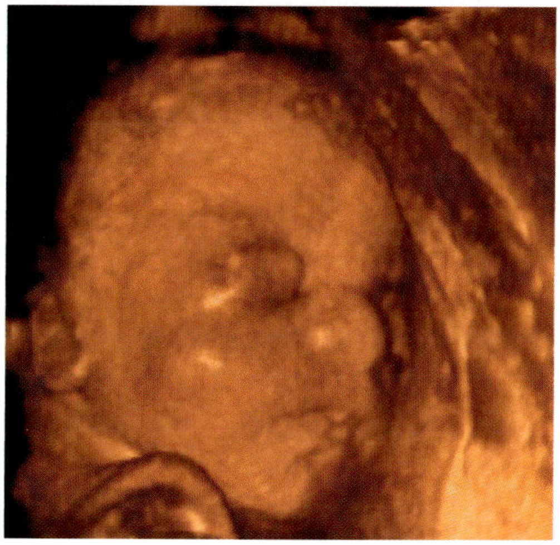

FIGURE 2-115 Third-trimester fetus with camptomelic dysplasia. (A) Three-dimensional surface rendering of the lower extremities shows pretzel configuration of the lower extremities, with legs folded upon each other because of severely bowed bones (not shown). (B) Relatively normal-appearing surface rendering of the upper extremity of the same fetus. (C) Surface rendering of the fetal face of the same fetus.

C

Pretorius DH, Rumack CM, Manco-Johnson ML, et al: Specific skeletal dysplasias in utero: sonographic diagnosis. *Radiology* 159:237–242, 1986.

Sanders RC, Greyson-Fleg RT, Hogge WA, et al: Osteogenesis imperfecta and camptomelic dysplasia: difficulties in prenatal diagnosis. *J Ultrasound Med* 13:691–700, 1994.

Sharony R, Browne C, Lachman RS, Rimoin DL: Prenatal diagnosis of the skeletal dysplasias. *Am J Obstet Gynecol* 169:668–675, 1993.

Slater CP, Ross J, Nelson MM, et al: The camptomelic syndrome—prenatal ultrasound investigations. *S Afr Med J* 67:863–866, 1985.

Tennstedt C, Bartho S, Bollmann R, et al: Osteochondrodysplasias. Prenatal diagnosis and pathological-anatomic findings. *Zentralbl Pathol* 139:71–80, 1993.

Tongsong T, Wanapirak C, Pongsatha S: Prenatal diagnosis of campomelic dysplasia. *Ultrasound Obstet Gynecol* 15:428–430, 2000.

Valcamonico A, Jeanty P: Camptomelic dysplasia. *Fetus* 2:1–4, 1992.

Wasant P, Waeteekul S, Rimoin DL, Lachman RS: Genetic skeletal dysplasia in Thailand: the Siriraj experience. *SE Asian J Trop Med Publ Health* 1:59–67, 1995.

CHONDRODYSPLASIA PUNCTATA

DESCRIPTION AND DEFINITION

Synonym: Conradi-Hünermann syndrome (in the case of the nonrhizomelic type of chondrodysplasia punctata)

This is a heterogeneous group of bone dysplasias; the two main types have different inheritance patterns, sonographic findings, and prognoses. The nonrhizomelic type is Conradi-Hünermann syndrome, which is characterized by asymmetric limb shortening. The rhizomelic type is associated with particularly short humeri and femora.

A third form of chondrodysplasia punctata, the tibia-metacarpal type, is due to the specifically short tibiae and second and third metacarpals. This disorder is associated with micrognathia, bowed femurs and humeri, and calcific stippling of the epitheses.

ABNORMALITIES DETECTABLE BY ULTRASOUND

Nonrhizomelic Type:

Abnormally early calcification of the proximal and distal epiphyses of the humerus and femur

Asymmetric shortening of the extremities

Spinal kyphoscoliosis, vertebral body abnormalities

Depressed or hypoplastic nasal bridge

Microphthalmos (occasional)

Cardiac defect (occasional)

Rhizomelic Type:

Ventriculomegaly

Microcephaly

Depressed or hypoplastic nasal bridge

Brachycephaly

Hypertelorism

Cataracts

Abnormal epiphyseal echogenicity

Symmetric, proximal shortening of the humerus and femur

Diaphragmatic hernia (occasional)

Cleft palate (occasional)

Hypospadias and cryptorchidism (occasional)

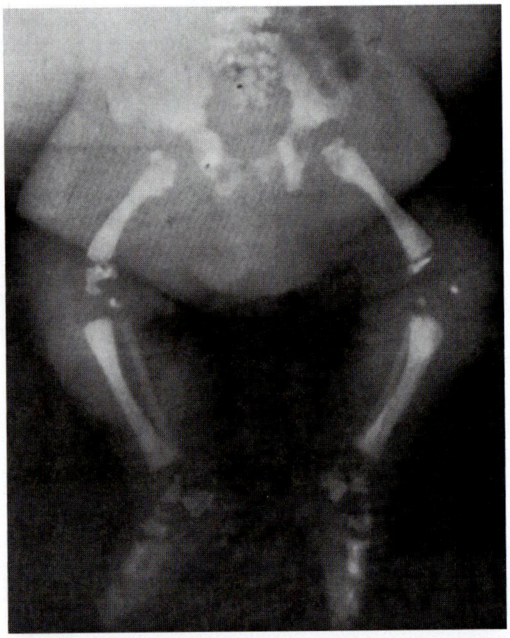

FIGURE 2-116 Radiograph shows punctate calcifications in the proximal and distal femoral epiphyses of the fetal lower extremities. (From Straub W, Zarabi M, Mazer J: *J Clin Ultrasound* 11:234–236, 1983.)

MAJOR DIFFERENTIAL DIAGNOSES

Although other skeletal dysplasias, including osteogenesis imperfect type II, may be considered in the differential diagnosis for chondrodysplasia punctata, the specific finding of abnormal, long bone with calcified epiphyses is crucial for the correct diagnosis.

ULTRASOUND DIAGNOSIS

Both types of chondrodysplasia punctata have been diagnosed sonographically in the early- to mid-second trimester. At 14 weeks' gestational age, the unusual appearance of the proximal femurs, with prematurely calcified epiphyses, has been detected in Conradi-Hünermann syndrome. Other features of the disorder recognized sonographically include nasal hypoplasia, hydrops, narrow thorax, and marked shortening of bones, with angular deformities similar to osteogenesis imperfecta type II seen at 16 weeks. Chondrodysplasia punctata is distinguished from osteogenesis imperfecta type II by the normally ossified calvaria in the former.

The rhizomelic type of chondrodysplasia punctata is detectable before 20 weeks' gestation, based on shortened long-bones and abnormally calcified epiphyses. There is one report of associated ascites and hydrocephalus and a case associated with cataracts. Antenatal diagnosis for affected families is available by amniocentesis using biochemical assays for a peroxisomal defect with deficient fibroblast plasmalogen synthesis enzymes.

HEREDITY

The Conradi-Hünermann syndrome has an X-linked dominant pattern of inheritance, although there also exists an X-linked recessive form of this syndrome. The rhizomelic type of chondromelic dysplasia is an autosomal recessive disorder.

NATURAL HISTORY AND OUTCOME

Conradi-Hünermann Syndrome:

Intelligence is normal. Problems include failure to thrive, respiratory infections in early childhood, and orthopedic problems, such as scoliosis. If the infant survives the first year of life, the outcome is good.

Rhizomelic Type:

While many infants survive beyond infancy, only 50% survive to age 6 years. Death occurs as a result of recurrent pulmonary problems. Most of those who survive past the first few months of life develop seizures, and have many orthopedic problems.

Suggested Reading

Basbug M, Serin IS, Ozcelik B, Gunes T, Akcakus M, Tayyar M: Prenatal ultrasonographic diagnosis of rhizomelic chondrodysplasia punctata by detection of rhizomelic shortening and bilateral cataracts. *Fetal Diagn Ther* 20:171–174, 2005.

Duff P, Harlass FE, Milligan DA: Prenatal diagnosis of chondrodysplasia punctata by sonography. *Obstet Gynecol* 76:497–500, 1990.

Furness ME, Haan EA, Hopkins PB, Chambers HM: Chondrodysplasia punctata, mild symmetric type, with echogenic coccyx in a 15-week fetus. *Fetus* 1:1–3, 1991.

Gendall PW, Baird CE, Becroft DM: Rhizomelic chondrodysplasia punctata: early recognition with antenatal ultrasonography. *J Clin Ultrasound* 22:271–274, 1994.

Goncalves L, Jeanty P: Fetal biometry of skeletal dysplasias: a multicentric study. *J Ultrasound Med* 13:767–775, 1994.

Hertzberg BS, Kliewer MA, Decker M, Miller CR, Bowie JD: Antenatal ultrasonographic diagnosis of rhizomelic chondrodysplasia punctata. *J Ultrasound Med* 18:715–718, 1999.

Hoeffler G, Hoeffler AB, Moser PA, et al: Prenatal diagnosis of rhizomelic chondrodysplasia punctata. *Prenat Diagn* 8:571–576, 1988.

Jansen V, Sarafoglou K, Rebarber A, Greco A, Genieser NB, Wallerstein R: Chondrodysplasia punctata, tibial-metacarpal type in a 16 week fetus. *J Ultrasound Med* 19:719–722, 2000.

Jones KL: *Smith's recognizable patterns of human malformations,* ed 6. Philadelphia, Elsevier, 2006.

Krakow D, Williams J 3rd, Poehl M, Rimoin DL, Platt LD: Use of three-dimensional ultrasound imaging in the diagnosis of prenatal-onset skeletal dysplasias. *Ultrasound Obstet Gynecol* 21:467–472, 2003.

Mayden Argo K, Toriello HV, Jelsema RD, Zuidema LJ: Prenatal findings in chondrodysplasia punctata, tibia-metacarpal type. *Ultrasound Obstet Gynecol* 8:350–354, 1996.

Pradhan GM, Chaubal NG, Chaubal JN, Raghavan J: Second-trimester sonographic diagnosis of nonrhizomelic chondrodysplasia punctata. *J Ultrasound Med* 21:345–349, 2002.

Ruano R, Molho M, Roume J, Ville Y: Prenatal diagnosis of fetal skeletal dysplasias by combining two-dimensional and three-dimensional ultrasound and intrauterine three-dimensional helical computer tomography. *Ultrasound Obstet Gynecol* 24:134–140, 2004.

Sastrowijoto SH, Vandenberghe K, Moerman P, Lauweryns JM, Fryns JP: Prenatal ultrasound diagnosis of rhizomelic chondrodysplasia punctata in a primigravida. *Prenat Diagn* 14:770–776, 1994.

Sharony R, Browne C, Lachman RS, Rimoin DL: Prenatal diagnosis of the skeletal dysplasias. *Am J Obstet Gynecol* 169:668–675, 1993.

Sherer DM, Glantz JC, Alien TA, Lonardo F, Metlay LA: Prenatal sonographic diagnosis of nonrhizomelic chondrodysplasia punctata. *Obstet Gynecol* 83:858–860, 1994.

Sidden CR, Filly RA, Norton ME, Kostiner DR: A case of chondrodysplasia punctata with features of osteogenesis imperfecta type II. *J Ultrasound Med* 20:699–703, 2001.

Straub W, Zarabi M, Mazer J: Fetal ascites associated with Conradi's disease (chondrodysplasia punctata): report of a case. *J Clin Ultrasound* 11:234–236, 1983.

Wasant P, Waeteekul S, Rimoin DL, Lachman RS: Genetic skeletal dysplasia in Thailand: the Siriraj experience. *SE Asian J Trop Med Publ Health* 1:59–67, 1995.

Wessels MW, Den Hollander NJ, De Krijger RR, et al: Fetus with an unusual form of nonrhizomelic chondrodysplasia punctata: case report and review. *Am J Med Genet A* 120:97–104, 2003.

Wester U, Brandberg G, Larsson M, Lonnerholm T, Anneren G: Chondrodysplasia punctata (CDP) with features of the tibia-metacarpal type and maternal phenytoin treatment during pregnancy. *Prenat Diagn* 22:663–668, 2002.

CLEIDOCRANIAL DYSOSTOSIS

DESCRIPTION AND DEFINITION

This is a skeletal disorder characterized mainly by hypoplasia or absence of the clavicle and ossification abnormalities of the skull.

ABNORMALITIES DETECTABLE BY ULTRASOUND

Common Findings:

Shortening of the clavicle (absence of the clavicle in 10% of affected infants)

Hypoplastic iliac bones with normal long-bones

Delayed mineralization of the pubic bone

Hypertelorism

Midface hypoplasia

Occasional Findings:

Cleft palate

Nasal hypoplasia

Micrognathia

MAJOR DIFFERENTIAL DIAGNOSES

Other Conditions Associated with Clavicular Hypoplasia:

Klippel-Feil sequence

Poland sequence with Sprengel anomaly

Other Conditions Associated with Clavicular Hypoplasia and Skeletal Dysplasia (Unlikely If Limbs Are of Normal Length and Configuration):

Achondrogenesis

Holt-Oram syndrome

Osteogenesis imperfecta

Roberts' syndrome

Thrombocytopenia–absent radius (TAR) syndrome

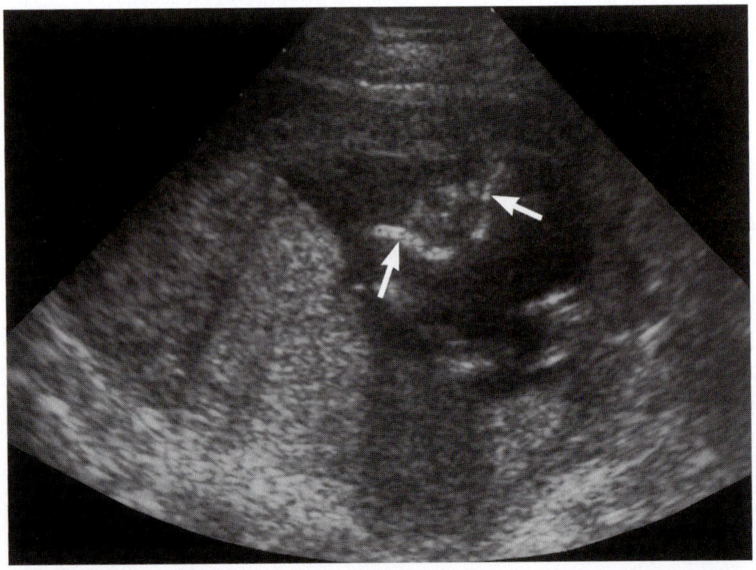

FIGURE 2-117 Transverse view through the fetal clavicles shows normal clavicles bilaterally *(arrows)*.

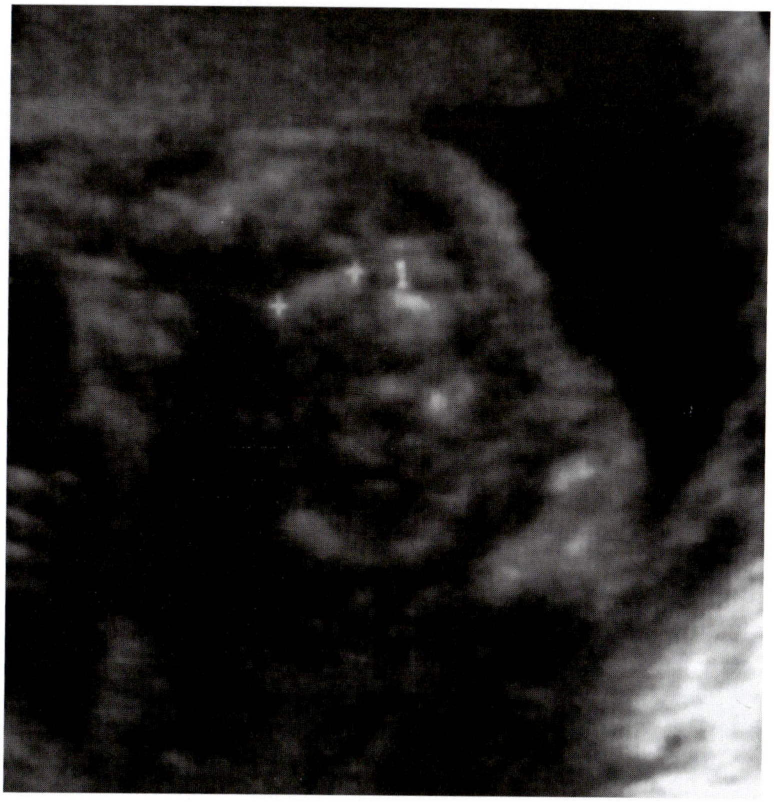

FIGURE 2-118 Short clavicle noted at 22 weeks' gestation in a fetus with cleidocranial dysostosis. (From Steele JR, Jeanty P: *Fetus* 4:1–5, 1994.)

ULTRASOUND DIAGNOSIS

The diagnosis of cleidocranial dysostosis has been established as early as 14 and 15 weeks' gestation, based on careful evaluation of the clavicles in fetuses at risk for the disorder. The clavicle was not identified at 15 weeks, and the diagnosis was confirmed at 20 weeks' gestational age. Hypoplasia of the nasal bone has been described with this disorder. Prenatal diagnoses have been established in patients having cleidocranial dysostosis, who are at increased risk (50%) for having affected offspring.

HEREDITY

The disorder has an autosomal dominant pattern of inheritance, with variable expression. The gene for this disorder has been mapped to chromosome 6p21.

NATURAL HISTORY AND OUTCOME

Affected individuals may have slightly shortened stature, but normal intelligence is anticipated. With increasing age, affected individuals may have postural deformities of the spine and pelvis. Some have deafness, dental problems, and a narrow thorax, leading to respiratory symptoms.

Suggested Reading

Chen CP, Hung HY, Chang TY, Lin SP, Wang W: Second-trimester nasal bone hypoplasia/aplasia associated with cleidocranial dysplasia. *Prenat Diagn* 24:399–400, 2004.

Hamner LH III, Fabbri EL, Browne PC: Prenatal diagnosis of cleidocranial dysostosis. *Obstet Gynecol* 83:856–857, 1994.

Hassan J, Sepulveda W, Teixeira J, Garrett C, Fisk NM: Prenatal sonographic diagnosis of cleidocranial dysostosis. *Prenat Diagn* 17:770–772, 1997.

Jones KL: *Smith's recognizable patterns of human malformations,* ed 6. Philadelphia, Elsevier, 2006.

Paladini D, Lamberti A, Agangi A, Martinelli P: Cleidocranial dysostosis. Prenatal ultrasound diagnosis of a late onset form. *Ultrasound Obstet Gynecol* 16:100–101, 2000.

Soule AB: Mutational dysostosis (cleidocranial dysostosis). *J Bone Joint Surg* 28:81, 1946.

Steele JR, Jeanty P: Cleidocranial dysplasia. *Fetus* 4:1–5, 1995.

Stewart PA, Wallerstein R, Moran E, Lee MJ: Early prenatal ultrasound diagnosis of cleidocranial dysplasia. *Ultrasound Obstet Gynecol* 15:154–156, 2000.

Wasant P, Waeteekul S, Rimoin DL, Lachman RS: Genetic skeletal dysplasia in Thailand: the Siriraj experience. *SE Asian J Trop Med Publ Health* 1:59–67, 1995.

Winer N, Le Caignec C, Quere MP, et al: Prenatal diagnosis of a cleidocranial dysplasia-like phenotype associated with a de novo balanced t(2q;6q)(q36;q16) translocation. *Ultrasound Obstet Gynecol* 22:648–651, 2003.

DIASTROPHIC DYSPLASIA

DESCRIPTION AND DEFINITION

This syndrome is characterized by micromelia, club feet, hand abnormalities, and scoliosis.

ABNORMALITIES DETECTABLE BY ULTRASOUND

Micrognathia

Cleft palate

Shortening of all long bones, with femurs measuring below the fifth percentile for gestational age

Hitchhiker thumb

Club feet

Kyphoscoliosis

Polyhydramnios

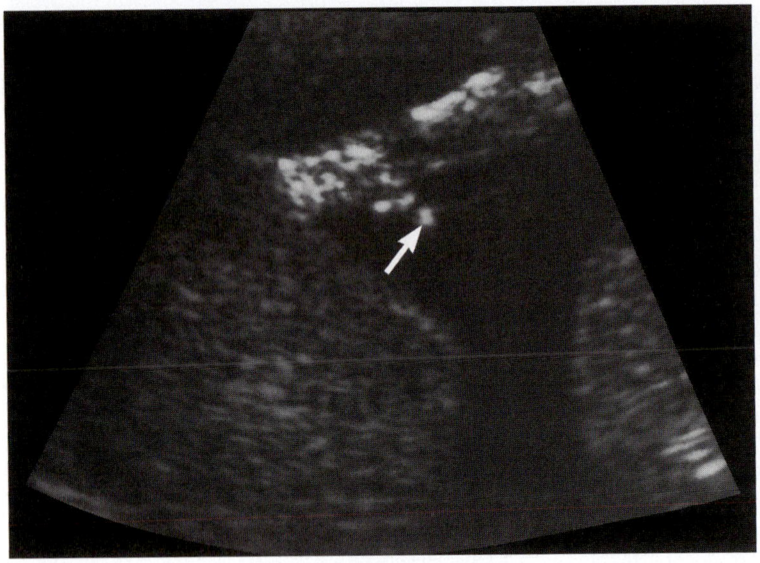

A

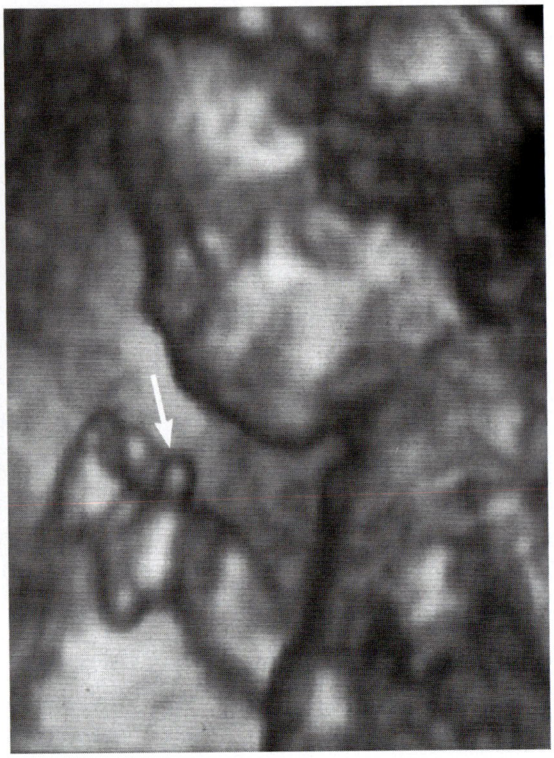

B

FIGURE 2-119 (A) View of the fetal hand shows the characteristic "hitchhiker thumb" *(arrow)*. (From Bromley B, Benacerraf B: *AJR Am J Roentgenol* 165:1239–1243, 1995.) (B) Three-dimensional surface rendering of a fetus with diastrophic dysplasia shows the hitchhiker thumb *(arrow)*.

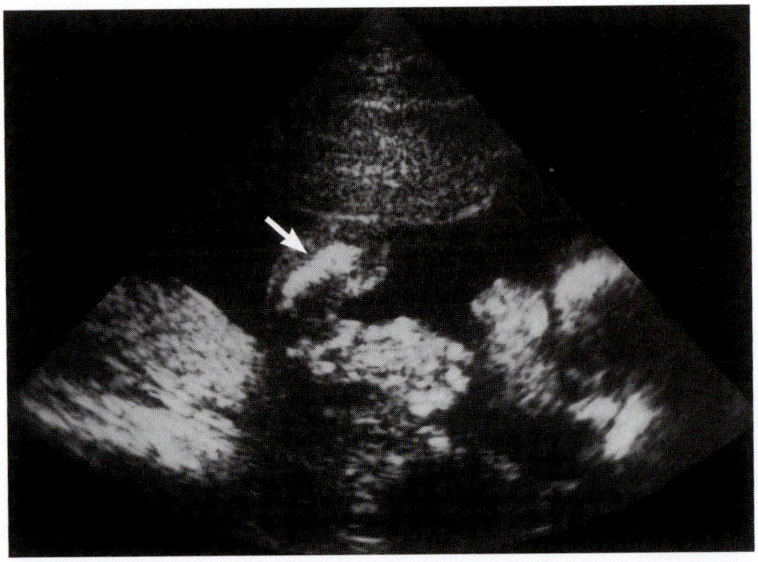

FIGURE 2-120 Upper extremity of a fetus with diastrophic dysplasia. Note bowing of the humerus *(arrow)*.

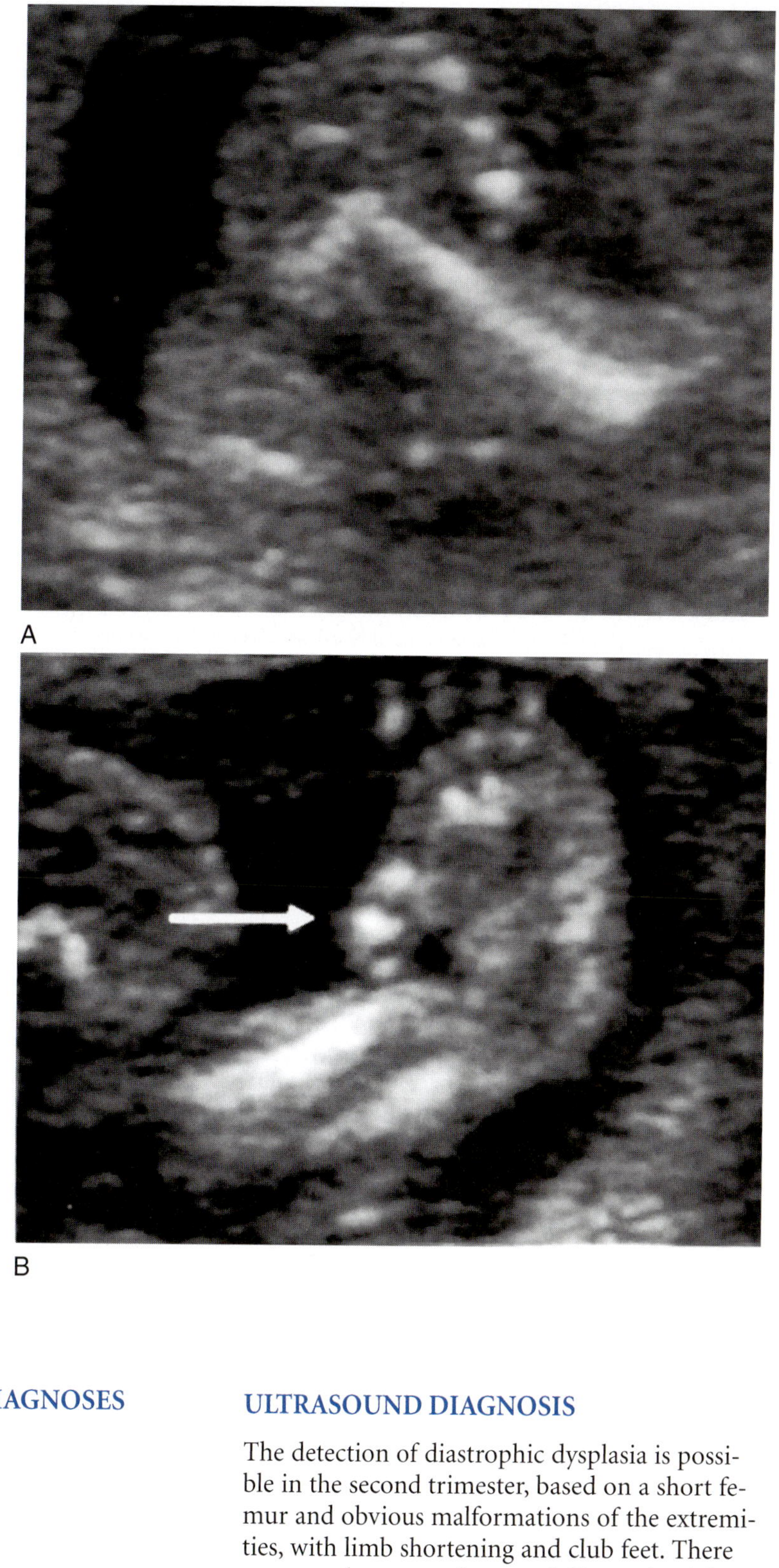

FIGURE 2-121 (A) Short tibia with clubbing of the foot in a fetus with diastrophic dysplasia. (B) Hitchhiker toe and club foot in the same fetus *(arrow)*. (From Babcook CJ, Filly RA: *Fetus* 3:19–22, 1993.)

MAJOR DIFFERENTIAL DIAGNOSES

Camptomelic dysplasia

Distal arthrogryposis

Larsen syndrome

Multiple pterygium syndrome

Roberts' syndrome

Spondyloepiphyseal dysplasia

Stickler syndrome

Thanatophoric dysplasia

ULTRASOUND DIAGNOSIS

The detection of diastrophic dysplasia is possible in the second trimester, based on a short femur and obvious malformations of the extremities, with limb shortening and club feet. There are several reports of prenatal diagnosis of the disorder as early 13 to 14 weeks' gestation, based on the presence of micromelia. Other prenatal ultrasound features that have been detected include thoracic scoliosis, hitchhiker thumb, micrognathia, ulnar deviation of the wrist, and polyhydramnios.

HEREDITY

The pattern of inheritance for diastrophic dysplasia is autosomal recessive. The mutation is mapped at 5q32-q33.1.

NATURAL HISTORY AND OUTCOME

Some affected infants die of respiratory complications, secondary to micrognathia, laryngeal stenosis, and kyphoscoliosis. In general, however, this is a nonlethal disorder associated with normal intelligence. Complications usually stem from the associated arthropathy and kyphoscoliosis, which lead to physical handicaps and require aggressive treatment.

Suggested Reading

Babcook CJ, Filly RA: Diastrophic dysplasia. *Fetus* 3:19–22, 1993.

Gembruch J, Niesen M, Kehrberg H, et al: Diastrophic dysplasia: a specific prenatal diagnosis by ultrasound. *Prenat Diagn* 8:539–545, 1988.

Gollop TR, Eigier A: Prenatal ultrasound diagnosis of diastrophic dysplasia at 16 weeks. *Am J Med Genet* 27:321–324, 1987.

Goncalves L, Jeanty P: Fetal biometry of skeletal dysplasias: a multicentric study. *J Ultrasound Med* 13:767–775, 1994.

Goncalves LF, Hill LM, Jeanty P: Diastrophic dysplasia. *Fetus* 2:7–10, 1992.

Jones KL: *Smith's recognizable patterns of human malformations,* ed 6. Philadelphia, Elsevier, 2006.

Jung C, Sohn C, Sergi C: Case report: prenatal diagnosis of diastrophic dysplasia by ultrasound at 21 weeks of gestation in a mother with massive obesity. *Prenat Diagn* 18:378–383, 1998.

Kaitila I, Ammala P, Karjalainen O, Liukkonen S, Rapola J: Early prenatal detection of diastrophic dysplasia. *Prenat Diagn* 3:237–244, 1983.

Mantagos S, Weiss RR, Mahoney M, Hobbins JC: Prenatal diagnosis of diastrophic dwarfism. *Am J Obstet Gynecol* 139:111–113, 1981.

O'Brien GD, Rodeck C, Queenan JT: Early prenatal diagnosis of diastrophic dwarfism by ultrasound. *Br Med J* 280:1300, 1980.

Sepulveda W, Sepulveda-Swatson E, Sanchez J: Diastrophic dysplasia: prenatal three-dimensional ultrasound findings. *Ultrasound Obstet Gynecol* 23:312–314, 2004.

Severi FM, Bocchi C, Sanseverino F, Petraglia F: Prenatal ultrasonographic diagnosis of diastrophic dysplasia at 13 weeks of gestation. *J Matern Fetal Neonatal Med* 13:282–284, 2003.

Sharony R, Browne C, Lachman RS, Rimoin DL: Prenatal diagnosis of the skeletal dysplasias. *Am J Obstet Gynecol* 169:668–675, 1993.

Tennstedt C, Bartho S, Bollmann R, et al: Osteochondrodysplasias. Prenatal diagnosis and pathological-anatomic findings. *Zentralbl Pathol* 139:71–80, 1993.

Tongsong T, Wanapirak C, Sirichotiyakul S, Chanprapaph P: Prenatal sonographic diagnosis of diastrophic dwarfism. *J Clin Ultrasound* 30:103–105, 2002.

Wax JR, Carpenter M, Smith W, et al: Second-trimester sonographic diagnosis of diastrophic dysplasia: report of 2 index cases. *J Ultrasound Med* 22:805–808, 2003.

Wladimiroff JW, Niermeijer MF, Laar J, Jahoda M, Stewart PA: Prenatal diagnosis of skeletal dysplasia by real-time ultrasound. *Obstet Gynecol* 63:360–364, 1984.

ELLIS-VAN CREVELD SYNDROME

DESCRIPTION AND DEFINITION

Synonym: Chondroectodermal dysplasia

First described in 1940, this skeletal dysplasia is characterized by disproportionate, short extremities; polydactyly; and cardiac defects.

ABNORMALITIES DETECTABLE BY ULTRASOUND

Common Findings:

Short long-bones

Polydactyly of the hands (and occasionally of the toes)

Narrow thorax with short ribs

Cardiac defects, most commonly atrial septal defects (50% of affected individuals)

Thickened nuchal translucency

Occasional Findings:

Dandy-Walker malformation

Club feet

Cryptorchidism

Renal agenesis

MAJOR DIFFERENTIAL DIAGNOSES

Other Syndromes and Conditions Associated with Short Ribs, Narrow Chest, and Polydactyly:

Asphyxiating thoracic dystrophy

Short rib–polydactyly syndrome, type I (Saldino-Noonan syndrome)

Short rib–polydactyly syndrome, type II (Majewski syndrome)

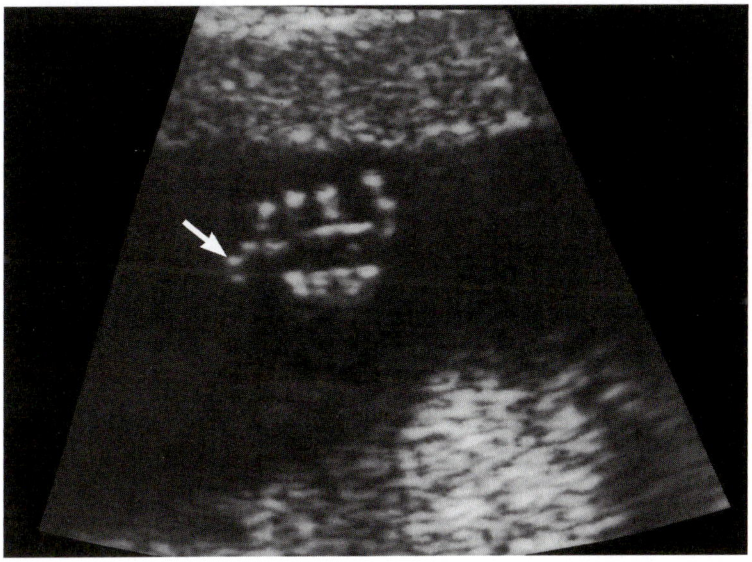

FIGURE 2-122 View of the fetal hand shows postaxial polydactyly *(arrow)*, as can be seen in fetuses with Ellis-van Creveld syndrome.

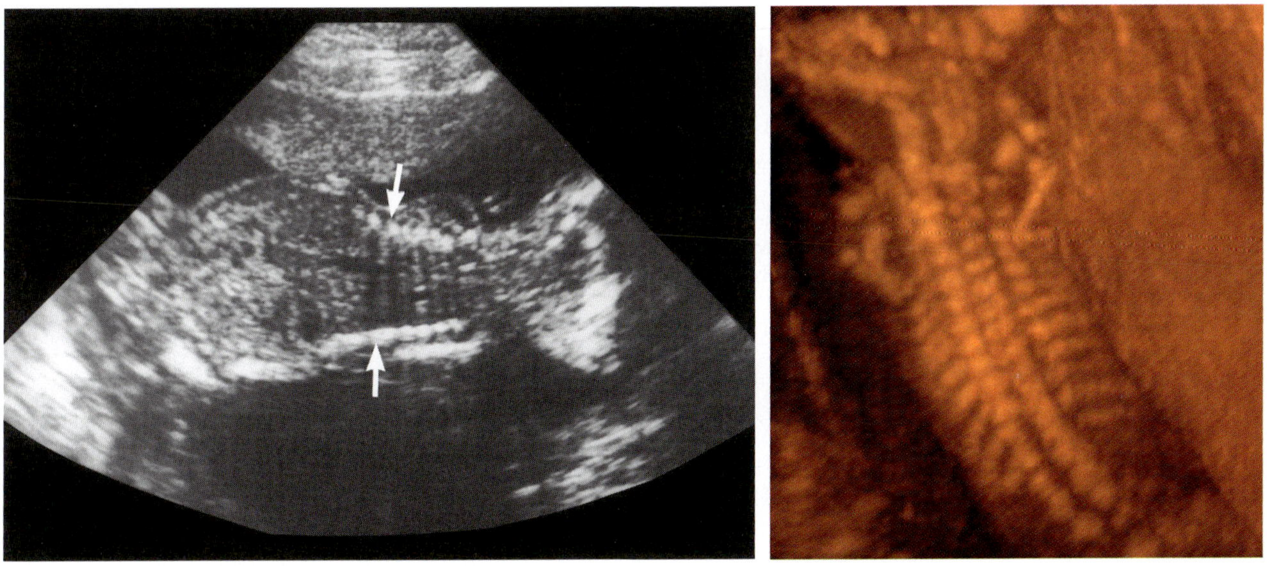

A B

FIGURE 2-123 (A) Long-axis view of the fetal chest and abdomen shows marked narrowing of the chest *(arrows)* compared with the fetal abdomen, as can be seen in fetuses with Ellis-van Creveld syndrome. (B) Three-dimensional surface rendering of a second-trimester fetus with marked shortening of the ribs and narrow chest, as can be seen in fetuses with Ellis-van Creveld syndrome.

Short rib–polydactyly syndrome, type III (Naumoff syndrome)

ULTRASOUND DIAGNOSIS

The diagnosis of Ellis-van Creveld syndrome has been established prenatally by both ultrasound and fetoscopy. The diagnosis is based on the findings of a narrow thorax/short ribs, short long-bones (including the femur), and polydactyly. There is a report of an affected fetus who presented with a thickened nuchal translucency at 13 weeks. At 18 weeks, the fetus had the typical anomalies, including narrow thorax, short long-bones, bowed femora, and polydactyly of hands and feet. Another report describes the diagnosis of Ellis-van Creveld syndrome at 12 weeks based on polydactyly and short long-bones in a family with a previously affected fetus. Atrial septal defects are difficult to detect early in pregnancy and may not be helpful in confirming the prenatal diagnosis.

HEREDITY

The disorder has an autosomal recessive pattern of inheritance. This disorder is a result of mutations at the locus 4p16.

NATURAL HISTORY AND OUTCOME

One third to half of affected infants die in the neonatal period as a result of pulmonary complications. Survivors have normal intelligence but very short stature.

Suggested Reading

Berardi JC, Moulis M, Laloux V, et al: Ellis-van Creveld syndrome: contribution of echography to prenatal diagnosis, apropos of a case. *J Gynecol Obstet Biol Reprod* 14:43–47, 1985.

Dugoff L, Thieme G, Hobbins JC: First trimester prenatal diagnosis of chondroectodermal dysplasia (Ellis-van Creveld syndrome) with ultrasound. *Ultrasound Obstet Gynecol* 17:86–88, 2001.

Ellis RWB, van Creveld S: A syndrome characterized by ectodermal dysplasia, polydactyly, chondro-dysplasia and congenital morbus cordis: report of three cases. *Arch Dis Child* 15:65–84, 1940.

Goncalves L, Jeanty P: Fetal biometry of skeletal dysplasias: a multicentric study. *J Ultrasound Med* 13:767–775, 1994.

Guschmann M, Horn D, Gasiorek-Wiens A, Urban M, Kunze J, Vogel M: Ellis-van Creveld syndrome: examination at 15 weeks' gestation. *Prenat Diagn* 19:879–883, 1999.

Jelic N, Vukovic-Mihuljec V, Jelic A: The Ellis-van Creveld syndrome. *Lijec Vjesn* 111:270–272, 1989.

Jones KL: *Smith's recognizable patterns of human malformations,* ed 6. Philadelphia, Elsevier, 2006.

Mahoney MJ, Hobbins JC: Prenatal diagnosis of chondroectodermal dysplasia (Ellis-van Creveld syndrome) with fetoscopy and ultrasound. *N Engl J Med* 297:258–260, 1977.

Muller LM, Cremin BJ: Ultrasonic demonstration of fetal skeletal dysplasia. *S Afr Med J* 67:222–226, 1985.

Sharony R, Browne C, Lachman RS, Rimoin DL: Prenatal diagnosis of the skeletal dysplasias. *Am J Obstet Gynecol* 169:668–675, 1993.

Tennstedt C, Bartho S, Bollmann R, et al: Osteochondrodysplasias. Prenatal diagnosis and pathological-anatomic findings. *Zentralbl Pathol* 139:71–80, 1993.

Tongsong T, Chanprapaph P: Prenatal sonographic diagnosis of ellis-van creveld syndrome. *J Clin Ultrasound* 28:38–41, 2000.

Torrente I, Mangino M, De Luca A, et al: First-trimester prenatal diagnosis of Ellis-van Creveld syndrome using linked microsatellite markers. *Prenat Diagn* 18:504–506, 1998.

Venkat-Raman N, Sebire NJ, Murphy KW, Carvalho JS, Hall CM: Increased first-trimester fetal nuchal translucency thickness in association with chondroectodermal dysplasia (Ellis-Van Creveld syndrome).*Ultrasound Obstet Gynecol* 25:412–414, 2005.

Wasant P, Waeteekul S, Rimoin DL, Lachman RS: Genetic skeletal dysplasia in Thailand: the Siriraj experience. *SE Asian J Trop Med Publ Health* 1:59–67, 1995.

Zangwill KM, Boal DKB, Ladda RL: Dandy-Walker malformation in Ellis-van Creveld syndrome. *Am J Med Genet* 31:123–129, 1988.

HYPOCHONDROPLASIA

DESCRIPTION AND DEFINITION

Characterized by mild-to-moderate limb shortening, this syndrome resembles classic achondroplasia but is less severe.

ABNORMALITIES DETECTABLE BY ULTRASOUND

Common Findings:

Macrocephaly

Shortened long-bones of all limbs, mainly in the third trimester

Occasional Findings:

Mild frontal bossing

Cataracts

Narrowing of the spinal canal in the lumbar region

Postaxial polydactyly of the feet

MAJOR DIFFERENTIAL DIAGNOSES

Other Skeletal Dysplasias Associated with Mild Limb Length Reduction and Macrocephaly:

Achondroplasia (heterozygous)

IUGR

Kniest syndrome

Trisomy 21 (Down syndrome)

ULTRASOUND DIAGNOSIS

Most of the prenatal sonographic diagnoses of hypochondroplasia have been established in the third trimester, based on long-bone shortening. As in achondroplasia, bone length shortening often is not apparent in the second trimester. The earliest diagnosis reported in the literature was at 22 weeks' gestation in a family at risk for the disorder. One case report describes normal

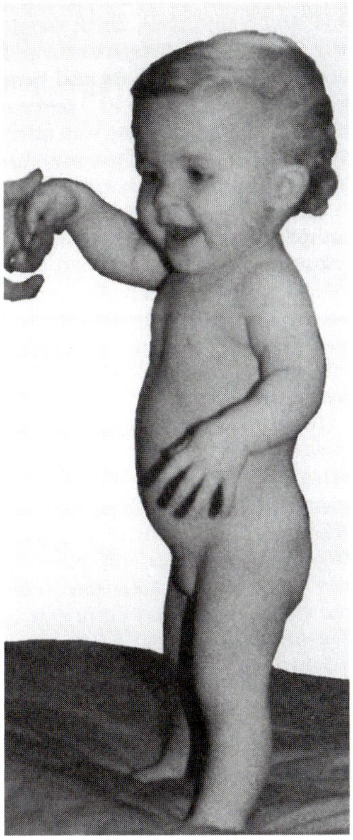

FIGURE 2-124 Thirteen-month-old child with hypochondroplasia has visible (but not striking) limb shortening and absence of the frontal bossing usually seen in achondroplasia. (From Allen SH, Jeanty P: *Fetus* 1:1–6, 1991.)

bone length at 16 weeks and up to 22 weeks in a fetus at risk for the syndrome. Only at 25 weeks were the long bones short enough to make the correct diagnosis.

HEREDITY

The pattern of inheritance for this disorder is autosomal dominant, although many cases are presumed to be fresh mutations and have been linked to advanced paternal age. Hypochondroplasia is considered to be an allele of achondroplasia, at locus 4p16.3 (FGFR3), suggesting that these two disorders result from mutations of the same gene.

NATURAL HISTORY AND OUTCOME

The prognosis for this condition is excellent. Although there is short stature, both life span and intelligence are normal.

Suggested Reading

Allen SH, Jeanty P: Hypochondroplasia. *Fetus* 1:1–6, 1991.

Goncalves L, Jeanty P: Fetal biometry of skeletal dysplasias: a multicentric study. *J Ultrasound Med* 13:767–775, 1994.

Goncalves L, Jeanty P: Fetal biometry of skeletal dysplasias: a multicentric study (corrected and republished). *J Ultrasound Med* 13:977–985, 1994.

Huggins MJ, Mernagh JR, Steele L, Smith JR, Nowaczyk MJ: Prenatal sonographic diagnosis of hypochondroplasia in a high-risk fetus. *Am J Med Genet* 87:226–229, 1999.

Jones KL: *Smith's recognizable patterns of human malformations,* ed 6. Philadelphia, Elsevier, 2006.

Jones SM, Robinson LK, Sperrazza R: Prenatal diagnosis of skeletal dysplasia identified postnatally as hypochondroplasia. *Am J Med Genet* 36:404–407, 1990.

Lemyre E, Azouz EM, Teebi AS, Glanc P, Chen MF: Bone dysplasia series. Achondroplasia, hypochondroplasia and thanatophoric dysplasia: review and update. *Can Assoc Radiol J* 50:185–197, 1999.

Stoll C, Manini P, Bloch J, Roth MP: Prenatal diagnosis of hypochondroplasia. *Prenat Diagn* 5:423–426, 1985.

Wasant P, Waeteekul S, Rimoin DL, Lachman RS: Genetic skeletal dysplasia in Thailand: the Siriraj experience. *SE Asian J Trop Med Publ Health* 1:59–67, 1995.

HYPOPHOSPHATASIA OF THE LETHAL TYPE

DESCRIPTION AND DEFINITION

This condition is characterized by severely demineralized bone and a congenital deficiency of alkaline phosphatase.

ABNORMALITIES DETECTABLE BY ULTRASOUND

Marked demineralization of the calvaria

Soft-appearing skull, with increased visualization of the brain within the skull

Bowed, tubular bones that are short and demineralized, with multiple fractures

First-trimester nuchal translucency

MAJOR DIFFERENTIAL DIAGNOSES

Osteogenesis imperfecta (similar in its associated bone demineralization, particularly of the skull, and bowed long-bones with apparent fractures)

Achondrogenesis

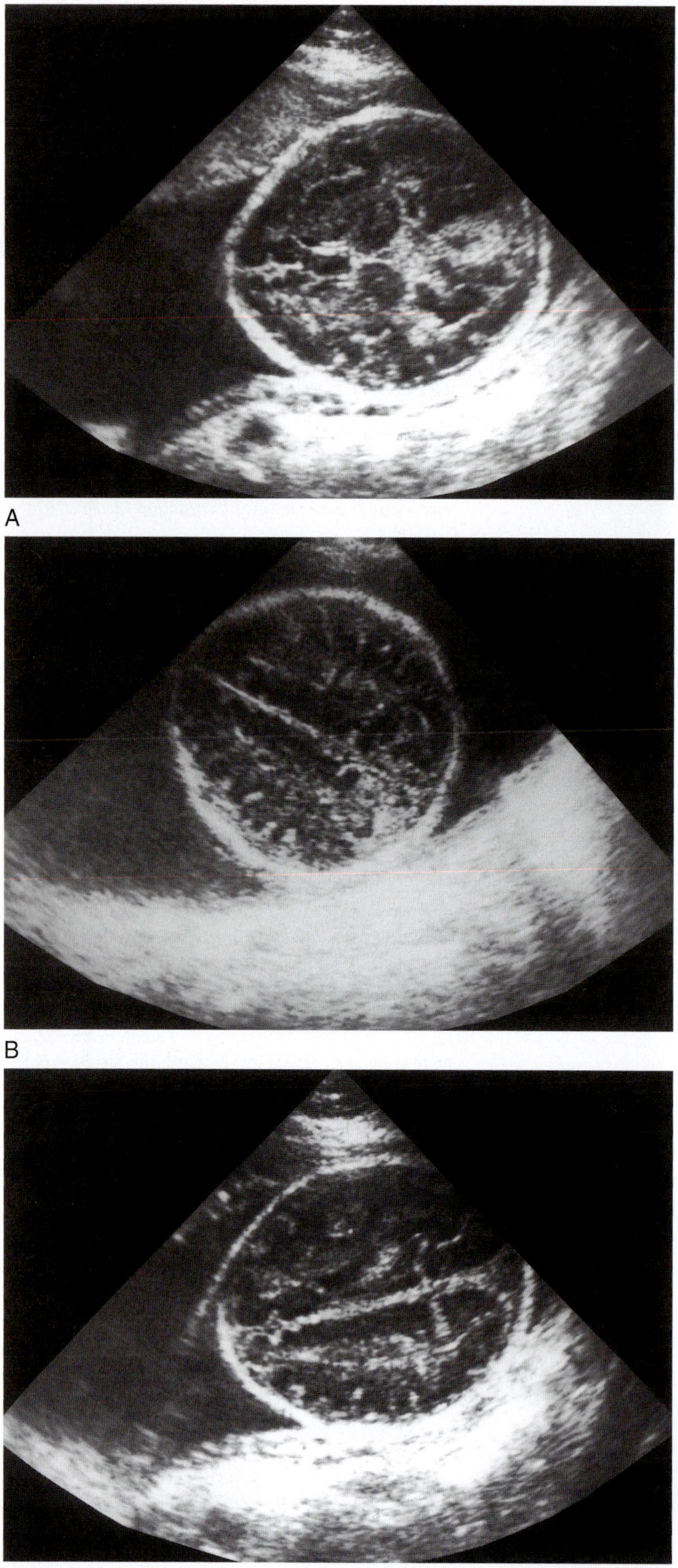

A

B

C

FIGURE 2-125 (A–C) Transverse views through the fetal head at three different levels. Note severe hypomineralization of the skull, as can be seen in fetuses with hypophosphatasia, allowing exceptionally clear imaging of the brain.

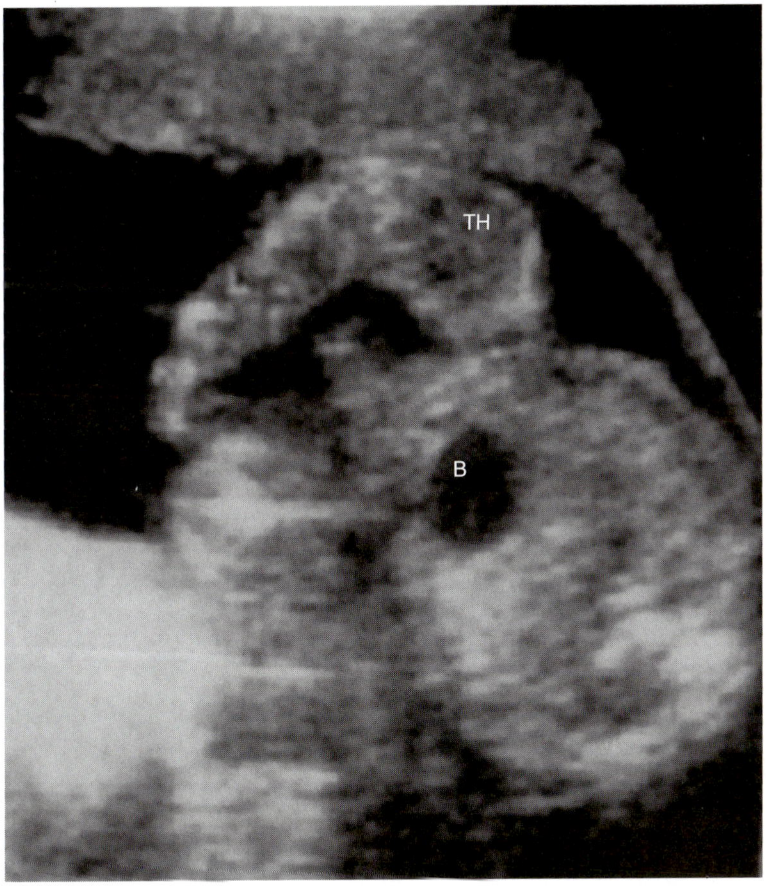

FIGURE 2-126 Longitudinal view of the lower extremity shows poorly ossified, shortened long-bones. (From Tongsong T, Sirichotiyakul S, Siriangkul S: *J Clin Ultrasound* 23:52–55, 1995.)

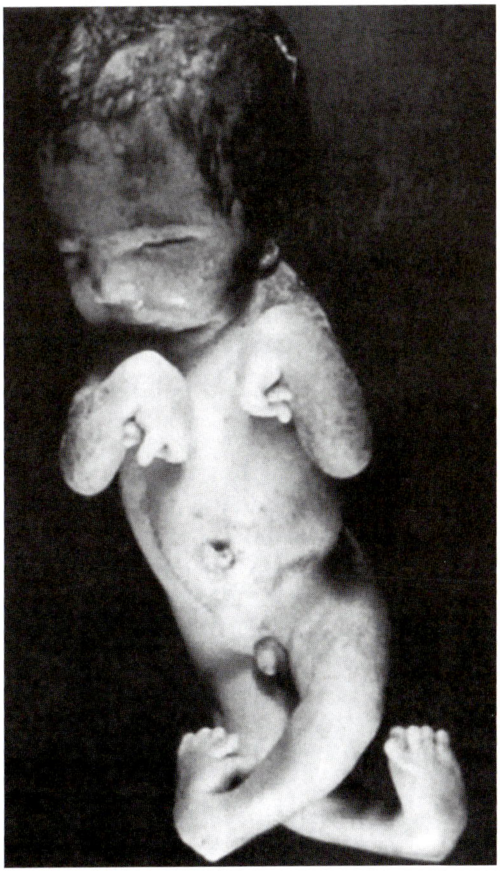

FIGURE 2-127 Postnatal appearance of a fetus with hypophosphatasia. Note marked contractures and limb shortening. (From Tongsong T, Sirichotiyakul S, Siriangkul S: *J Clin Ultrasound* 23:52–55, 1995.)

Atelosteogenesis

Chondrodysplasia punctata

ULTRASOUND DIAGNOSIS

Prenatal sonographic diagnosis of hypophosphatasia has been established several times by 14 weeks' gestation, based on the characteristic sonographic findings of a thin, sonolucent skull through which the gyri of the brain are well visualized; long bones that are delicate and poorly ossified; and bones of the hands and feet that are difficult to see. This disorder has been associated with a thickened nuchal translucency in the first trimester.

The diagnosis can be established in the first trimester by chorionic villus sampling assay of alkaline phosphatase.

HEREDITY

This disorder has an autosomal recessive pattern of inheritance resulting from mutations in the tissue-nonspecific alkaline phosphatase gene at 1p36.1-1.34.

NATURAL HISTORY AND OUTCOME

This is a lethal disorder, with death usually occurring as a result of respiratory insufficiency in the neonatal period. The occasional survivor has failure to thrive, seizures, and irritability.

Suggested Reading

DeLange M, Rouse GA: Prenatal diagnosis of hypophosphatasia. *J Ultrasound Med* 9:115–117, 1990.

Goncalves L, Jeanty P: Fetal biometry of skeletal dysplasias: a multicentric study. *J Ultrasound Med* 13:767–775, 1994.

Kleinman G, Uri M, Hull S, Keene C: Perinatal ultrasound casebook: antenatal findings in congenital hypophosphatasia. *J Perinatol* 11:282–284, 1991.

McGuire J, Manning F, Lange I, Lyons E, deSa DJ: Antenatal diagnosis of skeletal dysplasia using ultrasound. *Birth Defects Orig Artic Ser* 23:367–384, 1987.

Sharony R, Browne C, Lachman RS, Rimoin DL: Prenatal diagnosis of the skeletal dysplasias. *Am J Obstet Gynecol* 169:668–675, 1993.

Souka AP, Raymond FL, Mornet E, Geerts L, Nicolaides KH: Hypophosphatasia associated with increased nuchal translucency: a report of two affected pregnancies. *Ultrasound Obstet Gynecol* 20:294–295, 2002.

Tennstedt C, Bartho S, Bollmann R, et al: Osteochondrodysplasias. Prenatal diagnosis and pathological-anatomic findings. *Zentralbl Pathol* 139:71–80, 1993.

Tongsong T, Pongsatha S: Early prenatal sonographic diagnosis of congenital hypophosphatasia. *Ultrasound Obstet Gynecol* 15:252–255, 2000.

Tongsong T, Sirichotiyakul S, Siriangkul S: Prenatal diagnosis of congenital hypophosphatasia. *J Clin Ultrasound* 23:52–55, 1995.

van Dongen PW, Hamel BC, Nijhuis JG, de Boer CN: Prenatal follow-up of hypophosphatasia by ultrasound: case report. *Eur J Obstet Gynecol Reprod Biol* 34:283–288, 1990.

Witters I, Moerman P, Mornet E, Fryns JP: Positive maternal serum triple test screening in severe early onset hypophosphatasia. *Prenat Diagn* 24:494–497, 2004.

Wladimiroff JW, Niermeijer MF, Van der Harten JJ, et al: Early prenatal diagnosis of congenital hypophosphatasia: case report. *Prenat Diagn* 5:47–52, 1985.

JEUNE THORACIC DYSTROPHY

DESCRIPTION AND DEFINITION

Synonym: Asphyxiating thoracic dysplasia

Described by Jeune in 1955, this form of skeletal dysplasia, characterized by a very narrow rib cage and short ribs, results in severe respiratory failure and perinatal death.

ABNORMALITIES DETECTABLE BY ULTRASOUND

Common Findings:

Short, horizontal ribs that do not reach more than halfway around the thorax

Narrow chest in both anteroposterior diameter and width

Short long-bones, particularly in the late second or third trimester

Occasional Findings:

Polydactyly

Thickened nuchal translucency

MAJOR DIFFERENTIAL DIAGNOSES

Other Syndromes and Conditions Associated with Short Ribs and Polydactyly:

Ellis-van Creveld syndrome

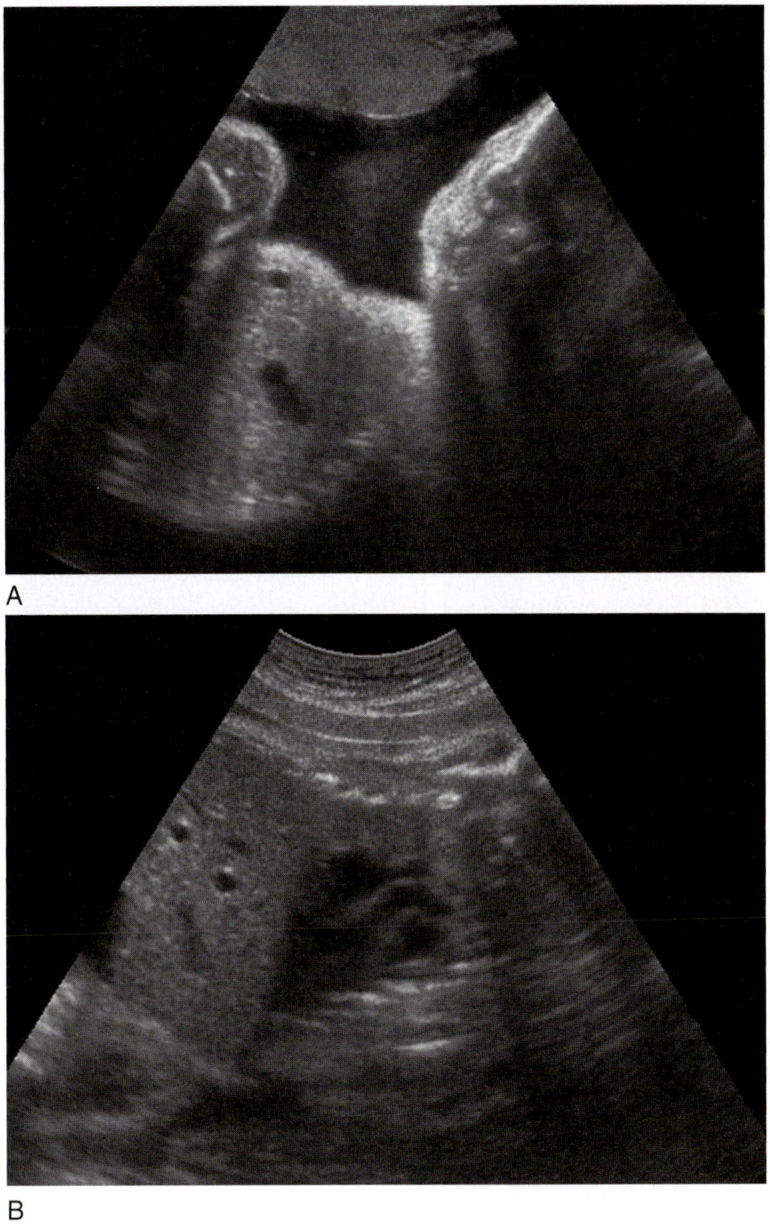

FIGURE 2-128 Thirty-two-week fetus with Lejeune thoracic dystrophy. (A) Longitudinal view of the fetal head, chest, and thoracic shows a very narrow chest. (B) Coronal view of the same fetus shows a narrow chest resulting from short ribs. Note that the width of the chest is narrow compared with the abdomen adjacent to it, and the space for the lungs is limited.

Short rib–polydactyly syndromes
- Saldino-Noonan syndrome (type I)
- Majewski syndrome (type II)
- Naumoff syndrome (type III)

ULTRASOUND DIAGNOSIS

Detection of this disorder has been reported in fetuses as young as 14 to 18 weeks, particularly in families with a history of a previously affected pregnancy. At 14 weeks, one report describes the femur below the fifth percentile and a narrow chest in a family with a previously affected child. The demonstration of short long-bones, however, is variable at that gestational age. Although in some cases the femoral measurement falls below the acceptable range, one of the reports at 17 weeks' gestational age revealed that the fetal limb lengths still were within 2 standard deviations below the mean. In most cases, the femoral length falls beyond 2 standard deviations below the mean by week 19. A family history of a previously affected pregnancy is helpful in the diagnosis of these cases, as is an abnormally flat and narrow thorax.

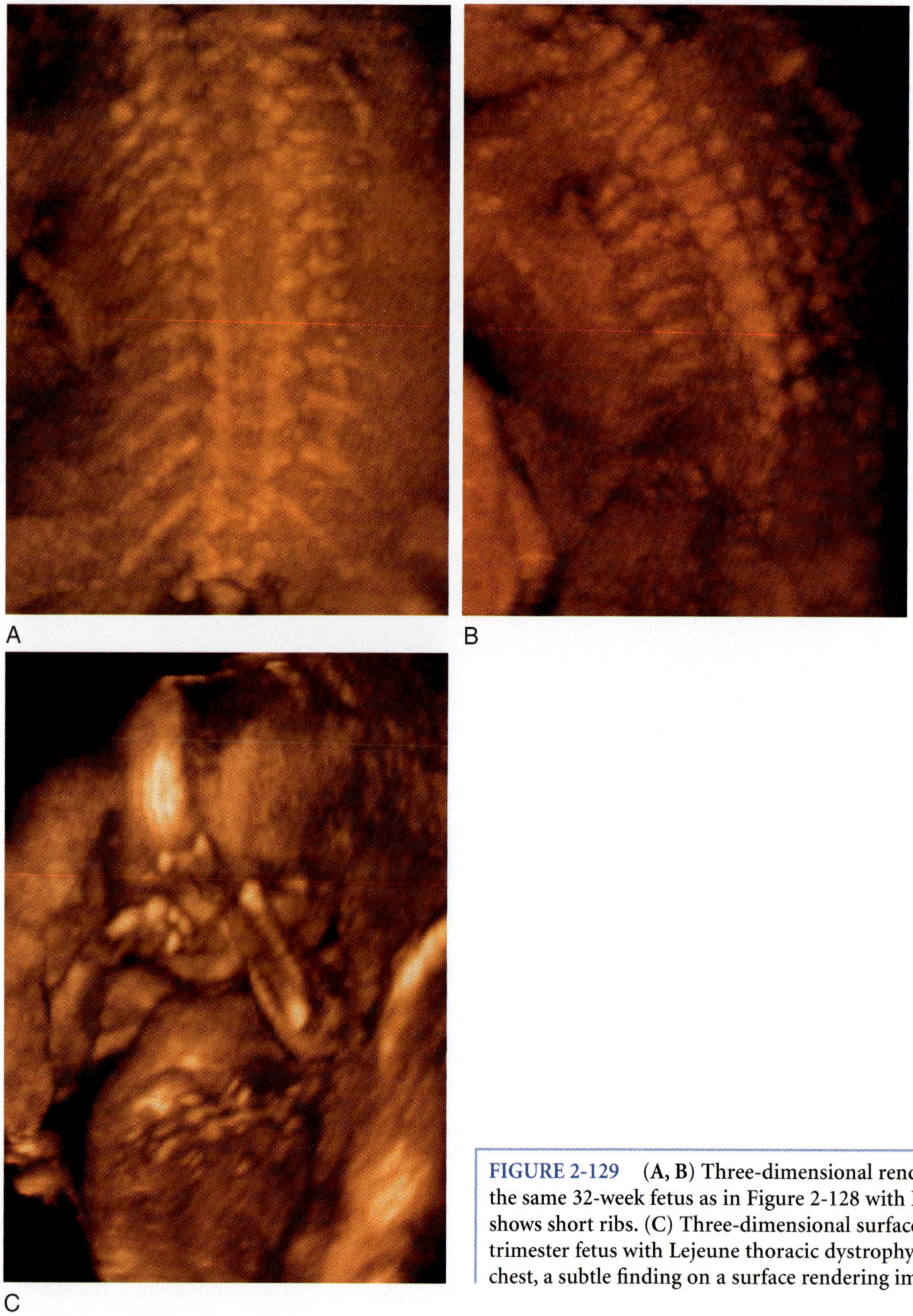

FIGURE 2-129 **(A, B) Three-dimensional rendering of the skeleton of the same 32-week fetus as in Figure 2-128 with Lejeune thoracic dystrophy shows short ribs. (C) Three-dimensional surface rendering of a second-trimester fetus with Lejeune thoracic dystrophy shows a relatively small chest, a subtle finding on a surface rendering image.**

There has been one report of pancreatic cysts identified prenatally in a fetus with this syndrome.

HEREDITY

The pattern of inheritance for Jeune thoracic dystrophy is autosomal recessive. The locus is 15q13.

NATURAL HISTORY AND OUTCOME

This is usually a lethal condition as a result of respiratory failure at birth. However, there have been occasional reports of long-term survivors, most of whom probably have a milder form of the disease. However, these individuals may be prone to renal or hepatic failure, both of which are features of this disorder's spectrum.

Suggested Reading

Ben Ami M, Perlitz Y, Haddad S, Matilsky M: Increased nuchal translucency is associated with asphyxiating thoracic dysplasia. *Ultrasound Obstet Gynecol* 10:297–298, 1997.

Chen CP, Lin SP, Liu FF, et al: Prenatal diagnosis of asphyxiating thoracic dysplasia (Jeune syndrome). *Am J Perinatol* 13:495–498, 1996.

Chen SH, Chung MT, Chang FM: Early prenatal diagnosis of Jeune syndrome in a low-risk pregnancy. *Prenat Diagn* 23:606–607, 2003.

den Hollander NS, Robben SG, Hoogeboom AJ, Niermeijer MF, Wladimiroff JW: Early prenatal sonographic diagnosis and follow-up of Jeune syndrome. *Ultrasound Obstet Gynecol* 18:378–383, 2001.

Elejalde BR, de Elejalde M, Pansch D: Prenatal diagnosis of Jeune syndrome. *Am J Med Genet* 21:433–438, 1985.

Herdman RC, Langer LO Jr: The thoracic asphyxiant dystrophy and renal disease. *Am J Dis Child* 116:192–201, 1968.

Hopper MS, Boultbee JE, Watson AR: Polyhydramnios associated with congenital pancreatic cysts and asphyxiating thoracic dysplasia: a case report. *S Afr Med J* 56:32–33, 1979.

Hudgins L, Rosengren S, Treem W, Hyams J: Early cirrhosis in survivors with Jeune thoracic dystrophy. *Am J Hum Genet* 47:A61, 1990.

Jeune M, Beraud C, Carron R: Dystrophie thoracique asphyxiante de caractere familial. *Arch Fr Pediatr* 12:886–891, 1955.

Jones KL: *Smith's recognizable patterns of human malformations,* ed 6. Philadelphia, Elsevier, 2006.

Lipson M, Waskey J, Rice J, et al: Prenatal diagnosis of asphyxiating thoracic dysplasia. *Am J Med Genet* 18:273–277, 1984.

Meinel K, Himmel D: Status of ultrasound and roentgen diagnosis in prenatal detection of osteochondrodysplasias. *Zentralbl Gynakol* 109:1303–1313, 1987.

Schinzel A, Savoldelli G, Briner J, Schubiger G: Prenatal sonographic diagnosis of Jeune syndrome. *Radiology* 154:777–778, 1985.

Shah KJ: Renal lesion in Jeune's syndrome. *Br J Radiol* 53:432–436, 1980.

Sharony R, Browne C, Lachman RS, Rimoin DL: Prenatal diagnosis of the skeletal dysplasias. *Am J Obstet Gynecol* 169:668–675, 1993.

Skiptunas SM, Weiner S: Early prenatal diagnosis of asphyxiating thoracic dysplasia (Jeune's syndrome): value of fetal thoracic measurement. *J Ultrasound Med* 6:41–43, 1987.

Tongsong T, Chanprapaph P, Thongpadungroj T: Prenatal sonographic findings associated with asphyxiating thoracic dystrophy (Jeune syndrome). *J Ultrasound Med* 18:573–576, 1999.

Wladimiroff JW, Niermeijer MF, Laar J, Jahoda M, Stewart PA: Prenatal diagnosis of skeletal dysplasia by real-time ultrasound. *Obstet Gynecol* 63:360–364, 1984.

Zimmer EZ, Weinraub Z, Raijman A, Pery M, Peretz BA: Antenatal diagnosis of a fetus with an extremely narrow thorax and short limb dwarfism. *J Clin Ultrasound* 12:112–114, 1984.

KNIEST SYNDROME

DESCRIPTION AND DEFINITION

Synonym: Metatropic dwarfism, type II

This is a nonlethal disorder characterized by platyspondyly leading to kyphoscoliosis, ophthalmologic complications, and shortened tubular bones.

ABNORMALITIES DETECTABLE BY ULTRASOUND

Common Findings:

Short long-bones in the third trimester, with some bowing and irregularity of the epiphyses

Lumbar kyphoscoliosis with platyspondyly

Inguinal hernia

Cleft palate

Occasional Finding:

Cataracts

MAJOR DIFFERENTIAL DIAGNOSES

Achondroplasia

Hypochondroplasia

Metatropic dysplasia, type I (although the face and thorax are normal in type I)

Russell-Silver syndrome

Shprintzen syndrome

Spondyloepiphyseal dysplasia (although the face is normal and the femora are not as profoundly affected as in Kniest syndrome)

ULTRASOUND DIAGNOSIS

We reported the ultrasound diagnosis of Kniest syndrome in 1991; the ultrasonogram that was obtained at 17 weeks' gestation appeared normal, with femoral length lagging by only 1 week (which was not suggestive of a skeletal dysplasia). Abnormalities became apparent at 31 weeks' gestation, when the fetal head size was 4

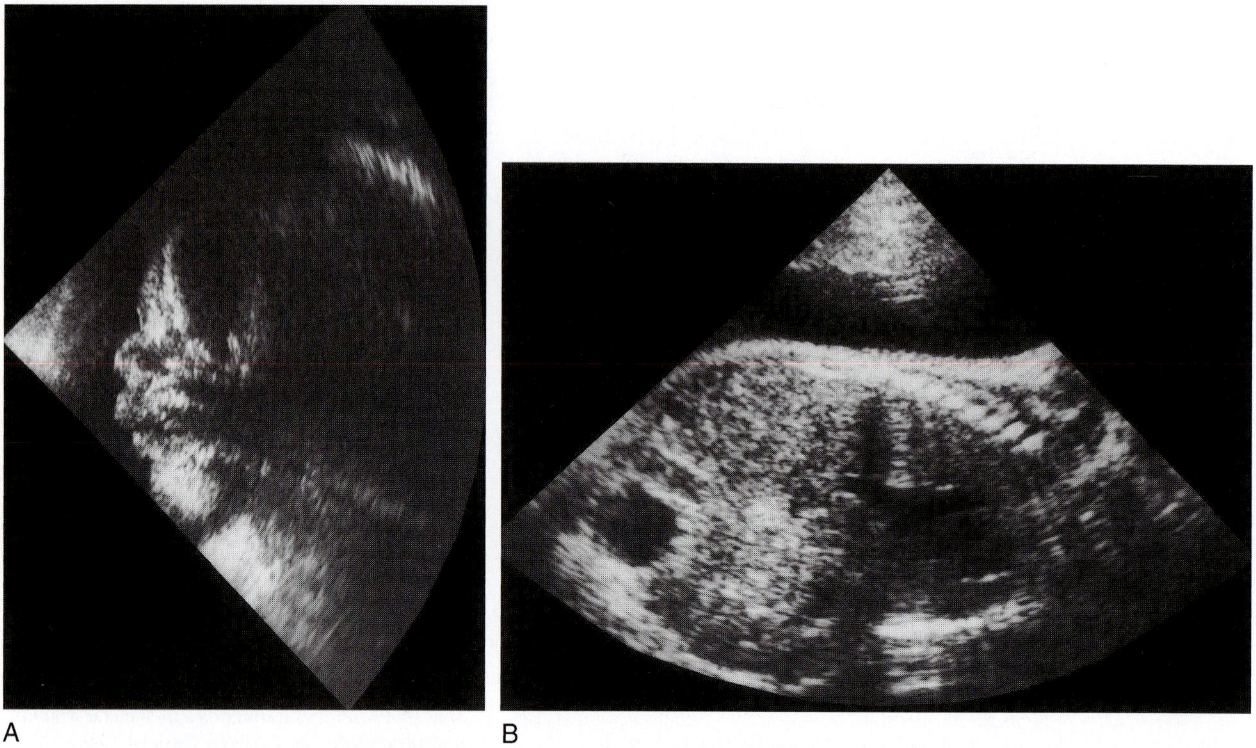

FIGURE 2-130 **(A) Long-axis view of the profile of a fetus with Kniest syndrome shows a depressed nasal bridge. (B) Coronal view of the chest and abdomen of the same fetus shows narrowing of the fetal chest compared with the abdomen.**

weeks ahead of dates and the femoral length was consistent with 25 weeks' gestation. The fetal profile was abnormal, characterized by a flat nose, short neck, and flat forehead. Chest size was normal, and there was polyhydramnios.

HEREDITY

Kniest syndrome results from a defect in the gene for type II collagen (COL2A1). Other syndromes caused by a defect in this gene include achondrogenesis type II, spondyloepiphyseal dysplasia, and Stickler syndrome. The pattern of inheritance is autosomal dominant, although most cases represent a fresh mutation.

NATURAL HISTORY AND OUTCOME

Although Kniest syndrome is compatible with life, there is significant disability secondary to deafness; ophthalmologic complications, such as cataracts, retinal detachment, and myopia; and orthopedic problems caused by kyphoscoliosis. There are flexion contractures of the extremities, particularly of the hips.

Suggested Reading

Bromley B, Miller W, Foster SC, Benacerraf BR: The prenatal sonographic features of Kniest syndrome. *J Ultrasound Med* 10:705–707, 1991.

Goncalves L, Jeanty P: Fetal biometry of skeletal dysplasias: a multicentric study. *J Ultrasound Med* 13:767–775, 1994.

Jones KL: *Smith's recognizable patterns of human malformations,* ed 6. Philadelphia, Elsevier, 2006.

Kniest W: Zur Abgrenzung der dysostosis enchondralis von der chondrodystrophie. *Z Kinderheilkd* 70:633, 1952.

Romero R: *Prenatal diagnosis of congenital anomalies.* East Norwalk, CT, 1988, Appleton & Lange.

Sconyers SM, Rimoin DL, Lachman RS, Adomian GE, Crandall BF: A distinct chondrodysplasia resembling Kniest dysplasia: clinical, roentgenographic, histologic, and ultrastructural findings. *J Pediatr* 103:898–904, 1983.

Sharony R, Browne C, Lachman RS, Rimoin DL: Prenatal diagnosis of the skeletal dysplasias. *Am J Obstet Gynecol* 169:668–675, 1993.

Tennstedt C, Bartho S, Bollmann R, et al: Osteochondrodysplasias. Prenatal diagnosis and pathological-anatomic findings. *Zentralbl Pathol* 139:71–80, 1993.

MAJEWSKI SYNDROME

DESCRIPTION AND DEFINITION

Synonym: Short rib–polydactyly syndrome, type II (SRPS II, Majewski type)

First described in 1971 by Majewski, this syndrome is a lethal form of short-limbed dwarfism.

ABNORMALITIES DETECTABLE BY ULTRASOUND

Common Findings:

Median facial cleft

Narrow thorax with short ribs

Short limbs, with shortening of all long bones

Preaxial and postaxial polysyndactyly of the hands and feet

Polydactyly

Polyhydramnios

Occasional Findings:

Small cerebellar vermis

Renal abnormalities

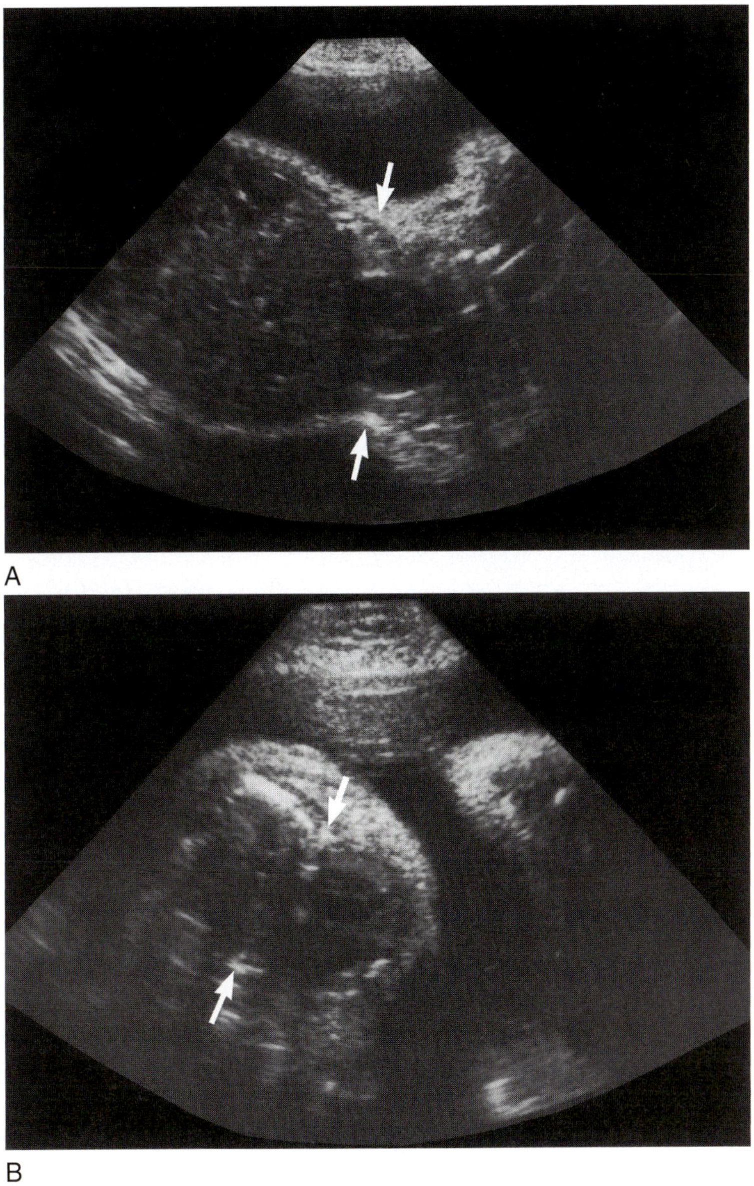

FIGURE 2-131 Coronal and transverse views through the chest of a fetus with Majewski syndrome. (A) Note narrow thorax *(arrows)* compared with the fetal abdomen, as well as the lack of space for lung development. (B) The ribs *(arrows)* extend only halfway around the chest. The volume of the heart takes up more of the volume of the chest than normal, which means that space for lung development is inadequate.

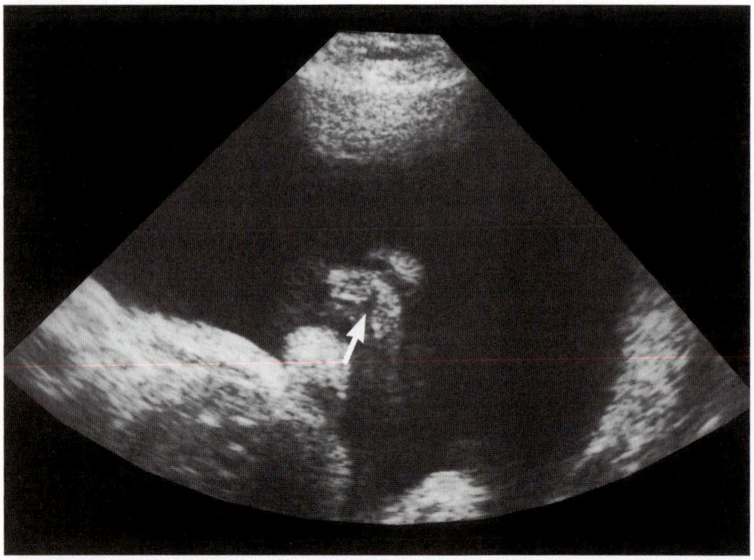

FIGURE 2-132 Coronal view of the upper lip of the same fetus as in Figure 2-116. Note midline facial cleft *(arrow)*.

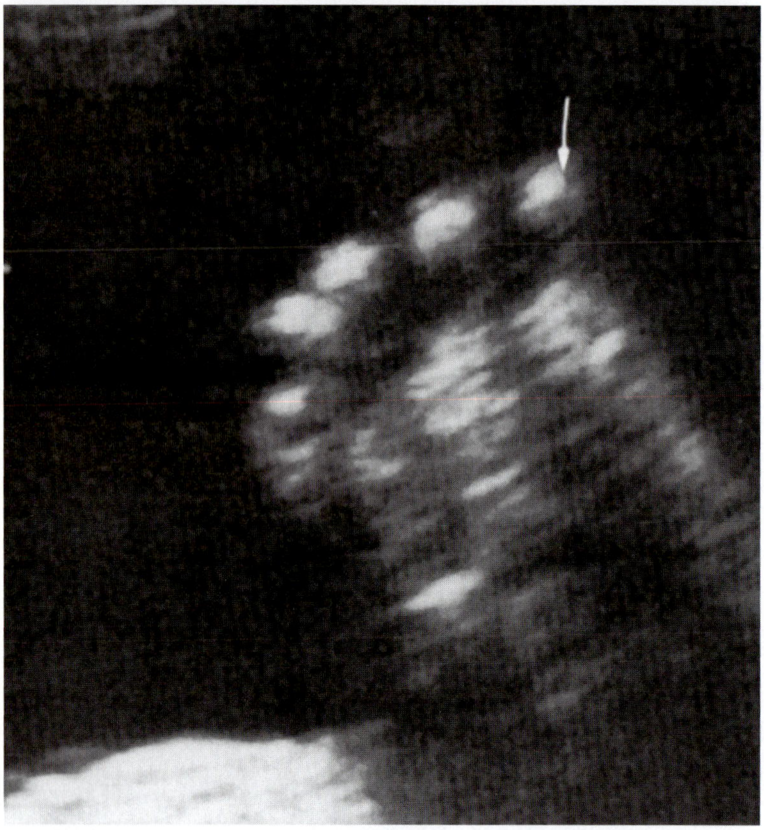

FIGURE 2-133 View of the fetal hand shows postaxial polydactyly *(arrow)* in the same fetus as in Figures 2-131 and 2-132. Note that the fetal thumb is not shown in this plane. (From Benacerraf BR: *J Ultrasound Med* 12:552–555, 1993.)

MAJOR DIFFERENTIAL DIAGNOSES

Other Skeletal Dysplasias Associated with Short Ribs and Polydactyly

Asphyxiating thoracic dystrophy (*not* associated with cleft lip and palate)

Ellis-van Creveld syndrome (associated with cardiac abnormalities in 60% of cases)

Oral-facial-digital syndrome (midline facial cleft and polydactyly)

Short rib–polydactyly syndrome, type I (Saldino-Noonan syndrome; *not* usually associated with cleft lip and palate)

Short rib–polydactyly syndrome, type III (Naumoff syndrome; *not* usually associated with cleft lip and palate)

Thanatophoric dysplasia (*not* usually associated with polydactyly)

ULTRASOUND DIAGNOSIS

Prenatal ultrasound diagnosis of Majewski syndrome has been established as early as 16 weeks, as well as in the third trimester in several cases. Findings are easily recognizable, even in the second trimester, and include polyhydramnios in association with postaxial polydactyly, relatively short long-bones, symmetric mesomelic brachymelia with disproportionately short tibiae, median cleft lip, and narrow chest with short ribs extending less than halfway around the chest in transverse section.

HEREDITY

Majewski syndrome has an autosomal recessive pattern of inheritance.

NATURAL HISTORY AND OUTCOME

This malformation leads to pulmonary hypoplasia and death shortly after birth.

Suggested Reading

Benacerraf BR: Prenatal sonographic diagnosis of short rib–polydactyly syndrome type II, Majewski type. *J Ultrasound Med* 12:552–555, 1993.

Chen CP, Chang TY, Tzen CY, Wang W: Second-trimester sonographic detection of short rib-polydactyly syndrome type II (Majewski) following an abnormal maternal serum biochemical screening result. *Prenat Diagn* 23:353–355, 2003.

Chen H, Yang SS, Gonzalez E, Fowler M, Al Saadi A: Short rib–polydactyly syndrome, Majewski type. *Am J Med Genet* 7:215–222, 1980.

Cooper CP, Hall CM: Lethal short rib–polydactyly syndrome of the Majewski type: a report of three cases. *Radiology* 144:513–517, 1982.

Gembruch U, Hansmann M, Fodisch HJ: Early prenatal diagnosis of short rib–polydactyly (SRP) syndrome type I (sic) (Majewski) by ultrasound in a case at risk. *Prenat Diagn* 5:357–362, 1985.

Goncalves L, Jeanty P: Fetal biometry of skeletal dysplasias: a multicentric study. *J Ultrasound Med* 13:767–775, 1994.

Majewski F, Pfeiffer RA, Lenz W: Polysyndaktylie, verkurzte gliedmaben und genital-fehlbildungen: kennzeichen eines selbstandigen syndroms? *Z Kinderheilkd* 111:118–138, 1971.

Montemarano H, Bulas DI, Chandra R, Tifft C: Prenatal diagnosis of glomerulocystic kidney disease in short rib–polydactyly syndrome type II, Majewski type. *Pediatr Radiol* 25:469–471, 1995.

Motegi T, Kusunoki M, Nishi T, et al: Short rib–polydactyly syndrome, Majewski type, in two male siblings. *Hum Genet* 49:269–275, 1979.

Naki MM, Gur D, Zemheri E, Tekcan C, Kanadikirik F, Has R: Short rib-polydactyly syndrome. *Arch Gynecol Obstet* 272:173–175, 2005.

Sharony R, Browne C, Lachman RS, Rimoin DL: Prenatal diagnosis of the skeletal dysplasias. *Am J Obstet Gynecol* 169:668–675, 1993.

Sirichotiyakul S, Tongsong T, Wanapirak C, Chanprapaph P: Prenatal sonographic diagnosis of Majewski syndrome. *J Clin Ultrasound* 30:303–307, 2002.

Thomson GSM, Reynolds CP, Cruickshank J: Antenatal detection of recurrence of Majewski dwarf (short rib–polydactyly syndrome type II Majewski). *Clin Radiol* 33:509–517, 1982.

Toftager-Larsen K, Benzie RJ: Fetoscopy in prenatal diagnosis of the Majewski and the Saldino-Noonan types of the short rib–polydactyly syndromes. *Clin Genet* 26:56–60, 1984.

Viora E, Sciarrone A, Bastonero S, Errante G, Botta G, Campogrande M: Three-dimensional ultrasound evaluation of short-rib polydactyly syndrome type II in the second trimester: a case report. *Ultrasound Obstet Gynecol* 19:88–91, 2002.

Wladimiroff JW, Neirmeijer MF, Laar J, et al: Prenatal diagnosis of skeletal dysplasia by realtime ultrasound. *Obstet Gynecol* 63:360–364, 1984.

METATROPIC DYSPLASIA

DESCRIPTION AND DEFINITION

First described in 1966 by Maroteaux, this form of dwarfism is characterized by progressive severe kyphoscoliosis, short-limbed skeletal abnormalities, and trumpet-shaped widening of the metaphyses.

ABNORMALITIES DETECTABLE BY ULTRASOUND

Common Findings:

Enlarged biparietal diameter

Elongated, narrow thorax

Platyspondyly with progressive kyphoscoliosis

Markedly shortened limbs, with disproportionately elongated hands and feet

Shortened femur

Metaphyseal flaring

Occasional Finding:

Ventriculomegaly

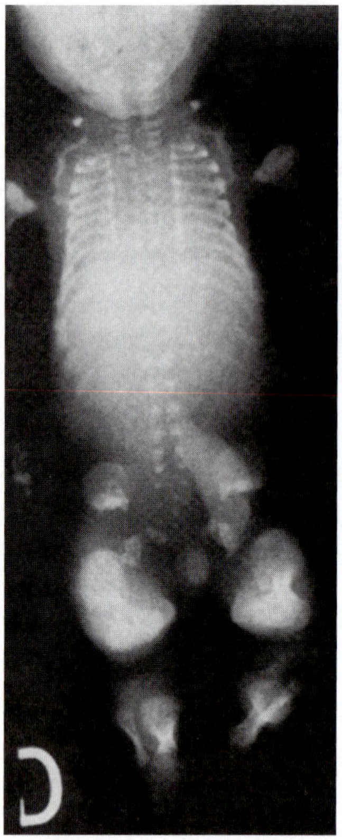

FIGURE 2-134 Fetal radiograph reveals the characteristic dumbbell appearance of the long bones and narrow thorax associated with metatropic dwarfism. (From Manouvrier-Hanu S, Devisme L, Zelasko MC, et al: *Prenat Diagn* 15:753–756, 1995.)

MAJOR DIFFERENTIAL DIAGNOSES

Skeletal Dysplasias Associated with Platyspondyly:

Atelosteogenesis

Kniest syndrome

Spondyloepiphyseal dysplasia

Thanatophoric dysplasia

ULTRASOUND DIAGNOSIS

Prenatal diagnosis of metatropic dysplasia has been established at 20 weeks' gestation, based on the detection of moderate polyhydramnios, dramatically foreshortened long-bones, elongated and narrow thorax, and macrocephaly. Radiographic studies of the pregnant uterus revealed the classic, dumbbell-like appearance of the fetal metaphyses, platyspondyly of the vertebral bodies, and enlargement of the hands and feet relative to the length of the limbs.

HEREDITY

The lethal form of this syndrome likely is autosomal recessive. Nonlethal forms are thought to be either autosomal recessive or autosomal dominant.

NATURAL HISTORY AND OUTCOME

Although this condition (nonlethal forms) is compatible with life, it is associated with severe disabilities secondary to progressive kyphoscoliosis. Some patients suffer cervical (C1–C2) subluxation, leading to spinal cord compression and instability of the spine.

Suggested Reading

Gordienko I, Grechanina E, Sopko NI, Tarapurova EN, Mikchailets LP: Prenatal diagnosis of osteochondrodysplasias in high risk pregnancy. *Am J Med Genet* 63:90–97, 1996.

Jones KL: *Smith's recognizable patterns of human malformations,* ed 6. Philadelphia, Elsevier, 2006.

Manouvrier-Hanu S, Devisme L, Zelasko MC, et al: Prenatal diagnosis of metatropic dwarfism. *Prenat Diagn* 15:753–756, 1995.

Maroteaux P, Spranger J, Wiedemann HR: Der metatropische zwergwuchs. *Arch Kinderheilkd* 173:211–226, 1966.

Nieves GA, Gonzalez ME, Martinez AMM, et al: Metatropic dysplasia: a case report. *Am J Perinatol* 12:129–131, 1995.

Sharony R, Browne C, Lachman RS, Rimoin DL: Prenatal diagnosis of the skeletal dysplasias. *Am J Obstet Gynecol* 169:668–675, 1993.

Tennstedt C, Bartho S, Bollmann R, et al: Osteochondrodysplasias. Prenatal diagnosis and pathological-anatomic findings. *Zentralbl Pathol* 139:71–80, 1993.

OSTEOPETROSIS (LETHAL TYPE)

DESCRIPTION AND DEFINITION

Synonym: Albers-Schönberg disease

Lethal osteopetrosis is a condition characterized by diffuse skeletal sclerosis secondary to osteoclastic dysfunction. Other than this autosomal recessive lethal form, less severe forms include the autosomal recessive form associated with renal tubular acidosis and a mild, autosomal dominant condition.

ABNORMALITIES DETECTABLE BY ULTRASOUND

Ventriculomegaly

Increased bone density

Bone fractures

Shortened long-bones

IUGR

MAJOR DIFFERENTIAL DIAGNOSES

Other Syndromes and Conditions Associated with Bone Sclerosis:

Pyknodysostosis (nonlethal)

Yunis-Varon syndrome (usually lethal)

ULTRASOUND DIAGNOSIS

Prenatal diagnosis of lethal osteopetrosis has been established as early as 18 weeks' gestation in a fetus known to be at risk for the disorder. Manifestations included ventriculomegaly and increased echogenicity of bone. Although the short long-bones initially were detected at 18 weeks, the abnormality was more obvious at 21 weeks' gestation, when they also exhibited a lack of adequate interval growth. Abnormal levels of fetal blood calcium, phosphorus, and alkaline phosphatase facilitated prenatal diagnosis.

In another case, a 35-week affected fetus had severe hydrocephalus, polyhydramnios, dense skeleton, and deformed humerus. Although bone density was difficult to determine (because of the lack of normal standards), hydrocephalus and increased bone density with rib fractures were demonstrated in the second trimester of a subsequent affected pregnancy in the same woman.

HEREDITY

This disorder has an autosomal recessive pattern of inheritance.

NATURAL HISTORY AND OUTCOME

Most fetuses with the most severe form of this disease die of anemia, bleeding, or overwhelming infection in the perinatal period. Approximately one third of affected individuals survive into early childhood, but there are no long-term survivors. Other complications include early blindness and deafness, secondary to cranial nerve palsy.

The pathogenesis of this disorder is thought to be failure of osteoclasts to resorb immature bone and calcified cartilage. As new bone is formed, excessive bone formation leads to obliteration of bone marrow. Consequently, there is

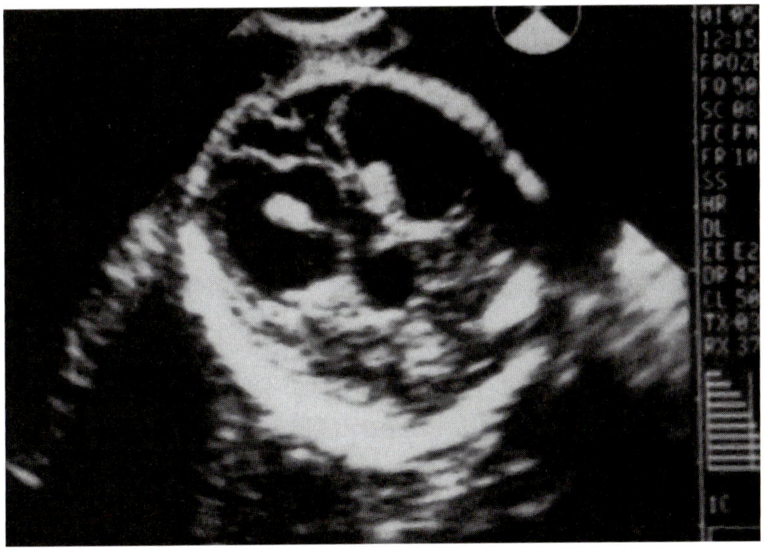

FIGURE 2-135 Transverse view through the fetal skull shows hydrocephalus and increased bone density in the calvaria. (From Sen C, Madazli R, Aksoy F, Ocak V: *Ultrasound Obstet Gynecol* 5:278–280, 1995.)

anemia and thrombocytopenia, as well as extramedullary hematopoiesis with hepatosplenomegaly and lymphadenopathy.

Suggested Reading

El Khazen N, Feverly D, Vamos E, et al: Lethal osteopetrosis with multiple fractures in utero. *Am J Med Genet* 23:811–819, 1986.

Jones KL: *Smith's recognizable patterns of human malformations,* ed 6. Philadelphia, Elsevier, 2006.

Malinger G, Ornoy A, El Shawwa R, Zakut H, Kohn G: Osteopetrosis. *Fetus* 4:15–17, 1994.

Sen C, Madazli R, Aksoy F, Ocak V: Antenatal diagnosis of lethal osteopetrosis. *Ultrasound Obstet Gynecol* 5:278–280, 1995.

Wasant P, Waeteekul S, Rimoin DL, Lachman RS: Genetic skeletal dysplasia in Thailand: the Siriraj experience. *SE Asian J Trop Med Publ Health* 1:59–67, 1995.

SHORT RIB–POLYDACTYLY SYNDROMES (SRPS): TYPES I (SALDINO-NOONAN) AND III (NAUMOFF)

DESCRIPTION AND DEFINITION

Originally thought to be two separate syndromes, these conditions now are considered part of a spectrum of one disorder with variable expression. Characterized by short ribs, polydactyly, and short limbs, these syndromes, unlike SRPS type II, are *not* associated with cleft lip and palate.

ABNORMALITIES DETECTABLE BY ULTRASOUND

Extremely short ribs

Distortion of the vertebral bodies, with underossification

Severe micromelia with metaphyseal flaring

Polydactyly

Cardiac defects

Double-outlet right ventricle

Endocardial cushion defect

Transposition of the great vessels

Imperforate anus

Intestinal atresia

Hypoplastic or polycystic kidneys

Ambiguous genitalia

MAJOR DIFFERENTIAL DIAGNOSES

Other Skeletal Dysplasias Associated with Short Ribs and Polydactyly:

Asphyxiating thoracic dystrophy

Ellis-van Creveld syndrome (most similar to SRPS I and III; all are associated with cardiac defects)

Short rib–polydactyly syndrome, type II (Majewski syndrome; associated with cleft lip and palate, however)

Thanatophoric dysplasia (*not* usually associated with polydactyly)

ULTRASOUND DIAGNOSIS

SRPS I has been diagnosed prenatally in different reports, at 13 and 16 weeks' gestation, based on findings of a narrow thorax, significant shortening of the long bones, and polydactyly.

SRPS III has been diagnosed prenatally at 20 weeks' gestation, based on the findings of severe micromelia with widened, flared, irregular, marginal spurs at the ends of the long bones and progressive, distal shortening of the tubular bones. The vertebral bodies of the spine were hypoplastic, with irregular margins. There was frontal bossing, narrow rib cage, and postaxial polydactyly.

Third-trimester sonographic diagnosis of SRPS often is prompted by polyhydramnios and fetal size greater than dates. The findings are similar throughout the second and third trimesters. Diagnosis of these syndromes also has been established using fetoscopy.

HEREDITY

The pattern of inheritance for these syndromes is autosomal recessive.

NATURAL HISTORY AND OUTCOME

These syndromes are lethal, with death occurring shortly after birth as a result of pulmonary hypoplasia.

Suggested Reading

Benacerraf BR: Prenatal sonographic diagnosis of short rib–polydactyly syndrome type II, Majewski type. *J Ultrasound Med* 12:552–555, 1993.

Bernstein R, Isdale J, Pinto M, et al: Short rib–polydactyly syndrome: a single or heterogeneous entity? A re-evaluation prompted by four new cases. *J Med Genet* 22:46–53, 1985.

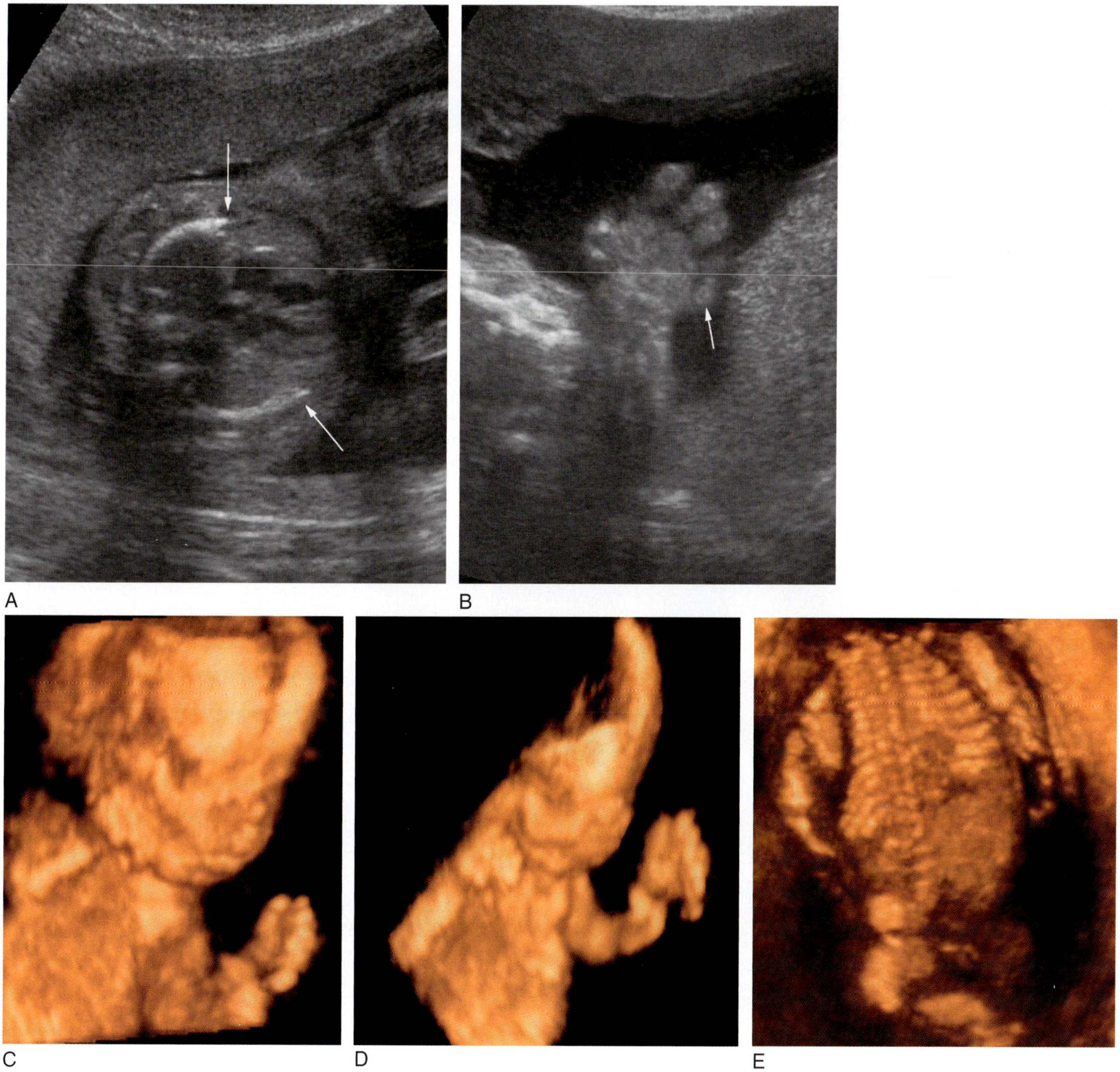

FIGURE 2-136 Short rib–polydactyly syndromes. (**A**) Second-trimester fetus with skeletal dysplasia, characterized by very short ribs *(arrows)*. (**B**) The same fetus has polydactyly *(arrow)* consistent with short rib–polydactyly syndrome, type I or III. This fetus did not have a facial cleft, indicating the fetus likely did not have short rib–polydactyly syndrome, type II. (**C, D**) Surface rendering of a second-trimester fetus with short ribs and polydactyly. Note short tubular bone and polydactyly. (**E**) Short ribs of the same fetus on surface rendering with bone settings.

Chen CP, Chang TY, Tzen CY, Lin CJ, Wang W: Sonographic detection of situs inversus, ventricular septal defect, and short-rib polydactyly syndrome type III (Verma-Naumoff) in a second-trimester fetus not known to be at risk. *Ultrasound Obstet Gynecol* 19:629–631, 2002.

Chen CP, Tzen CY: Short-rib polydactyly syndrome type III (Verma-Naumoff) in a third-trimester fetus with unusual associations of epiglottic hypoplasia, renal cystic dysplasia, pyelectasia and oligohydramnios. *Ultrasound Obstet Gynecol* 19:629–631, 2002.

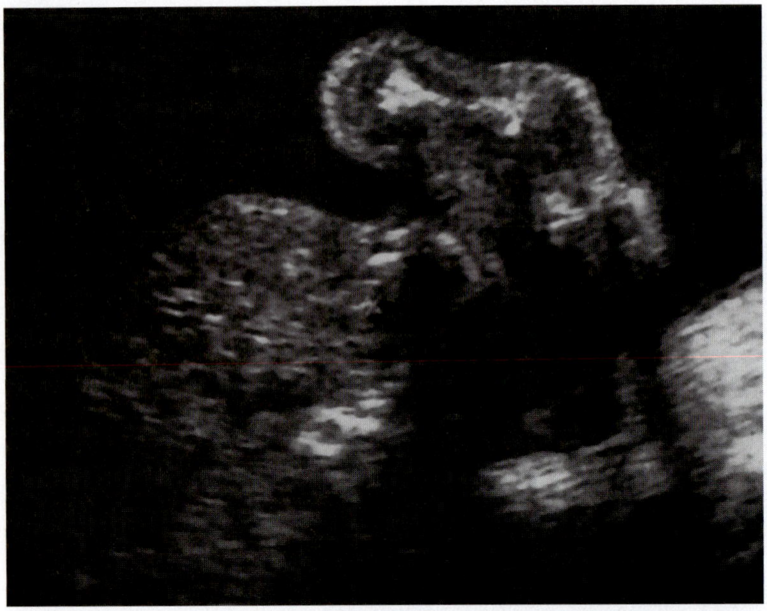

FIGURE 2-137 Shortened humerus with widened metaphyses typical of short rib–polydactyly syndrome, type III. (From Meizner I, Barnhard Y: *Prenat Diagn* 15:665–668, 1995.)

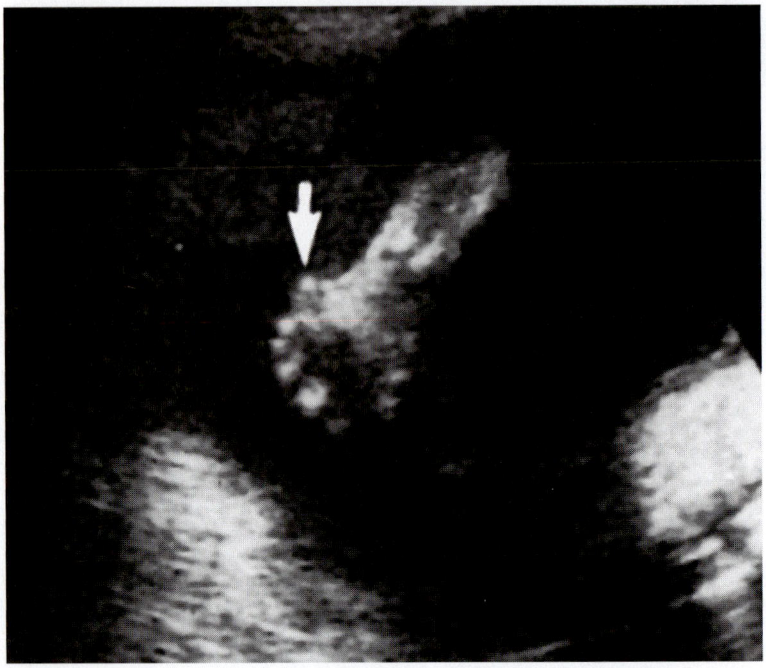

FIGURE 2-138 Evidence of polydactyly *(arrow)* in the same fetus as in Figure 2-122 with short rib–polydactyly syndrome, type III. (From Meizner I, Barnhard Y: *Prenat Diagn* 15:665–668, 1995.)

Gembruch U, Hansmann M, Fodisch HJ: Early prenatal diagnosis of short rib–polydactyly (SRP) syndrome type I (Majewski) by ultrasound in a case at risk. *Prenat Diagn* 5:357–362, 1985.

Golombeck K, Jacobs VR, von Kaisenberg C, et al: Short rib-polydactyly syndrome type III: comparison of ultrasound, radiology, and pathology findings. *Fetal Diagn Ther* 16:133–138, 2001.

Goncalves L, Jeanty P: Fetal biometry of skeletal dysplasias: a multicentric study. *J Ultrasound Med* 13:767–775, 1994.

Grote W, Weisner D, Janig U, Harms D, Wiedemann HR: Prenatal diagnosis of a short rib–polydactylia syndrome type Saldino-Noonan at 17 weeks' gestation. *Eur J Pediatr* 140:63–66, 1983.

Hill LM, Leary J: Transvaginal sonographic diagnosis of short-rib polydactyly dysplasia at 13 weeks' gestation. *Prenat Diagn* 18:1198–1201, 1998.

Johnson VP, Petersen LP, Holzwarth DR, Messner FD: Midtrimester prenatal diagnosis of short-limb dwarfism (Saldino-Noonan syndrome). *Birth Defects* 18(3 Pt A):133–141, 1982.

Jones KL: *Smith's recognizable patterns of human malformations,* ed 6. Philadelphia, Elsevier, 2006.

Kumru P, Aka N, Kose G, Vural ZT, Peker O, Kayserili H: Short rib polydactyly syndrome type 3 with absence of fibulae (Verma-Naumoff syndrome). *Fetal Diagn Ther* 20:410–414, 2005.

Meizner I, Barnhard Y: Short rib–polydactyly syndrome (SRPS) type III diagnosed during routine prenatal ultrasonographic screening. A case report. *Prenat Diagn* 15:665–668, 1995.

Meizner I, Bar-Ziv J: Prenatal ultrasonic diagnosis of short rib–polydactyly syndrome (SRPS) type III: a case report and a proposed approach to the diagnosis of SRPS and related conditions. *J Clin Ultrasound* 13:284–287, 1985.

Naumoff P, Young LW, Mazer J, Amortegui AJ: Short rib–polydactyly syndrome type 3. *Radiology* 122:443–447, 1977.

Richardson MM, Beaudet AL, Wagner ML, et al: Prenatal diagnosis of recurrence of Saldino-Noonan dwarfism. *J Pediatr* 91:467–471, 1977.

Saldino RM, Noonan CD: Severe thoracic dystrophy with striking micromelia, abnormal osseous development, including the spine, and multiple visceral anomalies. *AJR Am J Roentgenol* 114:257–263, 1972.

Sharony R, Browne C, Lachman RS, Rimoin DL: Prenatal diagnosis of the skeletal dysplasias. *Am J Obstet Gynecol* 169:668–675, 1993.

Tennstedt C, Bartho S, Bollmann R, et al: Osteochondrodysplasias. Prenatal diagnosis and pathological-anatomic findings. *Zentralbl Pathol* 139:71–80, 1993.

Toftager-Larsen K, Benzie RJ: Fetoscopy in prenatal diagnosis of the Majewski and the Saldino-Noonan types of the short rib–polydactyly syndromes. *Clin Genet* 26:56–60, 1984.

SPONDYLOEPIPHYSEAL DYSPLASIA CONGENITA

DESCRIPTION AND DEFINITION

This is a heterogeneous group of disorders involving the spine and proximal epiphyses and leading to a short trunk appearance.

ABNORMALITIES DETECTABLE BY ULTRASOUND

Short neck

Short spine with platyspondyly and narrow intervertebral distances, resulting in kyphoscoliosis and lordosis

No ossification of the pubis, calcaneus, or talus

Short long-bones, with a lag in mineralization of the epiphyses (although limbs may or may not be short, or they may be only mildly shortened)

Flared metaphyses

Clubfeet

Flat facies

MAJOR DIFFERENTIAL DIAGNOSES

Achondroplasia

Down syndrome

Hypochondroplasia

Kniest syndrome

Metatropic dysplasia

ULTRASOUND DIAGNOSIS

Kirk et al. have reported the prenatal sonographic findings associated with this disorder. Mild shortening of the femur and humerus for gestational age was the only sonographic finding at 16.5 weeks' gestation. Amniocentesis was performed to rule out Down syndrome because of the slightly shortened femur. By 27 weeks, the limb lengths were moderately short, although no bones were bowed. Polyhydramnios was present. In this particular case, spinal abnormalities were not well visualized sonographically but were present at birth.

HEREDITY

This syndrome has an autosomal dominant pattern of inheritance and is thought to result from alterations in type II collagen, secondary to an abnormal COL2A1 gene. Other conditions also thought to involve anomalies of the same gene include spondyloepimetaphyseal dysplasia, Kniest syndrome, achondrogenesis II, and Stickler syndrome.

NATURAL HISTORY AND OUTCOME

This condition is compatible with life, although affected adults usually are of short stature. Ophthalmologic complications, as well as progressive spinal deformities leading to kyphoscoliosis, are common.

Suggested Reading

Anderson IJ, Goldbert RB, Marion RW, Upholt WB, Tsipouras P: Spondyloepiphyseal dysplasia congenita: genetic linkage to type II collagen (COL2A1). *Am J Hum Genet* 46:896–901, 1990.

Jones KL: *Smith's recognizable patterns of human malformations,* ed 6. Philadelphia, Elsevier, 2006.

Kirk JS, Comstock CH: Antenatal sonographic appearance of Spondyloepiphyseal dysplasia congenita. *J Ultrasound Med* 9:173–175, 1990.

Murray LW, Rimoin DL: Abnormal type II collagen in the spondyloepiphyseal dysplasias. *Pathol Immunopathol Res* 7:99–103, 1988.

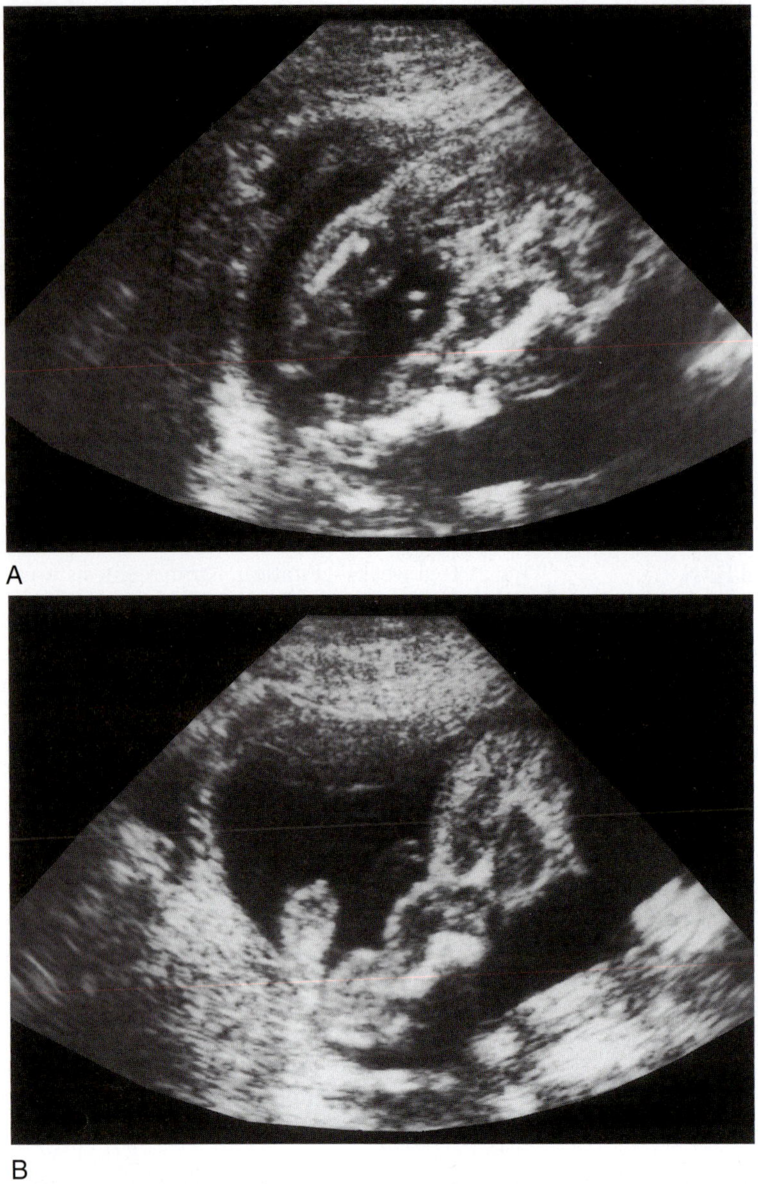

FIGURE 2-139 (**A, B**) Long-axis views of the lower extremities in a fetus with spondyloepiphyseal dysplasia. Note short tubular long-bones.

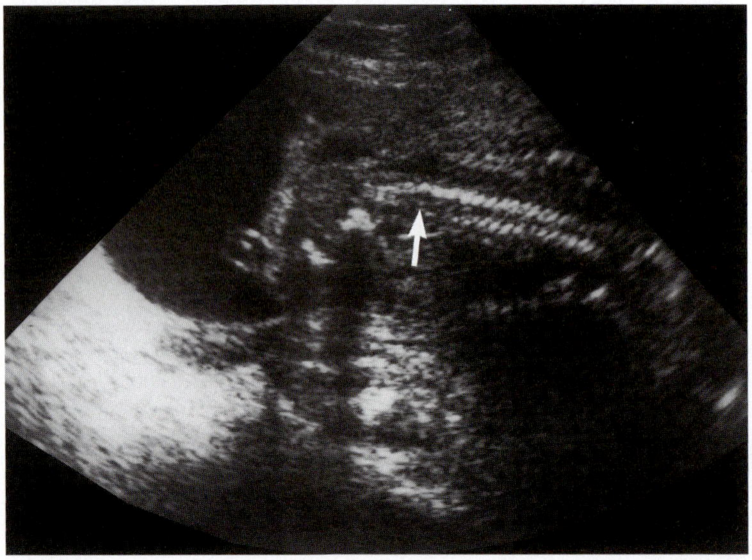

FIGURE 2-140 Coronal view of the spine of the same fetus as in Figure 2-139 shows decreased mineralization of the spine *(arrow)*.

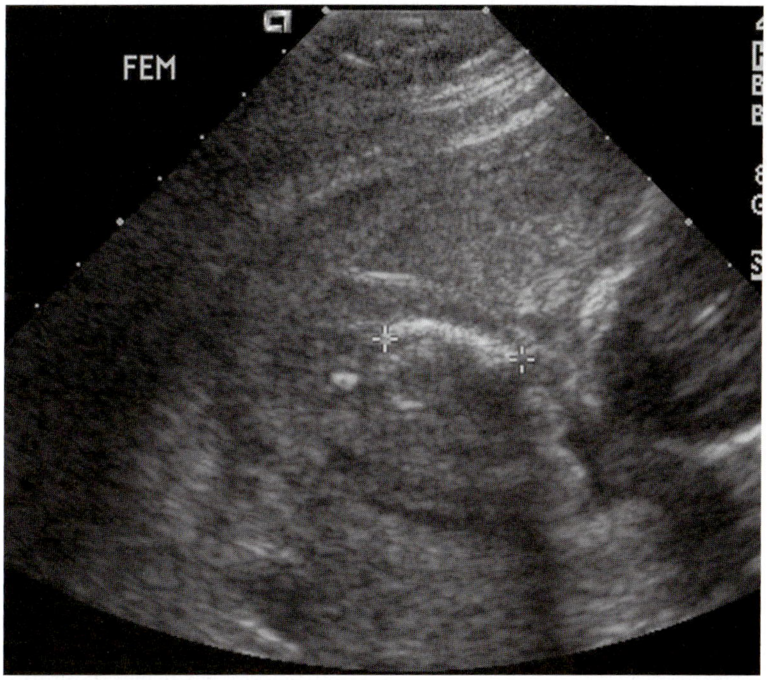

A

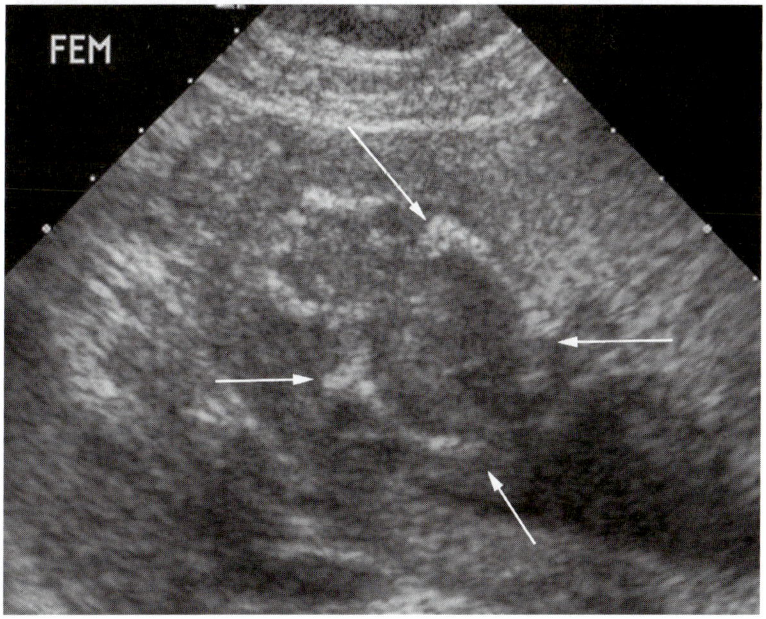

B

FIGURE 2-141 Spondyloepiphyseal dysplasia. (**A**) Image of the femur of a second-trimester fetus with spondyloepiphyseal dysplasia shows a bowed femur *(calipers)*. (**B**) View of both femurs, which are short and bowed *(arrows)*.

Parilla BV, Leeth EA, Kambich MP, Chilis P, MacGregor SN: Antenatal detection of skeletal dysplasias. *J Ultrasound Med* 22:255–258, 2003.

Sharony R, Browne C, Lachman RS, Rimoin DL: Prenatal diagnosis of the skeletal dysplasias. *Am J Obstet Gynecol* 169:668–675, 1993.

Spranger JW, Langer LO Jr: Spondyloepiphyseal dysplasia congenita. *Radiology* 94:313–322, 1970.

Wasant P, Waeteekul S, Rimoin DL, Lachman RS: Genetic skeletal dysplasia in Thailand: the Siriraj experience. *SE Asian J Trop Med Publ Health* 1:59–67, 1995.

THANATOPHORIC DYSPLASIA

DESCRIPTION AND DEFINITION

Derived from the Greek *thanatophoros*, meaning "death bearing," this lethal skeletal disorder is characterized by bowed, short long-bones; flat vertebral bodies; and a narrow chest.

ABNORMALITIES DETECTABLE BY ULTRASOUND

Common Findings:

Type I (most common)

- Curved and very short long-bones (particularly the femur), with a telephone receiver–like configuration; fibulae shorter than the tibiae
- Narrow, short ribs with small chest
- Platyspondyly
- Small facies
- Depressed nasal bridge
- Full forehead
- Polyhydramnios in the late second and third trimesters
- Ventriculomegaly

Type II

- Cloverleaf-shaped skull
- Curved and short long-bones (femora straighter than those found in type I)

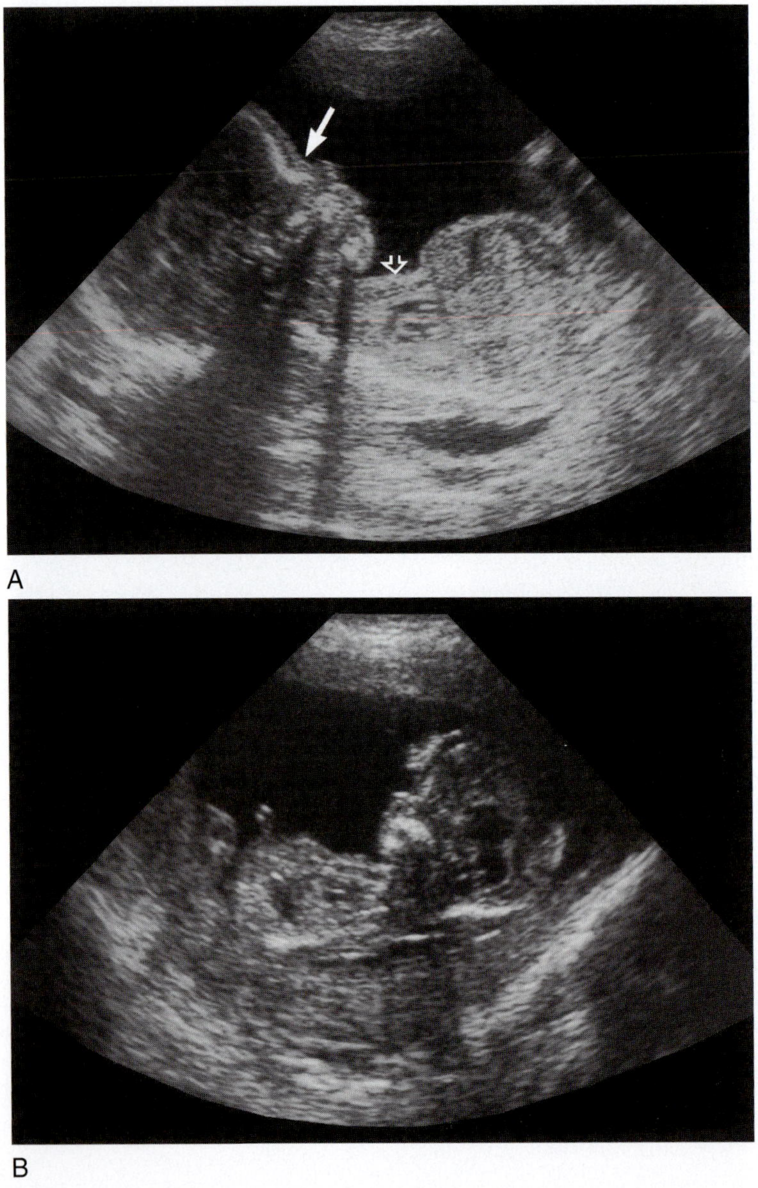

FIGURE 2-142 (A) Long-axis view of the head and body of a fetus with thanatophoric dysplasia. Note depressed nasal bridge *(solid arrow)* and very narrow chest *(open arrow)*. (B) The same features are evident in a late first-trimester/early second-trimester fetus with thanatophoric dysplasia.

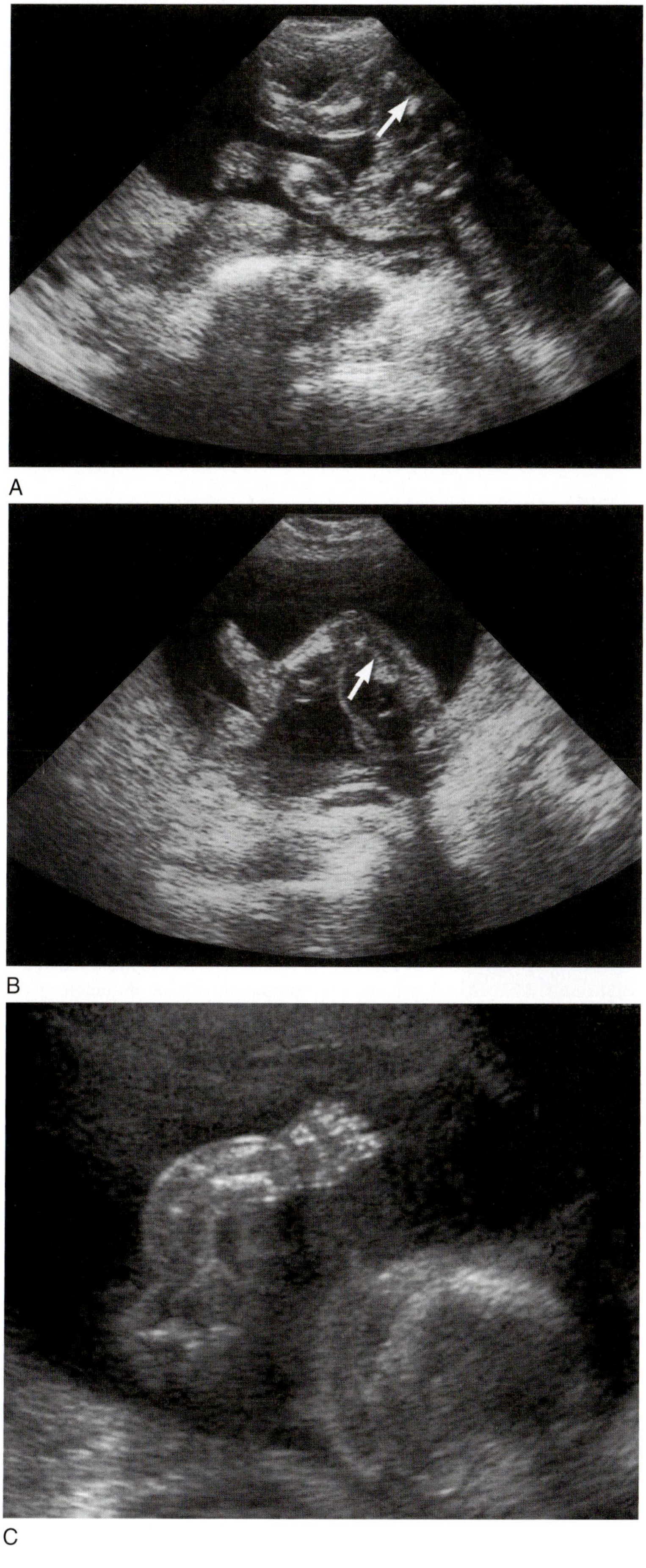

FIGURE 2-143 (A, B) Views of the lower extremities of a fetus with thanatophoric dysplasia show the characteristically bowed bones, particularly the femur *(arrow)*. (C) View of the upper extremity shows the short tubular bones.

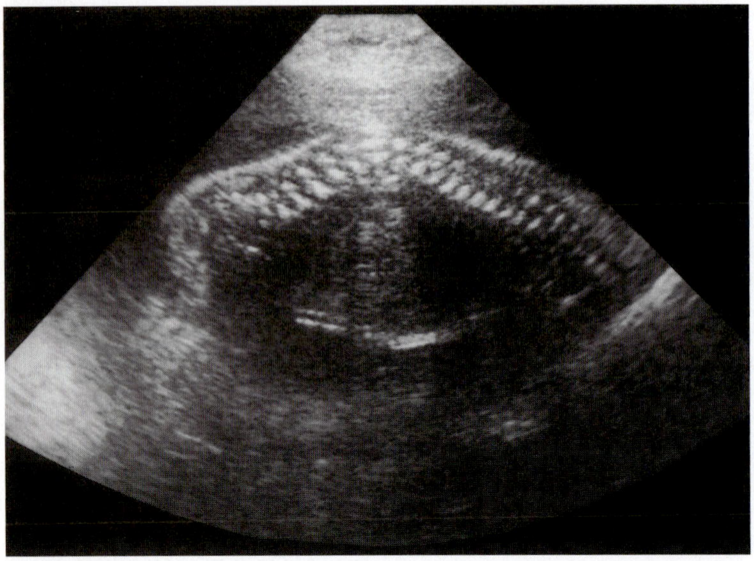

FIGURE 2-144 Longitudinal view of the fetal spine shows platyspondyly of the vertebral bodies, causing a slight kyphotic deformity.

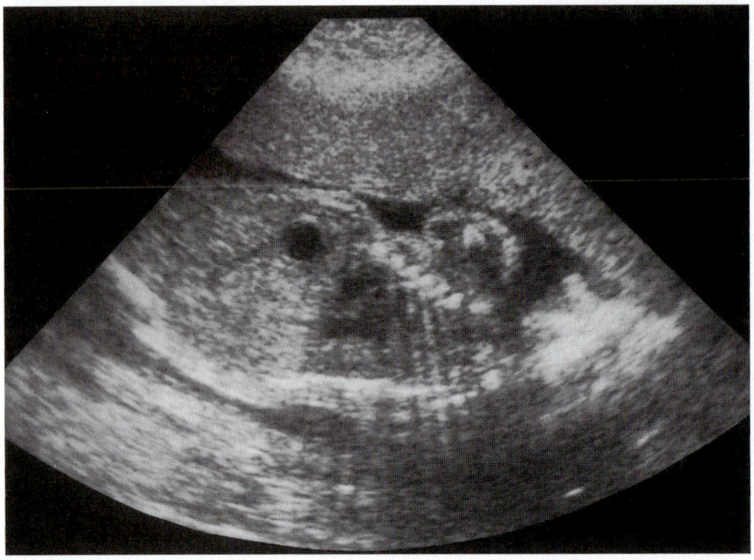

FIGURE 2-145 Longitudinal view of the chest of a fetus with thanatophoric dysplasia shows a narrow chest compared with the abdomen.

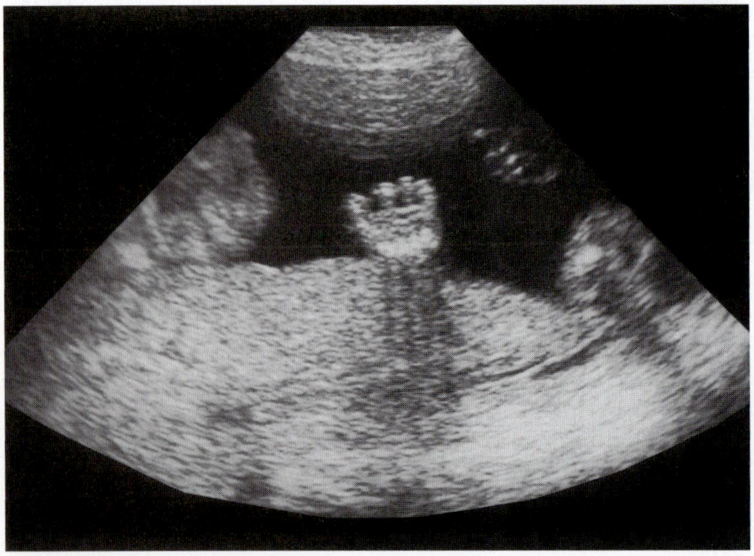

FIGURE 2-146 View of the hand of a fetus with thanatophoric dysplasia. Note trident appearance of the hand, with all fingers of the same length.

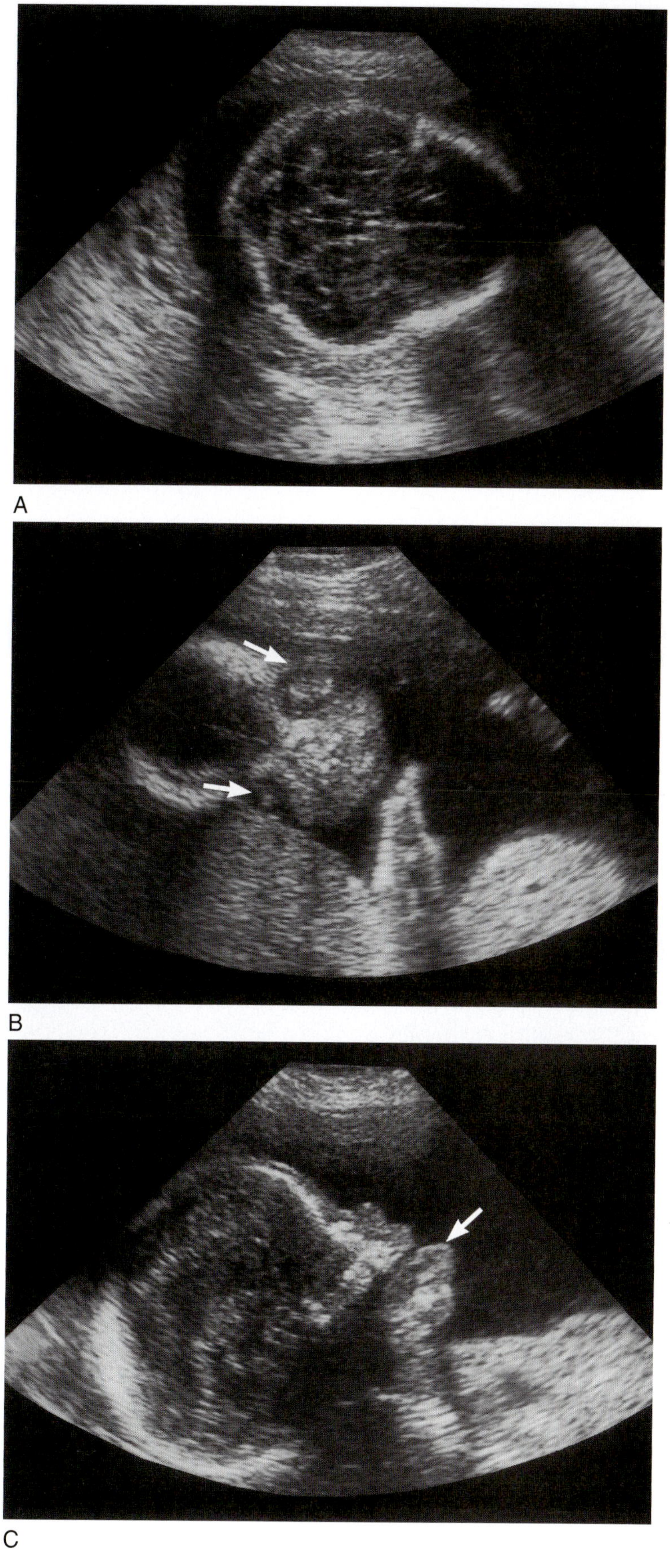

FIGURE 2-147 (A) Transverse view of the head of a fetus with thanatophoric dysplasia. Note unusual shape of the head, with some pointing of the frontal bones. (B) Coronal view of the face of the same fetus reveals hypertelorism, prominent forehead, and downsloping eyes *(arrows)*. (C) Longitudinal view of the fetal profile reveals a depressed nasal bridge and protruding tongue *(arrow)*.

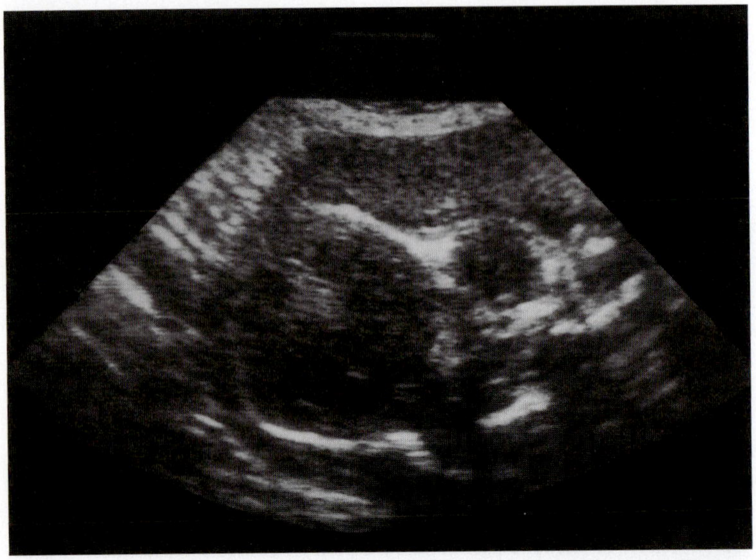

A

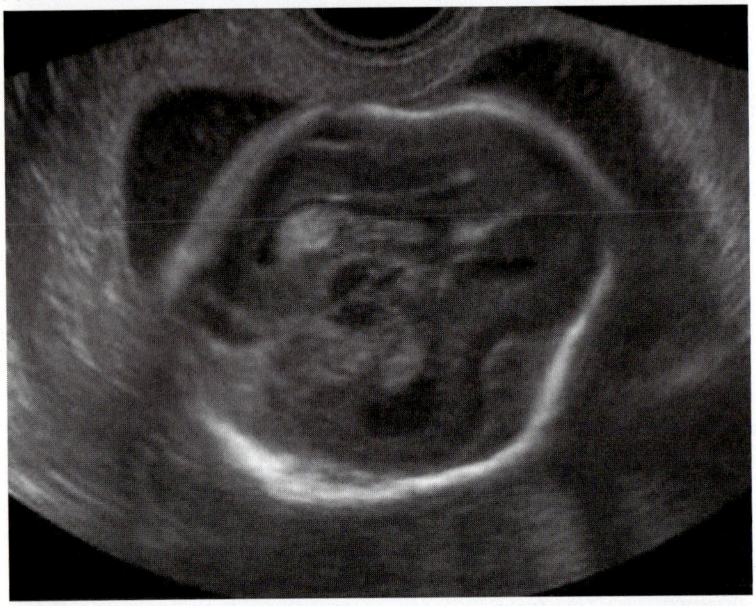

B

FIGURE 2-148 (A, B) Views of the heads of two different fetuses with thanatophoric dysplasia. Note unusual head shapes. (A) Classic cloverleaf-shaped head. (B) Two-dimensional image of a fetus with thanatophoric dysplasia type II shows the typical cloverleaf-shaped skull.

Platyspondyly (vertebral bodies taller than those found in type I)

Polyhydramnios in the late second and third trimesters

Occasional Findings:

Types I and II

Cardiac defects

Hydronephrosis

Agenesis of the corpus callosum

Nuchal translucency thickening, first trimester

MAJOR DIFFERENTIAL DIAGNOSES

Achondrogenesis (typically associated with more severe micromelia; tendency for affected fetuses to develop hydrops with polyhydramnios)

Asphyxiating thoracic dystrophy (associated with less bowing of the bones, although the features are similar)

Camptomelic dysplasia (associated with bowing of the femora and hypoplastic fibulae, although upper extremities are less affected)

Ellis-van Creveld syndrome (features similar to short rib–polydactyly syndromes)

Homozygous achondroplasia (usually occurs in families in which two parents have heterozygous achondroplasia)

Osteogenesis imperfecta (may be associated with bowing secondary to fractures of all the extremities but usually accompanied by decreased bone mineralization, which is not seen in thanatophoric dysplasia)

Short rib–polydactyly syndromes (associated with polydactyly, which is not a feature of thanatophoric dysplasia)

Although all of the following are associated with normal limb lengths, they should be considered as differential diagnoses for type II thanatophoric dysplasia because of their association with craniosynostosis and cloverleaf-shaped skull:

- Apert syndrome
- Carpenter syndrome
- Crouzon syndrome
- Kleeblattschädel anomaly
- Pfeiffer syndrome

ULTRASOUND DIAGNOSIS

Thanatophoric dwarfism has been identified sonographically in the early second trimester in fetuses as young as 14 to 15 weeks based on skeletal anomalies. In one case, normal-appearing limbs were evident at 13 weeks' gestation, but a thanatophoric dwarfism variant was diagnosed later in gestation. Usually, however, even in the early second trimester, the abnormal configuration of the long bones and the narrowness of the chest are quite characteristic. There are reports of thickened nuchal translucency in first-trimester fetuses with thanatophoric dysplasia.

The cloverleaf-shaped skull, frontal bossing, and large head size found in type II have been detected sonographically and become more pronounced with advancing gestation.

Polyhydramnios is a feature in the late second and third trimesters.

HEREDITY

This lethal disorder is thought to be autosomal dominant, with most cases representing new mutations of the FGFR3 gene.

NATURAL HISTORY AND OUTCOME

This is a uniformly lethal condition, with death resulting from pulmonary hypoplasia.

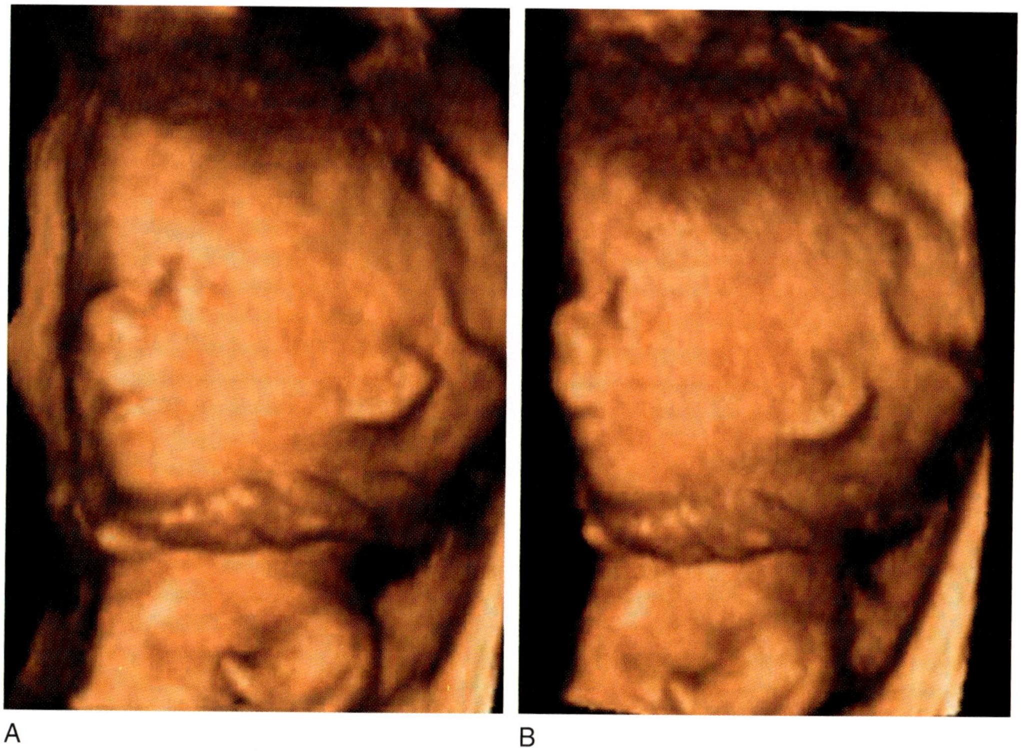

FIGURE 2-149 (**A, B**) Three-dimensional surface renderings of the fetal face with thanatophoric dysplasia show acrocephaly associated with the unusual head shape.

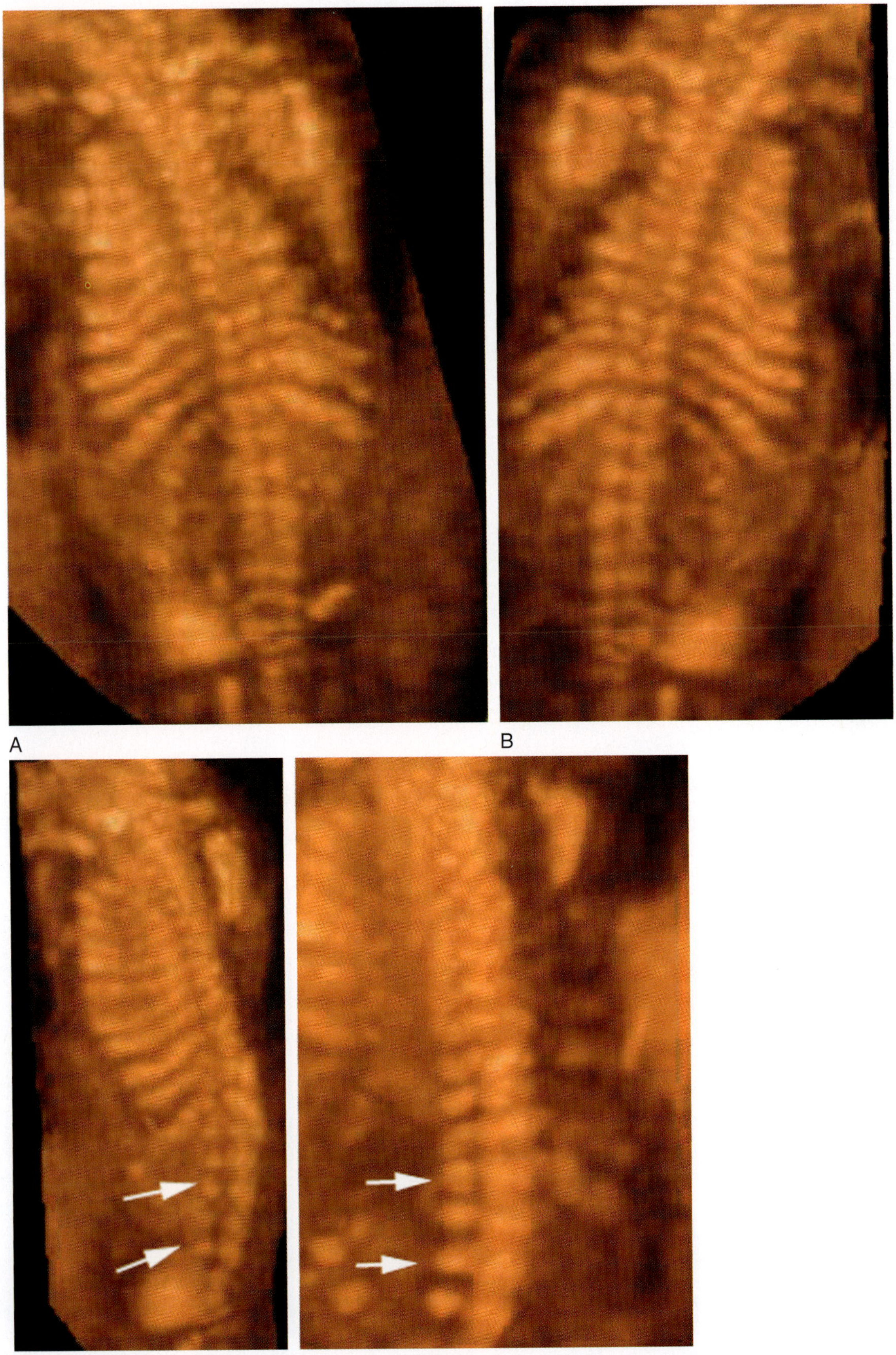

FIGURE 2-150 Three-dimensional renderings in skeletal mode of the same fetus as in Figure 2-149 show relatively short ribs (A–C), platyspondyly, and narrow vertebral bodies (C, D, *arrows*).

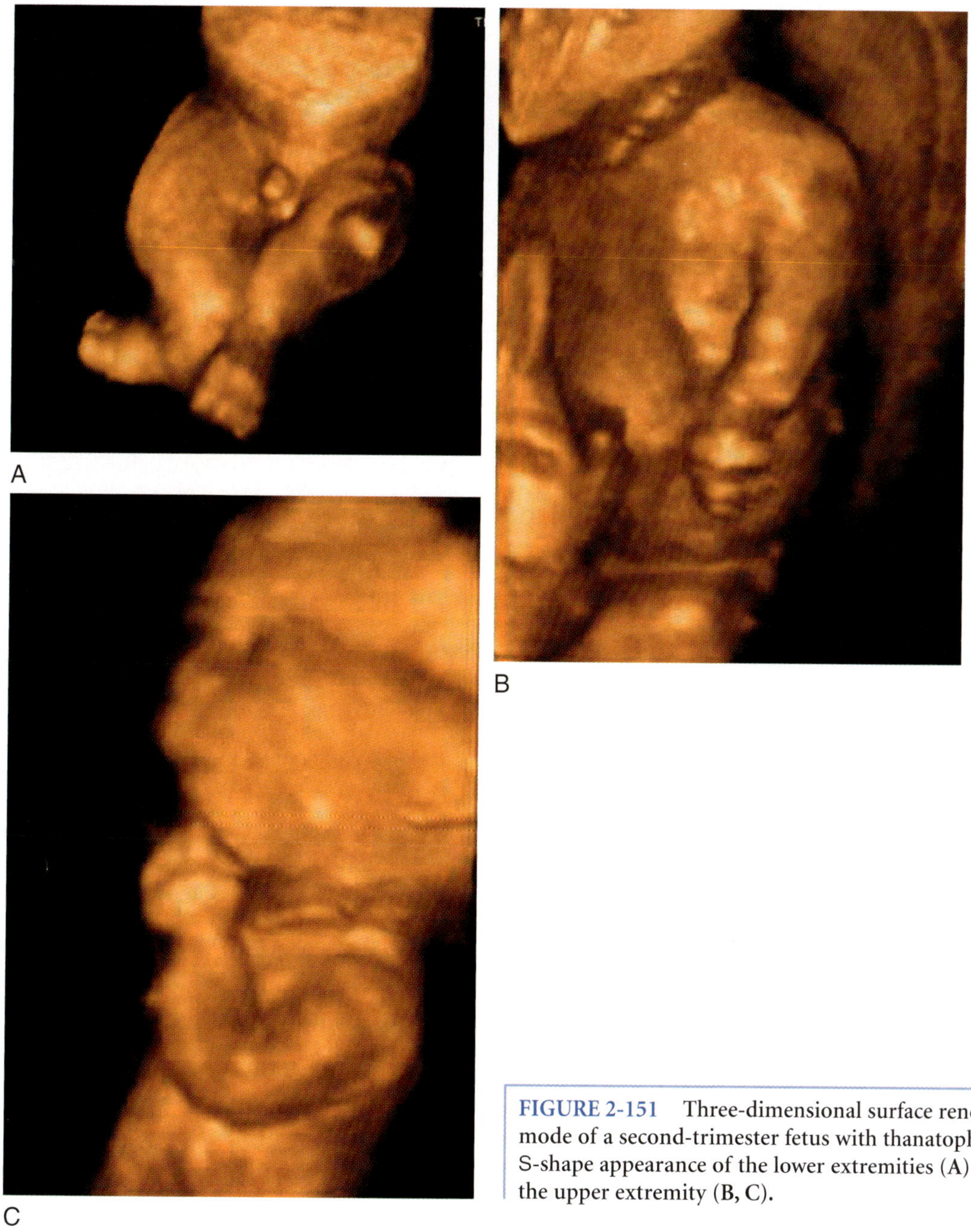

FIGURE 2-151 Three-dimensional surface renderings in soft-tissue mode of a second-trimester fetus with thanatophoric dysplasia. Note S-shape appearance of the lower extremities (A) and short appearance of the upper extremity (B, C).

Suggested Reading

Beetham FGT, Reeves JS: Early ultrasound diagnosis of thanatophoric dwarfism. *J Clin Ultrasound* 12:43–44, 1984.

Burrows PE, Stannard MW, Pearrow J, Sutterfield S, Baker ML: Early antenatal sonographic recognition of thanatophoric dysplasia with cloverleaf skull deformity. *AJR Am J Roentgenol* 143:841–843, 1984.

Camera G, Dodero D, De Pascale S: Prenatal diagnosis of thanatophoric dysplasia at 24 weeks. *Am J Med Genet* 18:39–43, 1984.

Campbell RE: Thanatophoric dwarfism in utero: a case report. *AJR Am J Roentgenol* 112:198–200, 1971.

Chen CP, Chern SR, Chang TY, Lin CJ, Wang W, Tzen CY: Second trimester molecular diagnosis of a stop codon FGFR3 mutation in a type I thanatophoric dysplasia fetus following abnormal ultrasound findings. *Prenat Diagn* 22:736–737, 2002.

Chervenak FA, Blakemore KJ, Isaacson G, Mayden K, Hobbins JC: Antenatal sonographic findings of thanatophoric dysplasia with cloverleaf skull. *Am J Obstet Gynecol* 146:984–985, 1983.

De Biasio P, Prefumo F, Baffico M, et al: Sonographic and molecular diagnosis of thanatophoric dysplasia type I at 18 weeks of gestation. *Prenat Diagn* 20:835–837, 2000.

Elejalde BR, de Elejalde M: Thanatophoric dysplasia: fetal manifestations and prenatal diagnosis. *Am J Med Genet* 22:669–683, 1985.

Ferreira A, Matias A, Brandao O, Montenegro N: Nuchal translucency and ductus venosus blood flow as early sonographic markers of thanatophoric dysplasia. A case report. *Fetal Diagn Ther* 19:241–245, 2004.

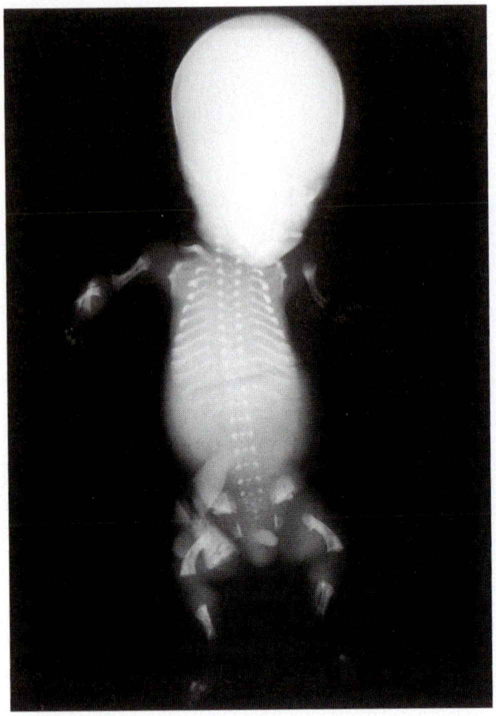

FIGURE 2-152 X-ray film of the skeleton of a fetus with thanatophoric dysplasia.

Fink IJ, Filly RA, Callen PW, Fiske CC: Sonographic diagnosis of thanatophoric dwarfism in utero. *J Ultrasound Med* 1:337–339, 1982.

Goncalves L, Jeanty P: Fetal biometry of skeletal dysplasias: a multicentric study. *J Ultrasound Med* 13:767–775, 1994.

Jones KL: *Smith's recognizable patterns of human malformations,* ed 6. Philadelphia, Elsevier, 2006.

Kalache KD, Lehmann K, Chaoui R, Kivelitz DE, Mundlos S, Bollmann R: Prenatal diagnosis of partial agenesis of the corpus callosum in a fetus with thanatophoric dysplasia type 2. *Prenat Diagn* 22:404–407, 2002.

Krakow D, Williams J 3rd, Poehl M, Rimoin DL, Platt LD: Use of three-dimensional ultrasound imaging in the diagnosis of prenatal-onset skeletal dysplasias. *Ultrasound Obstet Gynecol* 21:467–472, 2003.

Machado LE, Bonilla-Musoles F, Raga F, Bonilla F Jr, Machado F, Osborne NG: Thanatophoric dysplasia: ultrasound diagnosis. *Ultrasound Q* 17:235–243, 2001.

Macken MB, Grantmyre EB, Rimoin DL, Lachman RS: Normal sonographic appearance of a thanatophoric dwarf variant fetus at 13 weeks gestation. *AJR Am J Roentgenol* 156:149–150, 1991.

Mahony BS, Filly RA, Callen PW, Golbus MS: Thanatophoric dwarfism with the cloverleaf skull: a specific antenatal sonographic diagnosis. *J Ultrasound Med* 4:151–154, 1985.

Martinez-Frias ML, Ramos-Arroyo MA, Salvador J: Thanatophoric dysplasia: an autosomal dominant condition? *Am J Med Genet* 31:815–820, 1988.

Norman AM, Rimmer S, Landy S, Donnai D: Thanatophoric dysplasia of the straight-bone type (type 2). *Clin Dysmorph* 1:115–120, 1992.

Norris CD, Tiller G, Jeanty P, Malini S: Thanatophoric dysplasia in monozygotic twins. *Fetus* 4:27–32, 1994.

Parilla BV, Leeth EA, Kambich MP, Chilis P, MacGregor SN: Antenatal detection of skeletal dysplasias. *J Ultrasound Med* 22:255–258, 2003.

Pretorius DH, Rumack CM, Manco-Johnson ML, et al: Specific skeletal dysplasias in utero: sonographic diagnosis. *Radiology* 159:237–242, 1986.

Sahinoglu Z, Uludogan M, Gurbuz A, Karateke A: Prenatal diagnosis of thanatophoric dysplasia in the second trimester: ultrasonography and other diagnostic modalities. *Arch Gynecol Obstet* 269:57–61, 2003.

Schild RL, Hunt GH, Moore J, Davies H, Horwell DH: Antenatal sonographic diagnosis of thanatophoric dysplasia: a report of three cases and a review of the literature with special emphasis on the differential diagnosis. *Ultrasound Obstet Gynecol* 8:62–67, 1996.

Seymour R, Jones A: Strawberry-shaped skull in fetal thanatophoric dysplasia. *Ultrasound Obstet Gynecol* 4:434–436, 1994.

Sharony R, Browne C, Lachman RS, Rimoin DL: Prenatal diagnosis of the skeletal dysplasias. *Am J Obstet Gynecol* 169:668–675, 1993.

Tavormina PL, Shiang R, Thompson LM, et al: Thanatophoric dysplasia (types I and II) caused by distinct mutations in fibroblast growth factor receptor 3. *Nat Genet* 9:321–328, 1995.

Tennstedt C, Bartho S, Bollmann R, et al: Osteochondrodysplasias. Prenatal diagnosis and pathological-anatomic findings. *Zentralbl Pathol* 139:71–80, 1993.

Wasant P, Waeteekul S, Rimoin DL, Lachman RS: Genetic skeletal dysplasia in Thailand: the Siriraj experience. *SE Asian J Trop Med Publ Health* 1:59–67, 1995.

Weiner CP, Williamson RA, Bonsib SM: Sonographic diagnosis of cloverleaf skull and thanatophoric dysplasia in the second trimester. *J Clin Ultrasound* 14:463–465, 1986.

Syndromes Featuring Primarily Craniosynostosis

ANTLEY-BIXLER SYNDROME

DESCRIPTION AND DEFINITION

Synonyms: Trapezoidocephaly-synostosis syndrome, multisynostotic osteodysgenesis

This syndrome is characterized by craniosynostosis, resulting in severe brachycephaly, midfacial hypoplasia, multiple skeletal fusions, and contractures.

ABNORMALITIES DETECTABLE BY ULTRASOUND

Common Findings:

Craniosynostosis

Abnormally shaped head

Frontal bossing

Midfacial hypoplasia

Micrognathia

Choanal atresia

Radiohumeral synostosis

Joint contractures

Bowed bones (particularly the femur)

Rockerbottom feet

Polyhydramnios

Decreased activity

Occasional Findings:

Hydrocephalus

Renal anomalies

Cardiac anomalies

Ambiguous genitalia

MAJOR DIFFERENTIAL DIAGNOSES

Apert syndrome

Camptomelic dysplasia

Carpenter syndrome

Crouzon syndrome

Jacobsen syndrome

Pena Shokeir syndrome

Pfeiffer syndrome

Saethre-Chotzen syndrome

Thanatophoric dysplasia, type II

Trisomy 18

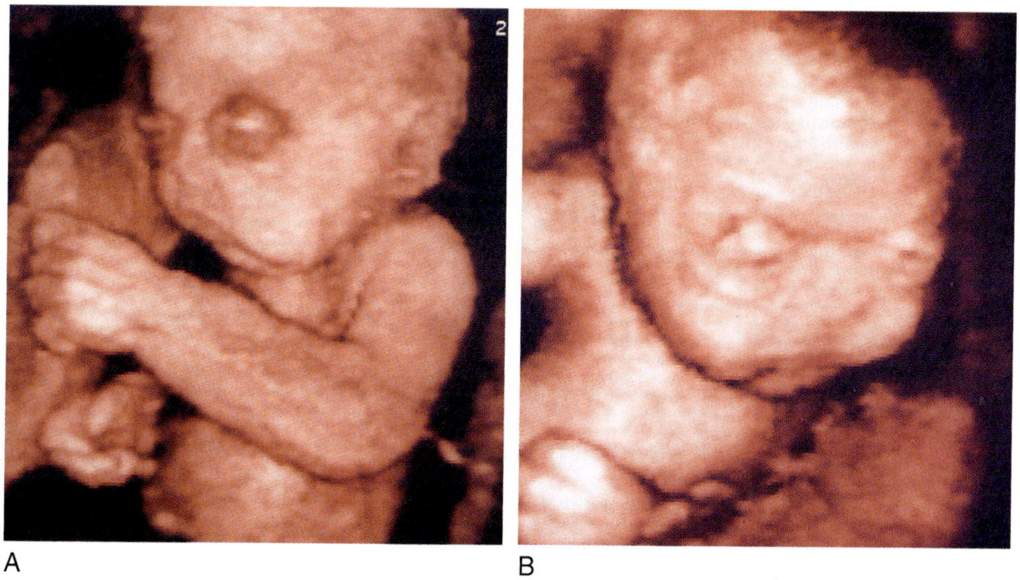

FIGURE 2-153 (A, B) Surface rendering of a third-trimester fetus with Antley-Bixler syndrome. Note abnormal forehead, exophthalmia, abnormal nasal bridge, and micrognathia. (From Machado LE, Osborne NG, Bonilla-Musoles F: *J Ultrasound Med* 23:73–77, 2001.)

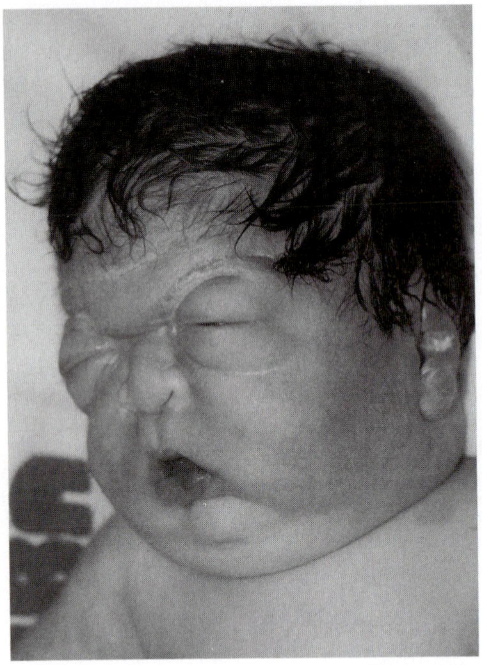

FIGURE 2-154 Postnatal photograph of the same fetus as Figure 2-153 shows hypertelorism, choanal atresia, acrocephaly, and frontal bossing from craniosynostosis. (From Machado LE, Osborne NG, Bonilla-Musoles F: *J Ultrasound Med* 23:73–77, 2001.)

ULTRASOUND DIAGNOSIS

This syndrome has been detected as early as 17 weeks' gestation, with fixed flexion contractures of the elbows, humeroradial synostosis, and bowed ulnae and femora. At 32 weeks, three-dimensional (3-D) ultrasound has shown the typical facies and head shape consistent with craniosynostosis and severe micrognathia.

HEREDITY

Antley-Bixler syndrome has multiple causes, which include an autosomal dominant form and an autosomal recessive form. The autosomal dominant form is associated with a mutation of the fibroblast growth factor receptor 2 (FGFR2). This disorder also can be caused by in utero exposure to fluconazole, which is an antifungal medication and a strong inhibitor of lanosterol 14-α-demethylase.

NATURAL HISTORY AND OUTCOME

There is a high incidence of neonatal mortality resulting from respiratory insufficiency. Those who survive are treated for orthopedic problems, choanal atresia, craniosynostosis (craniectomy), and other abnormalities. Brain development reportedly is normal.

Suggested Reading

Jones KL: *Smith's recognizable patterns of human malformations,* ed 6. Philadelphia, 2006, Elsevier.

Machado LE, Osborne NG, Bonilla-Musoles F: Antley-Bixler syndrome: report of a case. *J Ultrasound Med* 20:73–77, 2001.

Savoldelli G, Schinzel A: Prenatal ultrasound detection of humero-radial synostosis in a case of Antley-Bixler syndrome. *Prenat Diagn* 2:219–223, 1982.

Schinzel A, Savoldelli G, Briner J, Sigg P, Massini C: Antley-Bixler syndrome in sisters: a term newborn and a prenatally-diagnosed fetus. *Am J Med Genet* 14:139–147, 1983.

APERT SYNDROME

DESCRIPTION AND DEFINITION

Synonym: Acrocephalosyndactyly, type I

In 1906, Apert identified this syndrome, characterized by acrocephaly, craniosynostosis, and syndactyly.

ABNORMALITIES DETECTABLE BY ULTRASOUND

Common Findings:

Nuchal lucency (first trimester)

Brachycephaly and acrocephaly, with a high forehead and flat occiput

Craniosynostosis, usually involving the coronal suture

Flat face

Hypertelorism

Agenesis of the corpus callosum

Mild ventriculomegaly

Fusion of the cervical vertebrae at C5–C6

Syndactyly, both osseous and cutaneous (particularly involving the second, third, and fourth fingers)

Broad thumb

Broad hallux

Occasional Findings:

Long-bone abnormalities involving the upper extremities

Cardiac defects, such as tetralogy of Fallot

Diaphragmatic hernia

Genitourinary abnormalities, such as cystic kidneys, hydronephrosis, and cryptorchidism

MAJOR DIFFERENTIAL DIAGNOSES

Other Syndromes Associated with Craniosynostosis:

Carpenter syndrome

Crouzon syndrome

Kleeblattschädel anomaly (cloverleaf-shaped skull)

Pfeiffer syndrome

Saethre-Chotzen syndrome

Thanatophoric dysplasia (as a cause of cloverleaf-shaped skull)

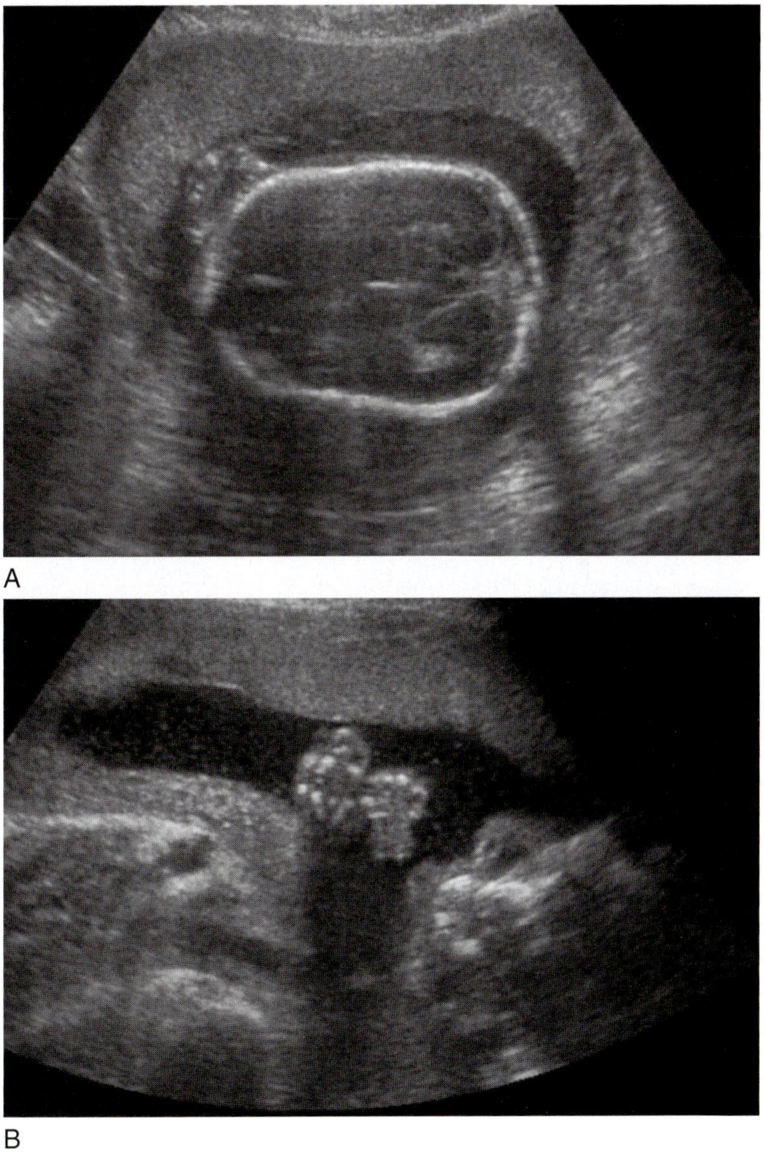

FIGURE 2-155 Second-trimester fetus with Apert syndrome. (A) Transverse view through the fetal head shows unusual head shape consistent with craniosynostosis. (B, C) Syndactyly of the fingers of both hands *(arrows)*. *Continued*

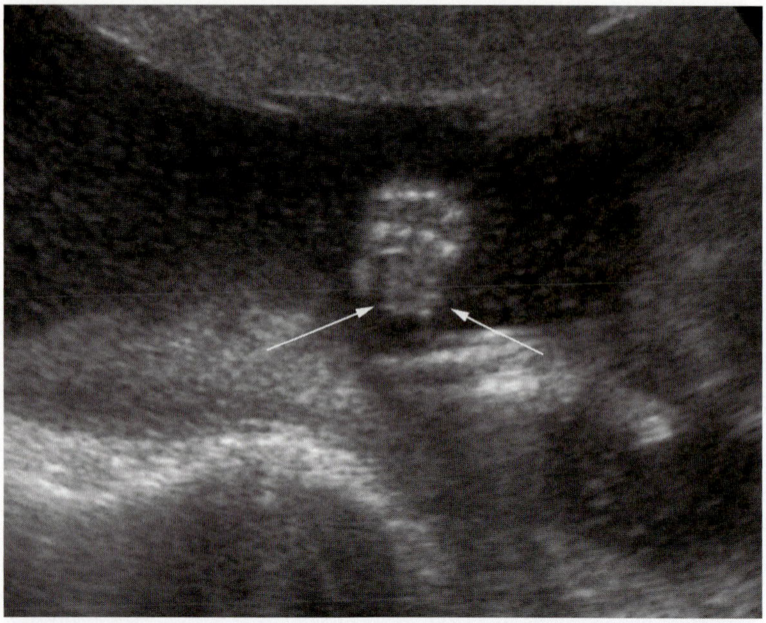

C

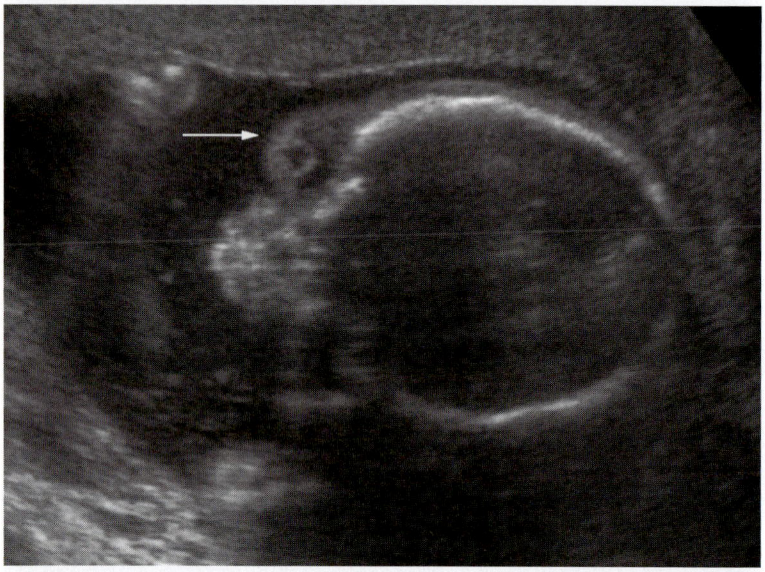

D

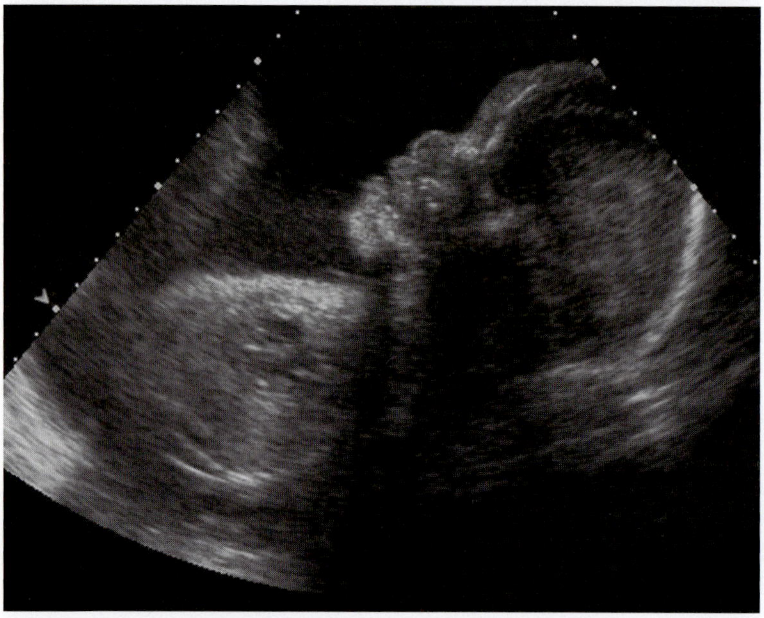

E

FIGURE 2-155, cont'd (**D**) Proptosis of the fetal orbit *(arrow)* in the same fetus with Apert syndrome. (**E**) Different third-trimester fetus with Apert syndrome shows the typical flat facies and high forehead associated with the syndrome.

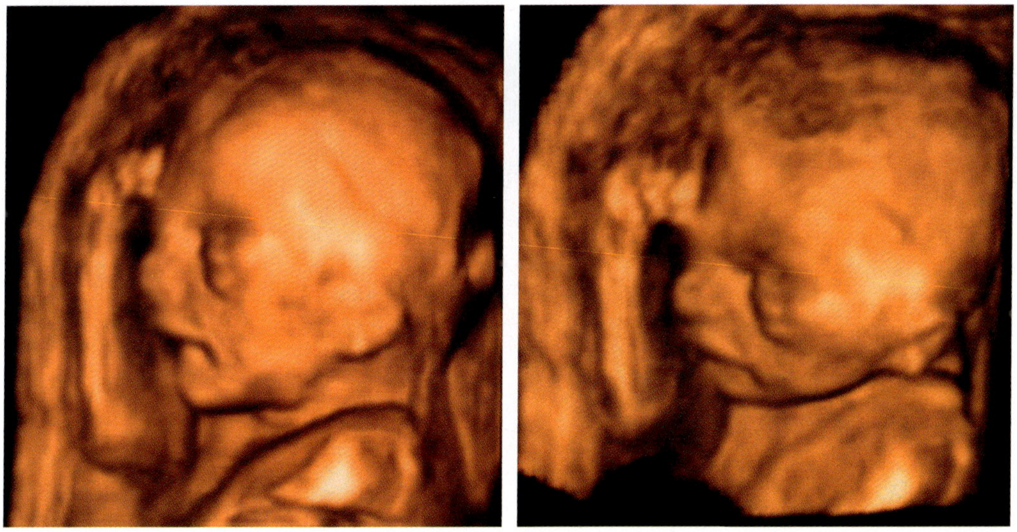

FIGURE 2-156 (A, B) Third-trimester fetus with Apert syndrome seen in three-dimensional surface rendering has low-set rotated ear, micrognathia, and ocular proptosis. A small portion of the hand can be seen, suggesting syndactyly.

Other Conditions Associated with Thickened Nuchal Translucency in the First Trimester:

See Differential Diagnosis for list, p. 50.

ULTRASOUND DIAGNOSIS

Prenatal diagnosis of Apert syndrome has been established several times. The earliest diagnosis was reported at 12 weeks' gestational age, based on the finding of a thickened nuchal fold. Although there have been several other reports of scans between 15 and 17 weeks' gestation, the diagnosis was not confirmed at that time. In one case, no abnormality was seen at 15 weeks other than a thickened nuchal fold; at 26 weeks' gestation, intracranial anatomy was abnormal, and ventriculomegaly, an abnormally shaped head, and a cardiac defect were noted. The earliest detection of Apert syndrome among families with no history of the condition was reported in several cases at 19 to 20 weeks, with the finding of abnormal head shape. Some of these cases had normal scans at 12–15 weeks. One of these cases had a 17-week scan in which mild ventriculomegaly and clenched hands were noted, prompting amniocentesis that was normal. The correct diagnosis was made with the finding of abnormal head shape at 19.5-week follow-up scan. In another case, the diagnosis of polyhydramnios, an acrocephalic shape of the cranium, and syndactyly prompted the prenatal diagnosis of Apert syndrome at 31 weeks' gestation. Several investigators have reported that 3-D ultrasound is helpful in these cases to demonstrate the sutures, notably the characteristically closed coronal suture and abnormally widened metopic suture.

In families at risk for the syndrome, earlier diagnosis is possible because of heightened suspicion of abnormal findings. The prenatal diagnosis of Apert syndrome was established at 17 weeks in a patient at risk for an affected child. "Mitten hand" deformities were noted bilaterally, as was lack of movement of individual fingers.

The abnormally shaped skull may not be apparent early in gestation. However, limb abnormalities are potentially detectable in the second trimester with careful detailed evaluation of the fetal hands, particularly in fetuses at increased risk for the disorder. Prenatal diagnosis has also been made by fetoscopy at 17 weeks' gestation.

HEREDITY

The pattern of inheritance for Apert syndrome is autosomal dominant, although most cases are fresh mutations. Apert syndrome has been associated with advanced paternal age.

The syndrome is considered to result from mutations in the gene encoding of FGFR2. It is located on gene map locus 10q25–10q26. The two

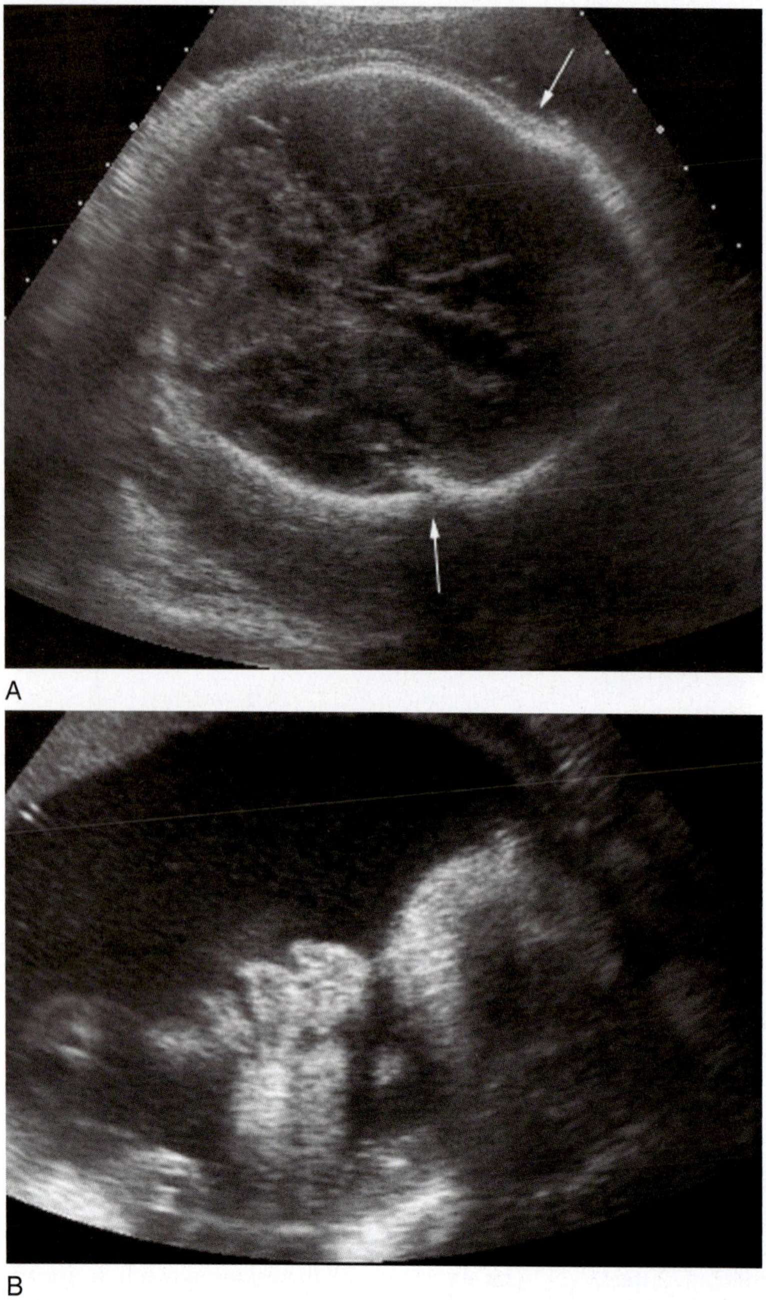

FIGURE 2-157 (**A**) Third-trimester fetus with Apert syndrome, with indentations at the temples of the skull consistent with fusion of the sutures *(arrows)*. The unusually shaped head is consistent with craniosynostosis. (**B**) Frontal view of the fetal face shows frontal bossing, typical of the syndrome. *Continued*

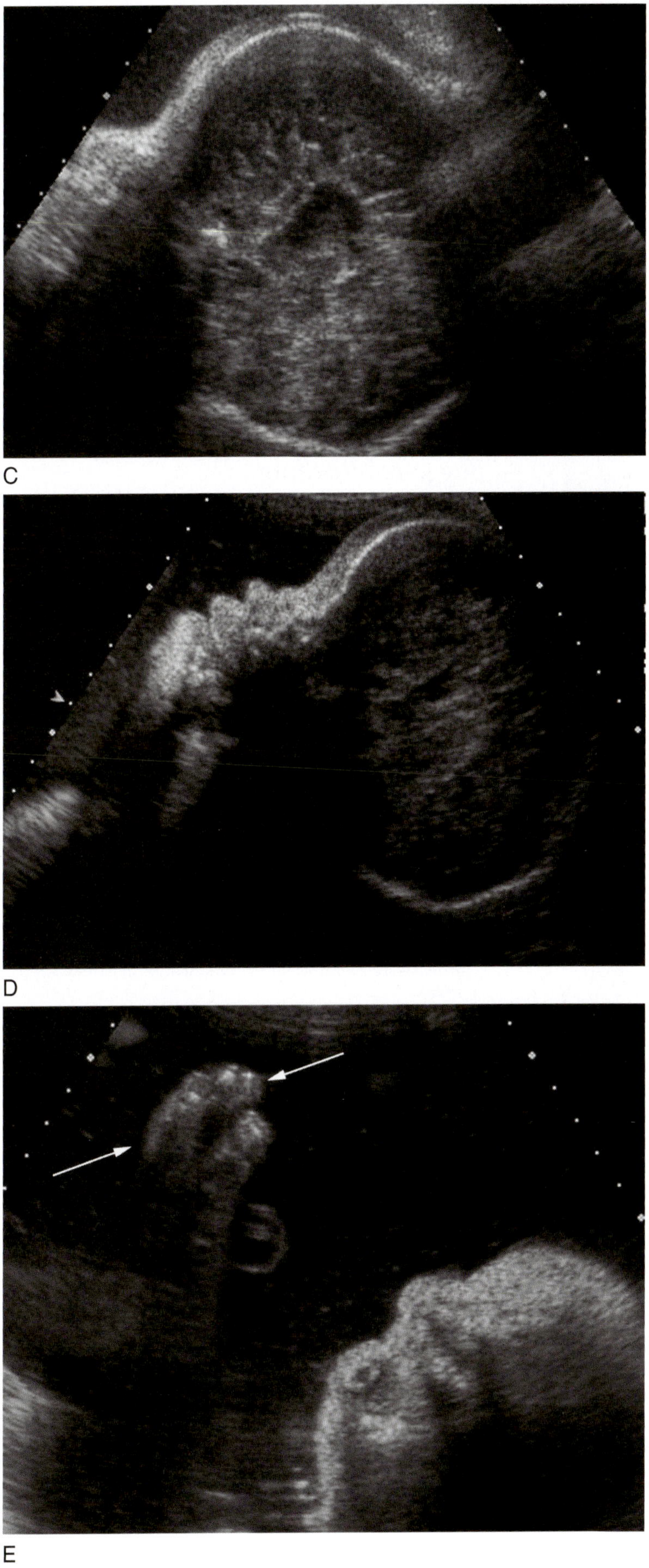

FIGURE 2-157, cont'd (C, D) Midline views of the fetal brain show agenesis of the corpus callosum in the same third-trimester fetus. (E) Mitten hand *(arrows)* of the same third trimester fetus with Apert syndrome. Note the proptosis of the orbit. (From Quintero-Rivera F, Robson CD, Reiss RE, et al: *Prenat Diagn* 26:966–972, 2006.)

alleles responsible for 98% of cases are S252W and P253R. Other mutations (alleles) in the same gene are thought to cause Crouzon and Pfeiffer syndromes.

NATURAL HISTORY AND OUTCOME

Varying degrees of mental retardation are associated with this syndrome. However, individuals may have normal intelligence.

Decompression of the craniosynostosis early in childhood may be necessary. Early orthopedic intervention is needed for management of the limb abnormalities associated with this syndrome.

Suggested Reading

Aleem S, Howarth ES: Apert syndrome associated with increased fetal nuchal translucency. *Prenat Diagn* 25:1066–1067, 2005.

Apert ME: De I-acrocephalosyndactylie. *Bull Mem Soc Med Hop Paris* 23:1310–1330, 1906.

Boog G, Le Vaillant C, Winer N, David A, Quere MP, Nomballais MF: Contribution of tridimensional sonography and magnetic resonance imaging to prenatal diagnosis of Apert syndrome at mid-trimester. *Fetal Diagn Ther* 14:20–23, 1999.

Chang CC, Tsai FJ, Tsai HD, et al: Prenatal diagnosis of Apert syndrome. *Prenat Diagn* 18:621–625, 1998.

Chenoweth-Mitchell C, Cohen GR: Prenatal sonographic findings of Apert syndrome. *J Clin Ultrasound* 22:510–514, 1994.

Cohen MM Jr: Craniosynostosis update 1987. *Am J Med Genet* 4:99–148, 1988.

Deliniere F, Lepinard C, Kerjean F, et al: Syndrome d'Apert. Diagnostic echographique, prise en charge obstetricale. *J Gynecol Obstet Biol Reprod* 24:613–617, 1995.

Esser T, Rogalla P, Bamberg C, Kalache KD: Application of the three-dimensional maximum mode in prenatal diagnosis of Apert syndrome. *Am J Obstet Gynecol* 193:1743–1745, 2005.

Faro C, Chaoui R, Wegrzyn P, Levaillant JM, Benoit B, Nicolaides KH: Metopic suture in fetuses with Apert syndrome at 22–27 weeks of gestation. *Ultrasound Obstet Gynecol* 27:28–33, 2006.

Ferreira JC, Carter SM, Bernstein PS, et al: Second-trimester molecular prenatal diagnosis of sporadic Apert syndrome following suspicious ultrasound findings. *Ultrasound Obstet Gynecol* 14:426–430, 1999.

Hansen WF, Rijhsinghani A, Grant S, Yankowitz J: Prenatal diagnosis of Apert syndrome. *Fetal Diagn Ther* 19:127–130, 2004.

Hill LM, Thomas ML, Peterson CS: The ultrasonic detection of Apert syndrome. *J Ultrasound Med* 6:601–604, 1987.

Humphreys RP: Apert syndrome: diagnosis and treatment of craniostenosis and intracranial anomalies. *Clin Plast Surg* 18:231–235, 1991.

Jones KL: *Smith's recognizable patterns of human malformations,* ed 6. Philadelphia, 2006, Elsevier.

Leonard CO, Daikoku NH, Winn K: Prenatal fetoscopic diagnosis of the Apert syndrome. *Am J Med Genet* 11:5–9, 1982.

Lyu KJ, Ko TM: Prenatal diagnosis of Apert syndrome with widely separated cranial sutures. *Prenat Diagn* 20:254–256, 2000.

Mahieu-Caputo D, Sonigo P, Amiel J, et al: Prenatal diagnosis of sporadic Apert syndrome: a sequential diagnostic approach combining three-dimensional computed tomography and molecular biology. *Fetal Diagn Ther* 16:10–12, 2001.

Narayan H, Scott FV: Prenatal ultrasound diagnosis of Apert's syndrome. *Prenat Diagn* 10:187–192, 1991.

Pooh RK, Nakagawa Y, Pooh KH, Nakagawa Y, Nagamachi N: Fetal craniofacial structure and intracranial morphology in a case of Apert syndrome. *Ultrasound Obstet Gynecol* 13:274–280, 1999.

Skidmore DL, Pai AP, Toi A, Steele L, Chitayat D: Prenatal diagnosis of Apert syndrome: report of two cases. *Prenat Diagn* 23:1009–1013, 2003.

Wilkie AOM, Slaney SF, Oldridge M, et al: Apert syndrome results from localized mutations of FGFR2 and is allelic with Crouzon syndrome. *Nat Genet* 9:165–172, 1995.

Witters I, Devriendt K, Moerman P, van Hole C, Fryns JP: Diaphragmatic hernia as the first echographic sign in Apert syndrome. *Prenat Diagn* 20:404–406, 2000.

CARPENTER SYNDROME

DESCRIPTION AND DEFINITION

Synonym: Acrocephalosyndactyly, type II

First described by Carpenter in 1901, this syndrome consists of acrocephaly, syndactyly, and preaxial polydactyly.

ABNORMALITIES DETECTABLE BY ULTRASOUND

Brachycephaly and acrocephaly, suggesting craniosynostosis that may occur at the coronal, sagittal, and/or lambdoid sutures

Depressed nasal bridge

Low-set ears

Micrognathia

Clinodactyly

Syndactyly and polydactyly

Preaxial polydactyly of the feet or wide hallux

Cardiac abnormalities, such as septal defect, tetralogy of Fallot, and transposition of the great arteries (in 50% of affected individuals)

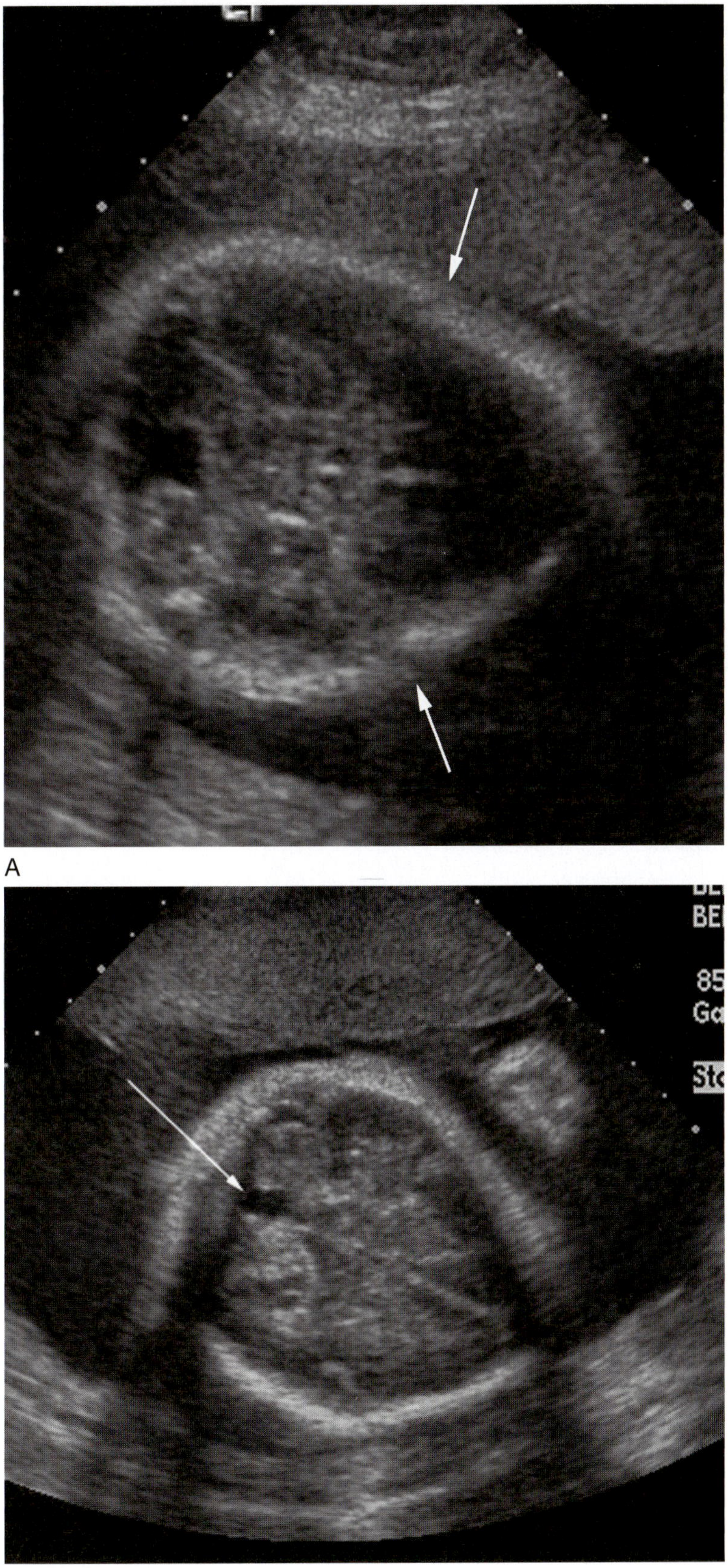

A

B

FIGURE 2-158 (A) Third-trimester fetus with Carpenter syndrome has unusual head shape associated with craniosynostosis. Indentation at the temples of the fetal skull *(arrows)* is present. Note evidence of Dandy-Walker abnormality. (B) Dandy-Walker abnormality better seen in this view shows hypoplasia of cerebellar vermis *(arrow)*.

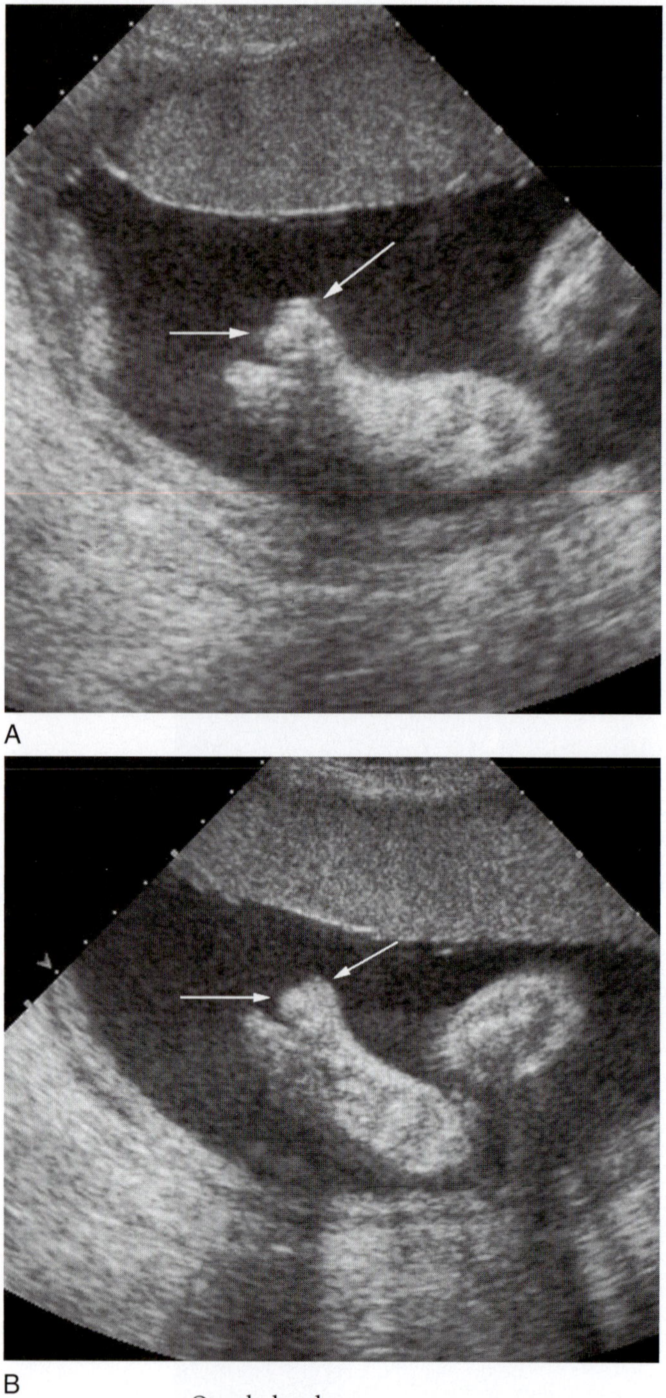

FIGURE 2-159 (A, B) Views of the plantar aspect of the fetal foot show a bifid hallux *(arrows)*.

Omphalocele

Hypogonadism

Cryptorchidism

MAJOR DIFFERENTIAL DIAGNOSES

Other Syndromes and Conditions Associated with Preaxial Polydactyly of the Feet:

Greig cephalopolysyndactyly

Hydrolethalus

Oral-facial-digital syndrome, type II (Mohr syndrome)

Saethre-Chotzen syndrome

Other Syndromes and Conditions Associated with Polydactyly:

Branchio-oculo-facial syndrome

Ellis-van Creveld syndrome

Hydrolethalus

Joubert syndrome

Meckel-Gruber syndrome

Oral-facial-digital syndrome, type I

Short rib–polydactyly syndromes

Trisomy 13 (Patau syndrome)

Other Syndromes and Conditions Associated with Acrocephaly and Cloverleaf-Shaped Skull:

Apert syndrome

Crouzon syndrome

Kleeblattschädel anomaly

Pfeiffer syndrome

Saethre-Chotzen syndrome

Thanatophoric dysplasia

Other Syndromes and Conditions Associated with Hypogenitalism:

CHARGE (**c**oloboma of the iris, **h**eart defect, choanal **a**tresia, intrauterine growth **r**estriction, **g**enital anomalies, and **e**ar anomalies) association

Smith-Lemli-Opitz syndrome

Camptomelic dysplasia

ULTRASOUND DIAGNOSIS

Prenatal diagnosis has been established at 17 weeks' gestation on the basis of detection of polydactyly and club-like hand deformities. At 20 weeks, the head shape begins to look abnormal. By 29 weeks, markedly abnormal head shape, flattening of the face, proptosis of the eyes, and apical peaking of the calvaria are apparent.

The later manifestation of the head shape abnormality, compared with the limb defects, should be kept in mind when seeking early prenatal diagnosis of this disorder.

HEREDITY

The pattern of inheritance for this syndrome is autosomal recessive.

NATURAL HISTORY AND OUTCOME

There is a wide range of mental deficiency associated with this syndrome, although normal intelligence is possible. Other features include obesity and hearing loss.

Suggested Reading

Ashby T, Rouse GA, De Lange M: Prenatal sonographic diagnosis of Carpenter syndrome. *J Ultrasound Med* 13:905–909, 1994.

Balci S, Onol B, Eryilmaz M, Haytoglu T: A case of Carpenter syndrome diagnosed in a 20–week-old fetus with postmortem examination. *Clin Genet* 51:412–416, 1997.

Carpenter G: Case of acrocephaly with other congenital malformations. *Proc R Soc Med* 2:45–53, 199–201, 1909.

Cohen MM Jr: Craniosynostosis update 1987. *Am J Med Genet* 4:99–148, 1988.

Eaton AP, Sommer A, Kontras SB, Sayers MP: Carpenter syndrome—acrocephalopolysyndactyly type II. *Birth Defects* 10:249–260, 1974.

Golwyn DH, Anderson TL, Jeanty P: Acrocephalopolysyndactyly. *Fetus* 4:1–4, 1994.

Robinson LK, James HE, Mubarak SJ, Allen EJ, Jones KL: Carpenter syndrome: natural history and clinical spectrum. *Am J Med Genet* 20:461–469, 1985.

CROUZON SYNDROME

DESCRIPTION AND DEFINITION

Synonym: Craniofacial dysostosis type I

Described in 1912 by Crouzon, this condition is characterized by premature closure of the coronal sutures, midface hypoplasia, and ocular proptosis.

ABNORMALITIES DETECTABLE BY ULTRASOUND

Common Findings:

Abnormally shaped skull, consistent with craniosynostosis and premature closure of coronal, lambdoid, and/or sagittal sutures

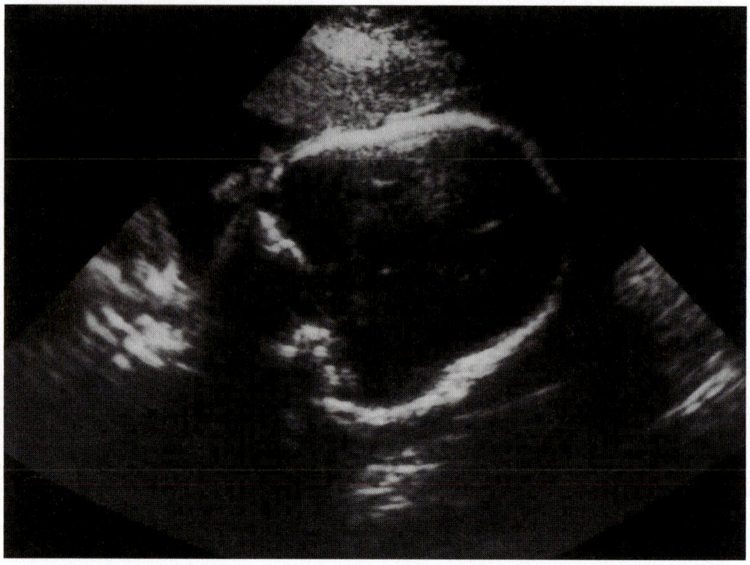

FIGURE 2-160 Coronal view of the head of a third-trimester fetus with Crouzon syndrome. Note unusual shape of the head, caused by acrocephaly, which is consistent with craniosynostosis.

Abnormal facial features

Hypertelorism or hypotelorism

Beaked nose

Micrognathia

Occasional Findings:

Cloverleaf-shaped skull (in severe cases)

Ventriculomegaly

Agenesis of the corpus callosum

Cleft lip and palate

MAJOR DIFFERENTIAL DIAGNOSES

Other Syndromes and Conditions Associated with Craniosynostosis:

Apert syndrome

Carpenter syndrome

Kleeblattschädel anomaly (cloverleaf-shaped skull)

Pfeiffer syndrome

Saethre-Chotzen syndrome

Thanatophoric dysplasia

ULTRASOUND DIAGNOSIS

The diagnosis of this condition has been established in the late second trimester (20–23 weeks' gestation), based on an abnormally shaped cranium, hypertelorism, ocular proptosis, and mild ventriculomegaly. Hypertelorism and a cloverleaf-shaped skull were apparent at 20 weeks in one case. A trilobar (cloverleaf-shaped) skull was apparent by 23 weeks in another case. The *absence* of limb abnormalities, in conjunction with craniosynostosis, is indicative of Crouzon syndrome.

In another case, a sonogram at 16 weeks' gestation showed normal binocular distance and interorbital diameters. It was only at 21 weeks that these measurements became questionable and at 24 weeks that the diagnosis of Crouzon syndrome was suggested.

Clearly, the finding of craniosynostosis is *not* a feature of the early second trimester but rather of the mid-to-late second trimester.

First-trimester diagnosis of this disorder has been possible, using DNA isolated from chorionic villus sampling, in a family known to be at risk for the disorder. There are no known first-trimester sonographic findings of this syndrome.

HEREDITY

This syndrome has an autosomal dominant pattern of inheritance, although 25% of reported cases occur in families without family history. This condition is thought to be attributable to mutations in the FGFR2 gene, mapping to 10q25–q26. Mutations (alleles) at that gene locus are also thought to cause Pfeiffer and Apert syndromes.

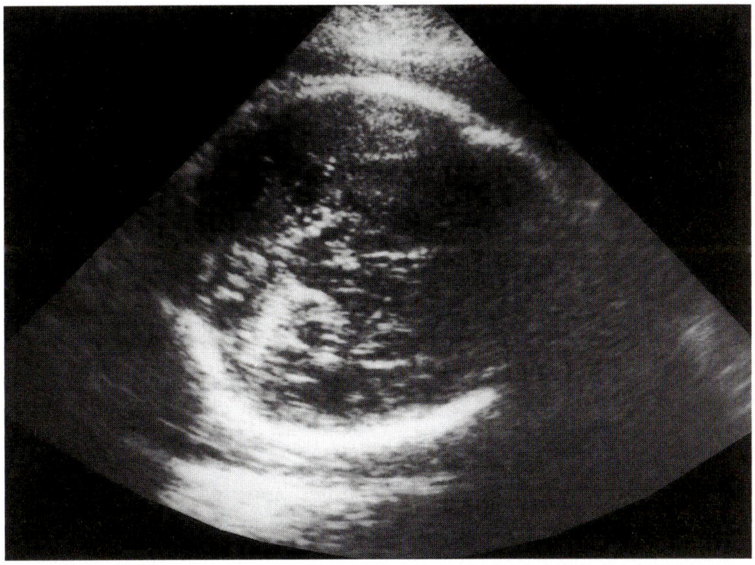

A

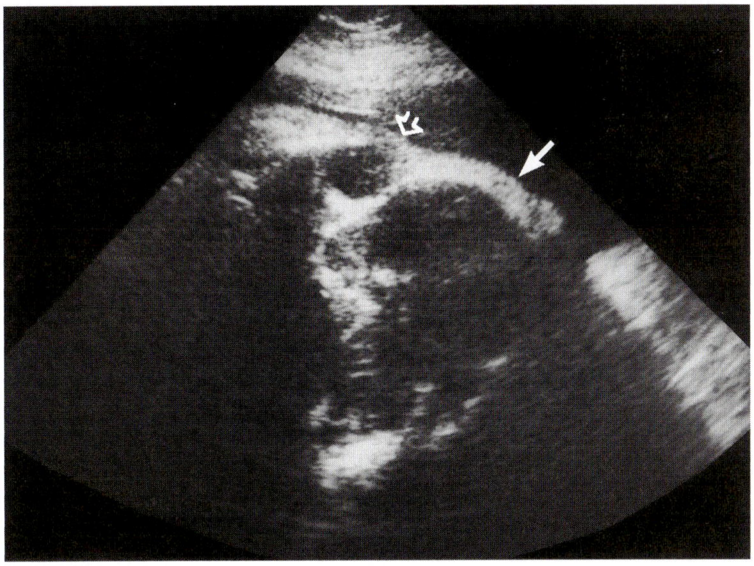

B

FIGURE 2-161 Transverse and coronal views of the head of a fetus with Crouzon syndrome show evidence of craniosynostosis. (A) Note brachycephalic configuration of the fetal head in transverse section. (B) Prominence of the frontal aspect of the skull *(solid arrow)*, just above the fetal orbit *(open arrow)*, is characteristic of the condition.

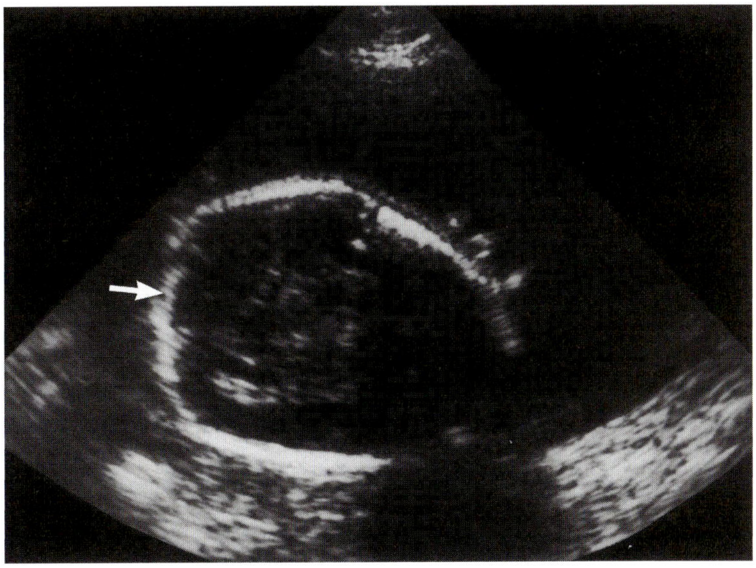

FIGURE 2-162 Transverse view through the head of a second-trimester fetus with Crouzon syndrome. Craniosynostosis and an abnormally shaped head are apparent, although less so than in the third trimester. Note flattening of the posterior aspect of the skull *(arrow)* and angulation at the parietal level.

NATURAL HISTORY AND OUTCOME

Surgery for craniosynostosis may be necessary after birth. Occasionally, features of the disorder include upper airway (nasal) obstruction, mental retardation, and seizures.

Suggested Reading

Crouzon O: Dysostose cranio-faciale hereditaire. *Bull Mem Hop Paris* 33:545–555, 1912.

Gollin YG, Abuhamad AZ, Inati MN, et al: Sonographic appearance of craniofacial dysostosis (Crouzon syndrome) in the second trimester. *J Ultrasound Med* 12:625–628, 1993.

Jones KL: *Smith's recognizable patterns of human malformations,* ed 6. Philadelphia, 2006, Elsevier.

Leo MV, Suslak L, Ganesh VL, Adhate A, Apuzzio JJ: Crouzon syndrome: prenatal ultrasound diagnosis by binocular diameters. *Obstet Gynecol* 78:906–908, 1991.

Menashe Y, Ben Baruch G, Rabinovitch O, et al: Exophthalmus—prenatal ultrasonic features for diagnosis of Crouzon syndrome. *Prenat Diagn* 9:805–808, 1989.

Miller C, Losken HW, Towbin R, Bowen A, Mooney MP, Towbin A, Faix RS: Ultrasound diagnosis of craniosynostosis. *Cleft Palate Craniofac J* 39:73–80, 2002.

Morris HW, Hurtt MR, Mulvihill JJ, Ehrlich GD: A gene for Crouzon craniofacial dysostosis maps to the long arm of chromosome 10. *Nat Genet* 7:149–153, 1994.

Reardon W, Winter RM, Rutland P, et al: Mutations in the fibroblast growth factor receptor 2 gene cause Crouzon syndrome. *Nat Genet* 8:98–103, 1994.

Schwartz M, Kreiborg S, Skovby F: First-trimester prenatal diagnosis of Crouzon syndrome. *Prenat Diagn* 16:155–158, 1996.

PFEIFFER SYNDROME

DESCRIPTION AND DEFINITION

Synonym: Acrofacial dysostosis

First reported by Pfeiffer in 1964, this condition is characterized by an acrocephalic skull, syndactyly of the hands and feet, and large thumbs.

ABNORMALITIES DETECTABLE BY ULTRASOUND

Common Findings:

Brachycephaly and acrocephaly, along with craniosynostosis (particularly of the coronal suture and sometimes the sagittal suture)

Hypertelorism

Depressed nasal bridge

Partial syndactyly

Broad thumb

Broad hallux

Occasional Findings:

Ventriculomegaly

Cloverleaf-shaped skull

Choanal atresia

Fused vertebrae

Tracheal abnormalities

Cardiac defect

MAJOR DIFFERENTIAL DIAGNOSES

Other Syndromes and Conditions Associated with Craniosynostosis:

Apert syndrome

Carpenter syndrome

Crouzon syndrome

Kleeblattschädel anomaly (cloverleaf-shaped skull)

Saethre-Chotzen syndrome

Thanatophoric dysplasia (as a cause of cloverleaf-shaped skull)

ULTRASOUND DIAGNOSIS

Ultrasound diagnosis has been established at 20 weeks' gestational age in a fetus with craniosynostosis, hypertelorism, proptosis, and broad thumbs. Another case was deemed abnormal at 18 weeks (no family history) upon finding of abnormal temporal indentations. Follow-up scans at 21 and 26 weeks showed progressive skull shape abnormality and mild ventriculomegaly. Ocular proptosis and craniosynostosis were demonstrated using 3-D ultrasound leading to the correct diagnosis. Other cases have been diagnosed in the third trimester with findings of more pronounced cloverleaf-shaped deformities of the skull, hydrocephalus, cardiac abnormality, abnormal toes, and ocular proptosis. The abnormal skull shape of affected fetuses

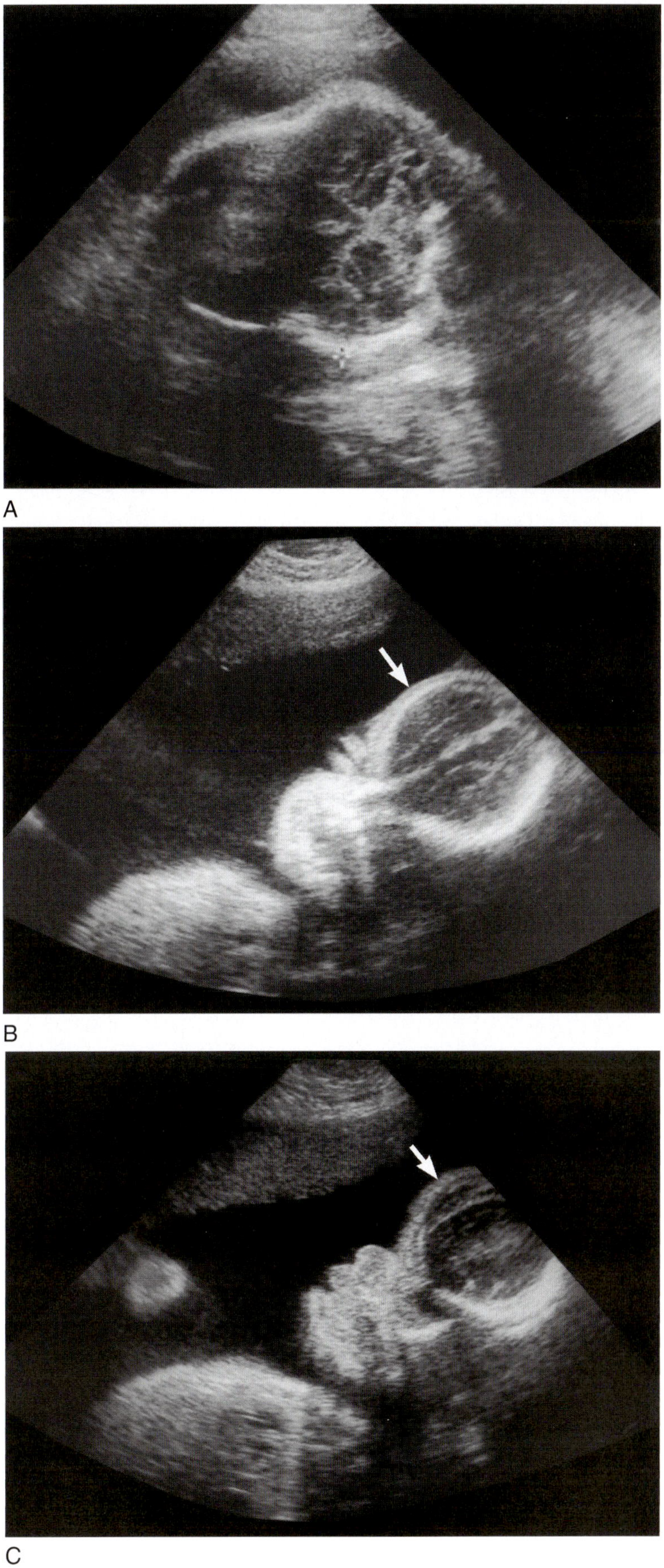

FIGURE 2-163 (A) Coronal view through the head of a third-trimester fetus reveals a cloverleaf-shaped skull, similar to that seen in Pfeiffer syndrome. (B) Frontal view of the same fetus shows marked prominence of the frontal region of the head *(arrow)*, consistent with findings in Pfeiffer syndrome. (C) Longitudinal view of the fetal profile shows marked frontal prominence *(arrow)* and a severely depressed nasal bridge, as can be seen in Pfeiffer syndrome.

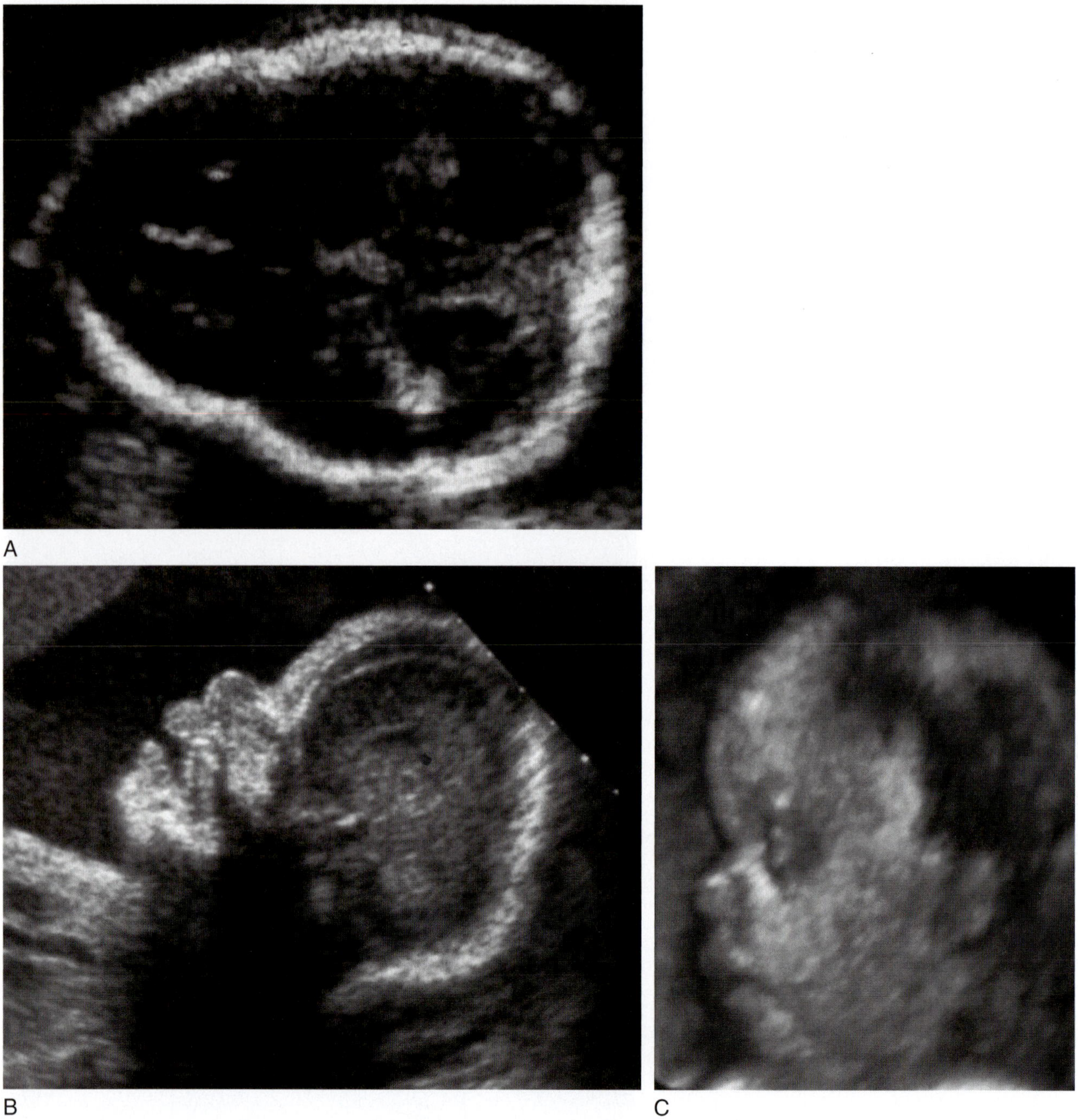

FIGURE 2-164 Pfeiffer syndrome. (A) Unusual head shape with squaring off at the temples of a late second-trimester fetus with Pfeiffer syndrome. (B) Longitudinal view of the fetal profile of the same fetus with Pfeiffer syndrome. (C) Surface rendering of the same fetus in the late second trimester shows an unusual facies with acrocephaly and dysmorphic appearance. *Continued*

may not be apparent or may be subtle in the early second trimester.

HEREDITY

Type I Pfeiffer syndrome is thought to be autosomal dominant, although often it may be the result of fresh mutations. Types II and III are sporadic.

This condition is thought to be attributable to mutations in the FGFR2 gene, mapping to 10q25–q26. Mutations (alleles) at that gene locus are also thought to cause Crouzon and Apert syndromes. The fibroblast growth factor receptor 1 gene, mapping to 8p11.22–p12, is another locus for some fetuses with this condition.

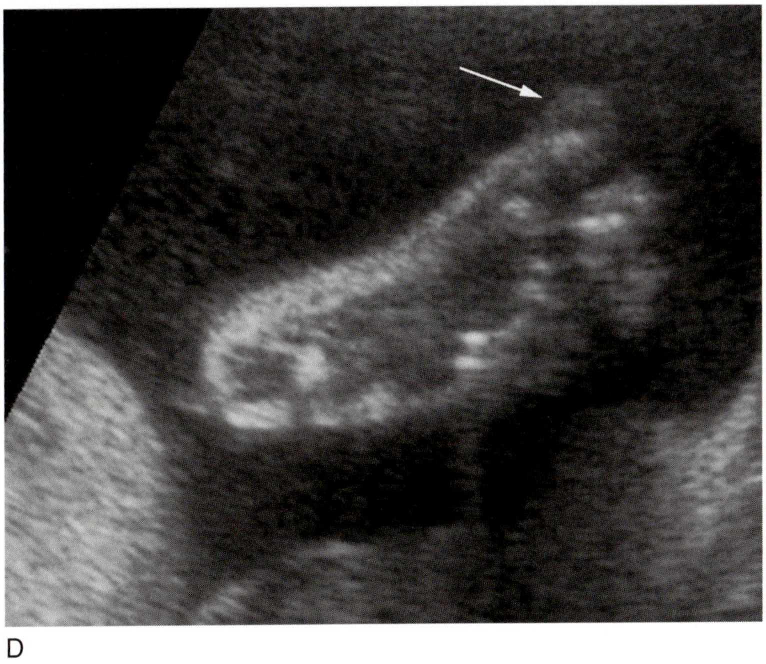

FIGURE 2-164, cont'd (**D**) Prominent hallux of the foot of a fetus with Pfeiffer syndrome.

NATURAL HISTORY AND OUTCOME

Type I Pfeiffer syndrome is compatible with life. It is characterized by normal intelligence and a classic phenotype of craniosynostosis, broad thumbs, and syndactyly.

Types II and III are sporadic in occurrence, with more severe involvement of the central nervous system (CNS) than in type I. Type II is associated with the classic cloverleaf-shaped skull. Neurologic compromise is common in both types II and III.

Suggested Reading

Bellus GA, Gaudenz K, Zackai EH, et al: Identical mutations in three different fibroblast growth factor receptor genes in autosomal dominant craniosynostosis syndromes. *Nat Genet* 14:174–176, 1996.

Benacerraf BR, Spiro R, Mitchell AG: Using three-dimensional ultrasound to detect craniosynostosis in a fetus with Pfeiffer syndrome. *Ultrasound Obstet Gynecol* 16:391–394, 2000.

Bernstain PS, Gross SJ, Cohen DJ, et al: Prenatal diagnosis of type 2 Pfeiffer syndrome. *Ultrasound Obstet Gynecol* 8:425–428, 1996.

Blaumeiser B, Loquet P, Wuyts W, Nothen MM: Prenatal diagnosis of Pfeiffer syndrome type II. *Prenat Diagn* 24:644–646, 2004.

Gorincour G, Rypens F, Grignon A, et al: Prenatal diagnosis of cloverleaf skull: watch the hands! *Fetal Diagn Ther* 20:296–300, 2005.

Hill LM, Grzybek PC: Sonographic findings with Pfeiffer syndrome. *Prenat Diagn* 14:47–49, 1994.

Itoh S, Nojima M, Yoshida K: Usefulness of magnetic resonance imaging for accurate diagnosis of Pfeiffer syndrome type II in utero. *Fetal Diagn Ther* 21:168–171, 2006.

Jones KL: *Smith's recognizable patterns of human malformations,* ed 6. Philadelphia, 2006, Elsevier.

Martsolf JT, Cracco JB, Carpenter GG, O'Hara AE: Pfeiffer syndrome: an unusual type of acrocephalosyndactyly with broad thumbs and great toes. *Am J Dis Child* 121:257–262, 1971.

Nazzaro A, Della Monica M, Lonardo F, et al: Prenatal ultrasound diagnosis of a case of Pfeiffer syndrome without cloverleaf skull and review of the literature. *Prenat Diagn* 24:918–922, 2004.

Pfeiffer RA: Dominant erbliche akrocephalosyndaktylie. *Z Kinderheilk* 90:301–320, 1964.

Rutland P, Pulleyn LJ, Reardon W, et al: Identical mutations in the FGFR2 gene cause both Pfeiffer and Crouzon syndrome phenotypes. *Nat Genet* 9:173–176, 1995.

Rutland P, Reardon W, Malcolm S, Winter RM: A common mutation in the fibroblast growth factor receptor 1 gene in Pfeiffer syndrome. *Nat Genet* 8:269–274, 1994.

Saldino RM, Steinbach HL, Epstein CJ: Familial acrocephalosyndactyly (Pfeiffer syndrome). *AJR Am J Roentgenol* 116:609–622, 1972.

Stone P, Trevenen CL, Mitchell I, Rudd N: Congenital tracheal stenosis in Pfeiffer syndrome. *Clin Genet* 38:145–148, 1990.

SAETHRE-CHOTZEN SYNDROME

DESCRIPTION AND DEFINITION

Synonym: Acrocephalosyndactyly, type III

This syndrome, first described by Saethre and Chotzen, is characterized by facial asymmetry, craniosynostosis of the coronal sutures, and digital abnormalities of the hands and feet.

ABNORMALITIES DETECTABLE BY ULTRASOUND

Craniosynostosis (particularly of the coronal suture)

Polysyndactyly of hands and feet

Duplicated hallux

Facial asymmetry, which may be caused by unilateral coronal synostosis

MAJOR DIFFERENTIAL DIAGNOSES

Apert syndrome

Carpenter syndrome

Crouzon syndrome

Kleeblattschädel anomaly (cloverleaf-shaped skull)

Pfeiffer syndrome

ULTRASOUND DIAGNOSIS

This syndrome has been diagnosed prenatally, first recognized at 12 weeks' gestational age, showing flat facies, high forehead, and unusual profile.

HEREDITY

This is an autosomal dominant syndrome resulting from a mutation of the TWIST transcription factor gene (7p21–p22).

NATURAL HISTORY AND OUTCOME

Some affected individuals may have mental deficiency, although most are of normal intelligence.

Suggested Reading

Chotzen F: Eine eigenartige familiare entwicklungsstoerung (akrocephalosyndaktylie, dysostosis craniofacialis und hypertelorismus). *Mschr Kinderheilk* 55:97–122, 1932.

Delahaye S, Bernard JP, Renier D, Ville Y: Prenatal ultrasound diagnosis of fetal craniosynostosis. *Ultrasound Obstet Gynecol* 21:347–353, 2003.

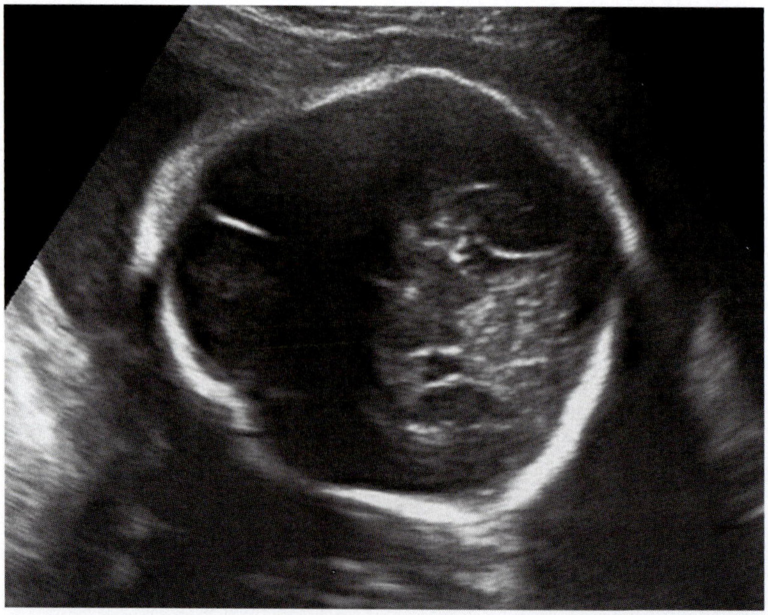

A

FIGURE 2-165 (A) Abnormally shaped skull in a fetus with craniosynostosis in the early third trimester.

Continued

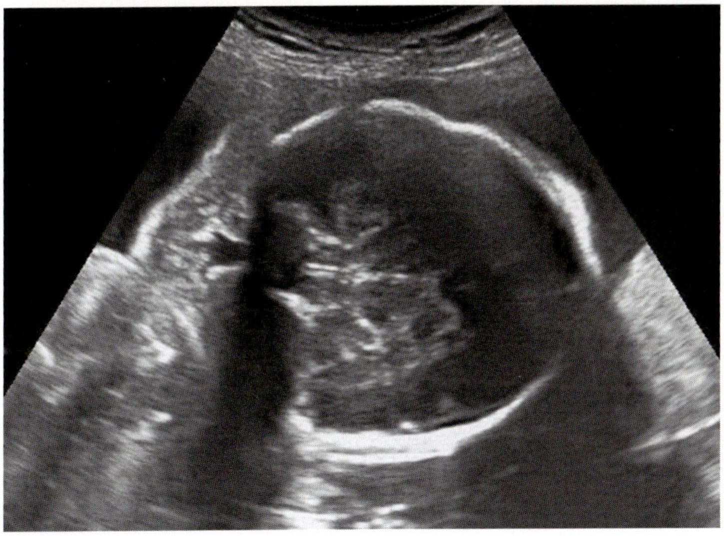
B

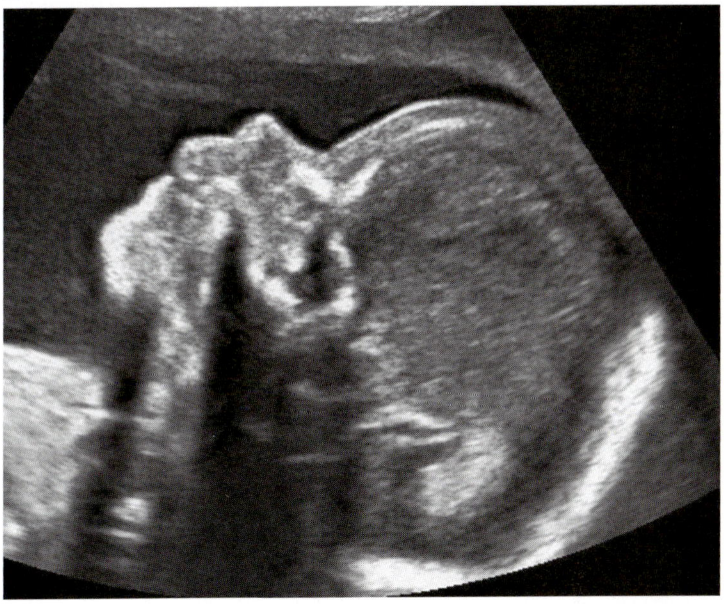
C

FIGURE 2-165, cont'd (B) Abnormally shaped skull in a fetus with craniosynostosis in the early third trimester. (C) Profile view of the same fetus with craniosynostosis shows acrocephaly.

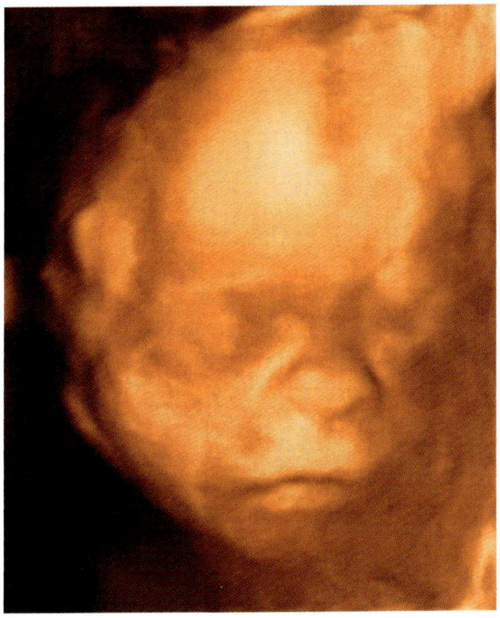
A

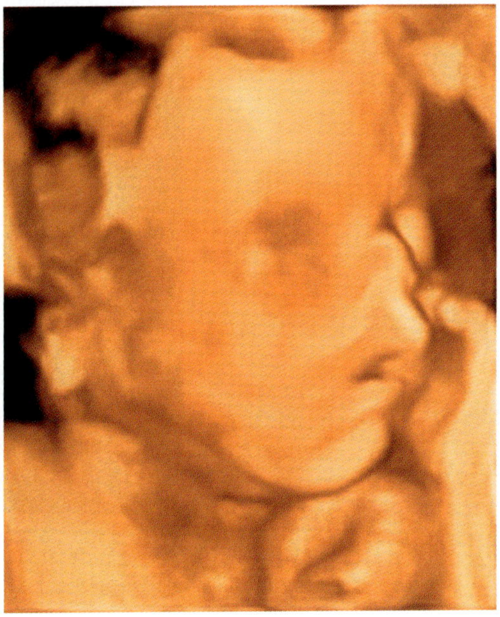
B

FIGURE 2-166 (A, B) Three-dimensional surface rendering of the fetal face of the same fetus as in Figure 2-165. Note that the metopic suture is not visible. Note the long philtrum, turned up nose, and high forehead of this fetus as a result of craniosynostosis.

Johnson D, Horsley SW, Moloney DM, et al: A comprehensive screen for TWIST mutations in patients with craniosynostosis identifies a new microdeletion syndrome of chromosome band 7p21.1 *Am J Hum Genet* 63:1282–1293, 1998.

Jones KL: *Smith's recognizable patterns of human malformations,* ed 6. Philadelphia, 2006, Elsevier.

Reardon W, Winter RM: Saethre-Chotzen syndrome. *J Med Genet* 31:393–396, 1994.

Saethre H: Ein beitrag zum turmschaedelproblem (pathogenese, erblichkeit und symptomatologie). *Dtsch Z Nervenheilk* 119:533–555, 1931.

Miscellaneous Syndromes

CYSTIC FIBROSIS

DESCRIPTION AND DEFINITION

This disorder is characterized by chronic obstruction and infection of the respiratory tract, exocrine pancreatic insufficiency, and elevated sweat chlorine levels.

ABNORMALITIES DETECTABLE BY ULTRASOUND

Hyperechoic bowel in the second and third trimesters

Dilated loops of bowel in the second and third trimesters

Fixed and mildly dilated loops of small bowel without obstruction (in the second trimester)

Meconium peritonitis

Polyhydramnios

MAJOR DIFFERENTIAL DIAGNOSES

Syndromes and Conditions Associated with Hyperechoic Bowel:

Alpha-thalassemia

Cytomegalovirus

Down syndrome

IUGR (onset in early second trimester)

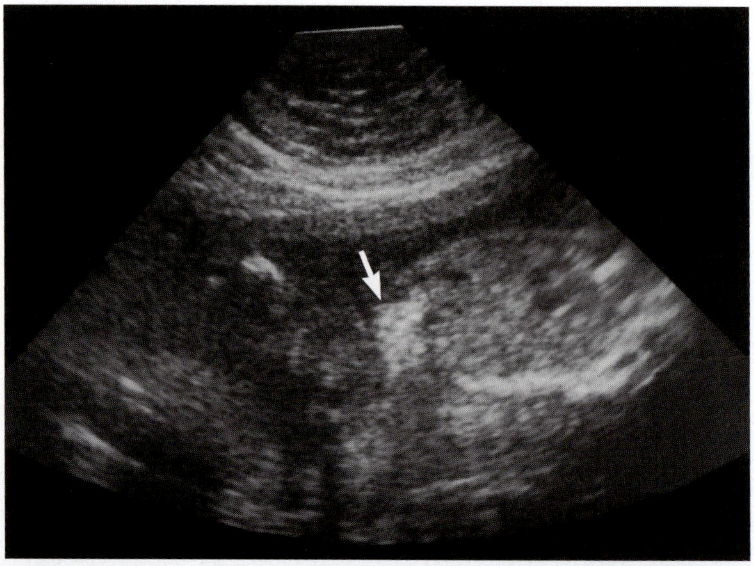

FIGURE 2-167 Longitudinal view of a second-trimester fetus shows a hyperechoic bowel *(arrow),* which sometimes is a feature of cystic fibrosis in the mid trimester. In fetuses with hyperechoic bowel, cystic fibrosis is uncommon; however, karyotyping for Down syndrome and parental testing for alleles of cystic fibrosis are recommended. Hyperechoic small bowel in the third trimester is much more suggestive of the diagnosis of cystic fibrosis.

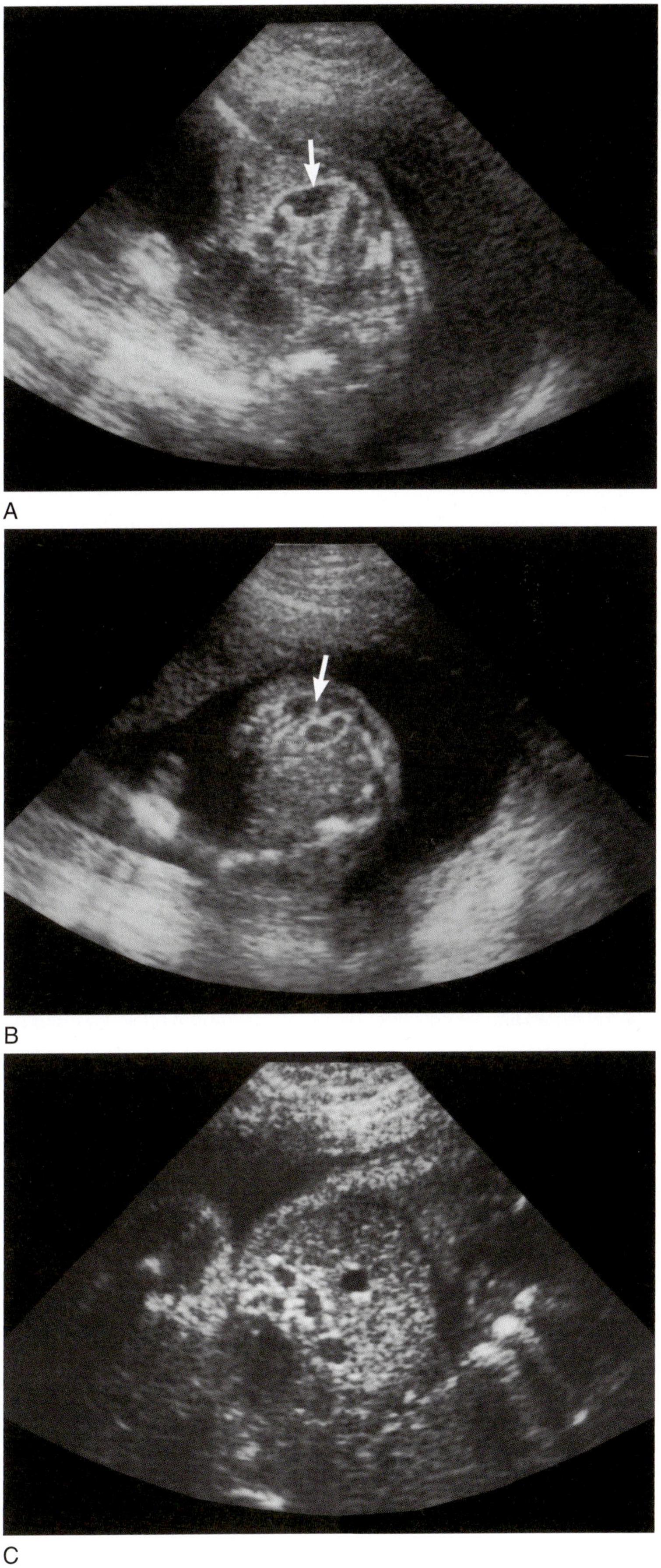

FIGURE 2-168 (A–C) Second-trimester fetus with cystic fibrosis. Note mild dilation of the bowel *(arrows)*, with some increased echogenicity of the surrounding nondilated, small bowel.

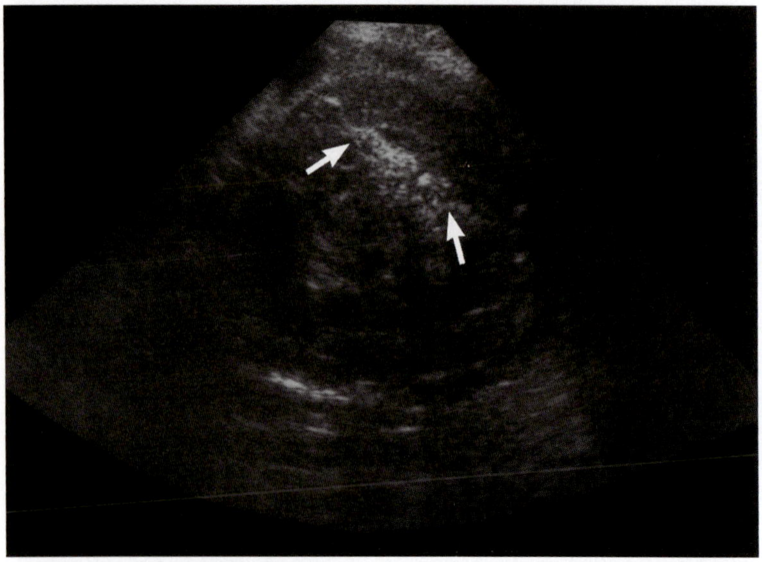

FIGURE 2-169 Bowel in a third-trimester fetus with cystic fibrosis. Note hyperechoic small bowel *(arrows)* with shadowing behind it. This is an uncommon feature in the third trimester and is highly suggestive of cystic fibrosis.

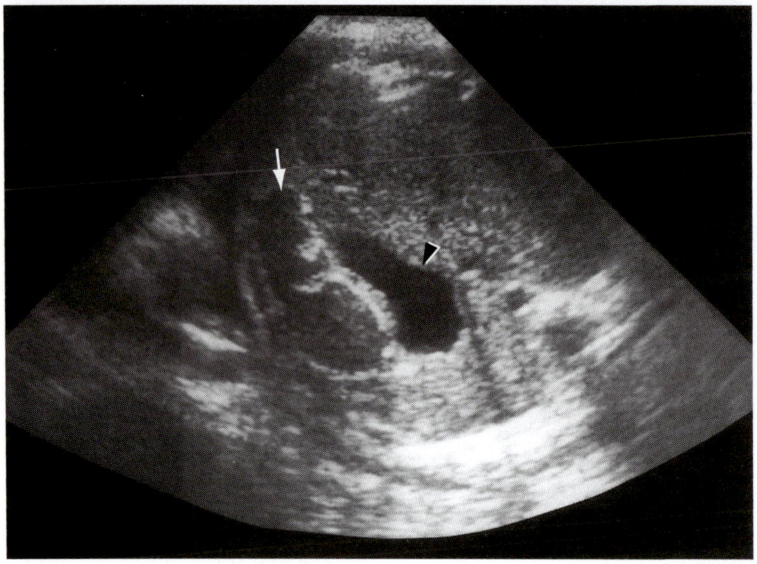

FIGURE 2-170 Third-trimester fetus with cystic fibrosis. Note dilated stomach *(arrowhead)*, which has been pushed medially by a dilated loop of bowel *(white arrow)*.

Syndromes and Conditions Associated with Dilatation of Intestinal Loops and/ or Meconium Peritonitis:

Bowel atresia

Idiopathic bowel perforations

Volvulus

ULTRASOUND DIAGNOSIS

In many cases, cystic fibrosis does not produce significant ultrasound findings. The sensitivity of ultrasound in the identification of cystic fibrosis has not been determined.

Prenatal sonographic findings are variable, but prenatal diagnosis of this condition has been established in the early second trimester, based on the presence of hyperechoic bowel. Several large studies have suggested that the incidence of cystic fibrosis in a population of fetuses with hyperechoic bowel is approximately 3%, although the additional presence of dilated bowel loops may raise the incidence to 17%. Other groups indicate a lower (1.3%) incidence of the disease when hyperechoic bowel is present and suggest that the risk of an affected fetus varies greatly with ethnic background.

The third-trimester fetus with cystic fibrosis may have a fixed, slightly dilated loop of bowel that is highly suggestive of the disorder and typically has hyperechogenicity with acoustic shadowing around the dilated loop.

Full-blown bowel obstruction, with severely dilated loops of bowel and polyhydramnios, may occur in the third trimester. Among fetuses with bowel obstruction in the third trimester, approximately one third also have cystic fibrosis.

Early detection can be achieved using fetal DNA derived from chorionic villus sampling or amniocentesis in previously affected families.

HEREDITY

The pattern of inheritance for cystic fibrosis is autosomal recessive.

The mutation responsible for this disorder is called "cystic fibrosis transmembrane conductance regulator (CFTR)." Currently, a panel of common mutations accounts for 85% of all CFTR mutations, the most common of which is delta F508. Testing for these mutations can be accomplished using parental blood and chorionic villus sampling or amniocentesis-derived fetal DNA.

NATURAL HISTORY AND OUTCOME

The mutation responsible for this disorder leads to altered epithelial cell electrolyte transport. The resultant viscous secretions cause obstruction of tubular structures, such as airways, pancreatic ducts, and bowel. Children with this disorder have chronic respiratory infections, pancreatic insufficiency, and meconium ileus.

Suggested Reading

Al-Kouatly HB, Chasen ST, Streltzoff J, Chervenak FA: The clinical significance of fetal echogenic bowel. *Am J Obstet Gynecol* 185:1035–1038, 2001.

Benacerraf BR, Chaudhury AK: Echogenic fetal bowel in the third trimester associated with meconium ileus secondary to cystic fibrosis. *J Reprod Med* 34:299–300, 1989.

Boyd PA, Chamberlain P, Gould S, et al: Hereditary multiple intestinal atresia—ultrasound findings and outcome of pregnancy in an affected case. *Prenat Diagn* 14:61–64, 1994.

Dankert-Roelse JE, te Meerman GJ, Martijn A, ten Kate LP, Knol K: Survival and clinical outcome in patients with cystic fibrosis with or without neonatal screening. *J Pediatr* 114:362–367, 1989.

Estroff JA, Bromley B, Benacerraf BR: Fetal meconium peritonitis without sequelae. *Pediatr Radiol* 22:277–278, 1992.

Estroff JA, Parad RB, Benacerraf BR: Prevalence of cystic fibrosis in fetuses with dilated bowel. *Radiology* 183:677–680, 1992.

Goldstein RB, Filly RA, Callen PW: Sonographic diagnosis of meconium ileus in utero. *J Ultrasound Med* 6:663–666, 1987.

Jouannic JM, Gavard L, Crequat J, et al: Isolated fetal hyperechogenic bowel associated with intra-uterine parvovirus B19 infection. *Fetal Diagn Ther* 20:498–500, 2005.

Kerem B, Rommens JM, Buchanan JA, et al: Identification of the cystic fibrosis gene: genetic analysis. *Science* 245:1073–1080, 1989.

Lemna WK, Feldman GL, Kerem B, et al: Mutation analysis for heterozygote detections and the prenatal diagnosis of cystic fibrosis. *N Engl J Med* 322:291–296, 1990.

Monaghan KG, Feldman GL: The risk of cystic fibrosis with prenatally detected echogenic bowel in an ethnically and racially diverse North American population. *Prenat Diagn* 19:604–609, 1999.

Moslinger D, Chalubinski K, Radner M, et al: Meconium peritonitis: intrauterine follow-up—postnatal outcome. *Wien Klin Wochenschr* 107:141–145, 1995.

Muller F, Simon-Bouy B, Girodon E, Monnier N, Malinge MC, Serre JL: French Collaborative Group. Predicting the risk of cystic fibrosis with abnormal ultrasound signs of fetal bowel: results of a French molecular collaborative study based on 641 prospective cases. *Am J Med Genet* 110:109–115, 2002.

Nyberg DA, Hastrup W, Watts H, Mack LA: Dilated fetal bowel: a sonographic sign of cystic fibrosis. *J Ultrasound Med* 6:257–260, 1987.

Riordan JR, Rommens JM, Kerem B, et al: Identification of the cystic fibrosis gene: cloning and characterization of complementary DNA. *Science* 245:1066–1072, 1989.

Samuel N, Dicker D, Landman J, Feldberg D, Goldman JA: Early diagnosis and intrauterine therapy of meconium plug syndrome in the fetus: risks and benefits. *J Ultrasound Med* 5:425–428, 1986.

Simon-Bouy B, Satre V, Ferec C, et al.; French Collaborative Group. Hyperechogenic fetal bowel: a large French collaborative study of 682 cases. *Am J Med Genet A* 121:209–213, 2003.

FRYNS SYNDROME

DESCRIPTION AND DEFINITION

Described in 1979 by Fryns, this syndrome is characterized by abnormal corneas, diaphragmatic defects, digital anomalies, and abnormal facies.

ABNORMALITIES DETECTABLE BY ULTRASOUND

Common Findings:

Cystic hygroma

Micrognathia

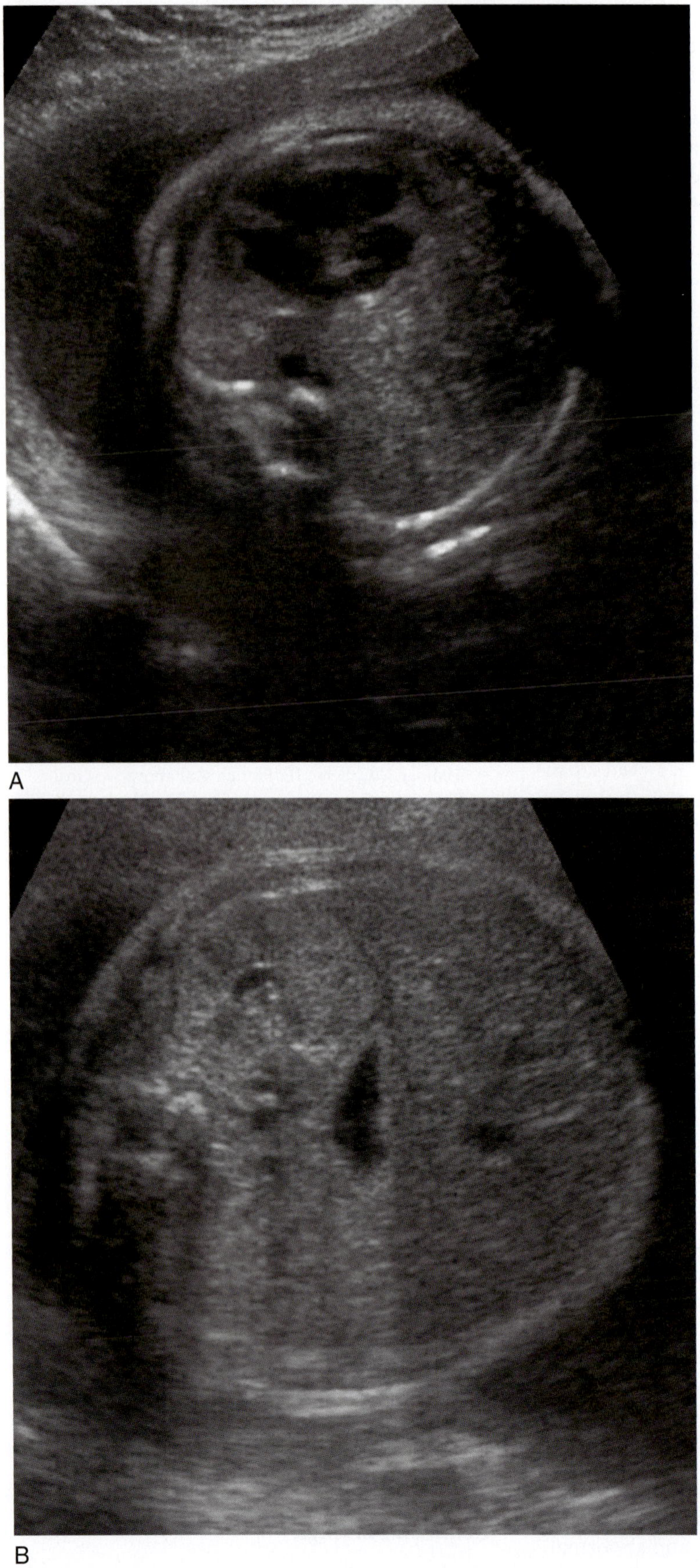

FIGURE 2-171 Third-trimester fetus with Fryns syndrome. (A) Evidence of a right diaphragmatic hernia with the fetal liver partly herniated above the diaphragm, pushing the heart to the left. (B) Abdominal diameter of the same fetus shows a midline stomach draped across the spine resulting from the diaphragmatic hernia. Note that the liver is midline.

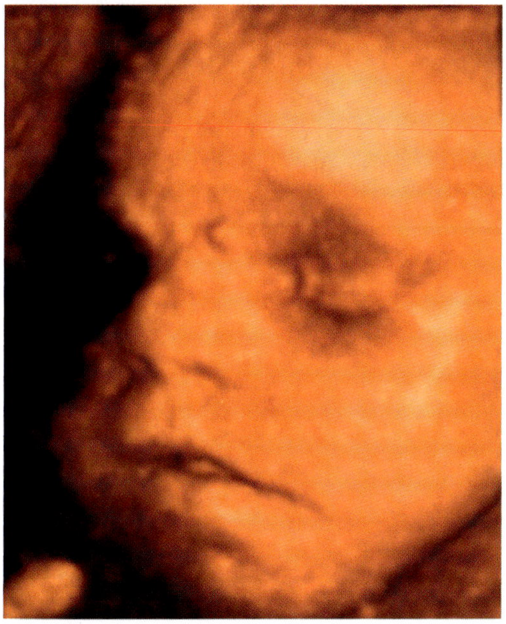

FIGURE 2-172 Surface rendering of the fetal face of the same fetus as in Figure 2-171 shows micrognathia but no cleft lip. (From Benacerraf BR, Barnewolt CE, Estroff JA, Sadow PM, Benson B: *J Ultrasound Obstet Gynecol* 27:566–570, 2006.)

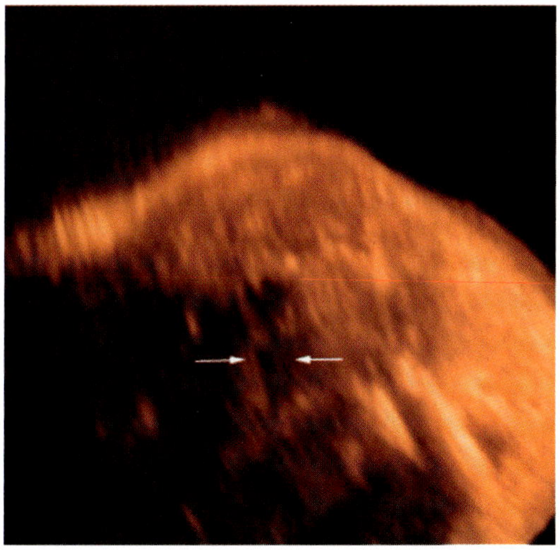

FIGURE 2-173 En face surface rendering of the fetal palate shows a cleft palate *(arrows)*.

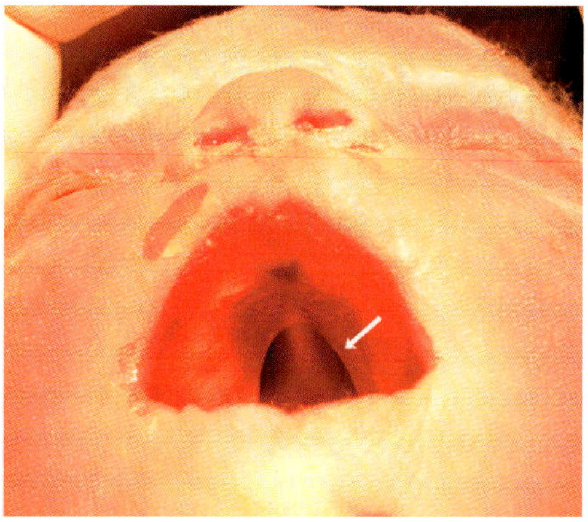

FIGURE 2-174 Postmortem view of cleft palate *(arrow)*. (From Benacerraf BR, Barnewolt CE, Estroff JA, Sadow PM, Benson B: *J Ultrasound Obstet Gynecol* 27:566–570, 2006.)

Broad nasal bridge

Cleft lip and palate

Diaphragmatic hernia

Abnormal ear shape

Ventriculomegaly

Dandy-Walker malformation

Agenesis of the corpus callosum

Intestinal malrotation

Distal digital hypoplasia

Renal cysts

Uterine abnormalities

Cryptorchidism

Hypospadias

Polyhydramnios

Occasional Findings:

Congenital cardiac defects (particularly ventricular septal defects)

Microphthalmia

Hydrops

MAJOR DIFFERENTIAL DIAGNOSES

Deletion 4p (Wolf-Hirschhorn syndrome) (CNS anomalies and diaphragmatic hernia)

Tetrasomy 12p (Pallister-Killian syndrome) (CNS anomalies and diaphragmatic hernia)

Trisomy 18 (Edwards' syndrome) (CNS anomalies, facial anomalies, diaphragmatic hernia)

Walker-Warburg syndrome (CNS and genital anomalies)

Other Syndromes and Conditions Associated with Early Nuchal Cystic Hygroma:

(See Differential Diagnosis section for complete list, p. 50)

Achondrogenesis

Apert syndrome

Cerebrocostomandibular syndrome

Chromosomal abnormalities (especially trisomies 18 and 21)

Cornelia de Lange syndrome

Cri du chat (5p-) syndrome

Kniest syndrome

Multiple pterygium syndrome

Noonan syndrome

Perlman syndrome

Roberts' syndrome

Smith-Lemli-Opitz syndrome

Turner syndrome

ULTRASOUND DIAGNOSIS

Prenatal detection of the features of Fryns syndrome was possible in a fetus as young as 12 weeks, based on the demonstration of cystic hygroma and diffuse lymphangiectasia. At 20 weeks, a diaphragmatic hernia was detected, with persistence of the diffuse lymphangiectasia. By 25 weeks' gestation, the cystic hygroma was less prominent and the diaphragmatic hernia persisted. Another case was detected at 16 weeks with findings of cystic hydromata and diaphragmatic hernia, echogenic kidneys, and normal karyotype. We had the opportunity to examine a fetus with this syndrome using both 2-D and 3-D ultrasound. At 18 weeks, the fetus had large kidneys, a thickened nuchal fold, and a diaphragmatic hernia. The patient was admitted to the hospital in preterm labor at 28 weeks because of polyhydramnios; at that time, 3-D scan showed a cleft palate with an intact lip. Considering the normal karyotype, the diagnosis of Fryns syndrome was suggested. The patient had an intrauterine fetal demise at 32 weeks.

Prenatal diagnosis of Fryns syndrome was also established in another fetus with polyhydramnios, a diaphragmatic hernia, cleft lip and palate, and mild ventriculomegaly at 28 weeks' gestation.

HEREDITY

The pattern of inheritance for Fryns syndrome is autosomal recessive.

NATURAL HISTORY AND OUTCOME

Fryns' syndrome usually is a lethal condition, with most affected fetuses stillborn or dying in the neonatal period. The few affected individuals who survive diaphragmatic hernia repair, or who do not have such a hernia, have mental retardation.

Suggested Reading

Ayme S, Julian C, Gambarelli D, et al: Fryns syndrome: Report on 8 new cases. *Clin Genet* 35:191–201, 1989.

Bamforth JS, Leonard CO, Chodirker BN, et al: Congenital diaphragmatic hernia, coarse facies, and acral hypoplasia: Fryns syndrome. *Am J Med Genet* 32:93–99, 1987.

Benacerraf BR, Barnewolt CE, Estroff JA, Sadow PM, Benson B: Cleft of the secondary palate without cleft lip diagnosed with 3–D ultrasound and fetal magnetic resonance imaging and in a fetus with Fryns syndrome. *J Ultrasound Obstet Gynecol* 27:566–570, 2006.

Bulas DI, Saal HM, Allen JF, et al: Cystic hygroma and congenital diaphragmatic hernia: early prenatal sonographic evaluation of Fryns' syndrome. *Prenat Diagn* 12:867–875, 1992.

Cunniff C, Jones KL, Saal HM, Stern HJ: Fryns syndrome: an autosomal recessive disorder associated with craniofacial anomalies, diaphragmatic hernia, and distal digital hypoplasia. *Pediatrics* 85:499–504, 1990.

Dillon E, Renwick M: Antenatal detection of congenital diaphragmatic hernias: the northern region experience. *Clin Radiol* 48:264–267, 1993.

Dix U, Beudt U: Langenbeck U. Fryns syndrome—pre- and postnatal diagnosis. *Z Geburtshilfe Perinatol* 195:280–284, 1991.

Fryns JP, Moerman F, Goddeeris P, Bossuyt C, van den Berghe H: A new lethal syndrome with cloudy corneae, diaphragmatic defects, and distal limb deformities. *Hum Genet* 50:65–70, 1979.

Gadow EC, Lippold S, Serafin E, et al: Prenatal diagnosis and long survival of Fryns' syndrome. *Prenat Diagn* 14:673–676, 1994.

Jelsema RD, Isada NB, Kazzi NJ, et al: Prenatal diagnosis of congenital diaphragmatic hernia not amenable to prenatal or neonatal repair: Brachmann-de Lange syndrome. *Am J Med Genet* 46:1022–1023, 1993.

Kershisnik MM, Craven CM, Jung AL, Carey JC, Knisely AS: Osteochondrodysplasia in Fryns syndrome. *Am J Dis Child* 145:656–660, 1991.

Manouvrier-Hanu S, Devisme L, Vaast P, Boute-Benejean O, Farriaux JP: Fryns' syndrome: report on 8 new cases. *Clin Genet* 35:191–201, 1989.

Pellissier MC, Philip N, Potier A, et al: Prenatal diagnosis of Fryns' syndrome. *Prenat Diagn* 12:299–303, 1992.

Sheffield JS, Twickler DM, Timmons C, Land K, Harrod MJ, Ramus RM: Fryns syndrome: prenatal diagnosis and pathologic correlation. *J Ultrasound Med* 17:585–589, 1998.

INFANTILE POLYCYSTIC KIDNEY DISEASE

DESCRIPTION AND DEFINITION

Synonym: Autosomal recessive polycystic kidney disease

Characterized by multiple tiny cysts of the fetal kidneys and liver, this disease leads to the development of oligohydramnios and neonatal death.

ABNORMALITIES DETECTABLE BY ULTRASOUND

Micrognathia

Congenital heart disease (such as ventricular septal defect)

Hepatic cysts (*not* usually seen on prenatal sonography)

Enlarged, echogenic kidneys with lack of normal renal architecture

Severe oligohydramnios (variable onset)

MAJOR DIFFERENTIAL DIAGNOSES

Other Syndromes and Conditions Associated with Enlarged, Echogenic Kidneys:

Adult or autosomal dominant polycystic kidney disease

Beckwith-Wiedemann syndrome (normal amniotic fluid and large fetus)

Bilateral renal dysplasia

Meckel-Gruber syndrome (polydactyly and encephalocele)

Trisomy 13 (Patau syndrome)

Echogenic kidneys can occur as a normal variant and with normal amniotic fluid volumes, in which case the fetus usually develop normally.

The onset of oligohydramnios is the most helpful differentiating factor in cases of infantile polycystic kidney disease.

ULTRASOUND DIAGNOSIS

In many cases, the fetal kidneys are enlarged and echogenic by 20 weeks' gestation. Early onset of oligohydramnios is helpful in establishing the diagnosis, particularly in previously affected families.

However, several reports cite delayed onset of any abnormal sonographic findings in this disorder, with normal-appearing kidneys until 24 weeks' gestation and late onset of oligohydramnios at 28 weeks. The outcome for these fetuses is equally grim, with neonatal death despite the late sonographic manifestations of the disease.

Thus far, liver cysts are *not* usually seen by prenatal sonography.

HEREDITY

This disease has an autosomal recessive pattern of inheritance.

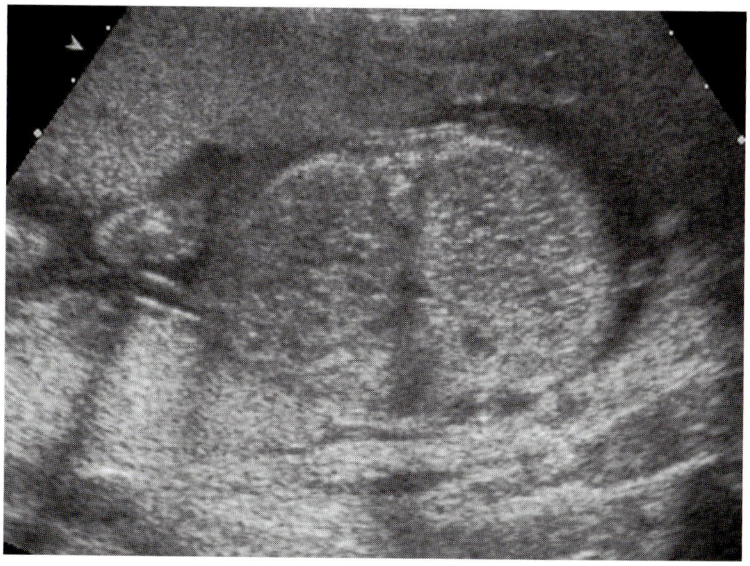

FIGURE 2-175 Infantile polycystic kidney disease. (A) Transverse and longitudinal views of a second-trimester fetus with markedly enlarged and echogenic kidneys, consistent with infantile polycystic kidney disease. *Continued*

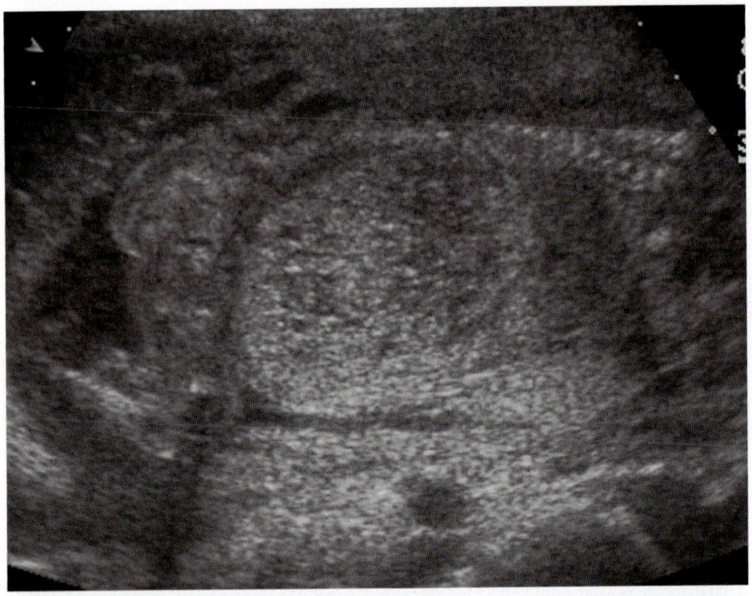

B

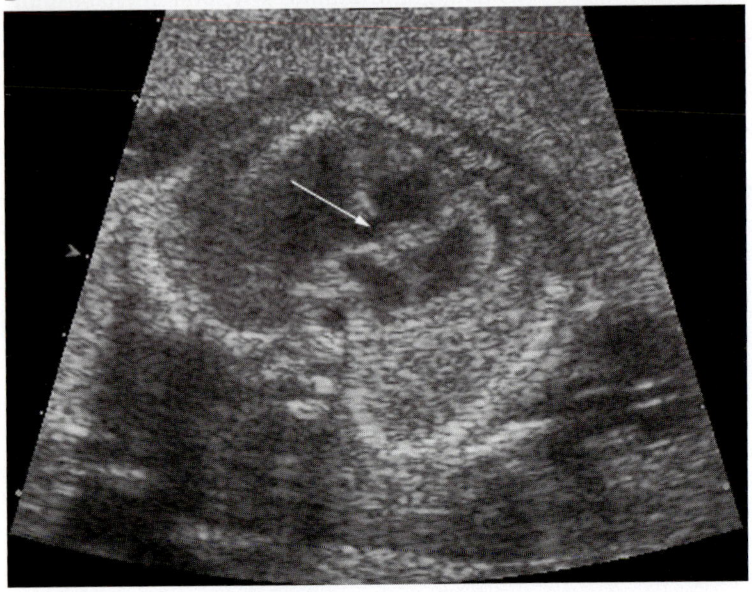

C

FIGURE 2-175, cont'd Infantile polycystic kidney disease. (B) Transverse and longitudinal views of a second-trimester fetus with markedly enlarged and echogenic kidneys, consistent with infantile polycystic kidney disease. (C) Transverse view through the fetal chest of the same fetus shows a ventricular septal defect *(arrow)*, narrow chest, and severe oligohydramnios.

NATURAL HISTORY AND OUTCOME

In cases in which sonography reveals oligohydramnios and large, echogenic kidneys, the outcome is dismal. Most fetuses with this condition are stillborn or die at birth. In rare cases, an infant survives the first year of life but eventually requires renal transplantation.

Suggested Reading

Bronshtein M, Bar-Hava I, Blumenfeld Z: Clues and pitfalls in the early prenatal diagnosis of "late onset" infantile polycystic kidney. *Prenat Diagn* 12:293–298, 1992.

Fong KW, Rahmani MR, Rose TH, Skidmore MB, Connor TP: Fetal renal cystic disease: sonographic-pathologic correlation. *AJR Am J Roentgenol* 146:767–773, 1986.

Lilford RJ, Irving HC, Allibone EB: A tale of two prior probabilities—avoiding the false-positive antenatal diagnosis of autosomal recessive polycystic kidney disease. *Br J Obstet Gynaecol* 99:216–219, 1992.

Luthy DA, Hirsch JH: Infantile polycystic kidney disease: observations from attempts at prenatal diagnosis. *Am J Med Genet* 20:505–517, 1985.

Romero R, Cullen M, Jeanty P, et al: The diagnosis of congenital renal anomalies with ultrasound. II. Infantile polycystic kidney disease. *Am J Obstet Gynecol* 150:259–262, 1984.

Tsatsaris V, Gagnadoux MF, Aubry MC, Gubler MC, Dumez Y, Dommergues M: Prenatal diagnosis of bilateral isolated fetal hyperechogenic kidneys. Is it possible to predict long term outcome? *Br J Obstet Gynaecol* 109:1388–1393, 2002.

Zerres K, Mucher G, Becker J, et al: Prenatal diagnosis of autosomal recessive polycystic kidney disease (ARPKD): molecular genetics, clinical experience, and fetal morphology. *Am J Med Genet* 76:137–144, 1998.

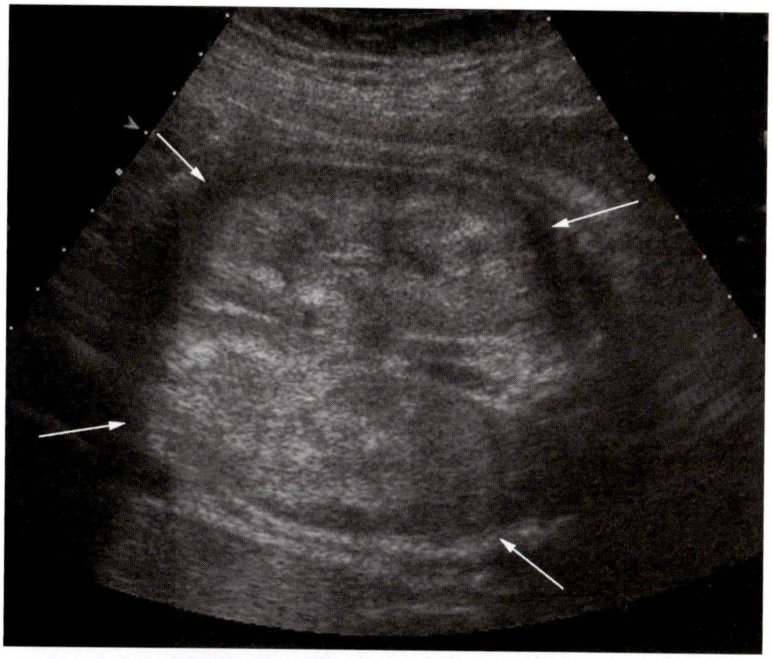

FIGURE 2-176 Third-trimester fetus with markedly enlarged and echogenic kidneys *(arrows)* in a fetus with autosomal recessive polycystic kidney disease.

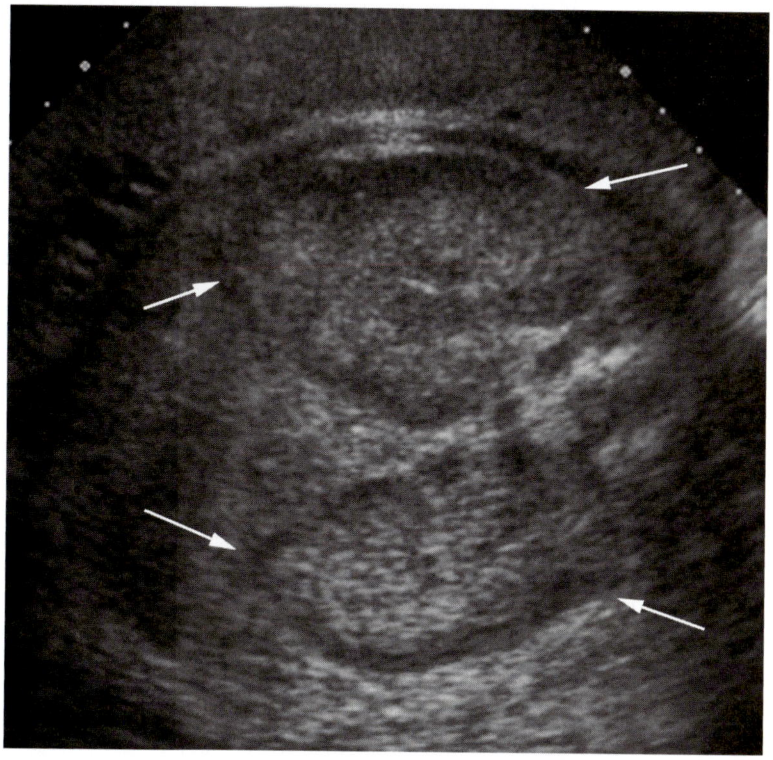

FIGURE 2-177 Transverse view through the fetal abdomen shows enlarged kidneys *(arrows)* with central increased echogenicity in a fetus with autosomal recessive polycystic kidney disease.

JARCHO-LEVIN SYNDROME

DESCRIPTION AND DEFINITION

Synonym: Spondylocostal dysostosis and spondylothoracic dysplasia (also covered here) are now considered separate entities with similar phenotypes.

Described by Jarcho and Levin in 1938, this disorder is characterized by vertebral and spinal defects, resulting in a very short thorax and spine with a protuberant abdomen.

ABNORMALITIES DETECTABLE BY ULTRASOUND

Common Findings:

Multiple abnormalities of the vertebral bodies throughout the spine (particularly the thoracic spine)

Crab-like flaring of the ribs and absence of some of the ribs

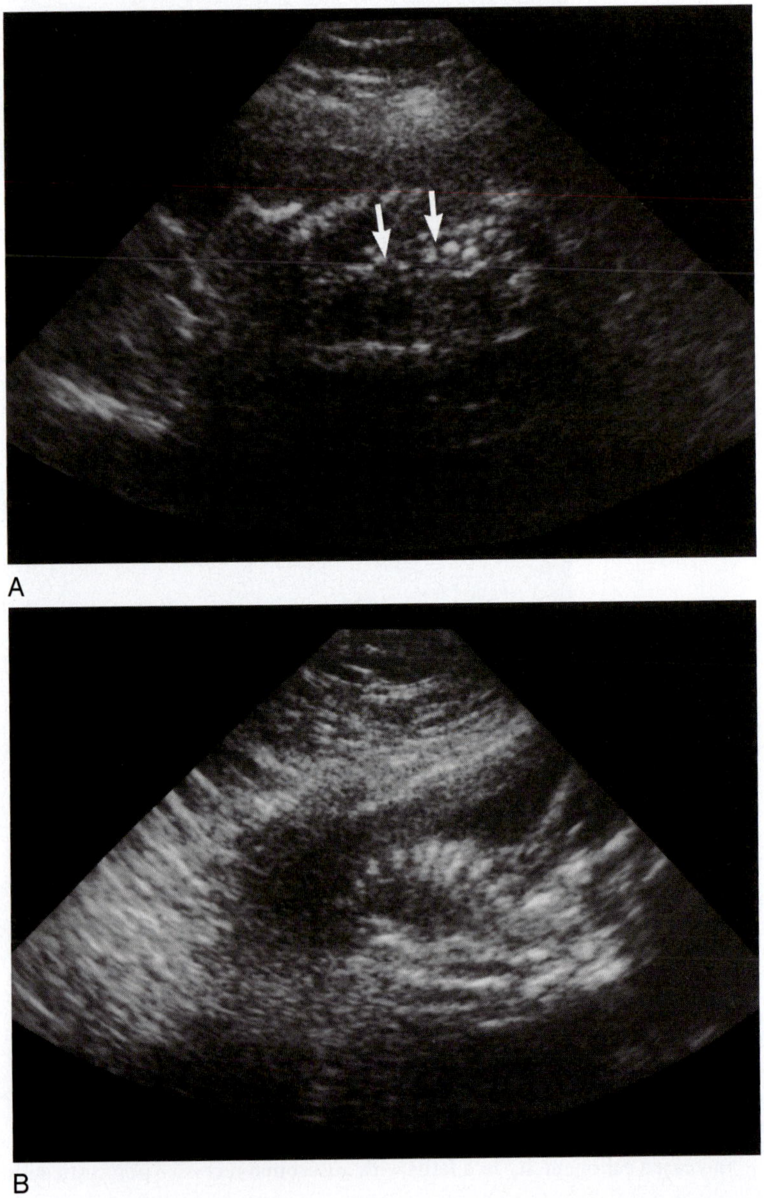

FIGURE 2-178 Spine of a second-trimester fetus with Jarcho-Levin syndrome. (A) Coronal view through the vertebral body ossification centers shows disorganization of the centers *(arrows)*. (B) Oblique view of the spine and ribs reveals multiple vertebral body abnormalities and some crowning of the ribs (crab-like), as can be seen in the syndrome.

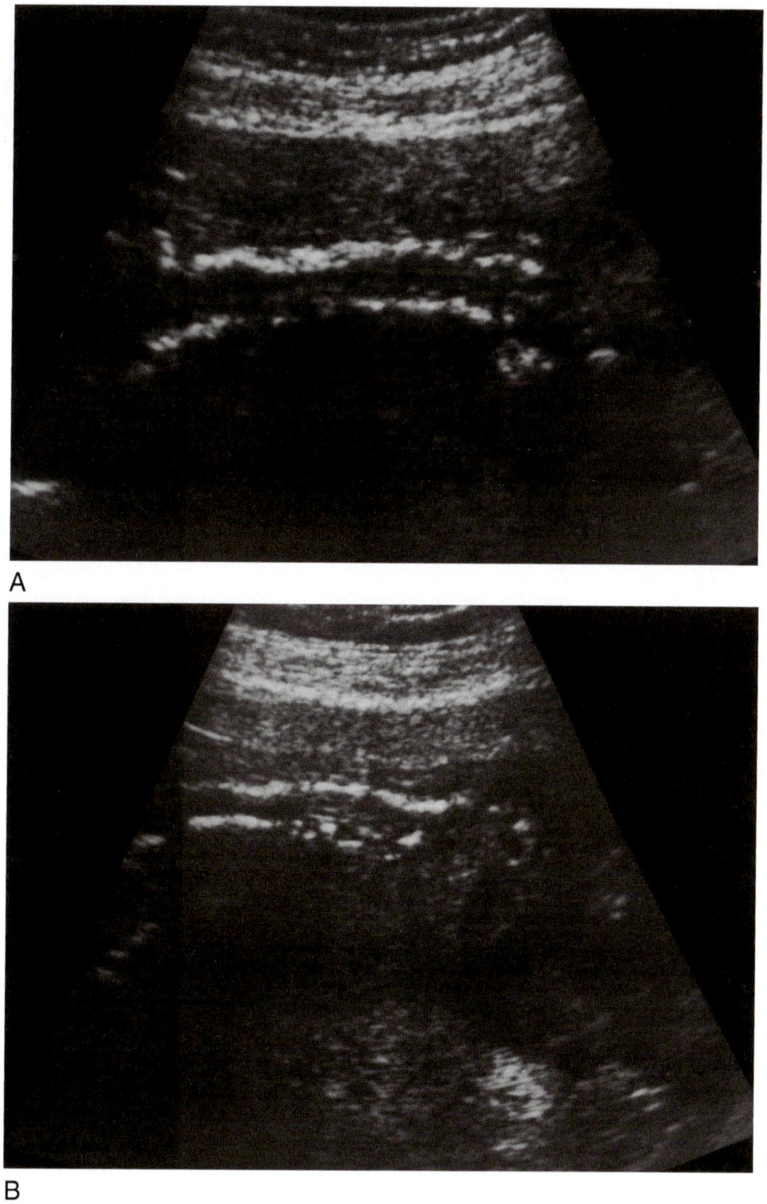

FIGURE 2-179 Coronal (A) and longitudinal (B) views of the foreshortened spine in a third-trimester fetus with Jarcho-Levin syndrome. Note that no normal vertebral bodies are visible.

Short neck

Lordosis and kyphoscoliosis

Protuberant abdomen, secondary to abnormal shortening of the spine

Nuchal translucency thickening

Occasional Findings:

Neural tube defect

Cleft palate

Hydronephrosis

Single umbilical artery

Cryptorchidism and abnormal genitals

MAJOR DIFFERENTIAL DIAGNOSES

Other Syndromes and Conditions Associated with Severe Segmental Vertebral Defects:

Caudal regression syndrome

Cerebrocostomandibular syndrome

Iniencephaly

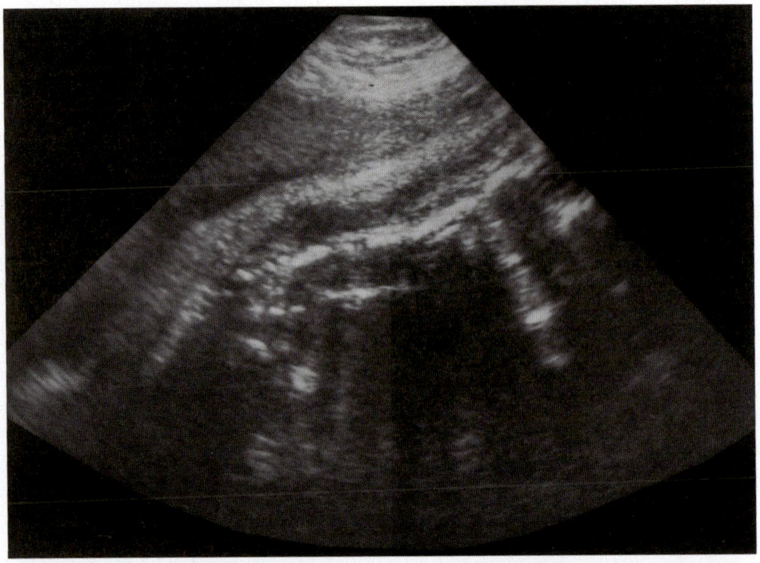
A

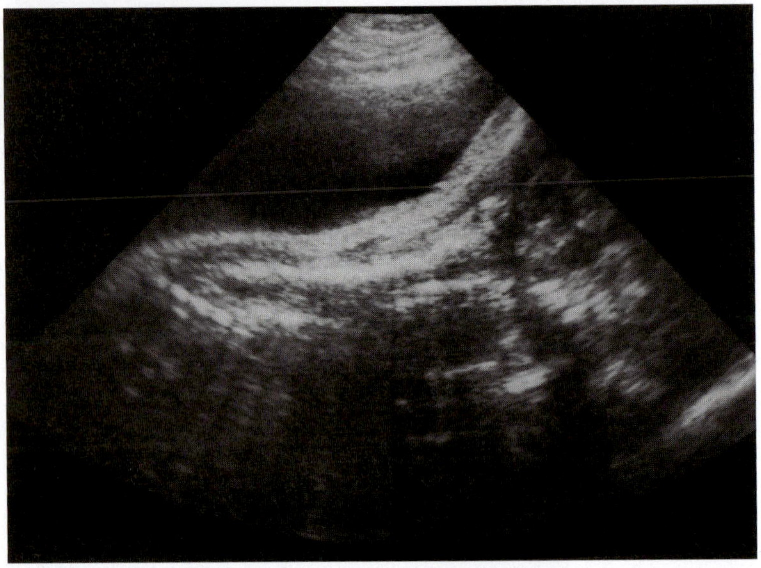
B

FIGURE 2-180 (A, B) Coronal views of the spine of a third-trimester fetus with Jarcho-Levin syndrome. Note extreme shortening of the spine. No normal ossification centers are visible.

Klippel-Feil sequence

MURCS (**mü**llerian duct aplasia, **r**enal aplasia, **c**ervicothoracic **s**omite dysplasia) association

Noonan syndrome

Sirenomelia

Spondylocostal dysostosis

Spondylothoracic dysostosis

VATER (**v**ertebral defects, **a**nal atresia, **t**racheo-esophageal fistula, **e**sophageal atresia, and **r**adial and renal dysplasias) association

ULTRASOUND DIAGNOSIS

Detection of this syndrome was first achieved by radiography in 1979 with demonstration of a crab-like deformity of the thorax. Prenatal ultrasound diagnosis was first established in 1987 and again in 1989. Since then, the syndrome has been detected by 12-week nuchal translucency thickening several times, both in previously affected families and de novo. The syndrome is characterized by multiple vertebral anomalies, abnormally short spine, unpaired dorsal vertebral centers, uneven ribs, and protuberant abdomen, all of which have been detected as early as 12 weeks' gestation.

Sonographic evidence of urogenital abnormalities and diaphragmatic hernia has been reported.

HEREDITY

Jarcho-Levin syndrome has an autosomal recessive pattern of inheritance. Two similar syndromes exist that often are lumped together with Jarcho-Levin syndrome. Some authors believe they are separate, with Jarcho-Levin being the most severe. Spondylothoracic dysostosis, also an autosomal recessive syndrome, has varying degrees of severity within a family; Spondylocostal dysostosis, an autosomal dominant condition, is considered the milder form of these vertebral segmentation syndromes, with resultant frequent kyphoscoliosis but normal lifespan.

NATURAL HISTORY AND OUTCOME

This disorder is most prevalent among Puerto Rican families. Most affected infants die early in infancy as a result of pulmonary complications and respiratory insufficiency caused by the small thorax. Survivors have moderately severe, restrictive pulmonary disease. Although the limbs are of normal length, shortening of the trunk causes a dwarf-like appearance. Spondylocostal dysostosis is thought to be an autosomal dominant disorder that is clinically similar to Jarcho-Levin syndrome but without the fan-like flaring of the ribs and with better survival.

Suggested Reading

Apuzzio JJ, Diamond N, Vigaya Ganesh MS, et al: Difficulties in the prenatal diagnosis of Jarcho-Levin syndrome. *Am J Obstet Gynecol* 156:916–918, 1987.

Ayme S, Preus M: Spondylocostal/spondylothoracic dysostosis: the clinical basis for prognosticating and genetic counseling. *Am J Med Genet* 24:599–606, 1986.

Comas AP, Castro JM: Prenatal diagnosis of OFC-TAD dysplasia or Jarcho-Levin syndrome. *Birth Defects* 15:39–44, 1979.

del Rio Holgado M, Martinez JM, Gomez O, et al: Ultrasonographic diagnosis of Jarcho-Levin syndrome at 20 weeks' gestation in a fetus without previous family history. *Fetal Diagn Ther* 20:136–140, 2005.

Eliyahu S, Weiner E, Lahav D, Shalev E: Early sonographic diagnosis of Jarcho-Levin syndrome: a prospective screening program in one family. *Ultrasound Obstet Gynecol* 9:314–318, 1997.

Hull AD, James G, Pretorius DH: Detection of Jarcho-Levin syndrome at 12 weeks' gestation by nuchal translucency screening and three-dimensional ultrasound. *Prenat Diagn* 21:390–394, 2001.

Jones KL: *Smith's recognizable patterns of human malformations,* ed 6. Philadelphia, 2006, Elsevier.

Kauffmann E, Roman H, Barau G, et al: Case report: a prenatal case of Jarcho-Levin syndrome diagnosed during the first trimester of pregnancy. *Prenat Diagn* 23:163–165, 2003.

Lam YH, Eik-Nes SH, Tang MH, Lee CP, Nicholls JM: Prenatal sonographic features of spondylocostal dysostosis and diaphragmatic hernia in the first trimester. *Ultrasound Obstet Gynecol* 13:213–215, 1999.

Lawson ME, Share J, Benacerraf B, Krauss CM: Jarcho-Levin syndrome: prenatal diagnosis, perinatal care, and follow-up of siblings. *J Perinatol* 17:407–409, 1997.

Marks F, Hernanz-Schulman M, Horii S, et al: Spondylothoracic dysplasia: clinical and sonographic diagnosis. *J Ultrasound Med* 8:1–5, 1989.

Poor MA, Alberti O, Griscom NT, et al: Nonskeletal malformations in one of three siblings with Jarcho-Levin syndrome of vertebral anomalies. *J Pediatr* 103:270–272, 1983.

Sallout BI, D'Agostini DA, Pretorius DH: Prenatal diagnosis of spondylocostal dysostosis with 3–dimensional ultrasonography. *J Ultrasound Med* 25:539–543, 2006.

Tolmie JL, Whittle MJ, McNay M, et al: Second trimester prenatal diagnosis of the Jarcho-Levin syndrome. *Prenat Diagn* 7:129–134, 1987.

Whittock NV, Turnpenny PD, Tuerlings J, Ellard S: Molecular genetic prenatal diagnosis for a case of autosomal recessive spondylocostal dysostosis. *Prenat Diagn* 23:575–579, 2003.

Wong G, Levine D: Jarcho-Levin syndrome: two consecutive pregnancies in a Puerto Rican couple. *Ultrasound Obstet Gynecol* 12:70–73, 1998.

Syndromes Featuring Primarily Soft-Tissue Anomalies

ALPHA-THALASSEMIA

DESCRIPTION AND DEFINITION

Homozygous alpha-thalassemia is an inherited disorder and is one of the major causes of non-immune hydrops among the Southeast Asian population. Anemia, portal hypertension, hypoproteinemia, and high-output cardiac failure are thought to cause hydrops in the affected fetus.

ABNORMALITIES DETECTABLE BY ULTRASOUND

Hepatosplenomegaly

Cardiomegaly

Hyperechoic bowel (early second trimester)

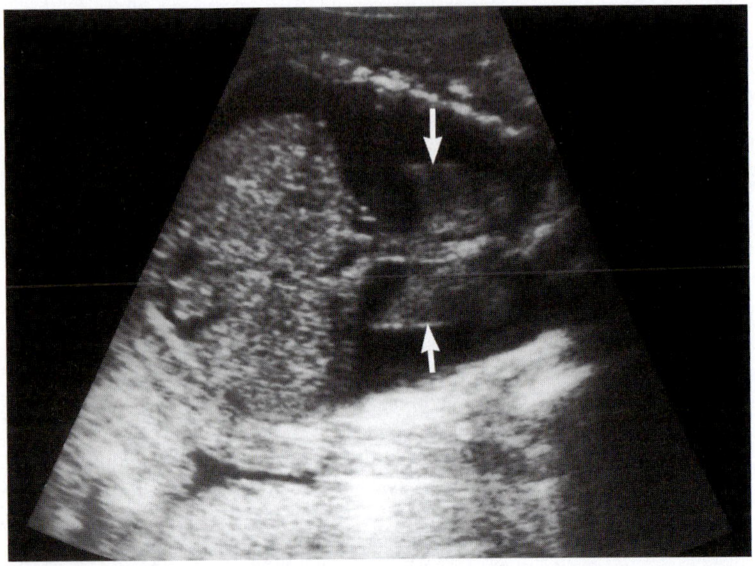

A

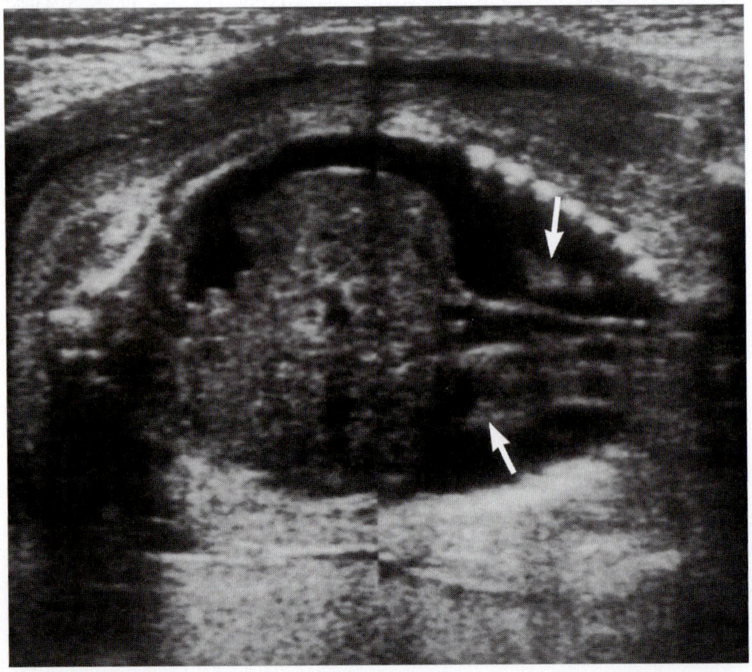

B

FIGURE 2-181 (A, B) Coronal views of the fetal chest and abdomen show diffuse hydrops. Note pleural effusions surrounding the lungs *(arrows)*, as well as the ascites.

Ascites

Edematous placenta

Subcutaneous edema with cord edema and enlarged umbilical vessels

Pericardial and pleural effusions

Oligohydramnios or polyhydramnios

MAJOR DIFFERENTIAL DIAGNOSES

Syndromes and Conditions Associated with Hydrops:

(see Differential Diagnosis for complete list, p. 111)

Achondrogenesis

Anemia

Arteriovenous shunt (aneurysm of the vein of Galen)

Cardiac arrhythmia (bradycardias and tachycardias)

Cardiomyopathy

Cardiovascular anomalies

Chest mass (causing mediastinal compression) (see Chapter 1, Intrathoracic Mass, p. 61, for differential diagnoses)

Chromosomal anomalies

Fetal–maternal hemorrhage

Fryns syndrome

Gastrointestinal obstruction

Glycogen storage disease

Idiopathic arterial calcification of infancy

Maternal infection

Multiple pterygium syndrome

Neu-Laxova syndrome

Noonan syndrome

Osteogenesis imperfecta

Tumors (fetal or placental)

Twin-to-twin transfusion syndrome

ULTRASOUND DIAGNOSIS

Fetuses with alpha-thalassemia have been detected at 12–13 weeks in families at risk, using an increased cardiothoracic ratio. The diagnosis of alpha-thalassemia has been established in fetuses in the mid second trimester, based on a thickened placenta, minimal ascites, and slight cardiomegaly. There is evidence that increased placental thickness may antedate the classic ultrasound findings of hydrops fetalis, as hydrops may not be present in the early second trimester of affected fetuses. With increasing gestational age, the findings of hydrops become more pronounced and recognizable.

A recent large study from France described 832 at-risk pregnancies, of which 168 (20.2%) were affected. The overall sensitivity and specificity of ultrasound (cardiothoracic ratio and placental thickness) for detecting the affected fetuses were 100% and 95.6%, respectively.

HEREDITY

Alpha-thalassemia has an autosomal recessive mode of inheritance. The frequency of the alpha-thalassemia gene among the Southeast Asian populations has been estimated to be 20% to 30%. As a result, alpha-thalassemia is the most common cause of hydrops in Thailand.

NATURAL HISTORY AND OUTCOME

Homozygous alpha-thalassemia is uniformly fatal for affected fetuses.

Suggested Reading

Bowman E, Watts J, Burrows R, Chui DH: Hemoglobin Barts hydrops fetalis syndrome. *Haematologia* 20:125–130, 1987.

Ko TM, Tseng LH, Hsu PM, et al: Ultrasonographic scanning of placental thickness and the prenatal diagnosis of homozygous alpha-thalassaemia 1 in the second trimester. *Prenat Diagn* 15:7–10, 1995.

Lam YH, Tang MH, Lee CP, Tse HY: Echogenic bowel in fetuses with homozygous alpha-thalassemia-1 in the first and second trimesters. *Ultrasound Obstet Gynecol* 14:180–182, 1999.

Lam YH, Tang MH, Lee CP, Tse HY: Prenatal ultrasonographic prediction of homozygous type 1 alpha-thalassemia at 12 to 13 weeks of gestation. *Am J Obstet Gynecol* 180:148–150, 1999.

Lam YH, Tang MH, Tse HY: Ductus venosus Doppler study in fetuses with homozygous alpha-thalassemia-1 at 12 to 13 weeks of gestation. *Ultrasound Obstet Gynecol* 17:30–33, 2001.

Leung KY, Liao C, Li QM, et al: A new strategy for prenatal diagnosis of homozygous alpha-thalassemia. *Ultrasound Obstet Gynecol* 28:173–177, 2006.

Petrou M, Brugiatelli M, Old J, et al: Alpha thalassaemia hydrops fetalis in the UK: The importance of screening pregnant women of Chinese, other South East Asian and Mediterranean extraction for alpha thalassaemia trait. *Br J Obstet Gynaecol* 99:985–989, 1992.

Tongsong T, Wanapirak C, Srisomboon J, Piyamongkol W, Sirichotiyakul S: Antenatal sonographic features of 100 alpha-thalassemia hydrops fetalis fetuses. *J Clin Ultrasound* 24:73–77, 1996.

APLASIA CUTIS CONGENITA (ACC)

DESCRIPTION AND DEFINITION

Skin denudation syndromes, such as aplasia cutis congenita (ACC), are manifested by bullae, blister formation, and in utero peeling of the skin.

ABNORMALITIES DETECTABLE BY ULTRASOUND

Common Findings:

"Snowflake effect" (pieces of skin float in the amniotic fluid when the skin is denuded in utero)

Skin irregularities on the surface of the fetus

Occasional Findings:

Pyloric atresia

MAJOR DIFFERENTIAL DIAGNOSES

Other skin denudation syndromes

Epidermolysis bullosa

Harlequin syndrome

ULTRASOUND DIAGNOSIS

Prenatal sonographic detection of ACC usually is possible in the second and third trimesters, especially among previously affected families. However, the diagnosis of ACC has been established as early as 19 weeks' gestation, based on the finding of multiple, small, echogenic particles floating in the amniotic cavity in a patient with a history of two previously affected gestations.

Pyloric atresia has been associated with ACC. At 16 weeks' gestation, the fetal ultrasound in one case was normal; at 26 weeks, a diagnosis of polyhydramnios, dilated stomach, and malformations of the ear and hand was established in a family at risk.

In some affected pregnant women, an elevated maternal serum alpha-fetoprotein level has been noted, possibly secondary to peeling of the fetal skin. A definitive diagnosis can be established by skin biopsy, through fetoscopy.

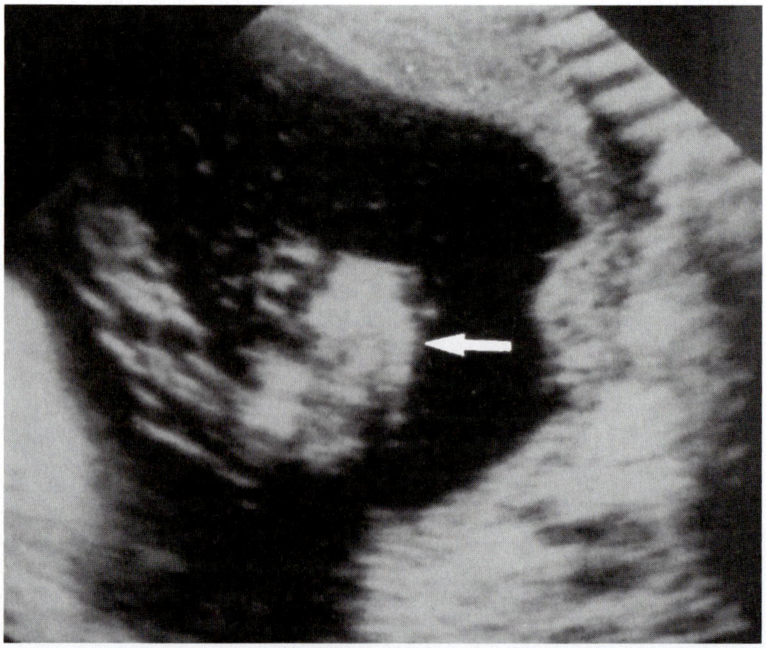

FIGURE 2-182 Numerous echogenic particles are seen floating in the amniotic fluid, near a fetal limb *(arrow)*. (From Meizner I, Carmi R: *J Ultrasound Med* 9:607–609, 1990.)

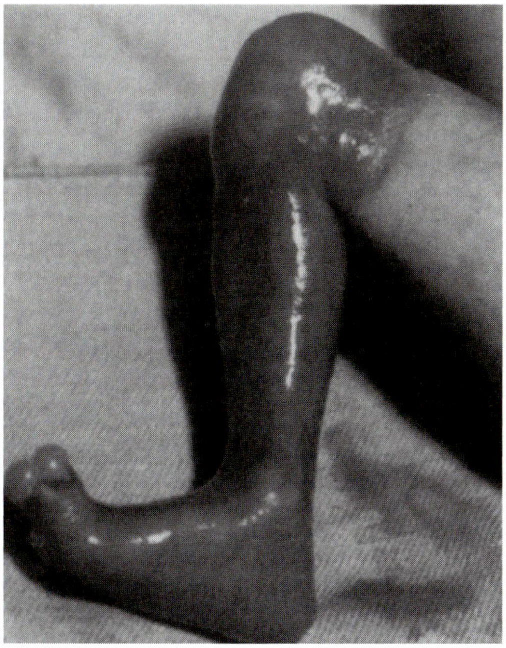

FIGURE 2-183 Postnatal photograph shows absence of skin on the right lower extremity. (From Meizner I, Carmi R: *J Ultrasound Med* 9:607–609, 1990.)

HEREDITY

The pattern of inheritance for ACC is autosomal recessive.

NATURAL HISTORY AND OUTCOME

The outcome of ACC is variable, depending on the severity of the generalized skin disorder. Fetuses with large blister formations throughout the skin (leaving large areas of the surface skinless) often die in the neonatal period.

Suggested Reading

Achiron R, Hamiel-Pinchas O, Engelberg S, et al: Aplasia cutis congenita associated with epidermolysis bullosa and pyloric atresia: the diagnostic role of prenatal ultrasonography. *Prenat Diagn* 12:765–771, 1992.

Meizner I, Carmi R: The snowflake sign: a sonographic marker for prenatal detection of fetal skin denudation. *J Ultrasound Med* 9:607–609, 1990.

HARLEQUIN SYNDROME

DESCRIPTION AND DEFINITION

Synonym: Ichthyosis congenita

This lethal condition is characterized by massive overgrowth of the keratin layers of skin, resulting in a parchment-like appearance and a clown-like appearance of the face (thus, the name "harlequin" fetus).

ABNORMALITIES DETECTABLE BY ULTRASOUND

Large, wide-open, oval mouth; tiny nose; protuberant eyes; micrognathia

Thick, anterior membrane consistent with desquamated skin

"Snowflake effect" (pieces of skin float in the amniotic fluid when skin is denuded in utero)

Fixed flexion of the extremities

Swollen hands and legs with short foot length

Markedly decreased fetal activity

Intrauterine growth restriction

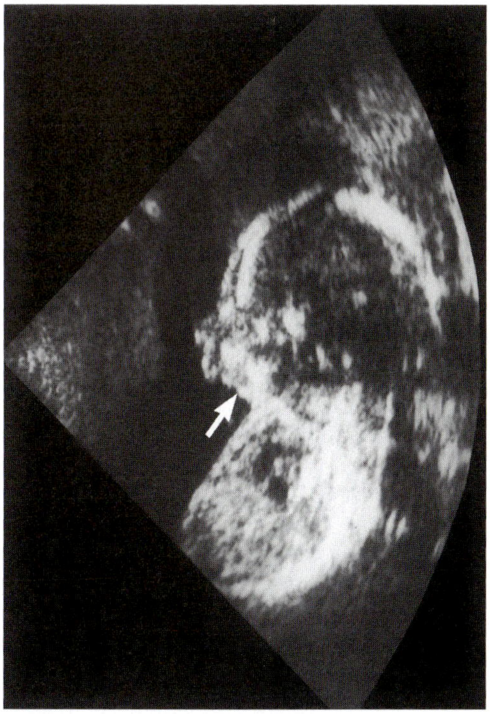

FIGURE 2-184 Longitudinal view of the face of a fetus with harlequin syndrome. Note severe micrognathia *(arrow)*.

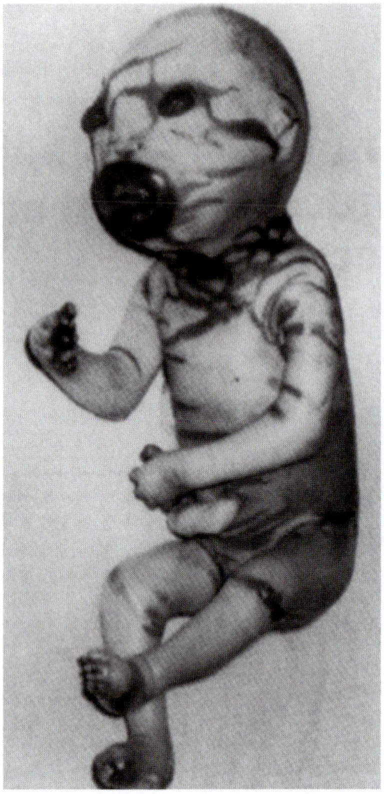

FIGURE 2-185 Photograph of a fetal body after birth shows the typical features of harlequin syndrome. (From Watson WJ, Mabee LM: *J Ultrasound Med* 14:241–243, 1995.)

MAJOR DIFFERENTIAL DIAGNOSES

Other Syndromes and Conditions Associated with Desquamating Skin Abnormalities:

Aplasia cutis congenita (ACC)

Bullous erythroderma ichthyosiform congenita

ULTRASOUND DIAGNOSIS

Prenatal diagnosis has traditionally been established by fetoscopy and skin biopsy. Recently, several reports of the sonographic appearance of harlequin fetuses have identified various characteristic features. In one report of a third-trimester fetal ultrasound, abnormal flexion contractures of the limbs, a fixed open mouth, and a mask-like face were noted. Although other reports also describe sonographic findings in the third trimester, early diagnosis of this condition is difficult. In one previously affected family, the 21-week sonogram of an affected fetus appeared normal. In another family at risk for the disorder, the 13-week scan was normal but the 17-week scan showed echogenic amniotic fluid and thick fetal lips with no other finding. The 22-week follow-up scan showed the characteristic flat profile, fixed open mouth, and thick lips consistent with recurrent Harlequin syndrome. This syndrome can be missed sonographically at the standard 16- to 18-week survey, particularly in families without a history of this disorder.

There is one report of first-trimester sonographic findings of a harlequin fetus. At 13 weeks' gestation, there was absence of fetal movement, and the arms and legs of the fetus appeared to be swollen but not to a measurable degree. Although no biometric abnormality could be identified, the fetal face appeared somewhat peculiar. The fetus died in utero shortly thereafter.

I established a diagnosis of harlequin syndrome in a mid–second-trimester fetus carried by a patient with a history of a previously affected pregnancy. The profile of the fetus was distinctly abnormal, there was no fetal movement, and the extremities were swollen.

HEREDITY

The pattern of inheritance for harlequin syndrome is autosomal recessive.

NATURAL HISTORY AND OUTCOME

This is a lethal condition, with death usually occurring in utero or in the newborn period.

Suggested Reading

Akiyama M, Suzumori K, Shimizu H: Prenatal diagnosis of harlequin ichthyosis by the examination of keratinized hair canals and amniotic fluid cells at 19 weeks' estimated gestational age. *Prenat Diagn* 19:167–171, 1999.

Arnold ML, Anton-Lamprecht I: Problems in prenatal diagnosis of the ichthyosis congenita group. *Hum Genet* 71:301–311, 1985.

Berg C, Geipel A, Kohl M, et al: Prenatal sonographic features of Harlequin ichthyosis. *Arch Gynecol Obstet* 268:48–51, 2003.

Blanchet-Bardon C, Dumez Y, Labbe F, Bernheim A, Brocheriou C: Prenatal diagnosis of a harlequin fetus using electron microscopy. *Ann Pathol (Paris)* 3:321–325, 1983.

Bongain A, Benoit B, Ejnes L, Lambert JC, Gillet JY: Harlequin fetus: three-dimensional sonographic findings and new diagnostic approach. *Ultrasound Obstet Gynecol* 20:82–85, 2002.

Elias S, Mazur M, Sabbagha R, Esterly NB, Simpson JL: Prenatal diagnosis of harlequin ichthyosis. *Clin Genet* 17:275–280, 1980.

Lattuada HP, Parker MS: Congenital ichthyosis. *Am J Surg* 82:236, 1951.

Meizner I: Prenatal ultrasonic features in a rare case of congenital ichthyosis (harlequin fetus). *J Clin Ultrasound* 20:132–134, 1992.

Mihalko M, Lindfors KK, Grix AW, Brant WE, McGahan JP: Prenatal sonographic diagnosis of harlequin ichthyosis. *AJR Am J Roentgenol* 153:827–828, 1989.

Suresh S, Vijayalakshmi R, Indrani S, Lata M: Short foot length: a diagnostic pointer for harlequin ichthyosis. *J Ultrasound Med* 23:1653–1657, 2004.

Suzumori K, Kanzaki T: Prenatal diagnosis of harlequin ichthyosis by fetal skin biopsy. Report of two cases. *Prenat Diagn* 11:451–457, 1991.

Thomson MS, Wakeley CPG: The harlequin foetus. *J Obstet Gynaecol Br Commw* 28:190–203, 1921.

Vohra N, Rochelson B, Smith-Levitin M: Three-dimensional sonographic findings in congenital (harlequin) ichthyosis. *J Ultrasound Med* 22:737–739, 2003.

Waring JJI: Early mention of a harlequin fetus in America. *Am J Dis Child* 43:442, 1932.

Watson WJ, Mabee LM: Prenatal diagnosis of severe congenital ichthyosis (harlequin fetus) by ultrasonography. *J Ultrasound Med* 14:241–243, 1995.

KLIPPEL-TRENAUNAY-WEBER SYNDROME

DESCRIPTION AND DEFINITION

This syndrome is characterized by large, cutaneous hemangiomata and lymphangiomas with hypertrophy of related bones and soft tissues, resulting in gigantism of the affected limb or part of the body.

ABNORMALITIES DETECTABLE BY ULTRASOUND

Common Findings:

Multiple cutaneous hemangiomata and lymphangiomas with complex texture and both anechoic and echogenic areas that may involve any part of the body (usually a single lower extremity, buttocks, or torso) and can vary from simple varicosities to cavernous hemangiomata

Limb hypertrophy secondary to vascular hamartoma of the limb

Long-bone asymmetry, with the affected limb being longer than its normal counterpart

Occasional Findings:

Gastrointestinal tract and retroperitoneal visceral involvement with hemangiomata

Lymphangiectasia

Asymmetric facial hypertrophy

MAJOR DIFFERENTIAL DIAGNOSES

Cystic hygromata

Disseminated hemangiomatosis syndrome

Maffucci syndrome

Proteus syndrome

Sacrococcygeal teratoma

XO syndrome (Turner syndrome)

ULTRASOUND DIAGNOSIS

Diagnosis is based on the identification of marked enlargement of the soft tissues of a limb or another part of the fetal body. This can be seen in the early second trimester. This syndrome has been diagnosed as early as 14 weeks' gestation, based on abnormal, mass-like tumors involving the sacrococcygeal region and chest wall. Several fetuses with this syndrome have been diagnosed at 15 and 17 weeks, based on cutaneous and subcutaneous cystic and complex lesions involving the lower extremity. These can progress rapidly in utero and lead to heart failure in severe cases.

HEREDITY

The pattern of inheritance for this syndrome is unknown, and its etiology has not yet been determined.

NATURAL HISTORY AND OUTCOME

This disorder is treated symptomatically and locally. Other than the specifically affected area, individuals with this disorder generally do well. Occasionally, however, a fetus develops hydrops, in which case the prognosis is far poorer.

Suggested Reading

Assimakopoulos E, Zafrakas M, Athanasiades A, Peristeri V, Tampakoudis P, Bontis J: Klippel-Trenaunay-Weber syndrome with abdominal hemangiomata appearing on ultrasound examination as intestinal obstruction. *Ultrasound Obstet Gynecol* 22:549–550, 2003.

Christenson L, Yankowitz J, Robinson R: Prenatal diagnosis of Klippel-Trenaunay-Weber syndrome as a cause for in utero heart failure and severe postnatal sequelae. *Prenat Diagn* 17:1176–1180, 1997.

Drose JA, Thickman D, Wiggins J, Haverkamp AB: Fetal echocardiographic findings in the Klippel-Trenaunay-Weber syndrome. *J Ultrasound Med* 10:525–527, 1991.

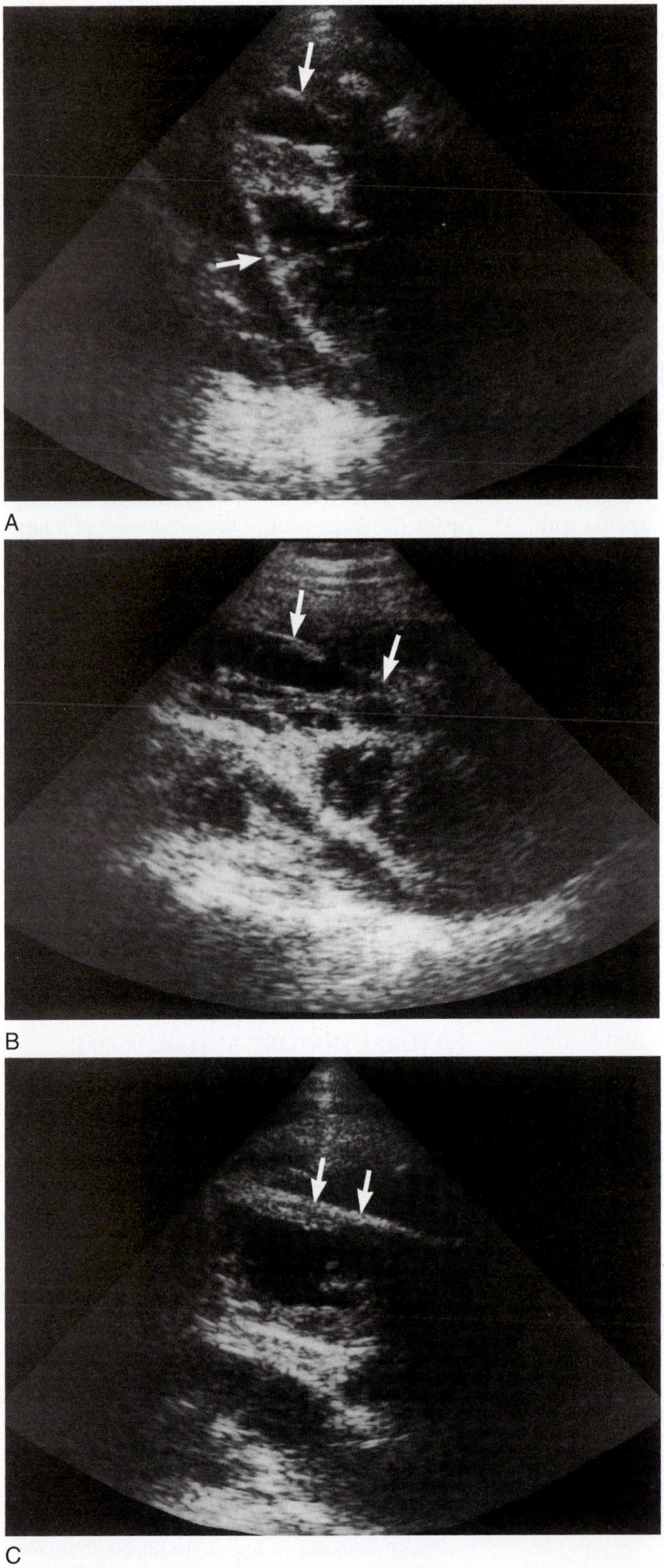

FIGURE 2-186 Fetal buttock (A) and thigh (B, C) of a third-trimester fetus diagnosed with Klippel-Trenaunay-Weber syndrome. Note multiple echolucencies *(arrows)* throughout the buttock and thigh.

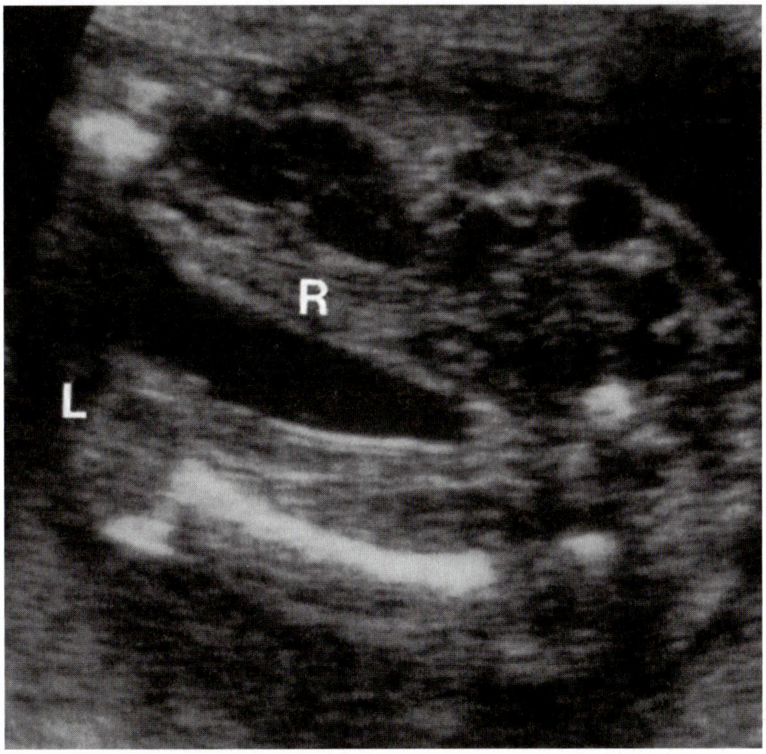

FIGURE 2-187 Longitudinal view of the fetal thighs. Note enlarged right thigh *(R)* and buttock and irregular cystic lesions throughout the soft tissues. (From Heydanus R, Wladi-Miroff JW, Brandenburg H, et al: *Ultrasound Obstet Gynecol* 2:360–363, 1992.)

Goncalves LF, Rojas MV, Vitorello D, Pereira ET, Pereima M, Saab Neto JA: Klippel-Trenaunay-Weber syndrome presenting as massive lymphangiohemangioma of the thigh: prenatal diagnosis. *Ultrasound Obstet Gynecol* 15:537–541, 2000.

Hatjis CG, Philip AG, Anderson GG, Mann LI: The in utero ultrasonographic appearance of Klippel-Trenaunay-Weber syndrome. *Am J Obstet Gynecol* 139:972–974, 1981.

Heydanus R, Wladimiroff JW, Brandenburg H, et al: Prenatal diagnosis of Klippel-Trenaunay-Weber syndrome: a case report. *Ultrasound Obstet Gynecol* 2:360–363, 1992.

Jones KL: *Smith's recognizable patterns of human malformations,* ed 6. Philadelphia, 2006, Elsevier.

Jorgenson RJ, Darby B, Patterson R, Trimmer KJ: Prenatal diagnosis of the Klippel-Trenaunay-Weber syndrome. *Prenat Diagn* 14:989–992, 1994.

Lewis BD, Doubilet PM, Heller VL, Bierre A, Bieber FR: Cutaneous and visceral hemangiomata in the Klippel-Trenaunay-Weber syndrome: antenatal sonographic detection. *AJR Am J Roentgenol* 147:598–600, 1986.

Martin WL, Ismail KM, Brace V, McPherson L, Chapman S, Kilby MD: Klippel-Trenaunay-Weber (KTW) syndrome: the use of in utero magnetic resonance imaging (MRI) in a prospective diagnosis. *Prenat Diagn* 21:311–313, 2001.

Meholic AJ, Freimanis AK, Stucka J, LoPiccolo ML: Sonographic in utero diagnosis of Klippel-Trenaunay-Weber syndrome. *J Ultrasound Med* 10:111–114, 1991.

Meizner I, Rosenak D, Nadjari M, Maor E: Sonographic diagnosis of Klippel-Trenaunay-Weber syndrome presenting as a sacrococcygeal mass at 14 to 15 weeks' gestation. *J Ultrasound Med* 13:901–904, 1994.

Paladini D, Lamberti A, Teodoro A, et al: Prenatal diagnosis and hemodynamic evaluation of Klippel-Trenaunay-Weber syndrome. *Ultrasound Obstet Gynecol* 12:215–217, 1998.

Roberts RV, Dickinson JE, Hugo PJ, Barker A: Prenatal sonographic appearances of Klippel-Trenaunay-Weber syndrome. *Prenat Diagn* 19:369–371, 1999.

Shalev E, Romano S, Nseir T, Zuckerman H: Klippel-Trenaunay syndrome: ultrasonic prenatal diagnosis. *J Clin Ultrasound* 16:268–270, 1988.

Shih JC, Shyu MK, Chang CY, et al: Application of the surface rendering technique of three-dimensional ultrasound in prenatal diagnosis and counselling of Klippel-Trenaunay-Weber syndrome. *Prenat Diagn* 18:298–302, 1998.

Warhit JM, Goldman MA, Sachs L, Weiss LM, Pek H: Klippel-Trenaunay-Weber syndrome. *J Ultrasound Med* 2:515–518, 1983.

Yancy MK, Lasley D, Richards DS: An unusual neck mass in a fetus with Klippel-Trenaunay-Weber syndrome. *J Ultrasound Med* 12:779–782, 1993.

Yang JI, Kim HS, Ryu HS: Prenatal sonographic diagnosis of Klippel-Trenaunay-Weber syndrome: a case report. *J Reprod Med* 50:291–294, 2005.

Yankowitz J, Slagel DD, Williamson R: Prenatal diagnosis of Klippel-Trenaunay-Weber syndrome by ultrasound. *Prenat Diagn* 14:745–749, 1994.

Zoppi MA, Ibba RM, Floris M, Putzolu M, Crisponi G, Monni G: Prenatal sonographic diagnosis of Klippel-Trenaunay-Weber syndrome with cardiac failure. *J Clin Ultrasound* 29:422–426, 2001.

MARFAN SYNDROME

DESCRIPTION AND DEFINITION

This connective tissue disorder, reported in 1896 by Marfan, is characterized by tall stature, long limbs, pectus deformities, ocular abnormalities, and congenital cardiac defects.

ABNORMALITIES DETECTABLE BY ULTRASOUND

Common Findings:

Cardiac abnormalities, primarily involving the ascending aorta, aortic valves, and, less commonly, the pulmonary artery or descending aorta

Tall stature (although biometric abnormalities may be difficult to detect sonographically)

Occasional Findings:

Cataracts

Cleft palate

Diaphragmatic hernia

Cardiac dysrhythmias

Scoliosis

Hemivertebrae

MAJOR DIFFERENTIAL DIAGNOSES

Other Syndromes and Conditions Associated with Aortic Abnormalities:

Isolated cardiac defects

XO syndrome (Turner syndrome) (with left heart abnormalities; however, fetuses with Turner syndrome tend to have slightly smaller biometry than normal)

ULTRASOUND DIAGNOSIS

Prenatal ultrasound diagnosis of Marfan syndrome has been established at 34 weeks' gestation, based on cardiomegaly with dilation of the aortic root and other valvar abnormalities.

Prenatal diagnosis also has been achieved using chorionic villus sampling in families with multiple affected members and informative linkage analysis.

HEREDITY

Marfan syndrome has an autosomal dominant pattern of inheritance, with wide variability of expression. This disorder is thought to result from mutations in the fibrillin gene (FBN1), located on chromosome 15q15–21.3, leading to altered fibrillin metabolism.

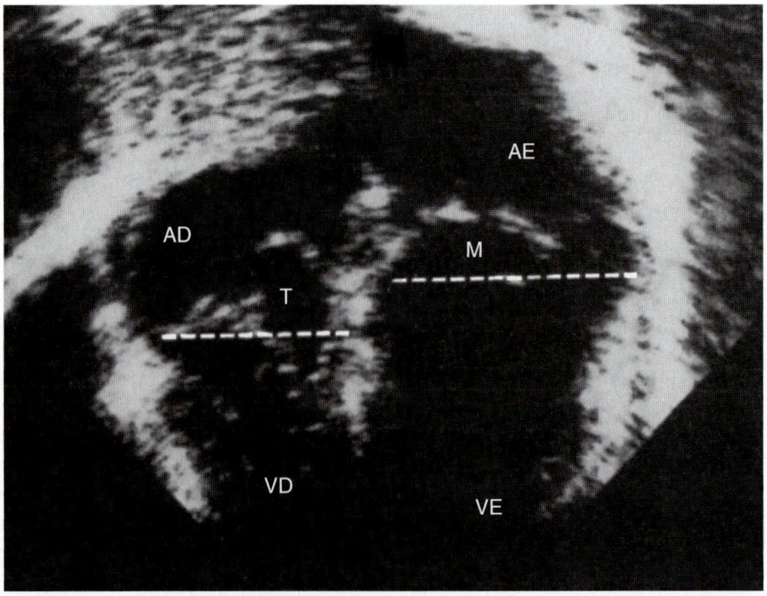

FIGURE 2-188 Fetal echocardiogram shows four-chamber view of the heart with prolapse of the tricuspid *(T)* and mitral valves *(M)*. *AD,* right atrium; *AE,* left atrium; *VD,* right ventricle; *VE,* left ventricle. (From Lopes LM, Cha SC, De Moraes EA, Zugaib M: *Prenat Diagn* 15:183–185, 1995.)

NATURAL HISTORY AND OUTCOME

Outcome depends on the severity of cardiac defects. Other medical problems that may arise in these individuals include lens subluxation, myopia, retinal detachment, chest deformity, micrognathia, scoliosis, and arachnodactyly. A more severe neonatal form of Marfan syndrome, usually diagnosed in infancy, features serious cardiac defects and contractures, as well as micrognathia, lens dislocation, arachnodactyly, and hyperextensible joints.

Suggested Reading

Godfrey M, Vandemark N, Wang M, et al: Prenatal diagnosis and a donor splice site mutation in fibrillin in a family with Marfan syndrome. *Am J Hum Genet* 53:472–480, 1993.

Jones KL: *Smith's recognizable patterns of human malformations,* ed 6. Philadelphia, 2006, Elsevier.

Koenigsberg M, Factor S, Cho S, Herskowitz A, Nitowsky H, Morecki R: Fetal Marfan syndrome: prenatal ultrasound diagnosis with pathological confirmation of skeletal and aortic lesions. *Prenat Diagn* 1:241–247, 1981.

Lopes LM, Cha SC, De Moraes EA, Zugaib M: Echocardiographic diagnosis of fetal Marfan syndrome at 34 weeks' gestation. *Prenat Diagn* 15:183–185, 1995.

Marfan AB: Un cas de deformation congenitales des quatre membres pus prononcee aux extremities characterisee par l'allongement des os avec un certain degre d'aminicissement. *Bull Mem Soc Med Hop* 13:220, 1896.

Pyeritz RE, McKusick VA: The Marfan syndrome: diagnosis and management. *N Engl J Med* 300:772–777, 1979.

Rantamaki T, Raghunath M, Karttunen L, et al: Prenatal diagnosis of Marfan syndrome: identification of a fibrillin-1 mutation in chorionic villus sample. *Prenat Diagn* 15:1176–1181, 1995.

OSTEOGENESIS IMPERFECTA

DESCRIPTION AND DEFINITION

Osteogenesis imperfecta is a heterogeneous group of conditions characterized by severe osseous fragility, defective ossification, and multiple fractures. There are six types. Type II (osteogenesis imperfecta congenita) is the most severe. Types I and IV have variable expression and may not present until after birth.

ABNORMALITIES DETECTABLE BY ULTRASOUND

Type I:

Usually none; onset of limb deformities often occurs after birth, so prenatal ultrasounds may be normal

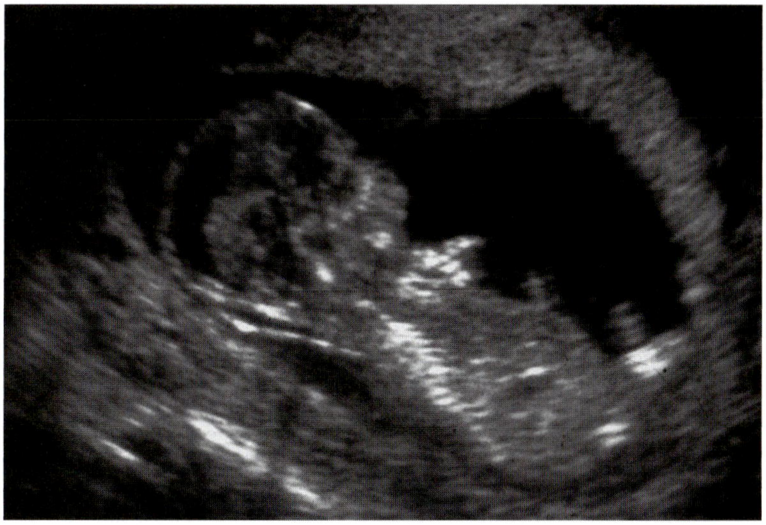

FIGURE 2-189 First-trimester fetus with osteogenesis imperfecta. Note lack of ossification of the skull and relatively short limbs.

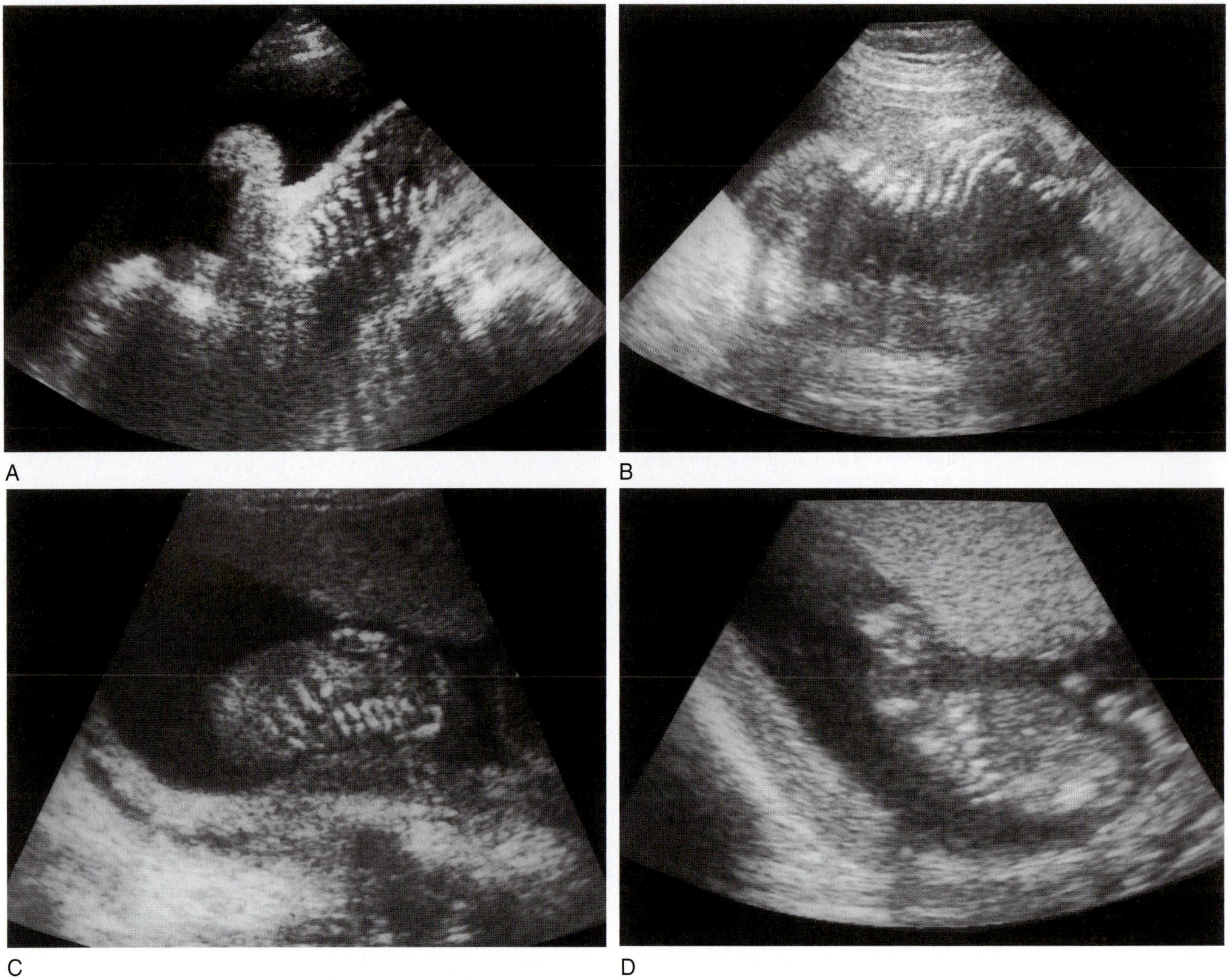

FIGURE 2-190 (A–D) Various views of the ribs of fetuses with osteogenesis imperfecta. Note unevenness of ribs and multiple fractures, which impart a beaded appearance.

Type II:

Limb shortening and angulation, secondary to severe fractures of all bones

Wrinkling of the cortical surface of the bones because of multiple fractures

Severe demineralization of the skull

Bell-shaped or narrow chest caused by rib fractures

Decreased fetal movements

Thickened nuchal translucency

Hydrops

Type III:

Multiple fractures usually detectable as early as the second trimester, of lesser severity than in type II

Type IV:

Usually none; this is the mildest form of the disease; bones tend to be normal in length, and in most cases the diagnosis is not made in utero

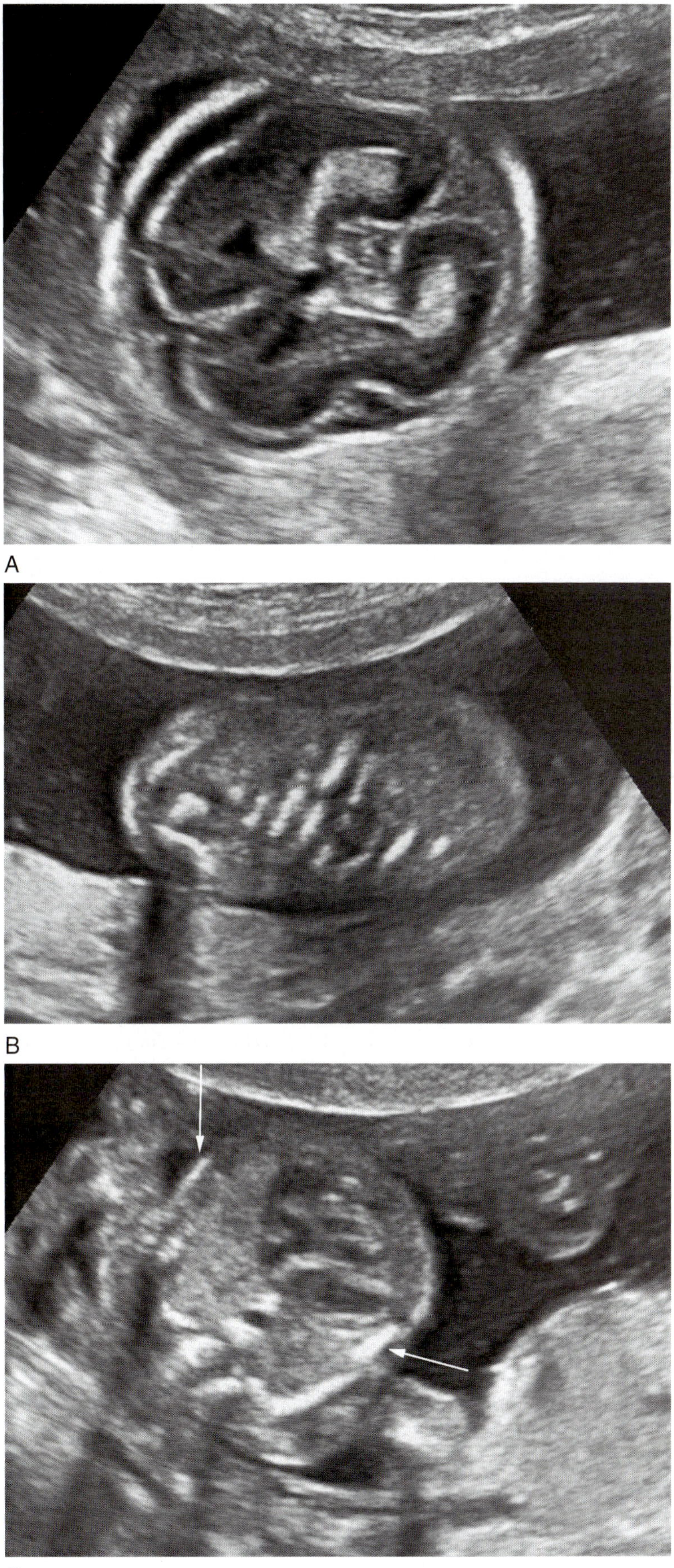

FIGURE 2-191 (A) Second-trimester fetus with osteogenesis imperfecta shows lack of ossification of the skull, permitting an unusually good evaluation of the fetal brain in the near field. (B) Tangential view of the fetal ribs of the same fetus shows multiple brakes in the ribs. (C) Transverse view of the fetal chest of the same fetus shows short ribs *(arrows)* resulting in a narrow chest caused by multiple fractured ribs.

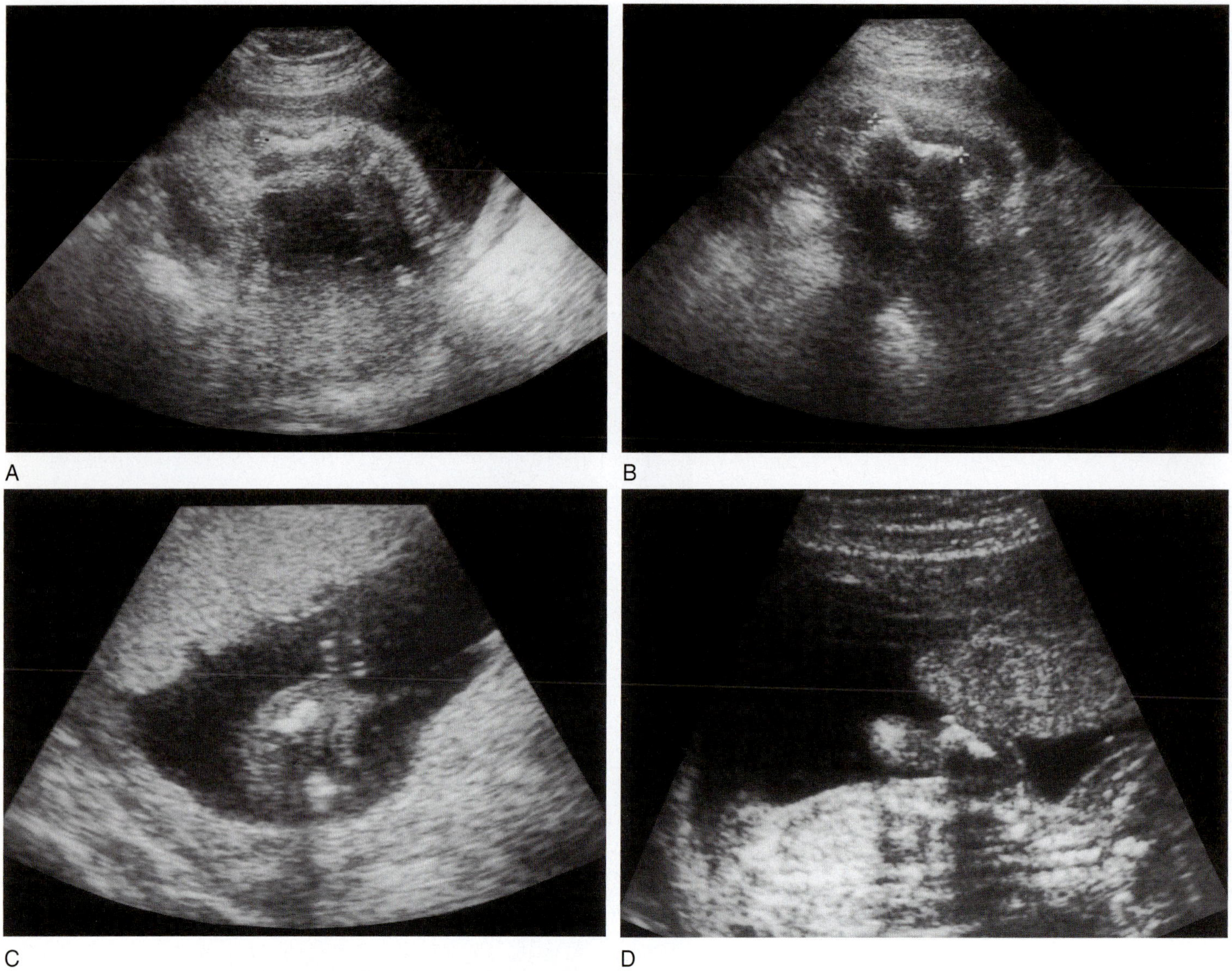

FIGURE 2-192 (A–D) Various views of the femur and humerus of fetuses with osteogenesis imperfecta. Note markedly foreshortened and beaded appearance of the bone, with evidence of fractures.

MAJOR DIFFERENTIAL DIAGNOSES

Other Syndromes and Conditions Associated with Decreased Bone Mineralization and Fractures:

Achondrogenesis

Atelosteogenesis

Chondrodysplasia punctata

Hypophosphatasia

Other Skeletal Dysplasias Associated with Bowing of the Extremities:

Camptomelic dysplasia

Diastrophic dysplasia

Thanatophoric dysplasia

ULTRASOUND DIAGNOSIS

Type II osteogenesis imperfecta, the form of this disorder most commonly diagnosed in utero, has been detected at as early as 13 weeks' gestation, based on the findings of micromelia, crumpled and bowed long bones, and beaded ribs. There are also several reports of thickened nuchal translucency in affected fetuses at 12 to 13 weeks. Abnormal skull ossification and severe shortening of the tubular bones, as well as fractures, are detectable early in the second trimester. The chest usually is narrow, indicating hypoplastic lungs and multiple rib fractures. All long bones are fractured, resulting in either angulation or rippling on the bone surface.

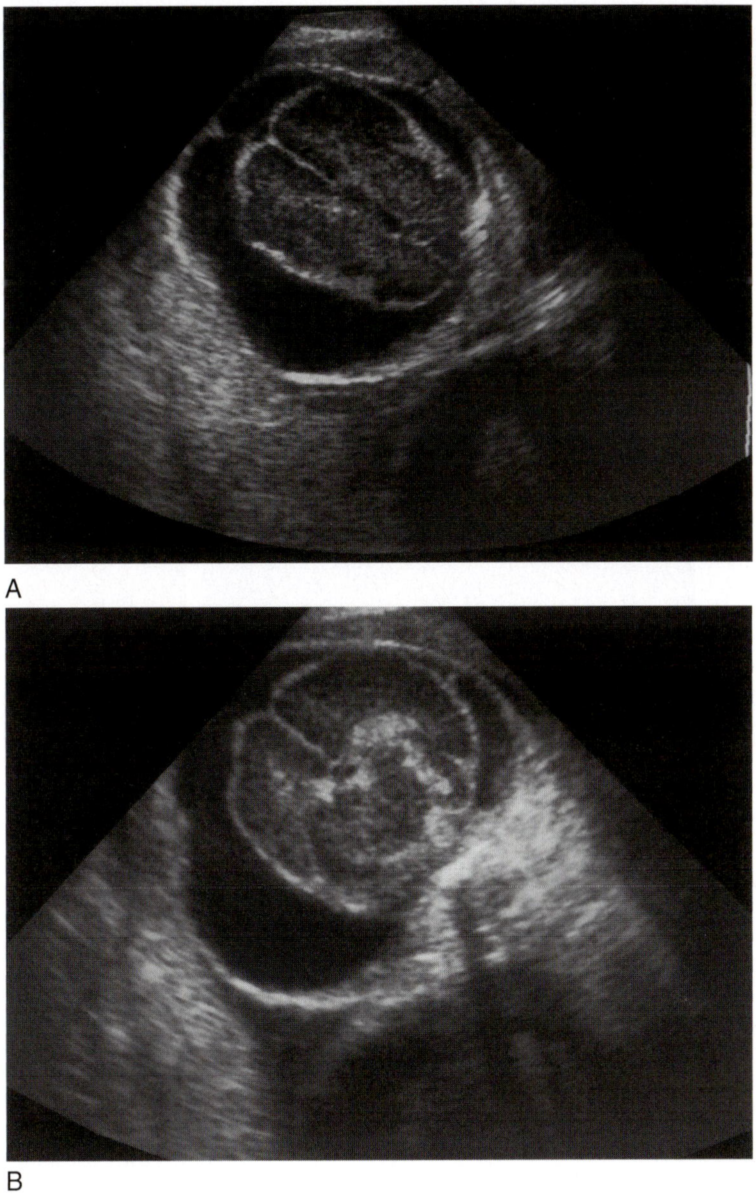

FIGURE 2-193 (A, B) Head of a third-trimester fetus with osteogenesis imperfecta. Note the almost complete lack of ossification of the skull, permitting unusually good visualization inside the head. A large amount of fluid surrounds the brain.

Osteogenesis imperfecta types I, III, IV, V, and VI are less severe than type II and vary in the onset of abnormalities detectable by ultrasound. The main sonographic findings are fractures of the long bones and bowing of the femurs. When fractures occur in utero, they can be detected by sonography. However, in many cases, the fractures may not occur in utero and so are not diagnosed until after birth. The type III form of this disorder has been diagnosed as early as 15 weeks' gestation, based on the findings of osteoporosis and macrocephaly. Type IV has been diagnosed in the late second and third trimesters, based on mild femoral bowing and slight shortening of the femurs (fifth percentile).

HEREDITY

Osteogenesis imperfecta is thought to be the result of abnormal type I collagen, produced as a result of a mutation in one of the two type I collagen genes (COL1A1 or COL1A2 locus). These mutations have been helpful in the prenatal diagnosis of various forms of osteogenesis imperfecta in which a parent is affected.

Type I has an autosomal dominant pattern of inheritance with variable expression. Type II,

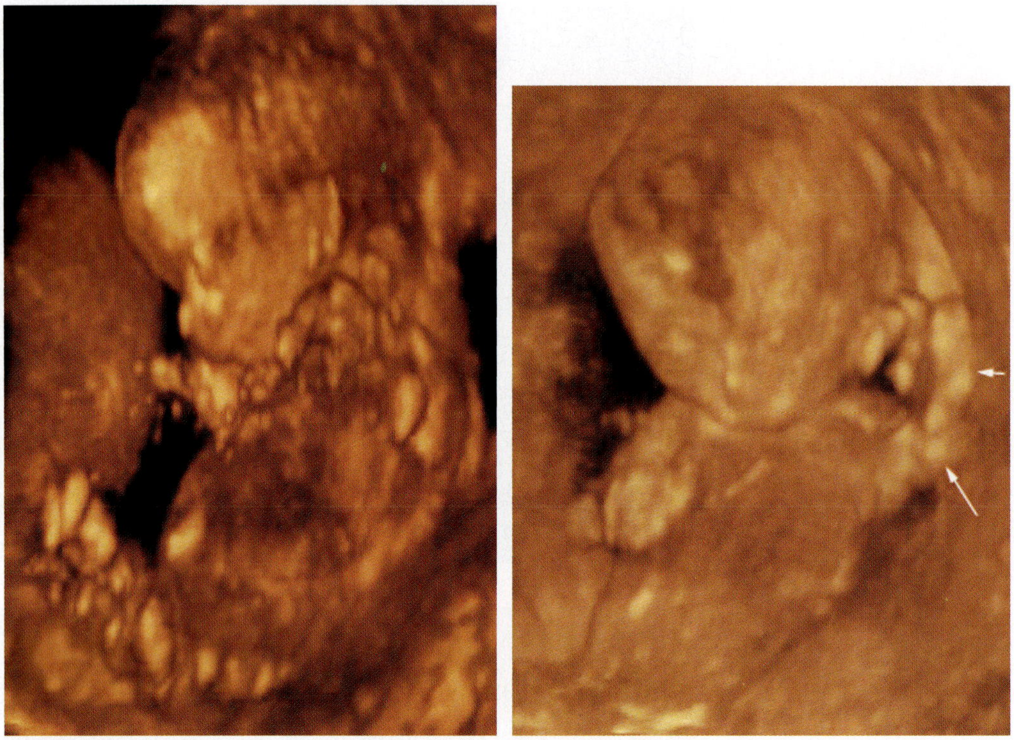

FIGURE 2-194 (A) Three-dimensional surface rendering of a first-trimester fetus with osteogenesis imperfecta shows markedly short limbs. (B) Second-trimester fetus with osteogenesis imperfecta has limbs that not only are short but are unusual in their position because of multiple fractures *(arrows)*.

the most severe, probably is a fresh autosomal dominant mutation in most cases. Type III has been reported as either an autosomal dominant or, less commonly, an autosomal recessive disorder. Type IV has an autosomal dominant pattern of inheritance. Types V and VI have unclear patterns of inheritance but are not thought to be the result of a mutation in the type I collagen genes.

NATURAL HISTORY AND OUTCOME

Type I:

Less than 10% of children with osteogenesis imperfecta type I have a fracture before birth. In most cases, affected children are ambulatory, with fractures occurring in childhood. Additional postnatal abnormalities include kyphoscoliosis and deafness.

Type II:

This form of osteogenesis imperfecta is lethal. Most fetuses have severe deformities of all bones and are stillborn or die at birth as a result of respiratory failure.

Type III:

Multiple fractures usually occur in utero, although they are not as severe as those in type II. Infants with type III disorder can have kyphoscoliosis and bowed and shortened long bones, with progressive deformity of the long bones and spine.

Type IV:

This is a milder form of the disease. It is associated with normal to moderately short stature and femoral bowing.

Types V and VI:

Types V and VI have not been described prenatally at this time. These two newer forms do not appear to be the result of the type I collagen genes and are not as severe as type II.

Suggested Reading

Aylsworth AS, Seeds JW, Guilford WB, Burns CB, Washburn DB: Prenatal diagnosis of a severe deforming type of osteogenesis imperfecta. *Am J Med Genet* 19:707–714, 1984.

Berge LN, Marton V, Tranebjaerg L, Kearney MS, Kiserud T, Oian P: Prenatal diagnosis of osteogenesis imperfecta. *Acta Obstet Gynecol Scand* 74:321–323, 1995.

Brons JTJ, van der Harten HJ, Wladimiroff JW, et al: Prenatal ultrasonographic diagnosis of osteogenesis imperfecta. *Am J Obstet Gynecol* 159:176–181, 1988.

Bronshtein M, Keret D, Deutsch M, Liberson A, Bar Chava I: Transvaginal sonographic detection of skeletal anomalies in the first and early second trimesters. *Prenat Diagn* 13:597–601, 1993.

Bronshtein M, Weiner Z: Anencephaly in a fetus with osteogenesis imperfecta: early diagnosis by transvaginal sonography. *Prenat Diagn* 12:831–834, 1992.

Bulas DI, Stern HJ, Rosenbaum KN, et al: Variable prenatal appearance of osteogenesis imperfecta. *J Ultrasound Med* 13:419–427, 1994.

Chang LW, Chang CH, Yu CH, Chang FM: Three-dimensional ultrasonography of osteogenesis imperfecta at early pregnancy. *Prenat Diagn* 22:77–78, 2002.

Chen FP, Chang LC: Prenatal diagnosis of osteogenesis imperfecta congenita by ultrasonography. *J Formos Med Assoc* 95:386–389, 1996.

Chervenak FA, Romero F, Berkowitz RL, et al: Antenatal sonographic findings of osteogenesis imperfecta. *Am J Obstet Gynecol* 143:228–230, 1982.

Constantine G, McCormack J, McHugo J, Fowlie A: Prenatal diagnosis of severe osteogenesis imperfecta. *Prenat Diagn* 11:103–110, 1991.

Dimaio MS, Earth R, Koprivnikar KE, et al: First-trimester prenatal diagnosis of osteogenesis imperfecta type II by DNA analysis and sonography. *Prenat Diagn* 13:589–596, 1993.

D'Ottavio G, Tamaro LF, Mandruzzato G: Early prenatal ultrasonographic diagnosis of osteogenesis imperfecta: a case report. *Am J Obstet Gynecol* 169:384–385, 1993.

Elejalde BR, de Elejalde MM: Prenatal diagnosis of perinatally lethal osteogenesis imperfecta. *Am J Med Genet* 14:353–359, 1983.

Garjian KV, Pretorius DH, Budorick NE, Cantrell CJ, Johnson DD, Nelson TR: Fetal skeletal dysplasia: three-dimensional US—initial experience. *Radiology* 214:717–723, 2000.

Hale AV, Medford E, Izquierdo LA, Curet L: Osteogenesis imperfecta. *Fetus* 2:5–10, 1992.

Jones KL: *Smith's recognizable patterns of human malformations,* ed 6. Philadelphia, 2006, Elsevier.

Kennon JC, Vitsky JL, Tiller GE, Jeanty P: Osteogenesis imperfecta. *Fetus* 4:11–14, 1994.

Lachman RS: Fetal imaging in the skeletal dysplasias: overview and experience. *Pediatr Radiol* 24:413–417, 1994.

Makrydimas G, Souka A, Skentou H, Lolis D, Nicolaides K: Osteogenesis imperfecta and other skeletal dysplasias presenting with increased nuchal translucency in the first trimester. *Am J Med Genet* 98:117–120, 2001.

McEwing RL, Alton K, Johnson J, Scioscia AL, Pretorius DH: First-trimester diagnosis of osteogenesis imperfecta type II by three-dimensional sonography. *J Ultrasound Med* 22:311–314, 2003.

Merz E, Goldhofer W: Sonographic diagnosis of lethal osteogenesis imperfecta in the second trimester: case report and review. *J Clin Ultrasound* 14:380–383, 1986.

Munoz C, Filly RA, Golbus MS: Osteogenesis imperfecta type II: prenatal sonographic diagnosis. *Radiology* 174:181–185, 1990.

Phillips OP, Shulman LP, Altieri LA, et al: Prenatal counseling and diagnosis in progressively deforming osteogenesis imperfecta: a case of autosomal dominant transmission. *Prenat Diagn* 11:705–710, 1991.

Ries L, Frydman M, Barkai G, Goldman B, Friedman E: Prenatal diagnosis of a novel COL1A1 mutation in osteogenesis imperfecta type I carried through full term pregnancy. *Prenat Diagn* 20:876–880, 2000.

Robinson LP, Worthen NJ, Lachman RS, Adomian GE, Rimoin DL: Prenatal diagnosis of osteogenesis imperfecta type III. *Prenat Diagn* 7:7–15, 1987.

Rouse GA, Filly RA, Toomey F, Grube GL: Short limb skeletal dysplasias: evaluation of the fetal spine with sonography and radiography. *Radiology* 174:177–180, 1990.

Ruano R, Molho M, Roume J, Ville Y: Prenatal diagnosis of fetal skeletal dysplasias by combining two-dimensional and three-dimensional ultrasound and intrauterine three-dimensional helical computer tomography. *Ultrasound Obstet Gynecol* 24:134–140, 2004.

Ruano R, Picone O, Benachi A, et al: First-trimester diagnosis of osteogenesis imperfecta associated with encephalocele by conventional and three-dimensional ultrasound. *Prenat Diagn* 23:539–542, 2003.

Sanders RC, Greyson-Fleg RT, Hogge WA et al: Osteogenesis imperfecta and camptomelic dysplasia: difficulties in prenatal diagnosis. *J Ultrasound Med* 13:691–700, 1994.

Viora E, Sciarrone A, Bastonero S, et al: Osteogenesis imperfecta associated with increased nuchal translucency as a first ultrasound sign: report of another case. *Ultrasound Obstet Gynecol* 21:200–202, 2003:

Viora E, Sciarrone A, Bastonero S, Errante G, Campogrande M, Botta G, Franceschini P: Increased nuchal translucency in the first trimester as a sign of osteogenesis imperfecta. *Am J Med Genet* 109:336–337, 2002.

Wax JR, Smith JF, Floyd RC: Lethal osteogenesis imperfecta: second trimester sonographic diagnosis in a twin gestation. *J Ultrasound Med* 13:711–713, 1994.

Woo JSK, Ghosh A, Liang ST, Wong VCW: Ultrasonic evaluation of osteogenesis imperfecta congenita in utero. *J Clin Ultrasound* 11:42–44, 1983.

PROTEUS SYNDROME

DESCRIPTION AND DEFINITION

This syndrome is characterized by asymmetric focal overgrowth, subcutaneous tumors (lipomas, hamartomatous, hemangiomas, lymphangiomas, nevi), and hemihypertrophy.

ABNORMALITIES DETECTABLE BY ULTRASOUND

Common Findings:

Limb enlargement with large, cystic spaces in the soft tissues

Overgrowth (may involve the entire body or may be localized in a limb or even a digit)

Focal lymphangiomata or hemangiomata

Macrocephaly

Macrodactyly

Occasional Findings:

Craniosynostosis

Ocular abnormalities

Renal anomalies

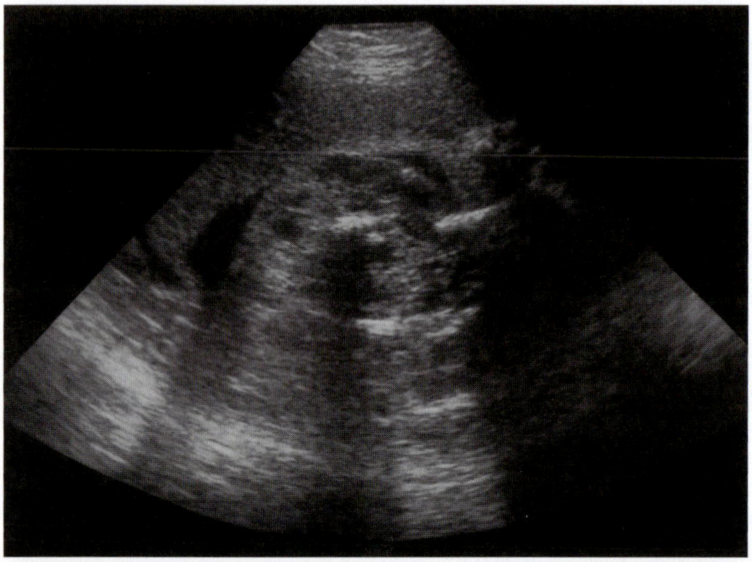

A

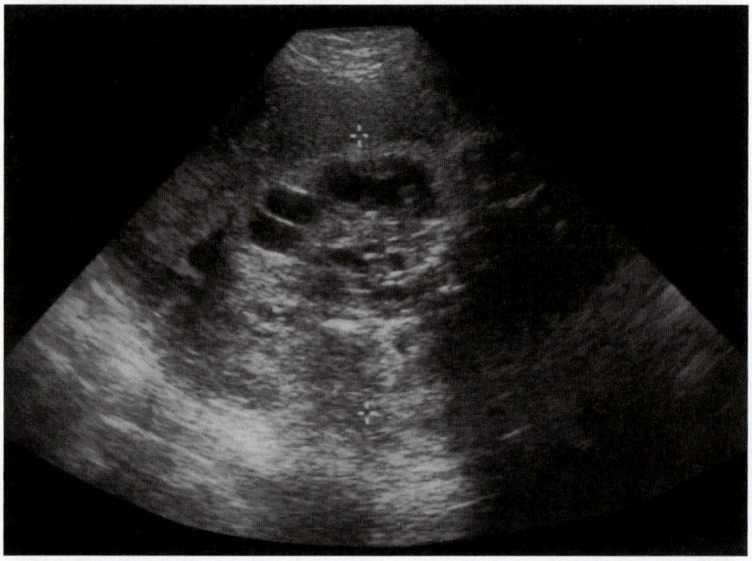

B

FIGURE 2-195 (A, B) Oblique views through the fetal buttock show a complex, cystic, solid mass originating from the buttock and sacral area. At delivery, this was found to be a large lymphangioma, as may be seen in fetuses with Proteus syndrome.

MAJOR DIFFERENTIAL DIAGNOSES

Other Syndromes and Conditions Associated with Cystic Enlargement of Subcutaneous Tissues:

Amniotic bands

Klippel-Trenaunay-Weber syndrome

Localized, subcutaneous lymphangiomata

Neurofibromatosis

ULTRASOUND DIAGNOSIS

Sonographic diagnosis of Proteus syndrome has been established in the third trimester, with the earliest diagnosis in two cases occurring at 26 and 29 weeks' gestation, respectively. It has not been determined how early in utero this condition manifests. In one of these two cases, a 17-week ultrasound showed a fixed abnormal positioning of two digits of one hand but no other anomaly. It was only at 26 weeks that the tumor involving the right side of the fetal abdomen and chest was discovered.

HEREDITY

The pattern of inheritance for this syndrome is indeterminate, and its etiology is unknown. All cases seem to occur sporadically.

NATURAL HISTORY AND OUTCOME

The manifestation of this syndrome is highly variable. Although the onset of tissue overgrowth abnormalities may occur in utero, it also may occur postnatally, and the newborn may look normal. Twenty percent of affected individuals have moderate mental deficiency. Other problems include localized abnormalities of the extremities, which usually require surgical procedures and, occasionally, amputation.

Suggested Reading

Jones KL: *Smith's recognizable patterns of human malformations,* ed 6. Philadelphia, 2006, Elsevier.

Richards DS, Williams CA, Cruz AC, Hendrickson JE: Prenatal sonographic findings in a fetus with Proteus syndrome. *J Ultrasound Med* 10:47–50, 1991.

Sigaudy S, Fredouille C, Gambarelli D, et al: Prenatal ultrasonographic findings in Proteus syndrome. *Prenat Diagn* 18:1091–1094, 1998.

Tissot H, Maugey B, Serville F, et al: Prenatal diagnosis of abdomino-pelvic cystic lymphangioma as part of Proteus syndrome. *J Gynecol Obstet Biol Reprod (Paris)* 20:335–340, 1991.

Wiedemann HR, Burgio GR, Aldenhoff P, et al: The Proteus syndrome: partial gigantism of the hands and/or feet, nevi, hemihypertrophy, subcutaneous tumors, macrocephaly or other skull anomalies, and possible accelerated growth and visceral affections. *Eur J Pediatr* 140:5, 1983.

TUBEROUS SCLEROSIS

DESCRIPTION AND DEFINITION

Tuberous sclerosis is characterized by the development of hamartomatous lesions throughout many tissues, particularly the brain, skin, heart, and kidneys.

ABNORMALITIES DETECTABLE BY ULTRASOUND

Cardiac rhabdomyomata (most commonly detected prenatal sonographic abnormality associated with tuberous sclerosis)

Brain lesions (particularly involving the basal ganglia and periventricular region; occasionally seen prenatally)

Fibroangiomatous skin lesions (probably undetectable prenatally)

Cystic bone changes (probably undetectable prenatally)

Renal angiomyolipomas (*not* yet reported on prenatal sonogram)

MAJOR DIFFERENTIAL DIAGNOSES

Because the primary sonographic feature of this syndrome is cardiac rhabdomyoma, the differential diagnosis revolves around other cardiac lesions, such as cardiac teratomas, myxomata, and fibromata.

ULTRASOUND DIAGNOSIS

Fetal cardiac tumors are the main abnormality characterizing tuberous sclerosis in utero. Reportedly, between 40% and 68% of fetuses with sonographically detected cardiac rhabdomyomas have tuberous sclerosis. Although usually diagnosed in the third trimester, cardiac rhabdomyomata have been detected as early as 22 weeks' gestation. They are characterized by echogenic masses in the heart, which are located

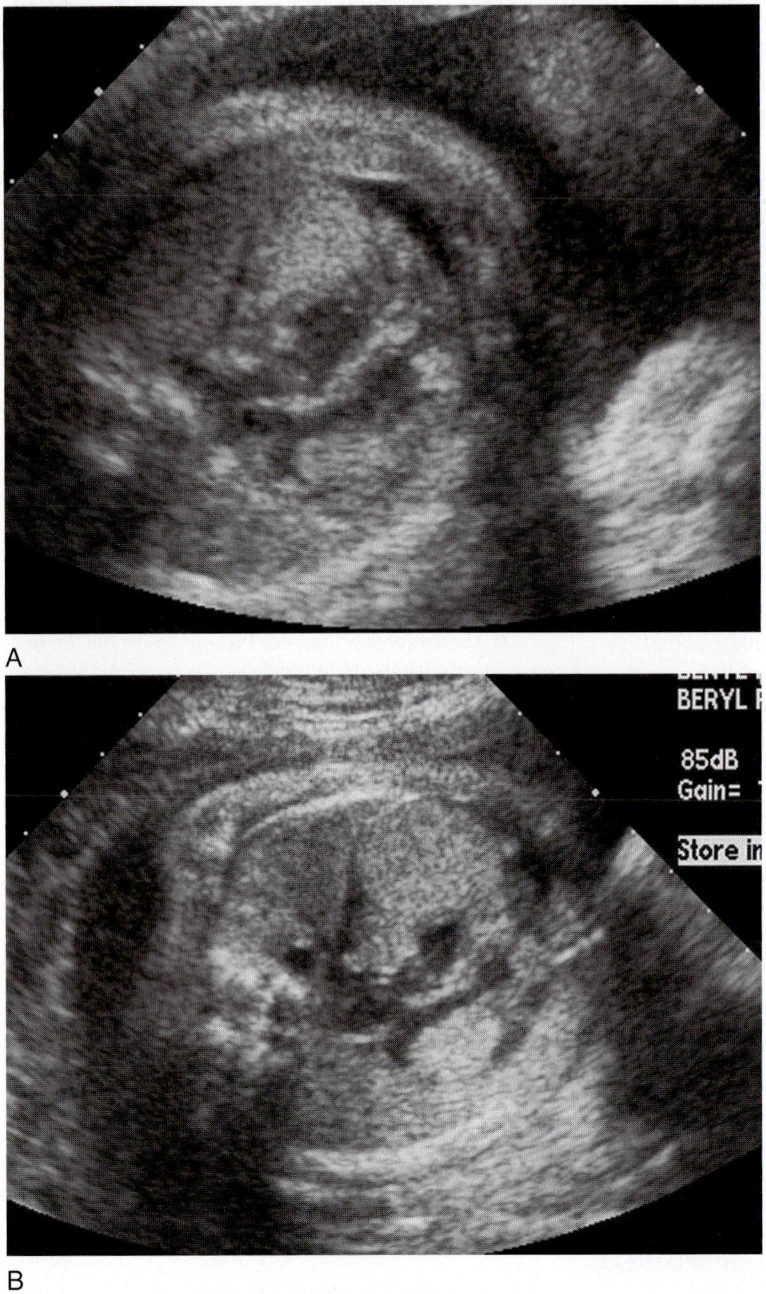

FIGURE 2-196 **(A, B) Tuberous sclerosis. Two views of the same third trimester fetus with bilateral severe involvement of the fetal heart with rhabdomyomas. This fetus had tuberous sclerosis at birth.**

in the ventricular walls and often protrude into the cardiac cavities. Fetal cardiac rhabdomyomata may lead to congestive heart failure and nonimmune hydrops. One case of monozygotic twins in which both fetuses were affected had evidence of cardiac tumors in only one twin at 22 weeks. The other twin was found to have cardiac masses only on follow-up scan at 29 weeks.

The earliest reported sonographic manifestation of a fetus with tuberous sclerosis was asymmetric lateral ventricles at 14 weeks in a family in which the father was affected. Another family at risk for the disease had an abnormal fetal echocardiogram at 21 weeks, with observation of cardiac masses. Prompted by these results, magnetic resonance imaging (MRI) was performed and showed a low-signal-intensity nodule in the subependymal region. After birth, more subependymal and cortical tubers were discovered.

In one case, a cystic neck mass was detected by ultrasound in an affected fetus of a pregnant woman with maternal tuberous sclerosis. There has also been a report of a large brain tumor detected prenatally by MRI at 26 weeks' gestation in a fetus with tuberous sclerosis. Brain and skin lesions usually are not identified, although a subependymal nodule has been detected prenatally by MRI in a fetus with cardiac rhabdomyomata.

HEREDITY

The pattern of inheritance for tuberous sclerosis is autosomal dominant, although two thirds of cases represent fresh mutations in unaffected families.

NATURAL HISTORY AND OUTCOME

Up to 80% of individuals with tuberous sclerosis have seizures and mental retardation, which are the most serious long-term complications of this disease. Sebaceous adenomata are among the classic manifestations. Additional abnormalities of the heart, kidneys, and eyes may require treatment, although many cardiac tumors regress after birth. Approximately 6% of patients develop brain tumors. There is wide variability in expression and manifestations of this disease.

Suggested Reading

Axt-Fliedner R, Qush H, Hendrik HJ, et al: Prenatal diagnosis of cerebral lesions and multiple intracardiac rhabdomyomas in a fetus with tuberous sclerosis. *J Ultrasound Med* 20:63–67, 2001.

Bader RS, Chitayat D, Kelly E, et al: Fetal rhabdomyoma: prenatal diagnosis, clinical outcome, and incidence of associated tuberous sclerosis complex. *J Pediatr* 143:620–624, 2003.

Brackley KJ, Farndon PA, Weaver JB, Dow DJ, Chapman S, Kilby MD: Prenatal diagnosis of tuberous sclerosis with intracerebral signs at 14 weeks' gestation. *Prenat Diagn* 19:575–579, 1999.

Dolkart LA, Reimers FT, Finnerty TC, Botti JJ, Weber HS: Cardiac rhabdomyoma. *Fetus* 3:5–9, 1993.

Gamzu R, Achiron R, Hegesh J, et al: Evaluating the risk of tuberous sclerosis in cases with prenatal diagnosis of cardiac rhabdomyoma. *Prenat Diagn* 22:1044–1047, 2002.

Gushiken BJ, Callen PW, Silverman NH: Prenatal diagnosis of tuberous sclerosis in monozygotic twins with cardiac masses. *J Ultrasound Med* 18:165–168, 1999.

Habbu JH, Hayman R, Roberts LJ: Tuberous sclerosis in an antenatally diagnosed cardiac rhabdomyoma. *J Obstet Gynaecol* 25:193–194, 2005:

Holley DG, Martin GR, Brenner JI, et al: Diagnosis and management of fetal cardiac tumors: A multicenter experience and review of published reports. *J Am Coll Cardiol* 26:516–520, 1995.

Jones KL: *Smith's recognizable patterns of human malformations,* ed 6. Philadelphia, 2006, Elsevier.

Journel H, Roussey M, Plais MH, et al: Prenatal diagnosis of familial tuberous sclerosis following detection of cardiac rhabdomyoma by ultrasound. *Prenat Diagn* 6:283–289, 1986.

Krapp M, Baschat AA, Gembruch U, Gloeckner K, Schwinger E, Reusche E: Tuberous sclerosis with intracardiac rhabdomyoma in a fetus with trisomy 21: case report and review of literature. *Prenat Diagn* 19:610–613, 1999.

Levine D, Barnes P, Korf B, Edelman R: Tuberous sclerosis in the fetus: second-trimester diagnosis of subependymal tubers with ultrafast MR imaging. *AJR Am J Roentgenol* 175:1067–1069, 2000.

Meyer WJ, Gauthier DW, Guillermo F: Cardiac rhabdomyoma. *Fetus* 3:11–14, 1993.

Monnier JC, Tiberghien B, Vaksmann G, et al: Bourneville's tuberous sclerosis: prenatal diagnosis of a case. *J Gynecol Obstet Biol Reprod (Paris)* 17:495–499, 1988.

Muller L, de Jong G, Falck V, et al: Antenatal ultrasonographic findings in tuberous sclerosis: report of 2 cases. *S Afr Med J* 69:633–638, 1986.

Platt LD, Devore GR, Horenstein J, et al: Prenatal diagnosis of tuberous sclerosis: the use of fetal echocardiography. *Prenat Diagn* 7:407–411, 1987.

Sgro M, Barozzino T, Toi A, Johnson J, Sermer M, Chitayat D: Prenatal detection of cerebral lesions in a fetus with tuberous sclerosis. *Ultrasound Obstet Gynecol* 14:356–359, 1999.

Sonigo P, Elmaleh A, Fermont L, et al: Prenatal MRI diagnosis of fetal cerebral tuberous sclerosis. *Pediatr Radiol* 26:1–4, 1996.

Tworetzky W, McElhinney DB, Margossian R, et al: Association between cardiac tumors and tuberous sclerosis in the fetus and neonate. *Am J Cardiol* 92:487–489, 2003.

van Oppen AC, Breslau-Siderius EJ, Stoutenbeek P, Pull Ter Gunne AJ, Merkus JM: A fetal cystic neck mass associated with maternal tuberous sclerosis. Case report and literature review. *Prenat Diagn* 11:915–920, 1991.

Sequences and Associations

AMNIOTIC BAND SEQUENCE

DESCRIPTION AND DEFINITION

The amniotic disruption complex is characterized by a destructive fetal process that is asymmetric and initiated by a rupture of the amnion. The fetus subsequently becomes adherent to, intertwined in, and tethered by fibrous bands. As the fetus grows, its anatomy is distorted, leading to cranial or body wall defects or limb abnormalities. Abnormalities can vary from a single digit abnormality to a lethal craniofacial or thoracoabdominal destructive evisceration.

ABNORMALITIES DETECTABLE BY ULTRASOUND

Abnormalities vary, depending on where the amniotic band comes into contact with the fetus, and may include the following:

Limb defects (asymmetric constriction of limbs or digits, amputations, club feet, clenched hands)

Anterior abdominal wall defects (gastroschisis, omphalocele)

Cranial abnormalities (encephalocele, asymmetric anencephaly)

Facial clefting

Micrognathia

MAJOR DIFFERENTIAL DIAGNOSES

Amniotic bands can mimic practically *any* asymmetric fetal malformation, including the following:

Adams-Oliver syndrome (transverse limb defects)

Club feet and/or clenched hands (see Chapter 1, pp. 104 and 91, for differential diagnoses)

Femoral hypoplasia

Gastroschisis

Limb defects (asymmetric; see Chapter 1 for differential diagnoses; see also p. 100)

Limb–body wall complex

Localized, subcutaneous lymphangiomata

Neural tube defects, such as anencephaly

Omphalocele, including those associated with Beckwith-Wiedemann syndrome

Pentalogy of Cantrell

Proteus or Klippel-Trenaunay-Weber syndrome

ULTRASOUND DIAGNOSIS

There are many reported instances of the prenatal diagnosis of this condition. It has been diagnosed as early as 9 weeks' gestation, with detection of a disruption of the anterior abdominal wall or skull or other parts of the fetal body.

The findings in amniotic band syndrome encompass such a broad constellation of anomalies that it is sometimes difficult to establish a definitive diagnosis unless more than two characteristic abnormalities are present in the same fetus. In some cases involving constrictive rings around the extremities or digits, the disorder has been difficult to detect sonographically, and some may even escape detection until after birth. In other cases, it may be possible, particularly when using a transvaginal ultrasound approach in the first trimester, to visualize the bands themselves tethered to the embryo of fetus, thus confirming the diagnosis.

HEREDITY

This is not considered a hereditary condition.

NATURAL HISTORY AND OUTCOME

The underlying mechanism for this condition is thought to be rupture of the amnion, with the fetus becoming adherent to and intertwined in fibrous bands that, in turn, damage the fetus. This amniotic rupture most likely occurs before 12 weeks' gestation, when the amnion and chorion are still completely separate membranes. It has been suggested that persistence of the amniotic/chorionic separation occasionally is a complication of amniocentesis. There are many reported cases, however, where amniotic/chorionic membrane separation occurred without invasive procedure.

Text continued on p. 361

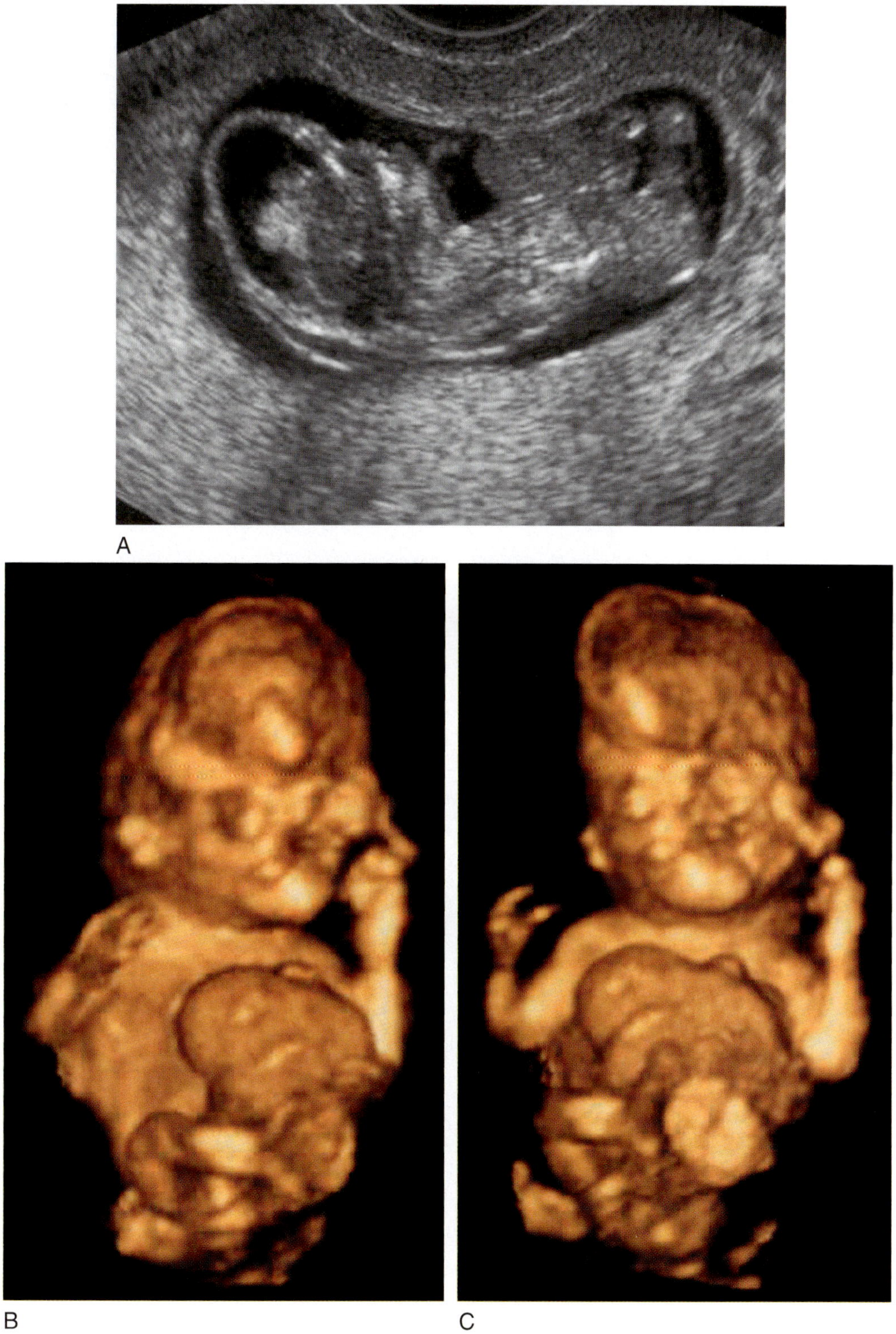

FIGURE 2-197 Longitudinal view of a first-trimester fetus with severe amniotic band syndrome. (A) Two-dimensional image shows complete disruption of the skull resulting in an encephalocele, as well as an anterior abdominal wall defect. (B, C) Three-dimensional surface rendering of the same fetus shows severe facial clefting , the encephalocele, and the anterior abdominal wall defect, which includes the liver and small bowel.

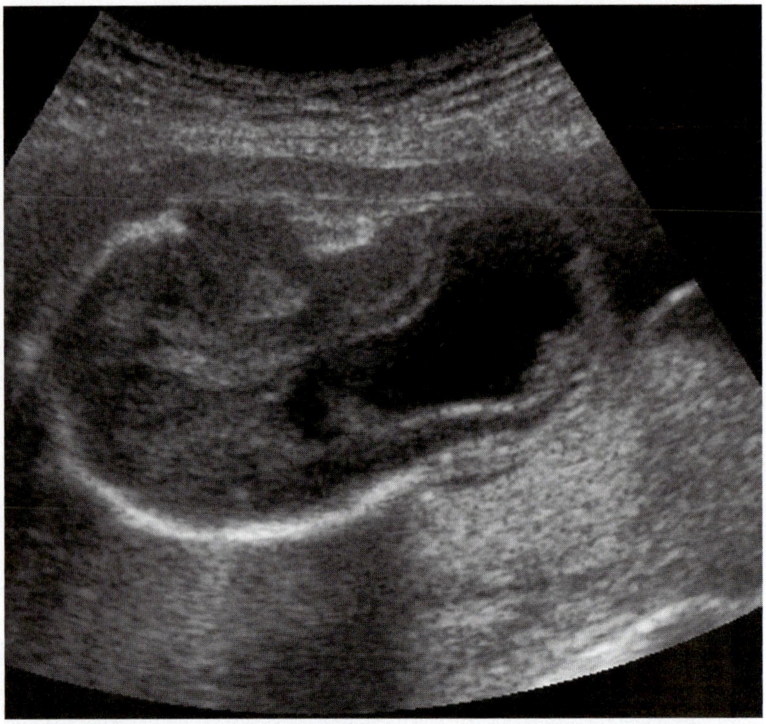

FIGURE 2-198 Second-trimester fetus with severe amniotic bands disrupting the occipital aspect of the fetal skull. A large encephalocele contains a dilated ventricle.

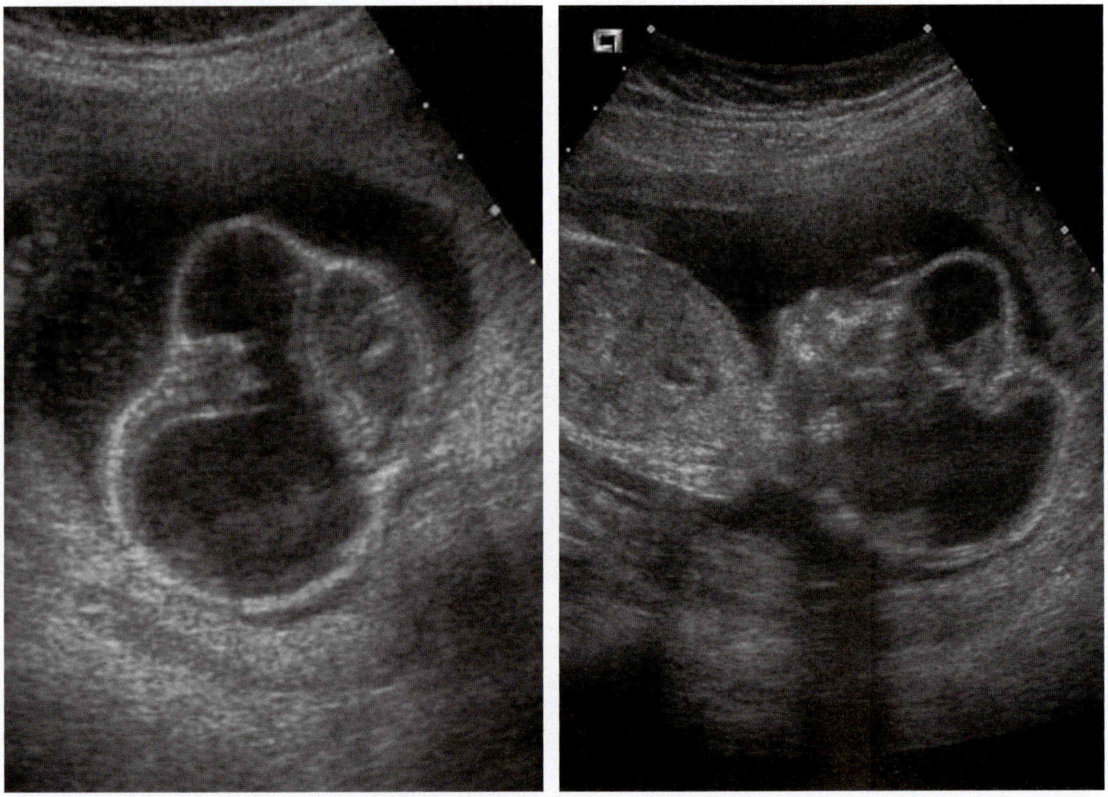

A B

FIGURE 2-199 Complete disruption of the fetal skull of a second-trimester fetus with amniotic band syndrome. Transverse (A) and longitudinal (B) views of complete disruption of the fetal skull.

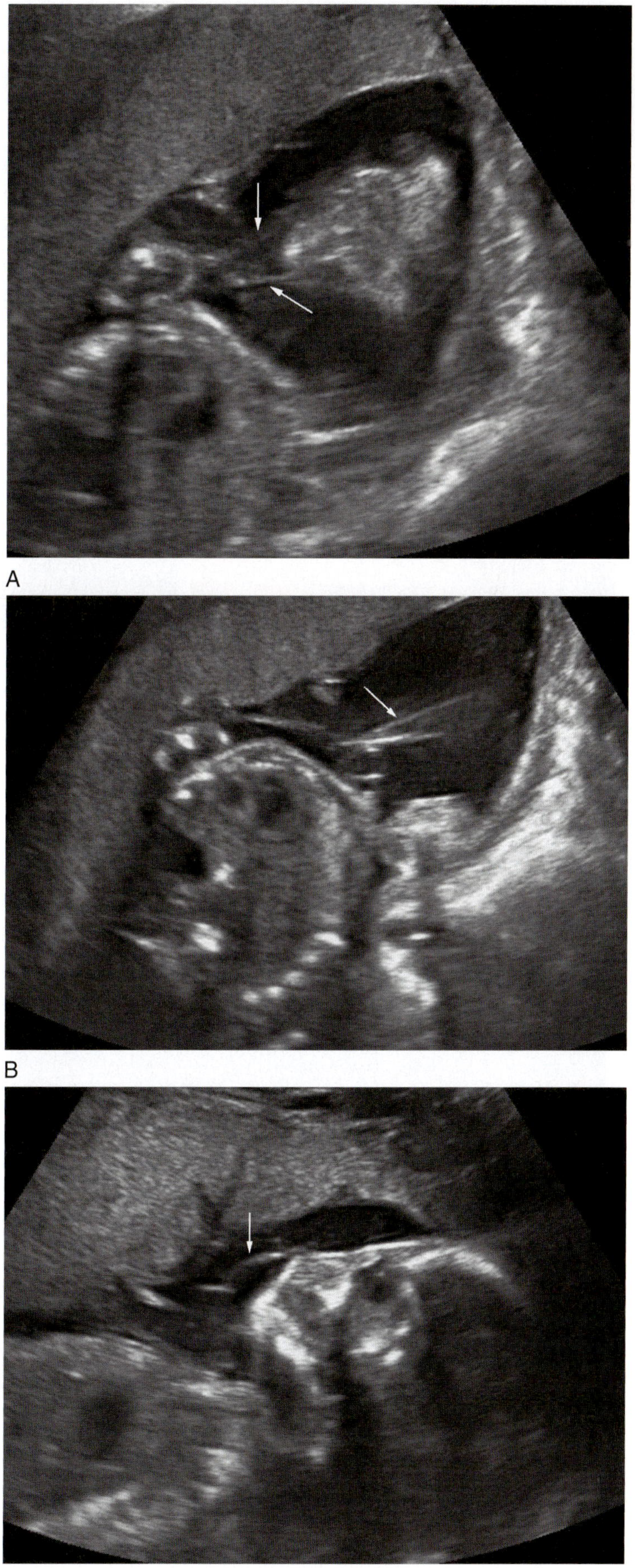

A B C

FIGURE 2-200 A 23-week fetus with amniotic band syndrome. (A) Note multiple bands *(arrows)* in front of the fetal face in close proximity to the nose and lips. (B) Amniotic bands *(arrow)* have collapsed down in front of the fetus, near the umbilical cord. (C) Longitudinal view of the fetal head of the same fetus shows the amniotic bands adherent to the fetal face *(arrow)*. *Continued*

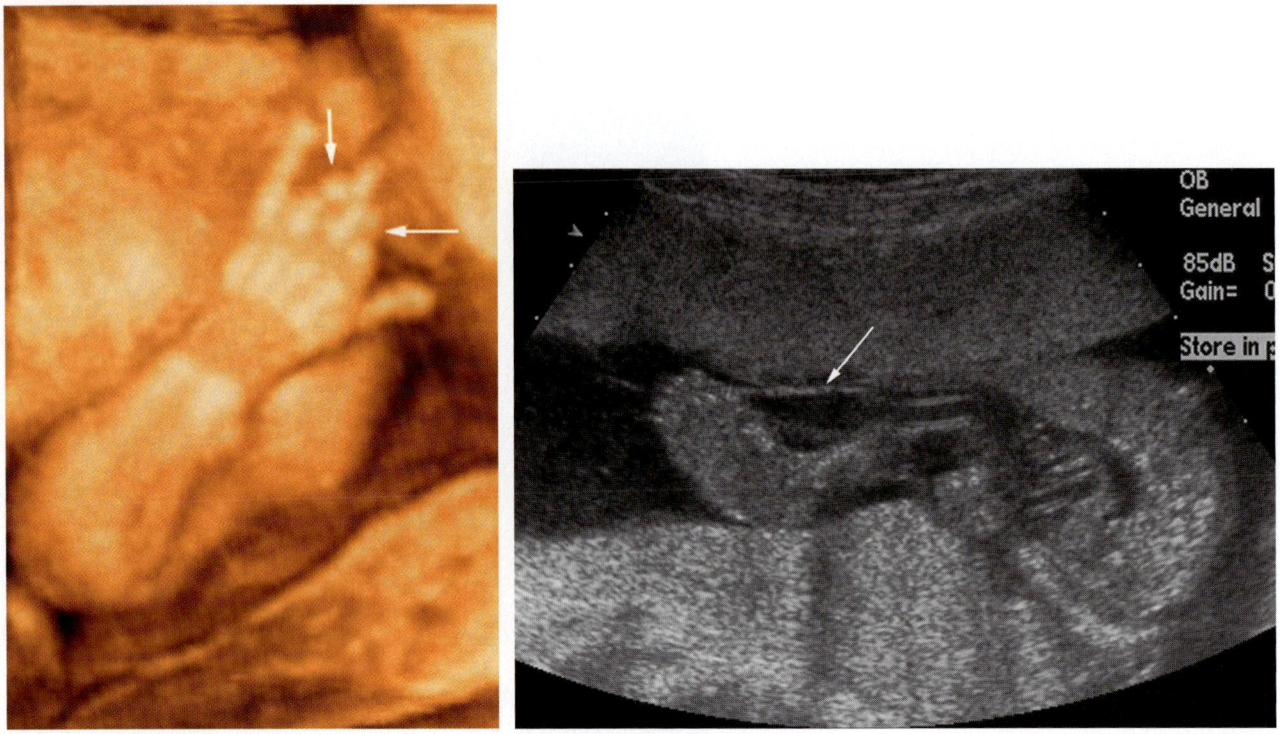

D E

FIGURE 2-200, cont'd (D) A 23-week fetus with amniotic band syndrome that has resulted in syndactyly of digits 2–4 of one hand *(arrows)*. (E) In an early second-trimester fetus with amniotic bands, bands *(arrow)* have tangled with the fetal foot, which appears to be club.

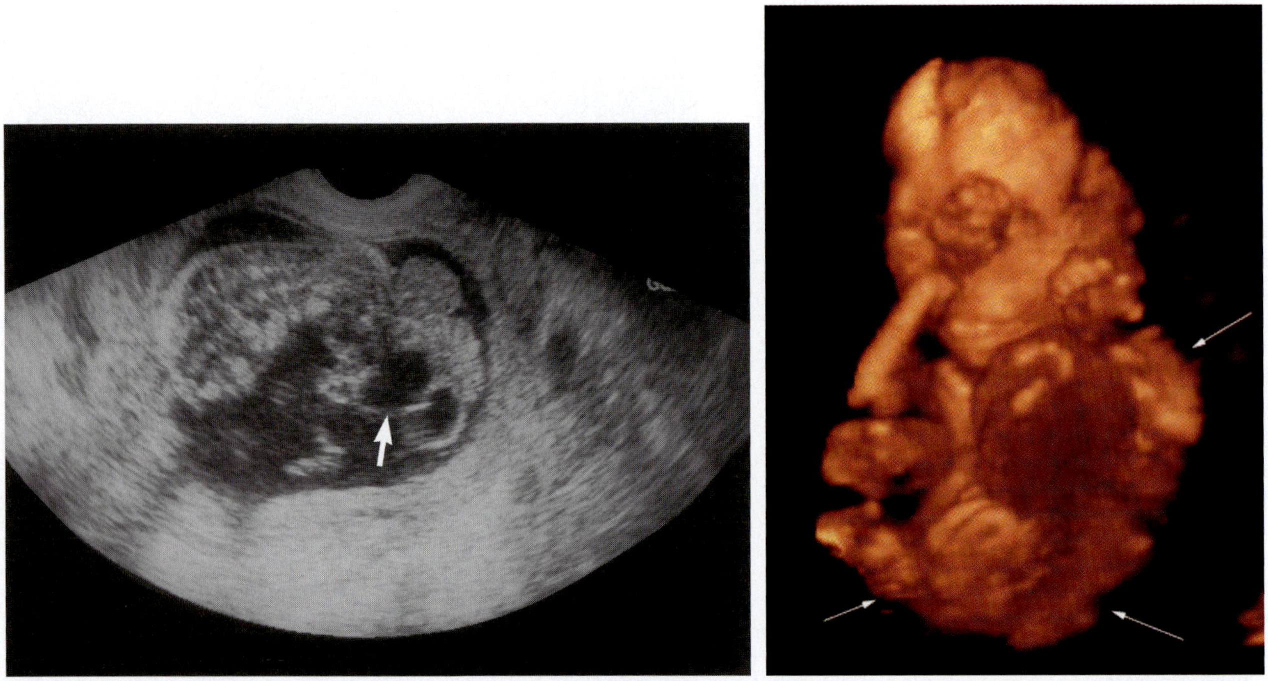

A B

FIGURE 2-201 (A) First-trimester fetus with body stalk abnormalities and complete disruption of the anterior abdominal wall and flank. The lower portion of the fetus is replaced by large masses *(arrow)*, which represent a combination of the extruded viscera and the short umbilical cord. Although this disorder is related to amniotic band syndrome and amniotic bands may be found in these defects, the initial etiology is thought to be different (see text for explanation). (B) Surface rendering of limb–body wall defect shows a large amount of the normally intraabdominal contents located outside the fetus *(arrows)*.

Fetal outcome depends on the severity of the lesion. Because this is a heterogeneous group of abnormalities, the outcome depends on the area affected, varying from a simple digit abnormality or amputation to a lethal condition involving complete disruption of the cranium or anterior abdominal wall. There are two isolated case reports describing in utero lysis of the bands around an affected limb with restoration of the circulation resulting in salvage of the limb.

RELATED SYNDROME

Limb–body wall complex is a clinically related lethal abnormality that consists of thoracoabdominoschisis with limb defects. Although its pathogenesis originally was thought to be secondary to amniotic rupture, recent evidence suggests that a disruption of the embryonic blood supply results in damage to the abdominal wall and viscera as well as lower limbs and neural tube. Adhesion of the amnion to these areas then may cause *secondary* amniotic bands. The ventral body wall fails to close because of vascular compromise and persistence of the extraembryonic coelom. This diagnosis has been made as early as 10 weeks, and the disruption of the fetal trunk is dramatic. Sonographic findings include complete evisceration of the abdominal viscera, including the liver, bowel, and other intraabdominal contents, resulting in a severe kyphoscoliosis and a very small abdominal cavity. Usually the umbilical cord is short, and there may be limb defects (particularly lower extremity) and occasionally neural tube defects.

Suggested Reading

Bolum KG: Amniotic band syndrome in second trimester associated with fetal malformations. *Prenat Diagn* 4:311–314, 1984.

Burton DJ, Filly RA: Sonographic diagnosis of the amniotic band syndrome. *AJR Am J Roentgenol* 156:555–558, 1991.

Chen CP: Prenatal sonographic diagnosis of limb-body wall complex with craniofacial defects. *Ultrasound Obstet Gynecol* 22:101, 2003.

Chen CP, Chang TY, Lin YH, Wang W: Prenatal sonographic diagnosis of acrania associated with amniotic bands. *J Clin Ultrasound* 32:256–260, 2004.

Chen CP, Shih JC, Chan YJ: Prenatal diagnosis of limb-body wall complex using two- and three-dimensional ultrasound. *Prenat Diagn* 20:1020, 2000.

Chen CP, Tzen CY, Chang TY, Yeh LF, Wang W: Prenatal diagnosis of acrania associated with facial defects, amniotic bands and limb-body wall complex. *Ultrasound Obstet Gynecol* 20:94–95, 2002.

Cincore V, Ninios AP, Pavlik J, Hsu CD: Prenatal diagnosis of acrania associated with amniotic band syndrome. *Obstet Gynecol* 102:1176–1178, 2003.

Daly CA, Freeman J, Weston W, Kovar I, Phelan M: Prenatal diagnosis of amniotic band syndrome in a methadone user: review of the literature and a case report. *Ultrasound Obstet Gynecol* 8:123–125, 1996.

De Catte L, Waterschoot T, Mares C, Goossens A, Foulon W: Umbilical cord, short umbilical cord syndrome. *Fetus* 3:5–10, 1992.

Fiedler JM, Phelan JP: The amniotic band syndrome in monozygotic twins. *Am J Obstet Gynecol* 146:864–865, 1983.

Finberg HJ, Glass M: Craniofacial damage from amniotic band syndrome subsequent to pathologic chorioamniotic separation at 10 weeks' gestation. *J Ultrasound Med* 15:665–668, 1996.

Fiske CE, Filly RA, Golbus MS: Prenatal ultrasound diagnosis of amniotic band syndrome. *J Ultrasound Med* 1:45–47, 1982.

Fried AM, Woodring JH, Shier RW, Falace PB: Omphalocele in limb/body wall deficiency syndrome: atypical sonographic appearance. *J Clin Ultrasound* 10:400–402, 1982.

Ginsberg NE, Cadkin A, Strom C: Prenatal diagnosis of body stalk anomaly in the first trimester of pregnancy. *Ultrasound Obstet Gynecol* 10:419–421, 1997.

Goldstein RB, Filly RA: Prenatal diagnosis of anencephaly: spectrum of sonographic appearances and distinction from the amniotic band syndrome. *AJR Am J Roentgenol* 151:547–550, 1988.

Goncalves LF, Jeanty P: Amniotic band syndrome. *Fetus* 2:1–8, 1992:

Gorczyca DP, Lindfors KK, McGahan JP, Hanson FW: Limb-body-wall complex: another cause for elevated maternal serum alpha fetoprotein. *J Clin Ultrasound* 18:198–201, 1990.

Hill LM, Kislak S, Jones N: Prenatal ultrasound diagnosis of a forearm constriction band. *J Ultrasound Med* 7:293–295, 1988.

Hughes RM, Benzie RJ, Thompson CL: Amniotic band syndrome causing fetal head deformity. *Prenat Diagn* 4:447–450, 1984.

Jeanty P, Laucirica R, Luna SK: Extra-amniotic pregnancy: a trip to the extraembryonic coelom. *J Ultrasound Med* 9:733–736, 1990.

Kancherla PL, Untawale G, Gabriel JB Jr, Chauhan PM: Intrauterine amputation in one monozygotic twin associated with amniotic band. *Am J Obstet Gynecol* 140:347–348, 1981.

Keswani SG, Johnson MP, Adzick NS, et al: In utero limb salvage: fetoscopic release of amniotic bands for threatened limb amputation. *J Pediatr Surg* 38:848–851, 2003.

Kohler HG, Jenkins DM: Extra-amniotic pregnancy: a case report. *Br J Obstet Gynaecol* 83:251–253, 1976.

Lin HH, Wu CC, Hsieh FJ, Hsieh CY, Lee TY: Amniotic rupture sequence: report of five cases. *Asia Oceania J Obstet Gynaecol* 15:343–350, 1989.

Liu IF, Yu CH, Chang CH, Chang FM: Prenatal diagnosis of limb-body wall complex in early pregnancy using three-dimensional ultrasound. *Prenat Diagn* 23:513–514, 2003.

Lockwood C, Ghidini A, Romero R: Amniotic band syndrome in monozygotic twins: prenatal diagnosis and pathogenesis. *Obstet Gynecol* 71:1012–1015, 1988.

Lockwood C, Ghidini A, Romero R, Hobbins JC: Amniotic band syndrome: reevaluation of its pathogenesis. *Am J Obstet Gynecol* 160:1030–1033, 1989.

Luehr B, Lipsett J, Quinlivan JA: Limb-body wall complex: a case series. *J Matern Fetal Neonatal Med* 12:132–137, 2002.

Mahony BS, Filly RA, Callen PW, Golbus MS: The amniotic band syndrome: antenatal sonographic diagnosis and potential pitfalls. *Am J Obstet Gynecol* 152:63–68, 1985.

Moessinger AC, Blanc WA, Byrne J, et al: Amniotic band syndrome associated with amniocentesis. *Am J Obstet Gynecol* 141:588–591, 1981.

Nevils BG, Maciulla JE, Izquierdo LA, et al: Umbilical cord, short umbilical cord syndrome. *Fetus* 3:1–4, 1993.

Nishi T, Nakano R: Amniotic band syndrome: serial ultrasonographic observations in the first trimester. *J Clin Ultrasound* 22:275–278, 1994.

Paladini D, Foglia S, Sglavo G, Martinelli P: Congenital constriction band of the upper arm: the role of three-dimensional ultrasound in diagnosis, counseling and multidisciplinary consultation. *Ultrasound Obstet Gynecol* 23:520–522, 2004.

Patten RM, Van Allen M, Mack LA, et al: Limb–body wall complex: In utero sonographic diagnosis of a complicated fetal malformation. *AJR Am J Roentgenol* 146:1019–1024, 1986.

Peer D, Moroder W, Delucca A: Prenatal diagnosis of the pentalogy of Cantrell combined with exencephaly and amniotic band syndrome. *Ultraschall Med* 14:94–95, 1993.

Perlman M, Tennenbaum A, Menashi M, Ron M, Ornoy A: Extramembranous pregnancy: maternal, placental, and perinatal implications. *Obstet Gynecol* 55:34S–37S, 1980.

Pumberger W, Schaller A, Bernaschek G: Limb-body wall complex: a compound anomaly pattern in body-wall defects. *Pediatr Surg Int* 17:486–490, 2001.

Quintero RA, Morales WJ, Phillips J, Kalter CS, Angel JL: In utero lysis of amniotic bands. *Ultrasound Obstet Gynecol* 10:316–320, 1997.

Seeds JW, Cefalo RC, Herbert WNP: Amniotic band syndrome. *Am J Obstet Gynecol* 144:243–248, 1982.

Sentilhes L, Verspyck E, Eurin D, et al: Favourable outcome of a tight constriction band secondary to amniotic band syndrome. *Prenat Diagn* 24:198–201, 2004.

Smrcek JM, Germer U, Krokowski M, et al: Prenatal ultrasound diagnosis and management of body stalk anomaly: analysis of nine singleton and two multiple pregnancies. *Ultrasound Obstet Gynecol* 21:322–328, 2003.

Weinstein L, Alien R: Extra-amniotic pregnancy. *S Med J* 73:796–797, 1980.

ARTHROGRYPOSIS

DESCRIPTION AND DEFINITION

Arthrogryposis is a sequence of neurologic, muscular, and connective tissue disorders, leading to limitation of joint mobility and fetal joint contractures and rigidity. Most cases of congenital joint contractures fall into three general categories: muscle diseases, connective tissue disorders, and central neurologic disease. Specific etiologies among neurologic disorders include congenital myotonic dystrophy, congenital myasthenia, and loss of anterior horn cells. The disorder can involve connective tissue disease, such as muscular and articular connective tissue dystrophy, or brain disorders, such as congenital encephalopathy. In an otherwise normal fetus, joint contractures can be caused by restrictive space in the uterus preventing fetal mobility.

ABNORMALITIES DETECTABLE BY ULTRASOUND

Fixed extremities

Flexed arms (frequent)

Hyperextension at the knee

Club feet

Clenched hands, with overlapping index fingers

Fetal immobility

Thickened nuchal translucency or cystic hygroma

Poor ossification of long bones (osteoporosis)

Polyhydramnios

CNS abnormalities (10% of cases)

Agenesis of the corpus callosum

Lissencephaly

Ventriculomegaly

Vermian agenesis

Renal defects

Fetuses with distal arthrogryposis usually have isolated orthopedic anomalies. Those with other types of arthrogryposis, such as neurologic arthrogryposis, may have the following associated anomalies:

- Facial defects
- Microcephaly

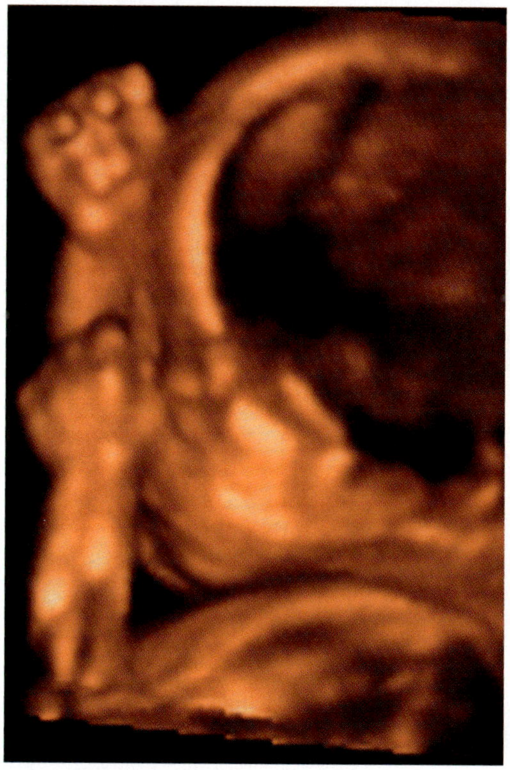

A

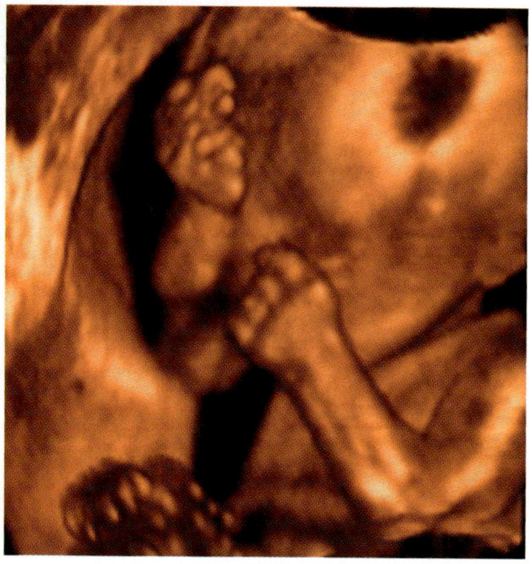

B

FIGURE 2-202 Arthrogryposis. (A, B) Surface renderings of the fetal hands in a fetus with arthrogryposis show contractures of the elbows, wrists, and fingers, with overlapping fingers.

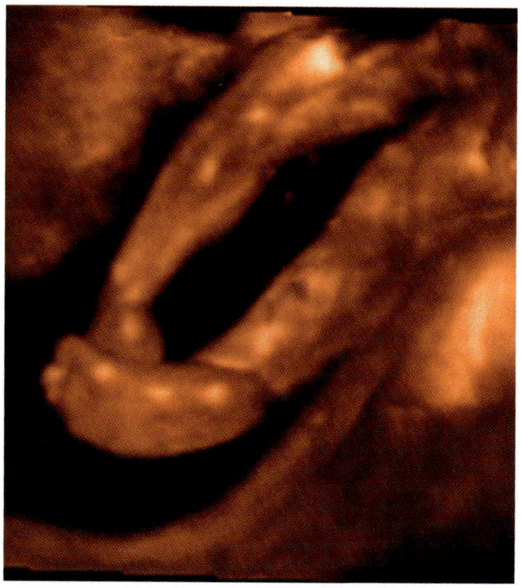

FIGURE 2-203 Lower extremities of the same fetus as in Figure 2-202 show bilateral club feet.

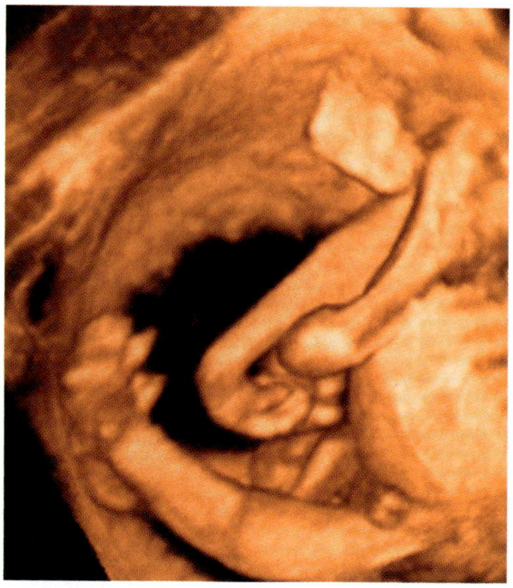

FIGURE 2-204 Fetus with severe arthrogryposis and contractures of upper and lower extremities. Note severe contractures at the elbows and wrists, hyperextended knees, and club feet.

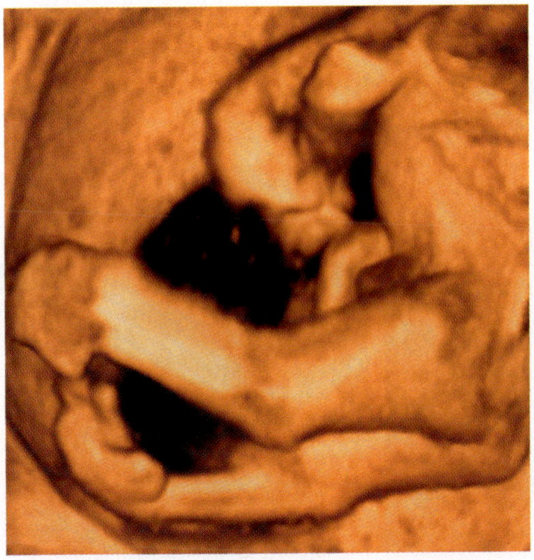

FIGURE 2-205 Different fetus with severe arthrogryposis has hyperextension at the knees and severely club feet. Contractures of the upper extremities are visible.

Agenesis of the corpus callosum

Cataracts

MAJOR DIFFERENTIAL DIAGNOSES*

Antley-Bixler syndrome

Cerebro-oculo-facio-skeletal (COFS) syndrome

Freeman-Sheldon syndrome (sometimes considered a variant of arthrogryposis)

Multiple pterygium syndrome (cystic hygroma, flexion contractures)

Pena Shokeir syndrome (severe growth deficiency, contractures of lesser severity)

Smith-Lemli-Opitz syndrome

Trisomy 18 (Edwards' syndrome, involving multiple abnormalities of other organ systems)

*See also Chapter 1, Club Feet and Contractures of the Extremities, pp. 104 and 91, for differential diagnoses.

ULTRASOUND DIAGNOSIS

One of the earliest manifestations of arthrogryposis multiplex congenital is a cystic hygroma at 13 weeks. In these cases, limb contractures did not become apparent until 17 to 18 weeks. One other case suspected to be due to scoliosis was seen sonographically at 15 weeks. In general, no more than 10% of cases of arthrogryposis are detected in the first trimester, and these tend to be the most severe cases.

In other cases, the diagnosis of arthrogryposis has been established by ultrasonography as early as 17 weeks' gestation on the basis of abnormal positioning of the extremities and decreased to absent fetal extremity movement.

HEREDITY

Arthrogryposis represents a heterogeneous group of disorders. Distal arthrogryposis syndrome is an autosomal dominant disorder with extensive variability of expression. In other forms of arthrogryposis, the pattern of inheritance is recessive or X-linked.

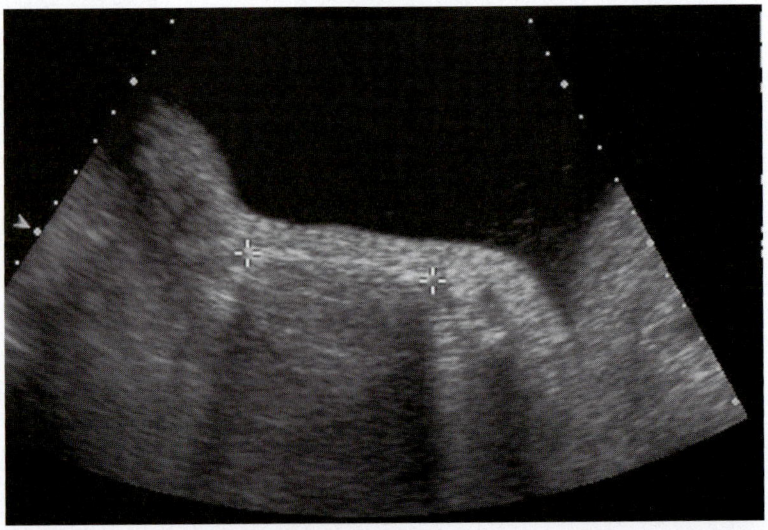

FIGURE 2-206 Third-trimester fetus with arthrogryposis. Bones (tibia) are faintly seen because of osteopenia, which likely is due to lack of activity for many weeks.

NATURAL HISTORY AND OUTCOME

Although a severe lethal form of this disease exists, less severe cases may involve only mild-to-moderate orthopedic limitations. The prognosis depends on the disorders associated with the arthrogryposis and the orthopedic limitations involved. There are many different types of distal arthrogryposis with different specific postnatal characteristics and prognoses. These types probably are nearly impossible to distinguish prenatally.

Suggested Reading

Baty BJ, Cubberley D, Morris C, Carey J: Prenatal diagnosis of distal arthrogryposis. *Am J Med Genet* 29:501–510, 1988.

Bendon R, Dignan P, Siddiqi T: Prenatal diagnosis of arthrogryposis multiplex congenita. *J Pediatr* 111:942–947, 1987.

Bonilla-Musoles F, Machado LE, Osborne NG: Multiple congenital contractures (congenital multiple arthrogryposis). *J Perinat Med* 30:99–104, 2002.

Bui TH, Lindholm H, Demir N, Thomassen P: Prenatal diagnosis of distal arthrogryposis type I by ultrasonography. *Prenat Diagn* 12:1047–1053, 1992.

Degani S, Shapiro I, Lewinsky R, Sharf M: Prenatal ultrasound diagnosis of isolated arthrogryposis of feet. *Acta Obstet Gynecol* Scand 68:461–462, 1989.

Dudkiewicz I, Achiron R, Ganel A: Prenatal diagnosis of distal arthrogryposis type 1. *Skel Radiol* 28:233–235, 1999.

Goldberg JD, Chervenak FA, Lipman RA, Berkowitz RL: Antenatal sonographic diagnosis of arthrogryposis multiplex congenita. *Prenat Diagn* 6:45–49, 1986.

Gorczyca DP, McGahan JP, Lindfors KK, Ellis WG, Grix A: Arthrogryposis multiplex congenita: prenatal ultrasonographic diagnosis. *J Clin Ultrasound* 17:40–44, 1989.

Gullino E, Abrate M, Zerbino E, Bricchi G, Rattazzi PD: Early prenatal sonographic diagnosis of neuropathic arthrogryposis multiplex congenita with osseous heterotopia. *Prenat Diagn* 13:411–416, 1993.

Hyett J, Noble P, Sebire NJ, Snijders R, Nicolaides KH: Lethal congenital arthrogryposis presents with increased nuchal translucency at 10–14 weeks of gestation. *Ultrasound Obstet Gynecol* 9:310–313, 1997.

Jones KL: *Smith's recognizable patterns of human malformations,* ed 6. Philadelphia, 2006, Elsevier.

Madazli R, Tuysuz B, Aksoy F, Barbaros M, Uludag S, Ocak V: Prenatal diagnosis of arthrogryposis multiplex congenita with increased nuchal translucency but without any underlying fetal neurogenic or myogenic pathology. *Fetal Diagn Ther* 17:29–33, 2002.

Mahieu-Caputo D, Salomon LJ, Dommergues M, et al: Arthrogryposis multiplex congenita and cerebellopontine ischemic lesions in sibs: recurrence of prenatal disruptive brain lesions with different patterns of expression? *Fetal Diagn Ther* 17:153–156, 2002.

Murphy JC, Neale D, Bromley B, Benacerraf BR, Copel JA: Hypoechogenicity of fetal long bones: a new ultrasound marker for arthrogryposis. *Prenat Diagn* 22:1219–1222, 2002.

Romero R. *Prenatal diagnosis of congenital anomalies.* East Norwalk, CT, 1988, Appleton & Lange.

Ruano R, Dumez Y, Dommergues M: Three-dimensional ultrasonographic appearance of the fetal akinesia deformation sequence. *J Ultrasound Med* 22:593–599, 2003.

Scott H, Hunter A, Bedard B: Non-lethal arthrogryposis multiplex congenita presenting with cystic hygroma at 13 weeks gestational age. *Prenat Diagn* 19:966–971, 1999.

Vuopala K, Herva R: Lethal congenital contracture syndrome: further delineation and genetic aspects. *J Med Genet* 31:521–527, 1994.

Witters I, Moerman P, Fryns JP: Fetal akinesia deformation sequence: a study of 30 consecutive in utero diagnoses. *Am J Med Genet* 113:23–28, 2002.

Yfantis H, Nonaka D, Castellani R, Harman C, Sun CC: Heterogeneity in fetal akinesia deformation sequence (FADS): autopsy confirmation in three 20–21-week fetuses. *Prenat Diagn* 22:42–47, 2002.

CARDIOSPLENIC SYNDROMES (ASPLENIA/POLYSPLENIA, HETEROTAXY)

DESCRIPTION AND DEFINITION

Heterotaxy syndromes involve bilateral left sidedness (polysplenia) and bilateral right sidedness (asplenia), which probably are two different manifestations of a defect in lateralization of normal body asymmetry.

ABNORMALITIES DETECTABLE BY ULTRASOUND

Both syndromes are associated with severe cardiac abnormalities, although those associated with asplenia may be more severe.

Asplenia (Bilateral Right Sidedness):

- Thickened nuchal translucency
- Bilateral, trilobed lungs
- Severe cardiac abnormalities
- Right-sided cardiac apex
- Anomalous pulmonary venous return
- Bilateral superior vena cava
- Endocardial cushion defect
- Transposition of the great arteries

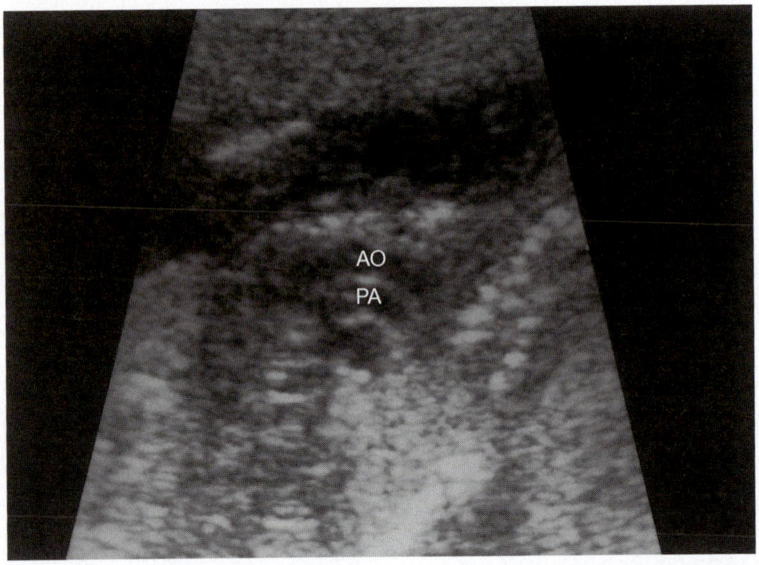

FIGURE 2-207 Long-axis view of the great vessels of a fetus with transposition of the great arteries. Note that the two great vessels are parallel, with the pulmonary artery *(PA)* located anterior and superior to the aorta *(AO)*.

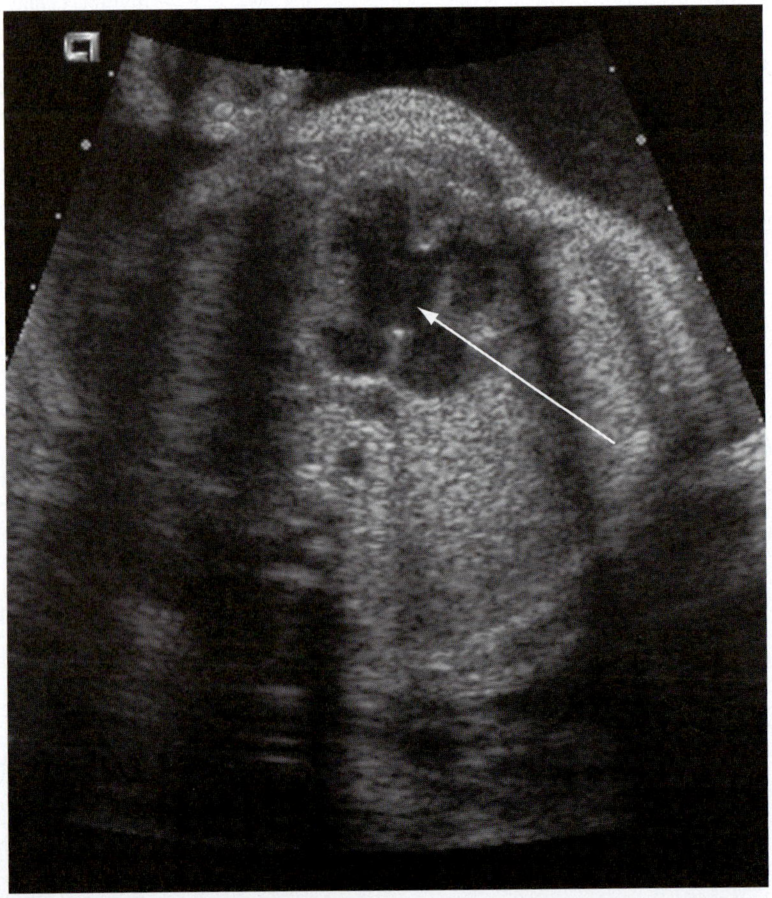

FIGURE 2-208 Transverse view through the fetal chest shows complete atrioventricular canal *(arrow)* in a fetus with heterotaxy syndrome.

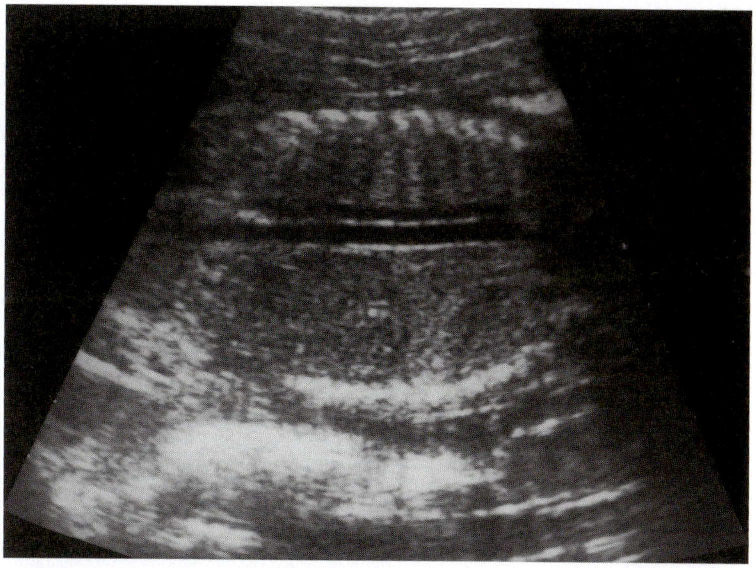

FIGURE 2-209 Long-axis view of the posterior aspect of the chest shows two parallel vessels, one of which is the aorta and the other the azygos vein. The fetus has an interrupted inferior vena cava with azygos continuation.

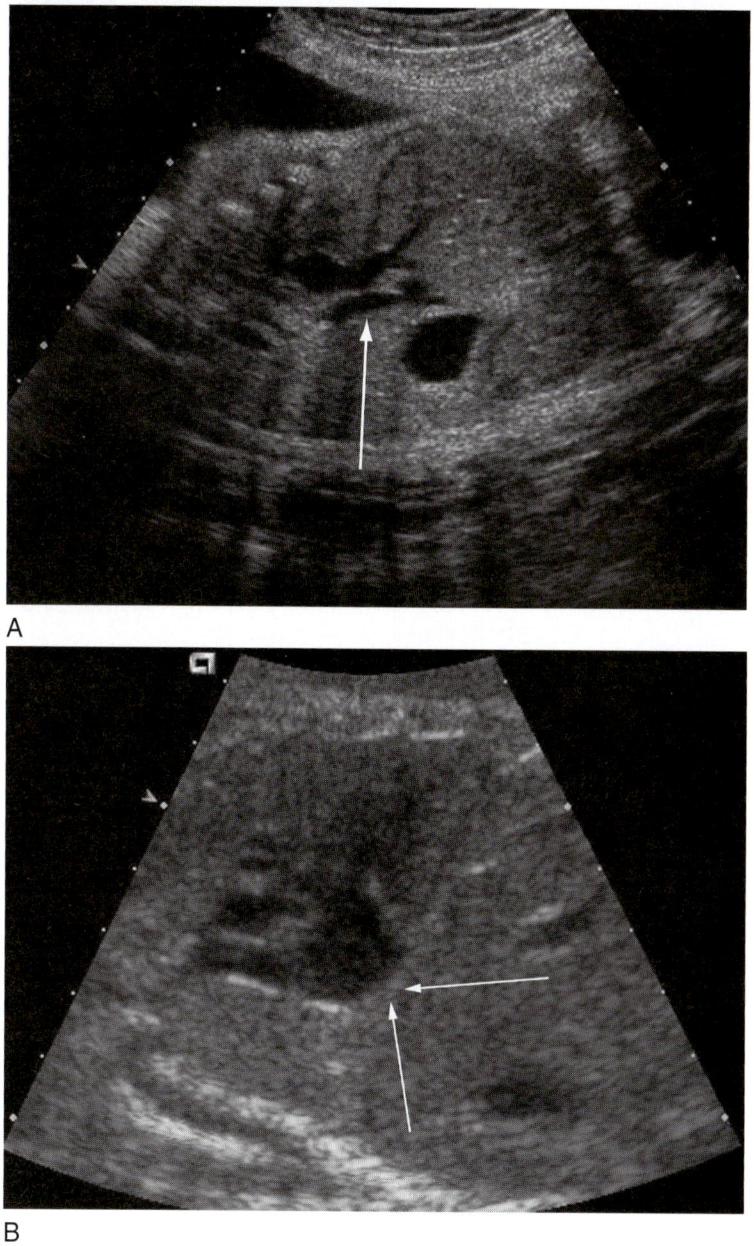

FIGURE 2-210 (A) Confluence of the hepatic veins in a fetus with heterotaxy syndrome. The hepatic veins enter the right atrium; however, there is no inferior vena cava. Continuation of the azygos is seen coursing behind the right atrium *(arrow)*. (B) Longitudinal view of a fetus with interrupted inferior vena cava shows a superior vena cava but no inferior vena cava entering the right atrium *(arrows)*.

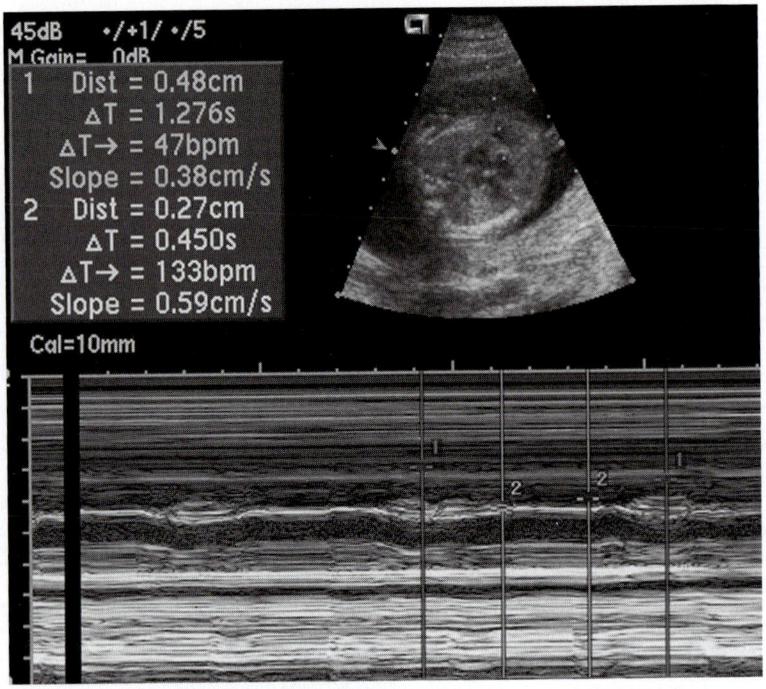

FIGURE 2-211 Fetus with heterotaxy syndrome who has complete heart block. Note that the atrial rate is 133, whereas the ventricular rate is 47. These rates are independent of each other.

Single ventricle

Pulmonic stenosis

Other complex cardiac abnormalities

Renal anomalies (25%)

Right-sided stomach

Midline liver

Polysplenia (Bilateral Left Sidedness):

Thickened nuchal translucency

Bilateral, bilobed lungs

Cardiac abnormalities

Azygos continuation of the inferior vena cava

Anomalous pulmonary venous return

Dextrocardia

Bilateral superior vena cava

Endocardial cushion defect

Other complex cardiac abnormalities

Right-sided stomach

Midline liver

MAJOR DIFFERENTIAL DIAGNOSES

Other Conditions Associated with Complex Cardiac Defects:

Anomalous pulmonary venous return associated with scimitar syndrome (dextroposition of the heart caused by right pulmonary hypoplasia)

Chromosomal abnormalities

Dextrocardia, as may be associated with Kartagener syndrome (situs inversus sinus abnormalities)

Dextrorotation of the heart, as may be associated with unilateral hypoplastic lung or intrathoracic masses

Syndromes associated with cardiac defects (see Chapter 1, p. 118, for differential diagnoses)

ULTRASOUND DIAGNOSIS

Prenatal detection of an abnormal nuchal translucency in the first trimester has been the first sonographic manifestation of some cases of cardiosplenic syndromes.

Ultrasound diagnosis of the cardiosplenic syndromes has been established numerous times at all gestational ages within the second and third trimesters, most frequently on the basis of sonographic detection of cardiac abnormalities. Azygos continuation of the inferior vena cava is easy to identify adjacent to the descending aorta in the chest, giving the easily recognized appearance of two vessels, side by side.

Other findings include abnormalities in the position of the cardiac axis, liver, and stomach bubble, as well as intrinsic abnormalities of the heart, seen on fetal echocardiogram.

Fetuses with these syndromes may have complete heart block, particularly in association with a complete endocardial cushion defect or double-outlet right ventricle. It may be helpful to identify the fetal spleen with Doppler, although the lack of a spleen (particularly in the second trimester) is sometimes difficult to detect. The experience of several large series (the largest is 35 cases of left isomerism) over 10- to 15-year periods suggests >90% correct prenatal diagnosis for these disorders. In the 35-patient study of left isomerism, 31 fetuses had interrupted inferior vena cava with azygos continuation, 22 had viscerocardiac heterotaxy, 13 had heart block, and 28 had major cardiac defects (including ventricular septal defect, double-outlet right ventricle, right ventricular outflow tract obstruction, and anomalous pulmonary venous return).

HEREDITY

Heredity is multifactorial and usually sporadic, although reports of autosomal dominant, autosomal recessive, and X-linked inheritance have been documented. Both of these syndromes have appeared within the same family, suggesting that they are manifestations of a primary defect in laterality.

Asplenia syndrome is more common among males than females.

NATURAL HISTORY AND OUTCOME

Prognosis depends on the severity of cardiac defects. A cardiac defect, such as an endocardial cushion defect, associated with complete heart block carries a poor prognosis. The mortality rate for these syndromes is high, with a 1-year survival rate of 50%. Only 25% of affected individuals are alive at 5 years, and only 10% live to adolescence.

Suggested Reading

Abuhamad AZ, Robinson JN, Bogdan D, Tannous RJ: Color Doppler of the splenic artery in the prenatal diagnosis of heterotaxic syndromes. *Am J Perinatol* 16:469–473, 1999.

Atkinson DE, Drant S: Diagnosis of heterotaxy syndrome by fetal echocardiography. *Am J Cardiol* 82:1147–1149, 1998.

Berg C, Geipel A, Kamil D, Knuppel M, et al: The syndrome of left isomerism: sonographic findings and outcome in prenatally diagnosed cases. *J Ultrasound Med* 24:921–931, 2005.

Berg C, Geipel A, Kohl T, et al: Fetal echocardiographic evaluation of atrial morphology and the prediction of laterality in cases of heterotaxy syndromes. *Ultrasound Obstet Gynecol* 26:538–545, 2005.

Berg C, Geipel A, Smrcek J, et al: Prenatal diagnosis of cardiosplenic syndromes: a 10-year experience. *Ultrasound Obstet Gynecol* 22:451–459, 2003.

Cesko I, Hajdu J, Marton T, Tarnai L, Papp Z: Polysplenia and situs inversus in siblings. Case reports. *Fetal Diagn Ther* 16:1–3, 2001.

Chitayat D, Lao A, Wilson RD, Fagerstrom C, Hayden M: Prenatal diagnosis of asplenia/polysplenia syndrome. *Am J Obstet Gynecol* 158:1085–1087, 1988.

Colloridi V, Pizzuto F, Ventriglia F, et al: Prenatal echocardiographic diagnosis of right atrial isomerism. *Prenat Diagn* 14:299–302, 1994.

Comstock CH, Smith R, Lee W, Kirk JS: Right fetal cardiac axis: clinical significance and associated findings. *Obstet Gynecol* 91:495–499, 1998.

DeVore GR, Steiger RM, Larson EJ: Fetal echocardiography: the prenatal diagnosis of a ventricular septal defect in a 14-week fetus with pulmonary artery hypoplasia. *Obstet Gynecol* 69:494–497, 1987.

DiSessa TG, Emerson DS, Felker RE, et al: Anomalous systemic and pulmonary venous pathways diagnosed in utero by ultrasound. *J Ultrasound Med* 9:311–317, 1990.

Fedrizzi RP, Bruner JP, Jeanty P: Polysplenia syndrome. *Fetus* 2:1–5, 1992.

Jones KL: *Smith's recognizable patterns of human malformations,* ed 6. Philadelphia, 2006, Elsevier.

Lin JH, Chang CI, Wang JK, et al: Intrauterine diagnosis of heterotaxy syndrome. *Am Heart J* 143:1002–1008, 2002.

Mauser I, Deutinger J, Bernaschek G: Prenatal diagnosis of a complex fetal cardiac malformation associated with asplenia. *Br Heart J* 65:293–295, 1991.

Shely RC, Nyberg DA, Kapur R: Azygous continuation of the interrupted inferior vena cava: a clue to prenatal diagnosis of the cardiosplenic syndromes. *J Ultrasound Med* 14:381–387, 1995.

Stewart PA, Becker AE, Wladimiroff JW, Essed CE: Left atrial isomerism associated with asplenia: prenatal echocardiographic detection of complex congenital cardiac malformations. *J Am Coll Cardiol* 4:1015–1020, 1984.

Winer-Muram HT, Tonkin IL: The spectrum of heterotaxic syndromes. *Radiol Clin North Am* 27:1147–1170, 1989.

Yasukochi S, Satomi G, Iwasaki Y: Prenatal diagnosis of total anomalous pulmonary venous connection with asplenia. *Fetal Diagn Ther* 12:266–269, 1997.

CAUDAL REGRESSION SYNDROME AND SIRENOMELIA

DESCRIPTION AND DEFINITION

Caudal regression syndrome originally was thought to encompass the severe sirenomelia sequence; however, now they are thought to have different etiologies.

Caudal regression syndrome has an increased incidence among diabetic mothers. It is associated with disruption in the caudal portion of the neural tube early in development, causing absence or dysplasia of the sacrum.

Sirenomelia, on the other hand, is thought to be produced by early vascular alteration, resulting in a single large intraabdominal artery that takes over the function of the umbilical arteries. This artery diverts blood flow from the lower extremities, leading to a "vitelline arterial steal phenomenon." It is associated with fusion of the lower extremities, as well as renal agenesis and absence of the sacrum, rectum, and bladder.

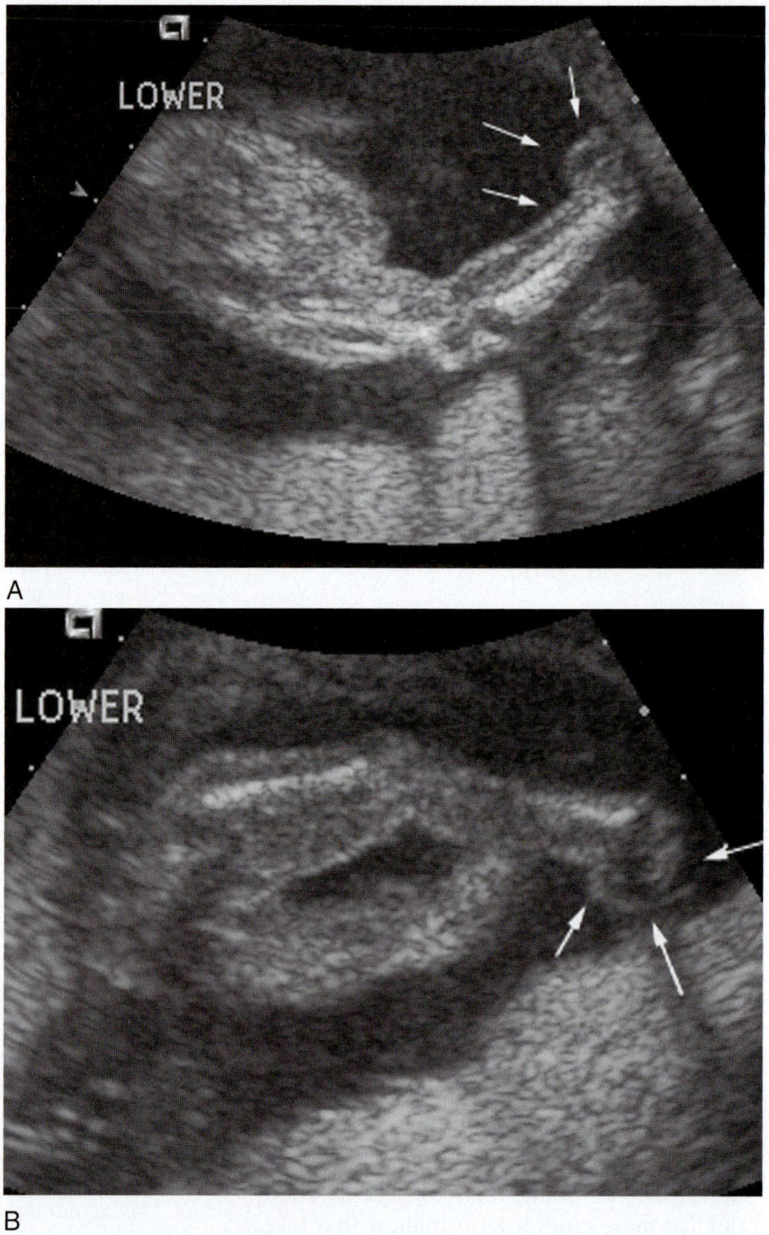

FIGURE 2-212 (A, B) Second-trimester fetus with caudal regression syndrome. Both lower extremities have contractures at the knees and ankles, most likely from lack of activity. Note the club feet *(arrows)*.

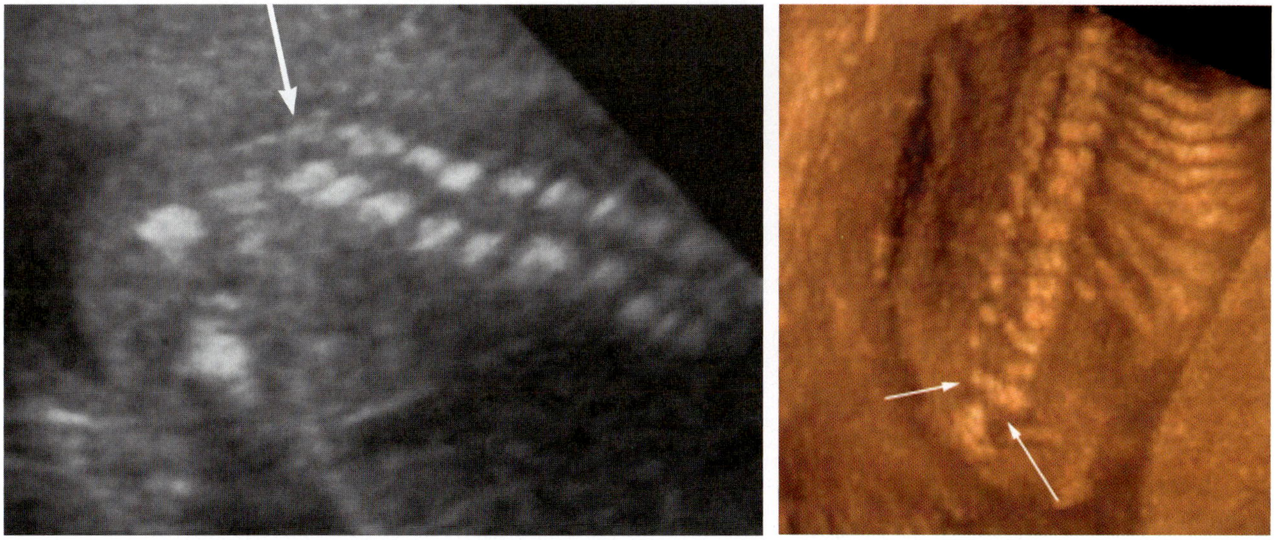

FIGURE 2-213 (A) Sacral agenesis in a late second-trimester fetus. Note absence of the spine below the lower lumbar region *(arrow)*. (B) Surface rendering with skeletal mode of the same fetus shows absence of the vertebral bodies past L5 *(arrows)*.

ABNORMALITIES DETECTABLE BY ULTRASOUND

Common Findings:

Caudal Regression Syndrome:

- Abnormal nuchal translucency
- Agenesis or dysgenesis of the sacrum
- Abnormal vertebral bodies of the lumbar spine
- Pelvic deformities
- Femoral hypoplasia
- Club feet
- Flexion contractures of the lower extremities
- Decreased movement of the lower extremities

Sirenomelia:

- Fusion and severe deformities of the lower extremities (mermaid syndrome)
- Oligohydramnios
- Bilateral renal agenesis
- Multiple abnormalities of the lower spine
- Cardiac anomalies
- Abdominal wall defects
- Chest deformities
- Lung hypoplasia
- Two-vessel umbilical cord with large intraabdominal artery
- Potter facies
- Absence of the genitals
- Imperforate anus

Occasional Findings:

Caudal Regression Syndrome:

- Renal agenesis or other anomaly
- Cardiac defect
- Pulmonary hypoplasia
- Neural tube defect
- Imperforate anus
- Facial cleft

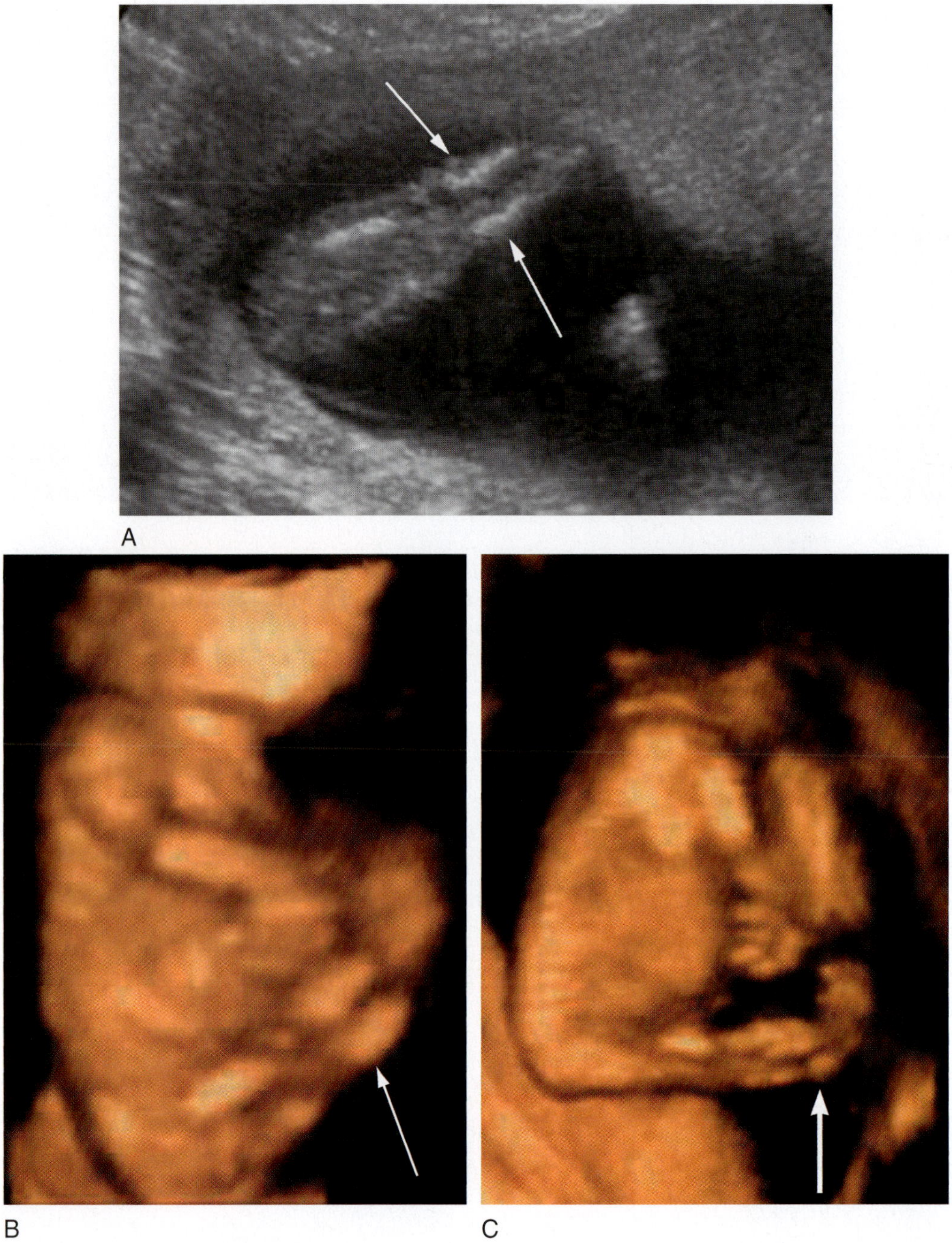

FIGURE 2-214 Late first-trimester fetus with sirenomelia. (A) Fused lower extremities *(arrows)* seen in two dimensions. (B, C) Three-dimensional surface renderings of the fused lower extremities *(arrow)*.

MAJOR DIFFERENTIAL DIAGNOSES

Other Syndromes and Conditions Associated with Abnormal Sacrum or Bilateral Renal Agenesis

Fraser syndrome

MURCS (**mü**llerian duct aplasia, **r**enal aplasia, **c**ervicothoracic **s**omite dysplasia) association

Renal agenesis (Potter syndrome)

VATER (**v**ertebral defects, **a**nal atresia, **t**racheo-esophageal fistula, **e**sophageal atresia, and **r**adial and renal dysplasias) syndrome

ULTRASOUND DIAGNOSIS

Both caudal regression syndrome and sirenomelia have been diagnosed sonographically, early in gestation.

The diagnosis of caudal regression syndrome has been established as early as 9 to 11 weeks' gestational age, based on an abnormal-appearing yolk sac and short crown–rump length. By 11 weeks, protuberance of the caudal region was noted. Thickened nuchal translucency has been reported in association with this syndrome. The diagnosis of caudal regression after the first trimester is based on the presence of a variety of abnormalities of varying degrees of severity. There may be abnormalities of the sacrum with essentially normal development of the lower extremities. Alternatively, there may be abnormalities of the entire lower lumbar spine and complete absence of the sacrum, along with abnormalities of the lower extremities (e.g., club feet and flexion contractures of the hips and knees because of inactivity). Amniotic fluid is normal in most cases, unlike the case of sirenomelia, which is associated with profound oligohydramnios. Because the sacrum is not well ossified in the late first trimester/early second trimester, not every case of caudal regression sequence can be identified early, particularly if it is a mild form of the disorder.

Sirenomelia has been detected in the first trimester transvaginally, seen as an abnormality of the lower extremities as well as the large single artery arising intraabdominally, stealing blood from the caudal part of the fetus. The normal amniotic fluid volume still present in the first trimester facilitates imaging at this stage. The correct diagnosis is sometimes difficult to make definitively in the second and third trimesters because of the severe oligohydramnios associated with renal agenesis. Detection of this disorder has been possible at 18 weeks' gestation, based on renal agenesis, abnormal lower extremities, and large abdominal artery best seen by Doppler. The diagnosis of sirenomelia has also been made in later pregnancy based on renal agenesis, cardiac defect, skeletal deformities of the lumbar spine, anterior abdominal wall defects, and a single abnormal lower extremity. Nevertheless, many cases of sirenomelia are misdiagnosed simply as Potter sequence based on absence of the kidneys and severe oligohydramnios. In those cases, the abnormal, fused extremity usually is overlooked.

HEREDITY

Neither caudal regression syndrome nor sirenomelia is thought to be hereditary, although the former has a strong association with maternal diabetes.

NATURAL HISTORY AND OUTCOME

The outcome for fetuses with caudal regression syndrome depends on the severity of associated anomalies and the extent of sacral defects. Urologic and orthopedic interventions usually are necessary.

Fetuses with sirenomelia do not survive because of the associated renal agenesis. There is only one prenatally diagnosed case of this condition, with survival of the child. The oligohydramnios was intermittent during the pregnancy, and only a small dysplastic kidney was present at birth, as were fused lower extremities and multiple other vascular and anatomic intraabdominal anomalies. The child survived after renal transplant.

Suggested Reading

Adra A, Cordero D, Mejides A, et al: Caudal regression syndrome: etiopathogenesis, prenatal diagnosis, and perinatal management. *Obstet Gynecol Surv* 49:508–516, 1994.

Baxi L, Warren W, Collins MH, Timor-Tritsch IE: Early detection of caudal regression syndrome with transvaginal scanning. *Obstet Gynecol* 75:486–489, 1990.

Chenoweth CK, Kellogg SJ, Abu-Yousef MM: Antenatal sonographic diagnosis of sirenomelia. *J Clin Ultrasound* 19:167–171, 1991.

Dordoni D, Freeman PC: Sirenomelia sequence. *Fetus* 1:1–3, 1991.

Fukada Y, Yasumizu T, Tsurugi Y, Ohta S, Hoshi K: Caudal regression syndrome detected in a fetus with increased nuchal translucency. *Acta Obstet Gynecol Scand* 78:655–656, 1999.

Honda N, Shimokawa H, Yamaguchi Y, Satoh S, Nakano H: Antenatal diagnosis of sirenomelia (sympus apus). *J Clin Ultrasound* 16:675–677, 1988.

Horikoshi T, Kikuchi A, Tatematsu M, Matsumoto Y, Hayashi A, Unno N: Two cases of a fetus with sirenomelia sequence. *Congenit Anom (Kyoto)* 45:93–95, 2005.

Jaffe R, Zeituni M, Fejgin M: Caudal regression syndrome. *Fetus* 1:1–3, 1991.

Loewy JA, Richards DG, Toi A: In-utero diagnosis of the caudal regression syndrome: report of three cases. *J Clin Ultrasound* 15:469–474, 1987.

Monteagudo A, Mayberry P, Rebarber A, Paidas M, Timor-Tritsch IE: Sirenomelia sequence: first-trimester diagnosis with both two- and three-dimensional sonography. *J Ultrasound Med* 21: 915–920, 2002.

Patel S, Suchet I: The role of color and power Doppler ultrasound in the prenatal diagnosis of sirenomelia. *Ultrasound Obstet Gynecol* 24:684–691, 2004.

Raabe RD, Harnsberger HR, Lee TG, Mukuno DH: Ultrasonographic antenatal diagnosis of "mermaid syndrome": fusion of the lower extremities. *J Ultrasound Med* 2:463–464, 1983.

Schiesser M, Holzgreve W, Lapaire O, et al: Sirenomelia, the mermaid syndrome—detection in the first trimester. *Prenat Diagn* 23:493–495, 2003.

Sirtori M, Ghidini A, Romero R, Bobbins JC: Prenatal diagnosis of sirenomelia. *J Ultrasound Med* 8:83–88, 1989.

Sonek JD, Gabbe SG, Landon MB, et al: Antenatal diagnosis of sacral agenesis syndrome in a pregnancy complicated by diabetes mellitus. *Am J Obstet Gynecol* 162:806–808, 1990.

Twickler D, Budorick N, Pretorius D, Grafe M, Currarino G: Caudal regression versus sirenomelia: sonographic clues. *J Ultrasound Med* 12:323–330, 1993.

CEREBRO-OCULO-FACIO-SKELETAL (COFS) SYNDROME

DESCRIPTION AND DEFINITION

Synonym: Neurogenic arthrogryposis

This syndrome was originally described by Pena and Shokeir in 1974 and is characterized by an autosomal recessive condition, with contractures of the joints of all the extremities and severe facial and brain abnormalities.

ABNORMALITIES DETECTABLE BY ULTRASOUND

Microcephaly

Micrognathia

Cataracts

Microphthalmia

Agenesis of the corpus callosum

Contractures of all extremities

Rockerbottom feet

MAJOR DIFFERENTIAL DIAGNOSES

Amniotic band syndrome

Arthrogryposis (contractures)

Freeman-Sheldon syndrome (flexion deformities)

Multiple pterygium syndrome (contractures)

Neu-Laxova syndrome (microcephaly)

Pena Shokeir syndrome (contractures)

Trisomy 18

ULTRASOUND DIAGNOSIS

This syndrome has been detected at 21 weeks' gestation, based on the presence of severe microphthalmia, micrognathia, contractures of the upper and lower extremities, and rockerbottom feet.

HEREDITY

This is an autosomal recessive condition, which has been localized to DNA repair genes CSB, XPG, and XPD.

NATURAL HISTORY AND OUTCOME

This disorder is characterized by neurogenic arthrogryposis, microcephaly, microphthalmia, and other severe abnormalities. It has an extremely poor prognosis, marked with severe failure to thrive and death within a few months to years of life.

Suggested Reading

Jones KL: *Smith's recognizable patterns of human malformations,* ed 6. Philadelphia, 2006, Elsevier.

Paladini D, D'Armiento M, Ardovino I, Martinelli P: Prenatal diagnosis of the cerebro-oculo-facio-skeletal (COFS) syndrome. *Ultrasound Obstet Gynecol* 16:91–93, 2000.

Pena SDJ, Shokeir MHK: Autosomal recessive cerebro-oculo-facio-skeletal (COFS) syndrome. *Clin Genet* 5:285–288, 1974.

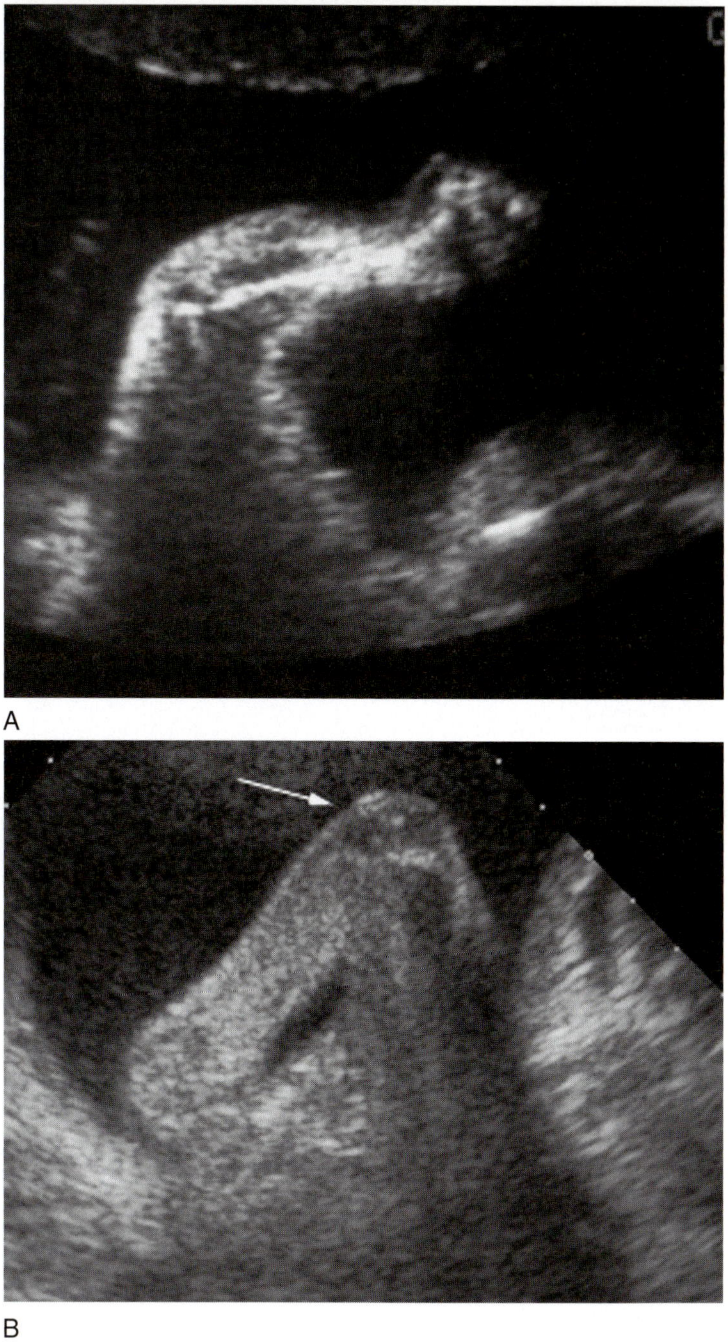

FIGURE 2-215 Severe contractions of the upper (A) and lower (B) extremities *(arrow)* of a third-trimester fetus, with features similar to cerebro-oculo-facio-skeletal syndrome (COFS).

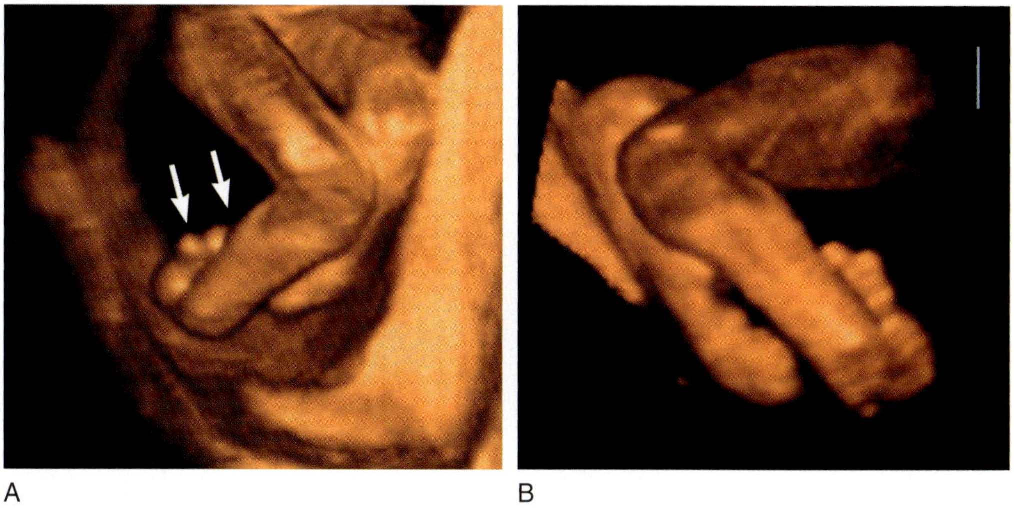

FIGURE 2-216 (A, B) Three-dimensional surface rendering of severely bilateral club feet shows that the feet are completely turned inward and posteriorly *(arrows)*. This is associated with lack of movement.

CHARGE ASSOCIATION

DESCRIPTION AND DEFINITION

This syndrome is characterized by abnormalities involving the eye, heart, nose, ear, and genitals. The acronym CHARGE stands for **c**oloboma of the iris, **h**eart defect, choanal **a**tresia, intrauterine growth **r**estriction, **g**enital anomalies, and **e**ar anomalies.

ABNORMALITIES DETECTABLE BY ULTRASOUND

Common Findings:

Cardiac defects:

- Tetralogy of Fallot
- Double-outlet right ventricle
- Endocardial cushion defect
- Ventricular septal defect
- Atrial septal defect

Hypoplastic nose resulting from choanal atresia

Ear abnormalities, which may not be detectable by ultrasound unless the ears are malformed

Growth deficiency (often first noted in the postnatal period; may not be apparent prenatally)

Genital hypoplasia involving the male genitals

Micropenis and small scrotum

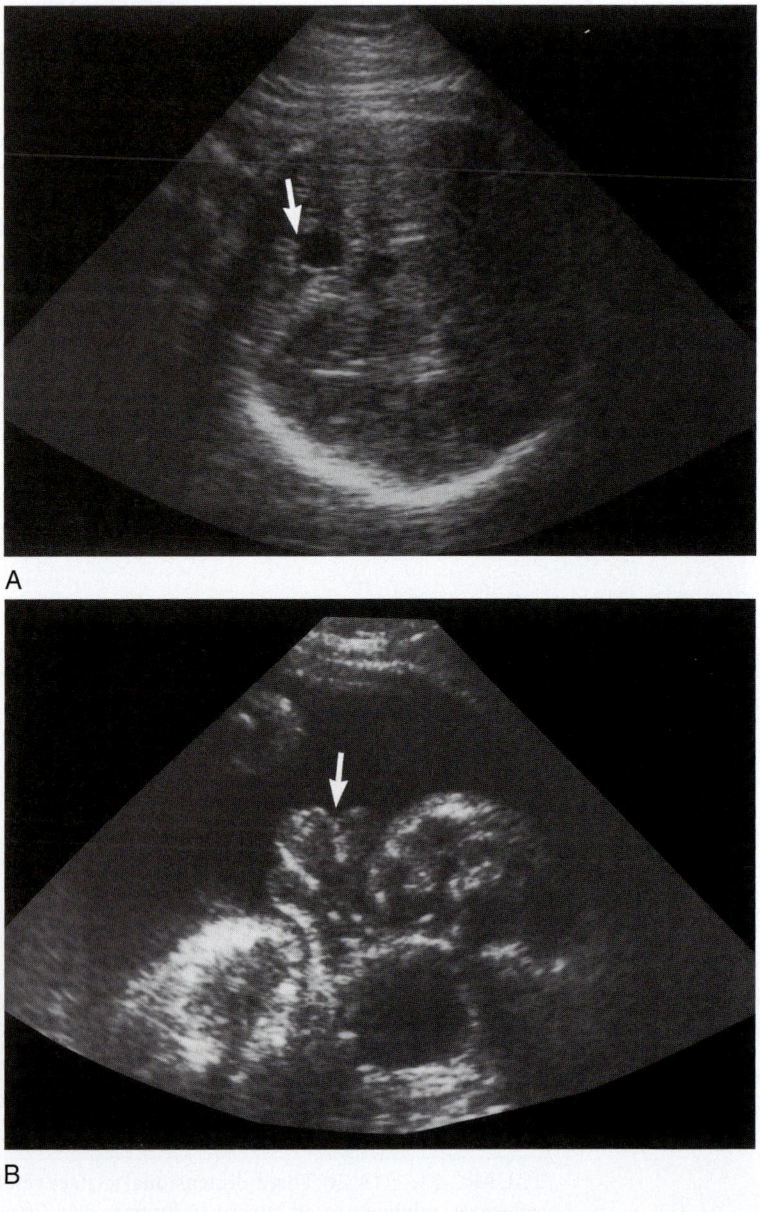

FIGURE 2-217 (A) View of the posterior fossa of a third-trimester fetus with CHARGE association reveals a Dandy-Walker variant. Note the connection *(arrow)* between the fourth ventricle and the cisterna magna. (B) Ambiguous genitalia *(arrow)* in a karyotypically male fetus, as may be seen in fetuses with CHARGE association.

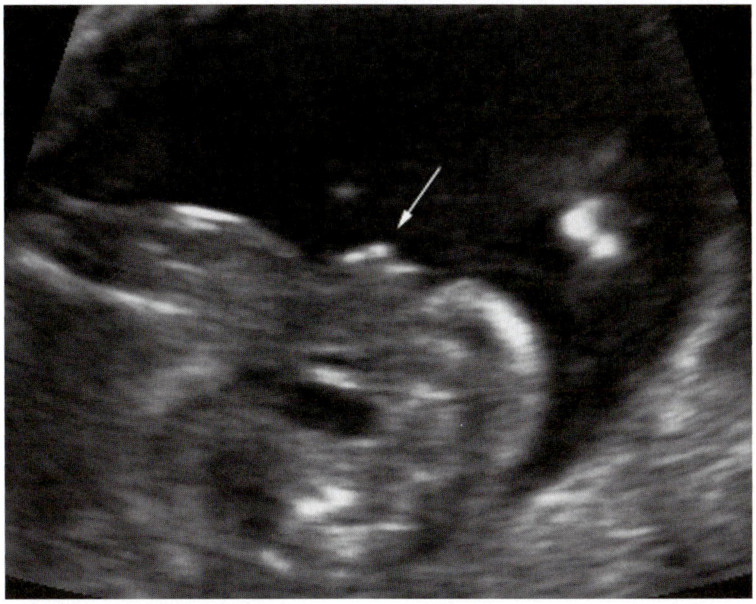

C

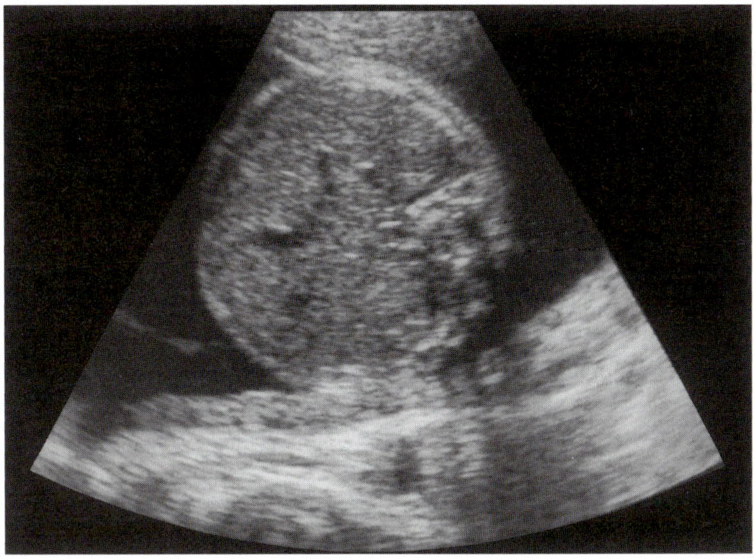

D

FIGURE 2-217, cont'd (C) Fetal genitals *(arrow)* of a second-trimester fetus with an XY karyotype. Note the apparent female phenotype for this genotypically male fetus. (D) Absent stomach bubble consistent with esophageal atresia in a different fetus. There is no connection between the mouth and the stomach pouch, as can occur in fetuses with CHARGE association.

Undescended testicles

Polyhydramnios

Occasional Findings:

Mild ventriculomegaly

Dandy-Walker malformation or variant

Microphthalmia

Hypertelorism

Micrognathia

Cleft lip and palate

Cystic hygroma

Hemivertebrae and scoliosis

Polydactyly and other hand abnormalities

Renal anomalies

Omphalocele

Tracheoesophageal fistula

Anal atresia

MAJOR DIFFERENTIAL DIAGNOSES

Chromosomal abnormalities:

- Deletion 4p (Wolf-Hirschhorn syndrome)
- Trisomy 13 (Patau syndrome)
- Trisomy 18 (Edwards' syndrome)

Congenital adrenal hyperplasia (genital anomalies)

Noonan syndrome (cardiac and genital anomalies)

Opitz syndrome (facial and genital anomalies)

Pena Shokeir syndrome (multiple anomalies)

Smith-Lemli-Opitz syndrome (IUGR, genital and cardiac anomalies)

Stickler syndrome (facial anomalies)

Treacher Collins syndrome (facial anomalies)

VATER (**v**ertebral defects, **a**nal atresia, **t**racheo-esophageal fistula, **e**sophageal atresia, and **r**adial and renal dysplasias) association

ULTRASOUND DIAGNOSIS

A fetus later found to have CHARGE syndrome presented in the first trimester with a cystic hygroma. In another case, intracranial abnormalities, including ventriculomegaly and cerebellar hypoplasia, were detected at 16 weeks; however, the final diagnosis was made postnatally. Diagnosis of the CHARGE association has been established in the third trimester, based on the detection of severe polyhydramnios, mild ventriculomegaly, Dandy-Walker variant, small phallus and scrotum, and small stomach. Although intracranial abnormalities such as ventriculomegaly and cerebellar anomalies are seen occasionally with this syndrome, affected fetuses detected prenatally seem to have a preponderance of these findings.

HEREDITY

Mutations in gene CHD7 are considered to be responsible for the disorder. This gene is important in the early development of the embryo because of its effect on chromatin structure.

NATURAL HISTORY AND OUTCOME

Outcome is dependent on the severity and type of abnormalities present in each individual case. In severe cases, neonatal death has resulted from respiratory insufficiency, intractable hypocalcemia, or congenital heart disease. Most survivors display CNS defects, as well as growth and mental deficiencies. Visual and auditory impairments are common complications.

Suggested Reading

Becker R, Stiemer B, Neumann L, Entezami M: Mild ventriculomegaly, mild cerebellar hypoplasia and dysplastic choroid plexus as early prenatal signs of CHARGE association. *Fetal Diagn Ther* 16:280–283, 2001.

Hall BD: Choanal atresia and associated multiple anomalies. *J Pediatr* 95:395–398, 1979.

Hertzberg BS, Kliewer MA, Lile RL: Antenatal ultrasonographic findings in the CHARGE association. *J Ultrasound Med* 13:238–242, 1994.

Jones KL: *Smith's recognizable patterns of human malformations,* ed 6. Philadelphia, 2006, Elsevier.

Kharrat R, Yamamoto M, Roume J, et al: Karyotype and outcome of fetuses diagnosed with cystic hygroma in the first trimester in relation to nuchal translucency thickness. *Prenat Diagn* 26:369–372, 2006.

CONGENITAL ADRENAL HYPERPLASIA

DESCRIPTION AND DEFINITION

Synonym: 21-hydroxylase deficiency

Congenital adrenal hyperplasia is an autosomal recessive syndrome characterized by a deficiency of one of the enzymes of cortisol biosynthesis. The majority of cases are due to 21-hydroxylase deficiency, resulting in defective cortisol synthesis. The consequent overproduction and accumulation of cortisol precursors causes excessive production of androgens, resulting in virilization of female fetuses.

ABNORMALITIES DETECTABLE BY ULTRASOUND

Common Findings:

Thickened nuchal translucency

Genital abnormalities, appearing as a phallus in a genotypically female fetus

Occasional Finding:

Enlarged adrenal glands

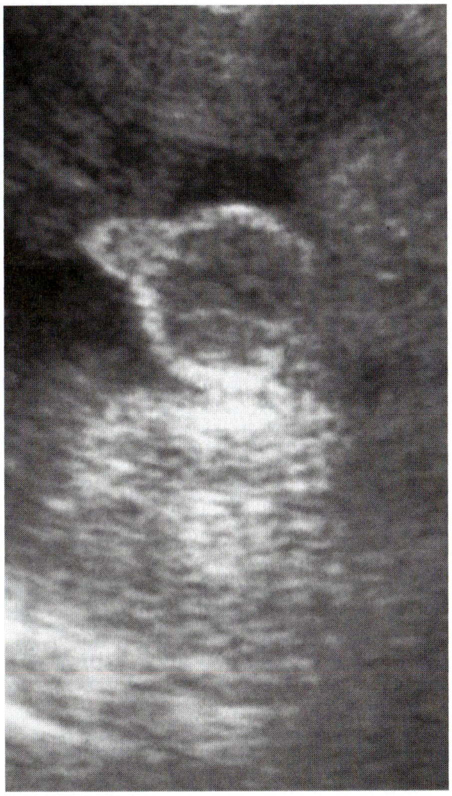

FIGURE 2-218 Third-trimester female fetus with congenital adrenal hyperplasia and severe masculinization of the genitals. Note that no testicles are visible in the presumed scrotum. The karyotype was XX with congenital adrenal hyperplasia noted after birth.

MAJOR DIFFERENTIAL DIAGNOSES

Other Syndromes Commonly Affecting the Appearance of the Genitals:

Antley-Bixler syndrome

CHARGE (**c**oloboma of the iris, **h**eart defect, choanal **a**tresia, intrauterine growth **r**estriction, **g**enital anomalies, and **e**ar anomalies) association

Cloacal exstrophy

Cornelia de Lange syndrome

MURCS (**mü**llerian duct aplasia, **r**enal aplasia, **c**ervicothoracic **s**omite dysplasia) association

Noonan syndrome

Opitz syndrome

Smith-Lemli-Opitz syndrome

ULTRASOUND DIAGNOSIS

The diagnosis of this syndrome has been made in the first trimester, seen as a thickened nuchal

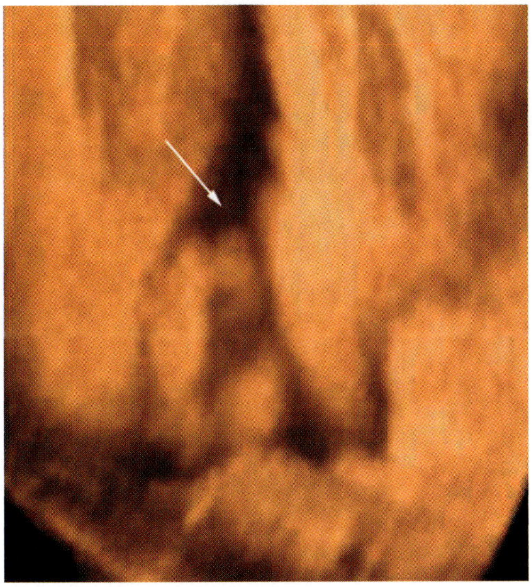

FIGURE 2-219 Three-dimensional surface rendering of mild masculinization of a fetus shows a prominent clitoris *(arrow)*.

translucency, and among female fetuses in the second trimester, seen as abnormal-appearing genitals and pseudo-phallus. Virilization of female fetuses has been noted as early as 18 weeks, when two female fetuses were mistaken for males in a set of affected twins. Enlarged adrenal glands in the second trimester also have been reported as a feature of this syndrome. There is some evidence that the measurement of 21-deoxycortisol and 17-hydroxyprogesterone in the amniotic fluid may be helpful in prenatal detection, particularly in the salt-wasting variant of this syndrome. There are no reported additional sonographic features of the salt-wasting variant of this disorder.

HEREDITY

This is an autosomal recessive disorder, with 90% of congenital adrenal hyperplasia cases resulting from 21-hydroxylase deficiency, which leads to 17-hydroxyprogesterone not being converted to 11-deoxycortisol. This causes excessive production of androgen, which virilizes female fetuses in utero.

NATURAL HISTORY AND OUTCOME

When a woman has a history of congenital adrenal hyperplasia in a previous pregnancy, it is important to establish the genotype with chorionic villus sampling or early amniocentesis so that affected female fetuses can be treated to prevent early masculinization in utero. A salt-wasting variant of this syndrome is caused by the lack of aldosterone. Untreated neonates with this variant are at risk for severe electrolyte imbalance and hypovolemic shock.

Suggested Reading

Bromley B, Mandell J, Gross G, Walzer TB, Benacerraf BR: Masculinization of female fetuses with congenital adrenal hyperplasia may already be present at 18 weeks. *Am J Obstet Gynecol* 17:264–265, 1994.

Chambier ED, Heinrichs C, Avni FE: Sonographic appearance of congenital adrenal hyperplasia in utero. *J Ultrasound Med* 21:97–100, 2002.

Esser T, Chaoui R: Enlarged adrenal glands as a prenatal marker of congenital adrenal hyperplasia: a report of two cases. *Ultrasound Obstet Gynecol* 23:293–297, 2004.

Fincham J, Pandya PP, Yuksel B, Loong YM, Shah J: Increased first-trimester nuchal translucency as a prenatal manifestation of salt-wasting congenital adrenal hyperplasia. *Ultrasound Obstet Gynecol* 20:392–394, 2002.

Gueux B, Fiet J, Couillin P, et al: Prenatal diagnosis of 21-hydroxylase deficiency congenital adrenal hyperplasia by simultaneous radioimmunoassay of 21-deoxycortisol and 17-hydroxyprogesterone in amniotic fluid. *J Clin Endocrinol Metab* 66:534–537, 1988.

Hughes IA, Dyas J, Riad-Fahmy D, Laurence KM: Prenatal diagnosis of congenital adrenal hyperplasia: reliability of amniotic fluid steroid analysis. *J Med Genet* 24:344–347, 1987.

Merkatz IR, New MI, Peterson RE, Seaman MP: Prenatal diagnosis of adrenogenital syndrome by amniocentesis. *J Pediatr* 75:977–982, 1969.

Pang S, Pollack MS, Loo M, et al: Pitfalls of prenatal diagnosis of 21-hydroxylase deficiency congenital adrenal hyperplasia. *J Clin Endocrinol Metab* 61:89–97, 1985.

Saada J, Grebille AG, Aubry MC, Rafii A, Dumez Y, Benachi A: Sonography in prenatal diagnosis of congenital adrenal hyperplasia. *Prenat Diagn* 24:627–630, 2004.

White PC, Speiser PW: Congenital adrenal hyperplasia due to 21-hydroxylase deficiency. *Endocr Rev* 21:245–291, 2000.

CONGENITAL HIGH AIRWAY OBSTRUCTION SYNDROME

DESCRIPTION AND DEFINITION

Synonym: CHAOS

Congenital high airway obstruction syndrome (CHAOS) is characterized by complete obstruction of the upper airway, secondary to either laryngeal or glottic atresia and leading to massive enlargement of the lungs.

ABNORMALITIES DETECTABLE BY ULTRASOUND

Common Findings:

Enlarged, echogenic lungs (bilateral)

Inverted diaphragm

Dilated trachea and bronchial tree

Ascites

Hydrops

Nuchal edema

Oligohydramnios

MAJOR DIFFERENTIAL DIAGNOSES

Bilateral cystic adenomatoid malformation of the lungs

Fraser syndrome

Intrathoracic teratoma

ULTRASOUND DIAGNOSIS

The diagnosis typically is made in the second trimester, having been described at 19 to 20 weeks' gestation. It is manifested by large, hyperechoic lungs, hydrops, nuchal edema, and oligohydramnios. Not only are the lungs large and echogenic, but the fluid-filled trachea and bronchial tree can be identified all the way up to the level of obstruction.

HEREDITY

CHAOS secondary to laryngeal atresia may be part of another syndrome such as Fraser syndrome. When CHAOS is *not* part of another syndrome (isolated glottal or tracheal atresia), then it is of unknown etiology and inheritance.

NATURAL HISTORY AND OUTCOME

Typically, laryngeal obstruction can be due to laryngeal atresia, tracheal atresia, or laryngeal webs, all of which give a similar picture of very large, echogenic lungs resulting from backup of secretions by the lungs. Tracheoesophageal fistula and hydrops often coexist. The outcome is guarded unless the diagnosis is made prenatally and the fetus undergoes an ex utero intrapartum treatment (EXIT) procedure at delivery. The EXIT procedure permits bronchoscopic control of the airway and placement of a

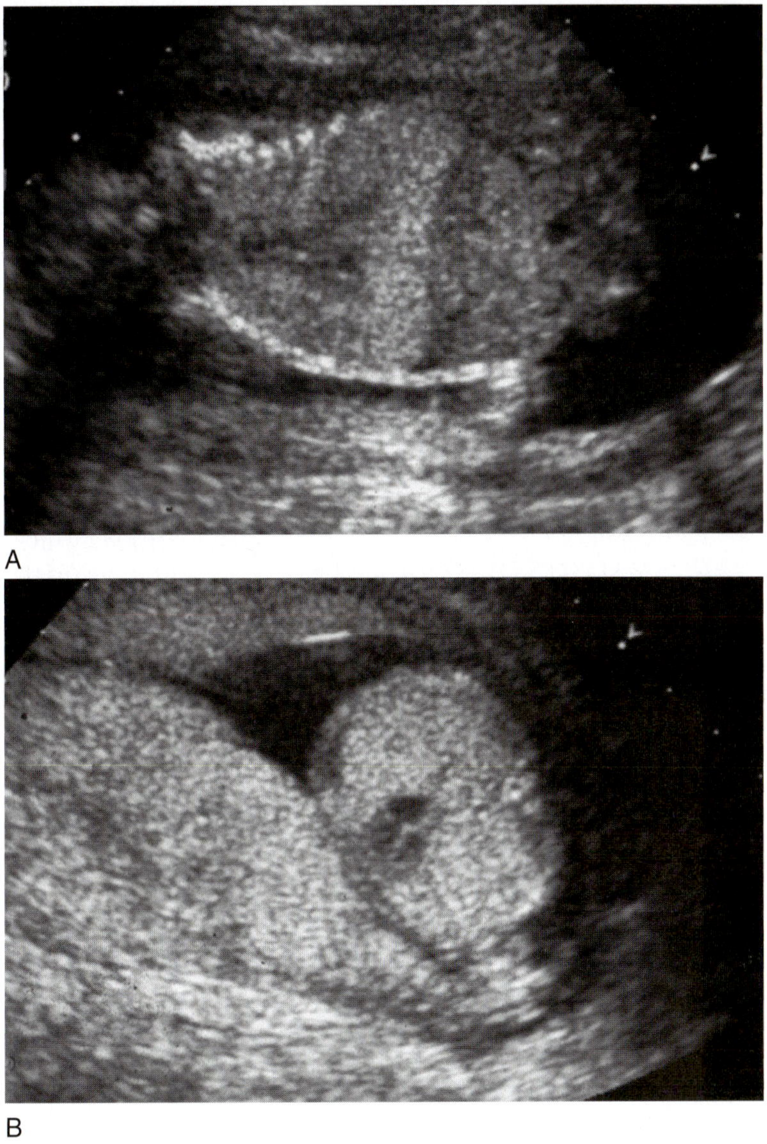

FIGURE 2-220 Second-trimester fetus with enlarged lungs. Longitudinal (A) and transverse (B) views through the chest show that the lungs are enlarged, making the heart small in a fetus with tracheal atresia.

tracheostomy to bypass the area of obstruction while the fetus is only halfway delivered and still connected to the placenta. This is essentially the only way that fetuses with high airway obstruction syndrome can survive past delivery.

Suggested Reading

Bouchard S, Johnson MP, Flakc AW, et al: The EXIT procedure: experience and outcome in 31 cases. *J Pediatr Surg* 37:418–426, 2002.

DeCou JM, Jones DC, Jacobs HD, Touloukian RJ: Successful ex utero intrapartum treatment (EXIT) procedure for congenital high airway obstruction syndrome (CHAOS) owing to laryngeal atresia. *J Pediatr Surg* 33:1563–1565, 1998.

Kalache KD, Chaouir, Tennstedt C, Bollmann R: Prenatal diagnosis of laryngeal atresia in two cases of congenital high airway obstruction syndrome (CHAOS) (short communication). *Prenat Diagn* 17:577–581, 1997.

Lim FY, Crombleholme TM, Hedrick HL, et al: Congenital high airway obstruction syndrome: natural history and management. *J Pediatr Surg* 38:940–945, 2003.

Oepkes D, Teunissen AKK, Van de Velde M, Devlieger H, Delaere P, Deprest J: Congenital high airway obstruction syndrome successfully managed with ex-utero intrapartum treatment (Picture of the month). *Ultrasound Obstet Gynecol* 22:437–439, 2003.

Onderoglu L, Karamursel S, Bulun A, Kale G, Tuncbilek E: Prenatal diagnosis of laryngeal atresia (Short communication). *Prenat Diagn* 23:277–280, 2003.

Zhang P, Herring D, Cook L, Mertz H: Fetal laryngeal stenosis/atresia and congenital high airway obstructive syndrome (CHAOS): a case report. *J Perinatol* 25:425–428, 2005.

CLOACAL EXSTROPHY SEQUENCE

DESCRIPTION AND DEFINITION

Synonyms: Omphalocele–exstrophy–imperforate anus–spinal defects, OEIS complex

This is a complex disorder characterized by a combination of defects that include omphalocele, imperforate anus, cloacal exstrophy, spinal defects, and genital abnormalities. The spectrum of genital and gastrointestinal defects varies from a mild case of epispadias to severe exstrophy of the bladder, cloacal exstrophy, and full-blown spinal defects with associated gastrointestinal anomalies.

ABNORMALITIES DETECTABLE BY ULTRASOUND

Common Findings:

Ventral wall defect

Absent bladder

Elephant trunk-like protrusion from the anterior abdominal wall (terminal ileum)

Neural tube defects

Genital abnormalities

Oligohydramnios

Cystic structures in the fetal pelvis

Occasional Findings:

Abnormalities of the lower extremities

Abnormalities of the kidneys

Ascites

Widened synthesis pubis

Single umbilical artery

MAJOR DIFFERENTIAL DIAGNOSES

Amniotic bands with disruption of the anterior abdominal wall

Gastroschisis

Limb–body wall defect

Omphalocele

Persistent cloaca (without anterior abdominal wall defect but with several cystic areas within the abdomen)

Simple bladder exstrophy

ULTRASOUND DIAGNOSIS

The diagnosis of cloacal exstrophy has been made in the early second trimester, seen as an anterior abdominal wall defect associated with urinary tract abnormalities and abnormal cystic spaces in the fetal abdomen. The accuracy of the ultrasound diagnosis varies according to the number of related malformations present. Milder cases are harder to recognize and may be missed sonographically until the third trimester.

Separate from cloacal exstrophy is simple bladder exstrophy, which is a milder defect characterized by inversion of the bladder, with exposure of the mucosa along the anterior abdominal wall. There are varying degrees of genital abnormalities as well as widening of the synthesis pubis. The ultrasound diagnosis of bladder exstrophy is generally made when fluid cannot be identified in the fetal bladder despite repeated attempts. Three-dimensional ultrasound may be helpful in identifying the bladder mucosa on the surface of the anterior abdominal wall.

HEREDITY

The etiology of this sequence is unknown, although there are some reports of OEIS occurring in monozygotic twins. In those cases, the disorder may be related to the abnormality of monozygotic twinning itself.

The heredity of bladder exstrophy is unknown, although there is some evidence of higher recurrence in affected families.

NATURAL HISTORY AND OUTCOME

Cloacal exstrophy is a severe exstrophy of the common cloaca, involving abnormalities of both the gastrointestinal and the genitourinary tracts, as well as incomplete development of the lumbosacral vertebral bodies, spinal dysraphism, imperforate anus, and müllerian duct abnormalities in females and epispadias in males. Because of the severity of these abnormalities, the outcome for an affected child is related to the success of surgical repair. There can be severe problems of urine incontinence, short bowel syndrome, and gender reassignment, with associated psychological issues. Although the quality of life may be negatively impacted by these problems, the prospect of survival is excellent.

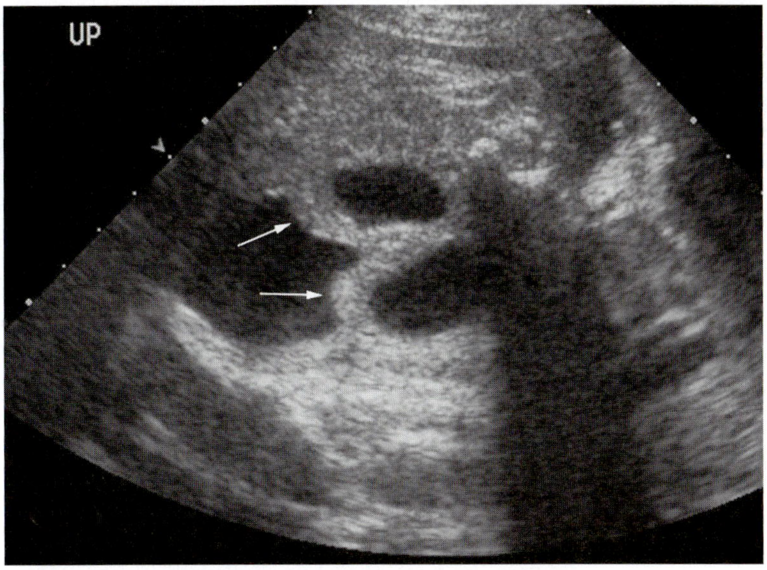

FIGURE 2-221 Transverse view through the fetal lower abdomen in a third-trimester fetus shows a cloacal abnormality. Note bilateral cystic structures *(arrows)*, which represent a bicornuate uterus with hematometra.

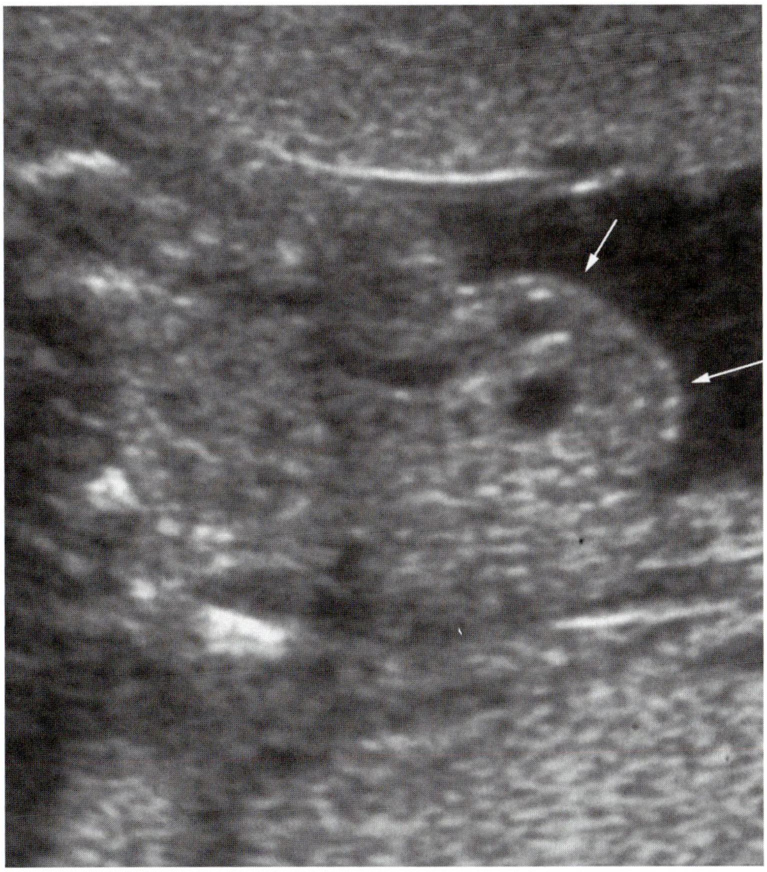

FIGURE 2-222 Note protrusion from the anterior abdominal wall *(arrows)* in a fetus with cloacal exstrophy.

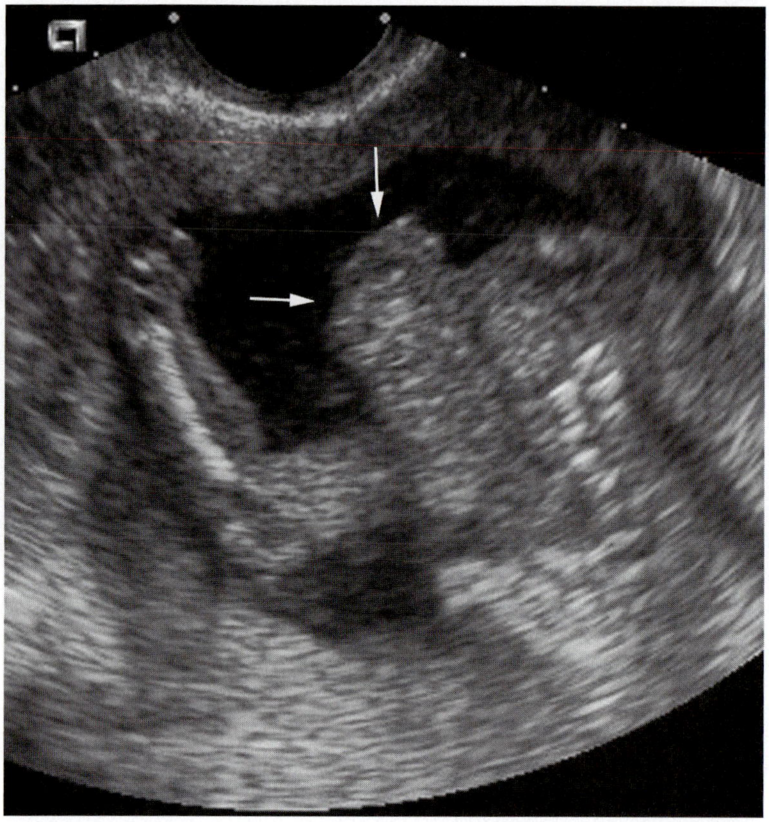

FIGURE 2-223 Trunk-like protrusion from the anterior abdominal wall *(arrows)* seen transvaginally in this early second-trimester fetus with cloacal exstrophy. Note the lower extremity on one side of the defect.

Bladder exstrophy with associated epispadias is considered a severe urologic birth defect because of its impact on the genitals, including incontinence and abnormal sexual function. The outcome is directly related to the success of surgery.

Suggested Reading

Carey JC, Greenbaum B, Hall BD: The OEIS complex (omphalocele, exstrophy, imperforate anus, spinal defects). *Birth Defects Orig Artic Ser* 14:253–263, 1978.

Chen CP, Shih SL, Liu FF, Jan SW, Jeng CJ, Lan CC: Perinatal features of omphalocele-exstrophy-imperforate anus-spinal defects (OEIS complex) associated with large meningomyeloceles and severe limb defects. *Am J Perinatol* 14:275–279, 1997.

Della MM, Nazzaro A, Lonardo F, Ferrara G, Di Blasi A, Scarano G: Prenatal ultrasound diagnosis of cloacal exstrophy associated with myelocystocele complex by the 'elephant trunk-like' image and review of the literature. *Prenat Diagn* 25:394–397, 2005.

Froster UG, Heinritz W, Bennek J, Horn LC, Faber R: Another case of autosomal dominant exstrophy of the bladder. *Prenat Diagn* 24:375–377, 2004.

Girz BA, Sherer DM, Atkin J, Venanzi M, Ahlborn L, Cestone L: First-trimester prenatal sonographic findings associated with OEIS (omphalocele-exstrophy-imperforate anus-spinal defects) complex: a case and review of the literature. *Am J Perinatol* 15:15–17, 1998.

Gosden C, Brock DJH: Prenatal diagnosis of exstrophy of the cloaca. *Am J Med Genet* 8:95–109, 1981.

Kutzner DK, Wilson WG, Hogge WA: OEIS complex (cloacal exstrophy): prenatal diagnosis in the second trimester. *Prenat Diagn* 8:247–253, 1988.

Lee DH, Cottrell JR, Sanders RC, Meyers CM, Wulfsberg EA, Sun CC: OEIS complex (omphalocele-exstrophy-imperforate anus-spinal defects) in monozygotic twins. *Am J Med Genet* 84:29–33, 1999.

Lee EH, Shim JY: New sonographic finding for the prenatal diagnosis of bladder exstrophy: a case report. *Ultrasound Obstet Gynecol* 21:498–500, 2003.

Myers C, Lee PA: Communicating with parents with full disclosure: a case of cloacal exstrophy with genital ambiguity. *J Pediatr Endocrinol Metab* 17:273–279, 2004.

Shapiro E, Lepor H, Jeffs RD: The inheritance of the bladder exstrophy-epispadias complex. *J Urol* 132:308–310, 1984.

Wu JL, Fang KH, Yeh GP, Chou PH, Hsieh CT: Using color Doppler sonography to identify the perivesical umbilical arteries: a useful method in the prenatal diagnosis of omphalocele-exstrophy-imperforate anus-spinal defects complex. *J Ultrasound Med* 23:1211–1215, 2004.

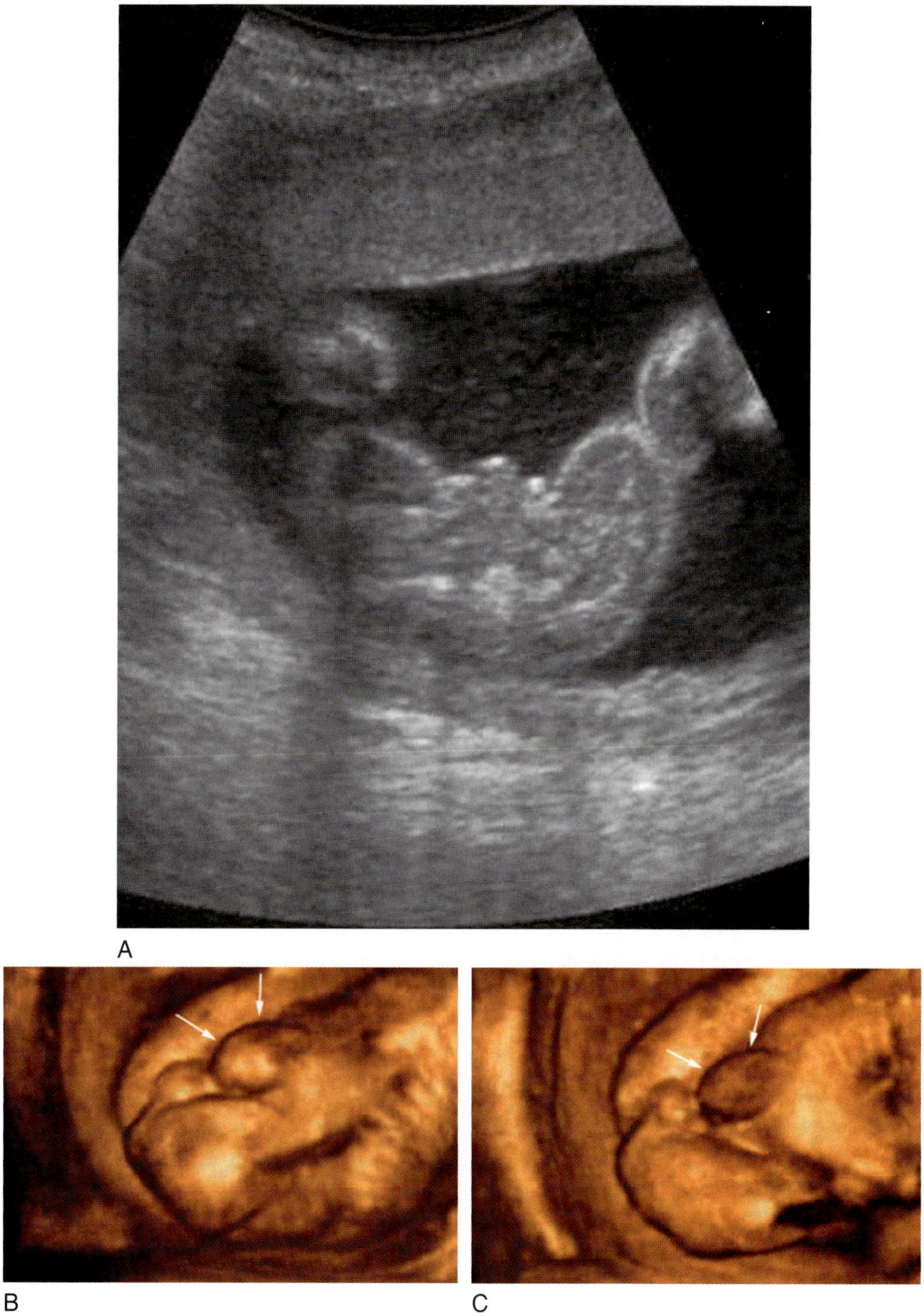

FIGURE 2-224 (A) Absence of the fetal bladder as well as unusual genitalia in a 20-week fetus with bladder exstrophy. (B, C) Three-dimensional surface rendering of the anterior abdominal wall shows a mass *(arrows)* protruding from the lower abdominal wall, consistent with the bladder. The bladder is splayed open on the anterior abdominal wall.

HOLOPROSENCEPHALY SEQUENCE

DESCRIPTION AND DEFINITION

Holoprosencephaly represents a spectrum of severe abnormalities in the cleavage of the prosencephalon, resulting in a monoventricle, fusion of the cerebellar hemispheres and thalami, and abnormalities of the optic and olfactory bulbs.

ABNORMALITIES DETECTABLE BY ULTRASOUND

Alobar Holoprosencephaly (Most Severe Form):

Absence of the inner hemispheric fissure

Single, central ventricle

Fused thalami

Absence of the third ventricle

Absence of the olfactory bulb

Major midfacial malformations

Cyclopia

Cebocephaly

Median cleft lip and palate

Hypotelorism

Maxillary hypoplasia or absence of the premaxilla with hypotelorism

First-trimester nuchal translucency thickening

Semilobar Holoprosencephaly:

Partially separated posterior cerebral hemispheres, with a single ventricle

Lobar Holoprosencephaly (Least Severe Form and Most Subtle in Terms of Prenatal Sonographic Findings):

Some fusion of the lateral ventricles and cingulate gyrus

Absence of the cavum septum pellucidum

Separate lateral ventricles, except for the frontal horns

Conditions Associated with Holoprosencephaly in General:

Microcephaly or macrocephaly

Dorsal cyst (representing expansion of the posterior aspect of the single ventricle)

Severe facial abnormalities

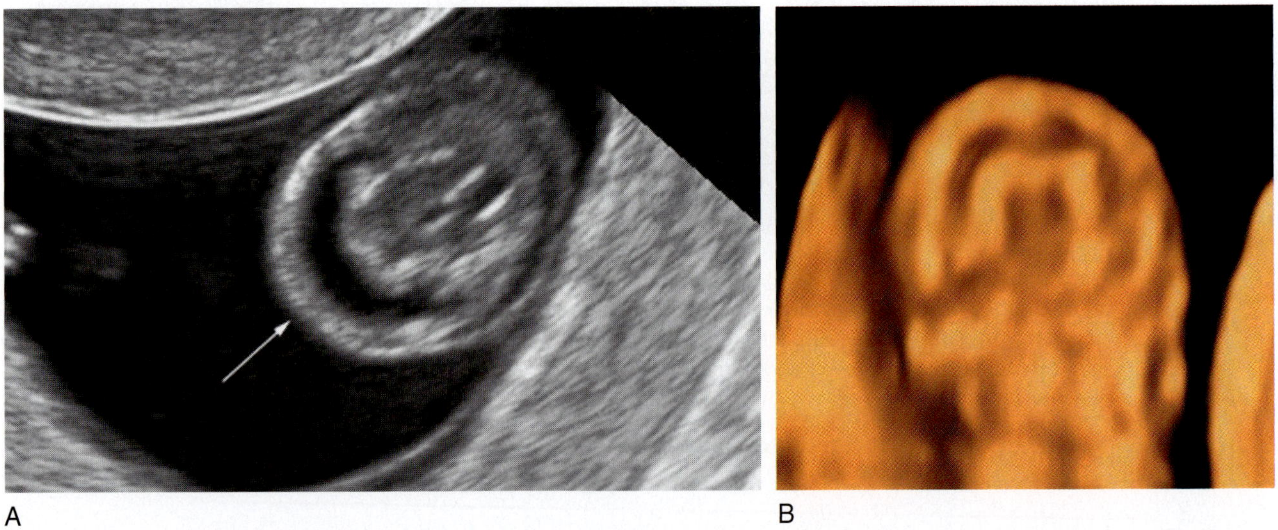

FIGURE 2-225 (A) Coronal view through the fetal head of a 13-week fetus with holoprosencephaly. Arrow indicates top of the head, at the level where the falx should originate. Note the monoventricle. (B) Surface-rendered coronal view of the monoventricle in the same fetus.

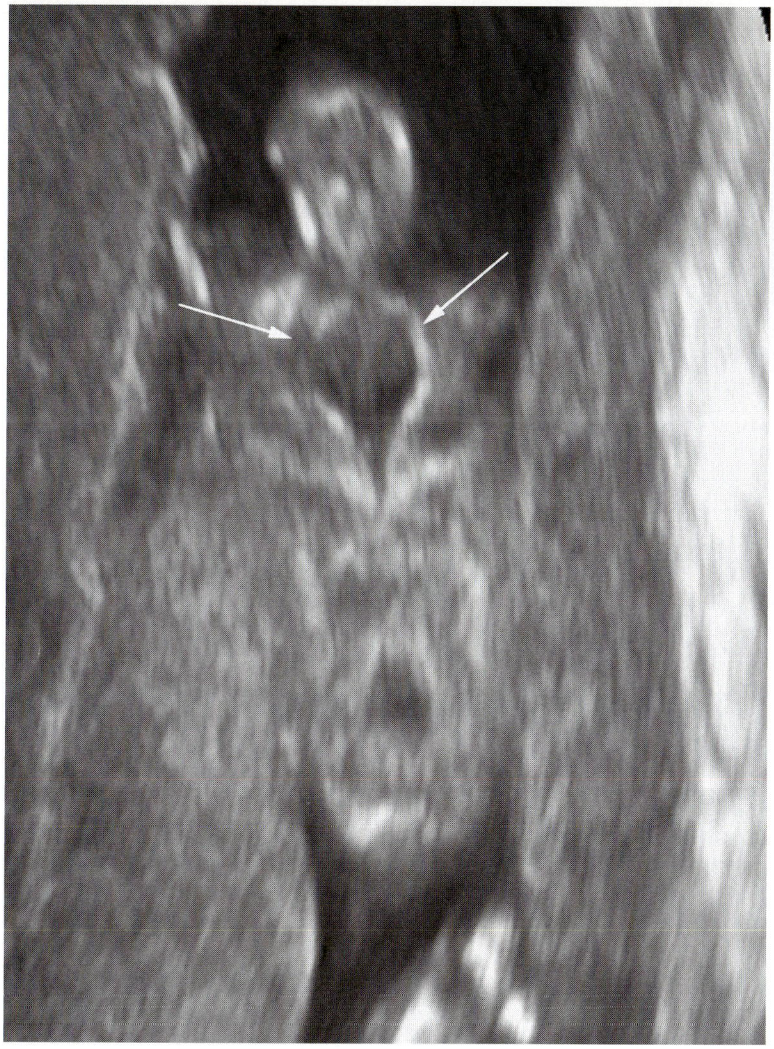

A

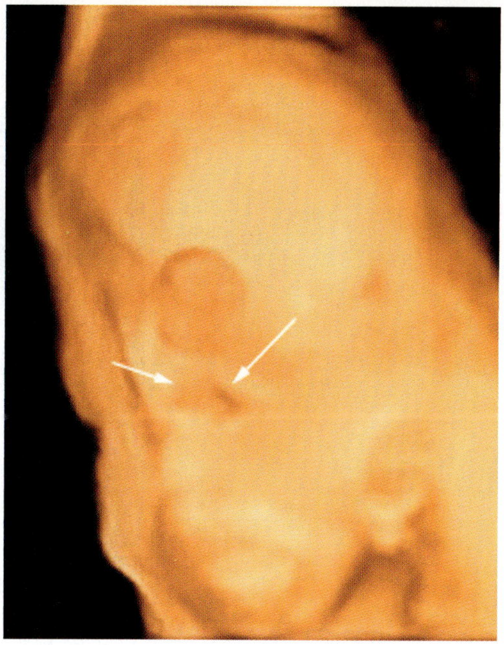

B

FIGURE 2-226 (A) Second-trimester fetus with cyclopia and holoprosencephaly. Coronal view through the fetal face shows the single orbit *(arrows)* and above it the proboscis. (B) Three-dimensional surface rendering of the same fetus shows the single orbit *(arrows)* with the proboscis directly above it. Note the low-set ear.

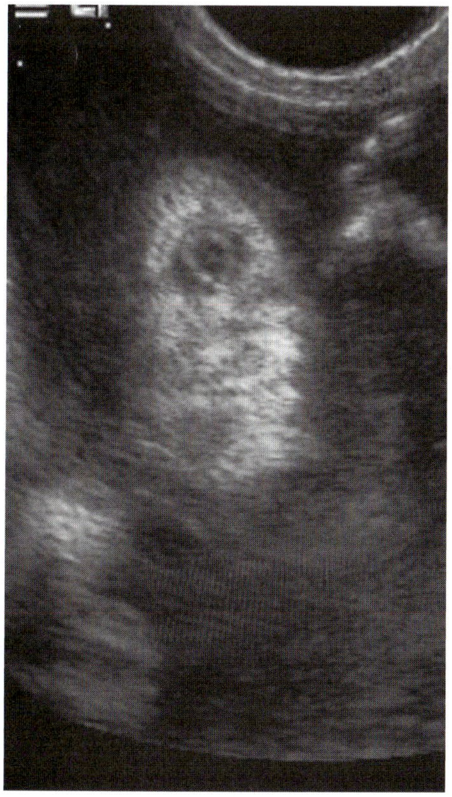

FIGURE 2-227 Second-trimester fetus with cyclopia and a single orbit. The lens of the eye is seen as the round circle within the orbit.

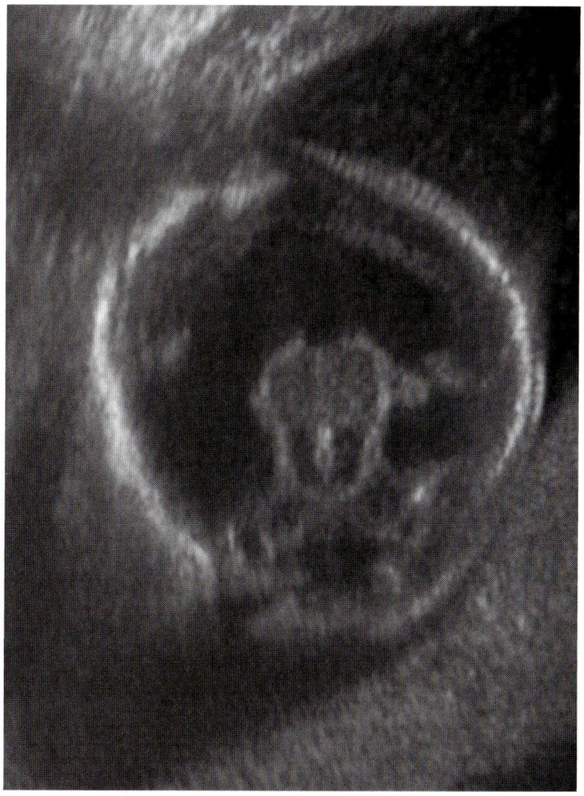

FIGURE 2-228 Coronal view of a fetus with alobar holoprosencephaly shows the fused thalami.

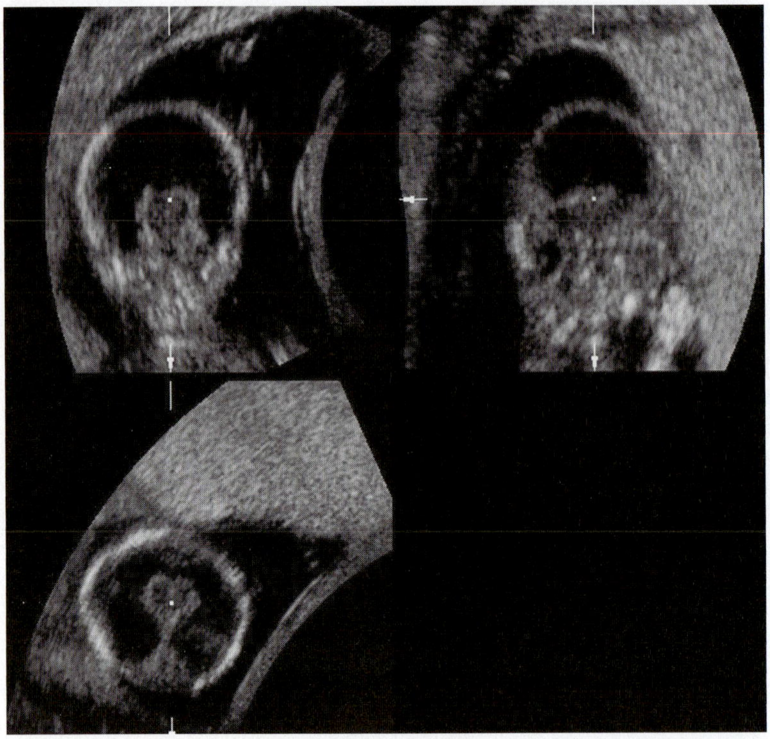

FIGURE 2-229 Three-dimensional multiplanar reconstruction of a fetus with alobar holoprosencephaly shows fused thalami in three orthogonal views through the monoventricle.

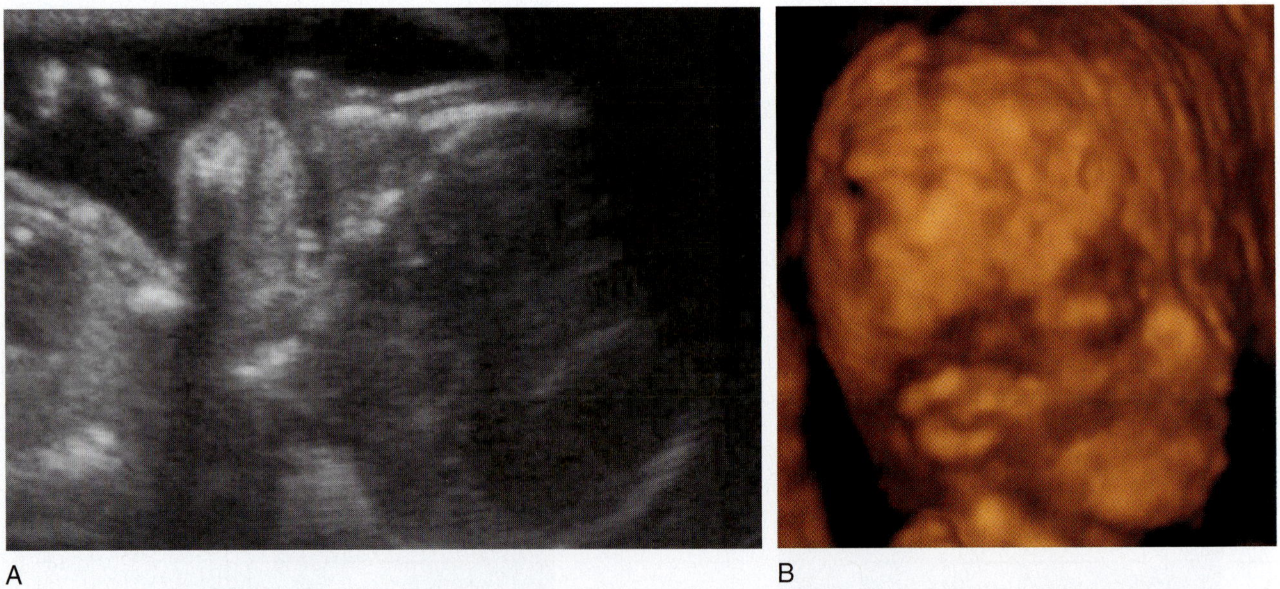

FIGURE 2-230 (A) Longitudinal view of a fetus with holoprosencephaly shows anophthalmia and no visible nose. (B) Three-dimensional surface rendering of the same fetus shows absence of the nose and the orbits consistent with anophthalmia.

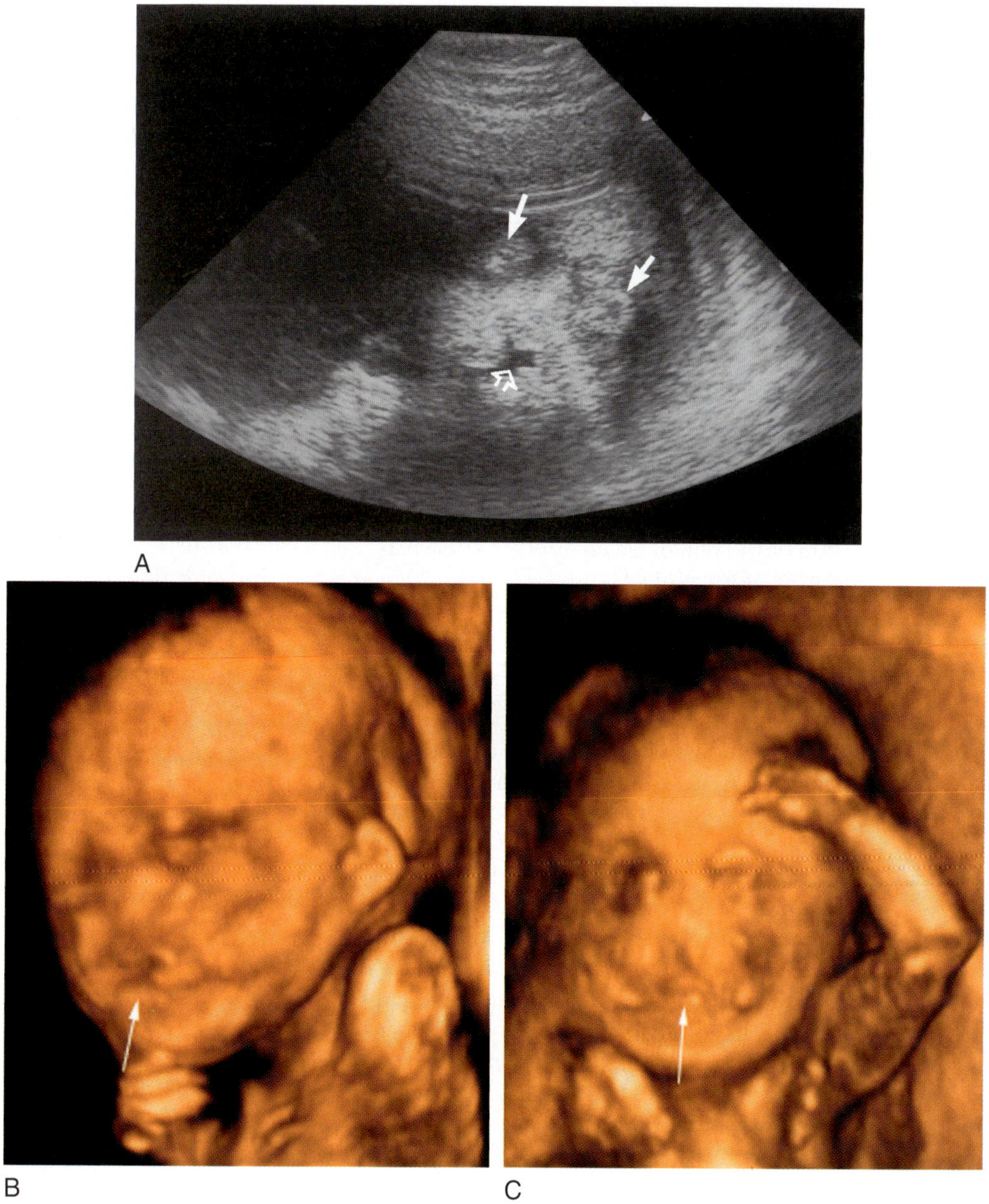

FIGURE 2-231 (A) Coronal view of the face of a fetus with hypotelorism. Solid arrows indicate the eyes. The nose is extremely hypoplastic, and there is a central median cleft lip and palate *(open arrow)* with severe maxillary hypoplasia. (B) Three-dimensional surface rendering of a second-trimester fetus with holoprosencephaly consistent with hypotelorism and a central-midline cleft lip and palate *(arrow)*. (C) Different fetus with holoprosencephaly, hypotelorism, and midline facial cleft *(arrow)*.

MAJOR DIFFERENTIAL DIAGNOSES

Syndromes and Conditions Associated with Holoprosencephaly:

Aicardi syndrome

Chromosomal abnormalities

- Trisomy 13 (Patau syndrome)
- Trisomy 18 (Edwards' syndrome)
- Triploidy

Ectrodactyly–ectodermal dysplasia–clefting (EEC) syndrome

Fetal hydantoin syndrome

Septo-optic dysplasia

Shprintzen syndrome

Smith-Lemli-Opitz syndrome

Syndromes and Conditions Associated with Central Fluid within the Brain:

Aneurysm of the vein of Galen

Arachnoid cysts

Asymmetric ventriculomegaly

Cystic teratomata

Hydranencephaly

Interhemispheric cysts associated with agenesis of the corpus callosum

Schizencephaly

Evaluation of the face is helpful in establishing a definitive diagnosis of holoprosencephaly. Doppler studies are necessary for detecting an aneurysm of the vein of Galen or other arteriovenous malformations.

ULTRASOUND DIAGNOSIS

Prenatal diagnosis of alobar holoprosencephaly has been established as early as 9 to 10 weeks' gestation and numerous times in the late first trimester based on severe intracranial and facial abnormalities and nuchal translucency abnormalities. Later in development, macrocephaly or microcephaly may be present, and the appearance of the monoventricle and fused thalami are characteristic of holoprosencephaly. In lobar holoprosencephaly, there are severe facial defects such as central clefts, hypotelorism, and cyclopia. In a study of 30 cases of holoprosencephaly, 18 were alobar, 5 semilobar, 2 lobar, 2 lobar variants, and 3 had associated anencephaly. Twenty of the 30 had associated non–CNS/facial anomalies. Eleven of the 20 had documented chromosomal anomalies, and 7 had nonchromosomal syndromes. The size and shape of the head were abnormal in 83% of these 30 cases.

HEREDITY

There is a familial alobar holoprosencephaly that is autosomal dominant (gene HPE3, located at 7q36 locus). Several other loci have been implicated in this disorder. Other etiologies for holoprosencephaly have their own patterns of heredity and recurrence risks. Trisomy 13 is the most common chromosomal abnormality associated with alobar holoprosencephaly.

NATURAL HISTORY AND OUTCOME

Most fetuses with alobar and semilobar holoprosencephaly die at birth. Survival in those with mild forms of the disorder, including lobar holoprosencephaly, is associated with mental retardation.

Suggested Reading

Achiron R, Achiron A: Transvaginal ultrasonic assessment of the early fetal brain. *Ultrasound Obstet Gynecol* 1:336–344, 1991.

Achiron R, Achiron A, Lipitz S, Mashiach S, Goldman B: Holoprosencephaly: alobar. *Fetus* 4:9–12, 1994.

Ardinger HH, Bartley JA: Microcephaly in familial holoprosencephaly. *J Craniofac Genet Dev Biol* 8:53–61, 1988.

Benke PJ, Cohen MM Jr: Recurrence of holoprosencephaly in families with a positive history. *Clin Genet* 24:324–328, 1983.

Bernard JP, Drummond CL, Zaarour P, Molho M, Ville Y: A new clue to the prenatal diagnosis of lobar holoprosencephaly: the abnormal pathway of the anterior cerebral artery crawling under the skull. *Ultrasound Obstet Gynecol* 19:605–607, 2002.

Blaas HG: Holoprosencephaly at 10 weeks 2 days (CRL 33 mm). *Ultrasound Obstet Gynecol* 15:86–87, 2000.

Blaas HG, Eik-Nes SH, Vainio T, Isaksen CV: Alobar holoprosencephaly at 9 weeks gestational age visualized by two- and three-dimensional ultrasound. *Ultrasound Obstet Gynecol* 15:62–65, 2000.

Blaas HG, Eriksson AG, Salvesen KA, et al: Brains and faces in holoprosencephaly: pre- and postnatal description of 30 cases. *Ultrasound Obstet Gynecol* 19:24–38, 2002.

Blin G, Rabbe A, Mandelbrot L: Prenatal diagnosis of lobar holoprosencephaly using color Doppler: three cases with the anterior cerebral artery crawling under the skull. *Ultrasound Obstet Gynecol* 24:476–478, 2004.

Bronshtein M, Wiener Z: Early transvaginal sonographic diagnosis of alobar holoprosencephaly. *Prenat Diagn* 11:459–462, 1991.

Cantu JM, Fragoso R, Garcia-Cruz D, Sanchez-Corona J: Dominant inheritance of holoprosencephaly. *Birth Defects* 14:215–220, 1978.

Cho FN, Kan YY, Chen SN, Lee TC, Hsu TJ, Hsu PH: Prenatal diagnosis of cyclopia and proboscis in a fetus with normal chromosome at 13 weeks of gestation by three-dimensional transabdominal sonography. *Prenat Diagn* 25:1059–1060, 2005.

Collins AL, Lunt PW, Garrett C, Dennis NR: Holoprosencephaly: a family showing dominant inheritance and variable expression. *J Med Genet* 30:36–40, 1993.

Corsello G, Buttitta P, Cammarata M, et al: Holoprosencephaly: examples of clinical variability and etiologic heterogeneity. *Am J Med Genet* 37:244–249, 1990.

Dallaire L, Fraser FC, Wigglesworth FW: Familial holoprosencephaly. *Birth Defects* 7:136–142, 1971.

DeMyer WE, Zeman W, Palmer CG: Familial alobar holoprosencephaly (arhinencephaly) with median cleft lip and palate: a report of a patient with 46 chromosomes. *Neurology* 13:913–918, 1963.

Faro C, Wegrzyn P, Benoit B, Chaoui R, Nicolaides KH: Metopic suture in fetuses with holoprosencephaly at 11 + 0 to 13 + 6 weeks of gestation. *Ultrasound Obstet Gynecol* 27:162–166, 2006.

Greene MF, Benacerraf BR, Frigoletto FD Jr: Reliable criteria for the prenatal sonographic diagnosis of alobar holoprosencephaly. *Am J Obstet Gynecol* 1546:687–689, 1987.
Grundy HO, Niemeyer P, Rupani MK, Ward VF, Wassman ER: Prenatal detection of cyclopia associated with interstitial deletion of 2p. *Am J Med Genet* 34:268–270, 1989.
Hockey A, Crowhurst J, Cullity G: Microcephaly, holoprosencephaly, hypokinesia—second report of a new syndrome. *Prenat Diagn* 8:683–686, 1988.
Jones KL: *Smith's recognizable patterns of human malformations,* ed 6. Philadelphia, 2006, Elsevier.
Joo GJ, Beke A, Papp C, Toth-Pal E, Szigeti Z, Ban Z, Papp Z: Prenatal diagnosis, phenotypic and obstetric characteristics of holoprosencephaly. *Fetal Diagn Ther* 20:161–166, 2005.
Kalache KD, Eder K, Esser T, et al: Three-dimensional ultrasonographic reslicing of the fetal brain to assist prenatal diagnosis of central nervous system anomalies. *J Ultrasound Med* 25:509–514, 2006.
Kuo HC, Chang FM, Wu CH, Yao BL, Liu CH: Antenatal ultrasonographic diagnosis of hypotelorism. *J Formos Med Assoc* 89:803–805, 1990.
Lehman CD, Nyberg DA, Winter TC III, et al: Trisomy 13 syndrome: prenatal US findings in a review of 33 cases. *Radiology* 194:217–222, 1995.
Lurie IW, Liyina HG, Podleschuk LV, Gorelik LB, Zaletajef DV: Chromosome 7 abnormalities in parents of children with holoprosencephaly and hydronephrosis. *Am J Med Genet* 35:286–288, 1990.
Martin AO, Perrin JCS, Muir WA, Ruch E, Schafer IA: An autosomal dominant midline cleft syndrome resembling familial holoprosencephaly. *Clin Genet* 12:65–72, 1977.
McGahan JP, Nyberg DA, Mack LA: Sonography of facial features of alobar and semilobar holoprosencephaly. *AJR Am J Roentgenol* 154:143–148, 1990.
Morse RP, Rawnsley E, Sargent SK, Graham JM: Prenatal diagnosis of a new syndrome: holoprosencephaly with hypokinesia. *Prenat Diagn* 7:631–638, 1987.
Nelson LH, King M: Early diagnosis of holoprosencephaly. *J Ultrasound Med* 11:57–59, 1977.
Nyberg DA, Mack LA, Bronshtein A, Hirsch J, Pagon RA: Holoprosencephaly: prenatal sonographic diagnosis. *AJR Am J Roentgenol* 149:1051–1058, 1987.
Papageorghiou AT, Avgidou K, Spencer K, Nix B, Nicolaides KH: Sonographic screening for trisomy 13 at 11 to 13(+6) weeks of gestation. *Am J Obstet Gynecol* 194:397–401, 2006.
Pilu G, Romero R, Rizzo N, et al: Criteria for the prenatal diagnosis of holoprosencephaly. *Am J Perinatol* 4:41–49, 1987.
Sepulveda W, Dezerega V, Be C: First-trimester sonographic diagnosis of holoprosencephaly: value of the "butterfly" sign. *J Ultrasound Med* 23:761–765, 2004.
Turner CD, Silva S, Jeanty P: Prenatal diagnosis of alobar holoprosencephaly at 10 weeks of gestation. *Ultrasound Obstet Gynecol* 13:360–362, 1999.
Wong HS, Lam YH, Tang MH, Cheung LW, Ng LK, Yan KW: First-trimester ultrasound diagnosis of holoprosencephaly: three case reports. *Ultrasound Obstet Gynecol* 13:356–359, 1999.

IDIOPATHIC ARTERIAL CALCIFICATION OF INFANCY

DESCRIPTION AND DEFINITION

Synonym: Occlusive infantile arterial calcification

First described by Bryant and White in 1901, this is a rare syndrome characterized by disruption and calcification of the internal elastic laminae of fetal arteries, with calcium deposits leading to fibrosis and occlusion of the arteries.

ABNORMALITIES DETECTABLE BY ULTRASOUND

Common Findings (Third Trimester Only):

Hydrops

Calcification of main vascular channels, particularly calcification of the aorta and pulmonary artery

Pericardial effusion

Polyhydramnios

MAJOR DIFFERENTIAL DIAGNOSES

Other Syndromes Associated with Hydrops but Not Characterized by Extensive Calcifications of the Vascular Channels:

Achondrogenesis

Alpha-thalassemia

Anemia

Arteriovenous shunt (aneurysm of the vein of Galen)

Bradycardia

Cardiac defect

Cardiomyopathy

Cardiovascular anomalies

Chest masses (causing mediastinal compression) (see Chapter 1, Intrathoracic Mass, p. 61, for differential diagnoses)

Chorioangioma

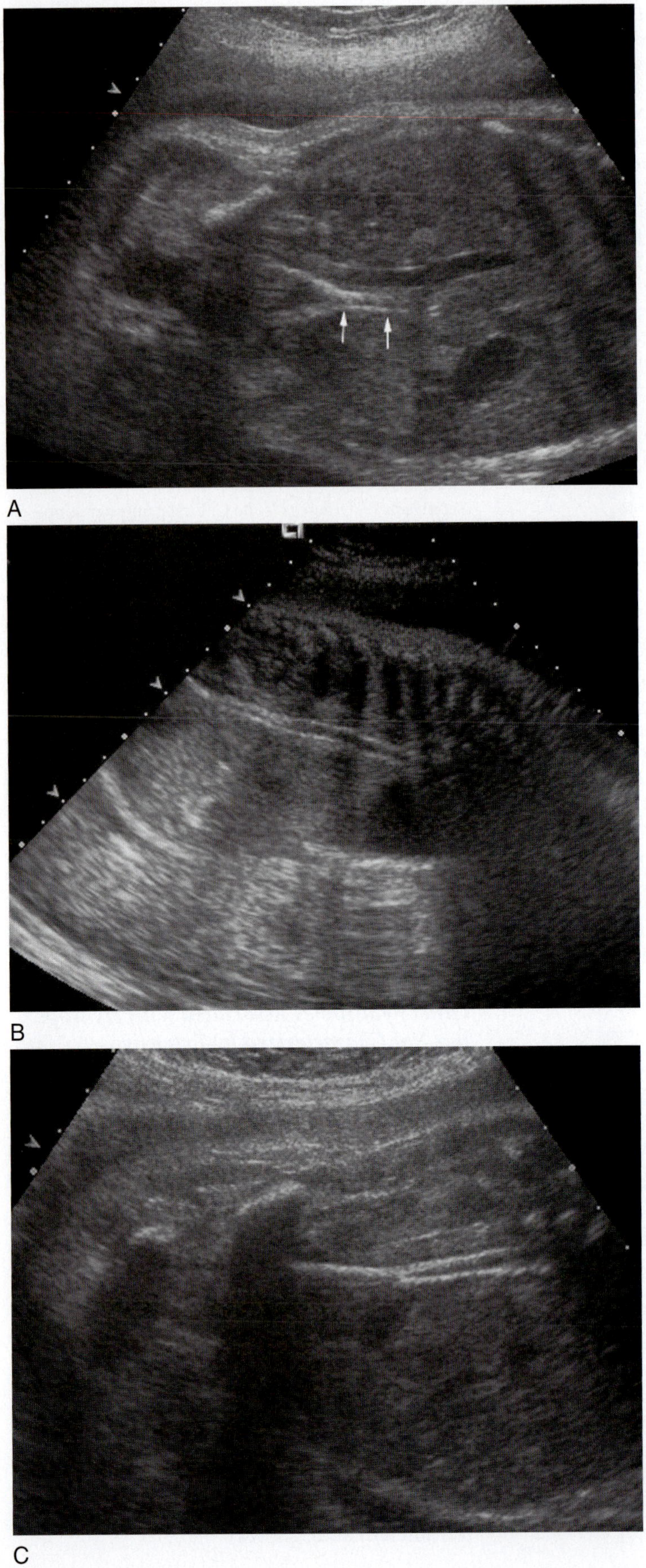

FIGURE 2-232 Idiopathic arterial calcification of infancy. (A) Calcification of a descending aorta and bifurcation with the iliac arteries *(arrows)* in a third-trimester fetus with the syndrome. (B, C) Longitudinal views of the fetal abdomen show calcification of the entire abdominal aorta. This finding was not apparent until after 24 weeks.

Chromosomal anomalies

Congenital high airway obstruction syndrome

Cri du chat syndrome

Cystic hygroma

CMV

Fetal–maternal hemorrhage

Fryns syndrome

Gastrointestinal obstructions

Glycogen storage diseases

Hepatic tumor (hemangioendothelioma)

Isoimmune parvovirus

Lymphangioma

Maternal infections

Multiple pterygium syndrome

Neu-Laxova syndrome

Noonan syndrome

Osteogenesis imperfecta

Parvovirus

Pena Shokeir syndrome

Short rib–polydactyly syndrome, types I and III

Syphilis

Tachycardia

Teratoma

Toxoplasmosis

Trisomy 21 (Down syndrome) (occasionally)

Tumors

Twin-to-twin transfusion syndrome

Varicella

Various other conditions (see Chapter 1, p. 111)

Various other trisomies

XO syndrome (Turner syndrome)

ULTRASOUND DIAGNOSIS

This syndrome has been diagnosed in the third trimester, from 28 to 30–32 weeks' gestation. It is manifested by severe hydrops associated with extensive calcifications of the ascending and descending aorta and central pulmonary artery.

HEREDITY

This is an autosomal recessive syndrome.

NATURAL HISTORY AND OUTCOME

This idiopathic syndrome of arterial calcification affects the arterial internal elastic lamina. Calcium hydroxyapatite is deposited into the layer of internal elastic lamina, leading to fibrosis and occlusion of these arteries. In turn, narrowing and occlusion of the arteries leads to hydrops fetalis, cardiac ischemia, vascular injury, neonatal infarction, and fetal or neonatal death.

Suggested Reading

Crade M, Lewis DF, Nageott MP: In utero appearance of idiopathic infantile arterial calcification: ultrasound study of a 28-week fetus. *Ultrasound Obstet Gynecol* 1:284–285, 1991.

Eronen M, Pohjavuori M, Heikkila P: Fatal outcome of 2 siblings with idiopathic arterial calcification of infancy diagnoses in utero. *Pediatr Cardiol* 22:167–169, 2001.

Levine JC, Campbell J, Nadal A: Prenatal diagnosis of idiopathic infantile arterial calcification. *Circulation* 103:325–326, 2001.

Nager AM, Hanchate V, Tandon A, Thakkar H, Chaubal NG: Antenatal detection of idiopathic arterial calcification with hydrops fetalis. *J Ultrasound Med* 22:653–659, 2003.

Rosenbaum DM, Blumhagen JD: Sonographic recognition of idiopathic arterial calcification of infancy. *AJR Am J Roentgenol* 146:249–250, 1986.

Samon LM, Ash KM, Murdison KA: Aorto-pulmonary calcification: an unusual manifestation of idiopathic calcification of infancy evident antenatally. *Obstet Gynecol* 85:863–865, 1995.

Spear R, Mack LA, Benedetti TJ, Cole RE: Idiopathic infantile arterial calcification in utero diagnosis. *J Ultrasound Med* 9:473–476, 1990.

KLIPPEL-FEIL SEQUENCE

DESCRIPTION AND DEFINITION

Originally described in 1912, this sequence includes abnormal cervical vertebrae, webbed neck, and facial asymmetry. It may be the result of a problem in early neural tube development and is found in association with cases of iniencephaly and syringomyelia.

ABNORMALITIES DETECTABLE BY ULTRASOUND

Common Findings:

Cervical vertebral anomalies

Short neck

Low-set ears

Facial asymmetry

Occasional Findings:

Cleft palate

Congenital cardiac defects

Rib defects

Sprengel abnormalities

Scoliosis

Renal anomalies

MAJOR DIFFERENTIAL DIAGNOSES

Other Syndromes and Conditions Associated with Segmental Vertebral Defects of the Upper Spine:

Apert syndrome (C5–C6)

Cerebrocostomandibular syndrome

Goldenhar syndrome (upper spine)

Gorlin syndrome

Jarcho-Levin syndrome

MURCS (**mü**llerian duct aplasia, **r**enal aplasia, **c**ervicothoracic **s**omite dysplasia) association (C5–T1)

Noonan syndrome

Spondylocostal dysplasia

VATER (**v**ertebral defects, **a**nal atresia, **t**racheo-esophageal fistula, **e**sophageal atresia, and **r**adial and renal dysplasias) association

ULTRASOUND DIAGNOSIS

Although prenatal diagnosis of this syndrome has not been officially reported, I had a recent case that was consistent with the sequence and is illustrated here. Findings included a very

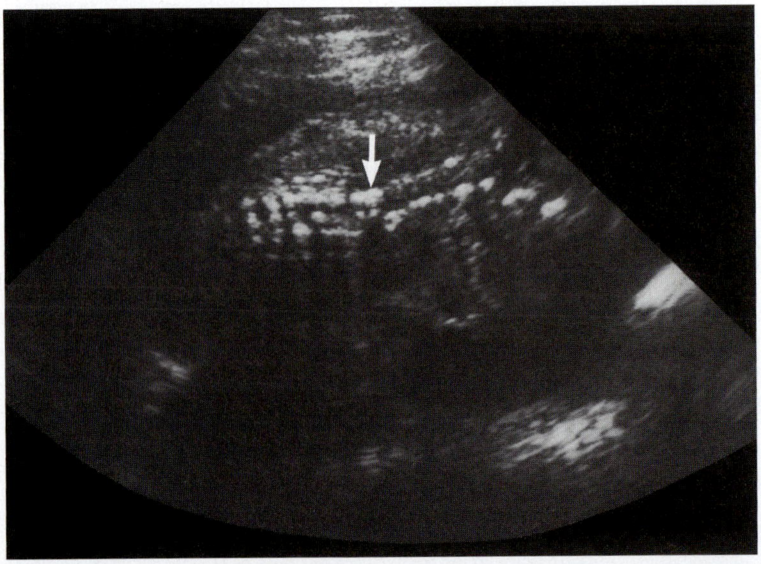

FIGURE 2-233 Oblique view through the fetal cervical and upper thoracic vertebrae shows a hemivertebra at the junction of the cervical and thoracic spine *(arrow)* in a fetus presumed to have Klippel-Feil syndrome.

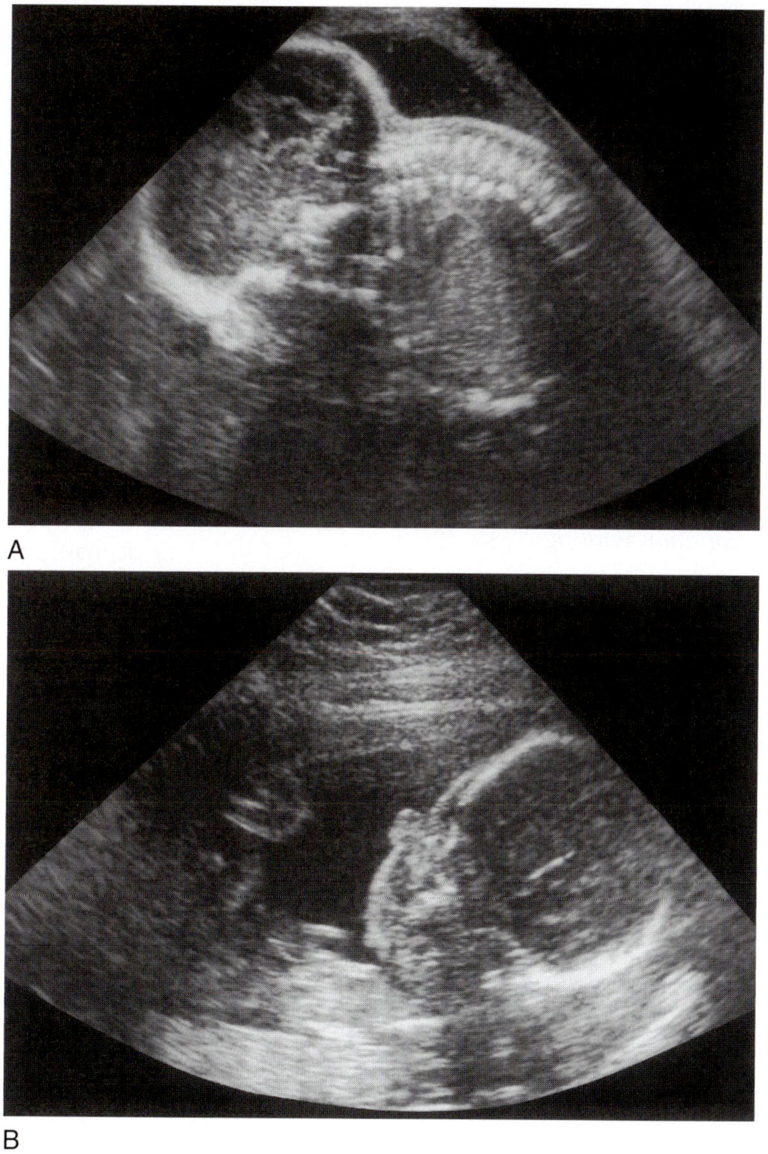

FIGURE 2-234 (A) Longitudinal view of the cervical spine of the same fetus as in Figure 2-233 shows a short neck, with the occipital aspect of the fetal head in close proximity to the first thoracic vertebra. The fetal shoulders are located just below the level of the head, with no visible neck area. (B) View of the fetal ear shows a malformed, small external ear. This fetus was presumed to have Klippel-Feil syndrome, although a full evaluation of the products of conception was not possible because of the method of termination.

short neck, with the inferior aspect of the cranium practically resting on the fetal shoulders.

HEREDITY

The sequence occurs sporadically, and its etiology is unknown. There have been reports of autosomal dominant inheritance with variable penetrance.

NATURAL HISTORY AND OUTCOME

Some mobility problems of the neck may be encountered. Those with hypermobility may be at risk for neurologic complications. Deafness is noted in up to 30% of affected individuals.

Suggested Reading

Bauman GI: Absence of the cervical spine: Klippel-Feil syndrome. *JAMA* 98:129–132, 1932.

Clemmesen V: Congenital cervical synostosis (Klippel-Feil's syndrome): four cases. *Acta Radiol* 17:480–490, 1936.

Gunderson CH, Greenspan RH, Glaser GH, Lubs HA: The Klippel-Feil syndrome: genetic and clinical reevaluation of cervical fusion. *Medicine* 46:491–512, 1967.

Jones KL: *Smith's recognizable patterns of human malformations,* ed 6. Philadelphia, 2006, Elsevier.

Klippel M, Feil A: Un cas d'absence des vertebres cervicales, avec cage thoracique remontant jusqu'a la base du crane (cage thoracique cervicale). *Mouv Inconogr Salpet* 25:223, 1912.

MEGACYSTIS–MICROCOLON–INTESTINAL HYPOPERISTALSIS SYNDROME

DESCRIPTION AND DEFINITION

Synonym: MMIHS

This lethal syndrome is characterized by a dilated urinary bladder resulting from lack of muscle tone in the urinary tract and hypoperistalsis of the gastrointestinal tract.

ABNORMALITIES DETECTABLE BY ULTRASOUND

Common Findings:

Dilated bladder, with a keyhole appearance of the posterior urethra

Enlarged stomach

Hydronephrosis

Amniotic fluid volume may vary between oligohydramnios and polyhydramnios

Occasional Finding:

Omphalocele

MAJOR DIFFERENTIAL DIAGNOSES

Cloacal abnormality

Posterior urethral valves

Prune-belly syndrome

ULTRASOUND DIAGNOSIS

The diagnosis of megacystis–microcolon–intestinal hypoperistalsis has been made at 26 weeks' gestation, with detection of multiple anomalies such as dilated bladder, enlarged stomach, dilated bowel, and hydronephrosis. However, the syndrome has been detected as early as 19 and 20 weeks' gestation, seen as a cystic mass in the fetus, a small omphalocele, and bilateral fetal hydronephrosis. The volume of amniotic fluid was normal.

HEREDITY

This is an autosomal recessive condition.

NATURAL HISTORY AND OUTCOME

This is a lethal syndrome, with most affected infants dying in the neonatal period. There is a predominance of affected females versus males. This syndrome is caused by decreased muscle tone in the intestinal and urinary tracts, leading to pseudo-obstruction of both the urinary and gastrointestinal tracts.

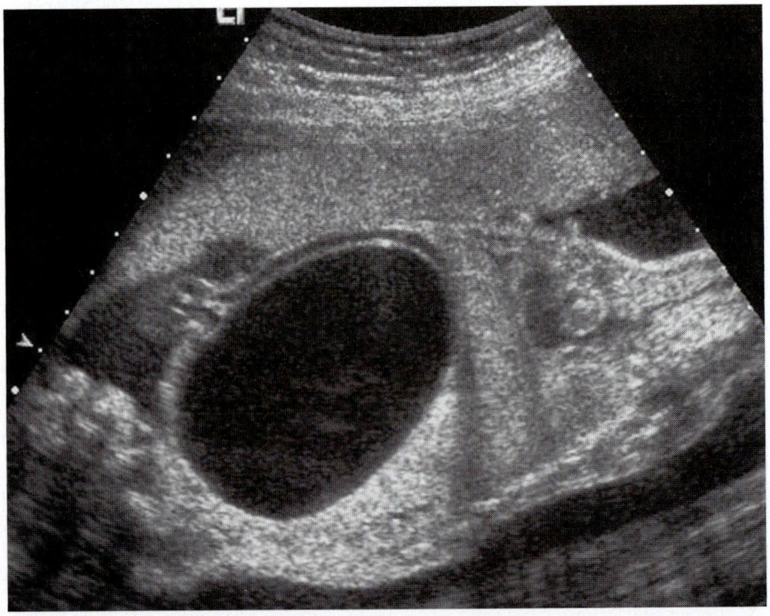

A

FIGURE 2-235 Megacystis–microcolon–intestinal hypoperistalsis syndrome (A) Longitudinal view of the fetal chest and abdomen shows a severely dilated bladder.

Continued

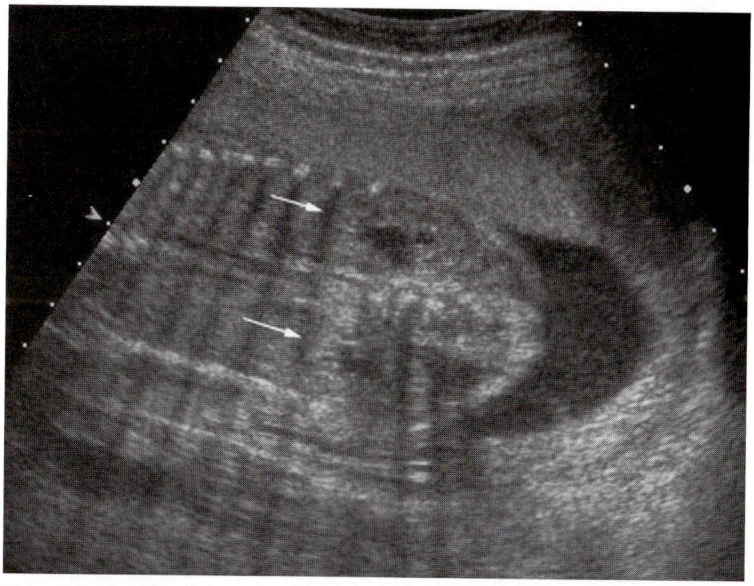

B

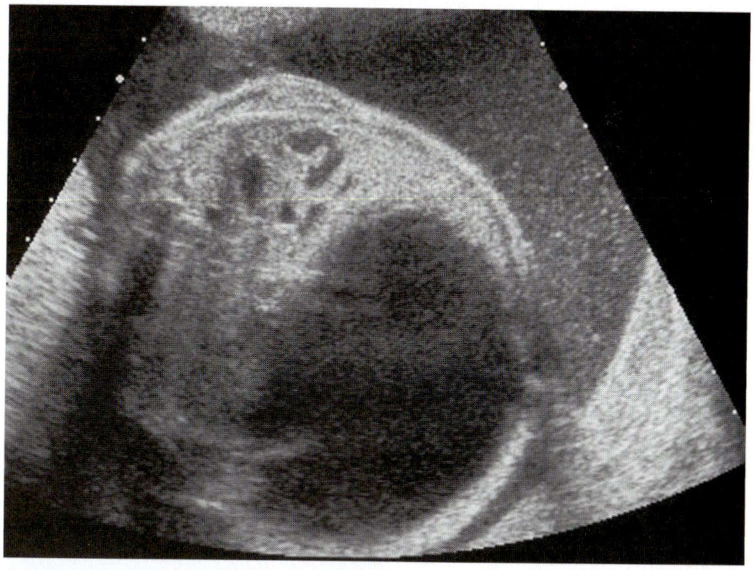

C

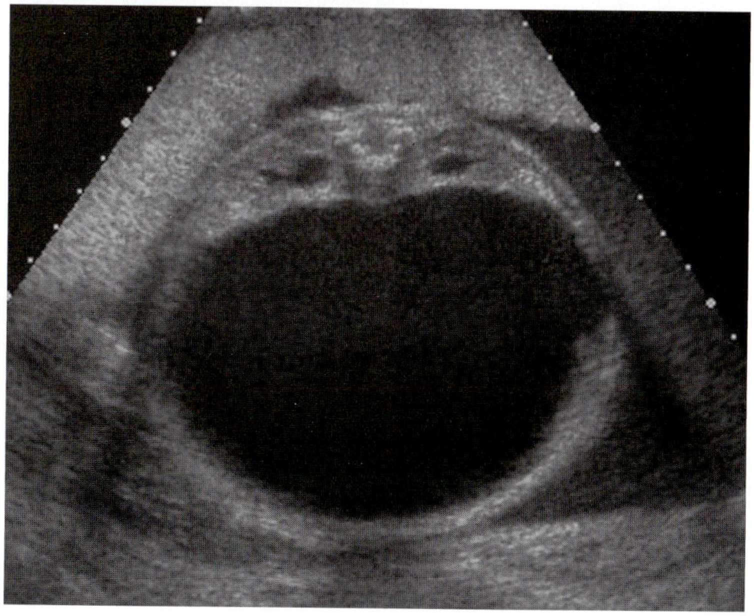

D

FIGURE 2-235, cont'd (B) Coronal view through the fetal kidneys *(arrows)* shows bilateral hydronephrosis. (C) Cross-section through the fetal abdomen shows a distended bladder and fetal hydronephrosis. (D) Transverse view through the back of the fetus at the level of the kidneys shows a severely dilated bladder and bilateral fetal hydronephrosis in the third trimester. Note that these images show the presence of amniotic fluid.

Suggested Reading

Annernen G, Meurling S, Olsen L: Megacystis-microcolon-intestinal hypoperistalsis syndrome (MMIHS), an autosomal recessive disorder: clinical reports and review of the literature. *Am J Med Genet* 441:251–254, 1991.

Farrel SA: Intrauterine death in megacystis-microcolon-intestinal hypoperistalsis syndrome. *J Med Genet* 25:350–352, 1988.

Hsu CD, Craig C, Pavlik J, Ninios A: Prenatal diagnosis of megacystis-microcolon-intestinal hypoperistalsis syndrome in one fetus of a twin pregnancy. *Am J Perinatol* 20:215–218, 2003.

Manco LG, Psterdahl P: the antenatal sonographic features of megacystis-microcolon-intestinal hypoperistalsis syndrome. *J Clin Ultrasound* 12:595–598, 1984.

Muller F, Dreux S, Vaast P, et al.; Study Group of the French Fetal Medicine Society. Prenatal diagnosis of megacystis-microcolon-intestinal hypoperistalsis syndrome: contribution of amniotic fluid digestive enzyme assay and fetal urinalysis. *Prenat Diagn* 25:203–209, 2005.

Nelson LH, Reiff RH: Megacystis-microcolon-intestinal hypoperistalsis syndrome and anechoic areas in the fetal abdomen. *Am J Obstet Gynecol* 144:464–467, 1982.

Penman DG, Lilford RJ: Megacystis-microcolon-intestinal hypoperistalsis syndrome: a fatal autosomal recessive condition. *J Med Genet* 26:66–67, 1989.

Stamm E, King G, Thickman D: Megacystis-microcolon-intestinal hypoperistalsis syndrome: prenatal identification in siblings and review of the literature. *J Ultrasound Med* 10:599–602, 1991.

Verbruggen SC, Wijnen RM, van den Berg P: Megacystis-microcolon-intestinal hypoperistalsis syndrome: a case report. *J Matern Fetal Neonatal Med* 16:140–141, 2004.

Vezina WC, Morin FR, Winsberg F: Megacystis-microcolon-intestinal hypoperistalsis syndrome: antenatal ultrasound appearance. *AJR Am J Roentgenol* 133:749–750, 1979.

Vinograd I, Mogle P, Lernau OZ, Nissan S: Megacystis-microcolon-intestinal hypoperistalsis syndrome. *Arch Dis Child* 59:169–171, 1984.

White SM, Chamberlain P, Hitchcock R, Sullivan PB, Boyd PA: Megacystis-microcolon-intestinal hypoperistalsis syndrome: the difficulties with antenatal diagnosis. Case report and review of the literature. *Prenat Diagn* 20:697–700, 2000.

Young ID, McKeever PA, Brown LA, Lang GD: Prenatal diagnosis of the megacystis-microcolon-intestinal hypoperistalsis syndrome. *J Med Genet* 26:403–406, 1989.

MURCS ASSOCIATION

DESCRIPTION AND DEFINITION

Described in 1979, this sequence comprises **m**üllerian duct aplasia, **r**enal aplasia, and **c**ervicothoracic **s**omite dysplasia.

ABNORMALITIES DETECTABLE BY ULTRASOUND

Common Findings:

Vertebral abnormalities of the lower cervical/upper thoracic region (C5–T1)

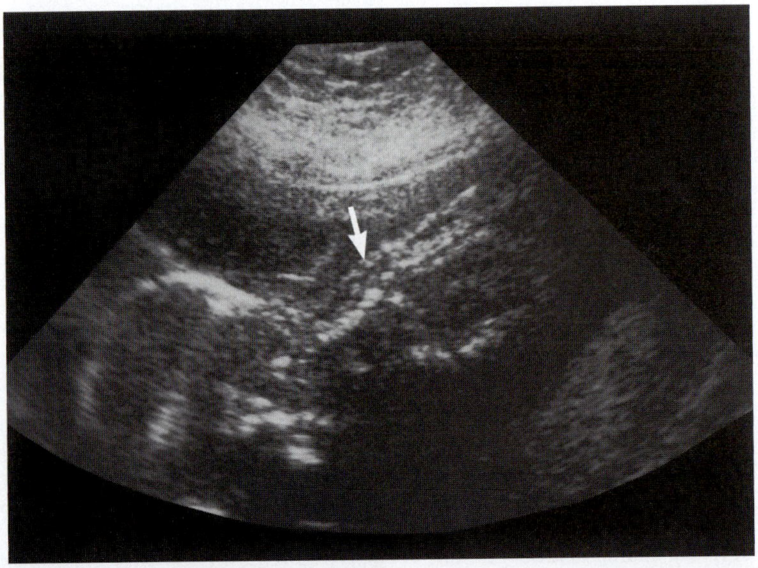

FIGURE 2-236 Longitudinal view of the fetal upper thoracic spine. Note the vertebral abnormalities involving the upper part of the spine *(arrow)*, as can be seen in fetuses with MURCS association.

Hypoplasia of the uterus and part of the vagina

Renal agenesis or ectopia

Occasional Findings:

Cerebellar cysts

Facial and external ear anomalies

Cleft lip and palate

Micrognathia

Rib deformities

Upper limb and scapular abnormalities

MAJOR DIFFERENTIAL DIAGNOSES

Because the manifestations of this association differ among individuals, the differential diagnosis varies according to the types of defects included.

Syndromes and Conditions Associated with Vertebral Defects of the Lower Cervical Spine:

Apert syndrome

Cerebrocostomandibular syndrome

Goldenhar syndrome

Gorlin syndrome

Jarcho-Levin syndrome

Klippel-Feil malformation sequence

Noonan syndrome

Syndromes and Conditions Associated with Vertebral Anomalies and/or Renal Agenesis:

Caudal regression sequence

Fraser syndrome

Sacral agenesis

Sirenomelia

VATER (**v**ertebral defects, **a**nal atresia, **t**racheoesophageal fistula, **e**sophageal atresia, and **r**adial and renal dysplasias) association

ULTRASOUND DIAGNOSIS

MURCS association has been identified sonographically at 21 weeks' gestation, based on severe oligohydramnios; dilated urinary bladder; cystic anterior mass (superior to the bladder dome) consistent with patent urachus; unilateral absence of a kidney; cystic umbilical cord; and vertebral abnormality of the upper thoracic region.

HEREDITY

The pattern of inheritance and the etiology of this association are unknown.

NATURAL HISTORY AND OUTCOME

The outcome depends on the severity and types of abnormalities present in each individual case. Rokitansky malformation, a condition included in the MURCS association, includes atretic vagina, rudimentary uterus, and lack of menstruation. When the MURCS association includes renal agenesis or urethral agenesis, no survival is possible.

Suggested Reading

Duncan PA, Shapiro LR, Stangel JJ, et al: The MURCS association: Müllerian duct aplasia, renal aplasia, and cervicothoracic somite dysplasia. *J Pediatr* 95:399–402, 1979.

Fernandez CO, McFarland RD, Timmons C, Ramus R, Twickler DM: MURCS association: ultrasonographic findings and pathologic correlation. *J Ultrasound Med* 15:867–870, 1996.

Jones KL: *Smith's recognizable patterns of human malformations,* ed 6. Philadelphia, 2006, Elsevier.

OPITZ SYNDROME

DESCRIPTION AND DEFINITION

Synonyms: Opitz G/BBB syndrome, hypospadias-dysphagia syndrome

This syndrome is characterized by ocular hypertelorism and, in males, hypospadias.

ABNORMALITIES DETECTABLE BY ULTRASOUND

Common Findings:

Ocular hypertelorism

Cleft lip and/or palate

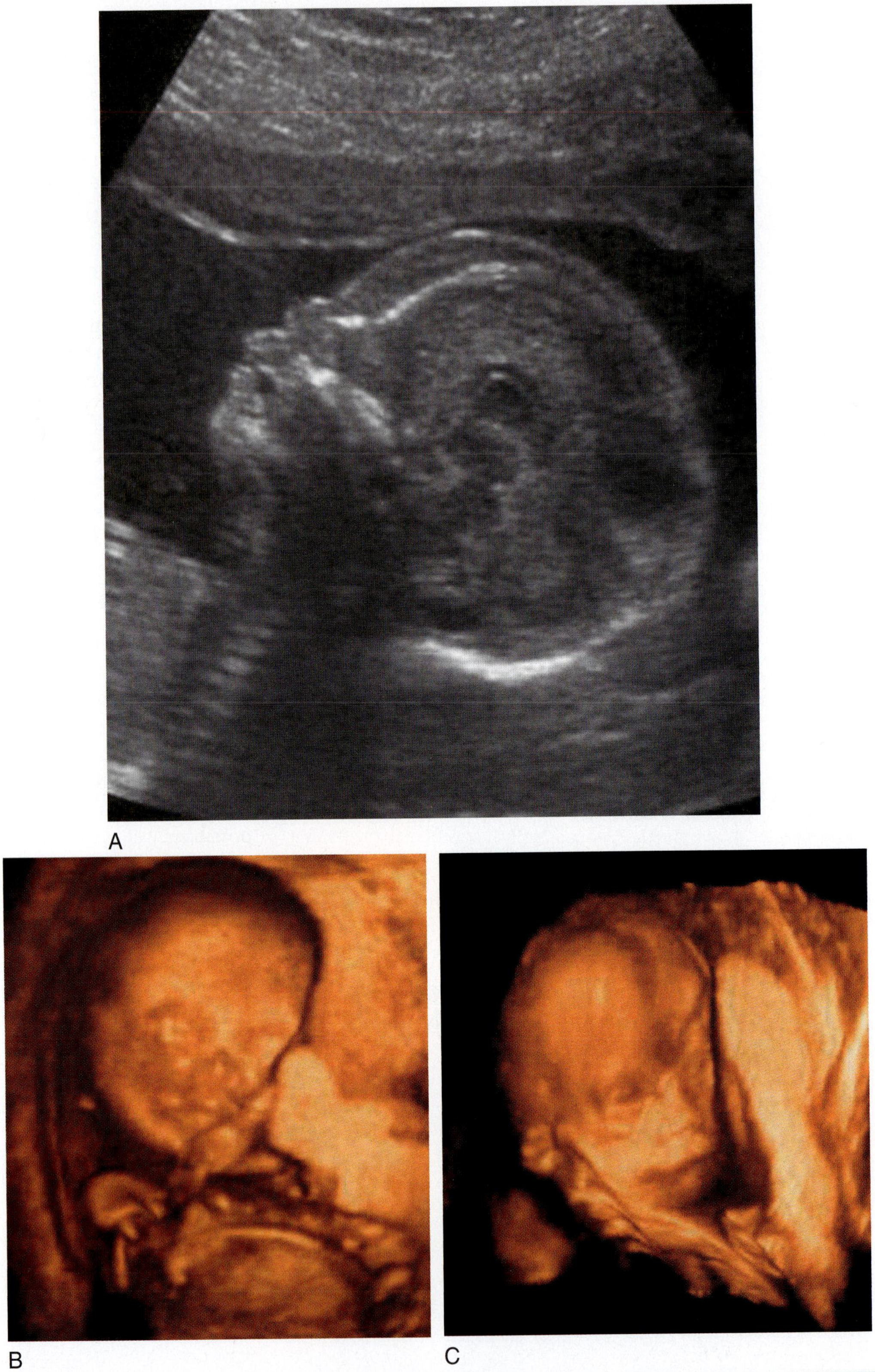

FIGURE 2-237 Opitz syndrome. (A) Longitudinal view of the fetal profile shows thickened soft tissues at the level of the forehead. (B, C) Three-dimensional surface image of the fetal face shows a high forehead associated with apparent hypertelorism, typical of the syndrome.

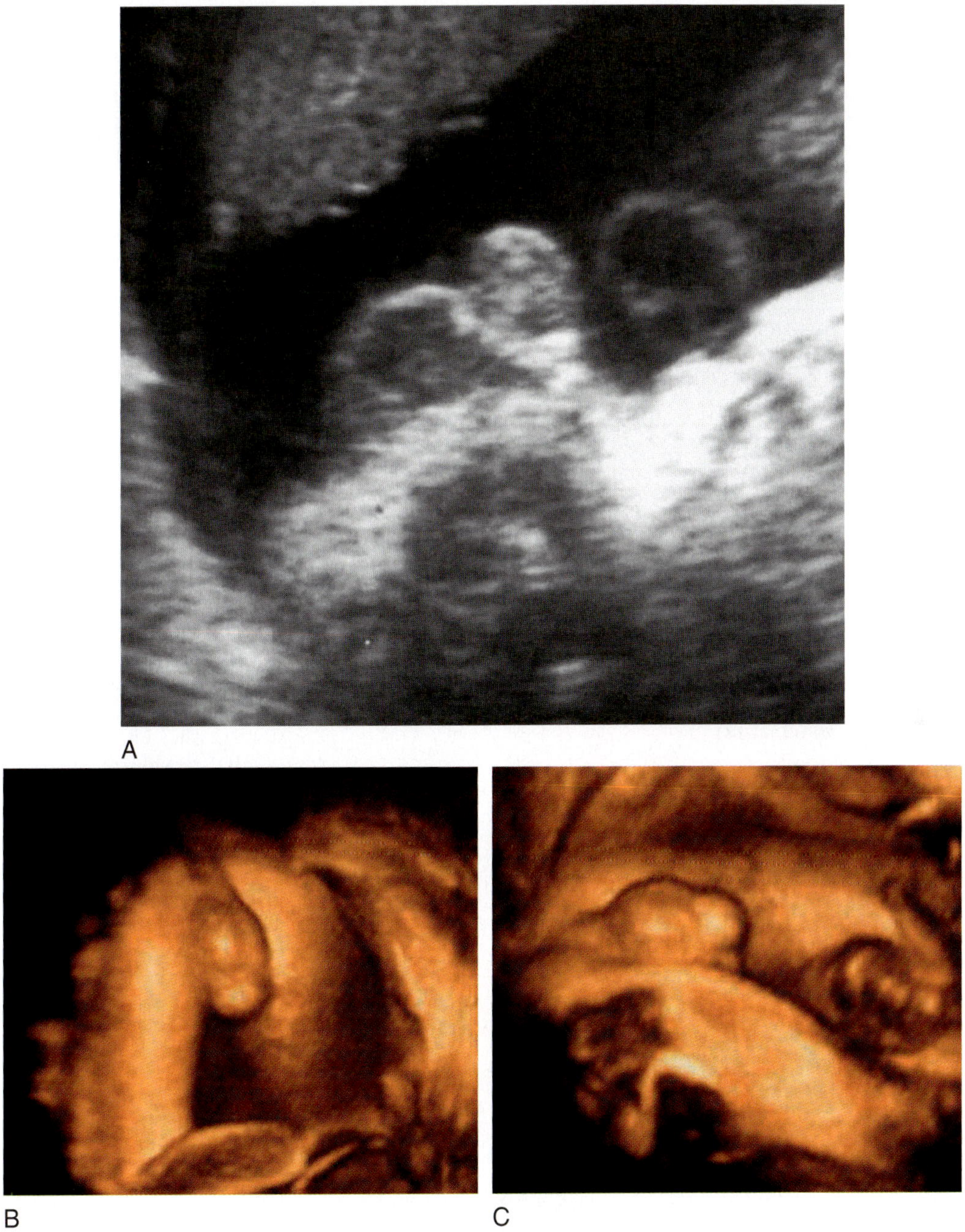

FIGURE 2-238 (A) Hypospadias, as evidenced by the chordee of the penis, indicating displacement of the urethral opening. (B, C) Surface rendering of the genitals of a fetus with hypospadias show the bend in the penis, making it appear short because of the chordee.

Micrognathia

Hypospadias

Cryptorchidism

Occasional Findings:

Agenesis of the corpus callosum

Ventriculomegaly

Cerebellar vermian hypoplasia

Cardiac defect

Renal abnormalities

MAJOR DIFFERENTIAL DIAGNOSES

Apert syndrome

CHARGE (**c**oloboma of the iris, **h**eart defect, choanal **a**tresia, intrauterine growth **r**estriction, **g**enital anomalies, and **e**ar anomalies) association

Crouzon syndrome

Median cleft face (hypertelorism)

Noonan syndrome

Smith-Lemli-Opitz syndrome (genital abnormalities)

ULTRASOUND DIAGNOSIS

The diagnosis of Opitz syndrome is possible in the third trimester, based on the presence of abnormal genitalia and hypertelorism with a flat facies.

HEREDITY

There are several forms of this syndrome, including an X-linked form that maps to locus Xp22.3 (MID1). There is also an autosomal dominant form, linked to 22q11.2.

NATURAL HISTORY AND OUTCOME

Because these individuals have malformations of the larynx and tracheoesophageal fistulas, their symptoms are related to swallowing issues and aspiration. In severe cases, early mortality usually is related to problems with potentially lethal laryngoesophageal defects.

Suggested Reading

Cox TC, Allen LR, Cox LL, et al: New mutations in MID1 provide support for loss of function as the cause of X-linked Opitz syndrome. *Hum Mol Genet* 9:2553–2562, 2000.

De Falco F, Cainarca S, Andolfi G, et al: X-linked Opitz syndrome: novel mutations in the MID1 gene and redefinition of the clinical spectrum. *Am J Med Genet* 120A:222–228, 2003.

Jones KL: *Smith's recognizable patterns of human malformations,* ed 6. Philadelphia, 2006, Elsevier.

PENA SHOKEIR SYNDROME

DESCRIPTION AND DEFINITION

Synonyms: Fetal akinesia/hypokinesia sequence, neurogenic arthrogryposis

Described by Pena and Shokeir in 1974, this syndrome is characterized by IUGR, polyhydramnios, multiple joint contractures, facial anomalies, and pulmonary hypoplasia.

ABNORMALITIES DETECTABLE BY ULTRASOUND

Common Findings:

Limb abnormalities

Multiple contractures and ankylosis

Ulnar deviation of the hands

Cardiac defect

Clenched hands

Club feet

Camptodactyly

Facial abnormalities

Hypertelorism

Micrognathia

Depressed nasal bridge

Hypoplastic lungs

Cryptorchidism

Polyhydramnios

Occasional Findings:

Cleft palate

Cardiac anomalies

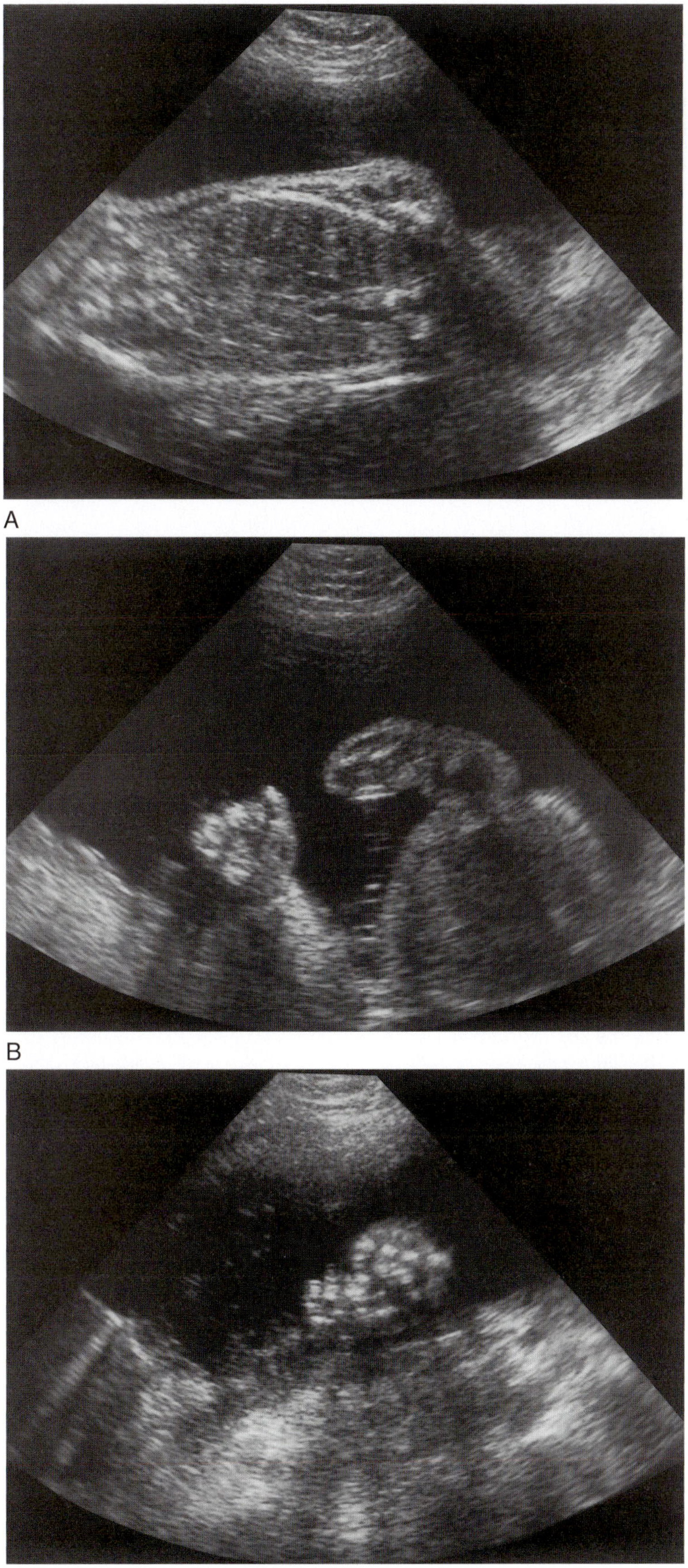

FIGURE 2-239 (A–C) Fetus with Pena Shokeir syndrome has evidence of polyhydramnios and clenched hands. (B, C) Both hands clearly are clenched. This fetus exhibited very little activity.

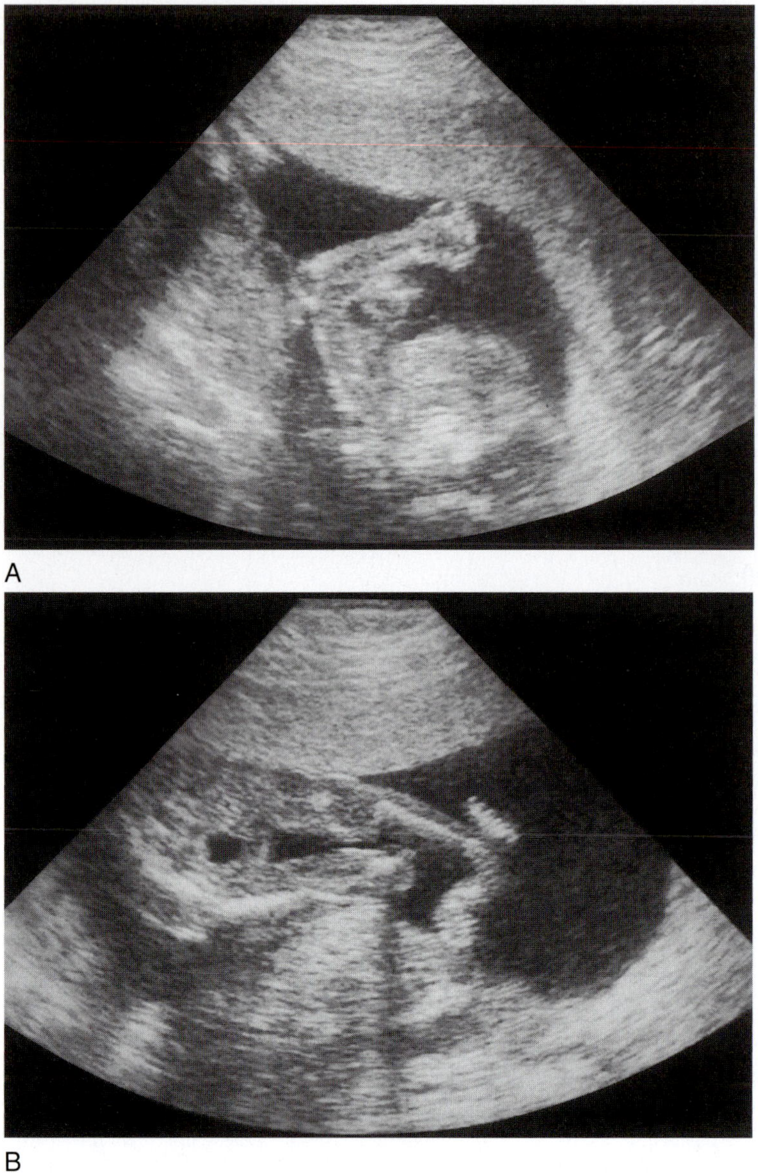

FIGURE 2-240 Views of the upper (A) and lower (B) extremities of a fetus with multiple contractures and little, if any, activity. Note that the feet are club and the hands are clenched. There is hyperextension at the knees and flexion contractures at the elbow.

MAJOR DIFFERENTIAL DIAGNOSES*

Antley-Bixler syndrome (contractures)

Arthrogryposis (contractures of greater severity)

Cerebro-oculo-facio-skeletal (COFS) syndrome (contractures)

Freeman-Sheldon syndrome (contractures)

Multiple pterygium syndrome (cystic hygroma, flexion contractures)

Smith-Lemli-Opitz syndrome (clenched hands)

Stickler syndrome (micrognathia)

*See also Chapter 1, Club Foot and Contractures of the Extremities, pp. 104 and 91, for differential diagnoses.

Trisomy 18 (Edwards' syndrome) (multiple organ system abnormalities)

ULTRASOUND DIAGNOSIS

Prenatal ultrasound diagnosis has been established at 12 weeks' gestation, based on an abnormal movement profile and abnormal limb position in a patient at risk for the syndrome. Other cases have been detected as limb position anomalies, lack of movement, hypertelorism, and micrognathia at 14 to 16 weeks initially, confirmed later in pregnancy. Limb positioning is similar to that found in trisomy 18, and karyotyping is needed to distinguish the two conditions. Other sonographic findings associated with Pena Shokeir syndrome include narrow chest, cryptorchidism, camptodactyly, micrognathia, polyhydramnios (usually third trimester), nonimmune hydrops, and IUGR.

HEREDITY

The pattern of heredity for this syndrome is autosomal recessive, although there have been a few sporadic cases.

NATURAL HISTORY AND OUTCOME

Most affected fetuses are stillborn or die shortly after birth. Ninety-two percent of affected liveborn infants die within the first month of life.

Suggested Reading

Ajayi RA, Keen CE, Knott PD: Ultrasound diagnosis of the Pena Shokeir phenotype at 14 weeks of pregnancy. *Prenat Diagn* 15:762–764, 1995.

Bacino CA, Platt LD, Garber A, et al: Fetal akinesia/hypokinesia sequence: prenatal diagnosis and intrafamilial variability. *Prenat Diagn* 13:1011–1019, 1993.

Cardwell MS: Pena-Shokeir syndrome: prenatal diagnosis by ultrasonography. *J Ultrasound Med* 6:619–621, 1987.

Chen H, Blumberg B, Immken L, et al: The Pena-Shokeir syndrome: report of five cases and further delineation of the syndrome. *Am J Med Genet* 16:213–224, 1983.

Davis JE, Kalousek DK: Fetal akinesia deformation sequence in previable fetuses. *Am J Med Genet* 29: 77–87, 1988.

Genkins SM, Hertzberg BS, Bowie JD, Blow O: Pena-Shokeir type I syndrome: in utero sonographic appearance. *J Clin Ultrasound* 17:56–61, 1989.

Grischke EM, Stolz W, Linderkamp O, Bastert G: Pena-Shokeir syndrome, type I. *Fetus* 1:1–3, 1991.

Hageman G, Willemse J, van Ketel BA, Barth PG, Lindhout D: The heterogeneity of the Pena-Shokeir syndrome. *Neuropediatrics* 18:45–50, 1987.

Herva R, Leisti J, Kirkinen P, Seppanen U: A lethal autosomal recessive syndrome of multiple congenital contractures. *Am J Med Genet* 20:431–439, 1985.

Jones KL: *Smith's recognizable patterns of human malformations,* ed 6. Philadelphia, 2006, Elsevier.

MacMillan RH, Harbert GM, Davis WD, Kelly TE: Prenatal diagnosis of Pena-Shokeir syndrome type I. *Am J Med Genet* 21:279–284, 1985.

Mulder EJ, Nikkels PG, Visser GH: Fetal akinesia deformation sequence: behavioral development in a case of congenital myopathy. *Ultrasound Obstet Gynecol* 18:253–257, 2001.

Muller LM, de Jong G: Prenatal ultrasonographic features of the Pena-Shokeir I syndrome and the trisomy 18 syndrome. *Am J Med Genet* 25:119–129, 1986.

Ochi H, Kobayashi E, Matsubara K, Katayama T, Ito M: Prenatal sonographic diagnosis of Pena-Shokeir syndrome type I. *Ultrasound Obstet Gynecol* 17:546–547, 2001.

Ohlsson A, Fong KW, Rose TH, Moore DC: Prenatal sonographic diagnosis of Pena-Shokeir syndrome type I, or fetal akinesia deformation sequence. *Am J Med Genet* 29:59–65, 1988.

Paladini D, Tartaglione A, Agangi A, Foglia S, Martinelli P, Nappi C: Pena-Shokeir phenotype with variable onset in three consecutive pregnancies. *Ultrasound Obstet Gynecol* 17:163–165, 2001.

Paluda SM, Comstock CH, Kirk JS, Lee W, Smith RS: The significance of ultrasonographically diagnosed fetal wrist position anomalies. *Am J Obstet Gynecol* 174:1834–1839, 1996.

Persutte WH, Lenke RR, Kurczynski TW, Brinker RA: Shokeir syndrome (type I) with ultrasonography and magnetic resonance imaging. *Obstet Gynecol* 72:472–475, 1988.

Shenker L, Reed K, Anderson C, Hauck L, Spark R: Syndrome of camptodactyly, ankyloses, facial anomalies, and pulmonary hypoplasia (Pena-Shokeir syndrome): obstetric and ultrasound aspects. *Am J Obstet Gynecol* 152:303–307, 1985.

Tongsong T, Chanprapaph P, Khunamornpong S: Prenatal ultrasound of regional akinesia with Pena-Shokeir phenotype. *Prenat Diagn* 20:422–425, 2000.

PENTALOGY OF CANTRELL

DESCRIPTION AND DEFINITION

In 1958, Cantrell described a combination of five anomalies recognized as a syndromic complex characterized by thoracoabdominal ectopia cordis. These five defects included ectopia cordis, omphalocele, and disruption of the distal sternum, anterior diaphragm, and diaphragmatic pericardium.

ABNORMALITIES DETECTABLE BY ULTRASOUND

Common Findings:

Large abdominal wall defect, consisting of a combination of an omphalocele and ectopia cordis (appears on ultrasound as a huge thoracoabdominal wall defect containing the heart and much of the abdominal contents)

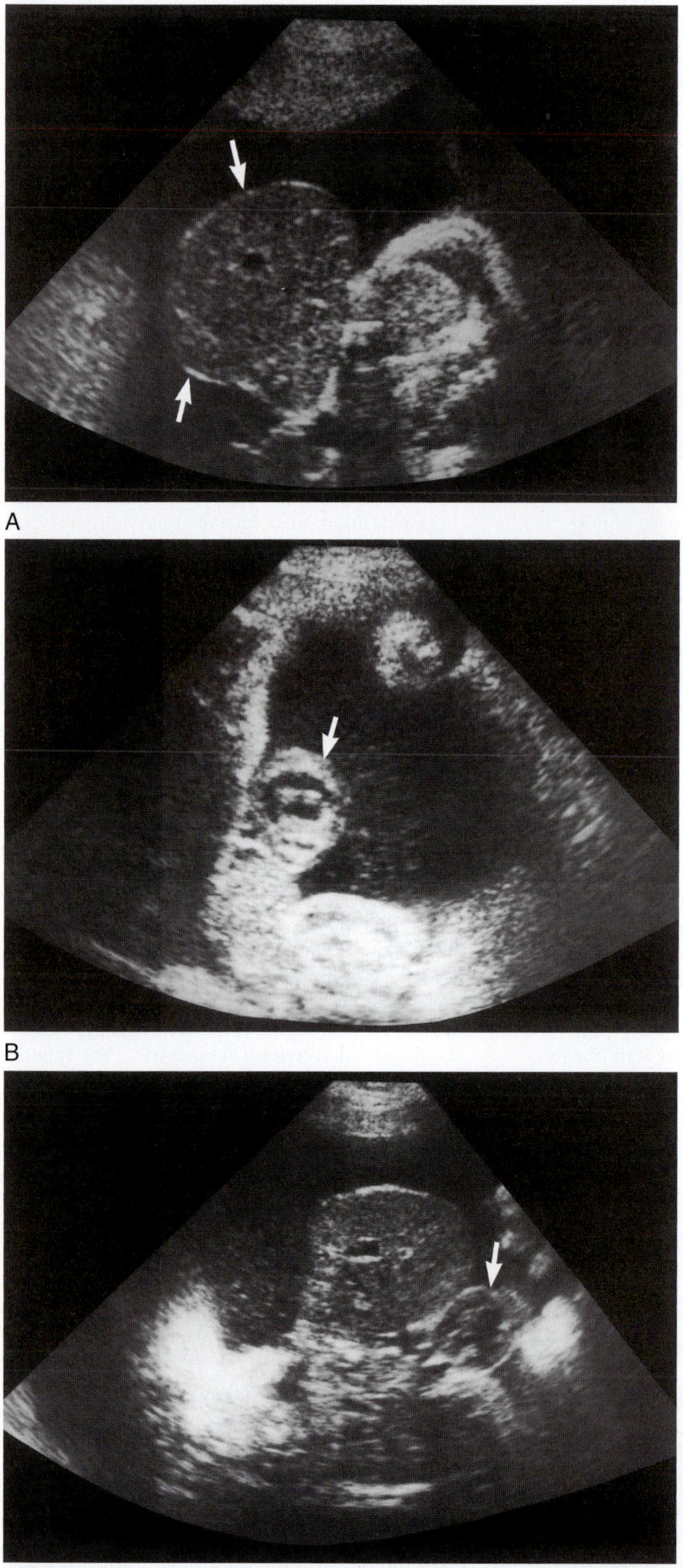

A

B

C

FIGURE 2-241 Third-trimester fetus with pentalogy of Cantrell shows evisceration of the liver, heart, and bowel. (A) Entire liver *(arrows)* is extruded into the amniotic cavity. (B, C) Heart is exteriorized *(arrow)*, and polyhydramnios is evident.

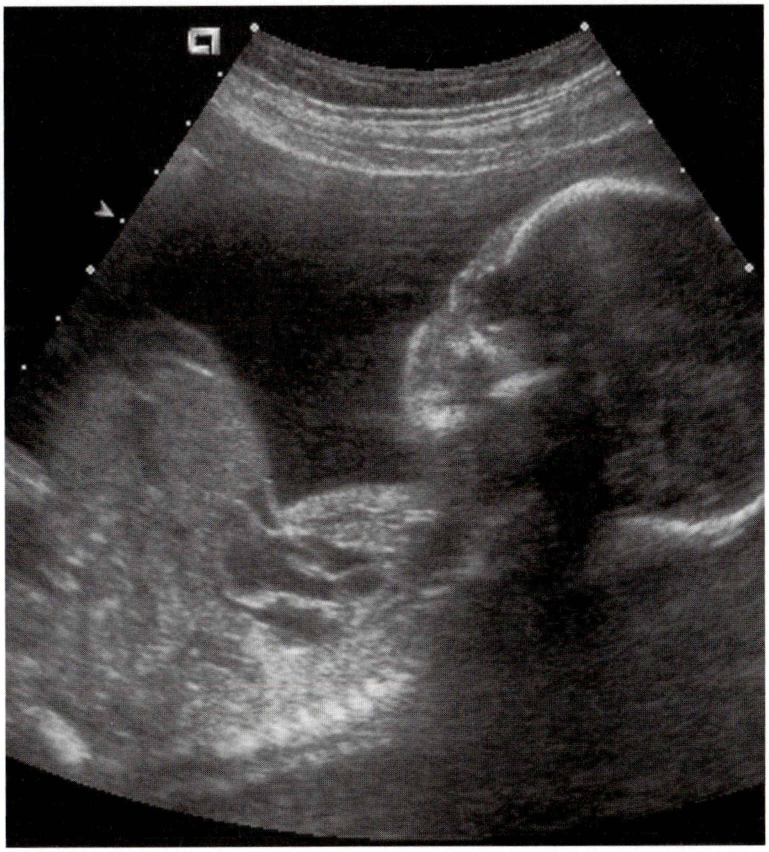

FIGURE 2-242 Pentalogy of Cantrell. Longitudinal view of a late second-trimester fetus with a large high thoracoabdominal defect that includes a defect in the sternum. This situation allows the liver and a portion of the heart to enter the defect.

Intracardiac abnormalities

Tetralogy of Fallot

Thickened nuchal translucency

Occasional Findings:

Neural tube defects

Facial defects

Club feet

Cystic hygroma

Exencephaly

MAJOR DIFFERENTIAL DIAGNOSES*

Amniotic band syndrome

Beckwith-Wiedemann syndrome

Chromosomal abnormalities (with omphalocele)

Isolated omphalocele (see Chapter 1, Omphalocele, p. 55, for differential diagnoses)

Limb–body stalk abnormality

ULTRASOUND DIAGNOSIS

Diagnosis has been established by 10 weeks because of complete disruption of the anterior abdominal and chest walls. Reportedly, the finding of thoracoabdominal ectopia cordis has led to diagnosis in all three trimesters. This syndrome is easily confused with limb–body wall defect and severe cases of amniotic band syndrome.

HEREDITY

The etiology of this condition is unknown. Pathogenesis suggests developmental failure of a segment of the lateral mesoderm in early development, resulting in failure of the ventral wall to close and failure of the sternal primordial bands to fuse. In these cases, defects in the diaphragm, pericardium, and sternum permit protrusion of the cardiac and abdominal structures.

*See also Chapter 1, Anterior Abdominal Wall Defects and Omphalocele, pp. 52, 55, for differential diagnoses.

NATURAL HISTORY AND OUTCOME

Severe cases, involving extrusion of the heart and intraabdominal contents, carry an extremely poor prognosis. Most cases with limb–body wall disruption are lethal. Minor degrees of ectopia cordis, which arise from failure of the sternum to close, are amenable to surgical repair.

Suggested Reading

Abu-Yousef MM, Wrat AB, Williamson RA, Bonsib SM: Antenatal ultrasound diagnosis of variant of pentalogy of Cantrell. *J Ultrasound Med* 6:535–538, 1987.

Craigo SD, Gillieson MS, Cetrulo CL: Pentalogy of Cantrell. *Fetus* 2:1–4, 1992.

Denath FM, Romano W, Solez M, Donnelly D: Ultrasonographic findings of exencephaly in pentalogy of Cantrell: case report and review of the literature. *J Clin Ultrasound* 22:351–354, 1994.

Emanuel PG, Garcia GI, Angtuaco TL: Prenatal detection of anterior abdominal wall defects with US. *Radiographics* 15:517–530, 1995.

Ghidini A, Sirtori M, Romero R, Hobbins JC: Prenatal diagnosis of pentalogy of Cantrell. *J Ultrasound Med* 7:567–572, 1988.

Jochems L, Jacquemyn Y, Blaumeiser B: Prenatal diagnosis of pentalogy of Cantrell: a case report. *Clin Exp Obstet Gynecol* 31:141–142, 2004.

Liang RI, Huang SE, Chang FM: Prenatal diagnosis of ectopia cordis at 10 weeks of gestation using two-dimensional and three-dimensional ultrasonography. *Ultrasound Obstet Gynecol* 10:137–139, 1997.

Peer D, Moroder W, Delucca A: Prenatal diagnosis of the pentalogy of Cantrell combined with exencephaly and amniotic band syndrome. *Ultraschall Med* 14:94–95, 1993.

Polat I, Gul A, Aslan H, et al: Prenatal diagnosis of pentalogy of Cantrell in three cases, two with craniorachischisis. *J Clin Ultrasound* 33:308–311, 2005.

Sarkar P, Bastin J, Katoch D, Pal A: Pentalogy of Cantrell: diagnosis in the first trimester. *J Obstet Gynaecol* 25:812–813, 2005.

Siles C, Boyd PA, Manning N, Tsant T, Chamberlain P: Omphalocele and pericardial effusion: possible sonographic markers for the pentalogy of Cantrell or its variants. *Obstet Gynecol* 87:840–842, 1996.

PRUNE-BELLY SYNDROME

DESCRIPTION AND DEFINITION

Synonym: Eagle-Barrett syndrome

This condition consists of the triad of abdominal wall distention with deficiency of abdominal wall musculature, urinary tract obstruction, and cryptorchidism.

ABNORMALITIES DETECTABLE BY ULTRASOUND

Distended bladder and ureters

Cryptorchidism

Megalourethra

Oligohydramnios (of varying degree)

MAJOR DIFFERENTIAL DIAGNOSES

Megacystis megaureter

Megacystis–microcolon–intestinal hypoperistalsis syndrome

Neurogenic bladder

Obstructive uropathy, such as posterior urethral valves or other types of urethral obstruction

Primary vesicoureteral reflux

ULTRASOUND DIAGNOSIS

Prenatal detection of this condition has been reported at 11 and 12 weeks, as well as through the rest of gestation. Diagnosis is based on finding a distended urinary tract with marked distention of the bladder, ureterohydronephrosis, and varying degrees of oligohydramnios. Some fetuses have megalourethra; in those cases, the specific diagnosis of prune-belly syndrome can be made more definitive antenatally. Some of these cases have evidence of undescended testes in the third trimester. Sonography cannot distinguish between obstructive uropathy, such as posterior urethral valves, and prune-belly syndrome in cases of urinary tract distention with oligohydramnios.

HEREDITY

The pattern of inheritance for this syndrome is unknown.

NATURAL HISTORY AND OUTCOME

The pathogenesis of this disorder is unclear. However, it may be explained by transient early urethral obstruction, leading to massive distention of the urinary tract that results in pressure atrophy of the anterior abdominal

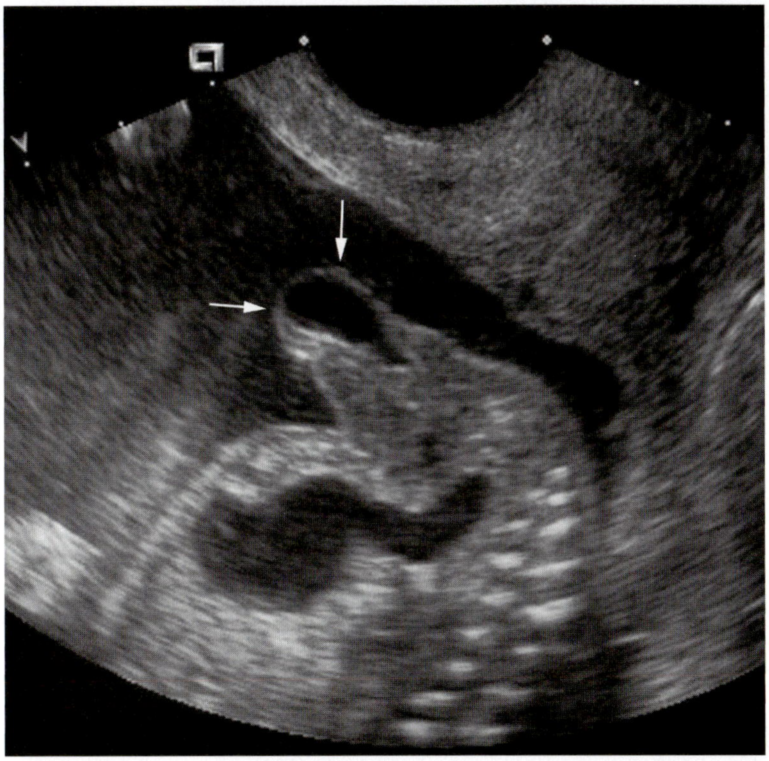

FIGURE 2-243 Longitudinal view of a fetus with prune-belly syndrome shows the fetal bladder and genitals. Note that the bladder is distended and tubular. Fluid in the fetal penile urethra is consistent with megalourethra *(arrows),* typical of this syndrome.

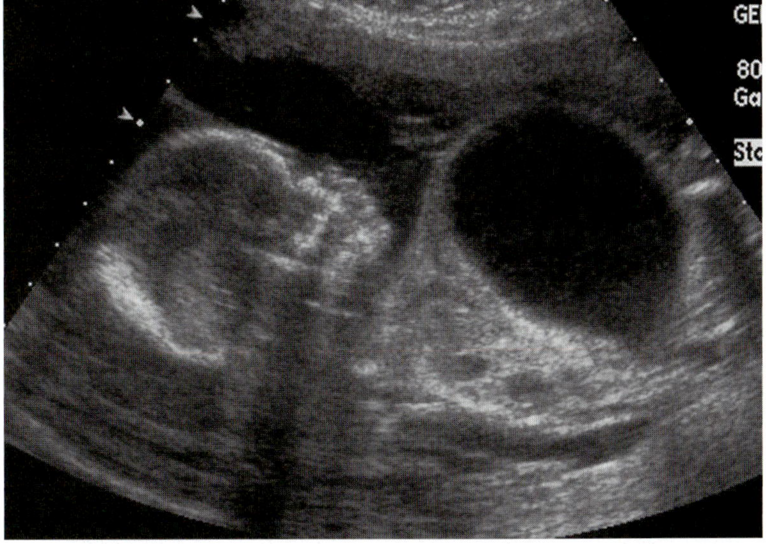

A

FIGURE 2-244 (A) Second-trimester fetus with prune-belly syndrome shows marked distention of the fetal bladder. *Continued*

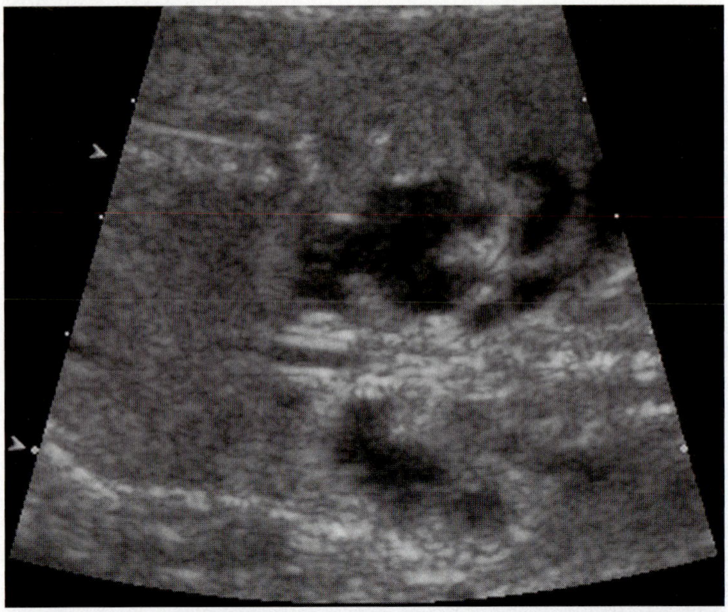

B

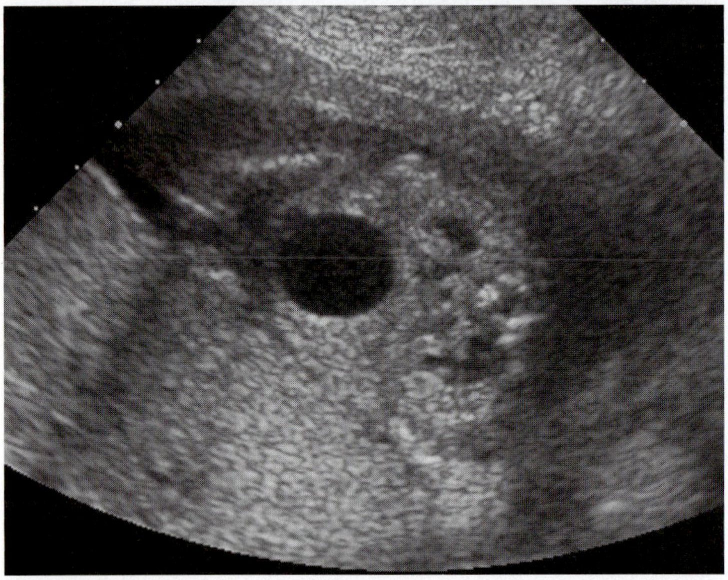

C

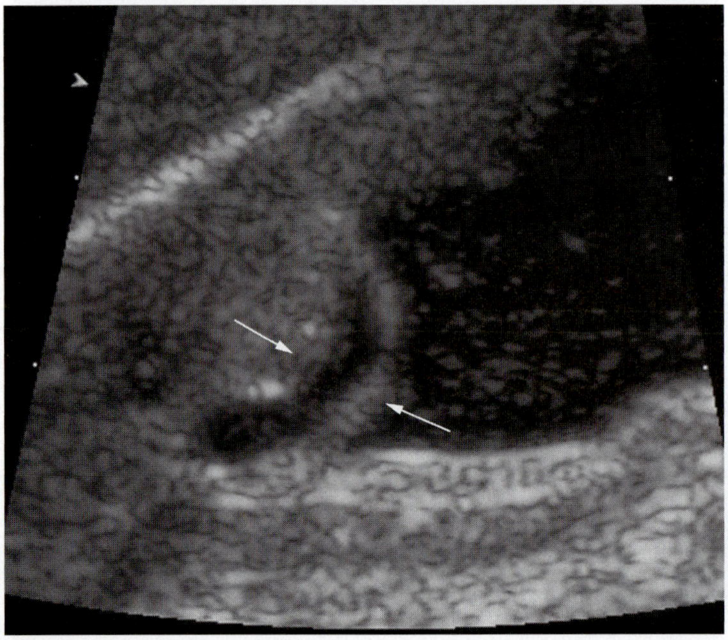

D

FIGURE 2-244, cont'd (B) Coronal view through the fetal kidneys of the same fetus shows bilateral hydronephrosis. (C) Cross-sectional view through the fetal bladder and kidneys of the same fetus shows a distended bladder and hydronephrosis. (D) Genitals of the same fetus show megalourethra *(arrows)*, with fluid in the penile urethra.

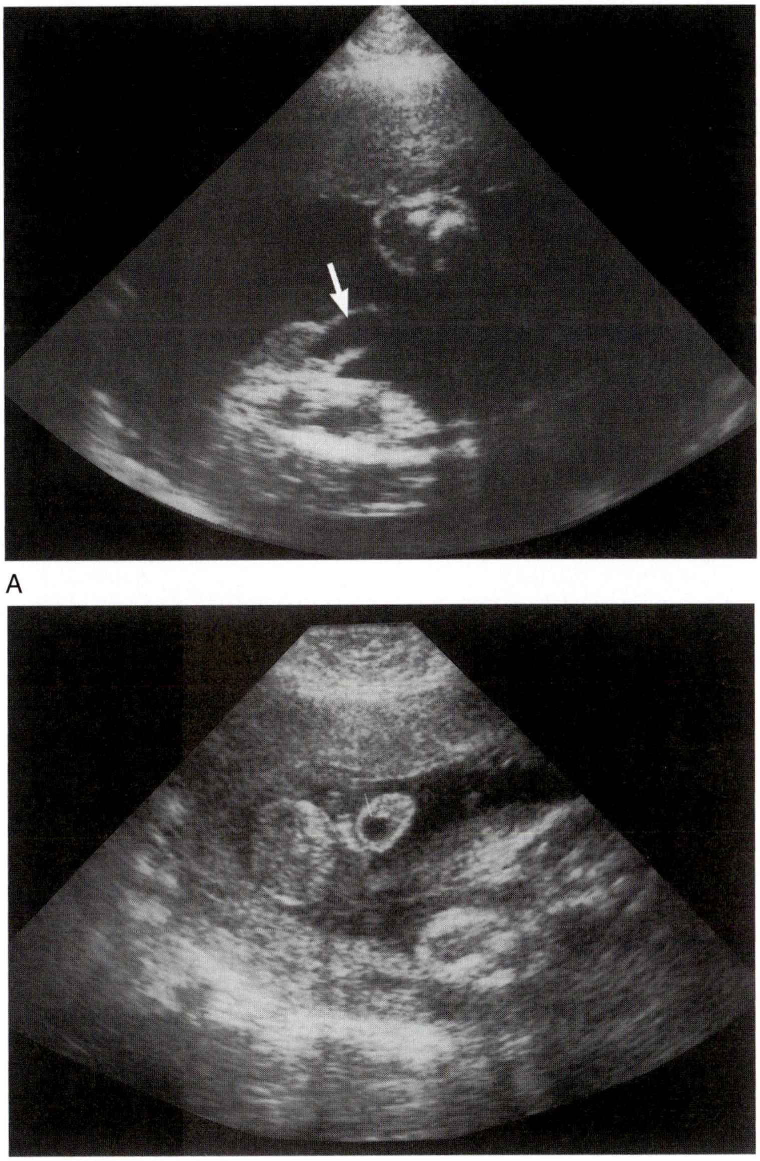

FIGURE 2-245 (A, B) Longitudinal views of the genitals of two fetuses with megalourethra *(arrow)*. Note that the penis is filled with fluid.

wall musculature. Bladder distention also interferes with descent of the testes, and ureteral obstruction results in oligohydramnios. The mesodermal theory suggests that a primary defect in the mesoderm of the anterior abdominal wall and urinary tract causes this syndrome.

The outcome of fetuses with prune-belly syndrome varies according to the types and severity of associated defects. Infants with severe oligohydramnios die secondary to pulmonary hypoplasia. There are reports of successful in utero shunting of the distended fetal bladder in some severe cases. However, at the other end of the spectrum, fetuses may have only mild hydronephrosis and megalourethra as a manifestation of the disorder. Infants who survive may have renal failure secondary to renal dysplasia in the neonatal period. Therefore, survival depends entirely on the severity of urinary distention, its effect on the kidneys in utero, and whether or not severe oligohydramnios prevented fetal lung development.

Suggested Reading

Aqua KA, McCurdy CM, Reed KL, Seeds JW: Prune-belly syndrome. *Fetus* 4:5–9, 1994.

Christopher CR, Spinelli A, Severt D: Ultrasonic diagnosis of prune-belly syndrome. *Obstet Gynecol* 59:391–394, 1982.

Fisk NM, Dhillon HK, Ellis CE, et al: Antenatal diagnosis of megalourethra in a fetus with the prune belly syndrome. *J Clin Ultrasound* 18:124–128, 1990.

Hoshino T, Ihara Y, Shirane H, Ota T: Prenatal diagnosis of prune belly syndrome at 12 weeks of pregnancy: case report and review of the literature. *Ultrasound Obstet Gynecol* 12:362–366, 1998.

Leeners B, Sauer I, Schefels J, Cotarelo CL, Funk A: Prune-belly syndrome: therapeutic options including in utero placement of a vesicoamniotic shunt. *J Clin Ultrasound* 28:500–507, 2000.

Lubinsky M, Rapoport P: Transient fetal hydrops and "prune belly" in one identical female twin. *N Engl J Med* 308:256–257, 1983.

Meizner I, Bar-Ziv J, Katz M: Prenatal ultrasonic diagnosis of the extreme form of prune belly syndrome. *J Clin Ultrasound* 13:581–583, 1985.

Perez-Brayfield MR, Gatti J, Berkman S, et al: In utero intervention in a patient with prune-belly syndrome and severe urethral hypoplasia. *Urology* 57:1178, 2001.

Perrotin F, Ayeva-Derman M, Lardy H, Cloarec S, Lansac J, Body G: Prenatal diagnosis and postnatal outcome of congenital megalourethra. Report of two cases. *Fetal Diagn Ther* 16:123–128, 2001.

Romero R: *Prenatal diagnosis of congenital anomalies.* East Norwalk, CT, 1988. Appleton & Lange.

Salihu HM, Tchuinguem G, Aliyu MH, Kouam L: Prune belly syndrome and associated malformations. A 13-year experience from a developing country. *West Indian Med J* 52:281–284, 2003.

Shigeta M, Nagata M, Shimoyamada H, et al: Prune-belly syndrome diagnosed at 14 weeks' gestation with severe urethral obstruction but normal kidneys. *Pediatr Nephrol* 13:135–137, 1999.

Shih WJ, Greenbaum LD, Baro C: In utero sonogram in prune belly syndrome. *Urology* 20:102–105, 1982.

Wachtel TJ, Hall S: Fetal hydrops and "prune belly" in one identical twin (letter). *N Engl J Med* 309:52–53, 1983.

Yamamoto H, Nishikawa S, Hayashi T, Sagae S, Kudo R: Antenatal diagnosis of prune belly syndrome at 11 weeks of gestation. *J Obstet Gynaecol Res* 27:37–40, 2001.

RENAL AGENESIS (POTTER SYNDROME)

DESCRIPTION AND DEFINITION

Synonym: Potter sequence, oligohydramnios sequence

Renal agenesis indicates bilateral absence of the kidneys, which is discussed in this section.

Potter syndrome also denotes severe oligohydramnios resulting from absent renal function caused by other etiologies, including bilateral cystic dysplastic kidneys and autosomal recessive polycystic kidney disease.

ABNORMALITIES DETECTABLE BY ULTRASOUND

Common Findings:

Oligohydramnios, usually of early onset (by 16–18 weeks' gestation)

Absent kidneys (although the adrenal glands may mimic kidneys; this is a pitfall in the early diagnosis of this condition)

Narrow chest (secondary to compression by the oligohydramnios), appearing later in gestation

Occasional Findings:

Vertebral defects

Complex cardiac defects (14%)

Skeletal anomalies (40%), such as sirenomelia, absent radius, and vertebral anomalies

CNS anomalies (11%), such as ventriculomegaly and neural tube defects

Other anomalies, such as imperforate anus, duodenal atresia, tracheoesophageal fistula, and single umbilical artery

MAJOR DIFFERENTIAL DIAGNOSES

Syndromes and Conditions Associated with Bilateral Renal Agenesis:

Caudal regression syndrome

Fraser syndrome

MURCS (**mü**llerian duct aplasia, **r**enal aplasia, **c**ervicothoracic **s**omite dysplasia) association

Sirenomelia

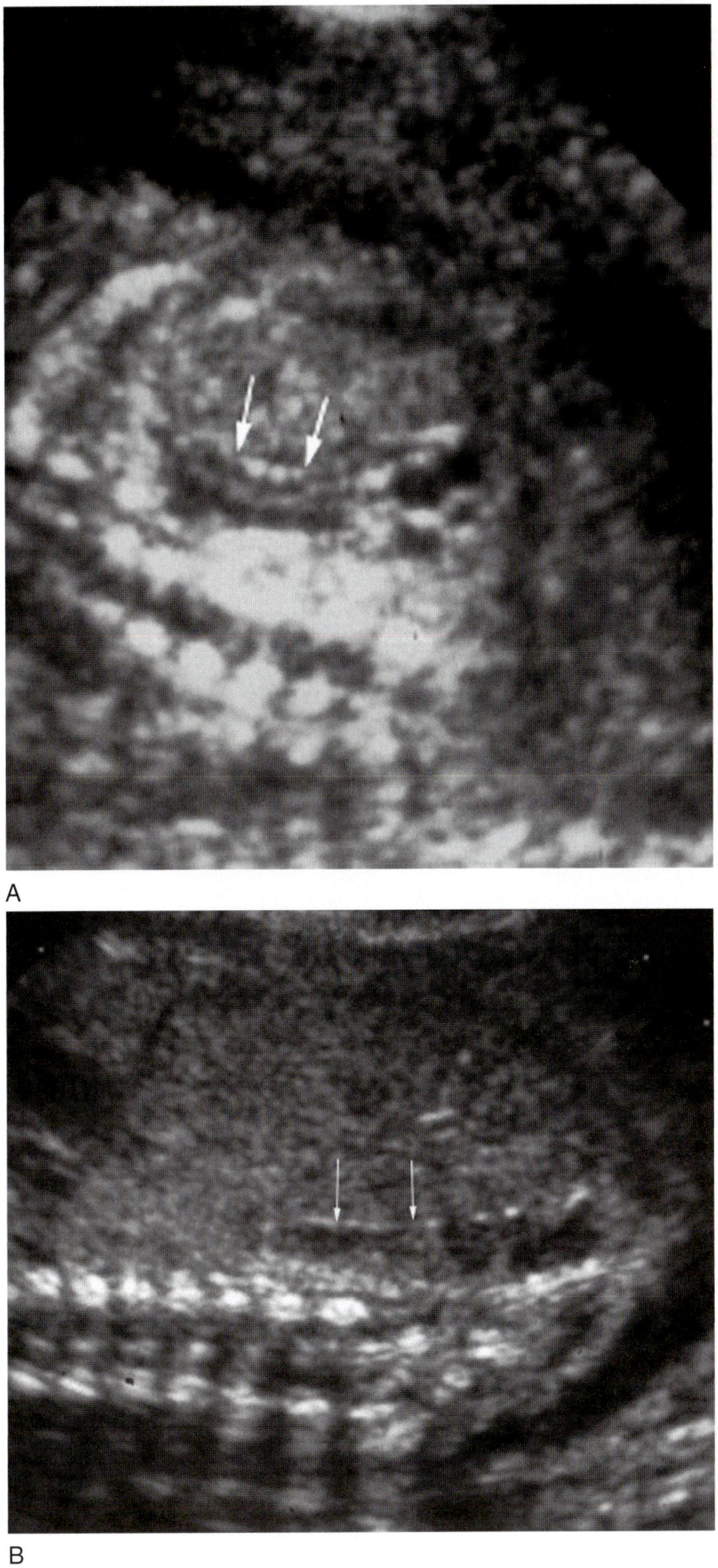

FIGURE 2-246 (**A, B**) Two different fetuses with absence of the kidney show the "lying down" adrenal sign *(arrows)*, which is consistent with complete absence of the kidney.

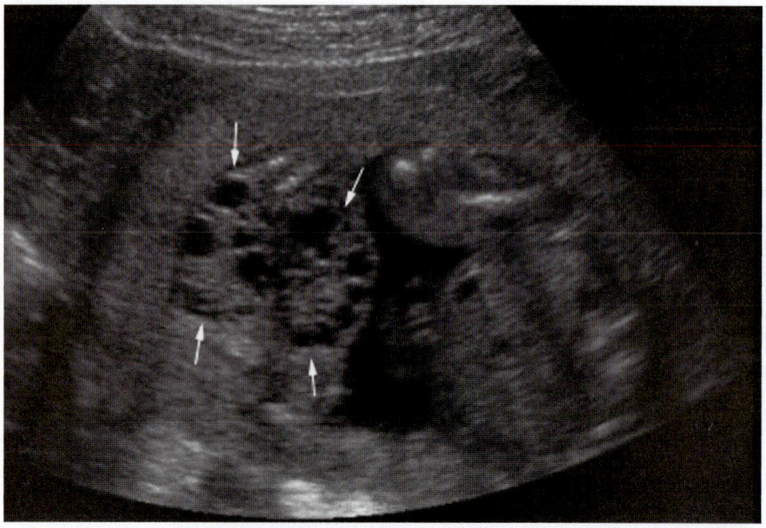

FIGURE 2-247 Twin pregnancy in which one twin has bilateral multicystic dysplastic kidneys *(arrows)*. This twin is seen in cross-section at the level of the kidneys and is confined to one side of the uterus by severe oligohydramnios.

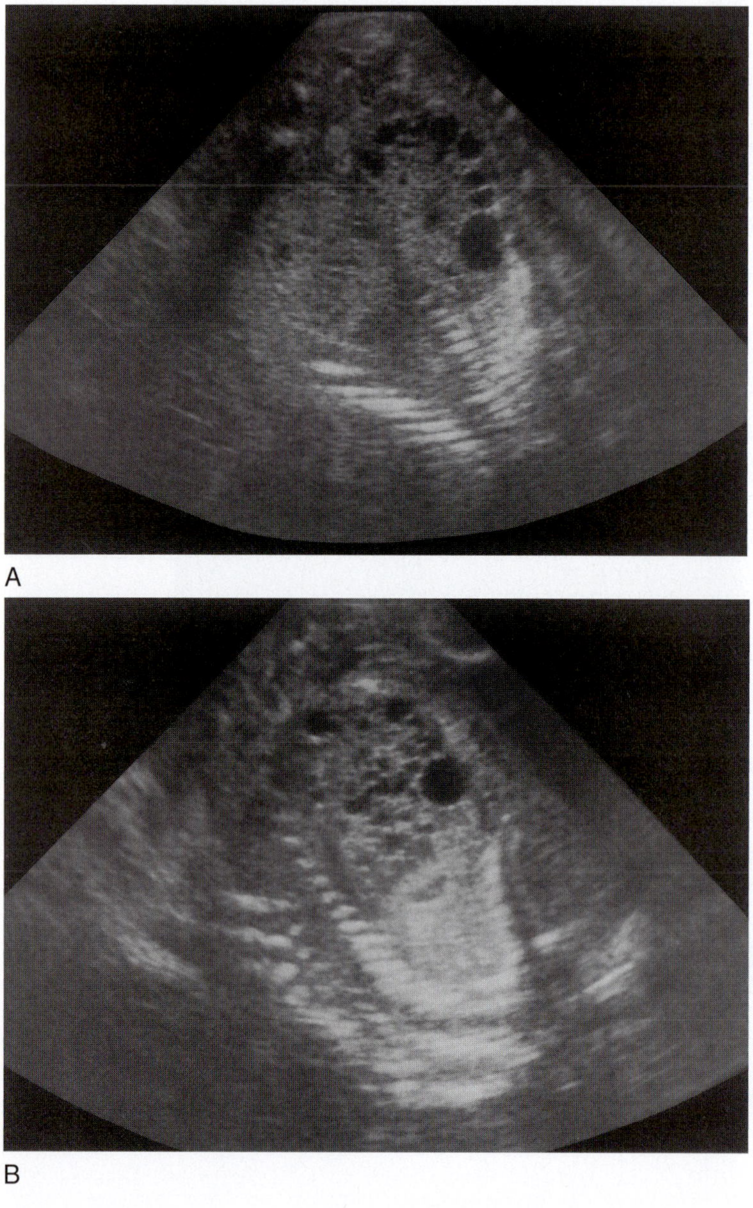

FIGURE 2-248 Coronal view through both kidneys (A) and through one kidney (B) of a fetus with bilateral, multicystic dysplastic kidneys. Neither kidney is functioning, and there is profound oligohydramnios.

VATER (**v**ertebral defects, **a**nal atresia, **t**racheoesophageal fistula, **e**sophageal atresia, and **r**adial and renal dysplasias) syndrome

ULTRASOUND DIAGNOSIS

Obstruction of the developing kidneys early in gestation may lead to bilateral renal agenesis or dysplasia. Renal agenesis may be a primary defect.

Ultrasonographic detection is possible early in the second trimester, by 12 weeks' gestation, particularly if oligohydramnios is present and bilateral renal masses, such as multicystic dysplastic kidneys, are visualized. However, diagnosis may be missed at that stage because of hypoechoic adrenals, which may mimic the kidneys, as well as the frequent delay (until 16–18 weeks' gestation) in onset of oligohydramnios. The position of the adrenal gland lying parallel to the spine when the kidney is absent may be a helpful sign for diagnosing renal agenesis. Color Doppler can be used to look for the renal arteries.

The diagnosis of renal agenesis/dysplasia is facilitated when other associated structural defects, such as sirenomelia, Fraser syndrome, and others, are seen.

Transvaginal scanning may be helpful in the structural survey, because severe oligohydramnios makes transabdominal imaging difficult.

HEREDITY

The pattern of inheritance for this syndrome depends on whether renal agenesis is associated with a particular syndrome with its own pattern of heredity.

Nine percent of first-degree relatives of fetuses with bilateral renal abnormalities themselves have renal malformations, many of which are asymptomatic. If parents have two affected infants, the risk of silent renal anomaly among first-degree relatives increases to 30%.

With a history of an affected fetus, the risk of recurrence of renal agenesis in subsequent pregnancies is 3%. If one parent has unilateral renal agenesis, the risk increases.

NATURAL HISTORY AND OUTCOME

This is a lethal malformation. Approximately 50% of fetuses with renal agenesis are stillborn. The remainder die of respiratory insufficiency resulting from pulmonary hypoplasia associated with prolonged oligohydramnios shortly after birth.

Unilateral renal agenesis usually is asymptomatic and is compatible with normal life.

Suggested Reading

Bankier A, Sheffield LJ, Danks DM: Renal ultrasound examination of parents in dominantly inherited renal adysplasia: a note of caution. *Am J Med Genet* 29:695–696, 1988.

Bronshtein M, Amit A, Achiron R, Noy I, Blumenfeld Z: The early prenatal sonographic diagnosis of renal agenesis: techniques and possible pitfalls. *Prenat Diagn* 14:291–297, 1994.

Bronshtein M, Yoffe N, Brandes JM, Blumenfeld Z: First and early second-trimester diagnosis of fetal urinary tract anomalies using transvaginal sonography. *Prenat Diagn* 10:653–656, 1990.

Buchta RM, Viseskul C, Gilbert EF, Sarto GE, Opitz JM: Familial bilateral renal agenesis and hereditary renal adysplasia. *Z Kinderheilk* 115:111–129, 1973.

Dicker D, Samuel N, Feldberg D, Goldman JA: The antenatal diagnosis of Potter syndrome (Potter sequence). A lethal and not-so-rare malformation. *Eur J Obstet Gynecol Reprod Biol* 18:17–24, 1984.

Helin I, Persson PH: Prenatal diagnosis of urinary tract abnormalities by ultrasound. *Pediatrics* 78:879–883, 1986.

Hoffman CK, Filly RA, Callen PW: The "lying down" adrenal sign: a sonographic indicator of renal agenesis or ectopia in fetuses and neonates. *J Ultrasound Med* 11:533–536, 1992.

Keirse MJ, Meerman RH: Antenatal diagnosis of Potter syndrome. *Obstet Gynecol* 52:64S–67S, 1978.

Pallotta R, Bucci I, Celentano C, Liberati M, Bellati U: The "skipped generation" phenomenon in a family with renal agenesis. *Ultrasound Obstet Gynecol* 24:586–587, 2004.

Potter EL: Facial characteristics of infants with bilateral renal agenesis. *Am J Obstet Gynecol* 51:885–888, 1946.

Romero R: *Prenatal diagnosis of congenital anomalies.* East Norwalk, CT, 1988, Appleton & Lange.

Schmidt W, Schroeder TM, Buchinger G, Kubli F: Genetics, pathoanatomy and prenatal diagnosis of Potter I syndrome and other urogenital tract diseases. *Clin Genet* 22:105–127, 1982.

Sgro M, Shah V, Barozzino T, Ibach K, Allen L, Chitayat D: False diagnosis of renal agenesis on fetal MRI. *Ultrasound Obstet Gynecol* 25:197–200, 2005.

Wiesel A, Queisser-Luft A, Clementi M, Bianca S, Stoll C, EUROSCAN Study Group: Prenatal detection of congenital renal malformations by fetal ultrasonographic examination: an analysis of 709,030 births in 12 European countries. *Eur J Med Genet* 48:131–144, 2005.

Wilson RD, Baird PA: Renal agenesis in British Columbia. *Am J Med Genet* 21:153, 1985.

Yuksel A, Batukan C: Sonographic findings of fetuses with an empty renal fossa and normal amniotic fluid volume. *Fetal Diagn Ther* 19:525–532, 2004.

Zerres K, Volpel MC, Weiss H: Cystic kidneys: genetics, pathologic anatomy, clinical picture, and prenatal diagnosis. *Hum Genet* 38:104–135, 1984.

SCIMITAR SYNDROME

DESCRIPTION AND DEFINITION

Scimitar syndrome is a rare abnormality consisting of dextroposition of the heart and situs solitus, secondary to right pulmonary hypoplasia and anomalous pulmonary venous return.

ABNORMALITIES DETECTABLE BY ULTRASOUND

Common Findings:

Dextroposition of the heart

Anomalous pulmonary vein, draining into the inferior vena cava

Small right lung

Occasional Finding:

Cardiac defects

MAJOR DIFFERENTIAL DIAGNOSES

Dextrorotation with a small right lung may have a similar appearance to dextroposition of the heart, secondary to a left lung mass. Differential diagnosis should include the following:

Adenomatoid cystic malformation of the left lung

Asplenia/polysplenia syndromes

Cardiac defects, with levorotation of the heart (also associated with chromosomal anomalies)

Cardiosplenic syndromes

Kartagener syndrome

Left diaphragmatic hernia

Other syndromes associated with dextroposition of the heart, including the following:

ULTRASOUND DIAGNOSIS

The earliest detection of scimitar syndrome occurred at 20 weeks, seen as dextroposition of the heart with a left-sided apex, distended pulmonary artery compared to aorta, and persistent left superior vena cava draining into the coronary sinus. Although scimitar syndrome was among the differential diagnostic possibilities, the exact diagnosis was not made until after birth, when the pulmonary veins from the right lower lobe were noted to drain into the inferior

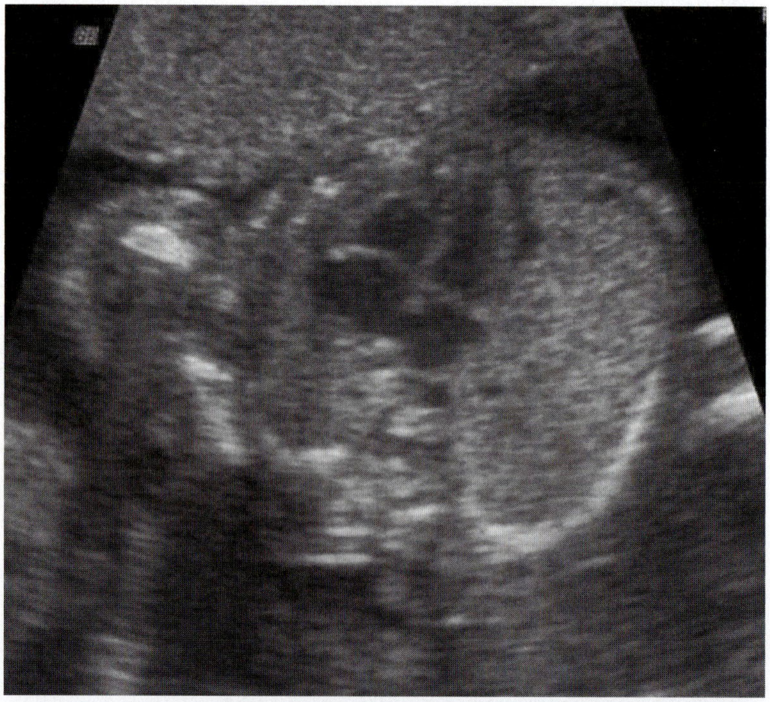

FIGURE 2-249 Transverse view through the chest of a fetus with hypoplasia of the right lung, as evidenced by rotation of the heart into the right side of the chest while the apex is still pointing to the left.

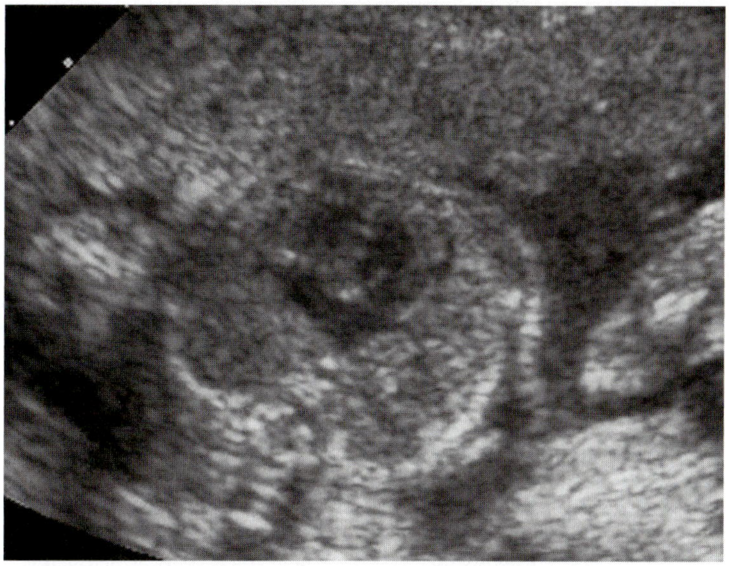

FIGURE 2-250 Scimitar syndrome in a 20-week fetus with a midline-appearing heart attributable to some hypoplasia of the right lung. (Courtesy Joshua Copel, MD.)

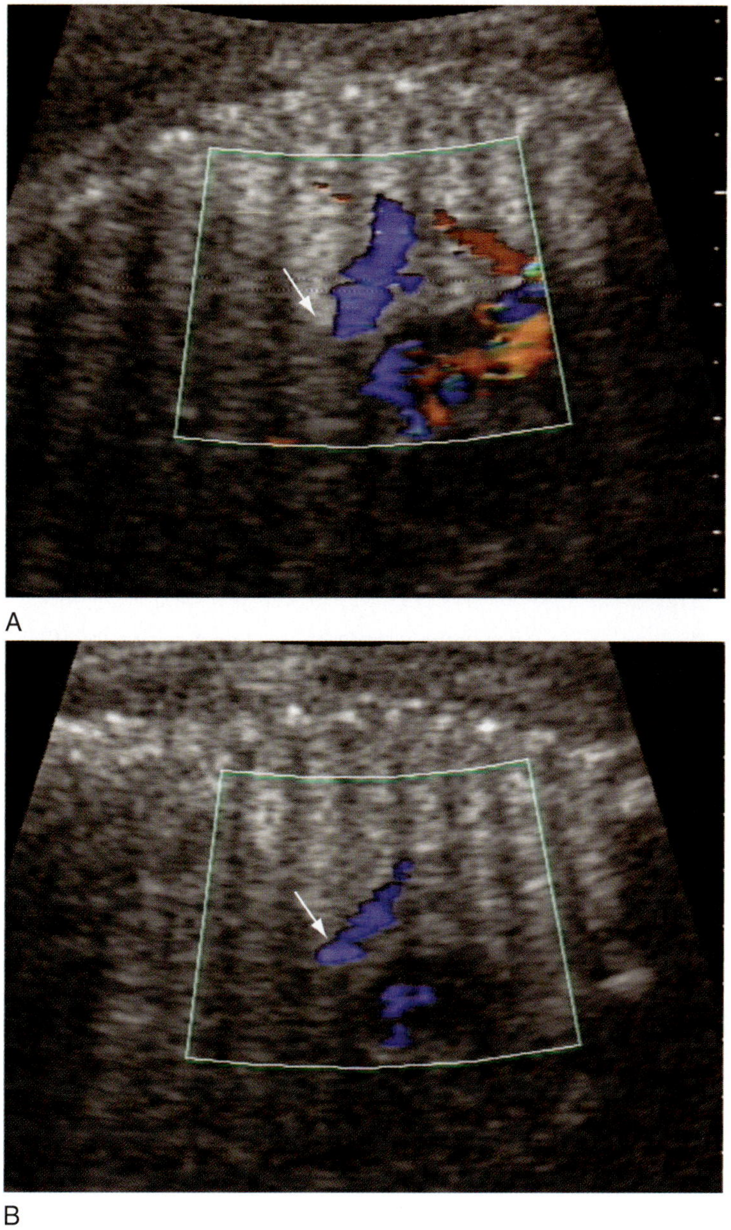

FIGURE 2-251 Anomalous pulmonary vein (**A, B** *arrows*) draining into the inferior vena cava. (Courtesy Joshua Copel, MD.)

vena cava, and an aberrant arterial vessel was seen to connect the aorta to that same lower lobe.

Sonographic detection of this syndrome was also reported at 21 weeks' gestation, based on the findings of dextroposition of the heart, mild dilation of the main pulmonary artery, and narrowing of the right pulmonary artery. At 24 weeks' gestation, polyhydramnios was evident. After birth, the findings of hypoplastic right lung with atrioventricular fistula and sequestration were noted, along with anomalous drainage of the right pulmonary vein into the inferior vena cava and persistent left superior vena cava.

Prenatal detection of this syndrome is based on identifying a dextroposition of the fetal heart in the absence of a thoracic mass, with a normal cardiac axis and reduced right lung size. In a study of 10 such cases, 3 had scimitar syndrome.

HEREDITY

The etiology and heredity of this syndrome are unknown.

NATURAL HISTORY AND OUTCOME

Many patients with scimitar syndrome do not come to medical attention until adulthood, particularly if no intrinsic cardiac abnormalities are present. Patients who are symptomatic in the neonatal period usually have congenital cardiac abnormalities, as well as the classic findings of dextrorotation of the heart, right pulmonary hypoplasia, and anomalous pulmonary venous drainage.

Suggested Reading

Abdullah MM, Lacro RV, Smallhorn J, et al: Fetal cardiac dextroposition in the absence of an intrathoracic mass: sign of significant right lung hypoplasia. *J Ultrasound Med* 19:669–676, 2000.

Grisaru D, Achiron R, Lipitz S, et al: Antenatal sonographic findings associated with scimitar syndrome. *Ultrasound Obstet Gynecol* 8:131–133, 1996.

Michailidis GD, Simpson JM, Tulloh RM, Economides DL: Retrospective prenatal diagnosis of scimitar syndrome aided by three-dimensional power Doppler imaging. *Ultrasound Obstet Gynecol* 17:449–452, 2001.

SPINAL DYSRAPHISM

DESCRIPTION AND DEFINITION

Synonym: Neural tube defect

Spinal dysraphism includes anencephaly, iniencephaly, encephalocele, and meningomyelocele as neural tube defects.

Anencephaly represents a defect in closure of the anterior portion of the neural groove, which normally is completed by 28 days' gestation. The unfused forebrain develops partially and then degenerates. Facial abnormalities, as well as cervical vertebral anomalies, are common.

Defects of closure of the cervical and upper thoracic spine can result in encephalocele and iniencephaly, which is associated with retroflexion of the upper spine and a short spine, relative to the anterior aspect of the body.

Defects in closure of the mid to caudal neural groove give rise to meningomyeloceles. These open defects usually are associated with Chiari II malformation and ventriculomegaly. The exception is the occasional closed defect, covered with skin.

ABNORMALITIES DETECTABLE BY ULTRASOUND

Anencephaly is the easiest ultrasound diagnosis among the neural tube defects, seen as the absence of the cranial vault. Iniencephaly also is easily detectable as the characteristically abnormal, retroflexed posture of the fetus, short neck, short spine, and dysraphism.

Meningomyelocele and encephalocele occur in a variety of sizes. Large defects, associated with a dorsal sac and severe disruption of the posterior elements of the spine, are easily identified sonographically. More subtle defects, involving only one or two segments or the sacrum, may be more difficult to detect, particularly if they are flat, without a dorsal sac. The diagnosis of open neural tube defects is most easily established by evaluating the head for evidence of either of the following signs, which are consistent with an Arnold-Chiari II malformation:

Banana sign—anterior bowing of the cerebellar hemispheres with obliteration of the

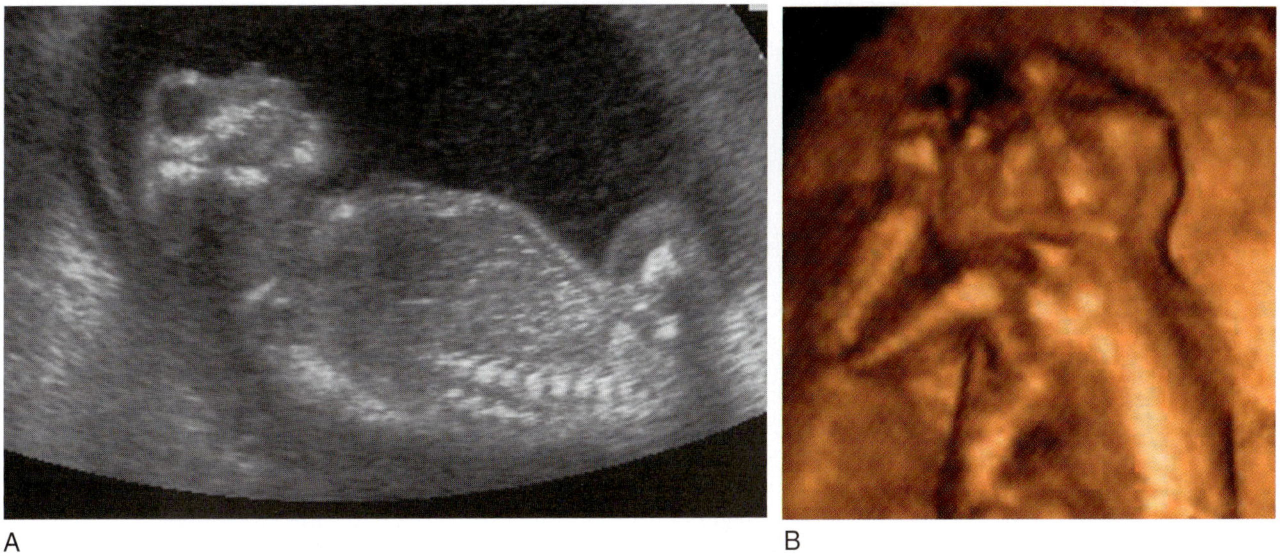

FIGURE 2-252 (A) Longitudinal view of a second-trimester fetus with anencephaly. (B) Three-dimensional surface rendering of the same fetus with anencephaly shows complete absence of the skull seen from behind.

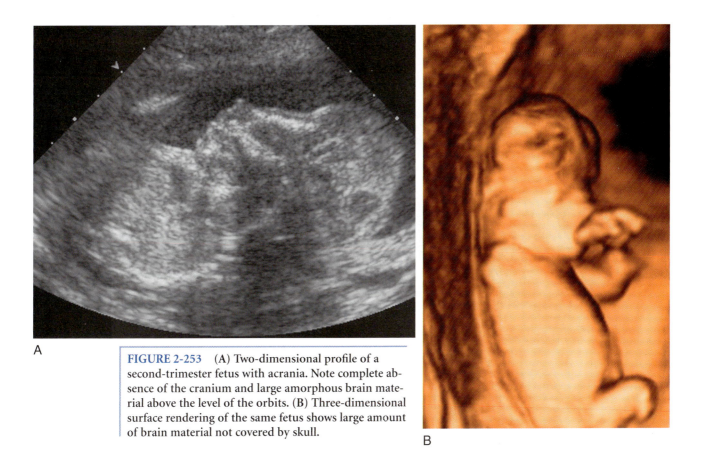

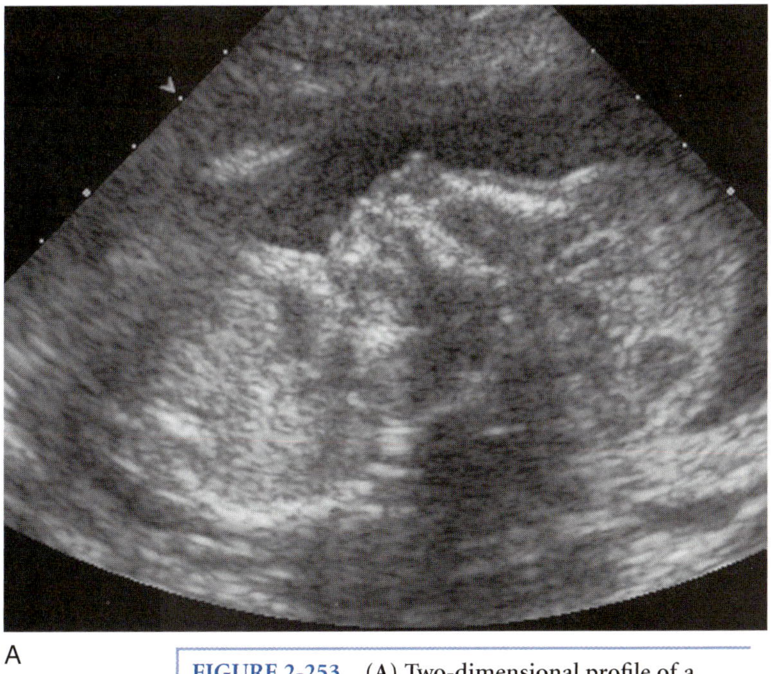

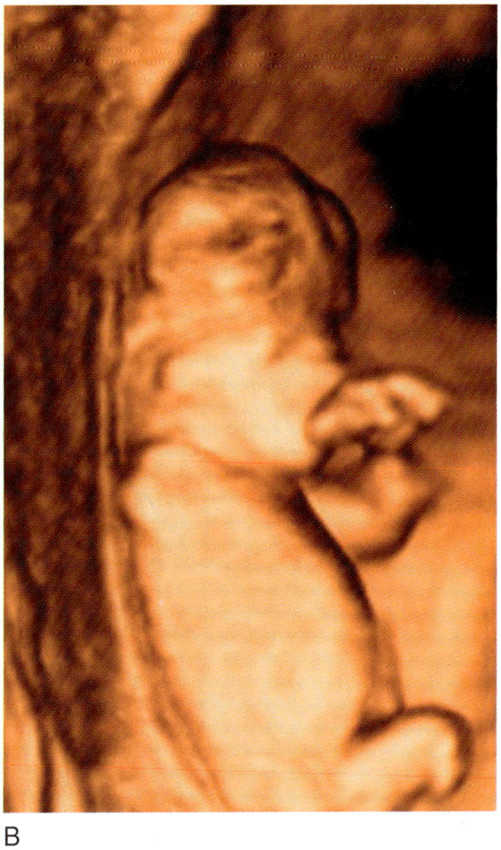

FIGURE 2-253 (A) Two-dimensional profile of a second-trimester fetus with acrania. Note complete absence of the cranium and large amorphous brain material above the level of the orbits. (B) Three-dimensional surface rendering of the same fetus shows large amount of brain material not covered by skull.

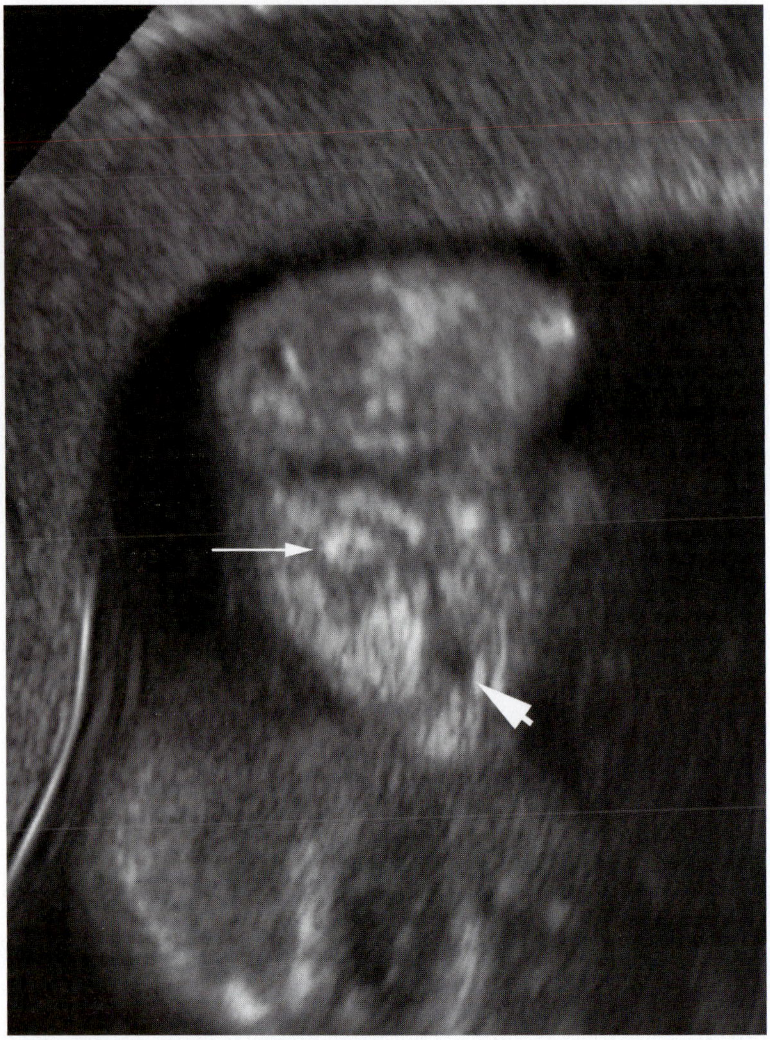

FIGURE 2-254 Second-trimester fetus with acrania has brain material above the level of the orbits. Note the cataract *(arrow)* and midline facial cleft *(arrowhead)*.

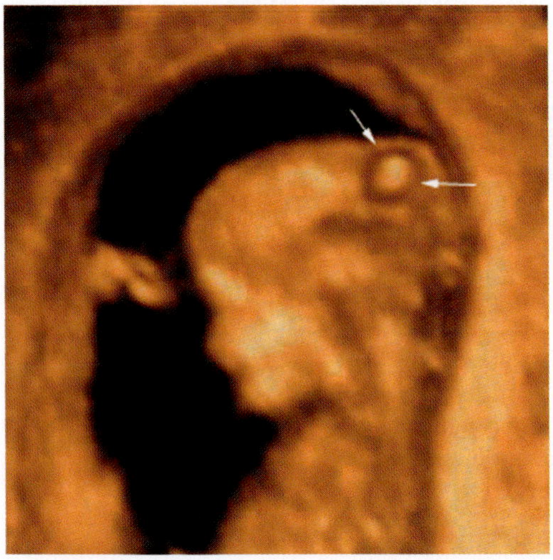

FIGURE 2-255 Three-dimensional surface rendering in the midline of a first-trimester fetus with an occipital encephalocele *(arrows)*.

cisterna magna secondary to an Arnold-Chiari type II malformation

Lemon sign—angulation of the frontal bones, often accompanied by mild ventriculomegaly and microcephaly

Other findings may include club feet (occasionally) and ventriculomegaly (frequently). Other anomalies that may be associated with a particular syndrome, such as chromosomal defects, include cardiac abnormalities, limb defects, and anterior abdominal wall defects.

MAJOR DIFFERENTIAL DIAGNOSES

Although the presence of a neural tube defect is unequivocal in most cases, occasional confusion may arise in distinguishing between a low, occipital encephalocele and a cystic hygroma or between a sacrococcygeal teratoma and a sacral

Text continued on p. 425

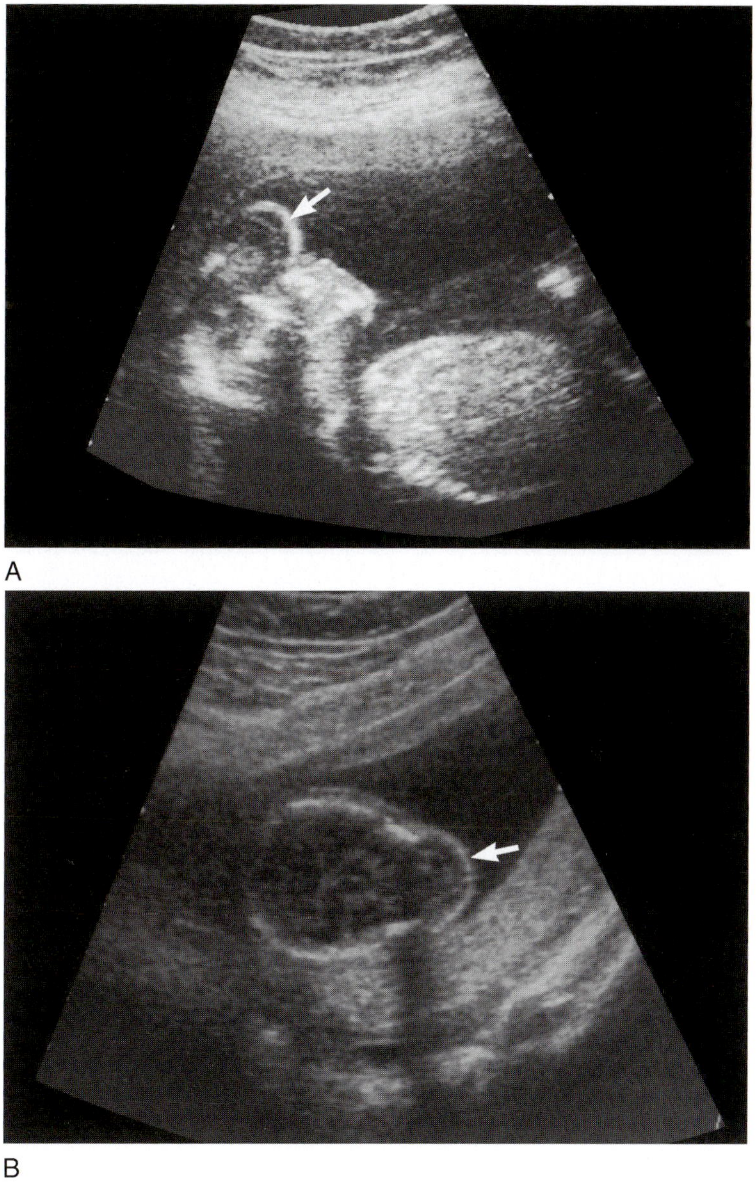

FIGURE 2-256 Longitudinal (A) and transverse (B) views of a fetus with a moderate-sized anterior encephalocele *(arrows)*. Note that part of the frontal lobes is extruded anteriorly through a defect in the skull.

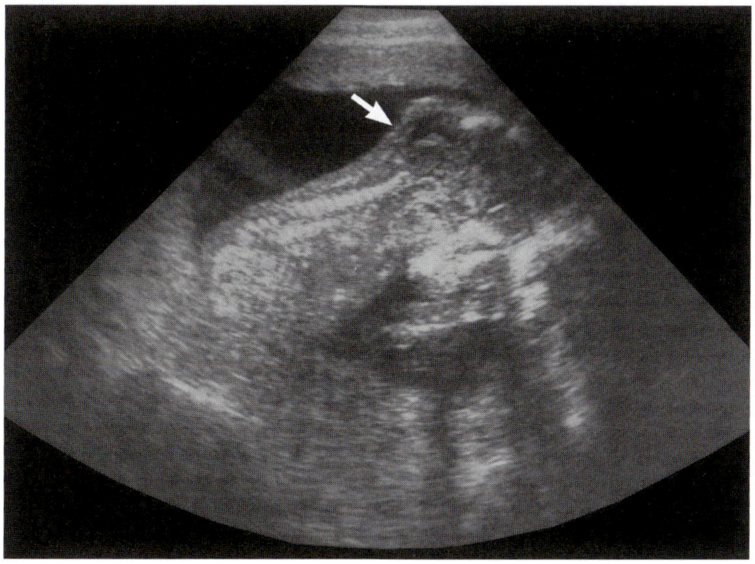

FIGURE 2-257 Early second-trimester fetus with a small posterior encephalocele *(arrow)*.

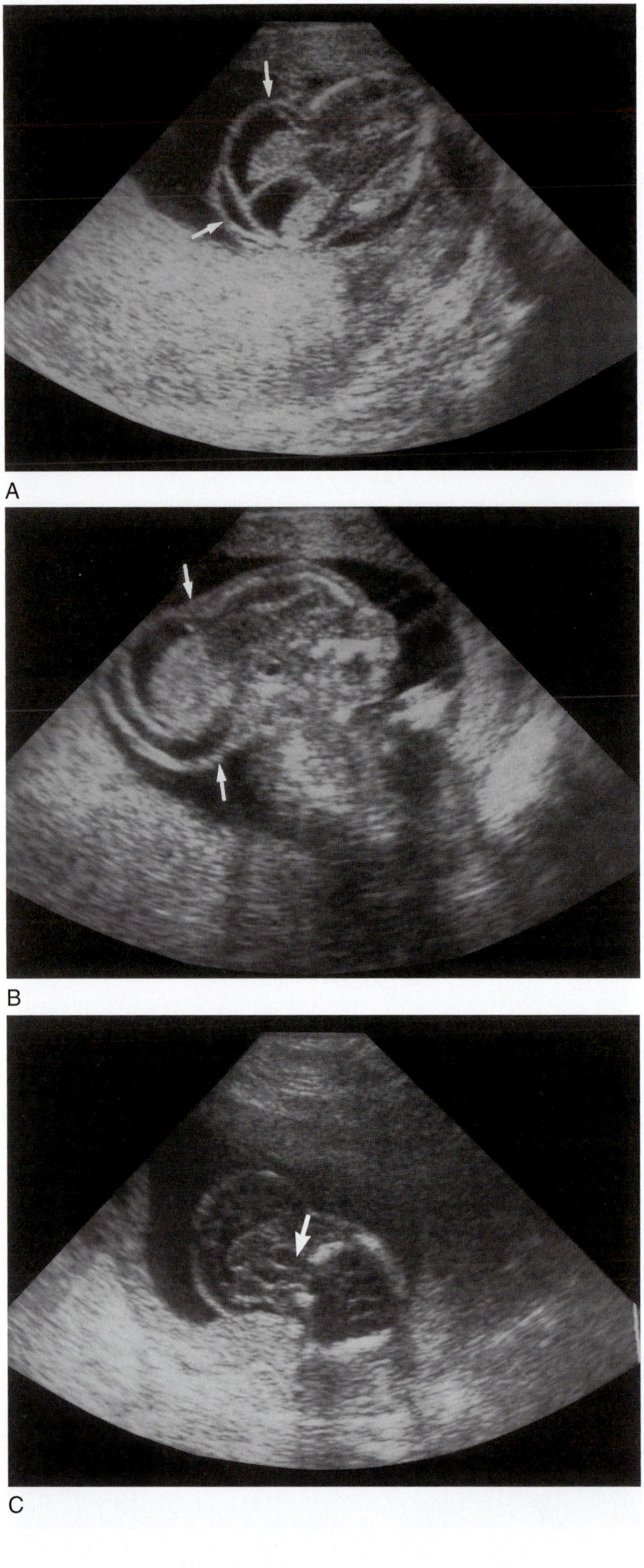

A

B

C

FIGURE 2-258 (A, B) Transverse and longitudinal views of a fetus with a large posterior encephalocele *(arrows)*. Most of the lateral hemispheres, ventricles, and choroid plexus are extruded posteriorly. (C, D) Transverse and longitudinal views of a fetus with a large encephalocele. (C) Transabdominal view show the brainstem *(arrow)* is partly outside the skull covering.

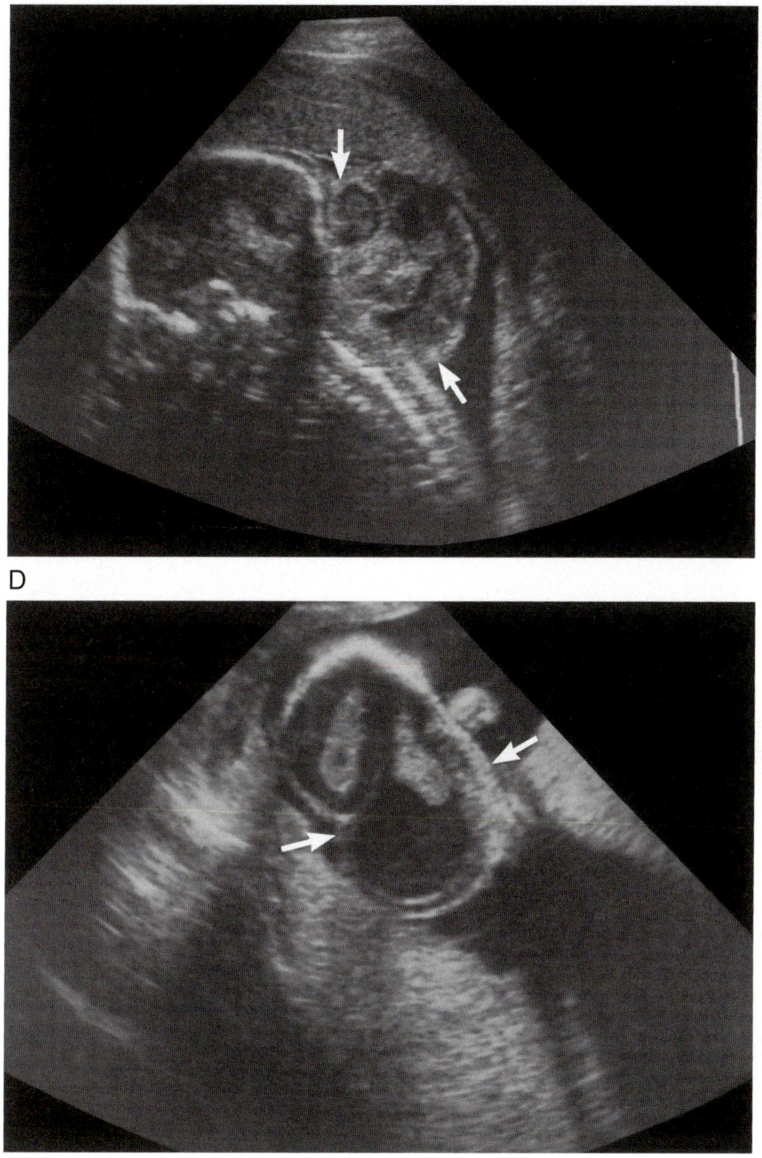

D

E

FIGURE 2-258 (D) Transvaginal scan shows a large amount of brain *(arrows)* extruded from the posterior aspect of the head. (E) Lateral parietal encephalocele *(arrows)*. Note the large defect in the parietal region of the skull, with extrusion of only one side of the brain, the lateral ventricle, and part of the choroid plexus.

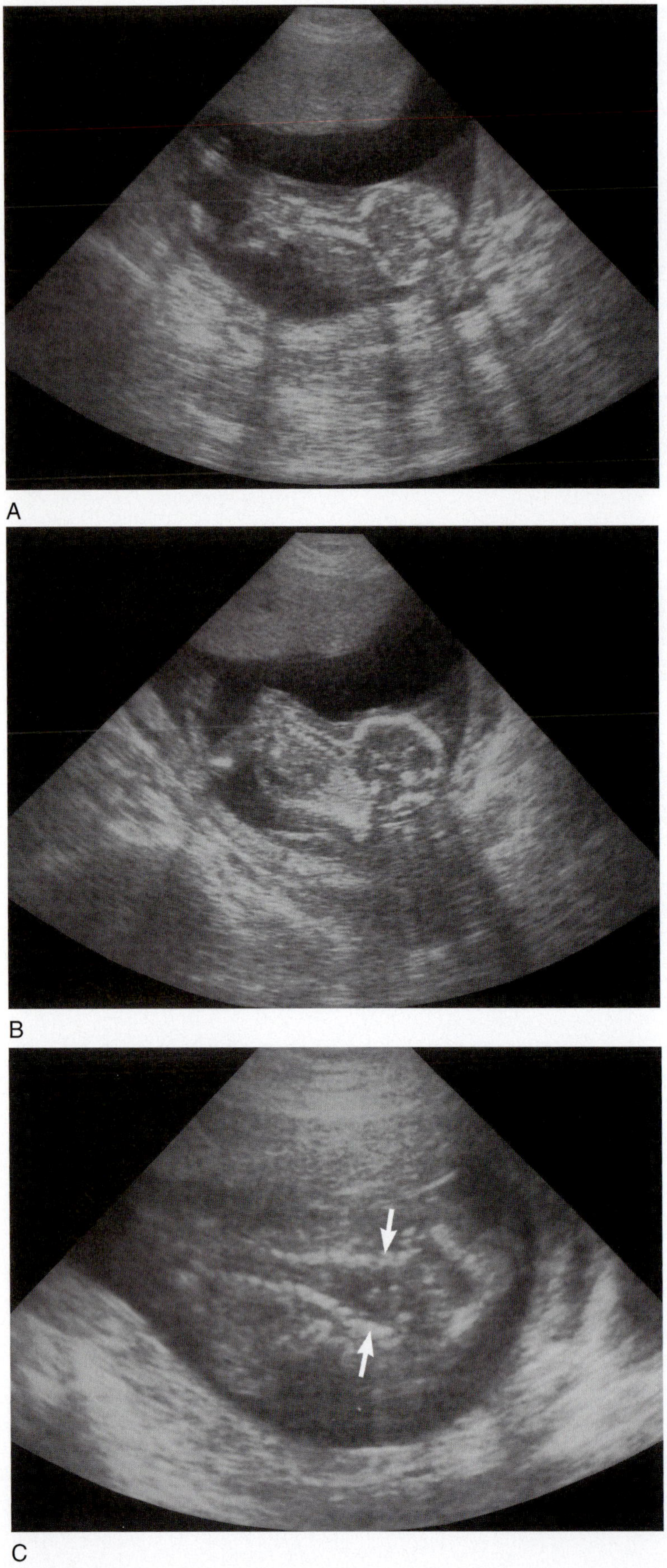

FIGURE 2-259 (**A, B**) Coronal and longitudinal views of a fetus with iniencephaly reveal a markedly foreshortened spine. The fetus is hyperextended as a result of foreshortening of the spine. (**C**) Magnification of the region of the upper spine. Note dysraphism *(arrows)*.

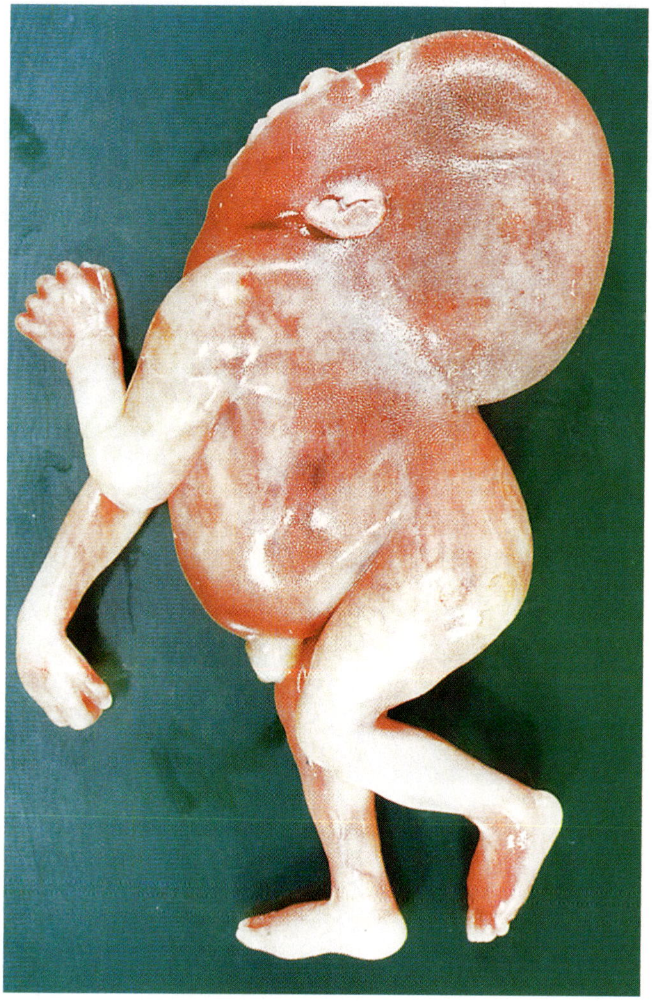
D

FIGURE 2-259 (D) Pathologic specimen of a fetus with iniencephaly. Note markedly hyperextended spine. (From Keeling J: *Fetal pathology.* London, 1994, Churchill Livingstone.)

neural tube defect. Careful sonographic evaluation of the lesion and the adjacent spine should enable the sonologist to arrive at the correct diagnosis.

Syndromes and Conditions Associated with Neural Tube Defects

(see Differential Diagnosis for complete list, p. 40)

Amniotic band syndrome (asymmetric)

Caudal regression syndrome/sirenomelia

Cloacal exstrophy

Cri du chat syndrome

Hydrolethalus

Jarcho-Levin syndrome

Joubert syndrome (encephalocele)

Maternal diabetes

Meckel-Gruber syndrome (encephalocele)

Median cleft face

Oral-facial-digital syndrome (Mohr syndrome)

Pentalogy of Cantrell

Renal agenesis

Triploidy

Trisomy 9

Trisomy 13 (Patau syndrome)

Trisomy 18 (Edwards' syndrome)

Walker-Warburg syndrome (encephalocele)

TERATOGENS

Aminopterin

Carbamazepine (Tegretol)

Clomiphene (Clomid)

Cytarabine

Dextroamphetamine

Hyperthermia

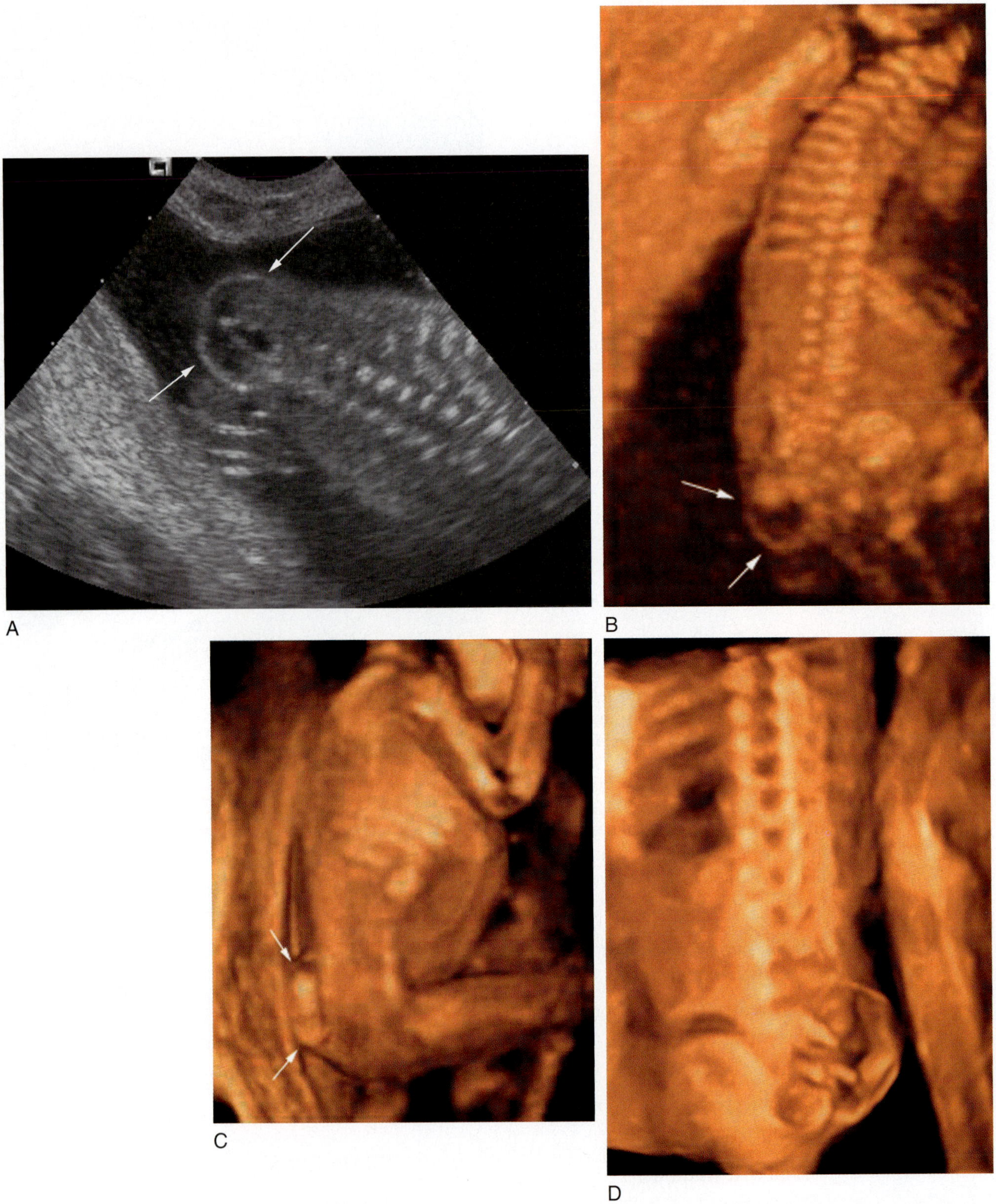

FIGURE 2-260 Lumbosacral neural tube defect. (A) Standard two-dimensional view of a neural tube defect involving the lower lumbar spine and sacrum *(arrows)*. (B) Three-dimensional surface rendering of a fetus with a sacral neural tube defect *(arrows)*. (C) Different view of the same fetus as in *A* shows the cystic area off the fetal back consistent with a meningomyelocele. (D) Three-dimensional surface rendering of a different second-trimester fetus with a lower lumbar sacral meningomyelocele.

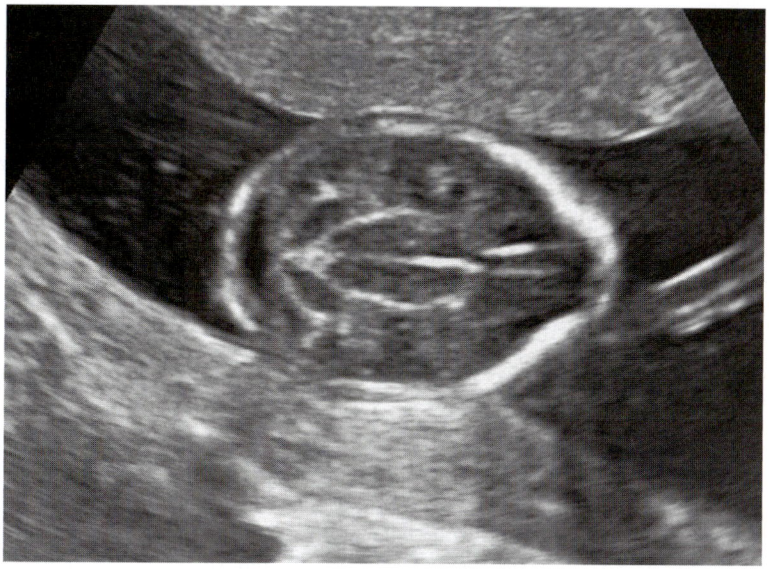

FIGURE 2-261 Axial view through the fetal head of a fetus with an open neural tube defect. Note compression of the cerebellum, obliteration of the cisterna magna (banana sign), and squaring of the frontal bone (lemon sign).

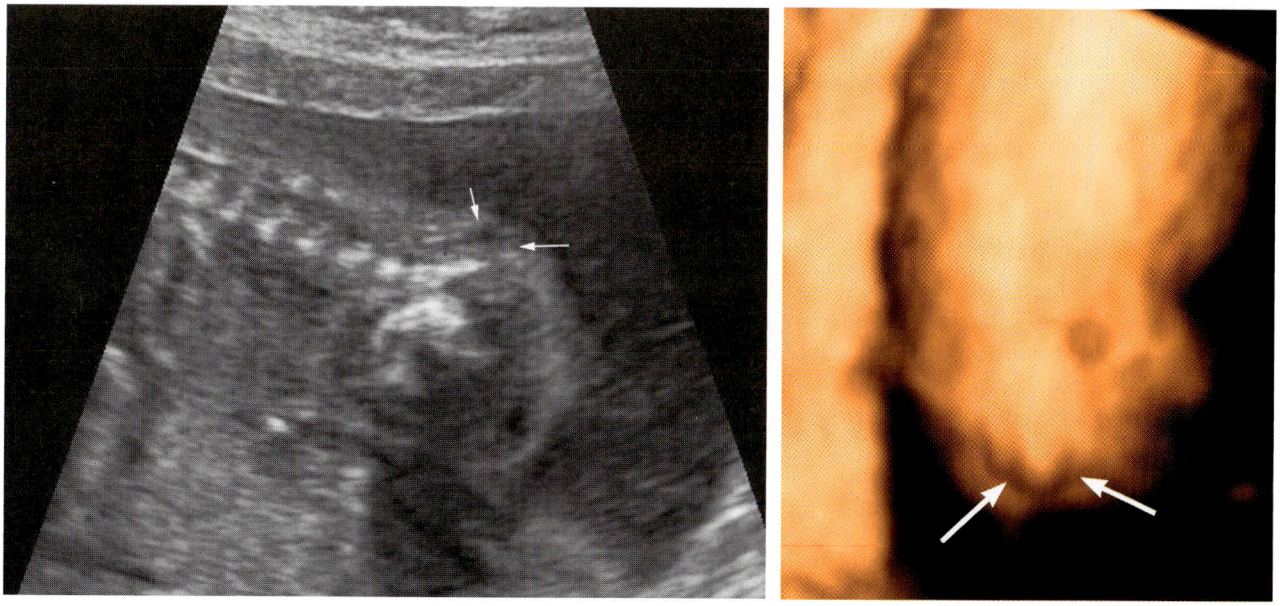

A

B

FIGURE 2-262 Tiny sacral neural tube defect. (A) Standard two-dimensional view of a tiny neural tube defect involving the end of the sacrum *(arrows)*. (B) Three-dimensional surface rendering of the same fetus shows a tiny bulge of the surface of the skin *(arrows)*.

Imipramine

Methotrexate

Progestin

Radiation

Valproic acid

Warfarin (Coumadin)

ULTRASOUND DIAGNOSIS

Sonographic diagnosis of anencephaly can be established as early as at 10 to 12 weeks' gestation, based on the abnormal shape of the head and the absence of the skull.

Diagnosis of iniencephaly also can be established early, based on the abnormal positioning of the fetus (marked hyperextension) caused by the short spine.

Meningomyeloceles may present more subtle findings. Although some encephaloceles and large meningomyeloceles can be detected in the later first/early second trimester, small, single-segment neural tube defects may not be visualized until 16 to 18 weeks' gestation. The lemon and banana signs, as well as mild ventriculomegaly, are more readily identifiable and usually can be seen prenatally by 15 to 16 weeks.

With the widespread use of serum alpha-fetoprotein (AFP) determinations, many pregnant women have been found to be carrying affected fetuses, based on an ultrasound scan prompted by an elevated maternal serum AFP level. Currently, the sensitivity of sonographic detection of neural tube defects is greater than 90%.

Three-dimensional ultrasound reportedly is slightly more accurate than standard two-dimensional ultrasound and MRI for diagnosing the exact level of the lesion. Identifying the exact level is precise in 80% of cases using standard ultrasound. Determining the level accurately is important for proper prenatal counselling.

HEREDITY

Inheritance of neural tube defects is thought to be multifactorial. The recurrence rate for parents with a previously affected child is approximately 2%. With more than one previously affected child, the recurrence rate may approach 10%.

NATURAL HISTORY AND OUTCOME

The outcome of infants with neural tube defects is highly variable, depending on the severity of the abnormality. In one study of 30 cases of neural tube defect, lower levels of defect and smaller ventricles sizes were predictive of a more favorable outcome. None of the infants with thoracic lesions was ambulatory, and all required shunts. All those with lesions at or below L4 were ambulatory, and 60% had ventriculomegaly. Among those with lesions at L1–L3, 50% were ambulatory.

Much work is being done to repair neural tube defect antenatally, with varying results. In general, in utero surgery seems to decrease the need for postnatal shunting of the ventricles but has not provided significant improvement in lower extremity function and other benchmarks. The results of a multicenter randomized trial are pending.

Suggested Reading

Aaronson OS, Hernanz-Schulman M, Bruner JP, Reed GW, Tulipan NB: Myelomeningocele: prenatal evaluation—comparison between transabdominal US and MR imaging. *Radiology* 227:839–843, 2003.

Aaronson OS, Hernanz-Schulman M, Bruner JP, Reed GW, Tulipan NB: Myelomeningocele: prenatal evaluation—comparison between transabdominal US and MR imaging. *Radiology* 227:839–843, 2003.

Adelberg A, Blotzer A, Koch G, et al: Impact of maternal-fetal surgery for myelomeningocele on the progression of ventriculomegaly in utero. *Am J Obstet Gynecol* 193(3 Pt 1):727–731, 2005.

Biggio JR Jr, Owen J, Wenstrom KD, Oakes WJ: Can prenatal ultrasound findings predict ambulatory status in fetuses with open spina bifida? *Am J Obstet Gynecol* 185:1016–1020, 2001.

Biggio JR Jr, Wenstrom KD, Owen J: Fetal open spina bifida: a natural history of disease progression in utero. *Prenat Diagn* 24:287–289, 2004.

Budorick NE, Pretorius DH, McGahan JP, et al: Cephalocele detection in utero: sonographic and clinical features. *Ultrasound Obstet Gynecol* 5:77–85, 1995.

Campbell J, Gilbert WM, Nicolaides KH, Campbell S: Ultrasound screening for spina bifida: cranial and cerebellar signs in a high-risk population. *Obstet Gynecol* 70:247–250, 1987.

Chervanek FA, Isaacson G, Mahoney MJ, et al: Diagnosis and management of fetal cephalocele. *Obstet Gynecol* 64:86–90, 1984.

Cortes RA, Farmer DL: Recent advances in fetal surgery. *Semin Perinatol* 28:199–211, 2004.

Cullen MT, Athanassiadis AP, Romero R: Prenatal diagnosis of anterior parietal encephalocele with transvaginal sonography. *Obstet Gynecol* 75:489–491, 1990.

Farmer DL, von Koch CS, Peacock WJ, et al: In utero repair of myelomeningocele: experimental pathophysiology, initial clinical experience, and outcomes. *Arch Surg* 138:872–878, 2003.

Goldstein RB, Filly RA: Prenatal diagnosis of anencephaly: spectrum of sonographic appearances and distinction from the amniotic band syndrome. *AJR Am J Roentgenol* 151:547–550, 1988.

Goldstein RB, LaPidus AS, Filly RA: Fetal cephaloceles: diagnosis with US. *Radiology* 180:803–808, 1991.

Goldstein RB, Podrasky AE, Filly RA, Callen PW: Effacement of the fetal cisterna magna in association with myelomeningocele. *Radiology* 172:409–413, 1989.

Johnson MP, Sutton LN, Rintoul N, et al: Fetal myelomeningocele repair: short-term clinical outcomes. *Am J Obstet Gynecol* 189:482–487, 2003.

Johnson SP, Sebire NJ, Snijders RJM, Tunkel S, Nicolaides KH: Ultrasound screening for anencephaly at 10–14 weeks of gestation. *Ultrasound Obstet Gynecol* 9:14–16, 1997.

Lee W, Chaiworapongsa T, Romero R, et al: A diagnostic approach for the evaluation of spina bifida by three-dimensional ultrasonography. *J Ultrasound Med* 21:619–626, 2002.

Lindfors KK, McGahan JP, Tennant FP, Hanson FW, Walter JP: Midtrimester screening for open neural tube defects: correlation of sonography with amniocentesis results. *AJR Am J Roentgenol* 149:141–145, 1987.

Lyon HM, Holmes LB, Huang T: Multiple congenital anomalies associated with in utero exposure of phenytoin: possible hypoxic ischemic mechanism? *Birth Defects Res A Clin Mol Teratol* 67:993–996, 2003.

Nishi T, Nakano R: First-trimester diagnosis of exencephaly by transvaginal ultrasonography. *J Ultrasound Med* 13:149–151, 1994.

Norem CT, Schoen EJ, Walton DL, et al: Routine ultrasonography compared with maternal serum alpha-fetoprotein for neural tube defect screening. *Obstet Gynecol* 106:747–752, 2005.

Penso C, Redline RW, Benacerraf BR: A sonographic sign which predicts which fetuses with hydrocephalus have an associated neural tube defect. *J Ultrasound Med* 6:307–311, 1987.

Peralta CF, Bunduki V, Plese JP, Figueiredo EG, Miguelez J, Zugaib M: Association between prenatal sonographic findings and post-natal outcomes in 30 cases of isolated spina bifida aperta. *Prenat Diagn* 23:311–314, 2003.

Robinson HP, Hood VD, Adam AH, et al: Diagnostic ultrasound: early detection of fetal neural tube defects. *Obstet Gynecol* 56:705–710, 1980.

VATER ASSOCIATION

DESCRIPTION AND DEFINITION

VATER association is an acronym for a nonrandom association of abnormalities that include **v**ertebral defects, **a**nal atresia, **t**racheoesophageal fistula, **e**sophageal atresia, and **r**adial and renal dysplasias.

ABNORMALITIES DETECTABLE BY ULTRASOUND

Common Findings:

Vertebral abnormalities

Hemivertebrae and other vertebral abnormalities

Scoliosis

Anal atresia (diagnosable if there is a rectovesical fistula, identified by the characteristic appearance of intraluminal calcifications [urine and meconium] in the distended loop of colon)

Tracheoesophageal fistula (usually accompanied by esophageal atresia, sometimes associated with a small or absent stomach and polyhydramnios)*

Cardiac defects

Renal anomalies

Hydronephrosis

Cystic kidneys

Radial ray abnormalities, with a short or absent radius and abnormal hands

Occasional Findings:

Spinal dysraphia

Lower extremity anomalies

Single umbilical artery

Genital defects

Polydactyly and syndactyly

MAJOR DIFFERENTIAL DIAGNOSES

Chromosomal Abnormalities:

Trisomy 13 (Patau syndrome)

Trisomy 18 (Edwards' syndrome)

Short Radial Ray Syndromes:

Ectrodactyly–ectodermal dysplasia–clefting (EEC) syndrome

Fanconi anemia

Holt-Oram syndrome

Nager syndrome

Roberts syndrome

Thrombocytopenia–absent radius (TAR) syndrome

Vertebral Body/Renal Anomalies:

Caudal regression syndrome

Cerebrocostomandibular syndrome

Jarcho-Levin syndrome and related syndromes

MURCS (**mü**llerian duct aplasia, **r**enal aplasia, **c**ervicothoracic **s**omite dysplasia) association

Sirenomelia

*Prenatal diagnosis may be difficult in many cases in which fluid *does* penetrate the stomach.

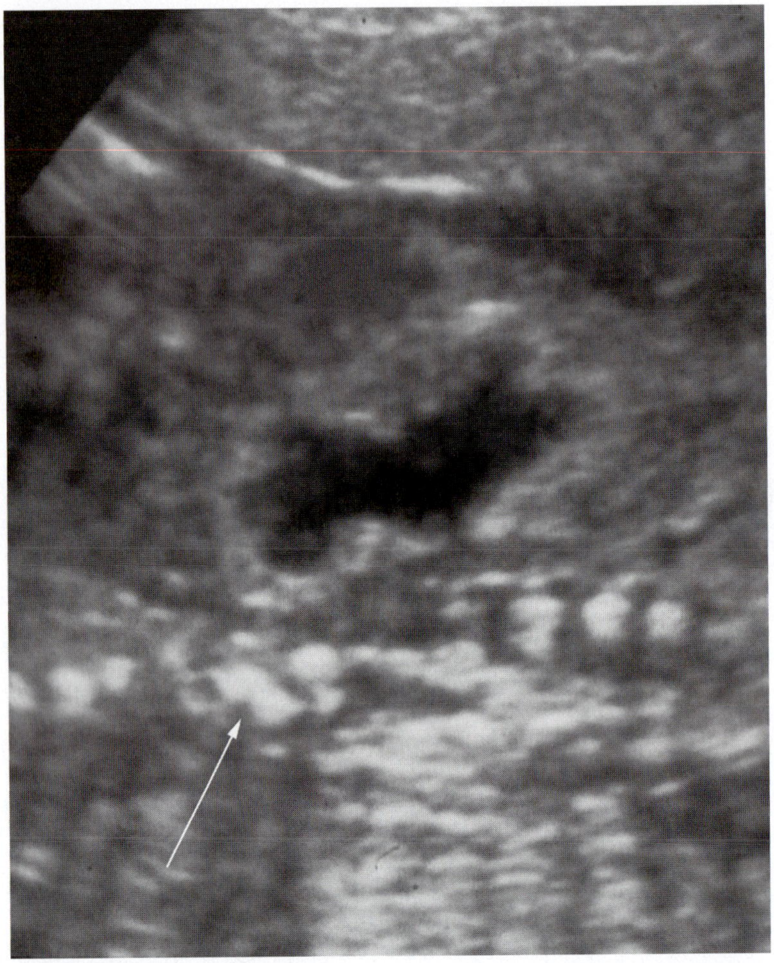

FIGURE 2-263 Hydronephrotic kidney in a fetus with multiple vertebral body abnormalities *(arrow)* consistent with VATER association.

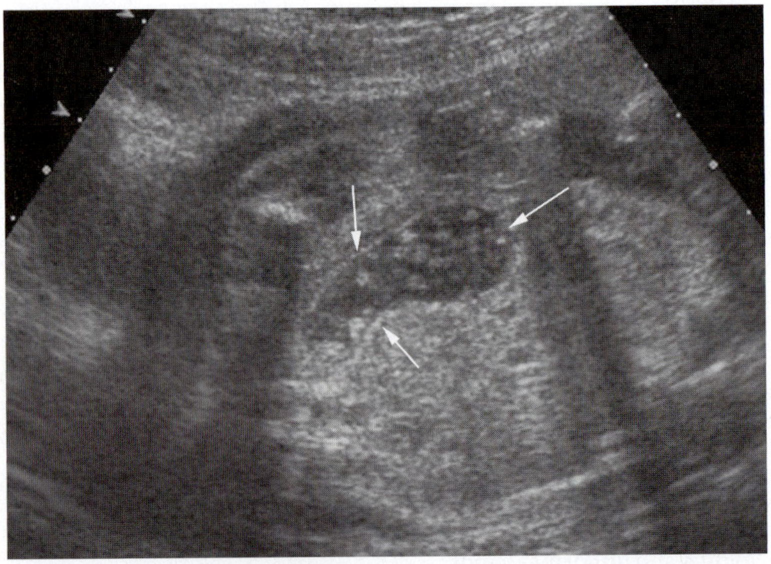

A

FIGURE 2-264 A 24-week fetus with VATER association. (A) View of the fetal abdomen shows a distended loop of bowel *(arrows),* which contains intraluminal calcifications consistent with the presence of a vesicorectal fistula.

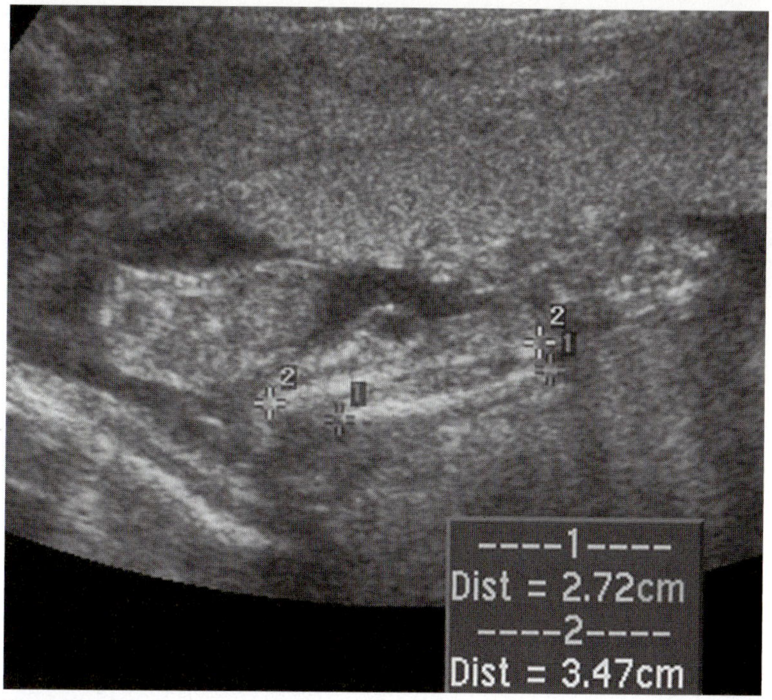

B

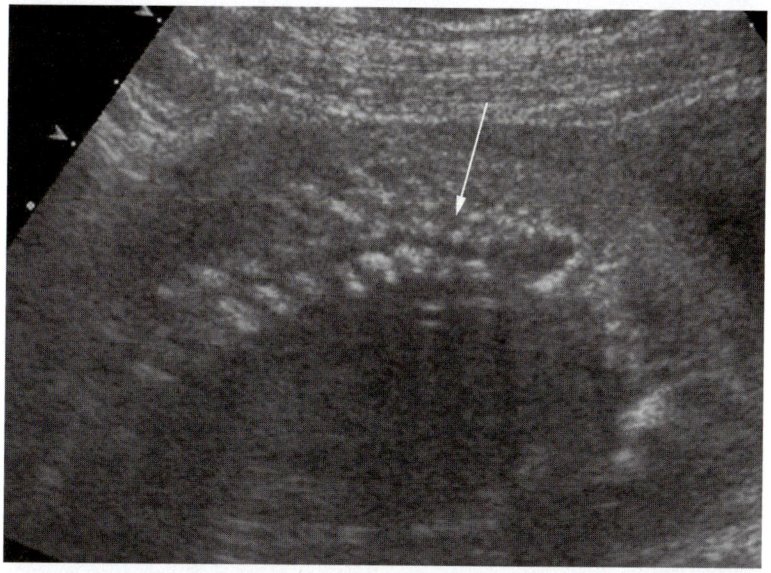

C

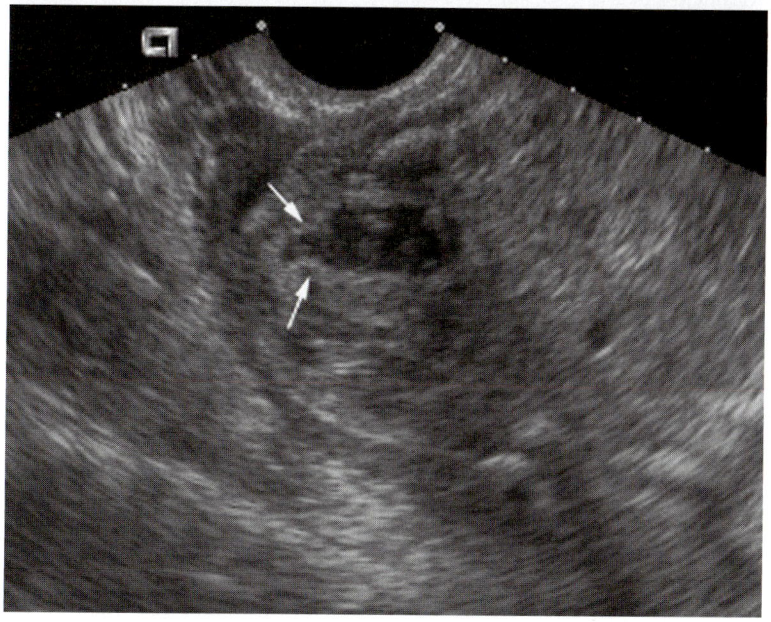

D

FIGURE 2-264, cont'd (B) Fetal forearm of the same fetus shows a shortened radius compared to the ulna. (C) Vertebral body abnormalities *(arrow)* in the thoracic spine of the same fetus. (D) Blindly ending rectosigmoid *(arrows)* in the same fetus with anal atresia.

Continued

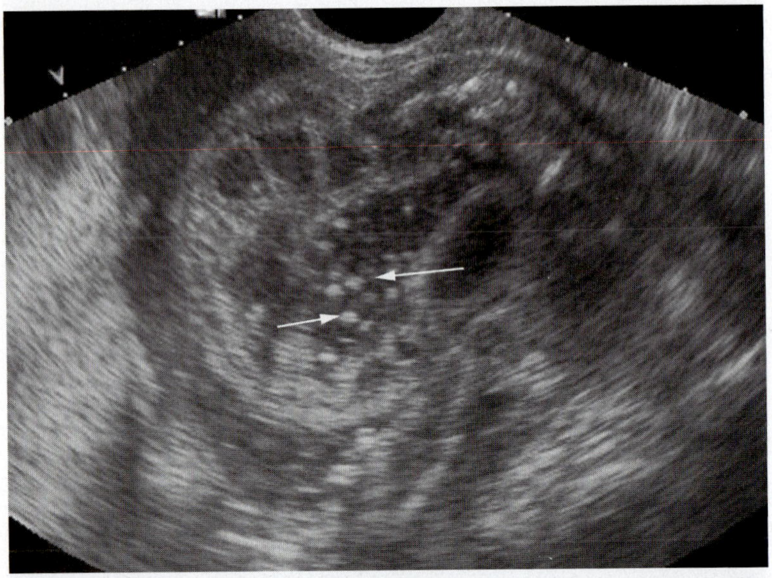

E

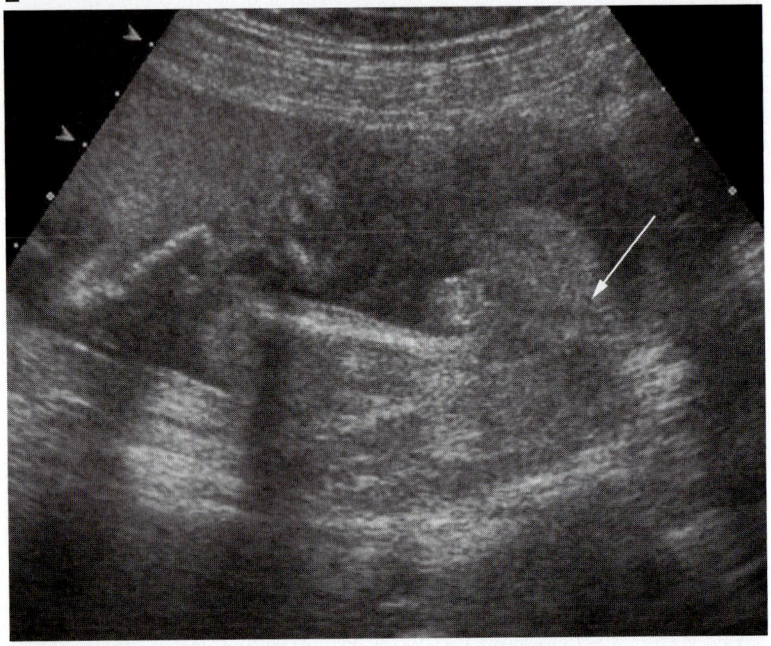

F

FIGURE 2-264, cont'd **(E) Dilated loop of bowel within the fetal abdomen has multiple intraluminal calcifications *(arrows)* consistent with mixture of meconium and urine through a fistula. (F) View of the fetal perineum of the same fetus shows absence of the anus *(arrow).***

ULTRASOUND DIAGNOSIS

Prenatal sonographic diagnosis of the VATER association has been established in the early- to mid-second trimester, based on an abnormal spine, kidneys, heart, and radial ray (although not all of these features will be present in each case). Esophageal atresia is detectable by ultrasound only if little or no fluid is present in the fetal stomach in association with polyhydramnios.

HEREDITY

The etiology and heredity pattern of this condition are unknown.

NATURAL HISTORY AND OUTCOME

The outcome depends on the severity of abnormalities. Most infants have normal intelligence and require surgical and rehabilitative intervention. VATER association can occur with ventriculomegaly secondary to aqueductal stenosis, which carries a poorer prognosis than other cases of the association.

Suggested Reading

Claiborne AK, Blocker SH, Martin CM, McAlister WH: Prenatal and postnatal sonographic delineation of gastrointestinal abnormalities in a case of the VATER syndrome. *J Ultrasound Med* 5:45–47, 1986.

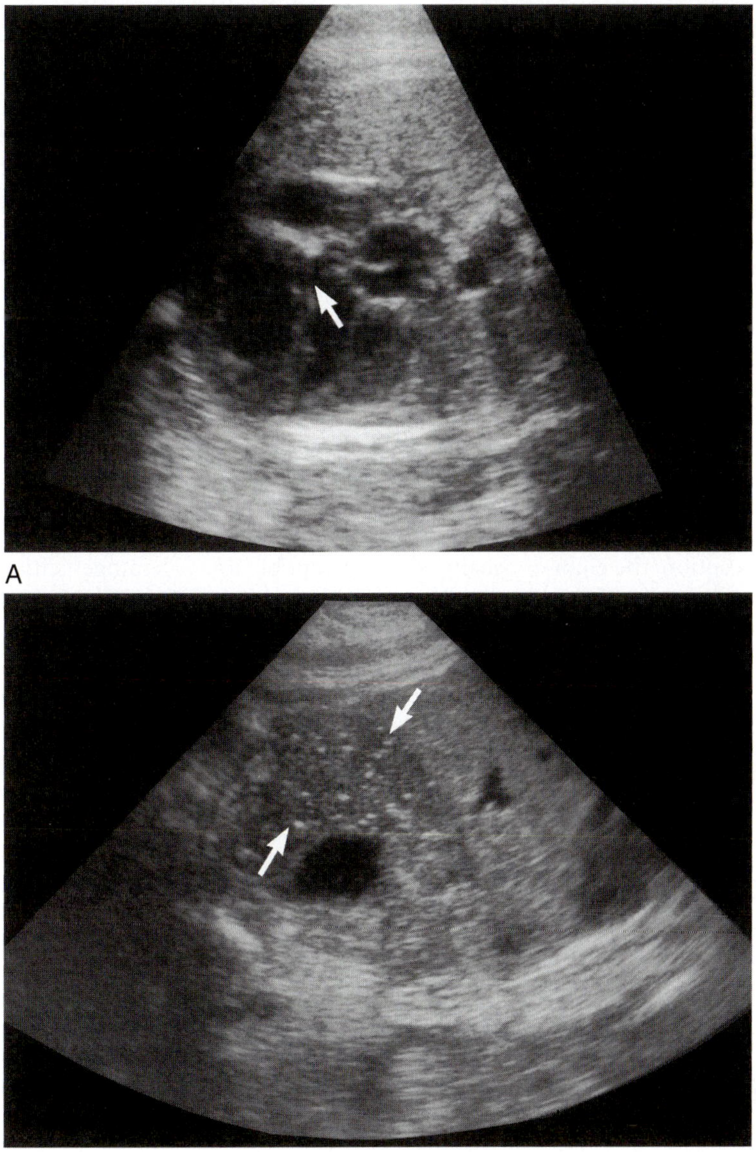

A

B

FIGURE 2-265 (**A**) Four-chamber view of the heart of a fetus with multiple abnormalities, including ventricular septal defect *(arrow)* and anal atresia with a vesicorectal fistula. (**B**) Multiple intraluminal calcifications in the same fetus are evident in the fetal bowel *(arrows),* indicating the mixture of urine and meconium seen with vesicorectal fistulas. This is a characteristic finding in cases of anal atresia, as can be seen in fetuses with VATER association.

Jones KL: *Smith's recognizable patterns of human malformations,* ed 6. Philadelphia, 2006, Elsevier.

Kaufman RL, Quinton BA, Ternberg JL: Imperforate anus, vertebral anomalies and preaxial limb abnormalities. *Birth Defects* 8:85–87, 1972.

McGahan JP, Leeba JM, Lindfors KK: Prenatal sonographic diagnosis of VATER association. *J Clin Ultrasound* 16:588–591, 1988.

Murr MM, Waziri MH, Schelper RL, Abu-Youself M: Case of multivertebral anomalies, cloacal dysgenesis, and other anomalies presenting prenatally as cystic kidneys. *Am J Med Genet* 42:761–765, 1992.

Quan L, Smith DW: The VATER association: vertebral defects, anal atresia, tracheoesophageal fistula with esophageal atresia, radial dysplasia. *Birth Defects* 8:75–78, 1972.

Tongsong T, Wanapirak C, Piyamongkol W, Sudasana J: Prenatal sonographic diagnosis of VATER association. *J Clin Ultrasound* 27:378–384, 1999.

Teratogens

Teratogenesis is the process by which genetic or environmental factors affect the development of the embryo. This section discusses the teratogenicity of some commonly used medications and maternal conditions and infections that cause serious fetal malformations. Environmental agents include medications, chemicals, infections, maternal conditions (e.g., phenylketonuria), radiation, and hyperthermia.

The susceptibility of the fetus depends on the developmental stage at the time of exposure, with the first trimester being the most sensitive. Specifically, during the first 2 weeks after conception, the embryo usually is not susceptible to teratogens. This is the predifferentiation stage, and damage to only a few cells can be overcome by the development of other cells that still are omnipotential. This allows the embryo to recover without anatomic defects. If all the cells are destroyed, the result is a miscarriage. Weeks 3 to 8 after conception (5–10 weeks' gestational age) is the most critical period for development and has the highest vulnerability to teratogenic insult. In weeks 3 and 4 after conception, the CNS and the eyes are most commonly affected by teratogens. In weeks 5 and 6 after conception, the heart, extremities, eyes, and ears may be affected, with major morphologic abnormalities. The impact of teratogens in weeks 7 and 8 after conception most commonly involves the eyes, palate, external genitalia, and ears. Subsequent to week 8, the embryo is less sensitive to teratogens. Although severe mental retardation still may occur in the 8- to 16-week postconception period, most of the other abnormalities that occur after 8 weeks tend to be minor morphologic or functional defects.

Teratogenicity is related to dosage; in most cases, a threshold dosage must be exceeded before damage occurs. Regarding pharmaceutical teratogenicity, a report by Levine et al. demonstrated a relatively low incidence of morphologic abnormality in fetuses of mothers exposed to a large variety of medications. Among 126 pregnancies with known exposure to drugs and other toxins, as well as to infections, only one fetal abnormality was identified: a duplicated kidney in a case of probably unrelated maternal parvovirus. The teratogens described in this chapter are based on anomalies associated with these chemicals reported in the literature. However, given an individual patient with a drug exposure, the likelihood of an abnormality remains relatively low for most exposures.

ANTIBIOTICS

METRONIDAZOLE (FLAGYL)

Midline facial defects

Possible increased risk for neuroblastoma

QUININE

Cardiac defects

Dysmelia

Facial defects

Ventriculomegaly

Vertebral anomalies

TETRACYCLINE

Enamel hypoplasia (teeth)

Hypospadias

Impaired bone growth

Limb hypoplasia

ANTICANCER AGENTS

AZATHIOPRINE

Hypospadias

Intrauterine growth restriction (IUGR)

Polydactyly

Pulmonary valvar stenosis

CYCLOPHOSPHAMIDE

Depressed nasal bridge

Finger and toe abnormalities

Ectrodactyly

Syndactyly

Tetralogy of Fallot

CYTARABINE

Anencephaly

IUGR

Lobster-claw deformities of the limbs

Tetralogy of Fallot

FLUOROURACIL

Esophageal and duodenal abnormalities

Radial aplasia

METHOTREXATE

Abnormal frontal and other cranial bones

Club feet

Dextrocardia

IUGR

Low-set ears

Mandibular hypoplasia

Microcephaly

Neural tube defects

Syndactyly

PROCARBAZINE

Cerebral hemorrhage

Oligodactyly

THIOGUANINE

IUGR

Missing digits or polydactyly

ANTICOAGULANTS

ACETYLSALICYLIC ACID (ASPIRIN)

Intracranial hemorrhage

IUGR (occasional)

Increased incidence of early spontaneous abortion (SAB) in first trimester

WARFARIN (COUMADIN)

Anencephaly

Blindness

Cardiac defects

Cataracts

Choanal atresia

Depressed nasal bridge

Encephalocele

IUGR

Nasal hypoplasia

Ophthalmic abnormalities

Rhizomelia

Scoliosis

Skeletal abnormalities

Spina bifida

Stippled epiphyses

ANTICONVULSANT DRUGS

CARBAMAZEPINE (TEGRETOL)

Ambiguous genitalia

Atrial septal defects

Cleft lip

Club feet

ETHOSUXIMIDE

Cardiac defects

Facial cleft

Hip dislocation

Hypertelorism

Meningomyelocele

Nasal hypoplasia

Patent ductus arteriosus

Possible mild developmental delays (occasional)

Short neck

Ventriculomegaly

HYDANTOIN

Cardiac defects (occasional)

Cleft lip and palate

Depressed nasal bridge

Genitourinary abnormalities (occasional)

Growth deficiency

Holoprosencephaly (occasional)

Hypertelorism

Hypoplasia of the distal phalanges

Microcephaly (occasional)

Rib anomalies

MECLIZINE

Hypoplastic left heart

PHENANTOIN

Craniofacial abnormalities:

- Broad nasal bridge
- Cleft lip and palate
- Hypertelorism
- Low-set ears
- Short nose

Cardiac disease

Hypoplastic distal phalanges

IUGR

Microcephaly

TRIMETHADION

High incidence of abnormalities involving many organ systems.

- Cardiac defects, particularly ventricular or atrial septal defects
- Facial anomalies:
  - Broad nasal bridge
  - Cleft lip and palate
  - Low-set ears
- Esophageal atresia
- Genital defects
- Hand and foot malformations
- IUGR
- Microcephaly

VALPROIC ACID

Cataracts

Depressed nasal bridge

Facial cleft

IUGR

Limb abnormalities

- Absence of the radial ray

Low-set ears

Meningomyelocele (1% to 2% incidence)

Microcephaly

Micrognathia

Septo-optic dysplasia and other brain abnormalities

Tetralogy of Fallot and other cardiac defects

Urogenital defects

ANTITHYROID AGENTS

Fetal goiter

HORMONES

CLOMIPHENE (CLOMID)

Anencephaly

Cardiac defects

Club feet

Esophageal atresia

Facial cleft

Hypospadias

Meningomyelocele

Microcephaly

Polydactyly

Syndactyly

CORTISONE

Cataract

Cleft lip and palate

Club feet

Coarctation of the aorta

IUGR

Ventricular septal defects

Ventriculomegaly

ESTROGEN

Cardiac disease

Eye and ear anomalies

Limb reductions

ORAL CONTRACEPTIVES

Genital abnormalities

Limb reduction defects

VATER (**v**ertebral defects, **a**nal atresia, **t**racheo-esophageal fistula, **e**sophageal atresia, and **r**adial and renal dysplasias) association

PROGESTIN

Anencephaly

Cardiac defects

Cataract

Genital anomalies (hypospadias)

Limb and thumb abnormalities

Spina bifida

Tetralogy of Fallot

Truncus arteriosus

Ventricular septal defects

Ventriculomegaly

THALIDOMIDE

Cardiac defects

Duodenal atresia

Limb reduction abnormalities

Microtia

Spine malformations

TRANQUILIZERS AND ANTIDEPRESSANTS

AMITRIPTYLINE

Hand and foot abnormalities

Limb reduction

Micrognathia

CHLORDIAZEPOXIDE (LIBRIUM)

Cardiac defects

Duodenal atresia

Microcephaly

CLONAZEPAM

One case of tetralogy and dysmorphic facies and IUGR

FLUOXETINE (PROZAC)

An occasional cluster of minor abnormalities is associated with use of this drug during pregnancy, but there is no increased risk for major abnormalities. Third-trimester fetal exposure to Prozac is associated with an increased rate of preterm delivery, poor neonatal adaptation, respiratory distress, jitteriness, and low birth weight.

FLUPHENAZINE

Facial cleft

Poor ossification of the frontal bone

HALOPERIDOL

Limb deformities

IMIPRAMINE

Cleft palate

Diaphragmatic hernia

Exencephaly

Limb reduction abnormalities

Renal cystic disease

MEPROBAMATE

Cardiac defects

Limb defects (bilateral)

Respiratory defects

NORTRIPTYLINE

Limb reduction

PHENOTHIAZINE (CHLORPROMAZINE)

Club feet

Syndactyly

MISCELLANEOUS

ACETAZOLAMIDE

IUGR

Sacrococcygeal teratoma

ALCOHOL

Cardiac and visceral malformations

Facial abnormalities:

- Cleft lip and palate
- Depressed nasal bridge
- Ear deformities
- Low forehead
- Micrognathia

IUGR

Microcephaly

Ophthalmic abnormalities

AMINOPTERIN (ANTIFOLATE)

Abnormalities of the extremities:

- Club feet
- Hypoplasia of the thumb and fibula
- Syndactyly

Anencephaly

Facial cleft

Incomplete skull ossification

IUGR

Low-set ears

Meningomyelocele

Microcephaly

Micrognathia

Ventriculomegaly

CARBON MONOXIDE

Cerebral atrophy

Stillbirth

Ventriculomegaly

CIPROFLOXACIN

Ventriculomegaly

CHLORPHENIRAMINE

Gastrointestinal abnormalities

Genital anomalies (females)

Hip dislocation

Polydactyly

Ventriculomegaly

CHLORPROPAMIDE

Dysmorphic hands

Ear abnormalities

Microcephaly

Prolonged hypoglycemia in neonate

COCAINE

Cardiac disease

Cranial defects

IUGR

Limb reduction anomalies

Placental abruption

Renal abnormalities

CODEINE

Cardiac defects

Dislocated hip

Facial cleft

Musculoskeletal malformations

Pyloric stenosis

Respiratory malformations

Ventriculomegaly

DEXTROAMPHETAMINE

Cardiac defects

Exencephaly

HYPERTHERMIA (MATERNAL BODY TEMPERATURE >102° F)

Hyperthermic exposure 14 to 28 days after conception may result in increased fetal risk for the following:

Facial defects

IUGR

Microcephaly

Neural tube defects

INDOMETHACIN

Closure of the ductus arteriosus in utero, resulting in pulmonary hypertension

Fetal hemorrhage

Phocomelia

Stillbirth

MATERNAL PHENYLKETONURIA

Maternal phenylketonuria (PKU) results in hyperphenylalaninemia, which is a teratogen for the fetus. First-trimester exposure to an increased maternal blood level of phenylalanine may result in the following:

Cardiac disease (in most cases, tetralogy of Fallot)

Microcephaly

Although the associated heart disease can be detected in the second trimester, in many cases the associated microcephaly may not be definitively diagnosed until after 22 weeks' gestational age.

PHENYLEPHRINE

Club feet

Eye and ear abnormalities

Hip dislocation

Syndactyly

Umbilical hernia

PHENYLPROPANOLAMINE

Hip dislocation

Pectus excavatum

Polydactyly

PROPRANOLOL*

Bradycardia

Decreased placental size

Hypoglycemia (postnatal)

IUGR

RADIATION

Radiation-induced defects are dose related. Irradiation with a dose <5 rad carries a negligible risk for malformations. Only large amounts of

*This drug has a long half-life, so it remains in the system long after its use has been discontinued.

ionizing radiation, as used in therapy for cervical cancer, are thought to cause fetal defects, such as the following:

Facial defects

IUGR

Microcephaly

Spina bifida

SMOKING

Abruption

Cardiac disease (two-fold increase in incidence)

Low birth weight

Perinatal death

Prematurity

Suggested Reading

Alsdorf R, Wyszynski DF: Teratogenicity of sodium valproate. *Expert Opin Drug Saf* 4:345–553, 2005.

Briggs GG, Freeman RK, Yaffe SJ: *Drugs in pregnancy and lactation.* Philadelphia, 2005, Lippincott Williams & Wilkins.

Chambers CD, Johnson KA, Dick LM, Felix RJ, Jones KL: Birth outcomes in pregnant women taking fluoxetine. *N Engl J Med* 335:1010–1015, 1996.

Chapa JB, Hibbard JU, Weber EM, Abramowicz JS, Verp MS: Prenatal diagnosis of methotrexate embryopathy. *Obstet Gynecol* 101(5 Pt 2):1104–1107, 2003.

Collins E: Maternal and fetal effects of acetaminophen and salicylates in pregnancy. *Obstet Gynecol* 58:57S–62S, 1981.

Gentile S: The safety of newer antidepressants in pregnancy and breastfeeding. *Drug Saf* 28:137–152, 2005.

Hill RM, Stern L: Drugs in pregnancy: effects on the fetus and newborn. *Drugs* 17:182–197, 1979.

Jacqz-Aigrain E, Koren G: Effects of drugs on the fetus. *Semin Fetal Neonatal Med* 10:139–147, 2005.

Janz D: Are antiepileptic drugs harmful when taken during pregnancy? *J Perinat Med* 22:367–377, 1994.

Jones KL: *Smith's recognizable patterns of human malformations.* Philadelphia, 2006, Elsevier.

Kelly-Buchanan C, ed: *Peace of mind during pregnancy.* Philadelphia, 1989, Dell.

Koren G, Edwards MB, Miskin M: Antenatal sonography of fetal malformations associated with drugs and chemicals: a guide. *Am J Obstet Gynecol* 156:79–85, 1987.

Kricker A, Elliott JW, Forrest JM, McCredie J: Congenital limb reduction deformities and use of oral contraceptives. *Am J Obstet Gynecol* 155:1072–1078, 1986.

Levine D, Filly RA, Goldberg JD: Teratogen exposure: lack of morphological abnormalities by detailed fetal sonography. *Ultrasound Obstet Gynecol* 4:452–456, 1994.

Levy HL, Lobbregt D, Platt LD, Benacerraf BR: Fetal ultrasonography in maternal phenylketonuria (PKU). *Prenat Diagn* 16:587–598, 1996.

Levy HL, Waisbren SE: Effects of untreated maternal phenylketonuria and hyperphenylalaninemia on the fetus. *N Engl J Med* 309:1269–1274, 1983.

Lindhout D, Omtzigt JG, Cornel MC: Spectrum of neural-tube defects in 34 infants prenatally exposed to antiepileptic drugs. *Neurology* 42:111–118, 1992.

Matalon ST, Ornoy A, Lishner M: Review of the potential effects of three commonly used antineoplastic and immunosuppressive drugs (cyclophosphamide, azathioprine, doxorubicin on the embryo and placenta). *Reprod Toxicol* 18:219–230, 2004.

Mitchell M, Sabbagha RE, Keith L, et al: Ultrasonic growth parameters in fetuses of mothers with primary addiction to cocaine. *Am J Obstet Gynecol* 159:1104–1109, 1988.

Moore KL: *The developing human*, ed 4. Philadelphia, 1988, WB Saunders.

Nahum GG, Uhl K, Kennedy DL: Antibiotic use in pregnancy and lactation: what is and is not known about teratogenic and toxic risks. *Obstet Gynecol* 107:1120–1138, 2006.

Omtzigt JG, Los FJ, Hagenaars AM, et al: Prenatal diagnosis of spina bifida aperta after first-trimester valproate exposure. *Prenat Diagn* 12:893–897, 1992.

Rosenberg L, Mitchell AA, Parsells JL, et al: Lack of relation of oral clefts to diazepam use during pregnancy. *N Engl J Med* 309:1282–1285,1983.

Schardern JL, ed: *Chemically induced birth defects,* ed 2. New York, 1993, Marcel Dekker.

Sharony R, Garber A, Viskochil D, et al: Preaxial ray deduction defects as part of valproic acid embryofetopathy. *Prenat Diagn* 13:909–918, 1993.

Thapa PB, Whitlock JA, Brockman Worrell KG, et al: Prenatal exposure to metronidazole and risk of childhood cancer: a retrospective cohort study of children younger than 5 years. *Cancer* 1;85:2494–2495, 1999.

Townsend RR, Laing FC, Jeffrey RB: Placental abruption associated with cocaine abuse. *AJR Am J Roentgenol* 150:1339–1340, 1988.

Wood BP, Young LW: Pseudohyperphalangism in fetal Dilantin syndrome. *Radiology* 131:371–372, 1979.

Ylagan LR, Budorick NE: Radial ray aplasia in utero: a prenatal finding associated with valproic acid exposure. *J Ultrasound Med* 13:408–411, 1994.

MATERNAL INFECTIONS

Antenatal sonography can demonstrate a number of abnormalities associated with in utero infection involving multiple organ systems. When sonographic findings indicate a fetal infection, usually the prognosis is poor.

In a study by Drose et al. of 19 fetuses with known congenital infections, multiple organ systems were affected in 47%, intracranial abnormalities in 42%, cardiac abnormalities in 37%, and parenchymal calcifications of the brain in 32%. Thirty-two percent of affected fetuses had large placentas, 37% had oligohydramnios, and another 37% had polyhydramnios. Sixty-three percent died at birth. All of the 37% who survived are developmentally impaired.

There are wide differences in the degree of teratogenicity and possibilities for treatment among fetuses with in utero infections. In the following sections, the six most common infections are discussed.

CYTOMEGALOVIRUS

Description and Definition

Cytomegalovirus (CMV) is caused by a double-stranded DNA herpes virus infection that

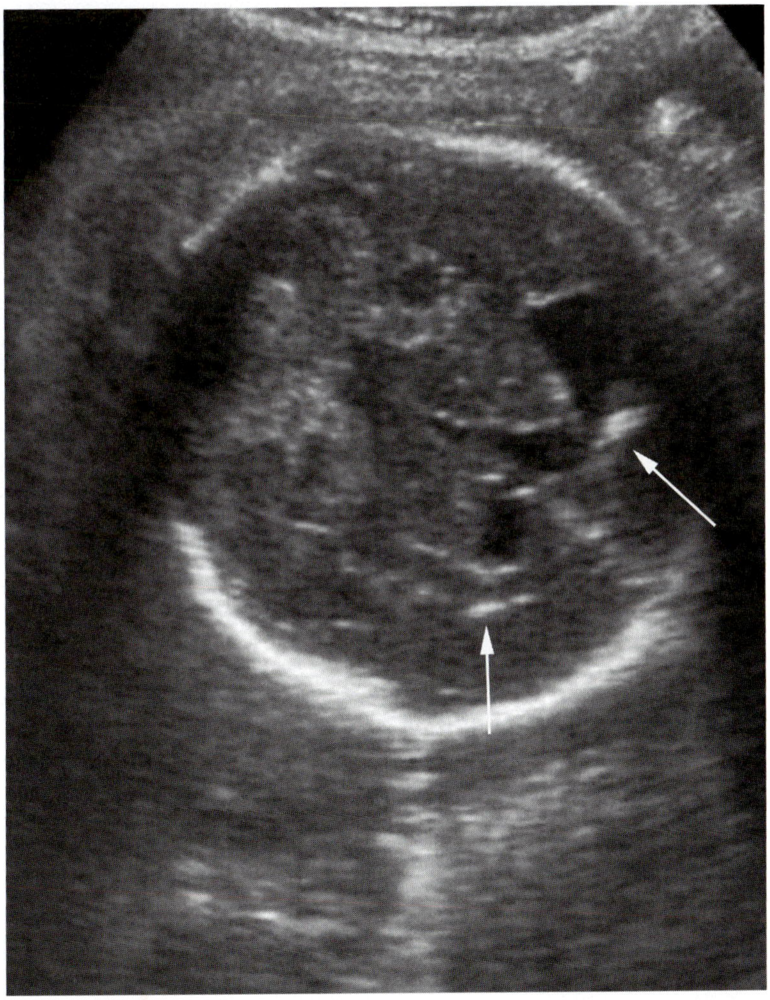

A

FIGURE 2-266 Third-trimester fetus with cytomegalovirus. (A, B) Third-trimester fetus with intrauterine infection has multiple intracerebral calcifications *(arrows)*.

Continued

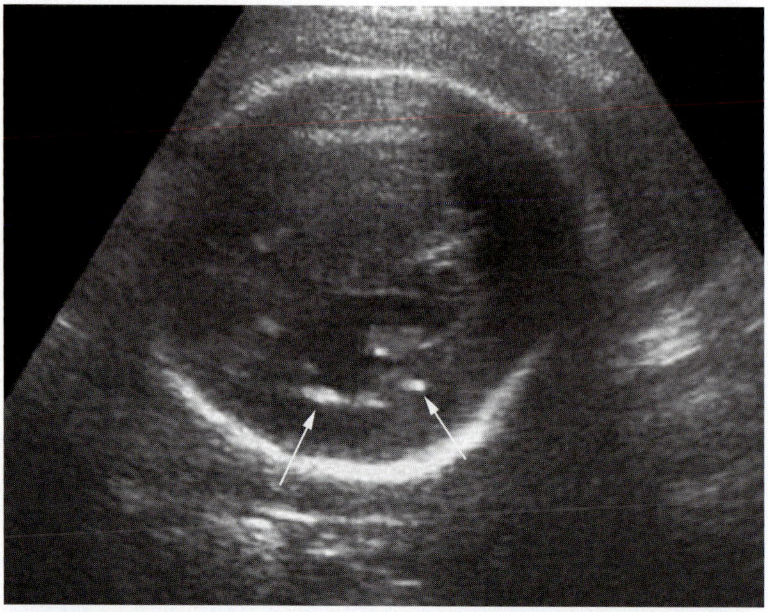

B

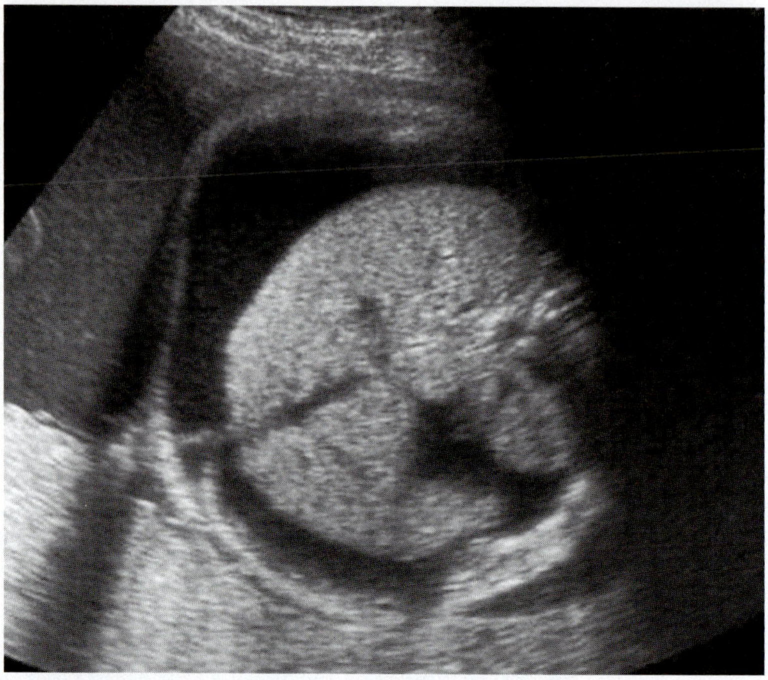

C

FIGURE 2-266, cont'd Third-trimester fetus with cytomegalovirus. (**A, B**) Third-trimester fetus with intrauterine infection has multiple intracerebral calcifications *(arrows)*. (**C**) Transverse view through the fetal abdomen of the same fetus shows marked ascites caused by intrauterine infection.

results in a mononucleosis-type illness. This is the most common cause of congenital infection.

Abnormalities Detectable by Ultrasound

Ventriculomegaly

Intracranial calcifications

Microcephaly

Brain atrophy

Hyperechoic bowel

Ascites, hydrops

Cardiomegaly

Intrahepatic calcifications

IUGR

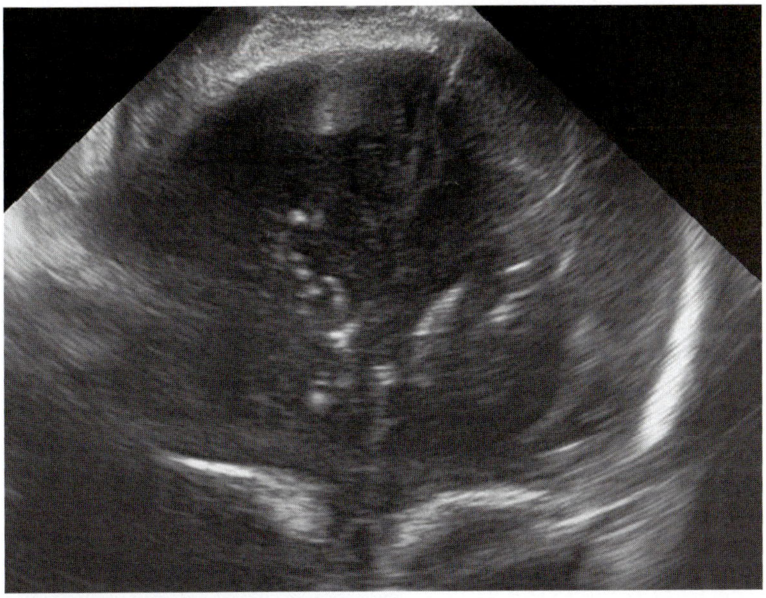

A

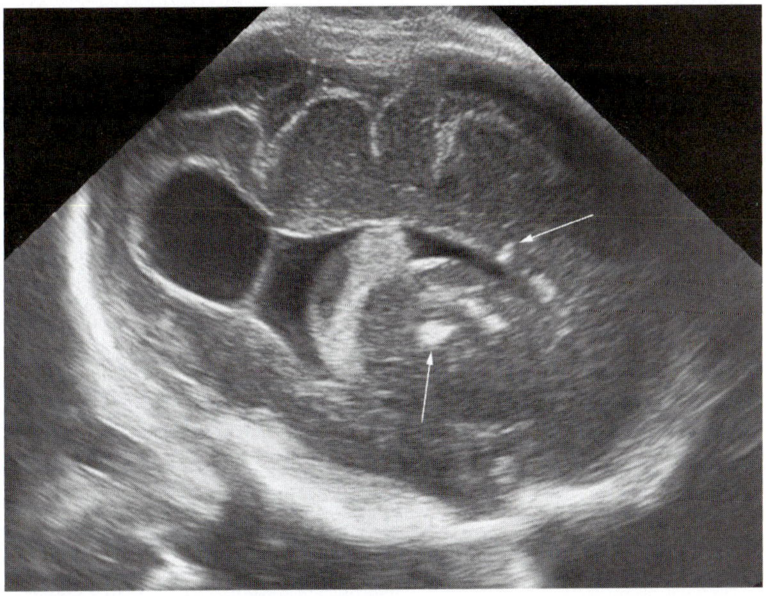

B

FIGURE 2-267 Third-trimester fetus with cytomegalovirus. (A) Coronal view through the frontal horns shows multiple calcifications in the region of the thalami and basal ganglia . (B) Transvaginal scan of the same fetus shows multiple calcifications *(arrows)* in the basal ganglia and an intraventricular adhesion in the posterior horn.

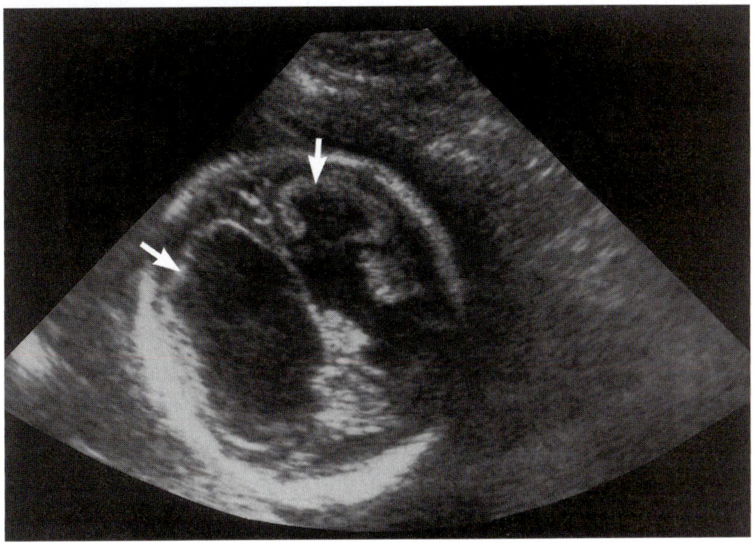

FIGURE 2-268 Oblique view through the head of a fetus with cytomegalovirus. Note marked ventricular dilation and periventricular calcifications *(arrows)*.

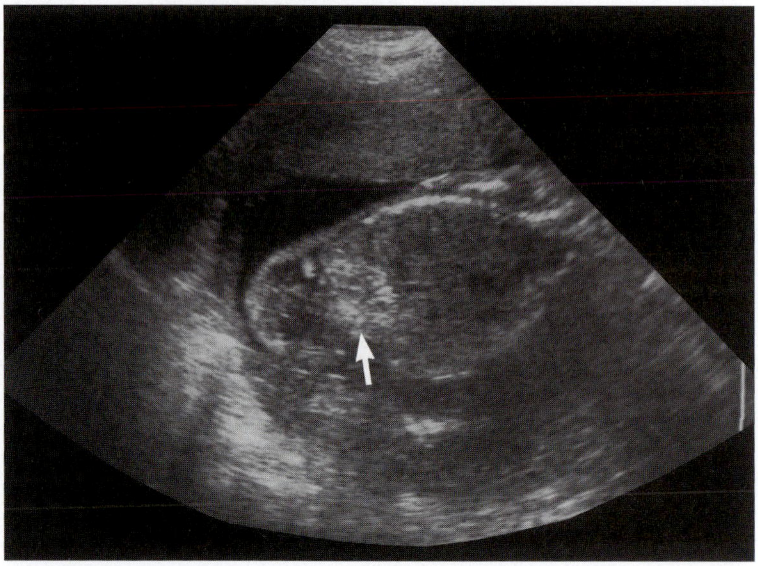

FIGURE 2-269 Longitudinal view of the fetal abdomen shows hyperechoic bowel *(arrow)*, which can be seen in some fetuses with cytomegalovirus.

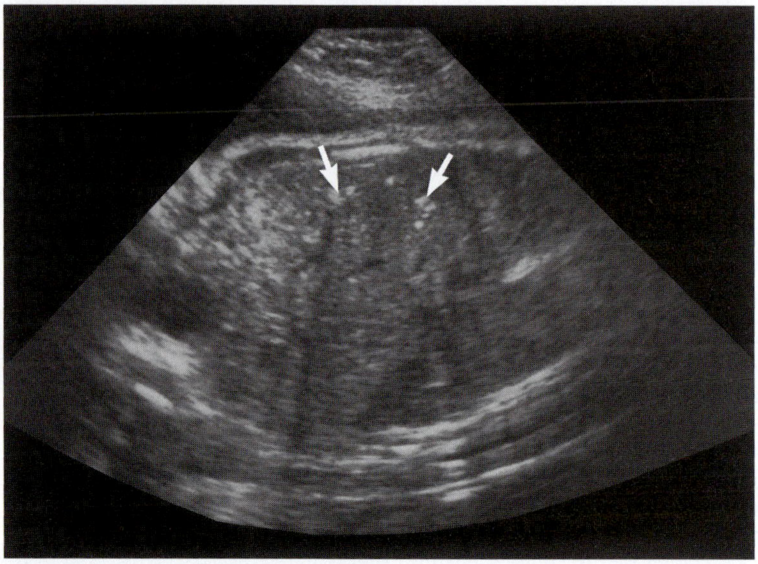

FIGURE 2-270 Coronal view through the fetal liver shows multiple calcifications *(arrows)* within the liver parenchyma. This fetus had cytomegalovirus with microcephaly at birth.

Enlarged placenta

Oligohydramnios

Polyhydramnios

Major Differential Diagnoses

Syndromes and Conditions Associated with Intracranial Calcifications:

Other congenital fetal infections, such as toxoplasmosis

Tuberous sclerosis

Syndromes and Conditions Associated with Hyperechoic Bowel:

Alpha-thalassemia with hydrops

Cystic fibrosis

Down syndrome

Early IUGR

Ingestion of blood by the fetus

Varicella infection

Ultrasound Diagnosis

In general, the diagnosis is most often established after 20 weeks' gestational age. Ultrasound seems to be less sensitive than amniocentesis or fetal blood sampling for detection of this disease. On the rare occasion when the diagnosis is established before 20 weeks' gestation, hyperechoic bowel appears to be a helpful finding. Normal findings at 22 weeks do not exclude an abnormal ultrasound examination later or a severely affected neonate.

In a group of 16 infected fetuses, the combination of ultrasound examination, amniocentesis, and fetal blood sampling resulted in the diagnosis in 13 (sensitivity of 81%). Amniocentesis allowed the diagnosis of 12 of these 13, and immunoglobulin M (IgM) antibody detection was evident in the fetal blood of 69%. Ultrasound findings were abnormal in only 5 of the 16 infected fetuses, with abnormalities including ventriculomegaly, hyperechoic bowel, and IUGR (see the study by Donner et al.). In another study of fetuses with CMV, 42% had intracranial calcification, 37% cardiac anomalies, 32% intraabdominal calcifications, and 32% large placentas.

Heredity

Heredity is not a factor in this fetal infection. Fetal infection occurs in approximately 30% of women with primary or recurrent infection.

Natural History and Outcome

Approximately 0.2% to 1% of liveborn infants are infected with congenital CMV infection, although only approximately 10% of these are symptomatic at birth. Among those who are symptomatic, mortality is as high as 30%. Symptoms include growth restriction, hepatosplenomegaly, jaundice, thrombocytopenia, anemia, chorioretinitis, microcephaly, ventriculomegaly, and intracranial calcifications.

Long-term effects include mental retardation, motor handicaps, and hearing loss.

Suggested Reading

Achiron R, Pinhas-Hamiel O, Lipitz S, et al: Prenatal ultrasonographic diagnosis of fetal cerebral ventriculitis associated with asymptomatic maternal cytomegalovirus infections. *Prenat Diagn* 14:523–526, 1994.

Adams JH, Corsellis JAN, Cuchen LW, eds. *Greenfield's neuropathology.* New York, 1985, Wiley.

Al-Kouatly HB, Chasen ST, Streltzoff J, Chervenak FA: The clinical significance of fetal echogenic bowel. *Am J Obstet Gynecol* 185:1035–1038, 2001.

Ben-Ami T, Yousefzadeh D, Backus M, et al: Lenticulostriate vasculopathy in infants with infections of the central nervous system: sonographic and Doppler findings. *Pediatr Radiol* 20:575–579, 1990.

Binder ND, Buckmaster JW, Benda GI: Outcome for fetus with ascites and cytomegalovirus infection. *Pediatrics* 82:100–103, 1988.

Butt W, Mackay RJ, de Crespigny LC, Murton LJ, Roy RND: Intracranial lesions of congenital cytomegalovirus infection detected by ultrasound scanning. *Pediatrics* 73:61–104, 1984.

Catanzarite V, Dankner WM: Prenatal diagnosis of congenital cytomegalovirus infection: false negative amniocentesis at 20 weeks' gestation. *Prenat Diagn* 13:1021–1025, 1993.

Chriss-Price D, Lawrence SK, Jeanty P: Cytomegalovirus, splenomegaly. *Fetus* 4:5–9, 1994.

Daffos F, Forestier F, Capella-Pavlovsky M, et al: Prenatal management of 746 pregnancies at risk for congenital toxoplasmosis. *N Engl J Med* 318:271–275, 1988.

Degani S: Sonographic findings in fetal viral infections: a systematic review. *Obstet Gynecol Surv* 61:329–336, 2006.

Donner C, Liesnard C, Content J, et al: Prenatal diagnosis of 52 pregnancies at risk for congenital cytomegalovirus infection. *Obstet Gynecol* 82:481–486, 1993.

Drose JA, Dennis MA, Thickman D: Infection in utero: US findings in 19 cases. *Radiology* 178:369–374, 1991.

Fakhry J, Khoury A: Fetal intracranial calcifications: the importance of periventricular hyperechoic foci without shadowing. *J Ultrasound Med* 10:51–54, 1991.

Fan-Havara P, Nanata MC, Brady MT: Ganciclovir—a review of pharmacology, therapeutic efficacy and potential use for treatment of congenital cytomegalovirus infection. *J Clin Pharm Ther* 14:329–340, 1989.

Forouzan I: Fetal abdominal echogenic mass: an early sign of intrauterine cytomegalovirus infection. *Obstet Gynecol* 80:535–537, 1992.

Graham D, Guidi SM, Sanders RC: Sonographic features of in utero periventricular calcification due to cytomegalovirus infection. *J Ultrasound Med* 1:171–172, 1982.

Hohlfeld P, Vial Y, Maillard-Brignon C, Vaudaux B, Fawer CL: Cytomegalovirus fetal infection: prenatal diagnosis. *Obstet Gynecol* 78:615–618, 1991.

Hughes P, Weinberger E, Shaw DWW: Linear areas of echogenicity in the thalami and basal ganglia of neonates: an expanded association. *Radiology* 179:103–105, 1991.

Koga Y, Mizumoto M, Matsumoto Y, et al: Prenatal diagnosis of fetal intracranial calcifications. *Am J Obstet Gynecol* 163:1543–1545, 1990.

Lamy ME, Mulongo KN, Gadisseux JF, et al: Prenatal diagnosis of fetal cytomegalovirus infection. *Am J Obstet Gynecol* 166:91–94, 1992.

Lynch L, Daffos F, Emanuel D, et al: Prenatal diagnosis of fetal cytomegalovirus infection. *Am J Obstet Gynecol* 165:714–718, 1991.

Malinger G, Ben-Sira L, Lev D, Ben-Aroya Z, Kidron D, Lerman-Sagie T: Fetal brain imaging: a comparison between magnetic resonance imaging and dedicated neurosonography. *Ultrasound Obstet Gynecol* 23:333–340, 2004.

Mazeron MC, Cordovi-Voulgaropoulos L, Perol Y: Transient hydrops fetalis associated with intrauterine cytomegalovirus infection: prenatal diagnosis. *Obstet Gynecol* 84:692–694, 1994.

Meisel RL, Alvarez M, Lynch L, et al: Fetal cytomegalovirus infection: a case report. *Am J Obstet Gynecol* 162:663–664, 1990.

Mittelmann-Handwerker S, Pardes JG, Post RC, et al: Fetal ventriculomegaly and brain atrophy in a woman with intrauterine cytomegalovirus infection. *J Reprod Med* 31:1061–1064, 1986.

Ortiz JU, Ostermayer E, Fischer T, Kuschel B, Rudelius M, Schneider KT: Severe fetal cytomegalovirus infection associated with cerebellar hemorrhage. *Ultrasound Obstet Gynecol* 2004;23:402–406.

Pletcher BA, Williams MK, Mulivor RA, et al: Intrauterine cytomegalovirus infection presenting as fetal meconium peritonitis. *Obstet Gynecol* 78:903–905, 1991.

Richards DS, Preziosi M, Sexton C: Fetal cytomegalovirus syndrome with ascites, hepatitis, and negative serology. *Fetus* 2:1–4, 1992.

Simchen MJ, Toi A, Bona M, Alkazaleh F, Ryan G, Chitayat D: Fetal hepatic calcifications: prenatal diagnosis and outcome. *Am J Obstet Gynecol* 187:1617–1622, 2002.

Stagno S, Pass RF, Cloud G, Britt WJ, et al: Primary cytomegalovirus infection in pregnancy: incidence, transmission to fetus and clinical outcome. *JAMA* 256:1904–1908, 1986.

Stagno S, Pass RF, Dworsky ME, et al: Congenital cytomegalovirus infection: the relative importance of primary and recurrent maternal infection. *N Engl J Med* 306:945–949, 1982.

Tassin GB, Maklad NF, Stewart RR, Bell ME: Cytomegalic inclusion disease: intrauterine sonographic diagnosis using findings involving the brain. *AJR Am J Roentgenol* 12:117–122, 1991.

Teele RL, Hernanz-Schulman M, Sotrel A: Echogenic vasculature in the basal ganglia of neonates: a sonographic sign of vasculopathy. *Radiology* 169:423–427, 1988.

Toma P, Magnano GM, Mezzano P, et al: Cerebral ultrasound images in prenatal cytomegalovirus infection. *Neuroradiology* 31:278–279, 1989.

Townsent JJ, Stroop WG, Baringer JR, et al: Neuropathology of progressive rubella panencephalitis after childhood rubella. *Neurology* 32:185–190, 1982.

Twickler DM, Perlman J, Mabeny MC: Congenital cytomegalovirus infection presenting as cerebral ventriculomegaly on antenatal sonography. *Am J Perinatol* 10:404–406, 1993.

Watt-Morse ML, Laifer SA, Hill LM: The natural history of fetal cytomegalovirus infection as assessed by serial ultrasound and fetal blood sampling: a case report. *Prenat Diagn* 15:567–570, 1995.

Weinbaum PJ, Cassidy AB, Vintzileos AM, et al: Prenatal detection of a neural tube defect after fetal exposure to valproic acid. *Obstet Gynecol* 67:31S–33S, 1986.

Yamashita Y, Iwanaga R, Goto A, et al: Congenital cytomegalovirus infection associated with fetal ascites and intrahepatic calcifications. *Acta Paediatr Scand* 78:965–967, 1989.

Yinon Y, Yagel S, Tepperberg-Dikawa M, Feldman B, Schiff E, Lipitz S: Prenatal diagnosis and outcome of congenital cytomegalovirus infection in twin pregnancies. *BJOG* 113:295–300, 2006.

Yow MD, Demmler GJ: Congenital cytomegalovirus disease—20 years is long enough. *N Engl J Med* 326:702–703, 1992.

PARVOVIRUS B19

Description and Definition

Synonym: Fifth disease

Infection with parvovirus B19 is common. It is innocuous in the general population but is a recognized threat to fetuses.

Abnormalities Detectable by Ultrasound

Hydrops

Ascites

Pericardial effusion

Nuchal thickening and skin edema

Cardiomegaly

Placental thickening

Polyhydramnios

Major Differential Diagnoses

Syndromes and Conditions Associated with Hydrops:

Anemia of various etiologies, such as isoimmune or nonimmune:

- Fetal–maternal hemorrhage
- Isoimmune parvovirus

Cardiovascular anomalies:

- Arteriovenous shunt (aneurysm of vein of Galen)
- Bradycardia
- Cardiac defects
- Cardiomyopathy
- Tachycardia

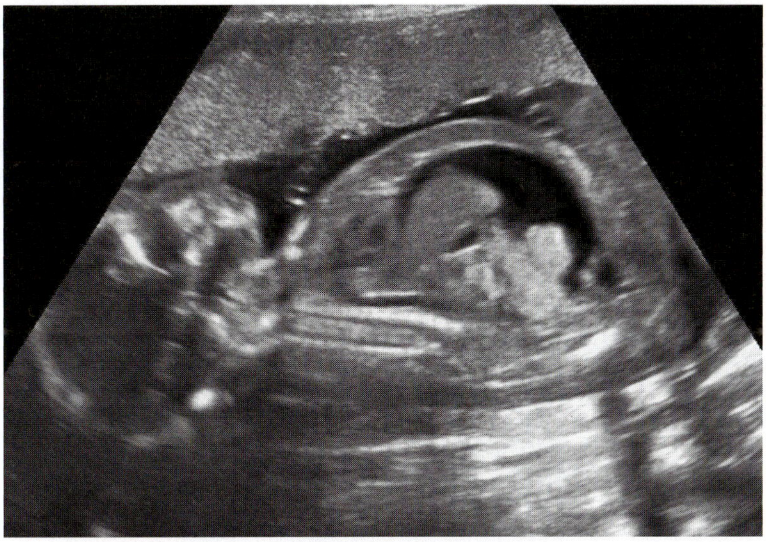

A

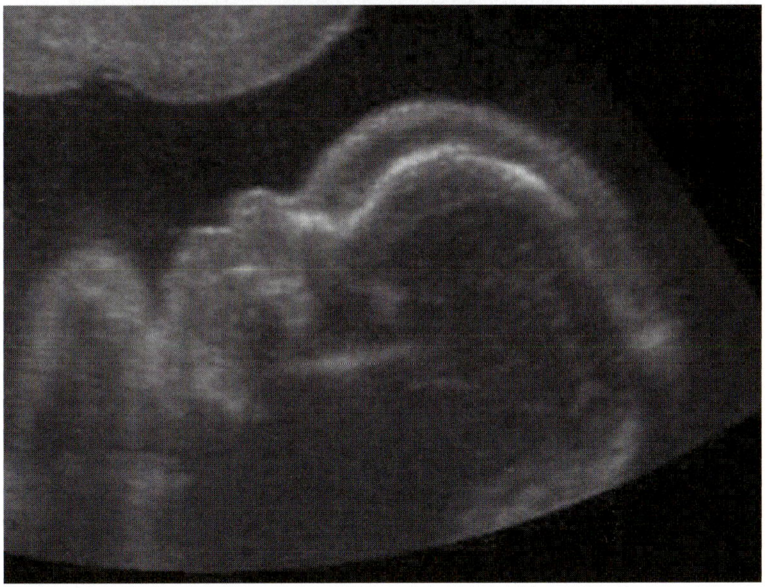

B

FIGURE 2-271 (A) Second-trimester fetus with nonimmune hydrops has overall skin edema of the body and ascites. Note that the ascitic fluid outlines the liver and multiple loops of bowel. (B) Longitudinal view of the fetal profile of the same fetus shows scalp edema.

Chest masses (causing mediastinal compression)*

Chromosomal anomalies

- Cri du chat syndrome
- Other trisomies
- Trisomy 21 (Down syndrome) (occasionally)
- XO syndrome (Turner syndrome)

Gastrointestinal obstructions

Maternal infection

- CMV
- Parvovirus
- Syphilis
- Toxoplasmosis
- Varicella

Tumors

- Chorioangioma
- Cystic hygroma
- Hepatic tumor (hemangioendothelioma)
- Lymphangioma
- Teratoma

*See Chapter 1, Nuchal Edema, p. 50, for differential diagnoses.

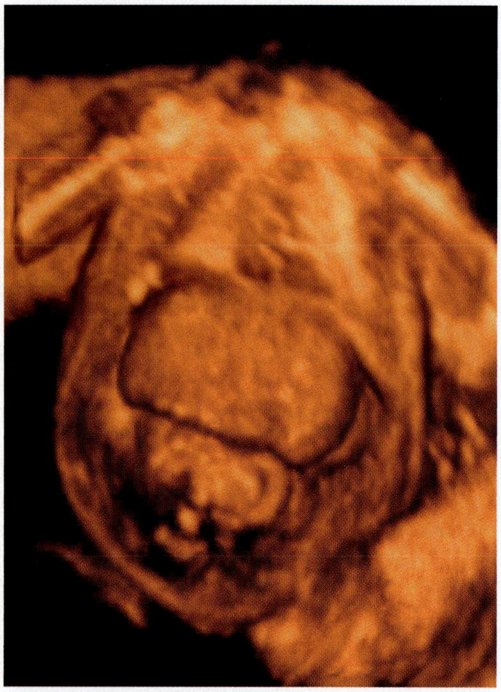

FIGURE 2-272 Three-dimensional surface rendering within the fetal abdomen of a second-trimester fetus with nonimmune hydrops.

Twin-to-twin transfusion syndrome

Other syndromes, such as:

- Achondrogenesis
- Alpha-thalassemia
- Congenital high airway obstruction syndrome
- Fryns syndrome
- Glycogen storage diseases
- Idiopathic arterial calcification of infancy
- Multiple pterygium syndrome
- Neu-Laxova syndrome
- Noonan syndrome
- Osteogenesis imperfecta
- Pena Shokeir syndrome
- Short rib–polydactyly syndrome, types I and III

Ultrasound Diagnosis

Most fetuses carried by women infected by parvovirus appear not to suffer any adverse outcome. Those who develop hydrops are in the minority. Hydrops secondary to parvovirus can occur at any gestational age and has been seen as early as 12 weeks' gestation, with subsequent spontaneous resolution. Parvovirus also has been known to cause early spontaneous abortion in first-trimester pregnancies. In most cases of hydrops, however, intrauterine transfusion is used to maintain the fetus until the anemia subsides spontaneously. Doppler velocimetry of the fetal middle cerebral artery is a very effective method for diagnosing fetal anemia severe enough to warrant consideration of in utero transfusion. Peak systolic velocity >1.5 multiples of the median for gestational age is a highly accurate method used for treatment of the disease, with a sensitivity of 93% for anemia.

There has been a report of a fetus with parvovirus infection and multiple congenital abnormalities, including abnormally flexed hands, cleft lip and palate, micrognathia, and flexion contractures. However, whether these abnormalities were attributable to the parvovirus or to a coincidental occurrence of anomalies and in utero infection is unclear.

Heredity

Heredity is not a factor in this fetal infection.

Natural History and Outcome

Fetal infection can lead to death in utero and reportedly is responsible for a 5% fetal loss rate among recently infected mothers. In a population of 1967 patients studied by Guidozzi et al., 64 (3.3%) tested positive for IgM, indicating recent infection. No adverse outcome was associated with these cases other than two fetuses who were born small for gestational age. Fetal anemia, secondary to parvovirus infection, is a rare but recognized cause of fetal hydrops among infected fetuses and typically is diagnosed using frequent Doppler velocimetry of the fetal middle cerebral artery. Treatment of profound fetal anemia with intrauterine transfusions may be lifesaving in affected fetuses. Intrauterine infection is associated with fetal hydrops secondary to fetal anemia, which occurs as a result of infection of the erythroid progenitor cells.

Suggested Reading

Bhal PS, Davies NJ, Westmoreland D, Jones A: Spontaneous resolution of non-immune hydrops fetalis secondary to transplacental parvovirus B19 infection. *Ultrasound Obstet Gynecol* 7:55–57, 1996.

Cosmi E, Mari G, Delle Chiaie L, et al: Noninvasive diagnosis by Doppler ultrasonography of fetal anemia resulting from parvovirus infection. *Am J Obstet Gynecol* 187:1290–1293, 2002.

Guidozzi F, Ballot D, Rothberg AD: Human B19 parvovirus infection in an obstetric population: a prospective study determining fetal outcome. *J Reprod Med* 39:36–38, 1994.

Hernandez-Andrade E, Scheier M, Dezerega V, Carmo A, Nicolaides KH: Fetal middle cerebral artery peak systolic velocity in the investigation of non-immune hydrops. *Ultrasound Obstet Gynecol* 23:442–445, 2004.

Jordan JA: Identification of human parvovirus B19 infection in idiopathic nonimmune hydrops fetalis. *Am J Obstet Gynecol* 174:37–42, 1996.

Mari G, Deter RL, Carpenter RL, Rahman F, et al: Noninvasive diagnosis by Doppler ultrasonography of fetal anemia due to maternal red-cell alloimmunization. Collaborative Group for Doppler Assessment of the Blood Velocity in Anemic Fetuses. *N Engl J Med* 342:9–14, 2000.

Marton T, Martin WL, Whittle MJ: Hydrops fetalis and neonatal death from human parvovirus B19: an unusual complication. *Prenat Diagn* 25:543–545, 2005.

Naides SJ, Weiner CP: Antenatal diagnosis and palliative treatment of nonimmune hydrops fetalis secondary to fetal parvovirus B19 infection. *Prenat Diagn* 9:105–114, 1989.

Petrikovsky BM, Baker D, Schneider E: Fetal hydrops secondary to human parvovirus infection in early pregnancy. *Prenat Diagn* 16:342–344, 1996.

Rodis JF, Quinn DL, Gary GW Jr, et al: Management and outcomes of pregnancies complicated by human B19 parvovirus infection: a prospective study. *Am J Obstet Gynecol* 163:1168–1171, 1990.

Tiessen RG, Van Elsaker-Niele AMW, Vermeij-Keers C, et al: A fetus with a parvovirus B19 infection and congenital anomalies. *Prenat Diagn* 14:173–176, 1994.

von Kaisenberg CS, Jonat W: Fetal parvovirus B19 infection. *Ultrasound Obstet Gynecol* 18:280–288, 2001.

RUBELLA

Description and Definition

Rubella infection in utero causes detectable defects in most fetuses exposed during the first 8 weeks of gestation. The rate of in utero infection drops to approximately 50% of fetuses exposed between 9 and 12 weeks' gestation and to <20% for those exposed between 12 and 20 weeks' gestational age.

Abnormalities Detectable by Ultrasound

Cardiac malformations (particularly septal defects)

Eye defects (particularly cataracts, microphthalmia)

Microcephaly

Enlarged liver and spleen

IUGR

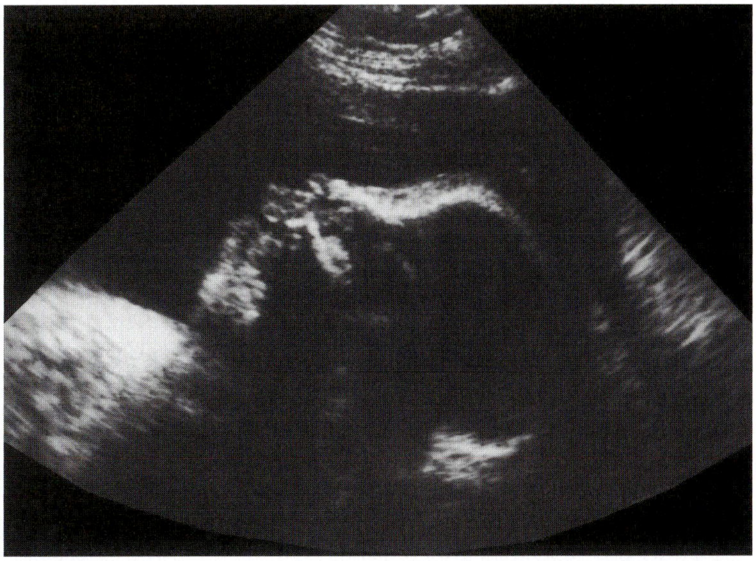

FIGURE 2-273 Longitudinal view of the face of a third-trimester fetus with microcephaly, as can be seen in fetuses with rubella infections. Note the small cranial vault compared with the size of the facial features.

Occasional:

Meconium peritonitis

Hyperechoic bowel

Intracranial calcification and subependymal pseudocysts

Major Differential Diagnoses

Conditions Associated with Hepatomegaly:

CMV

Fetal anemia of various etiologies (isoimmune, parvovirus, fetal–maternal hemorrhage)

Fetal liver tumor

Syphilis

Toxoplasmosis

Varicella

Some Syndromes and Conditions Associated with Cataracts:

Branchio-oculo-facial syndrome

Cerebro-oculo-facio-skeletal (COFS) syndrome.

Chondrodysplasia punctata

Neu-Laxova syndrome

Smith-Lemli-Opitz syndrome

Stickler syndrome

Varicella

Walker-Warburg syndrome

Ultrasound Diagnosis

Detection of fetal rubella infection is possible by fetal blood sampling and IgM assay. In 18 fetuses having blood samples tested at 20 to 26 weeks' gestation, 12 tested positive, 1 had a false-negative test result (presumably because of sampling too early in pregnancy), and 5 were confirmed to be normal at birth (Daffos et al.).

One fetus with congenital rubella was reported to have massive ventriculomegaly, with a calcified periventricular border seen prenatally.

Heredity

Heredity is not a factor in this fetal infection.

Natural History and Outcome

Postnatal effects of infection can include deafness, mental retardation, and hepatosplenomegaly, as well as cataracts, heart defects, and microcephaly.

Suggested Reading

Agarwal R, Kothari SS, Agarwal R: Ebstein's anomaly: a rare finding in congenital rubella syndrome. *Indian Pediatr* 38:1333–1335, 2001.

Daffos F, Forestier F, Grangeot-Keros L, et al: Prenatal diagnosis of congenital rubella. *Lancet* 2:1–3, 1984.

Degani S: Sonographic findings in fetal viral infections: a systematic review. *Obstet Gynecol Surv* 61:329–336, 2006.

Fakhry J, Khoury A: Fetal intracranial calcifications. The importance of periventricular hyperechoic foci without shadowing. *J Ultrasound Med* 10:51–54, 1991.

Makhoul IR, Zmora O, Tamir A, et al: Congenital subependymal pseudocysts: own data and meta-analysis of the literature. *Isr Med Assoc J* 3:178–183, 2001.

Parisot S, Droulle P, Feldmann M, Pinaud P, Marchal C: Unusual encephaloclastic lesions with paraventricular calcification in congenital rubella. *Pediatr Radiol* 21:229–230, 1991.

Radner M, Vergesslich KA, Weninger M, et al: Meconium peritonitis: a new finding in rubella syndrome. *J Clin Ultrasound* 21:346–349,1993.

Yamashita Y, Matshushi T, Murakami Y, et al: Neuroimaging findings (ultrasonography, CT, MRI) in 3 infants with congenital rubella syndrome. *Pediatr Radiol* 21:547–549, 1991.

SYPHILIS

Description and Definition

Syphilis, an infection caused by *Treponema pallidum*, can be transmitted to the fetus in utero. It is a recognized cause of nonimmune hydrops.

In utero syphilitic infection is rare, although the frequency of syphilis among young women of childbearing age is climbing. The reported incidence of congenital syphilis in the United States in 1992 was 4322.

Abnormalities Detectable by Ultrasound

Abnormal curvature of the long bones and bowing of the bones, simulating fractures in an otherwise normally mineralized skeleton

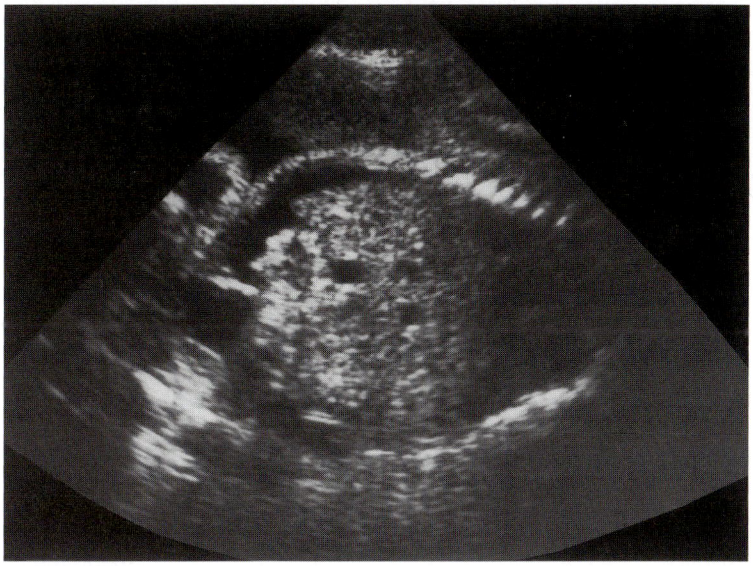

FIGURE 2-274 Longitudinal view of a third-trimester fetus shows ascites. This feature is seen in fetuses affected by syphilis.

Nonimmune hydrops, with focus on ascites

Abdominal enlargement secondary to ascites

Hepatosplenomegaly

Bowel obstruction

Placentomegaly

*Major Differential Diagnoses**

Syndromes and Conditions Associated with Ascites:

CMV

Meconium peritonitis

Parvovirus

Trisomy 21 (Down syndrome)

Urinary ascites secondary to genitourinary obstruction

XO syndrome (Turner syndrome)

Ultrasound Diagnosis

Congenital infection can be confirmed by demonstrating *T. pallidum* in fetal blood obtained by cordocentesis or in amniotic fluid. In a study of 21 patients in various stages of untreated syphilis (Nathan et al.), the diagnosis of fetal infection was established in 50% by amniotic fluid testing with a rabbit infectivity test. In these 21 patients, there was evidence of placental thickening in 13, enlarged fetal abdominal girth in 2, and fetal hepatomegaly in 12. In a study by Hollier et al., 66% of 24 cases with untreated syphilis had hepatomegaly, including 3 fetuses with ascites.

*See also Chapter 1, Hydrops, p. 111, for differential diagnoses.

Heredity

Heredity is not a factor in this fetal infection.

Natural History and Outcome

In the study by Nathan et al., 20 of the original 21 infants of mothers with syphilis were available for follow-up studies. Fifteen (75%) were reported to be normal at the time of neonatal examination, and 5 (25%) had evidence of congenital syphilis at birth. Seven of the 12 fetuses with hepatomegaly in utero were normal at birth, indicating successful treatment during gestation. However, the outcome was poor in cases involving fetal hydrops. In the study by Hollier et al., maternal treatment was successful in 83%, with a high risk of failure in cases with marked hepatomegaly and ascites.

Suggested Reading

Hallak M, Peipert JF, Ludomirsky A, Byers J: Nonimmune hydrops fetalis and fetal congenital syphilis. *J Reprod Med* 37:173–176, 1992.

Hollier LM, Harstad TW, Sanchez PJ, Twickler DM, Wendel GD Jr: Fetal syphilis: clinical and laboratory characteristics. *Obstet Gynecol* 97:947–953, 2001.

Nathan L, Twickler DM, Peters MT, Sanchez PJ, Wendel GD Jr: Fetal syphilis: correlation of sonographic findings and rabbit infectivity testing of amniotic fluid. *J Ultrasound Med* 2:97–101, 1993.

Raafat NA, Birch AA, Altieri LA, et al: Sonographic osseous manifestations of fetal syphilis: a case report. *J Ultrasound Med* 12:783–785, 1993.

Satin AJ, Twickler DM, Wendel GD Jr: Congenital syphilis associated with dilation of fetal small bowel. *J Ultrasound Med* 11:49–52, 1992.

TOXOPLASMOSIS

Description and Definition

Toxoplasma gondii is a parasite that crosses the placenta and infects the fetus in utero. Fetal infection occurs in approximately 1 in 3 cases of maternal infection.

Abnormalities Detectable by Ultrasound

The diagnosis of fetal toxoplasmosis usually involves sonography, amniocentesis, and fetal blood sampling. Parasitologic studies are performed on the fetal blood and amniotic fluid with the hope of instituting antibiotic treatment before significant malformations occur. Ultrasound findings include the following:

- Ventriculomegaly
- Microcephaly
- Intracranial calcifications
- Cataracts
- Liver calcifications
- Hepatomegaly
- Increased abdominal diameter
- Ascites

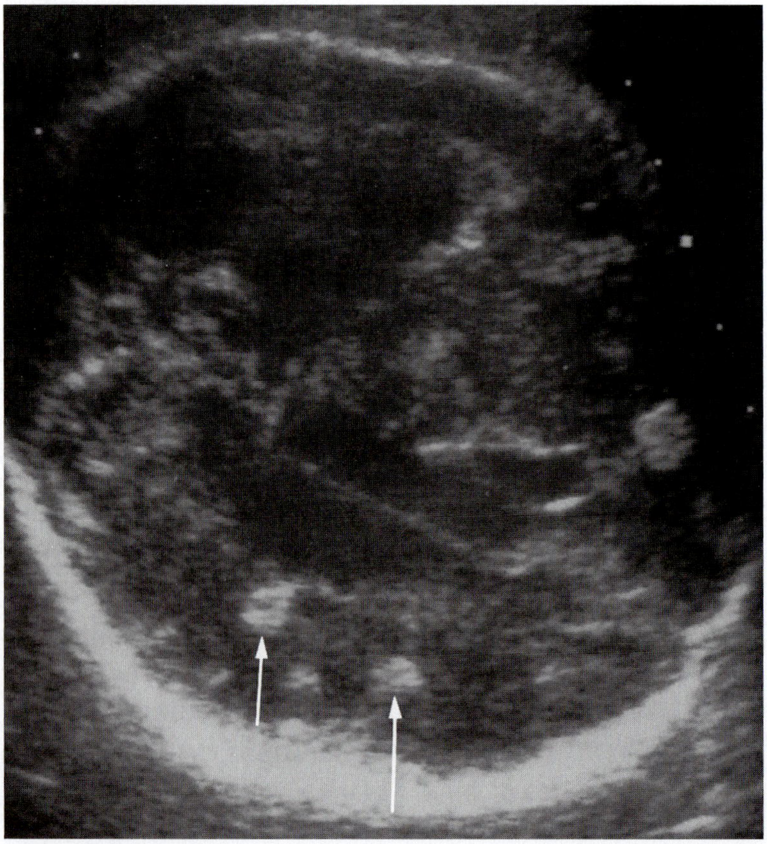

FIGURE 2-275 Periventricular hyperechoic areas *(arrows)* are seen at 33 weeks' gestation in a fetus with toxoplasmosis. (From Desai MB, Kurtz AB, Martin ME, Wapner RJ: *J Ultrasound Med* 13:60, 1994.)

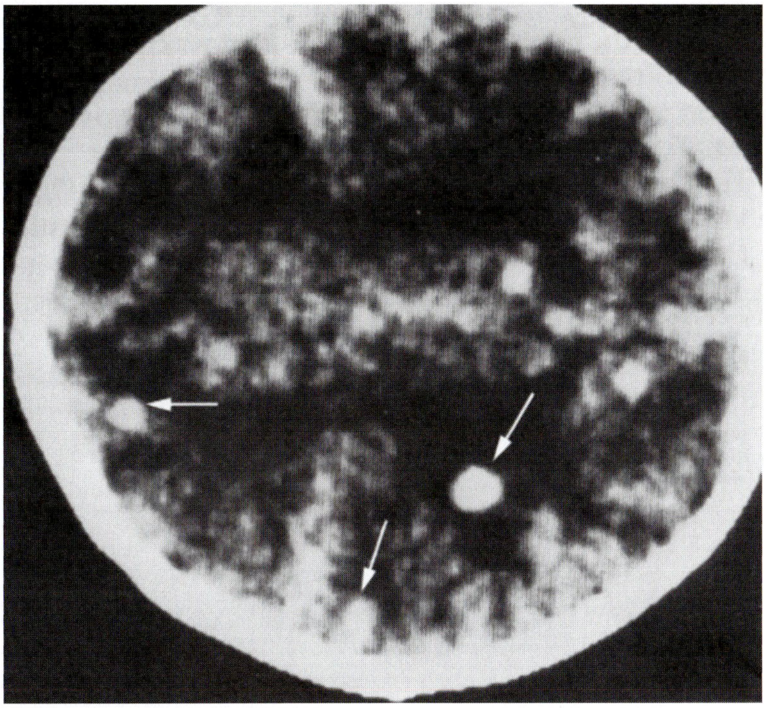

FIGURE 2-276 Computed tomographic scan shows brain calcifications *(arrows)* seen prenatally in a fetus with toxoplasmosis. (From Hohlfeld P, MacAleese J, Capella-Pavloski MC, et al: *Ultrasound Obstet Gynecol* 1:241–244, 1991.)

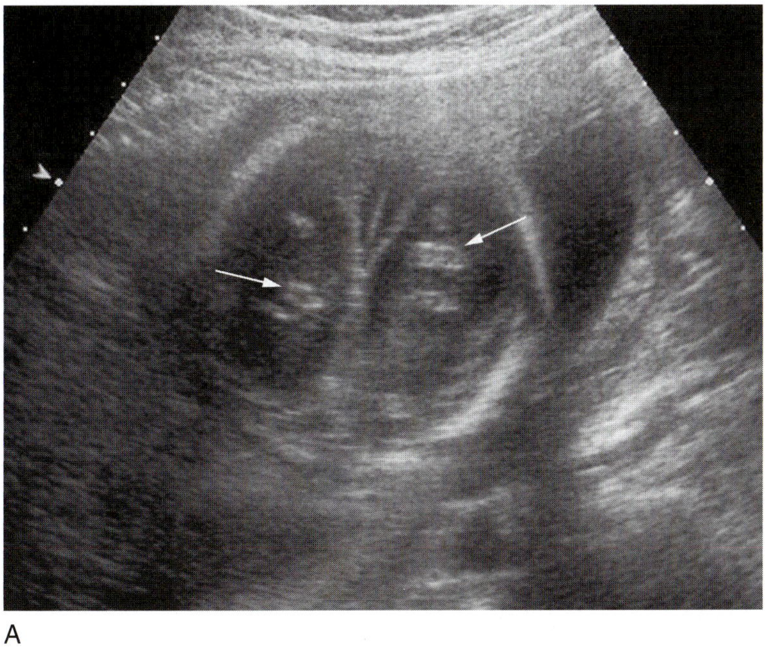

A

FIGURE 2-277 Third-trimester toxoplasmosis. (**A**) Third-trimester fetus with multiple intracerebral calcifications *(arrows)* consistent with toxoplasmosis. *Continued*

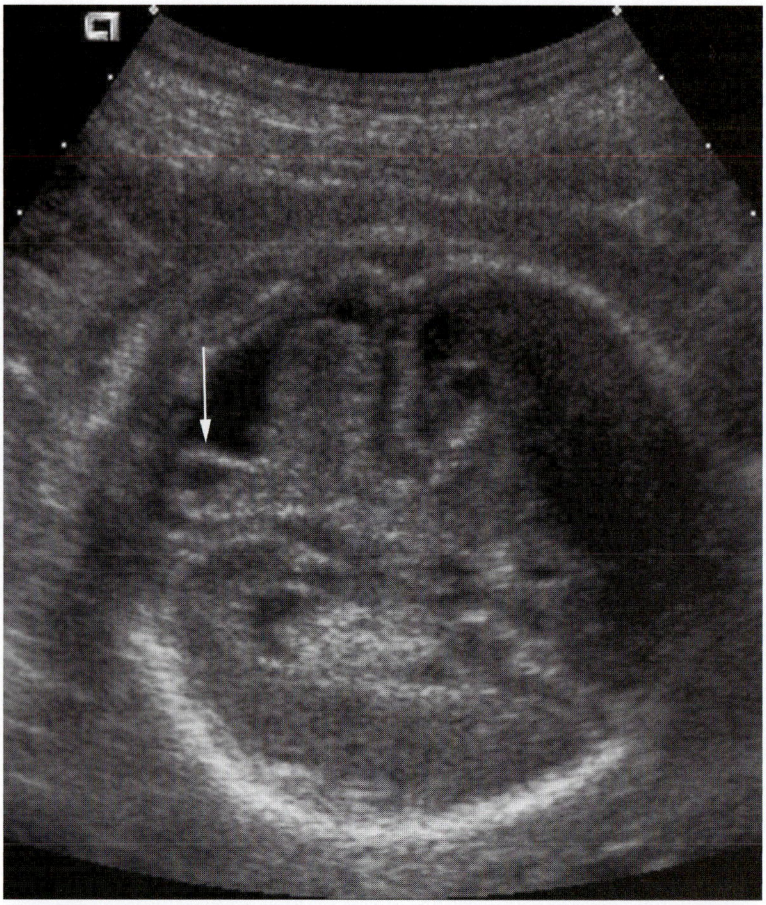

B

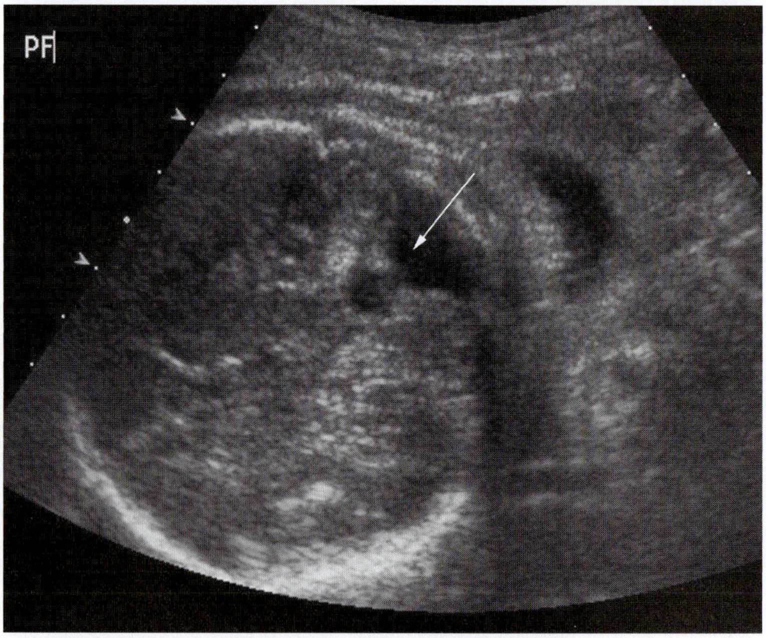

C

FIGURE 2-277, cont'd (B) Different third-trimester fetus with toxoplasmosis has an abnormal cerebellum with unilateral cerebellar hypoplasia *(arrow)*. (C) Same fetus as in B shows hypoplasia of the inferior cerebellar vermis *(arrow)*.

IUGR

Thickened placenta

Ultrasound findings indicative of infection usually can be demonstrated after 20 weeks' gestation. However, the absence of these findings does *not* rule out such an infection.

Major Differential Diagnoses

CMV infection is the main differential diagnosis, particularly in cases involving intrahepatic and intracranial calcifications and ventriculomegaly.

Ultrasound Diagnosis

In a study by Pratlong et al. in which infection was confirmed in 187 patients, fetal infection was diagnosed in 20 fetuses (10.5%); the remaining 89.5% were infection free. In the 20 cases with infection, diagnoses were made by amniocentesis, fetal blood sampling (using specific IgM, IgA), and ultrasound. However, ultrasound findings indicative of infection were identified in only 4 of the 20 infected fetuses (1 with hydrocephalus and 3 with hepatomegaly).

In another study, 32 of 89 infected fetuses had abnormal ultrasound examinations at 20 to 32 weeks' gestation. The sonographic signs were more prevalent in fetuses with early infections.

A third study describes 18 infected fetuses and showed that only 5 had sonographic abnormalities: 3 with ventriculomegaly and 2 with intrahepatic calcifications. The most sensitive diagnostic method (94% sensitive) is amniotic fluid sample for mouse inoculation and *T. gondii* DNA amplification by polymerase chain reaction (PCR).

Heredity

Heredity is not a factor in this fetal infection.

Natural History and Outcome

The earlier the fetal toxoplasmosis occurs, the more severe the congenital abnormalities. First-trimester infection may lead to miscarriage or severe neurologic deficits, including blindness. The majority of third-trimester exposures are associated with a good outcome.

Suggested Reading

Daffos F, Forestier F, Capella-Pavlovsky M, et al: Prenatal management of 746 pregnancies at risk for congenital toxoplasmosis. *N Engl J Med* 318:271–275, 1988.

Desai MB, Kurtz AB, Martin ME, Wapner RJ: Characteristic findings of toxoplasmosis in utero: a case report. *J Ultrasound Med* 13:60–62, 1994.

Foulon W, Naessens A, de Catte L, Amy JJ: Detection of congenital toxoplasmosis by chorionic villus sampling and early amniocentesis. *Am J Obstet Gynecol* 163:1511–1513, 1990.

Foulon W, Naessens A, Mahler T, et al: Prenatal diagnosis of congenital toxoplasmosis. *Obstet Gynecol* 76:769–772, 1990.

Friedman S, Ford-Jones LE, Toi A, Ryan G, Blaser S, Chitayat D: Congenital toxoplasmosis: prenatal diagnosis, treatment and postnatal outcome. *Prenat Diagn* 19:330–333,1999.

Gay-Andrieu F, Marty P, Pialat J, Sournies G, Drier de Laforte T, Peyron F: Fetal toxoplasmosis and negative amniocentesis: necessity of an ultrasound follow-up. *Prenat Diagn* 23:558–560, 2003.

Hohlfeld P, MacAleese J, Capella-Pavlovski MC, et al: Fetal toxoplasmosis: ultrasonographic signs. *Ultrasound Obstet Gynecol* 1:241–244, 1991.

Pedreira DA, Camargo ME, Leser PG: Toxoplasmosis: will the time ever come? *Ultrasound Obstet Gynecol* 17:459–463, 2001.

Pedreira DA, Diniz EM, Schultz R, Faro LB, Zugaib M: Fetal cataract in congenital toxoplasmosis. *Ultrasound Obstet Gynecol* 13:266–267,1999.

Pratlong F, Boulot P, Issert E, et al: Fetal diagnosis of toxoplasmosis in 190 women infected during pregnancy. *Prenat Diagn* 14:191–198, 1994.

Pratlong F, Boulot P, Villena I, et al: Antenatal diagnosis of congenital toxoplasmosis: evaluation of the biological parameters in a cohort of 286 patients. *Br J Obstet Gynaecol* 103:552–557, 1996.

Wilson CB, Remington JS, Stagno S, Reynolds DW: Development of adverse sequelae in children born with subclinical congenital toxoplasma infection. *Pediatrics* 66:767–774, 1980.

VARICELLA

Description and Definition

Synonym: Chickenpox

Herpesvirus varicella is responsible for both varicella and herpes zoster (shingles). Fetal varicella infection rarely occurs during pregnancy (incidence 0.7 per 1000 pregnancies). First- and second-trimester infections more often are linked to varicella fetal anomalies than is third-trimester infection.

Abnormalities Detectable by Ultrasound

Ventriculomegaly (one report of porencephalic cyst)

Microcephaly

Cataracts and microphthalmia

Club feet

Abnormally positioned hands and limb abnormalities

Decreased motion and cutaneous scars

Liver hyperechogenicity

Hyperechoic bowel

Two-vessel cord

Hydrops

Polyhydramnios

Major Differential Diagnoses

The fetal findings can be so variable that the differential diagnosis differs widely, depending on sonographic findings. However, amniotic bands can cause similar asymmetric head and limb defects.

Ultrasound Diagnosis

Sonographic findings indicative of infection can be seen at 15 weeks' gestation or later, which is generally 5 to 19 weeks after maternal infection. In most reported cases the time of exposure was between 10 and 20 weeks' gestation. The findings at 15 weeks have included hydrops and polyhydramnios.

In a study by Pretorius et al. of 37 fetuses exposed to varicella, 5 fetuses were reported to have sonographic findings indicative of infection. These findings included polyhydramnios, hydrops, and echogenic foci in the liver. A fatal outcome was reported in 4 of 5 of these cases. In this series, none of the other 32 fetuses was shown to have any infection at birth.

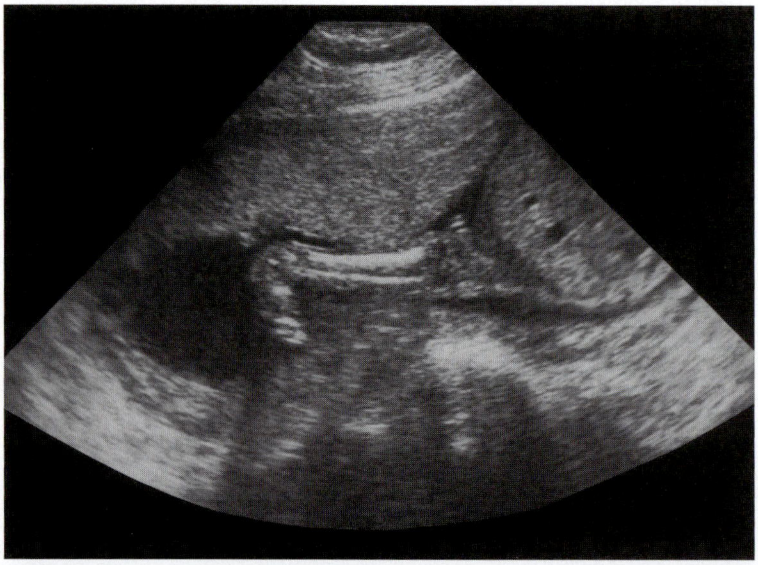

FIGURE 2-278 Longitudinal view of a deformed lower extremity in a second-trimester fetus, similar to what can be seen with a varicella infection. Note that the foot is abnormally oriented, and the fetal thigh is short. Varicella can affect the extremities in many different ways as a result of skin scarring.

Heredity

Heredity is not a factor in this fetal infection.

Natural History and Outcome

The incidence of fetal anomalies in fetuses of mothers infected with varicella prior to 20 weeks' gestation is 1% to 2%. Fifty percent of affected children die in early infancy. Survivors have a spectrum of problems ranging from mild cutaneous abnormalities to seizures, mental deficiency, and limb defects.

Suggested Reading

Hayward I, Pretorius DH: Varicella zoster. *Fetus* 2:5–6, 1992.

Higa K, Dan K, Manabe H: Varicella-zoster virus infections during pregnancy: hypothesis concerning the mechanisms of congenital malformations. *Obstet Gynecol* 69:214–222, 1987.

Jones KL: *Smith's recognizable patterns of human malformations.* Philadelphia, 2006, Elsevier.

Lebel RR, Fernandez BB, Gibson L: Varicella zoster; brain disruption. *Fetus* 2:1–4, 1992.

Lecuru F, Taurelle R, Bernard JP, et al: Varicella zoster virus infection during pregnancy: the limits of prenatal diagnosis. *Eur J Obstet Gynecol Reprod Biol* 56:67–68, 1994.

Ong CL, Daniel ML: Antenatal diagnosis of a porencephalic cyst in congenital varicella-zoster virus infection. *Pediatr Radiol* 28:94, 1998.

Petignat P, Vial Y, Laurini R, Hohlfeld P: Fetal varicella-herpes zoster syndrome in early pregnancy: ultrasonographic and morphological correlation. *Prenat Diagn* 21:121–124, 2001.

Pons JC, Vial P, Rozenberg F, et al: Prenatal diagnosis of fetal varicella in the second trimester of pregnancy. *J Gynecol Obstet Biol Reprod* 24:829–838, 1995.

Pretorius DH, Hayward I, Jones KL, Stamm E: Sonographic evaluation of pregnancies with maternal varicella infection. *J Ultrasound Med* 11:459–463, 1992.

Verstraelen H, Vanzieleghem B, Defoort P, Vanhaesebrouck P, Temmerman M: Prenatal ultrasound and magnetic resonance imaging in fetal varicella syndrome: correlation with pathology findings. *Prenat Diagn* 23:705–709, 2003.

Yaron Y, Hassan S, Geva E, Kupferminc MJ, Yavetz H, Evans MI: Evaluation of fetal echogenic bowel in the second trimester. *Fetal Diagn Ther* 14:176–180, 1999.

Syndromes Featuring Chromosomal Anomalies

CRI DU CHAT SYNDROME

DESCRIPTION AND DEFINITION

Synonym: Distal 5P deletion syndrome

This rare condition is associated with an abnormality of chromosome 5, characterized by microcephaly, hypertelorism, micrognathia, hydrops, and growth delay.

ABNORMALITIES DETECTABLE BY ULTRASOUND

Microcephaly

Hypertelorism

Micrognathia

Nasal bone hypoplasia

Cerebellar abnormality

Encephalocele

Ventriculomegaly

Thickened nuchal translucency

Cystic hygroma

Cardiac defects

Cardiomegaly

Hydrops

IUGR

MAJOR DIFFERENTIAL DIAGNOSES

The differential diagnosis is extremely varied because of the many abnormalities associated with the syndrome.

Other chromosomal abnormalities with similar findings include the following:

- Triploidy
- Trisomy 18
- Trisomy 9
- Turner syndrome

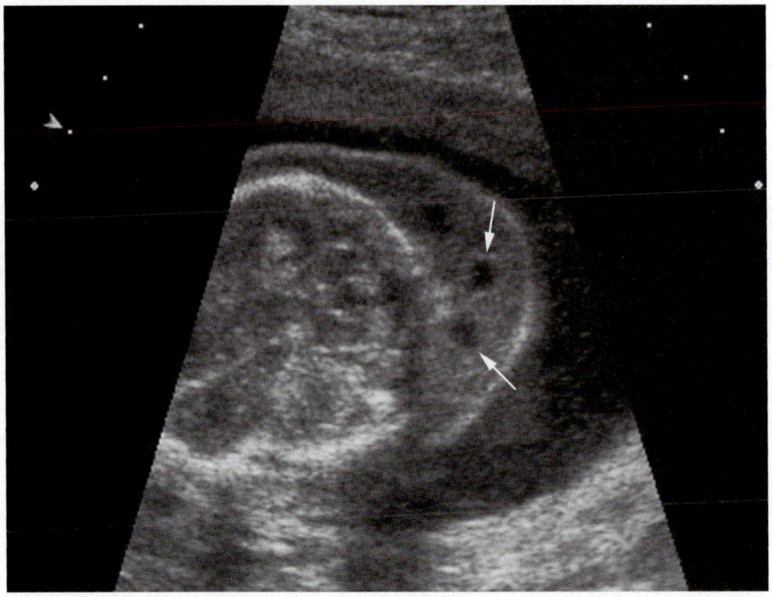

FIGURE 2-279 Transverse view through the fetal nuchal region shows a thickened nuchal fold with small cystic hygromas *(arrows)*.

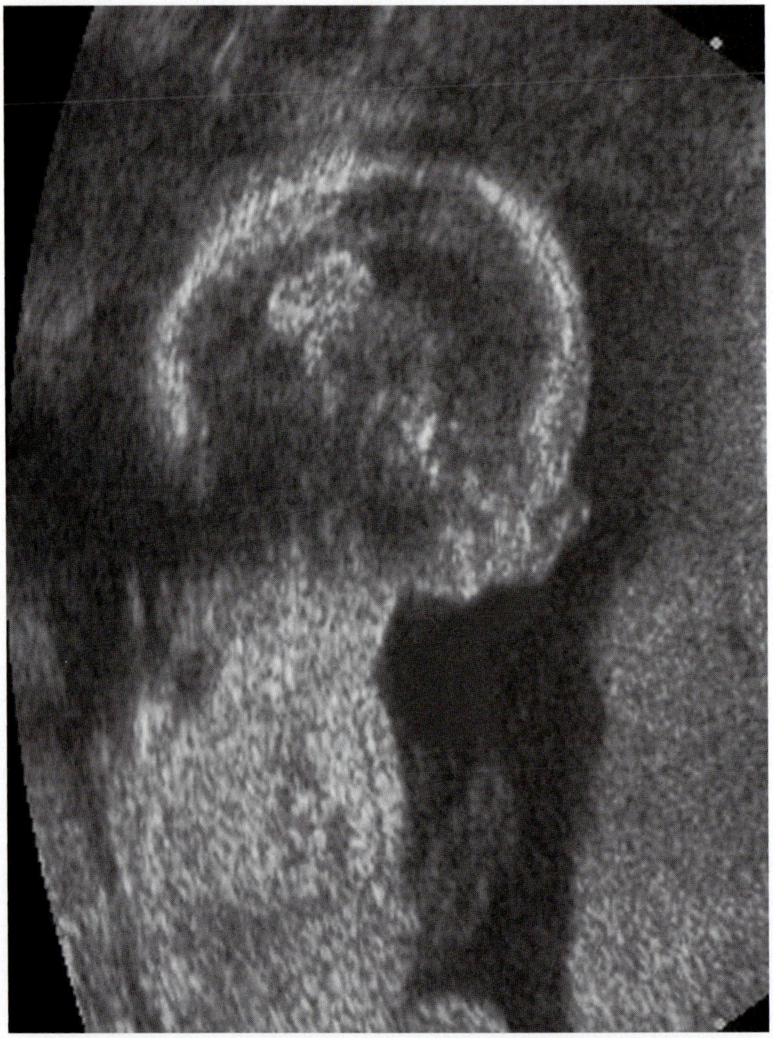

FIGURE 2-280 Longitudinal view of the fetal profile of a fetus with micrognathia.

ULTRASOUND DIAGNOSIS

This syndrome has been identified prenatally in the first trimester, with thickened nuchal translucency and cardiac defect, as well as in the second trimester, with multiple congenital abnormalities including neural tube defect (encephalocele); posterior fossa abnormalities; hydrocephalus; micrognathia; cystic hygromata; pleural effusions; and cardiac defects detected around 18 weeks. In the third trimester, other abnormalities include asymmetry of the skull, microcephaly, hypertelorism, hydrops, and ascites.

HEREDITY

This is a partial aneusomy of the short arm of chromosome 5. Although some cases are derived from a parental balanced translocation, most of the cases are new deletions. The deletions can vary, from involvement of only a small portion of the short arm to involvement of the entire short arm of chromosome 5.

NATURAL HISTORY AND OUTCOME

Cri du chat syndrome is characterized by a high-pitched, cat-like cry in a child with microcephaly and facial dysmorphic changes, hypertelorism, micrognathia, low-set ears, and severe mental and motor delays. Most affected individuals die in infancy or early childhood. Survivors are extremely handicapped.

Suggested Reading

Aoki S, Hata T, Hata K, Miyazaki K: Antenatal sonographic features of cri-du-chat syndrome (Letter). *Ultrasound Obstet Gynecol* 13:216–221, 1999.

Bakkum JN, Watson WJ, Johansen KL, Brost BC: Prenatal diagnosis of cri du chat syndrome with encephalocele. *Am J Perinatol* 22:351–352, 2005.

Chen CP, Lee CC, Chang TY, Town DD, Wang W: Prenatal diagnosis of mosaic distal 5p deletion and review of the literature. *Prenat Diagn* 24:50–57, 2004.

Jones KL: *Smith's recognizable patterns of human malformation,* ed 6. Philadelphia, 2006, Elsevier.

Paulick J, Tennstedt C, Schwabe M, Korner H, Bommer C, Chaoui R: Prenatal diagnosis of an isochromosome 5p in a fetus with increased nuchal translucency thickness and pulmonary atresia with hypoplastic right heart at 14 weeks (short communication). *Prenat Diagn* 24:371–374, 2004.

Sherer DM, Eugene P, Dalloul M, et al: Second-trimester diagnosis of cri du chat (5p-) syndrome following sonographic depiction of an absent fetal nasal bone. *J Ultrasound Med* 25:387–388, 2006.

Stefanou EGG, Hanna G, Foakes A, Crocker M, Fitchett M: Prenatal diagnosis of cri du chat (5p-) syndrome in association with isolated moderate bilateral ventriculomegaly (short communication). *Prenat Diagn* 22:64–66, 2002.

Vialard F, Robyr R, Hillion Y, Molina Gomes D, Selva J, Ville Y: Dandy-Walker syndrome and corpus callosum agenesis in 5p deletion. *Prenat Diagn* 25:311–313, 2005.

DELETION 4P (WOLF-HIRSCHHORN SYNDROME)

DESCRIPTION AND DEFINITION

Synonym: Wolf-Hirschhorn syndrome

Resulting from the deletion of the short arm of chromosome 4, this syndrome is characterized by IUGR, facial dysmorphology, cardiac defects, and hypospadias.

ABNORMALITIES DETECTABLE BY ULTRASOUND

Microcephaly

Cranial asymmetry

Agenesis of the corpus callosum

Micrognathia

Hypertelorism (with Greek warrior helmet appearance of forehead)

Cleft lip and palate

Cardiac defects

Ventricular septal defects

Diaphragmatic hernia

Hypospadias

Cryptorchidism

Club feet

IUGR (severe)

Occasional Findings:

Bladder exstrophy/renal anomalies

Dandy-Walker cyst (my case)

Polydactyly (my case)

Periventricular cystic abnormalities in brain

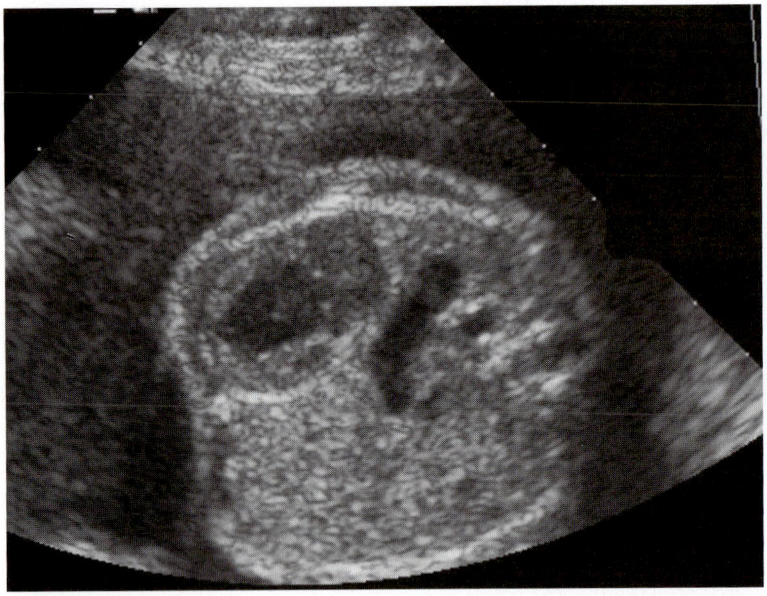

FIGURE 2-281 Transverse view through the fetal chest shows evidence of a diaphragmatic hernia with the fetal stomach draped across the spine and the fetal heart pushed over to the right. Note that only one cardiac ventricle is present.

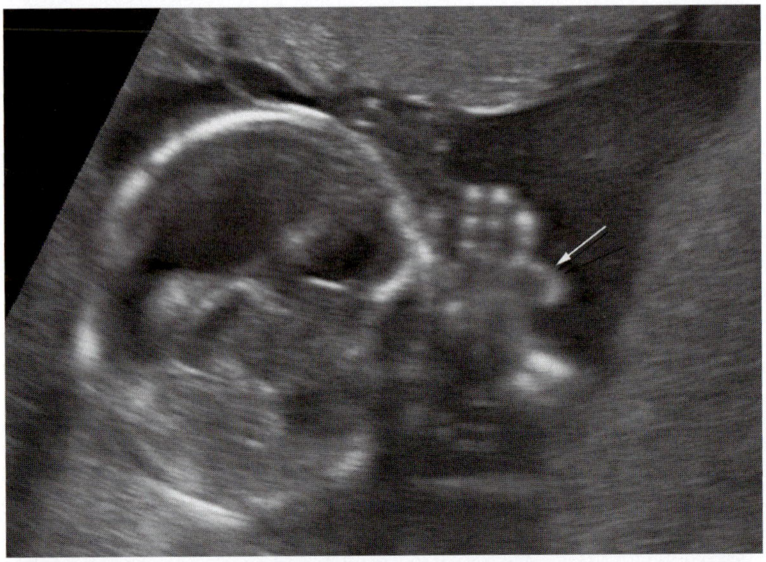

A

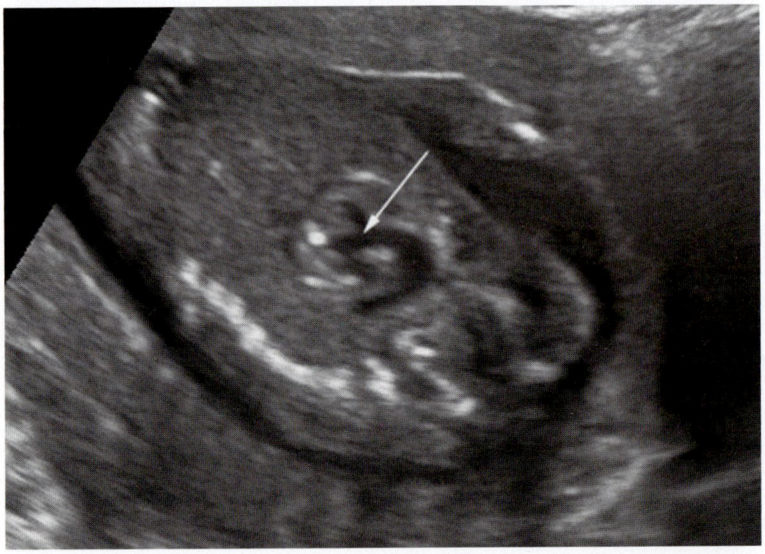

B

FIGURE 2-282 Second-trimester fetus with Wolf-Hirschhorn syndrome. (A) View of the fetal head shows evidence of ventriculomegaly and polydactyly *(arrow)*. (B) Long-axis view of the fetal heart shows an enlarged aortic root overriding a large ventricular septal defect *(arrow)*. *(Continued)*

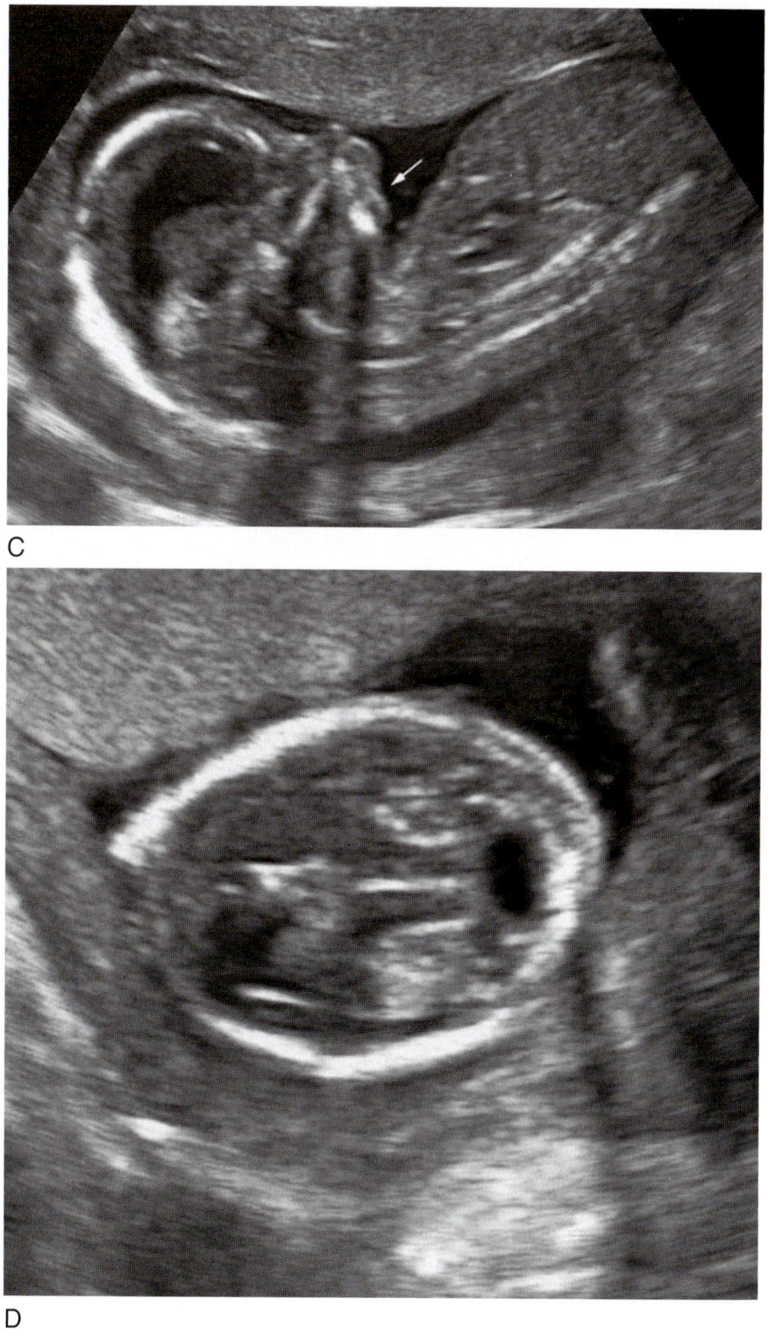

FIGURE 2-282, cont'd (C) Longitudinal view of the same fetus shows evidence of micrognathia *(arrow)*. (D) Transverse view through the fetal head of the same fetus shows a large Dandy-Walker cyst with hypoplasia of both cerebellar hemispheres.

Continued

MAJOR DIFFERENTIAL DIAGNOSES

Multiple abnormalities, including IUGR and diaphragmatic hernia, also can occur in the following syndromes and conditions:

- Fryns syndrome
- Deletion 11q (Jacobsen syndrome)
- Triploidy
- Trisomy 9
- Trisomy 18 (Edwards' syndrome)

The differential diagnosis for fetuses with this syndrome varies according to the findings in each specific case.

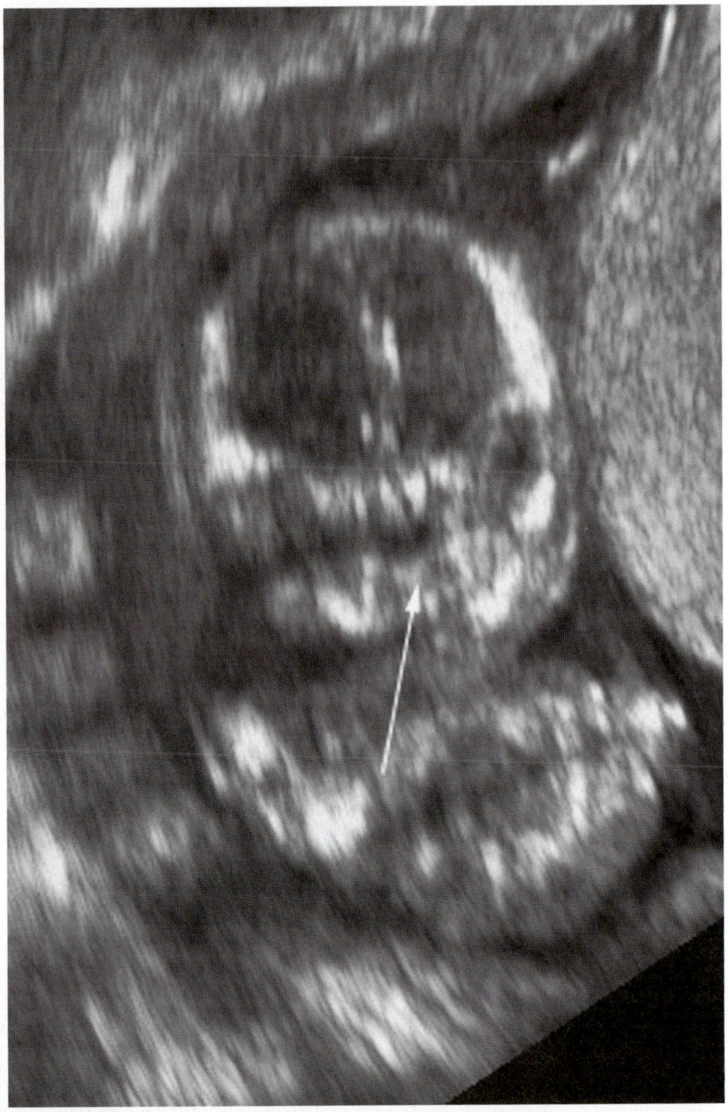

E

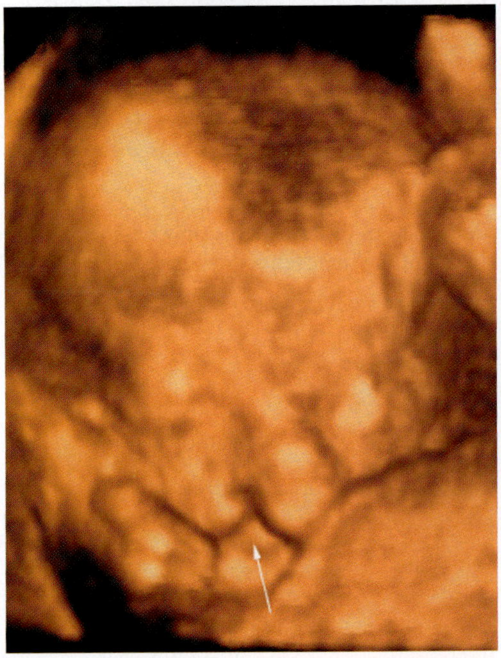

F

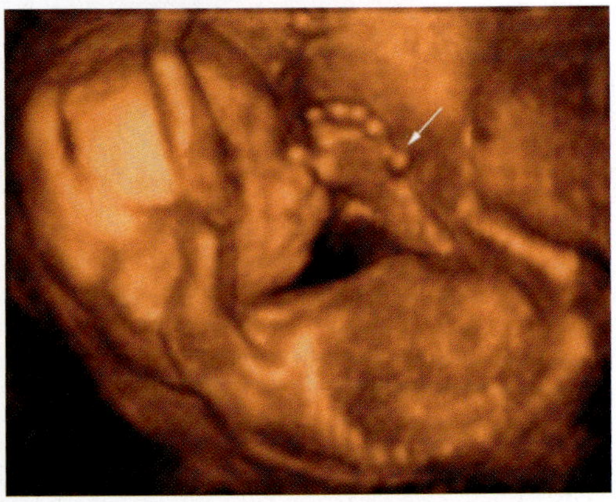

G

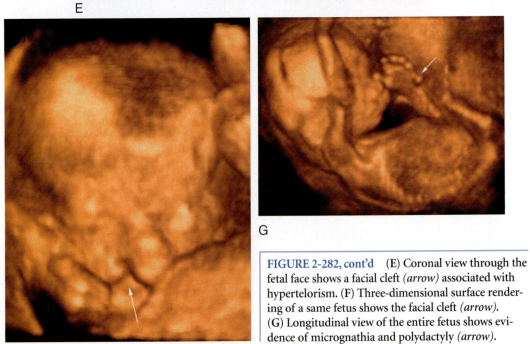

FIGURE 2-282, cont'd (E) Coronal view through the fetal face shows a facial cleft *(arrow)* associated with hypertelorism. (F) Three-dimensional surface rendering of a same fetus shows the facial cleft *(arrow)*. (G) Longitudinal view of the entire fetus shows evidence of micrognathia and polydactyly *(arrow)*.

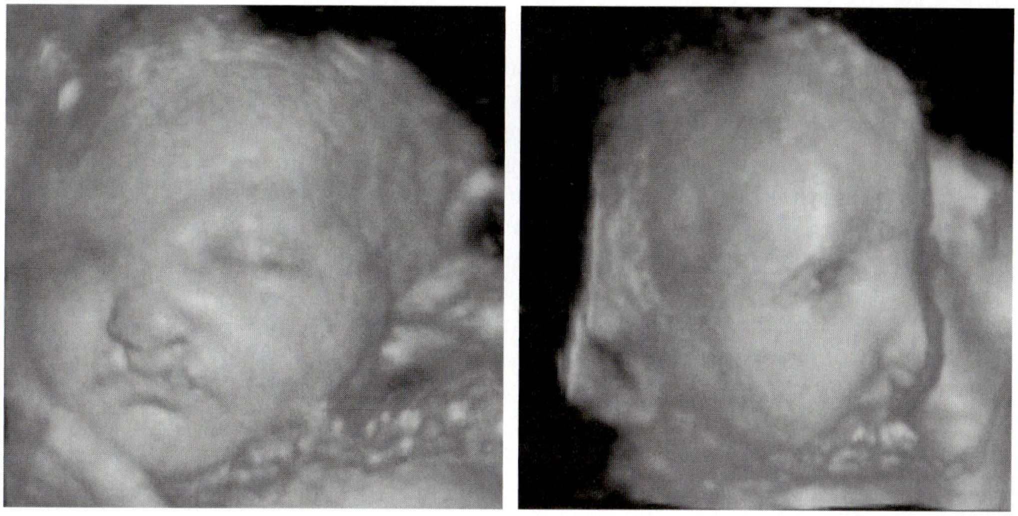
A B

FIGURE 2-283 (A, B) Three-dimensional surface rendering views of the fetal face of a 29-week fetus with Wolf-Hirschhorn syndrome. Note prominent glabella, bilateral cleft lip, and "Greek warrior helmet" appearance of the face. (From Sepulveda W: *J Ultrasound Med* 26:407–410, 2007.)

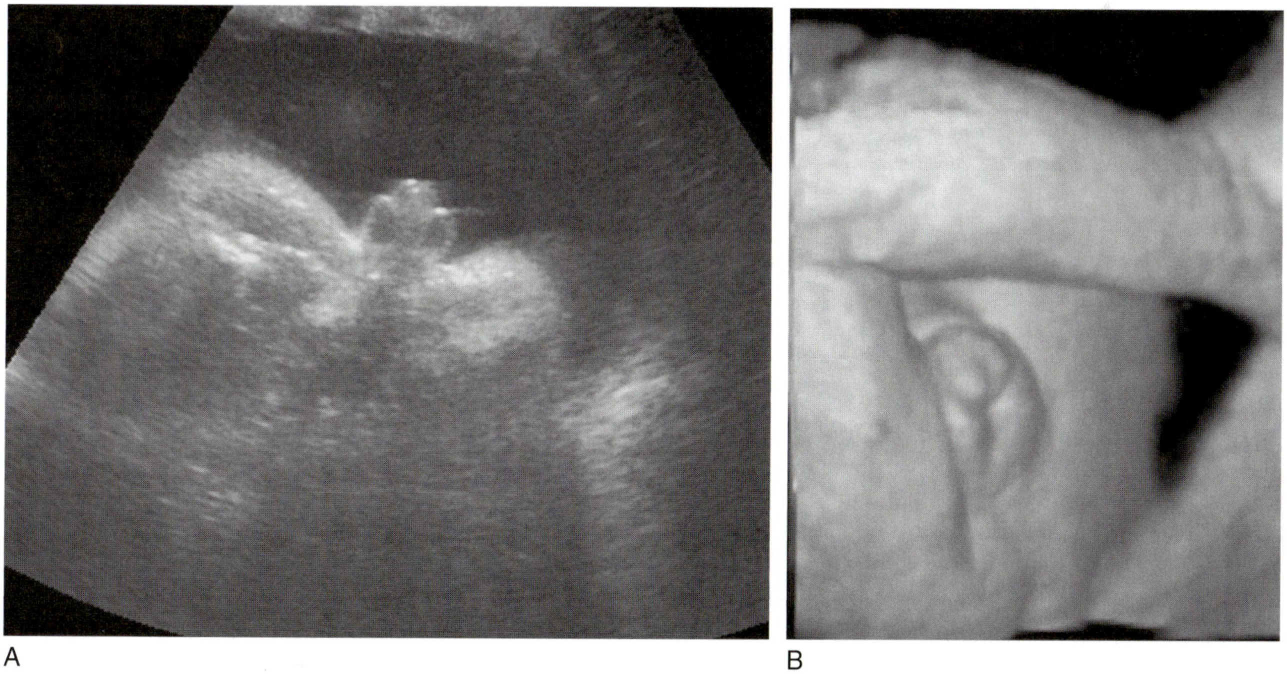
A B

FIGURE 2-284 (A) Two-dimensional sonography of the fetal genitalia shows the "tulip" sign, suggestive of severe hypospadias. (B) Three-dimensional sonography confirms the diagnosis of ambiguous genitalia attributable to severe penoscrotal hypospadias. (From Sepulveda W: *J Ultrasound Med* 26:407–410, 2007.)

ULTRASOUND DIAGNOSIS

Prenatal ultrasound diagnosis of deletion 4p syndrome has been established as early as 16 weeks' gestation. The literature contains several descriptions of prenatal findings associated with this syndrome; the most common are IUGR, facial clefting, hypospadias, and diaphragmatic hernia. I had the opportunity to see a case of this syndrome at 18 weeks (by prior ultrasound) in which the fetus measured 16 weeks' size and had micrognathia, hypertelorism, a cardiac defect, Dandy-Walker cyst of the posterior fossa, and polydactyly. The correct diagnosis was made by karyotype prompted by these findings.

HEREDITY

Partial deletion of the short arm of chromosome 4 occurs as a de novo deletion in most affected fetuses, although it can result from a balanced translocation carrier status in a parent.

NATURAL HISTORY AND OUTCOME

Affected individuals exhibit profound mental retardation and seizure disorder.

Suggested Reading

Beaujard MP, Jouannic JM, Bessieres B, et al: Prenatal detection of a de novo terminal inverted duplication 4p in a fetus with the Wolf-Hirschhorn syndrome phenotype. *Prenat Diagn* 25:451–455, 2005.

Boog G, Le Vaillant C, Collet M, et al: Prenatal sonographic patterns in six cases of Wolf-Hirschhorn (4p-) syndrome. *Fetal Diagn Ther* 19:421–430, 2004.

De Keersmaecker B, Albert M, Hillion Y, Ville Y: Prenatal diagnosis of brain abnormalities in Wolf-Hirschhorn (4p-) syndrome. *Prenat Diagn* 22:366–370, 2002.

Dietze I, Fritz B, Huhle D, Simoens W, Piecha E, Rehder H: Clinical, cytogenetic and molecular investigation in a fetus with Wolf-Hirschhorn syndrome with paternally derived 4p deletion. Case report and review of the literature. *Fetal Diagn Ther* 19:251–260, 2004.

Eiben B, Leipoldt M, Schubbe I, Ulbrich R, Hansmann I: Partial deletion of 4p in fetal cells not present in chorionic villi. *Clin Genet* 33:49–52, 1988.

Levaillant JM, Touboul C, Sinico M, et al: Prenatal forehead edema in 4p– deletion: the "Greek warrior helmet" profile revisited. *Prenat Diagn* 25:1150–1155, 2005.

Petek E, Wagner K, Steiner H, Schaffer H, Kroisel PM: Prenatal diagnosis of partial trisomy 4q26–qter and monosomy for the Wolf-Hirschhorn critical region in a fetus with split hand malformation. *Prenat Diagn* 20:349–352, 2000.

Phelan MC, Saul RA, Galley TA Jr, Skinner SA: Prenatal diagnosis of mosaic 4p– in a fetus with trisomy 21. *Prenat Diagn* 15:274–277, 1995.

Sase M, Hasegawa K, Honda R, et al: Ultrasonographic findings of facial dysmorphism in Wolf-Hirschhorn syndrome. *Am J Perinatol* 22:99–102, 2005.

Sepulveda W: Prenatal three-dimensional sonographic depiction of the Wolf-Hirschhorn phenotype: the "Greek warrior helmet" and "tulip" signs. *J Ultrasound Med* 26:407–410, 2007.

Tachdjian G, Fondacci C, Tapia S, et al: The Wolf-Hirschhorn syndrome in fetuses. *Clin Genet* 42:281–287, 1992.

Vamos E, Pratola D, Van Regemorter N, et al: Prenatal diagnosis and fetal pathology of partial trisomy 20p-monosomy 4p resulting from paternal translocation. *Prenat Diagn* 5:209–214, 1985.

Verloes A, Schaaps JP, Kerens C, et al: Prenatal diagnosis of cystic hygroma and chorioangioma in the Wolf-Hirschhorn syndrome. *Prenat Diagn* 11:129–132, 1991.

Vinals F, Sepulveda W, Selman E: Prenatal detection of congenital hypospadias in the Wolf-Hirschhorn (4p–) syndrome. *Prenat Diagn* 14:1166–1169, 1994.

DELETION 11Q (JACOBSEN SYNDROME)

DESCRIPTION AND DEFINITION

Synonym: Jacobsen syndrome

Deletion of the distal long arm of chromosome 11 was described in 1973 and is characterized by multiple congenital abnormalities and severe mental retardation.

ABNORMALITIES DETECTABLE BY ULTRASOUND

Common Findings:

Trigonocephaly (triangular-shaped frontal bones, similar to those found in a strawberry-shaped skull)

Microcephaly

Hypertelorism

Depressed nasal bridge

Micrognathia

Ear malformations

Joint contractures

Cardiac defects

Genital abnormalities

Hypospadias

Cryptorchidism

IUGR

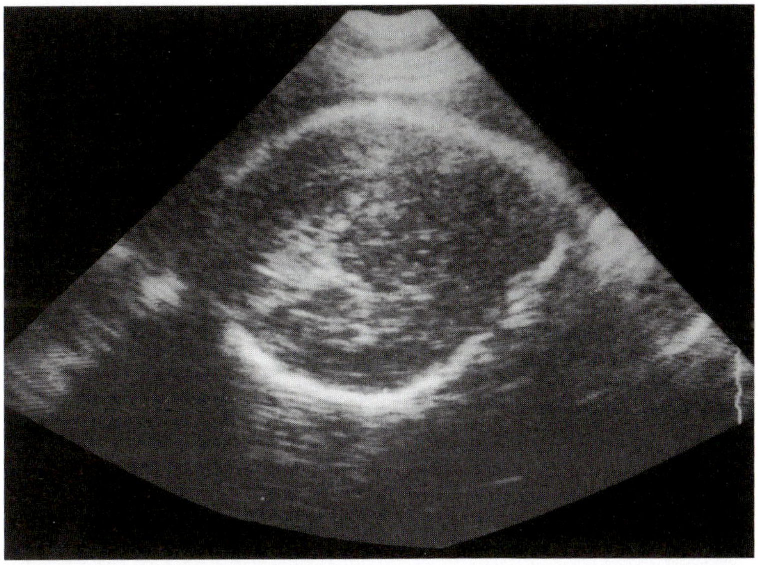

A

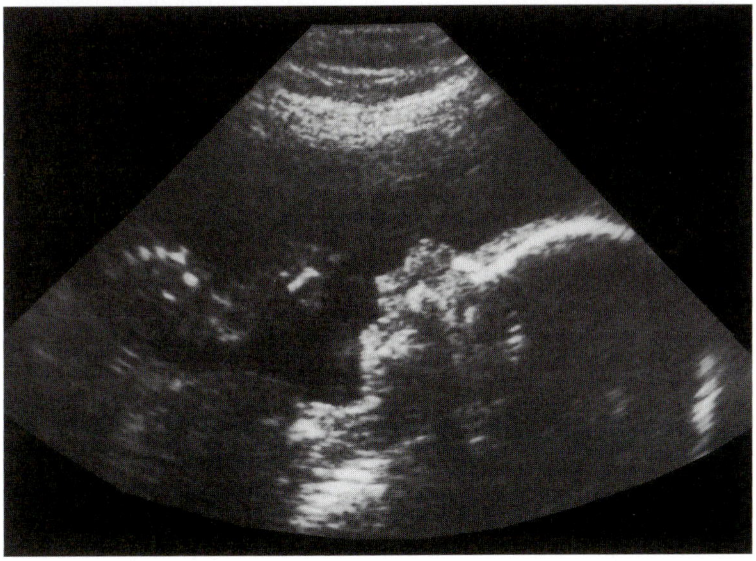

B

FIGURE 2-285 **(A) Transverse view through a fetal head shows trigonocephaly with acute angulation of the frontal bones, as can be seen in fetuses with Jacobsen syndrome. (B) Longitudinal view of the profile of a fetus with micrognathia, as can be seen in fetuses with Jacobsen syndrome.**

Occasional Findings:

Ventriculomegaly

Holoprosencephaly

Nuchal thickening

Facial cleft

Clinodactyly of the fifth finger

Renal anomalies

MAJOR DIFFERENTIAL DIAGNOSES

Other chromosomal abnormalities exhibiting similar findings include the following:

Trisomy 13 (Patau syndrome)

Trisomy 18 (IUGR, cardiac defects, abnormally shaped skull)

The head shape may bring to mind the lemon sign or strawberry-shaped skull, as may be seen in the following:

Craniosynostosis syndromes (see Chapter 1, Abnormal Head Shape/Craniosynostosis, p. 19, for differential diagnosis)

Spina bifida (lemon-shaped)

Trisomy 18 (Edwards' syndrome) (strawberry-shaped)

ULTRASOUND DIAGNOSIS

Prenatal sonographic findings associated with this syndrome have been seen in the third trimester, at 29 weeks' gestation, and have included fetal hydronephrosis, trigonocephalic head shape, hypotelorism, micrognathia, short femur, and polyhydramnios. An earlier scan at 20 weeks revealed only mild pyelectasis; other findings were not detectable until the third trimester. Other reports describe an affected fetus at 20 weeks diagnosed because of a thickened nuchal fold leading to an amniocentesis. Other fetuses with this syndrome have been described sonographically as having ventriculomegaly at 18 weeks, facial cleft and hydronephrosis at 20 weeks, and a short humerus and femur at 20 weeks.

HEREDITY

Deletion of the distal long arm of chromosome 11 involving 11q2-qter may arise de novo or may be the result of a balanced translocation in a parent. This is often a single deletion of part of a ring of chromosome 11.

NATURAL HISTORY AND OUTCOME

Fetuses with severe cardiac defects may not survive. The remainder have moderate-to-severe mental deficiency and hypotonia.

Suggested Reading

Boehm D, Laccone F, Burfeind P, et al: Prenatal diagnosis of a large de novo terminal deletion of chromosome 11q. *Prenat Diagn* 26:286–290, 2006.

Chen CP, Chern SR, Chang TY, et al: Prenatal diagnosis of the distal 11q deletion and review of the literature. *Prenat Diagn* 24:130–136, 2004.

Chen CP, Chern SR, Tzen CY, et al: Prenatal diagnosis of de novo distal 11q deletion associated with sonographic findings of unilateral duplex renal system, pyelectasis and orofacial clefts. *Prenat Diagn* 21:317–320, 2001.

Fryns JP, Kleczkowska A, Buttiens M, Marien P, van den Berghe H: Distal 11q monosomy: the typical 11q monosomy syndrome is due to deletion of subband 11q24.1. *Clin Genet* 30:255–260, 1986.

Jacobsen GK, Henriques UV: A fetal testis with intratubular germ cell neoplasia (ITGCN). *Mod Pathol* 5:547–549, 1992.

Jacobsen P, Hauge M, Henningsen K, et al: An (11, 21) translocation in four generations with chromosome 11 abnormalities in the offspring. *Hum Hered* 23:568–585, 1973.

McClelland SM, Smith AP, Smith NC, Gray ES, Diack JS, Dean JC: Nuchal thickening in Jacobsen syndrome. *Ultrasound Obstet Gynecol* 12:280–282, 1998.

Wax JR, Smith JF, Floyd RC, Eggleston MK: Prenatal ultrasonographic findings associated with Jacobsen syndrome. *J Ultrasound Med* 14:256–258, 1995.

DIGEORGE SYNDROME

Synonyms: Velocardiofacial syndrome, Shprintzen syndrome, CATCH 22 (**c**ardiac defect, **a**bnormal facies, **t**hymic hypoplasia, **c**left palate, **h**ypocalcemia), 22q11 deletion syndrome

This syndrome is characterized by cardiac abnormalities involving largely the great vessels, facial abnormalities, hypocalcemia, and hypoplasia or aplasia of the thymus. DiGeorge described this syndrome in 1965, and, in 1978, Shprintzen reported a group of patients with cleft palate and prominent nose. It was determined that both of these syndromes are actually manifestations of a deletion of chromosome 22q11.2.

See Shprintzen syndrome, p. 179.

ABNORMALITIES DETECTABLE BY ULTRASOUND

Common Findings:

Microcephaly

Micrognathia

Thickened nuchal translucency (first trimester)

Facial cleft

Short long-bones

Cardiac defect (tetralogy of Fallot, aortic arch abnormalities, ventricular septal defect)

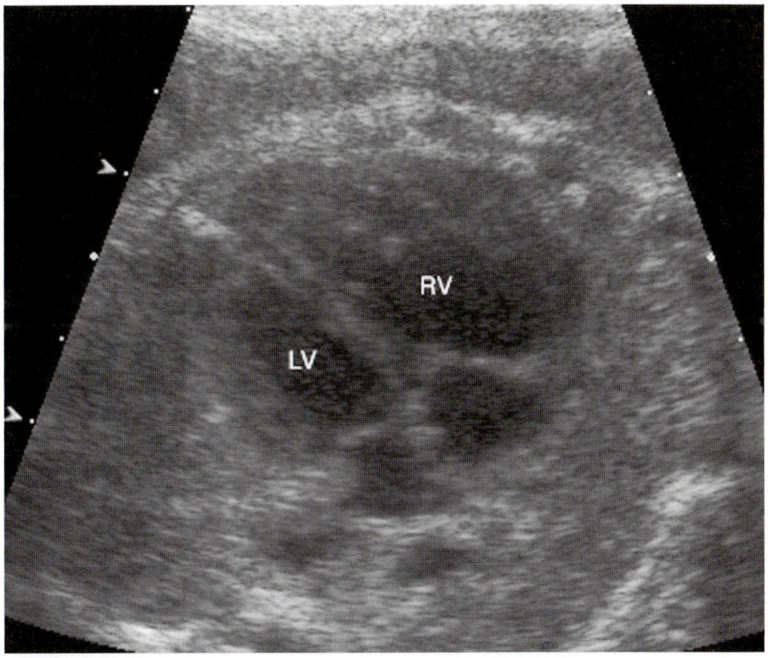

A

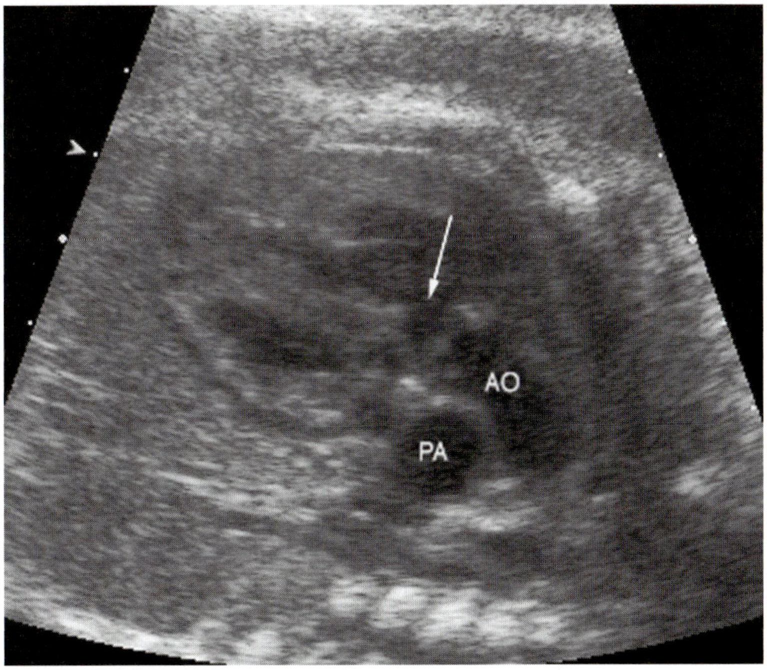

B

FIGURE 2-286 Tetralogy of Fallot with absent pulmonary valve. (**A**) Four-chamber view of a third-trimester fetus with tetralogy of Fallot and absent pulmonary valve shows a slightly larger right ventricle *(RV)* compared to the left ventricle *(LV)*. (**B**) Long-axis view of the same fetus shows a large ventricular septal defect *(arrow)* with an overriding aorta *(AO)*. *PA*, Pulmonary artery. Note that the pulmonary root is dilated.

Continued

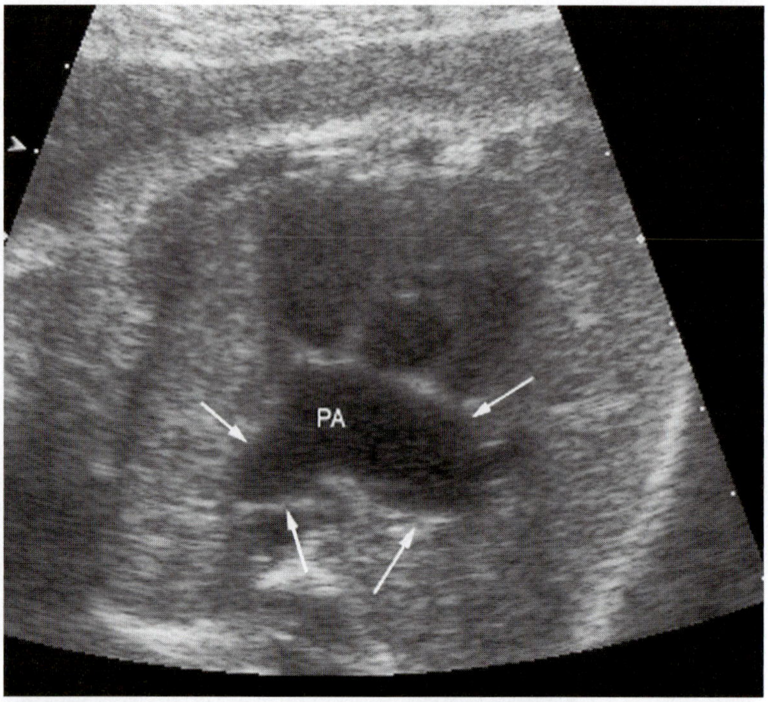

C

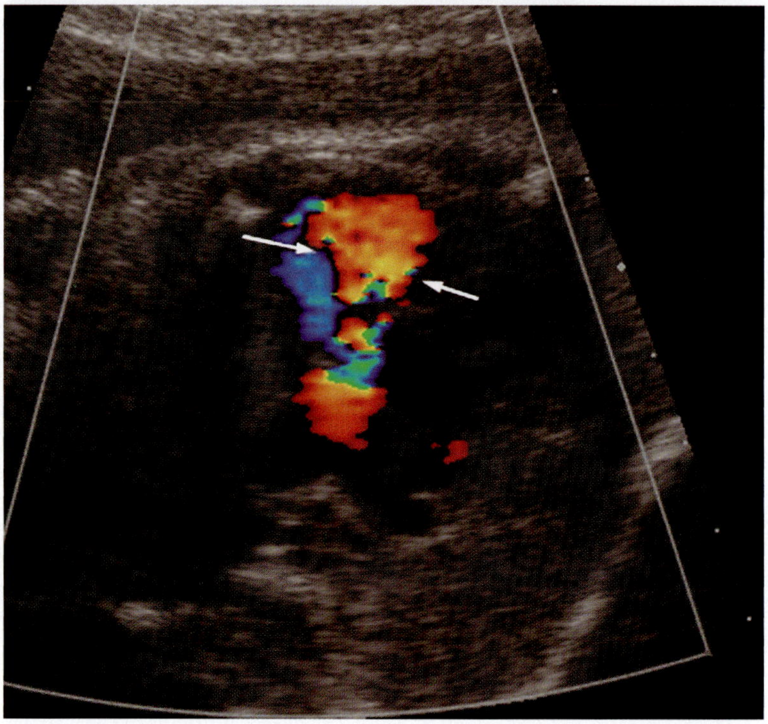

D

FIGURE 2-286, cont'd (C) View of the main pulmonary artery *(PA)* shows that it is dilated, with particular dilation of the branch pulmonary arteries *(arrows)*. (D) Color flow Doppler shows severe pulmonary valve regurgitation as evidenced by the orange flow coming back into the pulmonary artery outflow tract *(arrows)*.

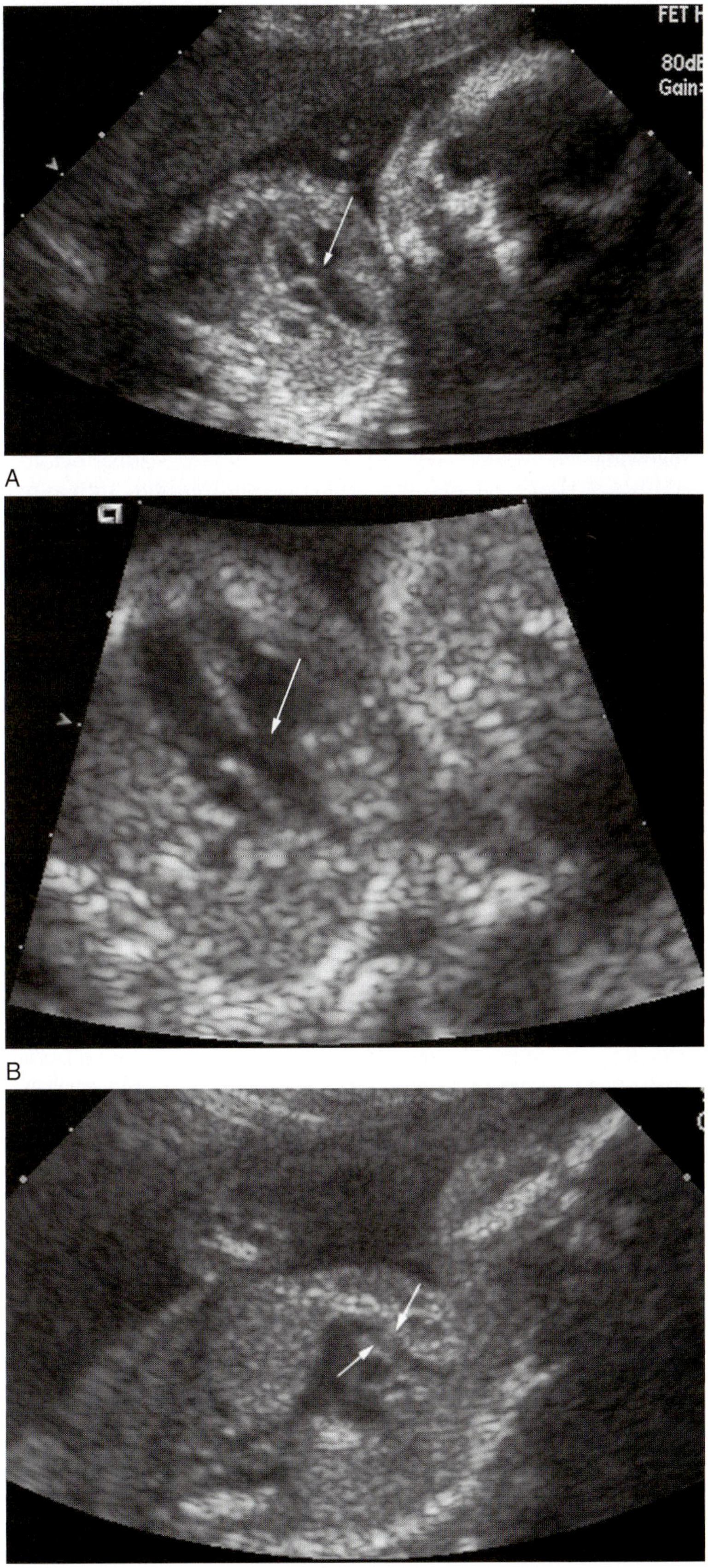

FIGURE 2-287 Second-trimester fetus with DiGeorge syndrome. (A, B) Note large ventricular septal defect *(arrows)* and enlarged overriding aortic root. (C) Longitudinal view of the pulmonary artery outflow tracts shows a narrow main pulmonary artery *(arrows)*.

Occasional Findings:

Pierre Robin syndrome

Brain abnormalities

Umbilical hernia

Cryptorchidism

Hypospadias

MAJOR DIFFERENTIAL DIAGNOSES

The differential diagnosis is extensive, depending on which feature of the syndrome is manifested. Major differential diagnoses include the following:

Chromosomal abnormalities, such as trisomy 18

Cornelia de Lange syndrome

Fanconi anemia

Goldenhar syndrome

Holt-Oram syndrome

Oral-facial-digital syndromes

Thrombocytopenia–absent radius (TAR) syndrome

VATER (**v**ertebral defects, **a**nal atresia, **t**racheoesophageal fistula, **e**sophageal atresia, and **r**adial and renal dysplasias) association

ULTRASOUND DIAGNOSIS

The diagnosis of this syndrome has been made in the first trimester (when affected fetuses have thickened nuchal translucency) and in the second trimester (when major cardiac defects are recognizable). In fetuses diagnosed with tetralogy of Fallot or other aortic arch abnormalities, deletion 22q11.2 is common enough that amniocentesis seeking this particular abnormality is indicated. Although most fetuses with DiGeorge syndrome are detected because of the cardiac defect, occasionally, the fetus is identified as having other, more apparent abnormalities, such as micrognathia and short long-bones. I saw a fetus at 16 weeks with micrognathia and slightly short long-bones who subsequently was born with features consistent with Shprintzen syndrome; a ventricular septal defect was identified only after birth. Some authors have been able to identify absence of the thymus in affected fetuses. Therefore, the 22q11 syndrome is highly diverse, with variable expression, rendering affected fetuses sonographically different from each other.

HEREDITY

The syndrome has an autosomal dominant pattern of inheritance and is caused by the interstitial deletion of chromosome 22q11.2. It can be a new mutation or an unbalanced translocation inherited from a parent with a balanced translocation.

NATURAL HISTORY AND OUTCOME

Cardiac defects must be addressed after birth, and prognosis depends on the severity of these cardiac defects and other associated abnormalities, such as renal anomalies. The issue of immune deficiency and hypocalcemia caused by hypoplasia of the parathyroid glands and seizures from hypocalcemia must be treated. There is a higher incidence of socialization, intellectual, and psychiatric problems. Occasional abnormalities include absent T-cell function secondary to the absent thymic tissue. Children with this disorder may have growth issues and failure to thrive, as well as endocrinologic, gastroenterologic, orthopedic, and urologic problems.

Suggested Reading

Achiron R, Hamiel-Pinchas O, Engelberg S, Barkai G, Reichman B, Mashiach S: Aplasia cutis congenita associated with epidermolysis bullosa and pyloric atresia: the diagnostic role of prenatal ultrasonography. *Prenat Diagn* 12:765–771, 1992.

Boudjemline Y, Fermont L, Le Bidois J, Villain E, Sidi D, Bonnet D: Can we predict 22q11 status of fetuses with tetralogy of Fallot? *Prenat Diagn* 22:231–234, 2002.

Chaoui R, Kalache KD, Heling KS, Tennstedt C, Bommer C, Korner H: Absent or hypoplastic thymus on ultrasound: a marker for deletion 22q11.2 in fetal cardiac defects. *Ultrasound Obstet Gynecol* 20:546–552, 2002.

Chen CP, Chern SR, Chang TY, et al: Prenatal diagnosis of mosaic ring chromosome 22 associated with cardiovascular abnormalities and intrauterine growth restriction. *Prenat Diagn* 23:40–43, 2003.

Jones KL: *Smith's recognizable patterns of human malformation,* ed 6. Philadelphia, 2006, Elsevier.

Lepinard C, Descamps P, Meneguzzi G, et al: Prenatal diagnosis of pyloric atresia-junctional epidermolysis bullosa syndrome in a fetus not known to be at risk. *Prenat Diagn* 20:70–75, 2000.

Machlitt A, Tennstedt C, Korner H, Bommer C, Chaoui R: Prenatal diagnosis of 22q11 microdeletion in an early second-trimester fetus with conotruncal anomaly presenting with increased nuchal translucency and bilateral intracardiac echogenic foci. *Ultrasound Obstet Gynecol* 19:510–513, 2002.

Moore JW, Binder GA, Berry R: Prenatal diagnosis of aneuploidy and deletion 22q11.2 in fetuses with ultrasound detection of cardiac defects. *Am J Obstet Gynecol* 191:2068–2073, 2004.

Nazzaro V, Nicolini U, De Luca L, Berti E, Caputo R: Prenatal diagnosis of junctional epidermolysis bullosa associated with pyloric atresia. *J Med Genet* 27:244–248, 1990.

Nyberg, DA, McGahan JP, Pretorius DH, Pilu G: *Diagnostic imaging of fetal anomalies.* Philadelphia, 2003, Lippincott Williams & Wilkins.

Sleurs E, De Catte L, Benatar A: Prenatal diagnosis of absent pulmonary valve syndrome in association with 22q11 deletion. *J Ultrasound Med* 23:417–422, 2004.

Volpe P, Marasini M, Caruso G, Gentile M: Prenatal diagnosis of interruption of the aortic arch and its association with deletion of chromosome 22q11. *Ultrasound Obstet Gynecol* 327–331, 2002.

Volpe P, Marasini M, Caruso G, et al: 22q11 deletions in fetuses with malformations of the outflow tacts or interruption of the aortic arch: impact of additional ultrasound signs. *Prenat Diagn* 23:752–757, 2003.

TETRASOMY 12p (PALLISTER-KILLIAN SYNDROME)

DESCRIPTION AND DEFINITION

Synonyms: Pallister-Killian syndrome, Killian/Teschler-Nicola syndrome, Pallister mosaic syndrome

This syndrome is a mosaic aneuploidy, consisting of tetrasomy 12p in skin fibroblasts but usually not in peripheral blood.

ABNORMALITIES DETECTABLE BY ULTRASOUND

Cerebellar hypoplasia

Ventriculomegaly

Facial dysmorphism

Hypertelorism

Low-set ears

Femoral and humeral shortening (micromelia)

Clinodactyly of the fifth digit

Diaphragmatic hernia

Cardiac abnormalities

Nuchal translucency thickening

Hydrops

Bilateral hydronephrosis

Omphalocele

Polyhydramnios

MAJOR DIFFERENTIAL DIAGNOSES

Polyhydramnios, short femurs, and diaphragmatic hernia (the most common abnormalities in this syndrome) are also seen in the following syndromes and conditions:

Deletion 4p (Wolf-Hirschhorn syndrome)

Fryns syndrome

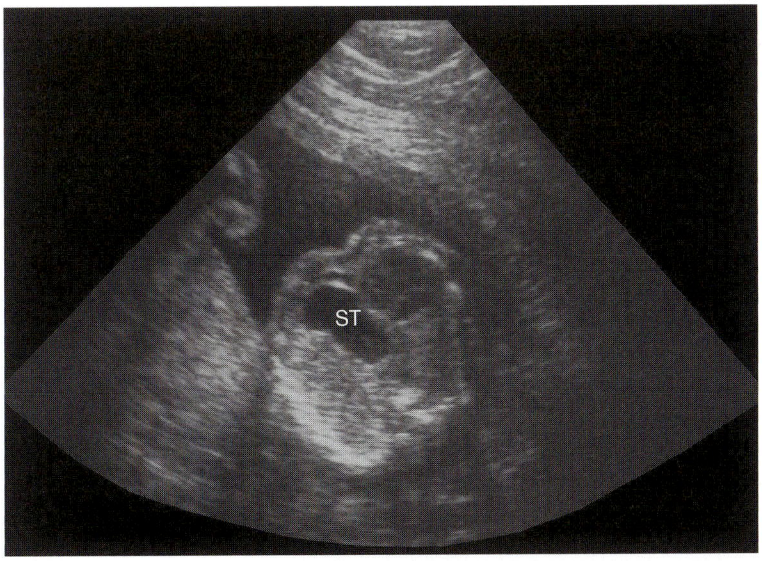

FIGURE 2-288 Transverse view through the fetal chest shows evidence of a left diaphragmatic hernia, as can be seen in fetuses with Pallister-Killian syndrome. Note that the fetal stomach *(ST)* is located adjacent to the heart.

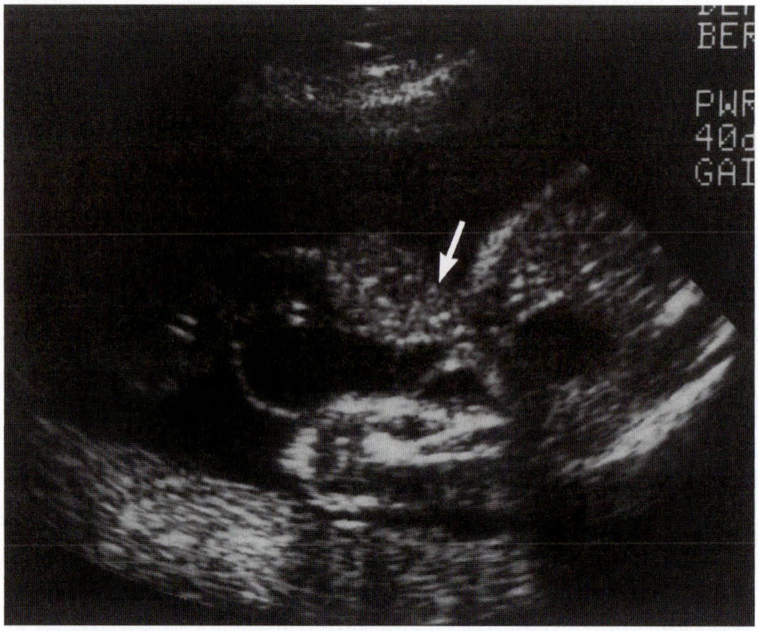

FIGURE 2-289 Tangential view of the cord insertion during the second trimester shows a small omphalocele *(arrow)*, as can be seen in fetuses with Pallister-Killian syndrome.

Trisomy 9

Trisomy 18 (Edwards' syndrome)

The differential diagnosis for first-trimester abnormal nuchal translucency also should be considered (see nuchal thickening; differential diagnosis section, p. 50).

ULTRASOUND DIAGNOSIS

An abnormal nuchal translucency measurement in first-trimester patients being screened for Down syndrome may be the first sonographic manifestation of the syndrome. Prenatal ultrasound diagnosis has been established at 16 weeks' gestation, primarily based on the presence of a diaphragmatic hernia, cardiac abnormality, and short femurs. Facial abnormalities such as a flat profile and protruding lower lip were noted at 21 weeks in another reported case with a diaphragmatic hernia and limb shortening. Polyhydramnios tends to be a later development.

HEREDITY

Tetrasomy 12p may be related to advanced maternal age.

NATURAL HISTORY AND OUTCOME

Many infants are stillborn or die neonatally. There is profound mental retardation, with seizures beginning during infancy.

Suggested Reading

Doray B, Girard-Lemaire F, Gasser B, et al: Pallister-Killian syndrome: difficulties of prenatal diagnosis. *Prenat Diagn* 22:470–477, 2002.

Hebenstreit K, Heyborne KD, Porreco RP: Sonographic and cytogenetic aspects of the prenatal diagnosis of mosaic tetrasomy 12p (Pallister-Killian syndrome): a case report and review of the literature. *J Matern Fetal Med* 2:176–178, 1993.

Jones KL: *Smith's recognizable patterns of human malformation,* ed 6. Philadelphia, 2006, Elsevier.

Langford K, Hodgson S, Seller M, Maxwell D: Pallister-Killian syndrome presenting through nuchal translucency screening for trisomy 21. *Prenat Diagn* 20:670–672, 2000.

Paladini D, Borghese A, Arienzo M, Teodoro A, Martinelli P, Nappi C: Prospective ultrasound diagnosis of Pallister-Killian syndrome in the second trimester of pregnancy: the importance of the fetal facial profile. *Prenat Diagn* 20:996–998, 2000.

Sharland M, Hill L, Patel R, Patton M: Pallister-Killian syndrome diagnosed by chronic villus sampling. *Prenat Diagn* 11:477–479, 1991.

Tejada MI, Uribarren A, Briones P, Vilaseca MA: A further prenatal diagnosis of mosaic tetrasomy 12p (Pallister-Killian syndrome). *Prenat Diagn* 12:529–534, 1992.

Wilson RD, Harrison LA, Clarke LA, Yong SL: Tetrasomy 12p (Pallister-Killian syndrome): ultrasound indicators and confirmation by interphase FISH. *Prenat Diagn* 14:787–792, 1994.

TRIPLOIDY

DESCRIPTION AND DEFINITION

Occurring as a result of a complete extra set of chromosomes, most triploid concepti are lost in miscarriage. Survival of the fetus beyond 20 weeks' gestation is rare.

ABNORMALITIES DETECTABLE BY ULTRASOUND

Severe, early-onset, asymmetric IUGR (affecting the skeleton more than the head)

Ventriculomegaly

Agenesis of the corpus callosum

Dandy-Walker malformation

Holoprosencephaly

Meningomyelocele

Hypertelorism

Microphthalmia

Micrognathia

Cardiac defect

Nuchal translucency thickening

Cystic hygroma

Omphalocele

Renal anomalies

Hydronephrosis

Hypospadias

Syndactyly of the third and fourth fingers

Club feet

Abnormal umbilical artery Doppler waveform showing a high-resistance pattern

Enlarged placenta or small, prematurely calcified placenta

Oligohydramnios, with or without a hydropic placenta

MAJOR DIFFERENTIAL DIAGNOSES

Deletion 4p (Wolf-Hirschhorn Syndrome) (early IUGR)

Maternal infections (early IUGR)

Neu-Laxova syndrome (early IUGR)

Russell-Silver syndrome (asymmetric, early IUGR)

Seckel syndrome (early IUGR)

Trisomy 9

Trisomy 18 (Edwards' syndrome)

Diagnosis in the first trimester, based on early, asymmetric IUGR is quite specific. If the diagnosis of syndactyly of the third and fourth digits can be established in such a fetus, triploidy is extremely likely.

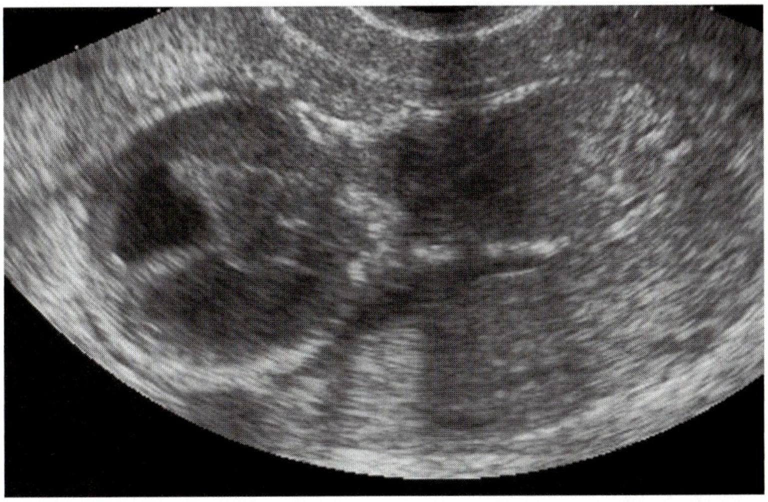

FIGURE 2-290 Late first-trimester fetus with triploidy shows evidence of ventriculomegaly and a small body for the size of the fetal head, indicating early-onset intrauterine growth restriction.

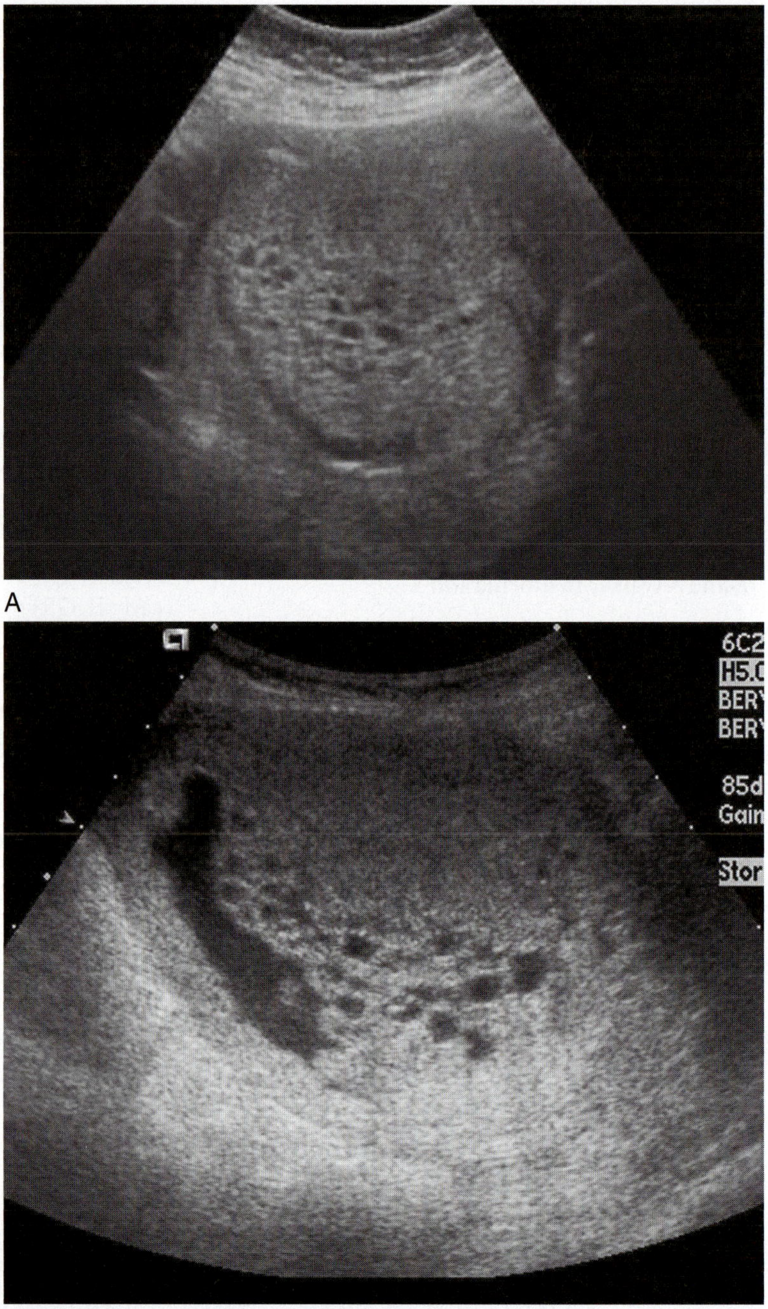

A

B

FIGURE 2-291 **(A, B) First-trimester pregnancy with multiple cystic spaces throughout a thickened placenta consistent with a molar pregnancy. These pregnancies often have a triploid karyotype.**

ULTRASOUND DIAGNOSIS

Diagnosis has been suspected as early as 11 weeks' gestational age, based on early, asymmetric IUGR. Other findings, such as hydropic placenta, major defects of multiple organ systems, and syndactyly of the fingers, may be helpful in making an early diagnosis. The findings of abnormal first-trimester nuchal translucency, free β-human chorionic gonadotropin (β-hCG), and pregnancy-associated plasma protein-A (PAPP-A) have been helpful in detecting fetuses with triploidy. Hydropic placenta that occurs with fetal triploidy is associated with preeclampsia and maternal HELLP (**h**emolysis, **e**levated **l**iver enzymes, **l**ow **p**latelet count) syndrome.

HEREDITY

In most cases (69%), the extra set of chromosomes are from paternal origin. Most of these

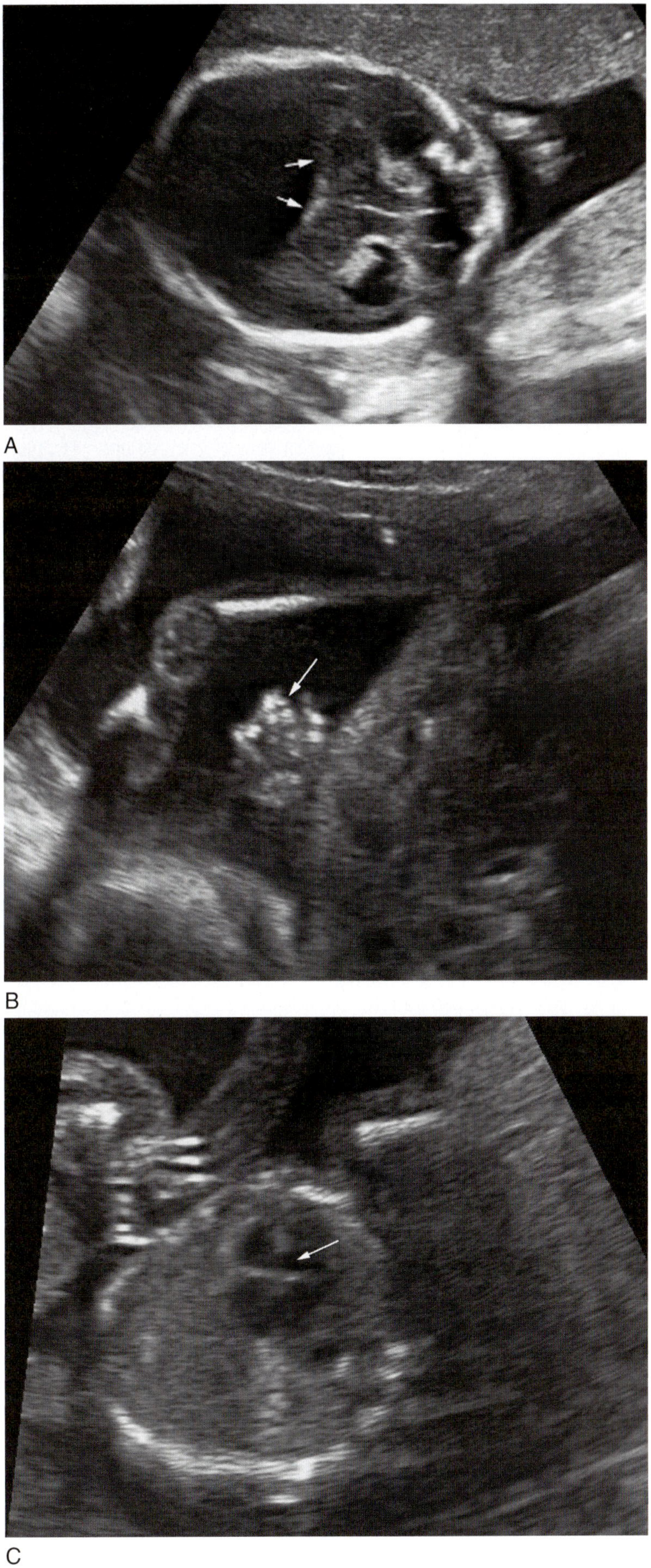

FIGURE 2-292 Second-trimester triploid fetus. (A) Coronal view through the fetal head shows holoprosencephaly with fused thalami *(arrows)*. (B) Fetal hand of the same fetus with triploidy shows characteristic syndactyly of the third and fourth digits *(arrow)*. (C) Four-chamber view of the heart of the same fetus shows a large ventricular septal defect *(arrow)*.

Continued

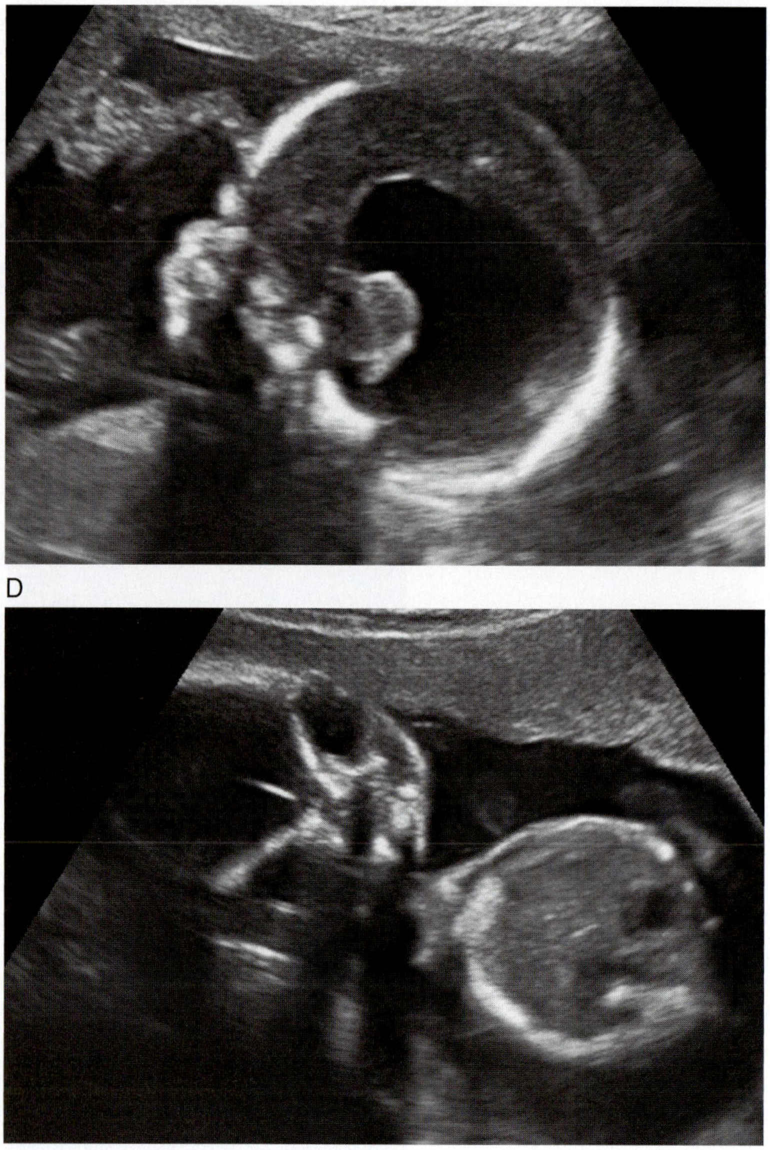

FIGURE 2-292, cont'd (D) Profile view of the fetal head and face shows the large monoventricle. (E) Cross section of the fetal face and abdomen shows the small size of the fetal abdomen compared to the width of the fetal head, consistent with early-onset intrauterine growth restriction. Note the associated hypertelorism.

cases occur secondary to fertilization of an ovum by two sperm; the others occur by fertilization with a diploid sperm. A minority of triploidy cases are the result of fertilization of a diploid egg. Some reports suggest that when the extra haploid set of chromosomes arises from the *maternal* side, the placenta is small and exhibits severe, early, placental insufficiency with fetal IUGR. In contrast, a *paternal* origin of the extra haploid set more likely leads to a large, cystic, hydropic-appearing placenta (often associated with appearance of a partial mole). Advanced maternal age is not reported as a risk factor.

NATURAL HISTORY AND OUTCOME

Most affected fetuses die during gestation or are stillborn. The longest recorded survival is 5 months.

Suggested Reading

Avrech OM, Jaffe R, Zabow PH, Weinraub Z, Caspi E: Triploidy, partial hydatiform mole. *Fetus* 1:1–3, 1991.

Benacerraf BR: Intrauterine growth retardation in the first trimester associated with triploidy. *J Ultrasound Med* 7:153–154, 1988.

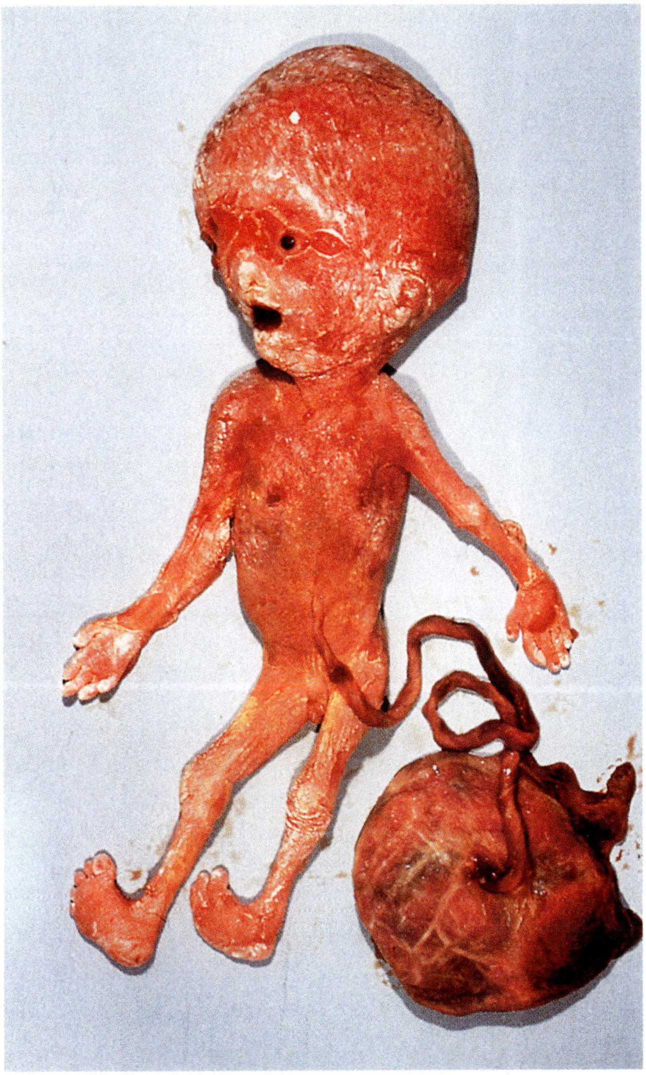

FIGURE 2-293 Pathology specimen shows severe, early-onset growth restriction with particular involvement of the fetal body. (From Keeling JW: *Fetal pathology.* London, 1994, Churchill Livingstone.)

Broekhuizen FF, Elejalde R, Hamilton PR: Early onset preeclampsia, triploidy and fetal hydrops. *J Reprod Med* 28:223–226, 1983.

Crane JP, Beaver HA, Cheung SW: Antenatal ultrasound findings in fetal triploidy syndrome. *J Ultrasound Med* 4:519–524, 1985.

Doshi N, Surti U, Szulman AE: Morphologic anomalies in triploid liveborn fetuses. *Hum Pathol* 14:716–723, 1983.

Edwards MT, Smith WL, Hanson J, Abu Yousef M: Prenatal sonographic diagnosis of triploidy. *J Ultrasound Med* 5:279–281, 1986.

Frates MC, Feinberg BB: Early prenatal sonographic diagnosis of twin triploid gestation presenting with fetal hydrops and theca-lutein ovarian cysts. *J Clin Ultrasound* 28:137–141, 2000.

Gassner R, Metzenbauer M, Hafner E, Vallazza U, Philipp K: Triploidy in a twin pregnancy: small placenta volume as an early sonographical marker. *Prenat Diagn* 23:16–20, 2003.

Jauniaux E, Brown R, Rodeck C, Nicolaides KH: Prenatal diagnosis of triploidy during the second trimester of pregnancy. *Obstet Gynecol* 88:983–989, 1996.

Jones KL: *Smith's recognizable patterns of human malformation,* ed 6. Philadelphia, 2006, Elsevier.

Lockwood C, Scioscia A, Stiller R, Hobbins J: Sonographic features of the triploid fetus. *Am J Obstet Gynecol* 157:285–287, 1987.

Philipp T, Grillenberger K, Separovic ER, Philipp K, Kalousek DK: Effects of triploidy on early human development. *Prenat Diagn* 24:276–281, 2004.

Pircon RA, Porto M, Towers CV, Drade M, Gocke SE: Ultrasound findings in pregnancies complicated by fetal triploidy. *J Ultrasound Med* 8:507–511, 1989.

Rubenstein JB, Swayne LC, Dise CA, et al: Placental changes in fetal triploidy syndrome. *J Ultrasound Med* 5:545–550, 1986.

Salomon LJ, Bernard JP, Nizard J, Ville Y: First-trimester screening for fetal triploidy at 11 to 14 weeks: a role for fetal biometry. *Prenat Diagn* 25:479–483, 2005.

Snijders RJM, Sherrod C, Gosden CM, Nicolaides KH: Fetal growth retardation: associated malformations and chromosomal abnormalities. *Am J Obstet Gynecol* 168:547–555, 1993.
Spencer K, Liao AW, Skentou H, Cicero S, Nicolaides KH: Screening for triploidy by fetal nuchal translucency and maternal serum free beta-hCG and PAPP-A at 10–14 weeks of gestation. *Prenat Diagn* 20:495–499, 2000.
Stefos T, Plachouras N, Mari G, Cosmi E, Lolis D: A case of partial mole and atypical type I triploidy associated with severe HELLP syndrome at 18 weeks' gestation. *Ultrasound Obstet Gynecol* 20:403–404, 2002.
Wu RT, Shyu MK, Lee CN, et al: Sonographic manifestation and Doppler blood flow study in fetal triploidy syndrome: report of two cases. *J Ultrasound Med* 14:555–557, 1995.

TRISOMY 9

DESCRIPTION AND DEFINITION

First described by Feingold and Atkins in 1973, this syndrome is associated with malformations of multiple organ systems.

ABNORMALITIES DETECTABLE BY ULTRASOUND

Microcephaly

Brain anomalies

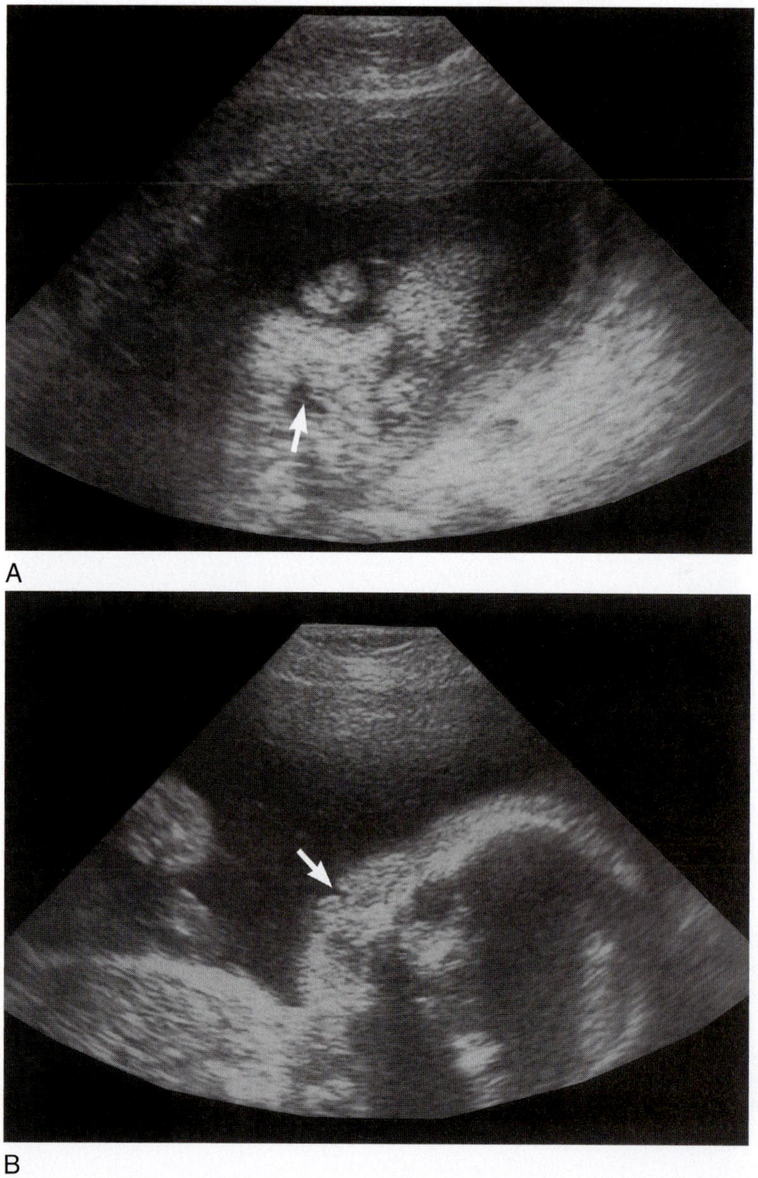

FIGURE 2-294 **(A, B)** Coronal and longitudinal views of the face of a fetus with trisomy 9. **(A)** Note severe hypotelorism and large median cleft lip and palate *(arrow)*. **(B)** View of the profile of the fetus shows malformation of the nose and lip area *(arrow)*, which corresponds to the cleft lip and palate.

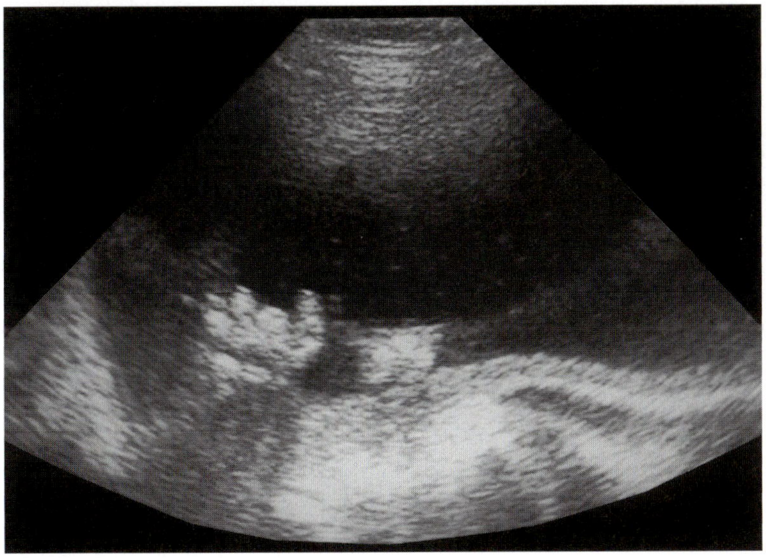

C

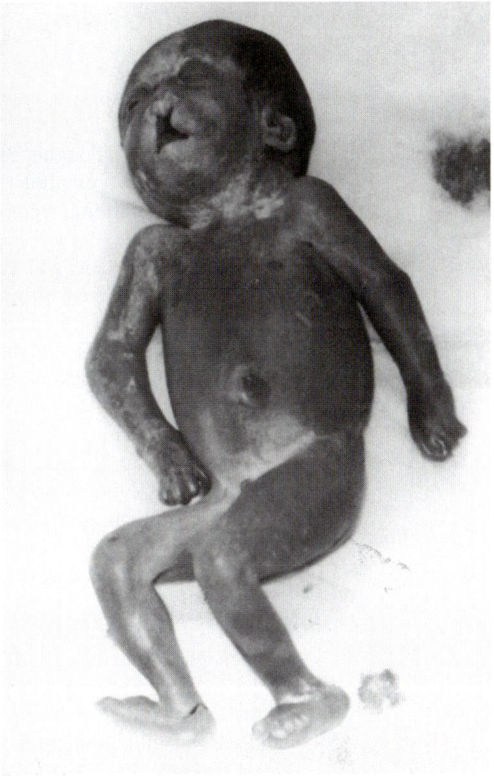

D

FIGURE 2-294, cont'd (C) Image of the hand of the same fetus shows an abnormally clenched hand. (D) Postmortem view of the same fetus with trisomy 9 shows the same features that were evident prenatally.

Cerebellar anomalies

Ventriculomegaly

Neural tube defect

Cleft lip and palate

Micrognathia

Microphthalmia

Nuchal translucency thickening

Cardiac defects

Diaphragmatic hernia

Renal anomalies

Multicystic kidneys

Hydronephrosis and hydroureter

Cryptorchidism

Flexion deformities of the fingers

Abnormal positioning of the feet

IUGR

MAJOR DIFFERENTIAL DIAGNOSES

Some other chromosomal anomalies with similar findings:

Deletion 4p (Wolf-Hirschhorn syndrome)

Triploidy

Trisomy 13 (Patau syndrome)

Trisomy 18 (Edwards' syndrome)

ULTRASOUND DIAGNOSIS

Prenatal diagnosis has been established in the early second trimester and is possible any time during the second and third trimesters, particularly among fetuses with multiple, severe abnormalities. The anomalies seen sonographically include brain abnormalities (Dandy-Walker cyst, ventriculomegaly, microcephaly); facial dysmorphism; renal anomalies; cardiac defects; limb anomalies; and growth restriction. The finding of abnormal first-trimester nuchal translucency has been the earliest sonographic finding, seen in two affected fetuses.

HEREDITY

This is an autosomal trisomic syndrome.

NATURAL HISTORY AND OUTCOME

Most affected fetuses die in the perinatal period. Survivors have profound mental and motor retardation. Among mosaics, the severity of malformations depends on the percentage of trisomic cells in the different tissues.

Suggested Reading

Benacerraf BR, Pauker S, Quade BJ, Bieber FR: Prenatal sonography in trisomy 9. *Prenat Diagn* 12:175–181, 1992.

Bureau YA, Fraser W, Fouquet B: Prenatal diagnosis of trisomy 9 mosaic presenting as a case of Dandy-Walker malformation. *Prenat Diagn* 13:79–85, 1993.

Chen CP, Chern SR, Cheng SJ, et al: Second-trimester diagnosis of complete trisomy 9 associated with abnormal maternal serum screen results, open sacral spina bifida and congenital diaphragmatic hernia, and review of the literature. *Prenat Diagn* 24:455–462, 2004.

de Grouchy J, Turleau C: *Clinical atlas of human chromosomes.* New York, 1984, John Wiley & Sons.

Diaz-Mares L, Molina B, Carnevale A: Trisomy 9 mosaicism in a girl with multiple malformations. *Ann Genet* 33:165–168, 1990.

Feingold M, Atkins L: A case of trisomy 9. *J Med Genet* 10:184–187, 1973.

Jones KL: *Smith's recognizable patterns of human malformation,* ed 6. Philadelphia, 2006, Elsevier.

Kurnick J, Atkins L, Feingold M, Hills J, Dvorak A: Trisomy 9: predominance of cardiovascular liver, brain and skeletal anomalies in the first diagnosed case. *Hum Pathol* 5:223–228, 1974.

Mace SE, Macintyre MN, Turk KB, Johnson WE: The trisomy 9 syndrome: multiple congenital anomalies and unusual pathological findings. *J Pediatr* 92:446–448, 1978.

Merino A, de Perdigo A, Nombalais F, et al: Prenatal diagnosis of trisomy 9 mosaicism: two cases. *Prenat Diagn* 13:1001–1007, 1993.

Murta C, Moron A, Avila M, Franca L, Vargas P: Reverse flow in the umbilical vein in a case of trisomy 9. *Ultrasound Obstet Gynecol* 16:575–577, 2000.

Nakagawa M, Hashimoto K, Ohira H, Hamanaka T, Ozaki M, Suehara N: Prenatal diagnosis of trisomy 9. *Fetal Diagn Ther* 21:68–71, 2006.

Pinette MG, Pan Y, Chard R, Pinette SG, Blackstone J: Prenatal diagnosis of nonmosaic trisomy 9 and related ultrasound findings at 11.7 weeks. *J Matern Fetal Med* 7:48–50, 1998.

Qazi QH, Masakawa A, Madahar C, Ehrlich R: Trisomy 9 syndrome. *Clin Genet* 12:221–226, 1977.

Quigg MH, Diment S, Roberson J: Second-trimester diagnosis of trisomy 9 associated with abnormal maternal serum screening results. *Prenat Diagn* 25:966–967, 2005.

Saura R, Traore W, Taine L, et al: Prenatal diagnosis of trisomy 9: six cases and a review of the literature. *Prenat Diagn* 15:609–614, 1995.

Sepulveda W, Wimalasundera RC, Taylor MJ, Blunt S, Be C, De La Fuente S: Prenatal ultrasound findings in complete trisomy 9. *Ultrasound Obstet Gynecol* 22:479–483, 2003.

Sherer DM, Wang N, Thompson HO, et al: An infant with trisomy 9 mosaicism presenting as a complete trisomy 9 by amniocentesis. *Prenat Diagn* 12:31–37, 1992.

Smart RD, Viljoen DL, Fraser B: Partial trisomy 9—further delineation of the phenotype. *Am J Med Genet* 31:947–951, 1988.

Stipoljev F, Kos M, Kos M, et al: Antenatal detection of mosaic trisomy 9 by ultrasound: a case report and literature review. *J Matern Fetal Neonatal Med* 14:65–69, 2003.

Sutherland GR, Carter RF, Morris LL: Partial and complete trisomy 9: delineation of a trisomy 9 syndrome. *Hum Genet* 32:133–140, 1976.

Yeo L, Waldron R, Lashley S, Day-Salvatore D, Vintzileos AM: Prenatal sonographic findings associated with nonmosaic trisomy 9 and literature review. *J Ultrasound Med* 22:425–430, 2003.

TRISOMY 10

DESCRIPTION AND DEFINITION

This is a rare chromosomal abnormality. Only those with *mosaic* trisomy 10 survive to infancy.

ABNORMALITIES DETECTABLE BY ULTRASOUND

Nuchal translucency thickening

Hypertelorism

Cardiac disease

Cryptorchidism

IUGR

With *complete* trisomy 10, findings also include the following:

- Cleft lip and palate
- Micrognathia
- Polydactyly (preaxial)
- Syndactyly of the toes
- Club feet

MAJOR DIFFERENTIAL DIAGNOSES

Nuchal thickening, the most easily detected feature of trisomy 10, is also seen in many other syndromes (see Chapter 1, p. 50, for nuchal thickening differential diagnosis), including the following:

- Apert syndrome
- Arthrogryposis
- Cardiosplenic syndromes
- Caudal regression syndrome

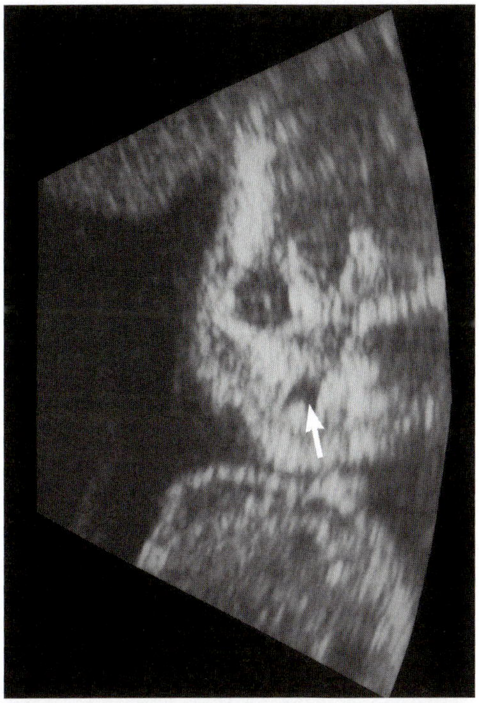

FIGURE 2-295 Coronal view of the face of a fetus with cleft lip and palate *(arrow)*, as can be seen in fetuses with trisomy 10.

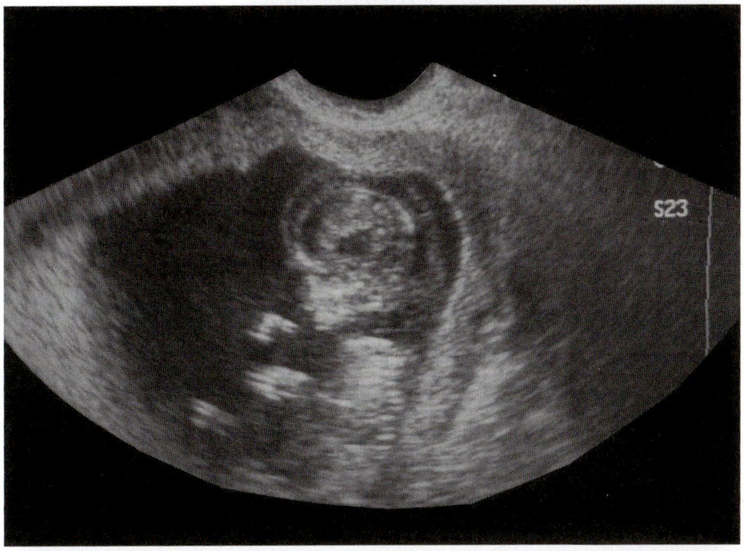

FIGURE 2-296 Longitudinal view of a late first-trimester/early second-trimester fetus with nuchal thickening involving the head and neck.

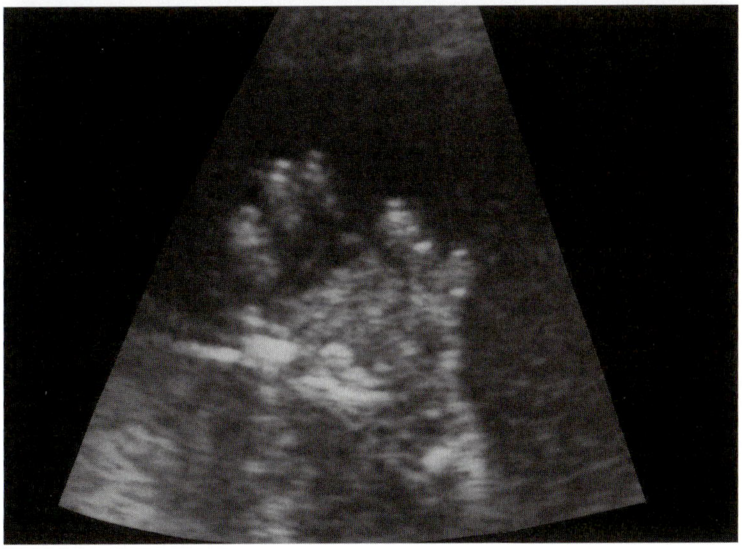

FIGURE 2-297 Palmar view of a fetal hand shows preaxial polydactyly, as seen in fetuses with trisomy 10.

Cerebrocostomandibular syndrome

CHARGE (**c**oloboma of the iris, **h**eart defect, choanal **a**tresia, intrauterine growth **r**estriction, **g**enital anomalies, and **e**ar anomalies) association:

Chromosomal anomalies

Congenital adrenal hyperplasia

Congenital high airway obstruction syndrome

Cornelia de Lange syndrome

DiGeorge syndrome

Ectrodactyly–ectodermal dysplasia–clefting (EEC) syndrome

Fanconi anemia

Fetal infections

Fryns syndrome

Holt-Oram syndrome

Hydrolethalus

Jarcho-Levin syndrome

Joubert syndrome

Multiple pterygium syndrome

Noonan syndrome

Osteogenesis Imperfecta

Pentalogy of Cantrell

Perlman syndrome

Roberts' syndrome

Skeletal dysplasias (several)

Smith-Lemli-Opitz syndrome

ULTRASOUND DIAGNOSIS

Prenatal ultrasound diagnosis has been established on the basis of finding a thickened nuchal fold measuring 7 mm at 15 weeks' gestation (by dates) in a 13-week gestation-sized fetus. On follow-up ultrasound study 1 week later, interval growth continued to lag while the nuchal thickening persisted. Another fetus was detected in the first trimester based on finding an abnormal nuchal translucency. Postmortem examination revealed facial cleft, contractures of extremities, diaphragmatic hernias, cardiac defect, and renal abnormality. Another fetus was noted to have nuchal thickening at 12 weeks, with hydrops, micrognathia, club feet, and cardiac defect. At 18 weeks, the fetus had severe IUGR and a facial cleft in addition to the other findings. By 31 weeks, a 7-week lag in growth was observed, associated with oligohydramnios and multiple anomalies. The fetus died in utero at 35 weeks.

HEREDITY

This is an autosomal trisomic syndrome.

NATURAL HISTORY AND OUTCOME

This condition is lethal in cases of complete trisomy 10.

Mosaic individuals have been reported to survive into infancy but have hypertelorism, cardiac defects, cryptorchidism, and mental and growth retardation.

Suggested Reading

Brizot ML, Schultz R, Patroni LT, Lopes LM, Armbruster-Moraes E, Zugaib M: Trisomy 10: ultrasound features and natural history after first trimester diagnosis. *Prenat Diagn* 21:672–675, 2001.

de France HF, Beemer FA, Senders RCH, Schaminee-Main SCE: Trisomy 10 mosaicism in a newborn boy. Delineation of the syndrome. *Clin Genet* 27:92–96, 1985.

Farrell SA, Sue-Chue-Lam A, Miskin M, Fan YS: Fetal nuchal oedema and antenatal diagnosis of trisomy 10. *Prenat Diagn* 14:463–467, 1994.

Knoblauch H, Sommer D, Zimmer C, et al: Fetal trisomy 10 mosaicism: ultrasound, cytogenetic and morphologic findings in early pregnancy. *Prenat Diagn* 19:379–382, 1999.

Schwarzler P, Moscoso G, Bernard JP, Hill L, Senat MV, Ville Y: Trisomy 10: first-trimester features on ultrasound, fetoscopy and postmortem of a case associated with increased nuchal translucency. *Ultrasound Obstet Gynecol* 13:67–70, 1999.

Vianello MG, Gemme G, Bonioli E, Olivo F: Trisomy of chromosome No. 10 in mosaic. *J Genet Hum* 26:185–191, 1978.

TRISOMY 13 (PATAU SYNDROME)

DESCRIPTION AND DEFINITION

Synonym: Patau syndrome

With an incidence of 1:5000 births, this syndrome is characterized by multiple congenital abnormalities involving virtually every organ system.

ABNORMALITIES DETECTABLE BY ULTRASOUND

Holoprosencephaly

Ventriculomegaly

Enlarged cisterna magna

Microcephaly

Agenesis of the corpus callosum

Cleft lip and palate

Midface hypoplasia

Cyclopia

Microphthalmia

Hypotelorism

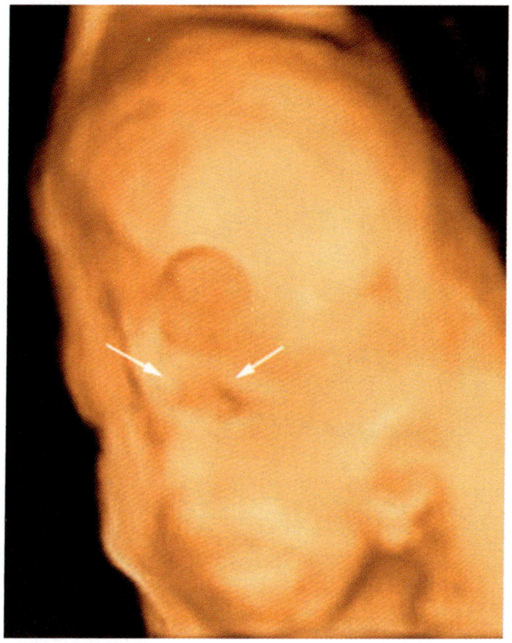

FIGURE 2-298 Three-dimensional surface rendering of a fetus with cyclopia (single orbit = arrows). Note the proboscis is located above the level of the orbit. This fetus had trisomy 13 and holoprosencephaly.

Nuchal thickening

Neural tube defect

Omphalocele

Echogenic, enlarged kidneys

Hyperechoic bowel

Echogenic chordae tendineae

Single umbilical artery

Cardiac defects

Radial aplasia

Polydactyly

Flexion deformity of the fingers

MAJOR DIFFERENTIAL DIAGNOSES

Meckel-Gruber syndrome is the main mimicker of trisomy 13 (polydactyly, neural tube defects, enlarged echogenic kidneys)

Other diagnostic possibilities vary, depending on the multiple abnormalities present in each affected fetus.

ULTRASOUND DIAGNOSIS

Prenatal sonographic detection has been established as early as 12 weeks' gestation, based on the presence of holoprosencephaly. Sonographic abnormalities (described earlier) are easily detectable because of the severity of defects and the multitude of organ systems involved. Sonographic detection of trisomy 13 has a reported sensitivity of 90% to 100% when a complete structural survey (including the heart) is accomplished.

It is possible, but unusual, for a fetus with trisomy 13 syndrome to have a completely normal structural sonographic survey early in the second trimester.

HEREDITY

This is an autosomal trisomic syndrome.

NATURAL HISTORY AND OUTCOME

Most neonates with trisomy 13 die within hours or days of delivery. Eighty percent of affected babies die within the first month of life. Occasionally, survivors are reported, but they have profound mental retardation, seizures, and failure to thrive.

Text continued on p. 490

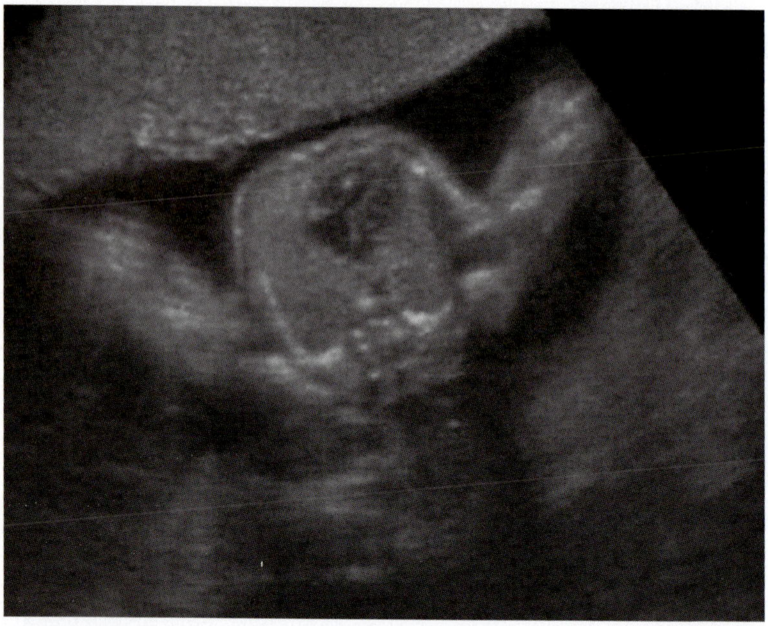

FIGURE 2-299 Four-chamber view of the fetal heart of a fetus with trisomy 13 shows an echogenic intracardiac focus as well as a small left ventricle compared to the right ventricle.

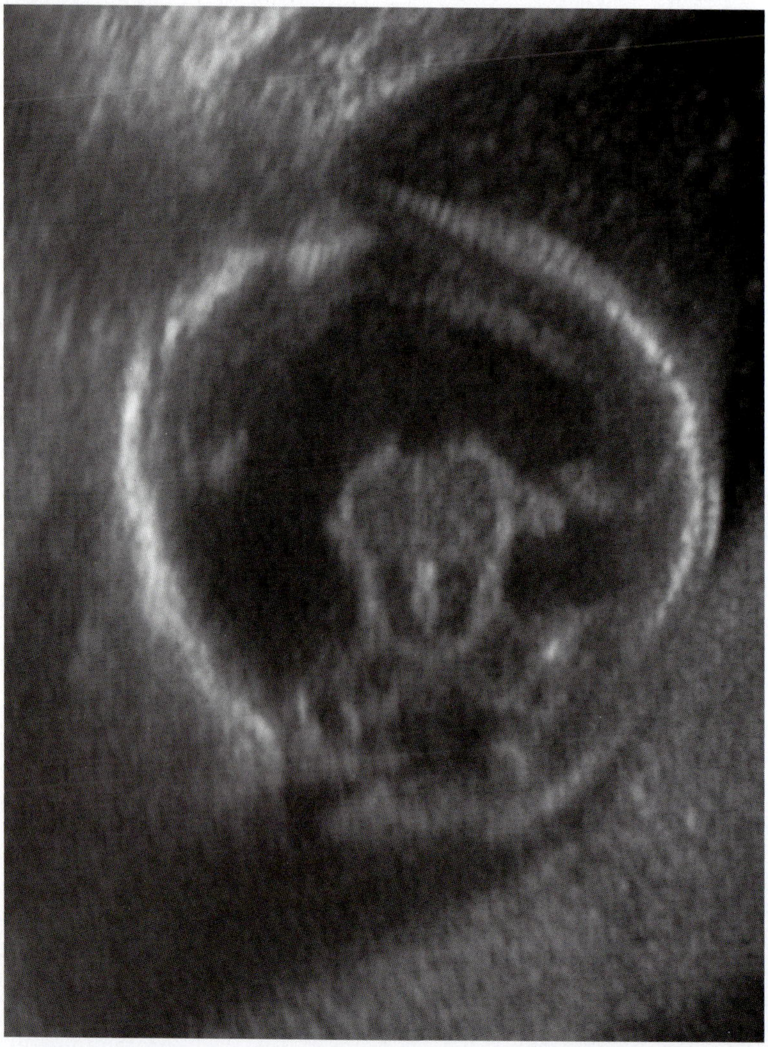

FIGURE 2-300 Coronal view of a second-trimester fetal head shows holoprosencephaly with a monoventricle surrounding the fused thalami.

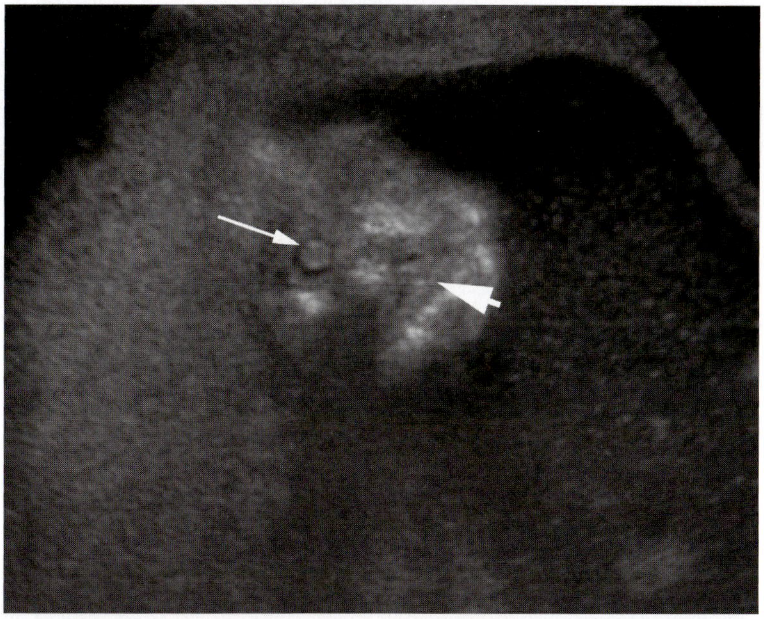

A

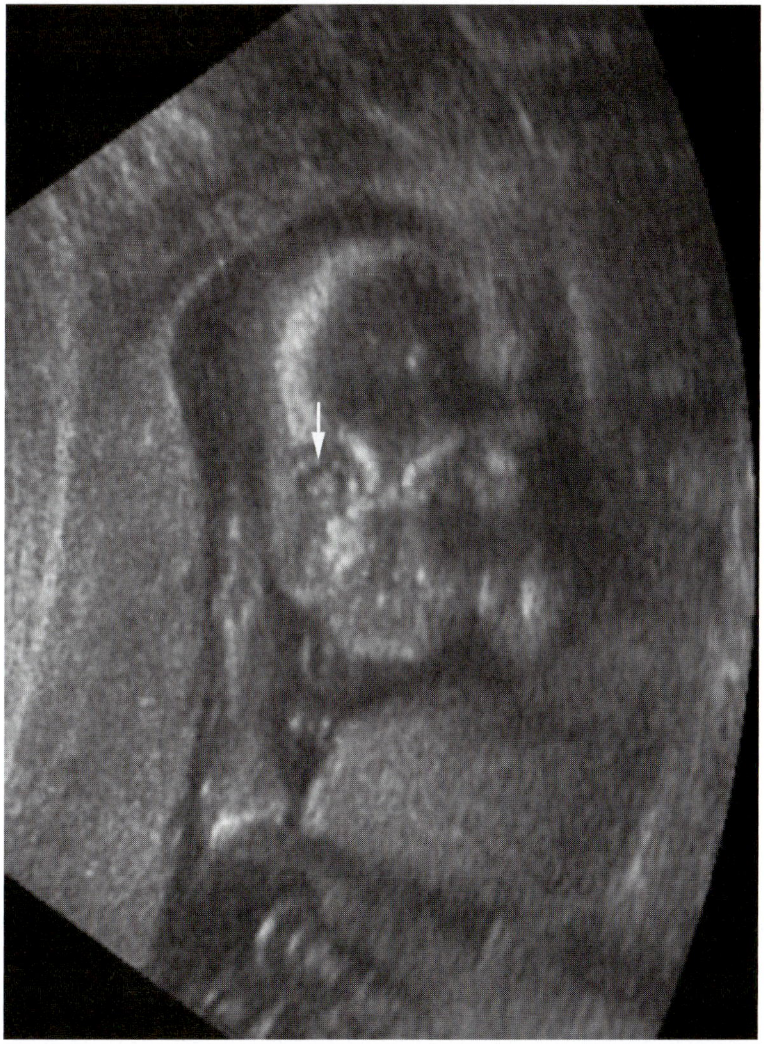

B

FIGURE 2-301 Second-trimester fetus with trisomy 13. (A) Coronal view through the fetal face shows a cataract in the eye *(arrow)* and a midline facial cleft *(arrowhead)*. (B) Coronal view of the same fetus shows cataracts *(arrow)*, cleft, and hypotelorism. *Continued*

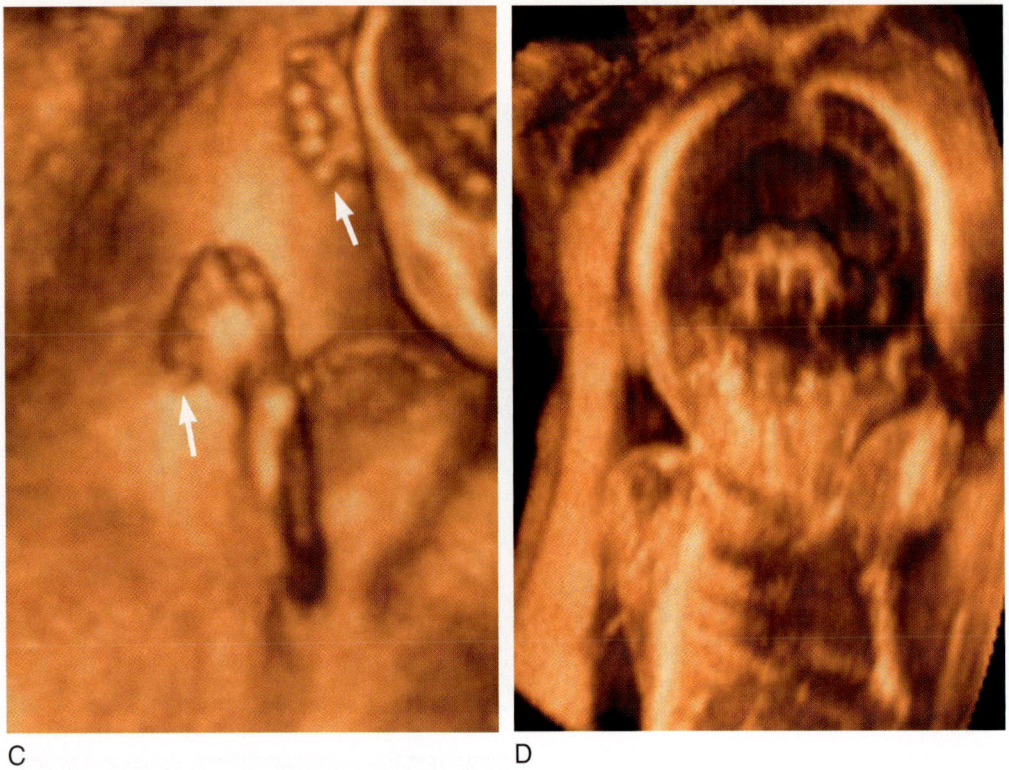

FIGURE 2-301, cont'd (C) Surface rendering of the fetal hands of the same fetus shows bilateral polydactyly *(arrows)* associated with trisomy 13. (D) Surface rendering of the inside of the fetal brain of the same fetus shows the monoventricle surrounding the fused thalami.

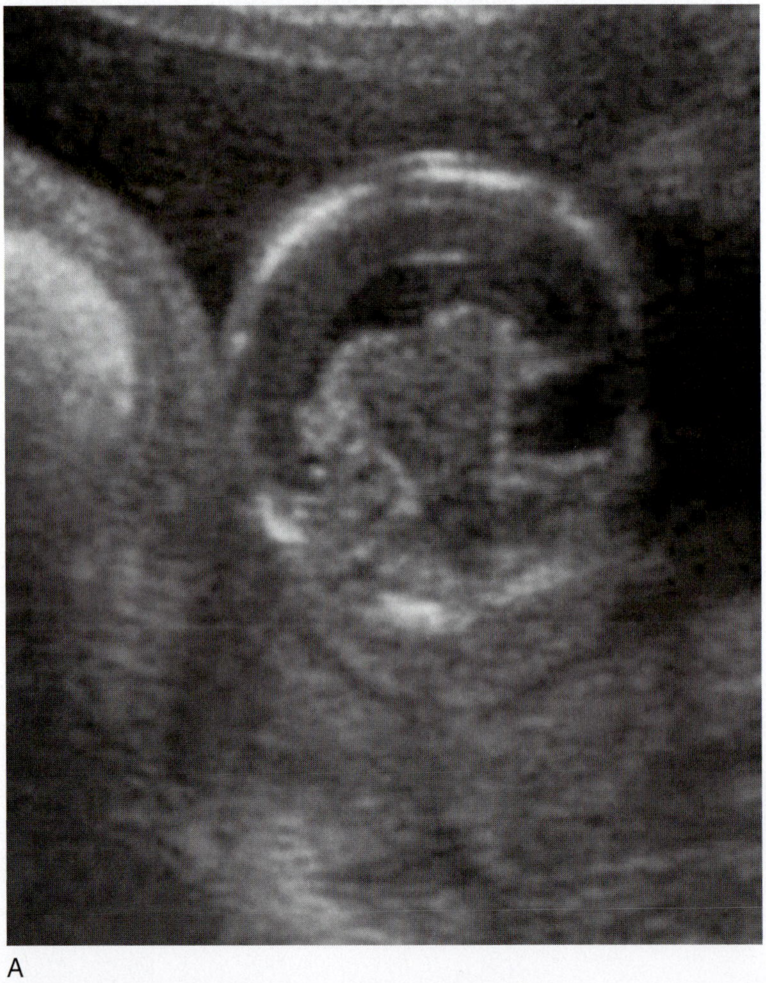

FIGURE 2-302 Second-trimester fetus with trisomy 13. (A) Coronal view through the fetal head shows holoprosencephaly.

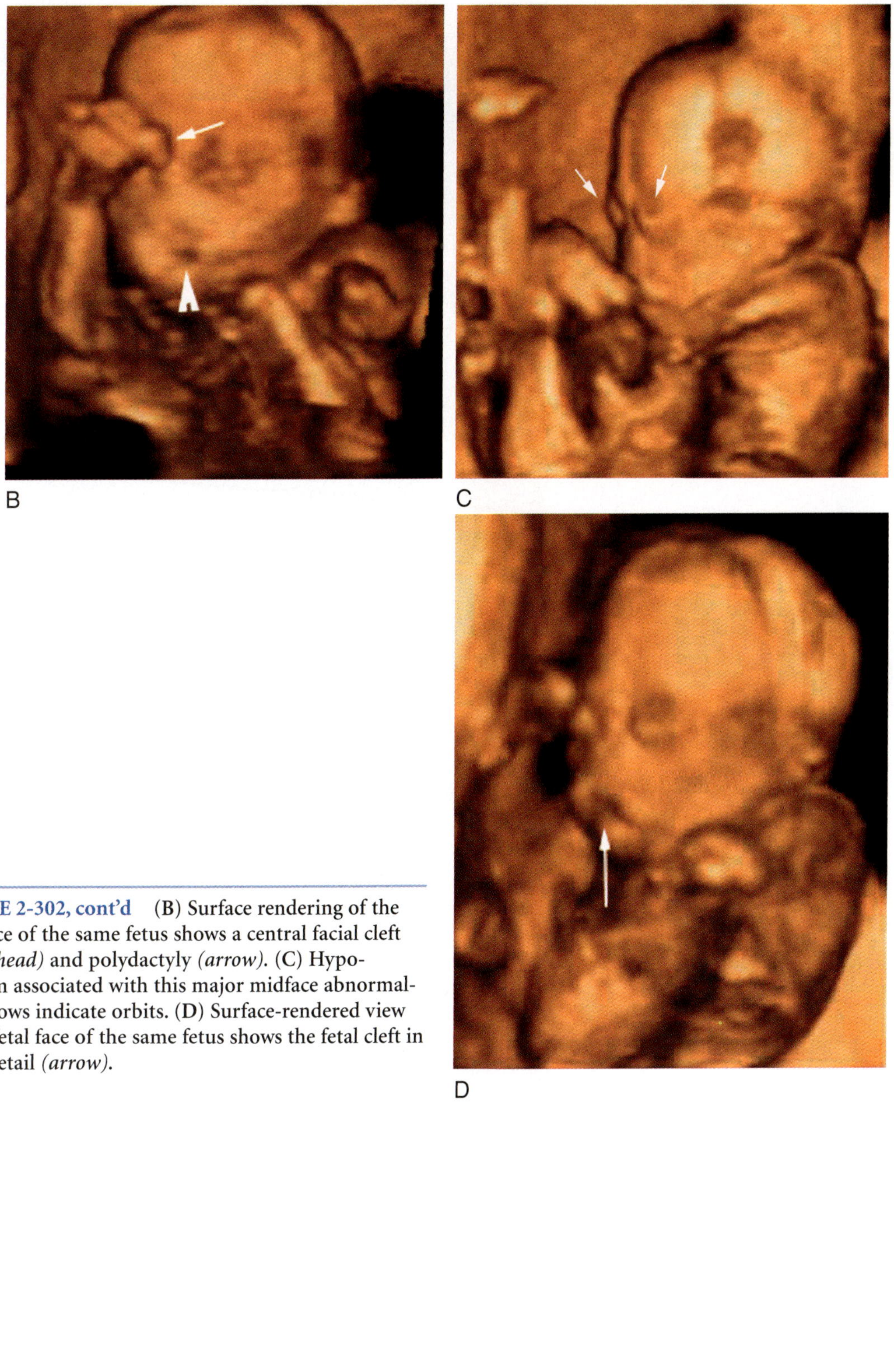

FIGURE 2-302, cont'd (B) Surface rendering of the fetal face of the same fetus shows a central facial cleft *(arrowhead)* and polydactyly *(arrow)*. (C) Hypotelorism associated with this major midface abnormality. Arrows indicate orbits. (D) Surface-rendered view of the fetal face of the same fetus shows the fetal cleft in more detail *(arrow)*.

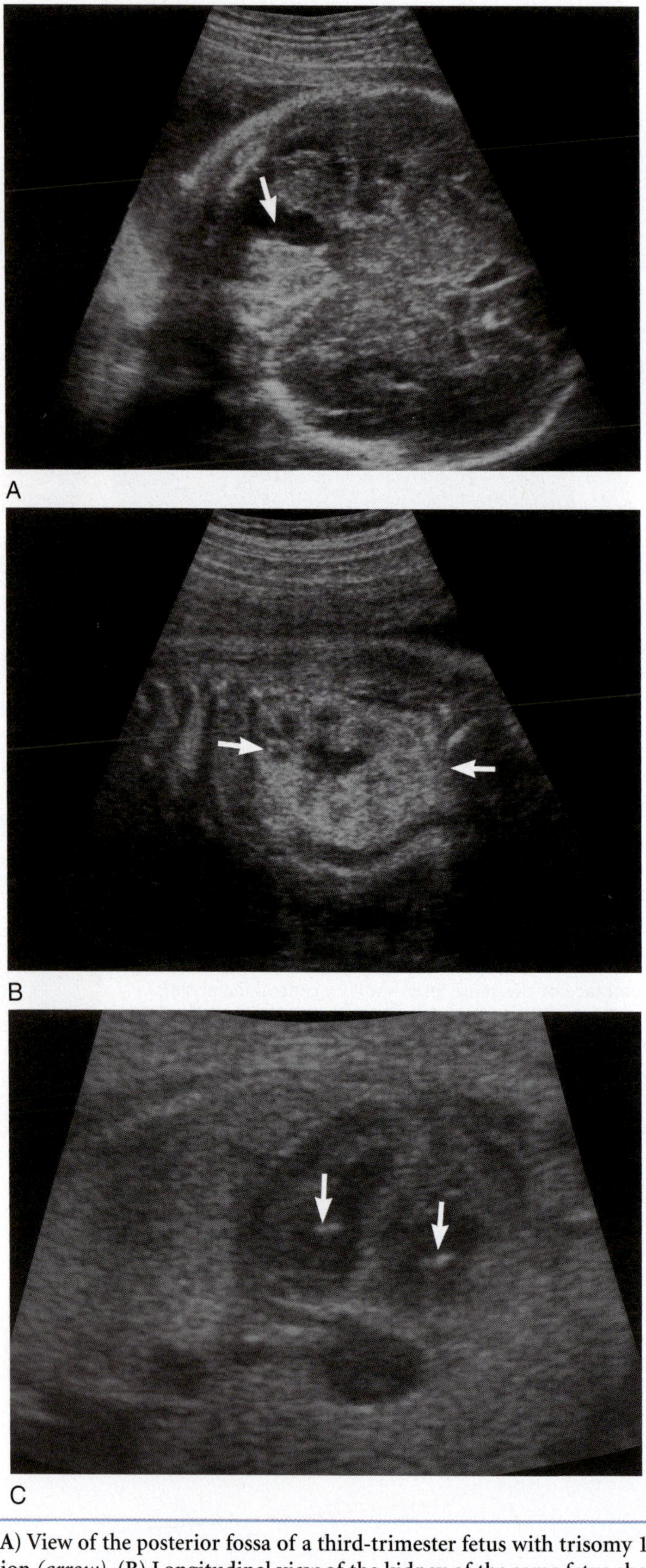

A B C

FIGURE 2-303 (A) View of the posterior fossa of a third-trimester fetus with trisomy 13 shows a Dandy-Walker malformation *(arrow)*. (B) Longitudinal view of the kidney of the same fetus shows an enlarged, echogenic kidney *(arrows)*. (C) Four-chamber view of the heart of the same fetus shows bilateral, echogenic, intracardiac foci *(arrows)*.

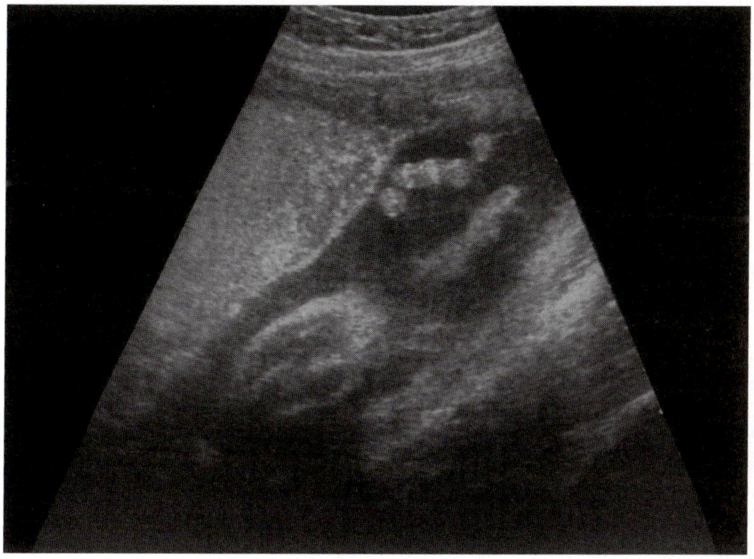

D

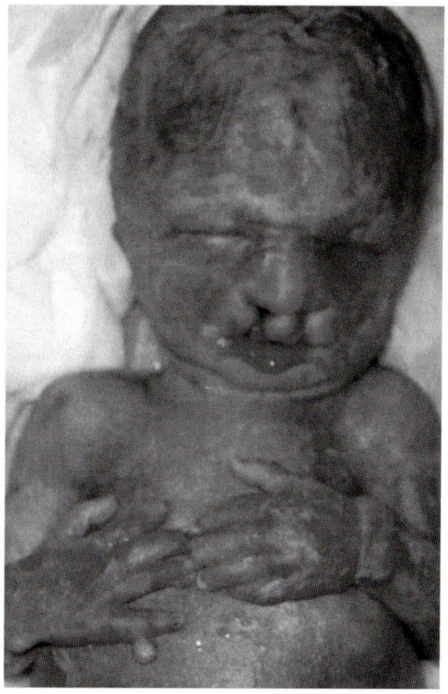

E

FIGURE 2-303, cont'd (D) View of the fingers of the same fetus shows postaxial polydactyly. (E) Postmortem photograph of the same infant shows anophthalmia, facial cleft, and polydactyly.

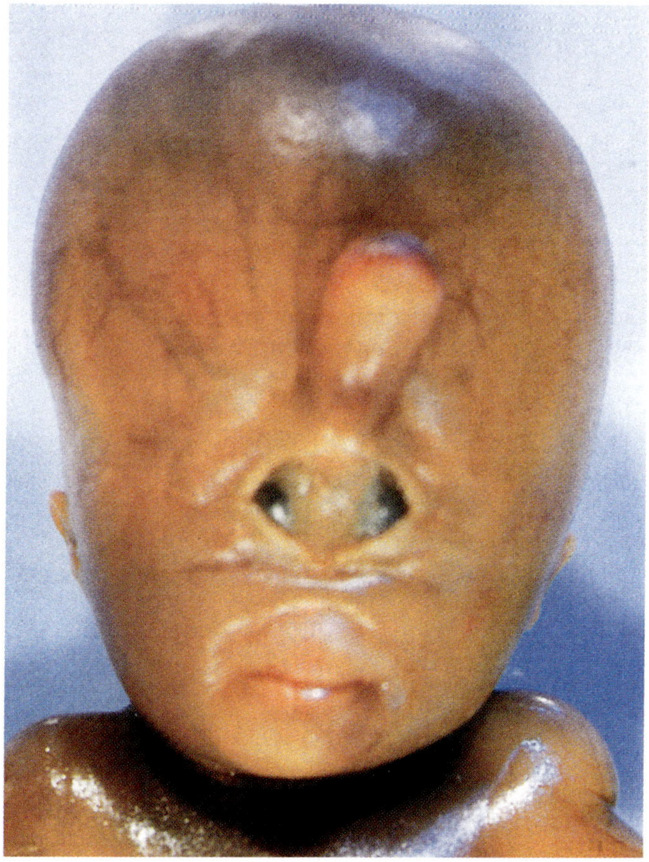

FIGURE 2-304 Postnatal view of fetus with trisomy 13 shows cyclopia. (From Keeling JW: *Fetal pathology.* London, 1994, Churchill Livingstone.)

Those with trisomy 13 mosaicism may have a less severe clinical picture, and usually survival is longer.

Suggested Reading

Benacerraf BR, Frigoletto FD, Greene MF: Abnormal facial features and extremities in human trisomy syndromes: prenatal US appearance. *Radiology* 159:243–246, 1986.

Benacerraf BR, Miller WA, Frigoletto FD: Sonographic detection of fetuses with trisomy 13 and 18: accuracy and limitations. *Am J Obstet Gynecol* 158:404–409, 1988.

Carter PE, Pearn JH, Bell J, et al: Survival in trisomy 13: life tables for use in genetic counseling and clinical pediatrics. *Clin Genet* 27:59–60, 1985.

Curtin WM, Marcotte MP, Myers LL, Brost BC: Trisomy 13 appearing as a mimic of a triploid partial mole. *J Ultrasound Med* 20:1137–1139, 2001.

Greene MF, Benacerraf BR, Frigoletto FD: Reliable criteria for the prenatal sonographic diagnosis of alobar holoprosencephaly. *Am J Obstet Gynecol* 156:687–689, 1987.

Heling KS, Tennstedt C, Chaoui R: Unusual case of a fetus with congenital cystic adenomatoid malformation of the lung associated with trisomy 13. *Prenat Diagn* 23:315–318, 2003.

Lehman CD, Nyberg DA, Winter TC III, et al: Trisomy 13 syndrome: prenatal US findings in a review of 33 cases. *Radiology* 194:217–222, 1995.

Papageorghiou AT, Avgidou K, Spencer K, Nix B, Nicolaides KH: Sonographic screening for trisomy 13 at 11 to 13(+6) weeks of gestation. *Am J Obstet Gynecol* 194:397–401, 2006.

Parker MJ, Budd JL, Draper ES, Young ID: Trisomy 13 and trisomy 18 in a defined population: epidemiological, genetic and prenatal observations. *Prenat Diagn* 23:856–860, 2003.

Rijhsinghani AG, Hruban RH, Stetten G: Fetal anomalies associated with an inversion duplication 13 chromosome. *Obstet Gynecol* 71:991–994, 1988.

Saltzman DH, Benacerraf BR, Frigoletto FD: Diagnosis and management of fetal facial clefts. *Am J Obstet Gynecol* 155:377–379, 1986.

Seoud MA, Alley DC, Smith DL, Levy DL: Prenatal sonographic findings in trisomy 13, 18, 21 and 22. *J Reprod Med* 39:781–787, 1994.

Sepulveda W, Dezerega V, Be C: First-trimester sonographic diagnosis of holoprosencephaly: value of the "butterfly" sign. *J Ultrasound Med* 23:761–765, 2004.

Spencer K, Nicolaides KH: A first trimester trisomy 13/trisomy 18 risk algorithm combining fetal nuchal translucency thickness, maternal serum free beta-hCG and PAPP-A. *Prenat Diagn* 22:877–879, 2002.

Wax JR, Pinette MG, Blackstone J, Cartin A: Isolated multiple bilateral echogenic papillary muscles: a unique sonographic feature of trisomy 13. *Obstet Gynecol* 99:902–903, 2002.

TRISOMY 18 (EDWARDS' SYNDROME)

DESCRIPTION AND DEFINITION

Synonym: Edwards' syndrome

Characterized by malformations of multiple organ systems, trisomy 18 has an incidence of 3:10,000 live births.

ABNORMALITIES DETECTABLE BY ULTRASOUND

Common Findings:

Agenesis of the corpus callosum

Choroid plexus cysts

Posterior fossa abnormalities

Micrognathia

Low-set ears

Microphthalmos

Hypertelorism

Short radial ray

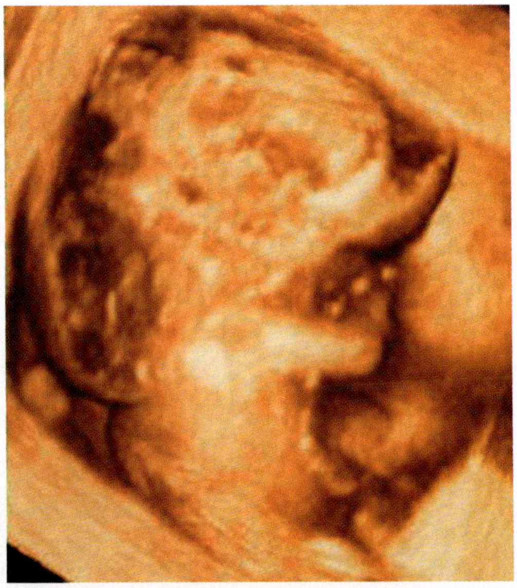

FIGURE 2-305 Three-dimensional surface rendering of a first-trimester fetus with cystic hygroma and lymphangiectasia of the fetal back, neck, and scalp. This fetus had trisomy 18.

Text continued on p. 494

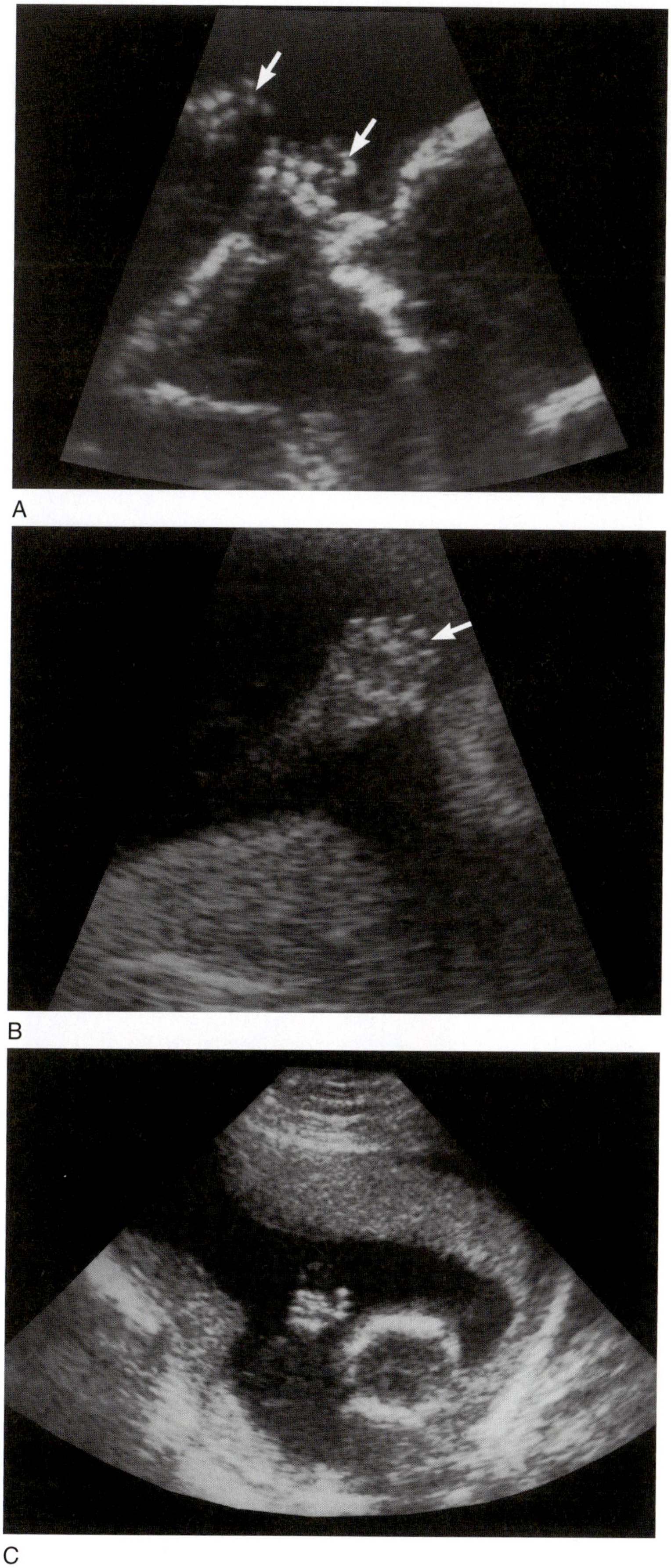

FIGURE 2-306 (A–C) Views of different fetuses with trisomy 18 (Edwards' syndrome) show the characteristic clenched hand with overlapping index finger (*arrows*, A, B) in each case. (A, from Bromley B, Benacerraf B: *AJR Am J Roentgenol* 165:1239–1243, 1995.) *Continued*

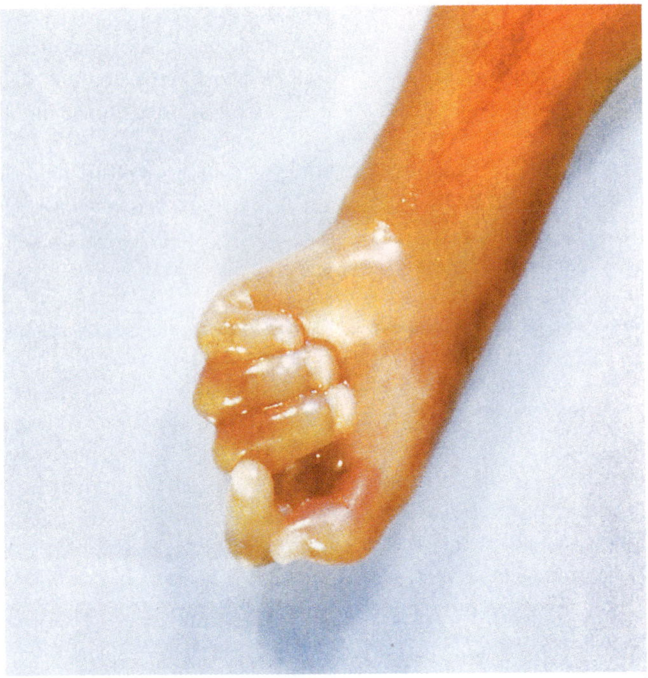

D

FIGURE 2-306, cont'd (D) Pathology specimen shows the characteristic clenched hand with overlapping index finger. (D, from Keeling J: *Fetal pathology.* London, 1994, Churchill Livingstone.)

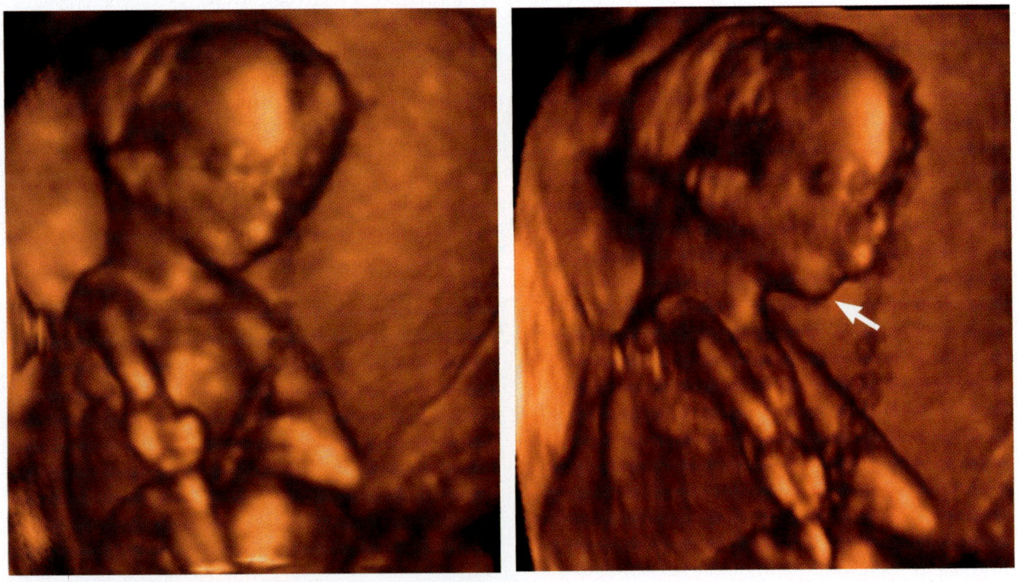

A B

FIGURE 2-307 (A, B) Second-trimester fetus with trisomy 18 shows bilateral abnormalities of the forearms with absent radii and club hands bilaterally. Note micrognathia in B *(arrow).*

Clenched hand with overlapping index finger

Club feet

Rockerbottom feet

Omphalocele

Diaphragmatic hernia

Renal anomalies

Hydronephrosis

Cardiac defects

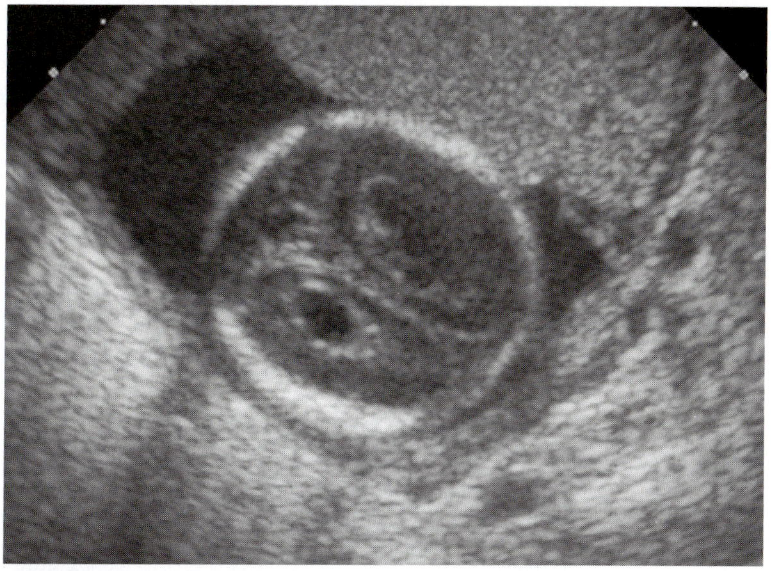

FIGURE 2-308 Transverse view through the fetal head of a fetus with trisomy 18 shows bilateral choroid plexus cysts.

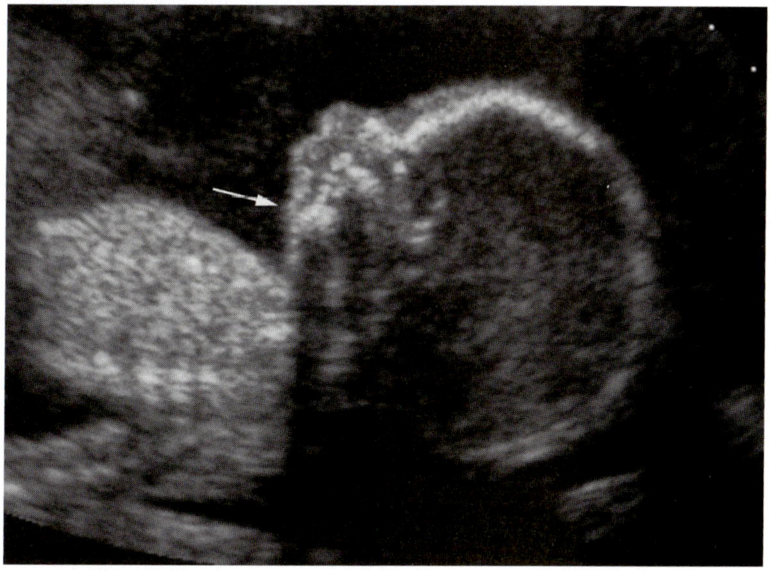

FIGURE 2-309 Second-trimester fetus with trisomy 18 shows micrognathia *(arrow)*.

Single umbilical artery

IUGR

Polyhydramnios

Nuchal lucency thickening

Cryptorchidism

Occasional Findings:

Meningomyelocele

Ventriculomegaly

Cleft lip and palate

MAJOR DIFFERENTIAL DIAGNOSES

Cerebro-oculo-facio-skeletal (COFS) syndrome (limb contractures and CNS anomalies)

Freeman-Sheldon syndrome (clenched hands and IUGR)

Pena Shokeir syndrome (pseudo-trisomy 18)

Smith-Lemli-Opitz syndrome (clenched hands and IUGR)

Triploidy (IUGR)

Trisomy 9

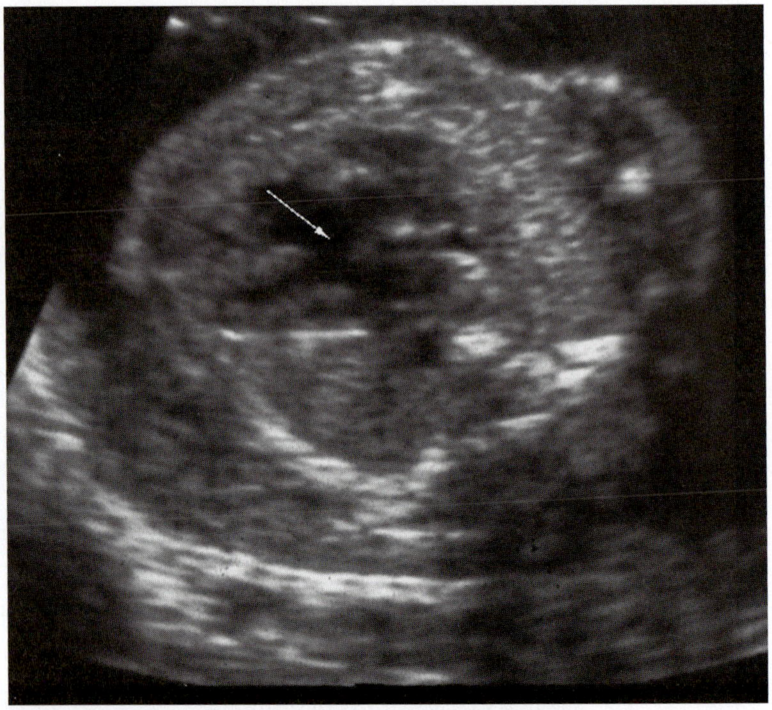

FIGURE 2-310 Transverse view through the fetal heart shows the four chambers of the heart and a large ventricular septal defect *(arrow)* in a second-trimester fetus with trisomy 18.

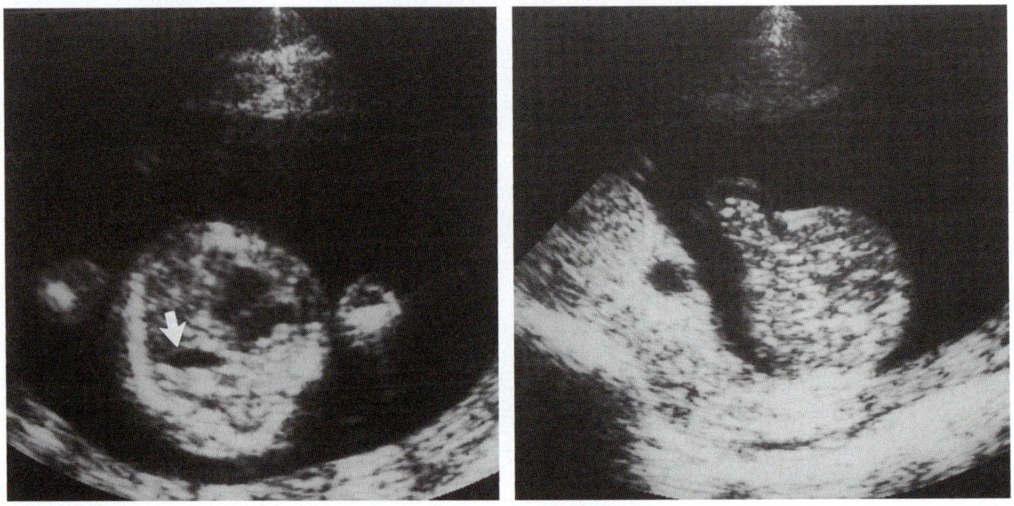

FIGURE 2-311 (A) Transverse view through the chest of a fetus with trisomy 18 shows evidence of a diaphragmatic hernia. Note that the fetal stomach *(arrow)* is located next to the fetal heart, posteriorly, in the fetal chest. (B) Transverse view through the umbilical insertion of a fetus with trisomy 18 shows a small, bowel-containing omphalocele typical of trisomy 18.

Other multiple malformation syndromes associated with intrauterine growth retardation, limb anomalies, and/or cardiac defects (see Chapter 1, specific anomalies, for differential diagnosis).

ULTRASOUND DIAGNOSIS

Prenatal ultrasound diagnosis has been established in the first trimester, based on the finding of a nuchal lucency. Detectable features in the early second trimester include abnormal forearms, clenched hands, club feet, omphalocele, and major cardiac defect.

Features of trisomy 18 are detectable in 80% of affected fetuses in the second trimester.

Sonography is often used to evaluate fetuses for the presence of trisomy 18 when choroid plexus cysts are present or when the serum screen results show a low level of maternal serum alpha-fetoprotein, estriol, and hCG combination. Although trisomy 18 occurs in 1:100 fetuses with choroid plexus cysts, if it is an isolated finding, the risk for trisomy 18 falls below 1:400. Documenting an open hand is very helpful, as most fetuses with trisomy 18 are unable to unclench their hands. Correlation with maternal serum testing for trisomy 18 is helpful to evaluate fetuses with choroid plexus cysts.

HEREDITY

This is an autosomal trisomic syndrome.

NATURAL HISTORY AND OUTCOME

Fetuses with trisomy 18 often die in utero. Ninety percent of liveborns with this abnormality die in the first year of life. The 10% who survive are profoundly mentally retarded and handicapped.

Suggested Reading

Achiron R, Barkai G, Katznelson B-M, Mashiach S: Fetal lateral ventricle choroid plexus cysts: the dilemma of amniocentesis. *Obstet Gynecol* 78:815–818, 1991.

Bahado-Singh RO, Choi SJ, et al: Early second-trimester individualized estimation of trisomy 18 risk by ultrasound. *Obstet Gynecol* 101:463–468, 2003.

Benacerraf B, Miller W, Frigoletto F: Sonographic detection of fetuses with trisomies 13 and 18: accuracy and limitations. *Am J Obstet Gynecol* 158:404–409, 1988.

Benacerraf BR, Harlow B, Frigoletto FD Jr: Are choroid plexus cysts an indication for second-trimester amniocentesis? *Am J Obstet Gynecol* 162:1001–1006, 1990.

Bronsteen R, Lee W, Vettraino IM, Huang R, Comstock CH: Second-trimester sonography and trisomy 18: the significance of isolated choroid plexus cysts after an examination that includes the fetal hands. *J Ultrasound Med* 23:241–245, 2004.

Bronsteen R, Lee W, Vettraino IM, Huang R, Comstock CH: Second-trimester sonography and trisomy 18. *J Ultrasound Med* 23:233–240, 2004.

Brumfield CG, Wenstrom KD, Owen J, Davis RO: Ultrasound findings and multiple marker screening in trisomy 18. *Obstet Gynecol* 95:51–54, 2000.

Bundy AL, Saltzman DH, Pober B, et al: Antenatal sonographic findings in trisomy 18. *J Ultrasound Med* 5:361–364, 1986.

Cheng PJ, Liu CM, Chueh HY, Lin CM, Soong YK: First-trimester nuchal translucency measurement and echocardiography at 16 to 18 weeks of gestation in prenatal detection for trisomy 18. *Prenat Diagn* 23:248–251, 2003.

Chervenak FA, Goldberg JD, Tsung-Hong C, Gilbert F, Berkowitz RL: The importance of karyotype determination in a fetus with ventriculomegaly and spina bifida discovered during the third trimester. *J Ultrasound Med* 5:405–406, 1985.

Chinn DH, Miller EI, Worthy LM, Towers CV: Sonographically detected fetal choroid plexus cysts: frequency and association with aneuploidy. *J Ultrasound Med* 10:255–258, 1991.

DeVore GR: Second trimester ultrasonography may identify 77 to 97% of fetuses with trisomy 18. *J Ultrasound Med* 19:565–576, 2000.

Feuchtbaum LB, Currier RJ, Lorey FW, Cunningham GC: Prenatal ultrasound findings in affected and unaffected pregnancies that are screen-positive for trisomy 18: the California experience. *Prenat Diagn* 20:293–299, 2000.

Gabrielli S, Reece A, Pilu G, et al: The clinical significance of prenatally diagnosed choroid plexus cysts. *Am J Obstet Gynecol* 160:1207–1210, 1989.

Gross SJ, Shulman LP, Tolley EA, et al: Isolated fetal choroid plexus cysts and trisomy 18: a review and meta-analysis. *Am J Obstet Gynecol* 172:83–87, 1995.

Gupta JK, Cave M, Lilford RF, et al: Clinical significance of fetal choroid plexus cysts. *Lancet* 346:724–729, 1995.

Hertzberg BS, Kay HH, Bowie JD: Fetal choroid plexus lesions: Relationship of antenatal sonographic appearance to clinical outcome. *J Ultrasound Med* 8:77–82, 1989.

Hill LM, Macpherson T, Rivello D, Peterson C: The spontaneous resolution of cystic hygromas and early fetal growth delay in fetuses with trisomy 18. *Prenat Diagn* 11:673–677, 1991.

Hill LM, Marchese S, Peterson C, Fries J: The effect of trisomy 18 on transverse cerebellar diameter. *Am J Obstet Gynecol* 165:72–75, 1991.

Izquierdo LA, Vill M, Jones D, et al: Trisomy 18. *Fetus* 2:1–6, 1992.

Jackson S, Porter H, Vyas S: Trisomy 18: first-trimester nuchal translucency with pathological correlation. *Ultrasound Obstet Gynecol* 5:55–56, 1995.

Kupferminc MJ, Tamura RK, Sabbagha RE, et al: Isolated choroid plexus cyst(s): an indication for amniocentesis. *Am J Obstet Gynecol* 171:1068–1071, 1994.

Kuwata T, Matsubara S, Izumi A, et al: Umbilical cord pseudocyst in a fetus with trisomy 18. *Fetal Diagn Ther* 18:8–11, 2003.

Lam YH, Tang MH: Sonographic features of fetal trisomy 18 at 13 and 14 weeks: four case reports. *Ultrasound Obstet Gynecol* 13:366–369, 1999.

Lin HY, Lin SP, Chen YJ, et al: Clinical characteristics and survival of trisomy 18 in a medical center in Taipei, 1988–2004. *Am J Med Genet A* 140:945–951, 2006.

Martinez Crespo JM, Comas C, Borrell A, et al: Reversed end diastolic umbilical artery velocity in two cases of trisomy 18 at 10 weeks' gestation. *Ultrasound Obstet Gynecol* 7:447–449, 1996.

Nava S, Godmilow L, Reeser S, Ludomirsky A, Donnenfeld AE: Significance of sonographically detected second-trimester choroid plexus cysts: a series of 211 cases and a review of the literature. *Ultrasound Obstet Gynecol* 4:448–451, 1994.

Nicolaides KH, Salvesen DR, Snijders RJM, Gosden CM: Strawberry-shaped skull in fetal trisomy 18. *Fetal Diagn Ther* 7:132–137, 1992.

Nyberg DA, Kramer D, Resta RG, et al: Prenatal sonographic findings in trisomy 18: review of 47 cases. *Fetal Diagn Ther* 2:103–113, 1993.

Nyberg DA, Mahony BS, Hegge FN, et al: Enlarged cisterna magna and the Dandy-Walker malformation: factors associated with chromosome abnormalities. *Obstet Gynecol* 77:436–442, 1991.

Ostlere SJ, Irving HC, Lilford RJ: Fetal choroid plexus cysts: a report of 100 cases. *Radiology* 175:753–755, 1990.

Oyelese Y, Vintzileos AM: Is second-trimester genetic amniocentesis for trisomy 18 ever indicated in the presence of a normal genetic sonogram? *Ultrasound Obstet Gynecol* 26:691–694, 2005.

Perpignano MC, Cohen HL, Klein VR, et al: Fetal choroid plexus cysts: beware the smaller cyst. *Radiology* 182:715–717, 1992.

Platt LD, Carlson DE, Medearis AL, Walla CA: Fetal choroid plexus cysts in the second trimester of pregnancy: a cause for concern. *Am J Obstet Gynecol* 161:1652–1656, 1991.

Porto M, Murata Y, Warneke LA, Keegan KA Jr: Fetal choroid plexus cysts: an independent risk factor for chromosomal anomalies. *J Clin Ultrasound* 21:103–108, 1993.

Ramirez P, Haberman S, Baxi L: Significance of prenatal diagnosis of umbilical cord cyst in a fetus with trisomy 18. *Am J Obstet Gynecol* 173:955–957, 1995.

Sepulveda W, Corral E, Kottmann C, Illanes S, Vasquez P, Monckeberg MJ: Umbilical artery aneurysm: prenatal identification in three fetuses with trisomy 18. *Ultrasound Obstet Gynecol* 21:292–296, 2003.

Sepulveda W, Treadwell MC, Fisk NM: Prenatal detection of preaxial upper limb reduction in trisomy 18. *Obstet Gynecol* 85:847–850, 1995.

Steiger RM, Porto M, Lagrew DC, Randall R: Biometry of the fetal cisterna magna: estimates of the ability to detect trisomy 18. *Ultrasound Obstet Gynecol* 5:384–390, 1995.

Thorpe-Beeston JG, Gosden M, Nicolaides KH: Choroid plexus cysts and chromosomal defects. *Br J Radiol* 63:783–786, 1990.

Thurmond AS, Nelson DW, Lowensohn RI, Young WP, Davis L: Enlarged cisterna magna in trisomy 18: prenatal ultrasonographic diagnosis. *Am J Obstet Gynecol* 161:83–85, 1989.

Tongsong T, Sirichotiyakul S, Wanapirak C, Chanprapaph P: Sonographic features of trisomy 18 at midpregnancy. *J Obstet Gynaecol Res* 28:245–250, 2002.

Tul N, Spencer K, Noble P, Chan C, Nicolaides K: Screening for trisomy 18 by fetal nuchal translucency and maternal serum free beta-hCG and PAPP-A at 10–14 weeks of gestation. *Prenat Diagn* 19:1035–1042, 1999.

Walkinshaw S, Pilling D, Spriggs A: Isolated choroid plexus cysts—the need for routine offer of karyotyping. *Prenat Diagn* 14:663–667, 1994.

Yang JH, Chung JH, Shin JS, Choi JS, Ryu HM, Kim MY: Prenatal diagnosis of trisomy 18: report of 30 cases. *Prenat Diagn* 25:119–122, 2005.

Yeo L, Guzman ER, Day-Salvatore D, Walters C, Chavez D, Vintzileos AM: Prenatal detection of fetal trisomy 18 through abnormal sonographic features. *J Ultrasound Med* 22:581–590, 2003.

Zerres K, Schuler H, Gembruch U, et al: Chromosomal findings in fetuses with prenatally diagnosed cysts of the choroid plexus. *Hum Genet* 89:301–304, 1992.

TRISOMY 21 (DOWN SYNDROME)

DESCRIPTION AND DEFINITION

Synonym: Down syndrome

The most common chromosomal abnormality among newborns, trisomy 21 has an incidence of 1:700 births.

ABNORMALITIES DETECTABLE BY ULTRASOUND

Thickened nuchal fold

Ventriculomegaly

Brachycephaly

Flat facies

Nasal bone hypoplasia

Small ears

Cardiac defects

- Ventricular septal defect
- Atrioventricular canal
- Tetralogy of Fallot

Echogenic intracardiac focus

Pyelectasis

Hyperechoic bowel

Hydrops (occasional)

Duodenal atresia (after 22 weeks' gestation)

Clinodactyly, with hypoplasia of the middle phalanx of the fifth digit

Short humerus

Short femur

Wide iliac angle

Sandal foot

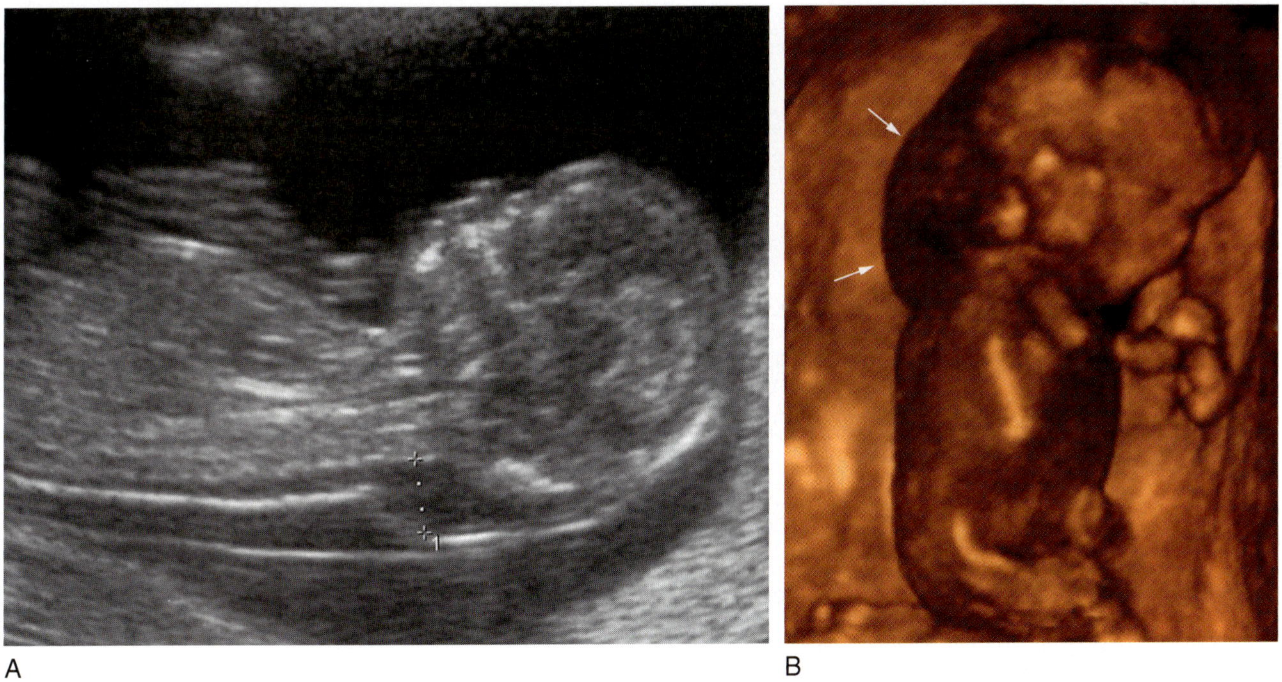

FIGURE 2-312 (A) Standard two-dimensional image of the fetal profile of a fetus with a cystic hygroma and thickened nuchal translucency. (B) Three-dimensional surface rendering of a similar fetus with cystic hygroma *(arrows)*.

MAJOR DIFFERENTIAL DIAGNOSES

A *thickened nuchal fold* is associated with multiple other chromosomal abnormalities such as trisomy 18. Noonan syndrome also is associated with a thickened nuchal fold and cardiac defect.

Other Nonkaryotypic Abnormalities Associated with Thickened Nuchal Fold:

Achondrogenesis

Apert syndrome

Cornelia de Lange syndrome

Ectrodactyly–ectodermal dysplasia–clefting (EEC) syndrome

Fryns syndrome

Joubert syndrome

Kniest syndrome

Multiple pterygium syndrome

Noonan syndrome

Roberts' syndrome

Smith-Lemli-Opitz syndrome

Syndromes Associated with Slightly Short Femur:

Achondroplasia, heterozygous

Femoral hypoplasia–unusual facies syndrome

Hypochondroplasia

IUGR (early-onset)

Jeune thoracic dystrophy

Neu-Laxova syndrome

Russell-Silver syndrome

Shprintzen syndrome

Spondyloepiphyseal dysplasia congenita

Tetrasomy 12p (Pallister-Killian syndrome)

XO syndrome (Turner syndrome)

Fetuses with Down syndrome can have ventriculomegaly or cardiac defects as a primary abnormality (see Chapter 1, pp. 27 and 118 for differential diagnosis)

ULTRASOUND DIAGNOSIS

First Trimester:

Prenatal diagnosis is possible in the *first trimester*, based on nuchal translucency thickening. Nicolaides led a landmark research initiative into the detection of chromosomal abnormalities—namely, Down syndrome—using nuchal translucency measurements, defined as multiples of the median for crown rump length. Nicolaides'

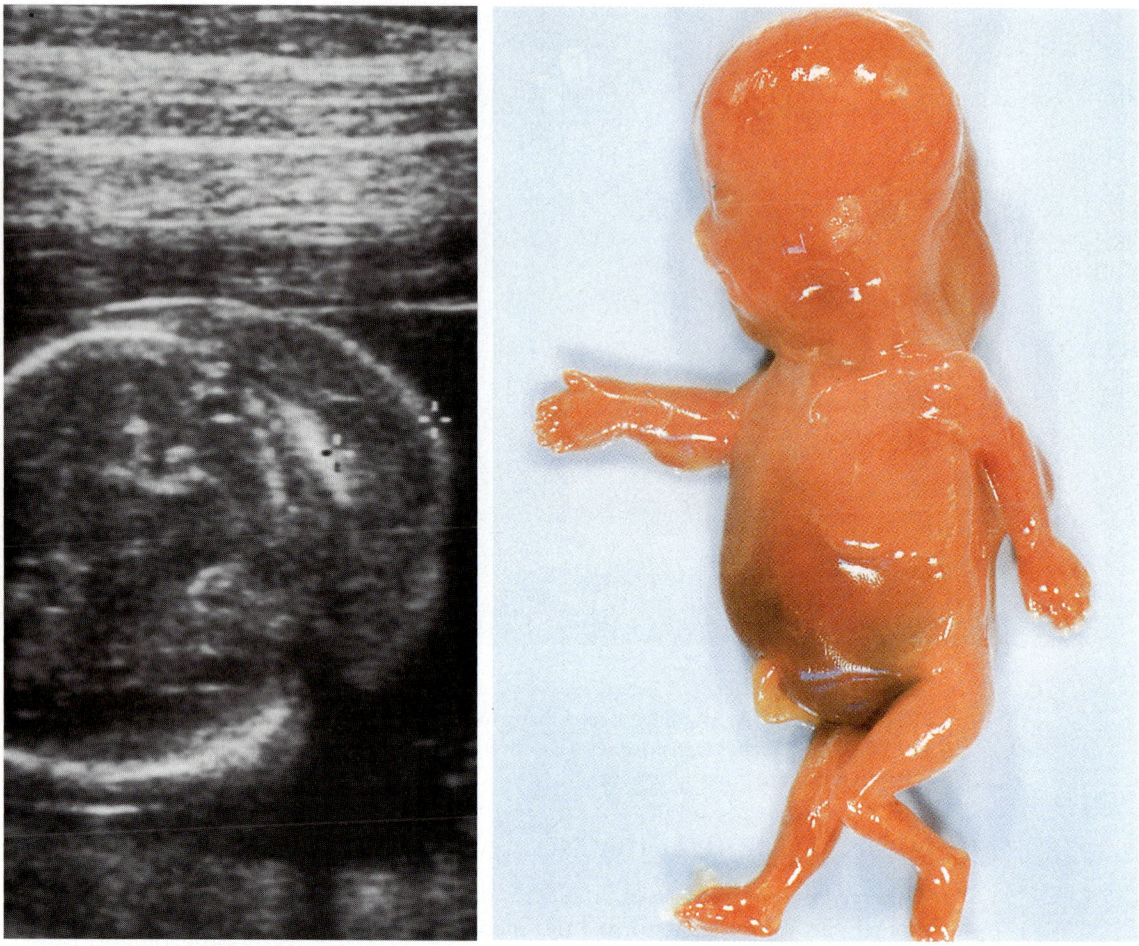

FIGURE 2-313 (**A**) Transverse view through the head of a second-trimester fetus with Down syndrome shows a thickened nuchal fold *(calipers)*. (**B**) Nuchal fold seen after delivery. (From Keeling JW: *Fetal pathology.* London, 1994, Churchill Livingstone.)

methods initially led to the identification of as many as 77% of trisomic fetuses, with a false-positive rate of 5% among normal fetuses. In a meta-analysis of 34 studies with 1355 cases of Down syndrome, the sensitivity and false-positive rates for detecting affected fetuses were 76.8% and 6.2%, respectively.

First-trimester serum markers (free β-hCG and PAPP-A) were added to the nuchal translucency and maternal age in various studies from England and the United States, resulting in an increase in sensitivity to 78% to 89% for a fixed 5% false-positive testing rate among normal fetuses. The FASTER trial in the United States also confirmed Nicolaides' findings, combining first-trimester serum and ultrasound screening with second-trimester serum testing to achieve a 90% sensitivity for a 5.4% false-positive rate. Different permutations of first- and second-trimester ultrasound and biochemistry can be used to determine the risk of Down syndrome for any individual patient. Although first-trimeter testing seems to have a superior detection rate compared with second-trimester testing, the spontaneous loss rate of first-trimester fetuses between the first and second trimesters must be considered so as not to overestimate the success of first-trimester screening.

Second Trimester:

The thickened nuchal fold that the author first described in 1985 as being associated with Down syndrome is the most sensitive and specific single marker for identification of Down

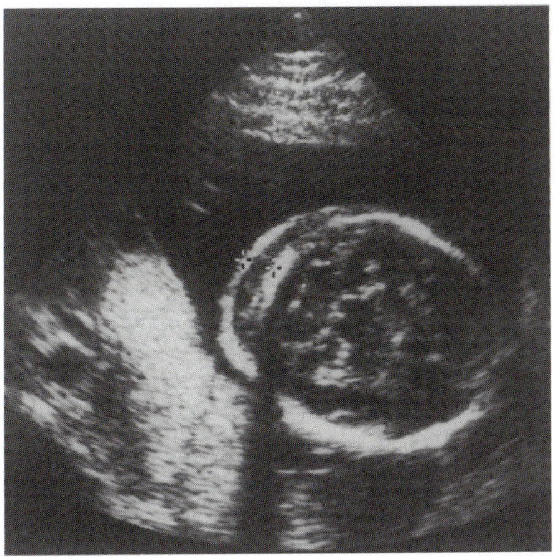

FIGURE 2-314 Transverse view through the head of a second-trimester fetus with Down syndrome shows a thickened nuchal fold *(calipers)*. Note that the view for making this measurement includes the cerebellum, posterior fossa, and occipital bone.

syndrome in the *second trimester*. The presence of a thickened nuchal fold (≥6 mm) has allowed detection of Down syndrome in 40% to 70% of affected fetuses, with a false-positive rate <1%. However, the nuchal fold tends to resolve with time, so it may not be as sensitive a marker in the late second trimester as it is in the first or early second trimester.

The advantage to using mid second-trimester scans is the capability of detecting additional features of Down syndrome, including major malformations (cardiac defects, ventriculomegaly) as well as sonographic markers (pyelectasis, nuchal fold, hyperechoic bowel, echogenic intracardiac focus, and abnormal long-bone biometry). Table 2-1 lists sensitivities and false-positive rates for the sonographic markers used in the detection of Down syndrome. A combination of markers seems to be the most desirable method for detecting fetuses with Down syndrome because of the increased sensitivity and specificity over any single marker. Table 2-1 also lists the scoring index that is arbitrarily assigned to the sonographic findings. A score ≥2 can result in a sensitivity of 75.5% and a false-positive rate of 5.7% for detection of Down syndrome. A multicenter study (eight centers) showed a detection rate for Down syndrome ranging from 63.6% to 80.0% using biometric data, presence or absence of major structural abnormalities, and six additional ultrasound markers.

More recently, Nyberg put forth the method of calculating likelihood ratios for each marker, which then could be used to modify the patient's individual a priori risk of Down syndrome based on maternal age of serum biochemistry. In our study, more than one marker conveyed much higher likelihood ratios. Two markers (even *minor* markers) and three markers resulted in likelihood ratios of 6.2 and 80, respectively (Tables 2-2 and 2-3). On the other hand, the absence of any marker on a genetic sonogram resulted in an 80% reduction in the risk of an affected fetus. The likelihood ratios from four large studies are listed in Table 2-3 and demonstrate that the nuchal fold still is the most efficient marker for detecting affected fetuses.

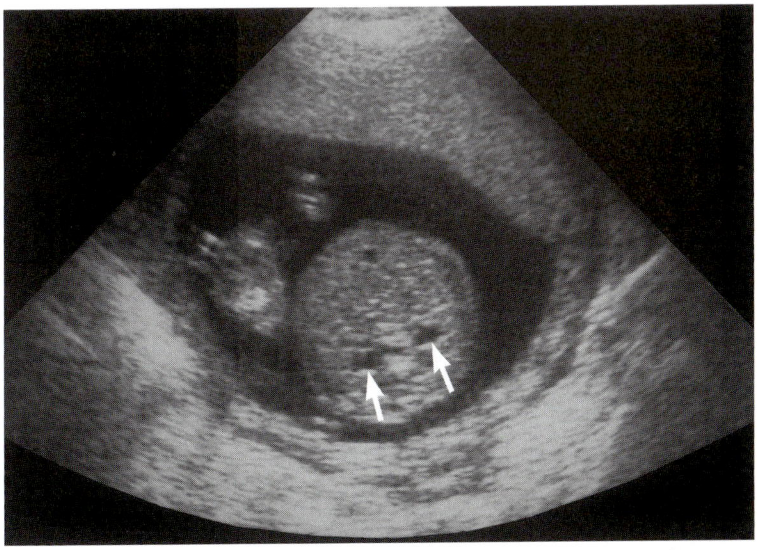

FIGURE 2-315 Transverse view through the fetal kidneys shows mild pyelectasis *(arrows)* in a fetus with Down syndrome.

TABLE 2-1

Sensitivity and False-Positive Rates for Sonographic Markers in Detection of Second-Trimester Fetuses with Trisomy 21

Finding	Trisomy 21	Non-Trisomy 21	Score
Anomaly	24.5%	2.8%	2
Nuchal fold	50.9%	0.6%	2
Short humerus	41.3%	3.4%	1
Short femur	47.2%	7.9%	1
Hyperechoic bowel	24.5%	2.3%	1
Echogenic intracardiac focus	30.2%	4.5%	1
Pyelectasis	22.6%	0.6%	1
Score ≥1 overall risk	83%	17.5%	≥1
Score ≥2 overall risk	75.5%	5.7%	≥2

Adapted from Bromley B, Lieberman E, Benacerraf BR: *Ultrasound Obstet Gynecol* 10:321–324, 1997.

TABLE 2-2

Sensitivity and Specificity for Individual Markers Based on 164 Down Syndrome Fetuses and 656 Control Fetuses in the Second Trimester

Marker	Trisomy 21	Controls
Nuchal fold ≥6 mm	71/164 (42.3%)	3/656 (0.5%)
Nuchal fold ≥5 mm	77/164 (47.0%)	5/656 (0.8%)
Anomaly	44/164 (26.8%)	6/656 (1.2%)
Humerus	73/150 (48.7%)	12/579 (2.1%)
Femur	88/164 (53.7%)	35/656 (5.3%)
Bowel	18/138 (13.0%)	5/552 (0.9%)
Echogenic intracardiac focus	38/111 (34.2%)	19/444 (4.3%)
Pyelectasis	35/164 (21.3%)	16/656 (2.4%)
Abnormal	132/164 (80.5%)	81/656 (12.3%)
Normal scan	32/164 (19.5%)	575/656 (87.7%)

Adapted from Benacerraf B: *Semin Perinatol* 29:386, 2005.

TABLE 2-3

Likelihood Ratios of Isolated Markers in Four Large Studies

Marker	Smith-Bindnam	AAURA	Nyberg	Bromley
None	NA	0.4	0.36	0.22
Nuchal fold	17	8.6	11	Infinite
Bright bowel	6.1	5.5	6.7	NA
Short humerus	7.5	2.5	5.1	5.8
Short femur	2.7	2.2	1.5	1.2
Echogenic intracardiac focus	2.8	2	1.8	1.4
Pyelectasis	1.9	1.5	1.5	1.5

Adapted from Benacerraf B: *Semin Perinatol* 29:386, 2005.

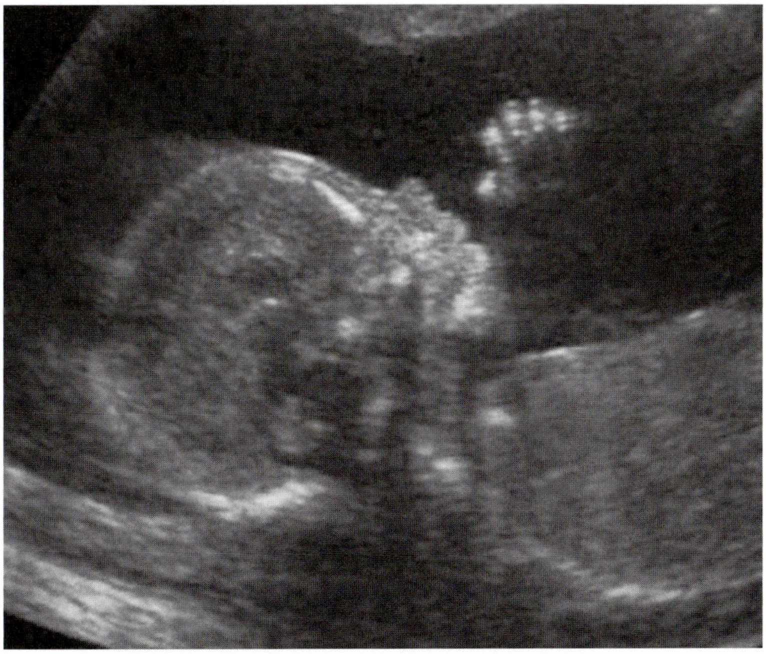

FIGURE 2-316 Longitudinal view of the fetal face of a second-trimester fetus with Down syndrome shows absence of nasal bone ossification.

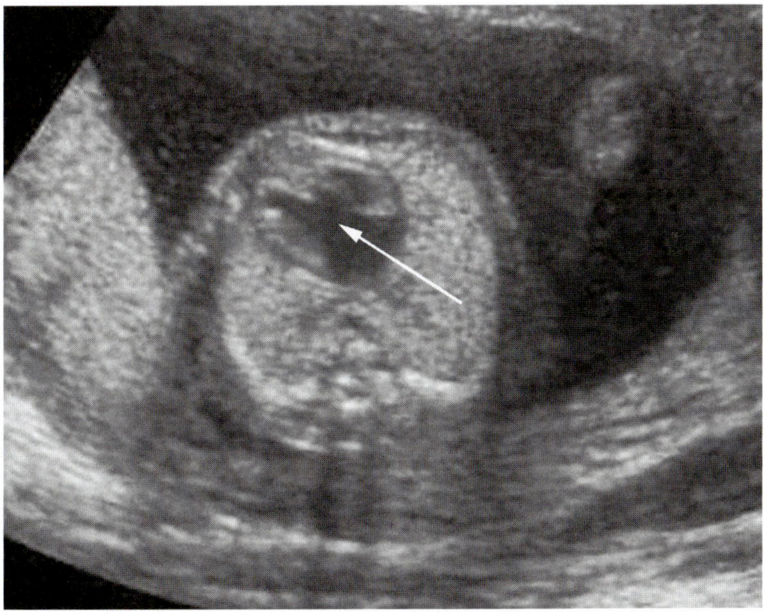

FIGURE 2-317 Four-chamber view of the same fetus as in Figure 2-316 shows a complete atrioventricular canal *(arrow)*.

Patients with a normal genetic sonogram and a normal maternal serum screen can lower their risk of having a fetus with trisomy 21, often prompting them to forego invasive testing. Many more patients who ordinarily would undergo amniocentesis because of advanced maternal age or abnormal serum screening have used the genetic sonogram to modify their risk.

Fetuses with Down syndrome have hypoplasia of the nasal bone in both the first and second trimesters. Cicero first showed that absent nasal bone ossification in fetuses at 11 to 14 weeks' gestation could identify 73% of fetuses with trisomy 21 with a 0.5% false-positive rate. This is an exciting new marker that promises to be an important part of first- and second-trimester

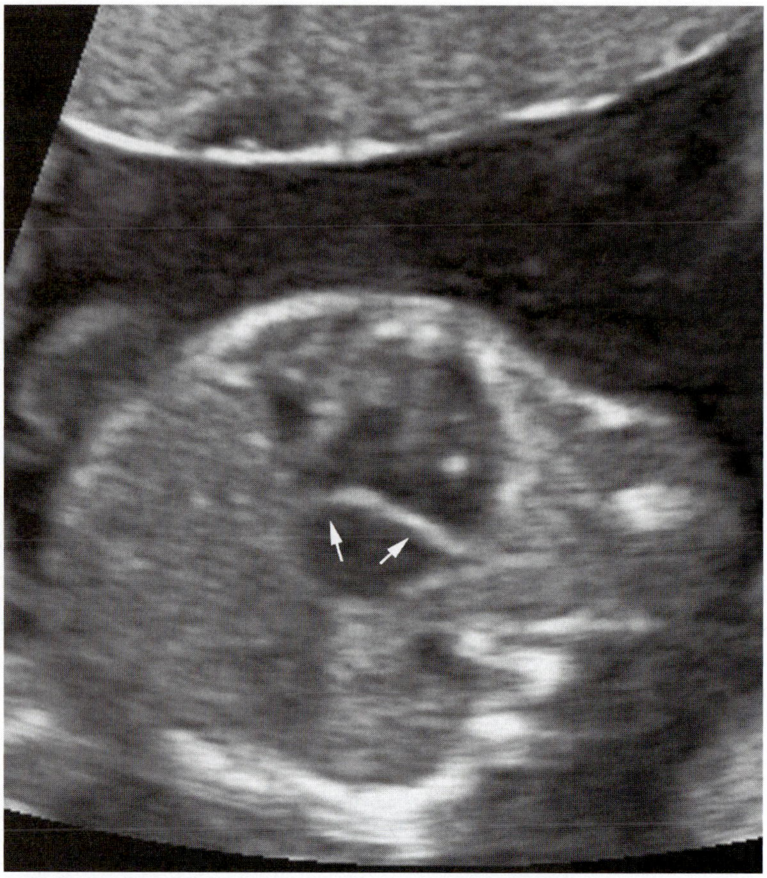

FIGURE 2-318 Transverse view through the fetal chest shows four chambers of the heart in a fetus with trisomy 21. Note the echogenic intracardiac focus and the straight line across the mitral and tricuspid valves *(arrows)*. The lack of demarcation of the medial insertion of these valves indicates an atrioventricular *(AV)* canal and common AV valve.

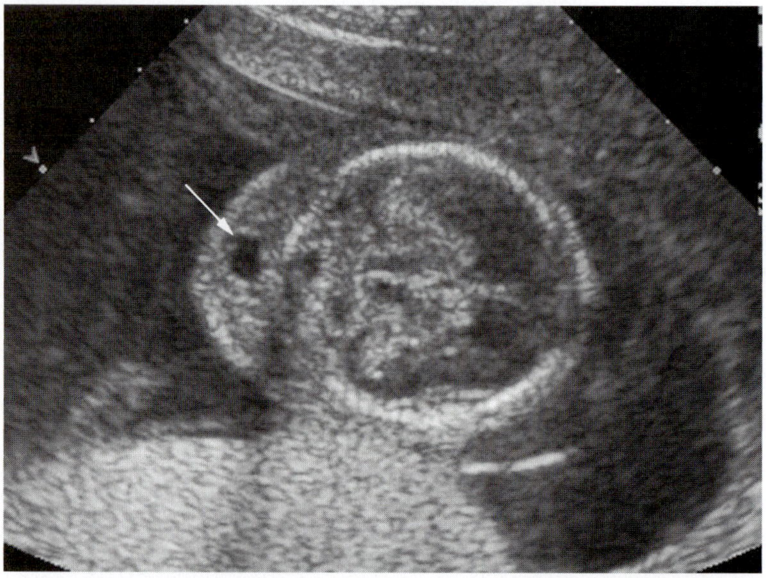

FIGURE 2-319 Second-trimester fetus with Down syndrome has a thickened nuchal fold and a small cystic hygroma within the thickened nuchal fold *(arrow)*.

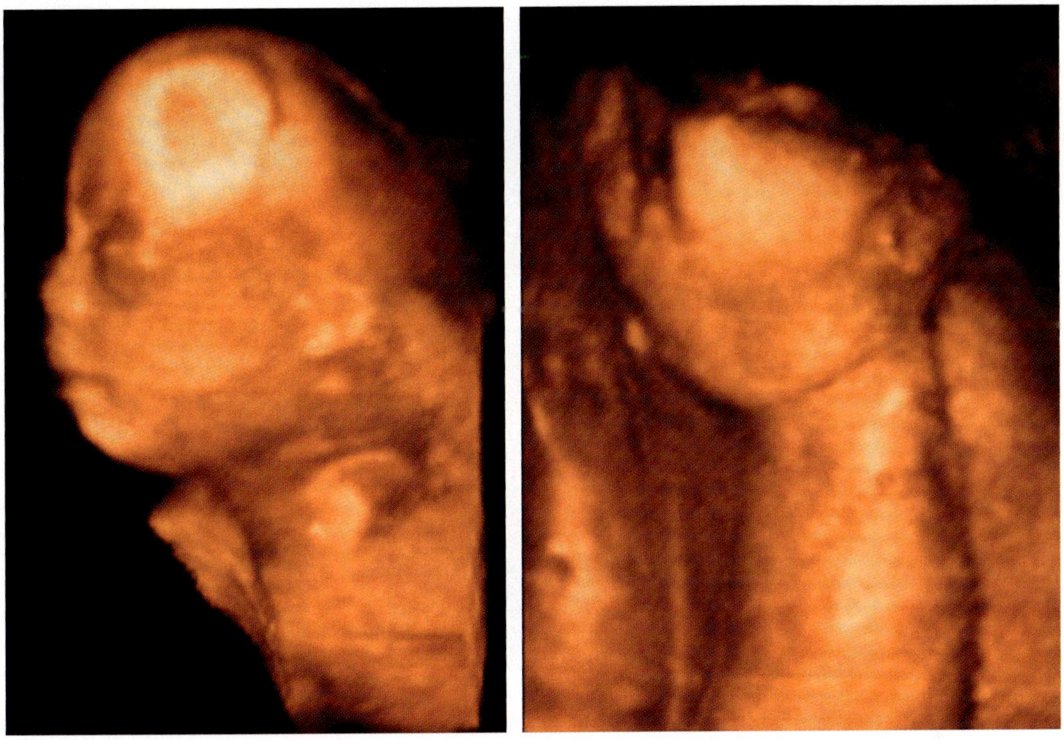

A B

FIGURE 2-320 (A) Three-dimensional surface rendering of a 22-week fetus with Down syndrome. Note the flat face, typical of this syndrome. (B) Surface rendering of the back of this fetus shows redundant skin at the back of the neck, considered a thickened nuchal fold.

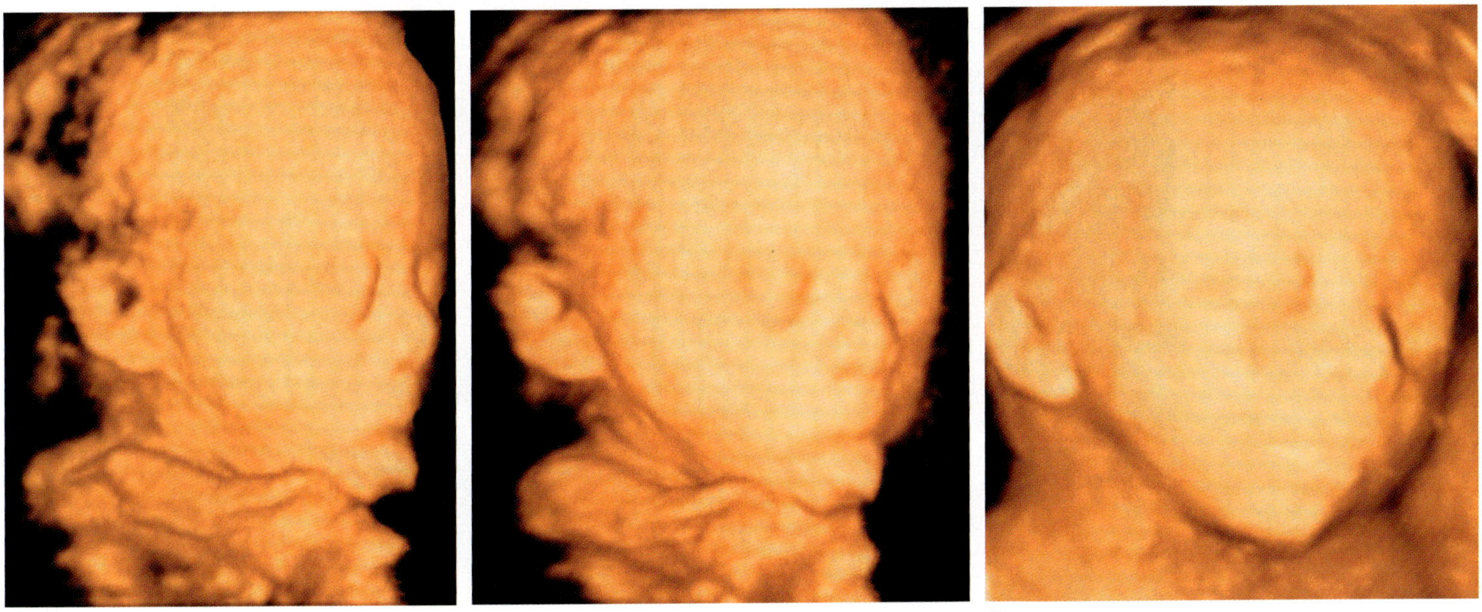

A B C

FIGURE 2-321 (A–C) Views of a 23-week fetus with Down syndrome obtained using three-dimensional surface rendering. Note the flat appearance of the face as well as the protruding tongue consistent with low tone. Note the forward rotated ear inferiorly.

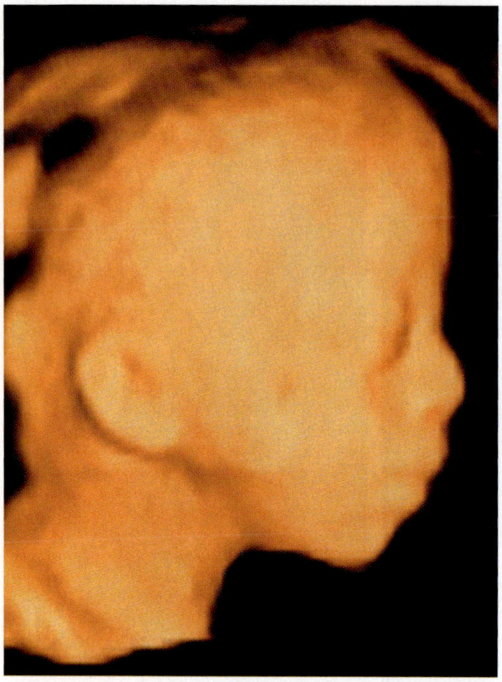

FIGURE 2-322 Three-dimensional surface rendering of the profile of the same fetus as in Figure 2-321 shows the abnormally rotated ear as well as the flat profile.

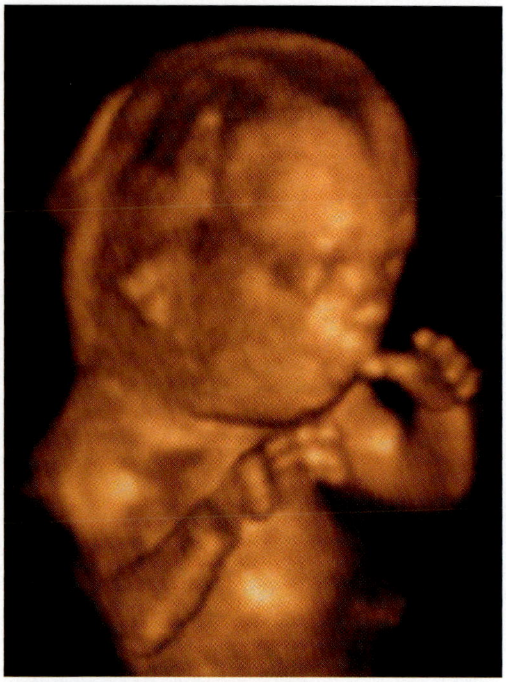

FIGURE 2-323 View of an 18-week fetus with Down syndrome obtained using three-dimensional surface rendering shows flat face, small ear, and redundant skin around the neck area.

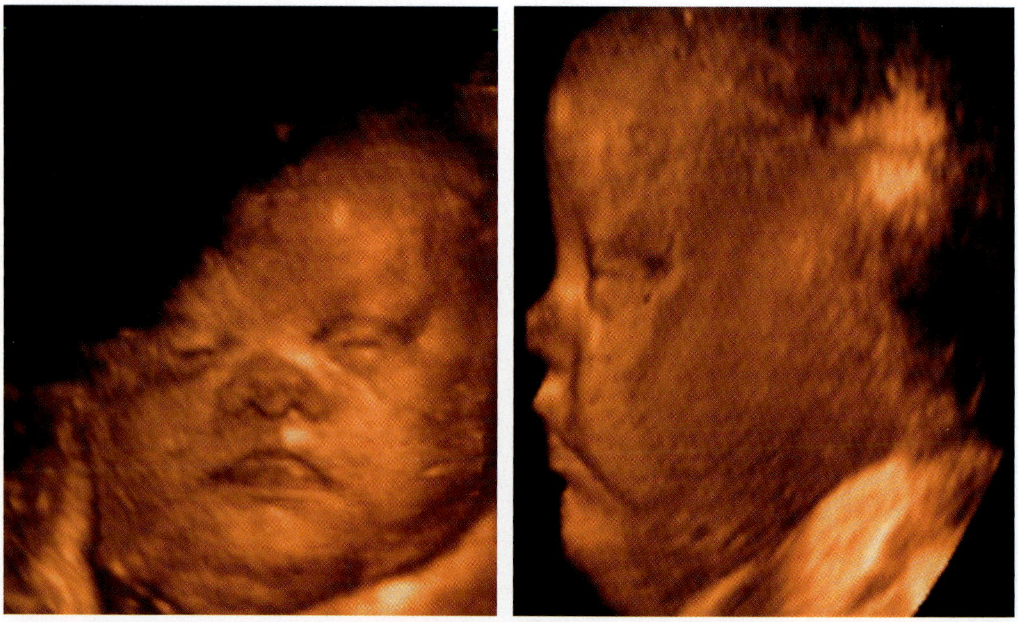

A B

FIGURE 2-324 Views of third-trimester fetus with Down syndrome obtained using three-dimensional surface rendering. (A) Frontal view of a fetus with mild hypotelorism and flat-appearing dysmorphic face. (B) Profile of the same fetus shows the typically flat face of Down syndrome phenotype.

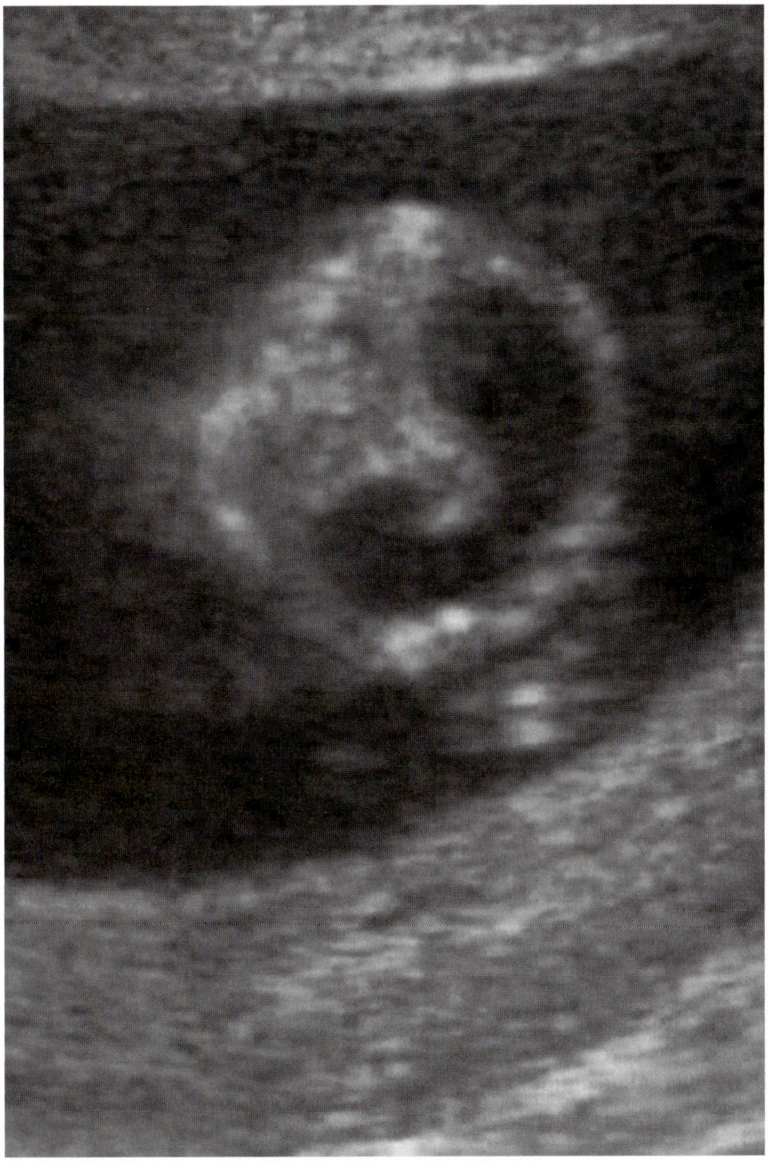

FIGURE 2-325 Late first-trimester fetus with Down syndrome who has duodenal and esophageal atresia. Note the large C-shaped fluid collection consistent with dilated stomach and duodenum on this transverse view through the fetal abdomen. The C-shaped appearance of the fluid collection is typical of a combination of duodenal and esophageal atresia.

screening for Down syndrome. In the second trimester, absent nasal bone and shortened nasal bone length both are criteria for this marker. Other new markers include tricuspid regurgitation and fetal heart rate; however, these are not currently in widespread use.

HEREDITY

This is an autosomal trisomic syndrome.

NATURAL HISTORY AND OUTCOME

Children with Down syndrome have reduced IQs, decreased muscle tone, and mental and physical developmental delays. Surgery may be needed for cardiac defects and occasional duodenal atresia. The major cause of mortality is cardiac defects.

Criteria for Markers:

- Anomaly: Any major fetal malformation
- Nuchal fold: $\geq$6 mm is abnormal at 15 to 20 weeks
- Short humerus: Expected humerus length = –7.9404 + 0.8492 (biparietal diameter [BPD]). The ratio of measured to expected

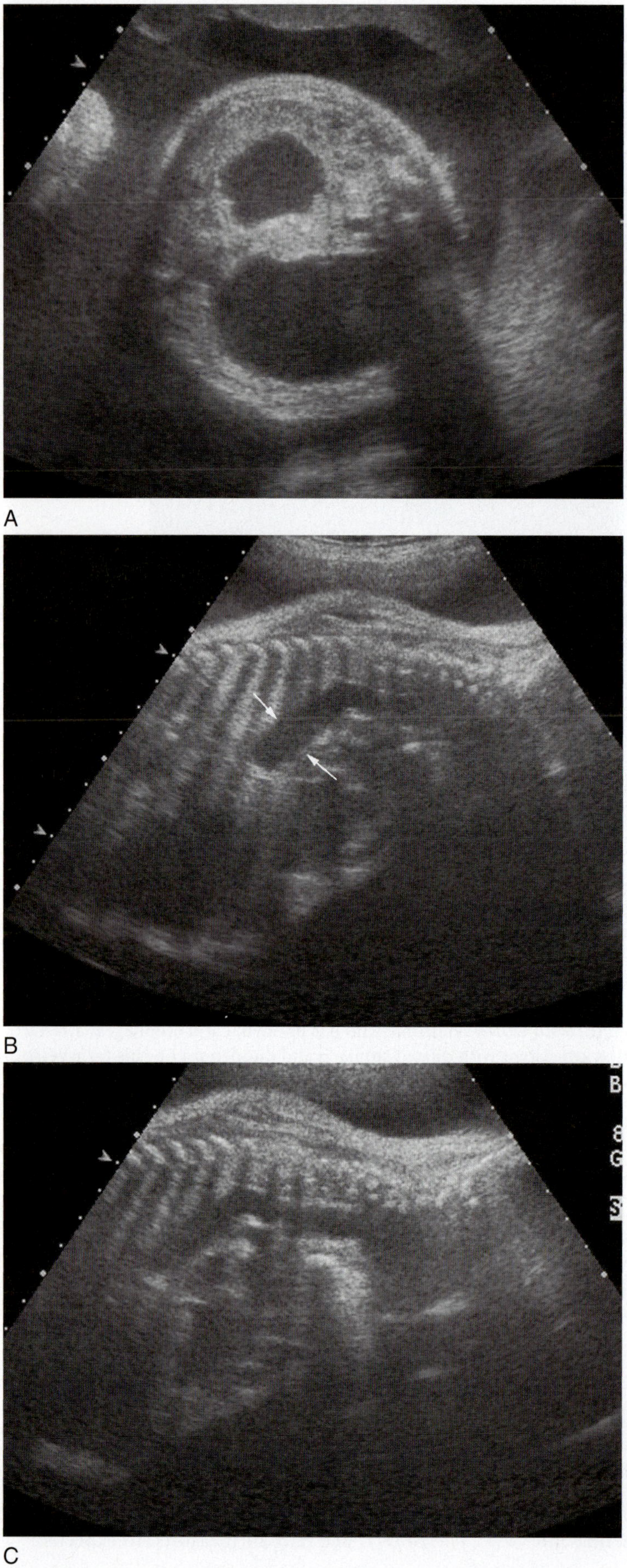

FIGURE 2-326 (**A**) Transverse view of the fetal abdomen of a third-trimester fetus with duodenal atresia. Note polyhydramnios and dilated stomach and duodenal bulb, known as the "double bubble." (**B, C**) Views of the same fetus show the dilated esophagus (*arrows* in **B**) coursing in fetal chest.

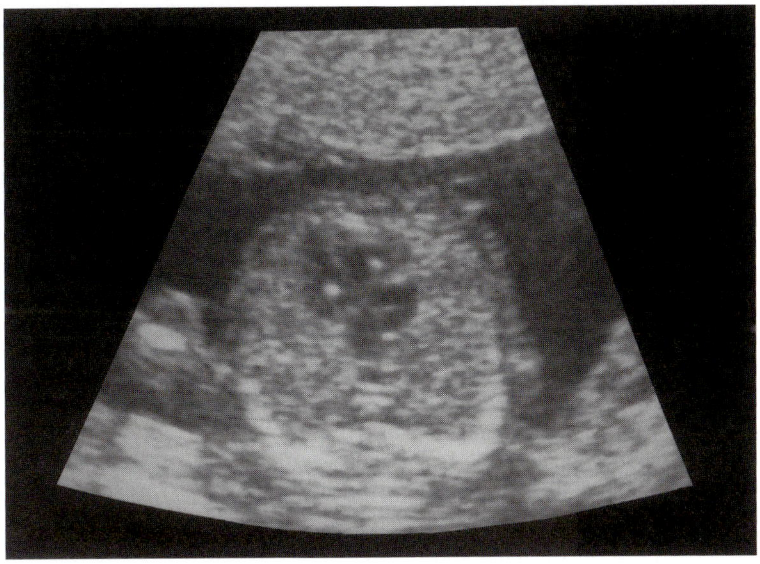

FIGURE 2-327 Four-chamber view of the heart shows an echogenic intracardiac focus in each ventricle. Fetuses with echogenic intracardiac foci have an increased risk for Down syndrome.

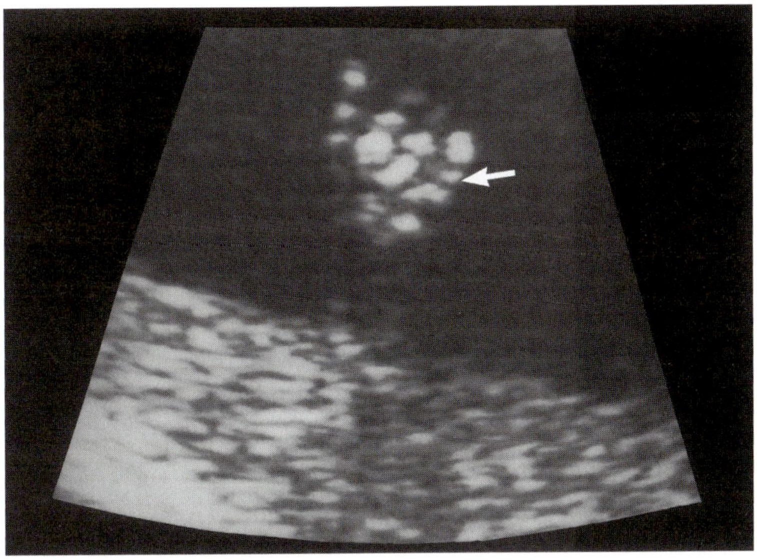

FIGURE 2-328 View of the fetal hand shows hypoplasia of the middle phalanx of the fifth digit *(arrow)*. Note clinodactyly of the fifth digit.

humerus length then is calculated. A ratio <0.90 is considered abnormal.

- Short femur: Expected femur length = –9.3105 + 0.9028 (BPD). The ratio of measured to expected femur length then is calculated. A ratio of ≤0.91 is considered abnormal.
- Hyperechogenic bowel: Hyperechoic bowel is as bright as bone.
- Echogenic intracardiac focus (EIF): Bright dot in the left and/or right ventricles of the heart, equal in brightness to that of bone.
- Pyelectasis: Anteroposterior diameter of renal pelvis 4 mm or more is considered a positive marker.
- Nasal bone: Absent or <2.5 mm, or BPD/nasal bone length >11 (Tables 2-2 and 2-3)

Suggested Reading

Abuhamad AZ, Kolm P, Mari G, Slotnick N, Evans AT III: Ultrasonographic fetal iliac length measurement in the screening for Down syndrome. *Am J Obstet Gynecol* 171:1063–1067, 1994.

Avgidou K, Papageorghiou A, Bindra R, Spencer K, Nicolaides KH: Prospective first-trimester screening for trisomy 21 in 30,564 pregnancies. *Am J Obstet Gynecol* 192:1761–1767, 2005.

Bahado-Singh RO, Goldstein I, Uerpairojkit B, et al: Normal nuchal thickness in the midtrimester indicates reduced risk of Down syndrome in pregnancies with abnormal triple-screen results. *Am J Obstet Gynecol* 173:1106–1110, 1995.

Benacerraf BR, Barss VA, Laboda LA: A sonographic sign for the detection in the second trimester of the fetus with Down's syndrome. *Am J Obstet Gynecol* 151:1078–1079, 1985.

Benacerraf BR, Gelman R, Frigoletto FD Jr: Sonographic identification of second trimester fetuses with Down syndrome. *N Engl J Med* 317:1371–1376, 1987.

Benacerraf BR, Harlow B, Frigoletto FD Jr: Hypoplasia of the middle phalanx of the fifth digit, a feature of the second trimester fetus with Down syndrome. *J Ultrasound Med* 9:389–394, 1990.

Benacerraf BR, Mandell J, Estroff JA, Harlow BL, Frigoletto FD Jr: Fetal pyelectasis, a possible association with Down syndrome. *Obstet Gynecol* 76:58–60, 1990.

Benacerraf BR, Nadel A, Bromley B: Identification of second trimester fetuses with autosomal trisomy by use of a sonographic scoring index. *Radiology* 193:135–140, 1994.

Benacerraf BR, Neuberg D, Frigoletto FD Jr: Humeral shortening in second-trimester fetuses with Down syndrome. *Obstet Gynecol* 77:223–227, 1991.

Biagiotti R, Periti E, Cariati E: Humerus and femur length in fetuses with Down syndrome. *Prenat Diagn* 14:429–434, 1994.

Bromley B, Doubilet P, Frigoletto FD Jr, et al: Is fetal hyperechoic bowel on second trimester sonogram an indication for amniocentesis? *Obstet Gynecol* 83:647–651, 1994.

Bromley B, Lieberman E, Benacerraf BR: Choroid plexus cysts: not associated with Down syndrome. *Ultrasound Obstet Gynecol* 8:232–235, 1996.

Bromley B, Lieberman E, Shipp T, Richardson M, Benacerraf BR: Echogenic intracardiac focus (EIF): association with aneuploidy in both high and low risk patients. *J Ultrasound Med* 17:127–131, 1998

Bromley B, Lieberman E, Shipp TD, Benacerraf BR: Fetal nose bone length: a marker for Down syndrome in the second trimester. *J Ultrasound Med* 21:1387–1394, 2002.

Bromley B, Lieberman E, Shipp TD, Benacerraf BR: The genetic sonogram, a method for risk assessment for Down syndrome in the mid trimester. *Ultrasound Med* 21:1087–1096, 2002.

Cicero S, Sonek JD, McKenna DS, Croom CS, Johnson L, Nicolaides KH: Nasal bone hypoplasia in trisomy 21 at 15–22 weeks' gestation. *Ultrasound Obstet Gynecol* 21:15–18, 2003.

Cicero S, Curcio P, Papageorghiou A, Sonek J, Nicolaides K: Absence of nasal bone in fetuses with trisomy 21 at 11–14 weeks of gestation: an observational study. *Lancet* 358:1665–1667, 2001.

Crane JP, Gray DL: Sonographically measured nuchal skinfold thickness as a screening tool for Down syndrome: results of a prospective clinical trial. *Obstet Gynecol* 77:533–536, 1991.

DeVore GR, Alfi O: The use of color Doppler ultrasound to identify fetuses at increased risk for trisomy 21, an alternative for high-risk patients who decline genetic amniocentesis. *Obstet Gynecol* 85:378–386, 1995.

DeVore GR, Romero R: Genetic sonography: an option for women of advanced maternal age with negative triple-marker maternal serum screening results. *J Ultrasound Med* 2003;22:1191–1199.

FitzSimmons J, Droste S, Shepard TH, et al: Longbone growth in fetuses with Down syndrome. *Am J Obstet Gynecol* 161:1174–1177, 1989.

Gill P, Vanhook J, FitzSimmons J, Pascoe-Mason J, Fantel A: Fetal ear measurements in the prenatal detection of trisomy 21. *Prenat Diagn* 14:739–743, 1994.

Grandjean H, Sarramon M, Association Francaise pour le Depistage et la Prevention des Handicaps de l'Enfant (AFDPHE) Study Group: Sonographic measurement of nuchal skinfold thickness or detection of Down syndrome in the second-trimester fetus: a multicenter prospective study. *Obstet Gynecol* 85:103–106, 1995.

Gray DL, Crane JP: Optimal nuchal skin-fold thresholds based on gestational age for prenatal detection of Down syndrome. *Am J Obstet Gynecol* 171:1282–1286, 1994.

Hobbins JC, Lezotte DC, Persutte WH, et al: An 8-center study to evaluate the utility of midterm genetic sonograms among high-risk pregnancies. *J Ultrasound Med* 22:33–38, 2003.

Johnson MP, Michaelson JE, Barr M Jr, et al: Combining humerus and femur length for improved ultrasonographic identification of pregnancies at increased risk for trisomy 21. *Am J Obstet Gynecol* 172:1229–1235, 1995.

Lee W, DeVore GR, Comstock CH, et al: Nasal bone evaluation in fetuses with Down syndrome during the second and third trimesters of pregnancy. *J Ultrasound Med* 22:55–60, 2003.

Lockwood C, Benacerraf B, Krinsky A, et al: A sonographic screening method for Down syndrome. *Am J Obstet Gynecol* 157:803–808, 1987.

Malone FD, Canick JA, Ball RH, et al., First- and Second-Trimester Evaluation of Risk (FASTER) Research Consortium: first-trimester or second-trimester screening, or both, for Down's syndrome. *N Engl J Med* 353:2001–2011, 2005.

Nicolaides KH: Nuchal translucency and other first-trimester sonographic markers of chromosomal abnormalities. *Am J Obstet Gynecol* 191:45–67, 2004.

Nicolaides KH: First-trimester screening for chromosomal abnormalities. *Semin Perinatol* 29:190–194, 2005.

Nicolaides KH, Azar G, Byrne D, Mansur C, Marks K: Fetal nuchal translucency: ultrasound screening for chromosomal defects in first trimester of pregnancy. *BMJ* 304:867–869, 1992.

Nyberg DA, Luthy DA, Cheng EY, et al: Role of prenatal ultrasonography in women with positive screen for Down syndrome on the basis of maternal serum markers. *Am J Obstet Gynecol* 173:1030–1035, 1995.

Nyberg DA, Luthy DA, Resta RG, Nyberg BC, Williams MA: Age-adjusted ultrasound risk assessment for fetal Down's syndrome during the second trimester:

description of the method and analysis of 142 cases. *Ultrasound Obstet Gynecol* 12:8–14, 1998.

Nyberg DA, Resta RG, Luthy DA, et al: Prenatal sonographic findings of Down syndrome: review of 94 cases. *Obstet Gynecol* 76:370–377, 1990.

Nyberg DA, Resta RG, Mahony BS, et al: Fetal hyperechogenic bowel and Down's syndrome. *Ultrasound Obstet Gynecol* 3:330–333, 1993.

Nyberg DA, Souter VL, El-Bastawissi A, Young S, Luthhardt F, Luthy DA: Isolated sonographic markers for detection of fetal Down syndrome in the second trimester of pregnancy. *J Ultrasound Med* 10:1053–1063, 2001.

Pandya PP, Kondylios A, Hilbert L, Snijders RJM Nicolaides KH: Chromosomal defects and outcome in 1015 fetuses with increased nuchal translucency. *Ultrasound Obstet Gynecol* 5:15–19, 1995.

Pandya PP, Snijders RJM, Johnson S, Nicholaides KH: Natural history of trisomy 21 fetuses with increased nuchal translucency thickness. *Ultrasound Obstet Gynecol* 5:381–383, 1995.

Platt LD, Medearis AL, Carlson DE, et al: Screening for Down syndrome with the femur length/biparietal diameter ratio—a new twist of the data. *Am J Obstet Gynecol* 167:124–128, 1992.

Roberts DJ, Genest D: Cardiac histologic pathology characteristic of trisomies 13 and 21. *Hum Pathol* 23:1130–1140, 1992.

Rotmensch S, Luo J, Liberati M, et al: Fetal humeral length to detect Down syndrome. *Am J Obstet Gynecol* 166:1330–1334, 1992.

Scioscia AL, Pretorius DH, Budorick NE, et al: Second-trimester hyperechoic bowel and chromosomal abnormalities. *Am J Obstet Gynecol* 167:889–894, 1992.

Shipp TD, Bromley B, Lieberman E, Benacerraf BR: The iliac angle as a sonographic marker for Down syndrome in second trimester fetuses. *Obstet Gynecol* 89:446–450, 1997.

Smith-Bindman R, Hosmer W, Feldstein V, Deeks JJ, Goldberg JD: Second-trimester ultrasound to detect fetuses with Down syndrome: a meta-analysis. *JAMA* 285:1044–1055, 2001.

Smulian JC, Vintzileos AM, Ciarleglio L, Rodis JF, Campbell WA: Gender-specific patterns of second trimester femur and humerus measurements in fetuses with Down's syndrome. *J Matern Fetal Med* 4:225–230, 1995.

Vintzileos A, Walters C, Yeo L: Absent nasal bone in the prenatal detection of fetuses with trisomy 21 in a high-risk population. *Obstet Gynecol* 101:905–908, 2003.

Vintzileos AM, Egan JFX: Adjusting the risk for trisomy 21 on the basis of second-trimester ultrasonography. *Am J Obstet Gynecol* 172:837–844, 1995.

Vintzileos AM, Guzman ER, Smulian JC, Yeo L, Scorza WE, Knuppel RA: Second-trimester genetic sonography in patients with advanced maternal age and normal triple screen. *Obstet Gynecol* 99:993–995, 2002.

Wapner R, Thom E, Simpson JL, et al., First Trimester Maternal Serum Biochemistry and Fetal Nuchal Translucency Screening (BUN) Study Group: First-trimester screening for trisomies 21 and 18. *N Engl J Med* 349:1405–1413, 2003.

Wapner RJ: First trimester screening: the BUN study. *Semin Perinatol* 29:236–239, 2005.

Watson WJ, Miller RC, Menard K, et al: Ultrasonographic measurement of fetal nuchal skin to screen for chromosomal abnormalities. *Am J Obstet Gynecol* 170:583–586, 1994.

Wilkins I: Separation of the great toe in fetuses with Down syndrome. *J Ultrasound Med* 13:229–231, 1994.

TRISOMY 22

DESCRIPTION AND DEFINITION

Trisomy 22 is a rare, lethal chromosomal abnormality, believed to be found in approximately 10% of spontaneous abortions.

ABNORMALITIES DETECTABLE BY ULTRASOUND

Common Findings:

Cardiac disease (100%)

Cleft lip and palate (80%)

Renal anomalies (80%)

Gastrointestinal abnormalities, usually imperforate anus (80%)

Occasional Findings:

Neck webbing

Hypoplastic digits

MAJOR DIFFERENTIAL DIAGNOSES

Caudal regression syndrome

CHARGE (**c**oloboma of the iris, **h**eart defect, choanal **a**tresia, intrauterine growth **r**estriction, **g**enital anomalies, and **e**ar anomalies) association

Triploidy

Trisomy 18 (Edwards' syndrome)

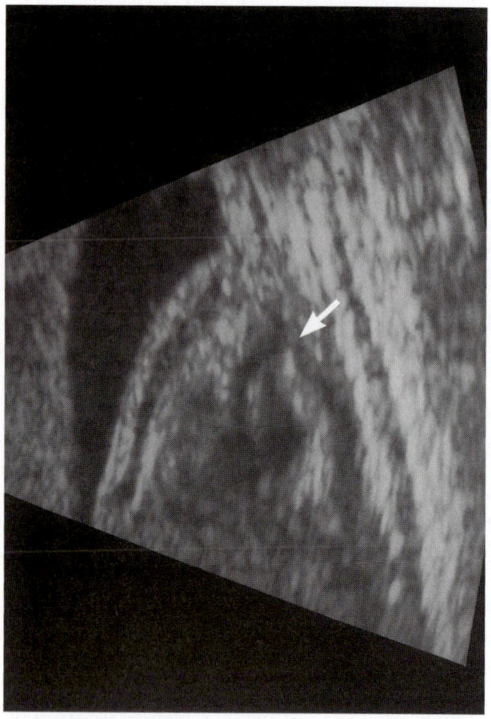

FIGURE 2-329 Longitudinal view of the aortic arch of a fetus with coarctation of the aorta *(arrow)*. Fetuses with trisomy 22 have cardiac defects, including aortic arch abnormalities similar to that shown.

VATER (**v**ertebral defects, **a**nal atresia, **t**racheo-esophageal fistula, **e**sophageal atresia, and **r**adial and renal dysplasias) association

ULTRASOUND DIAGNOSIS

Only a single case of ultrasound diagnosis has been reported, in a 19-week fetus with cardiac abnormality, bilateral cleft lip and palate, absence of stomach bubble, shortened great toes, absence of left kidney, and short femurs.

HEREDITY

This is an autosomal trisomic syndrome.

NATURAL HISTORY AND OUTCOME

This condition is invariably lethal.

Suggested Reading

Harding K, Freeman J, Weston W, Smith JR: Trisomy 22: prenatal diagnosis. A case report. *Ultrasound Obstet Gynecol* 5:136–137, 1995.

XO SYNDROME (TURNER SYNDROME)

DESCRIPTION AND DEFINITION

Synonym: Turner syndrome

Turner syndrome is characterized in early pregnancy by large cystic hygromata and lymphangiectasia, leading to fetal hydrops. Affected infants who survive gestation may represent Turner mosaic individuals.

ABNORMALITIES DETECTABLE BY ULTRASOUND

Large, septate cystic hygroma

Pleural effusions

Ascites

Severe lymphedema of all the soft tissues, consistent with lymphangiectasia

Cardiac defects (mostly left-sided)

Coarctation of the aorta

Renal abnormalities

Horseshoe kidneys

Short femur

MAJOR DIFFERENTIAL DIAGNOSES

Cystic hygromata in the first and second trimesters also can occur in multiple other chromosomal syndromes, including the following:

Cri du chat (5p-) syndrome

Down syndrome

Trisomy 10

Trisomy 18 (Edwards' syndrome)

Thick nuchal translucency suggesting cystic hygroma also is present among many nonkaryotypic abnormalities, including the following (see Chapter 1, p. 50, for differential diagnosis, thick nuchal translucency):

Achondrogenesis

Apert syndrome

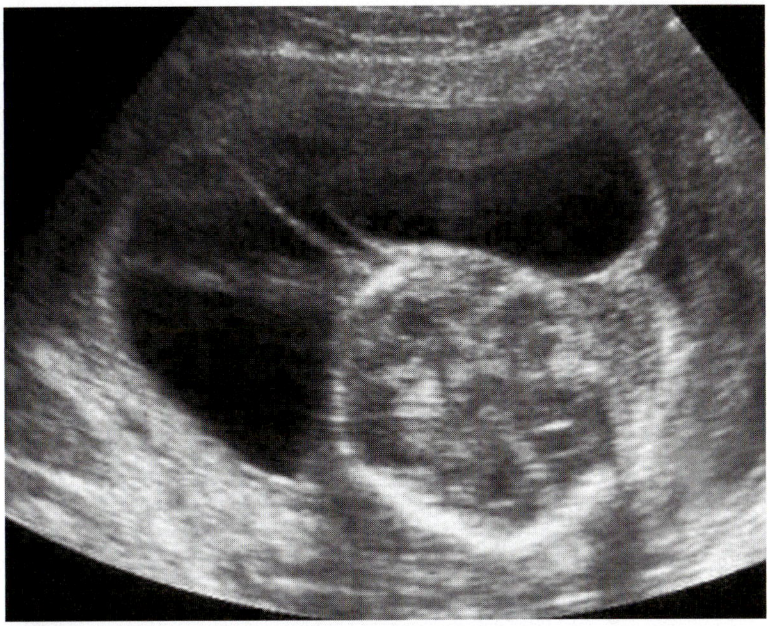

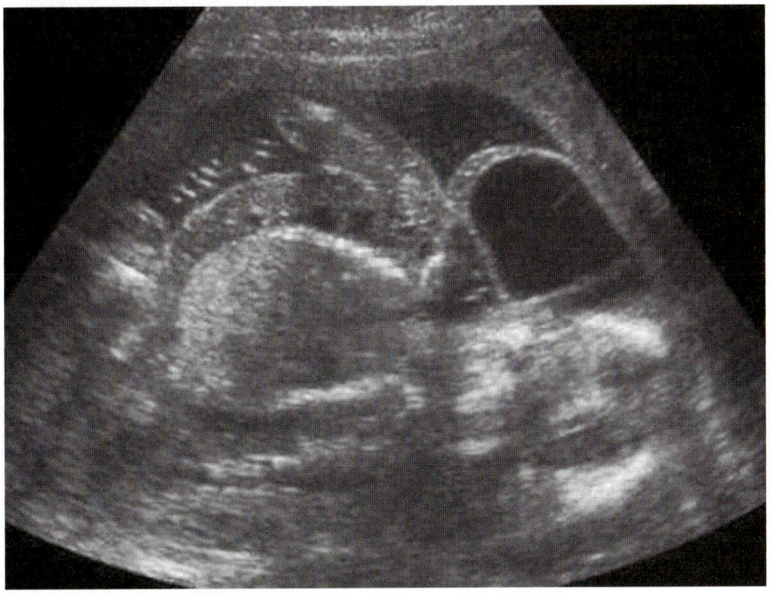

FIGURE 2-330 Large septate cystic hygromas typical of Turner syndrome. (A) Transverse view through the fetal head and the bulk of the cystic hygroma. (B) Longitudinal view of the fetus shows the cystic hygroma at the level of the neck as well as severe lymphangiectasia involving the entire rest of the body.

Cerebrocostomandibular syndrome

Cornelia de Lange syndrome

Ectrodactyly–ectodermal dysplasia–clefting (EEC) syndrome

Fryns syndrome

Joubert syndrome

Kniest syndrome

Multiple pterygium syndrome

Noonan syndrome

Perlman syndrome

Roberts' syndrome

Smith-Lemli-Opitz syndrome

ULTRASOUND DIAGNOSIS

When prenatal sonographic diagnosis is established in the late first and early second trimesters based on cystic hygroma formation, most

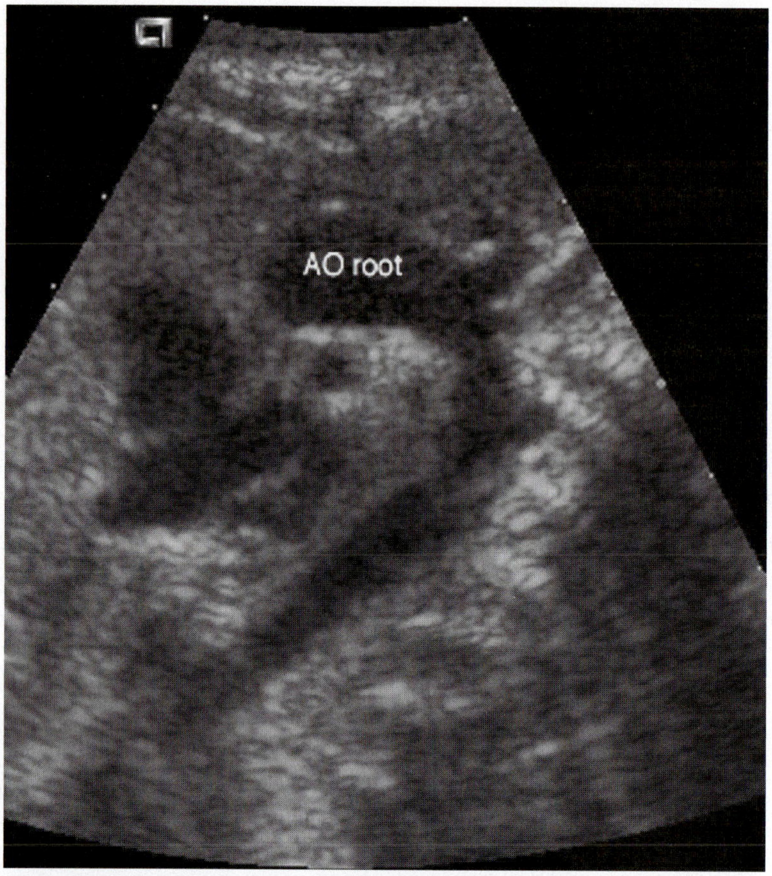

A

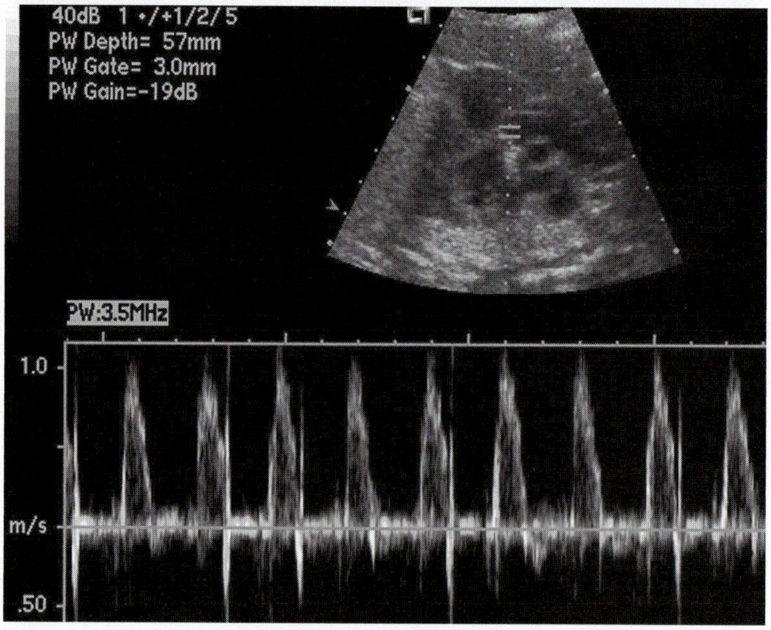

B

FIGURE 2-331 (A) View of the aortic arch of a fetus with aortic stenosis shows poststenotic dilation of the aortic root. *AO*, Aorta. (B) Doppler waveform taken in the aortic root shows a high-velocity jet consistent with aortic stenosis.

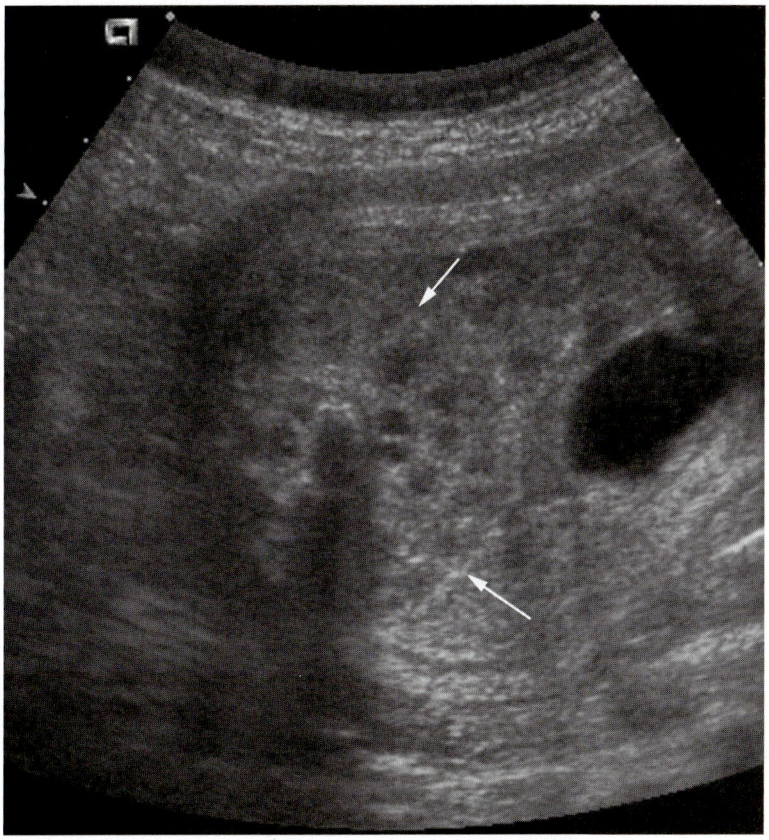

FIGURE 2-332 Transverse view through the fetal pelvis shows the fetal bladder. Just posterior to the fetal bladder is a horseshoe kidney *(arrows)*.

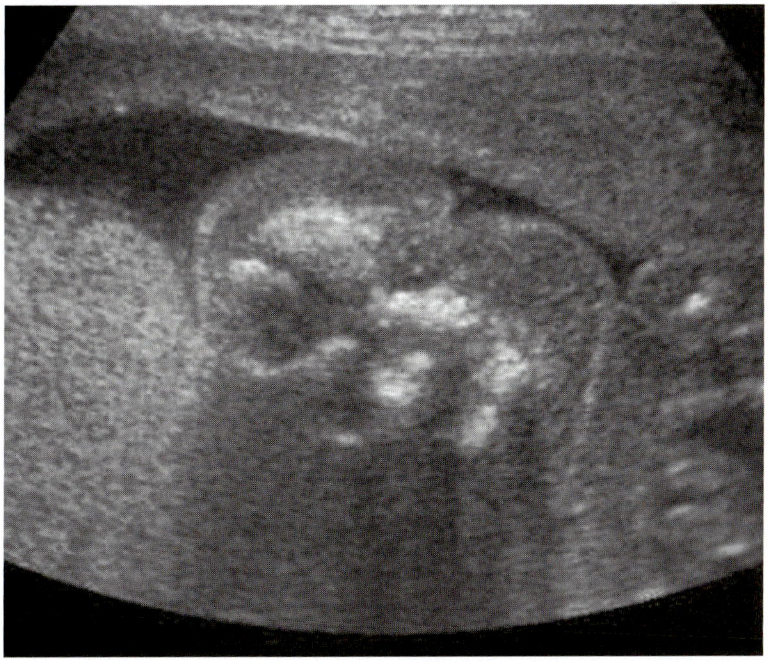

A

FIGURE 2-333 Turner syndrome with severe lymphangiectasia and cystic hygromas. (A) Fetal face with severe thickening of the soft tissues.

Continued

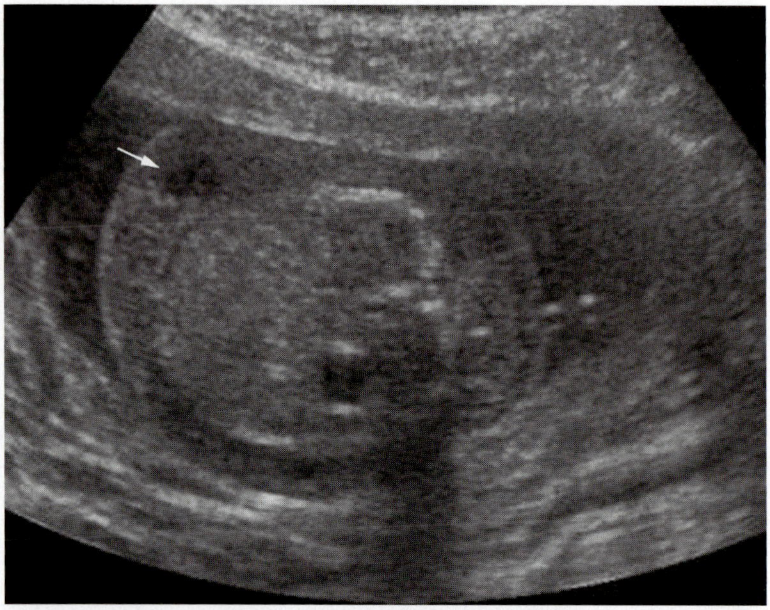

B

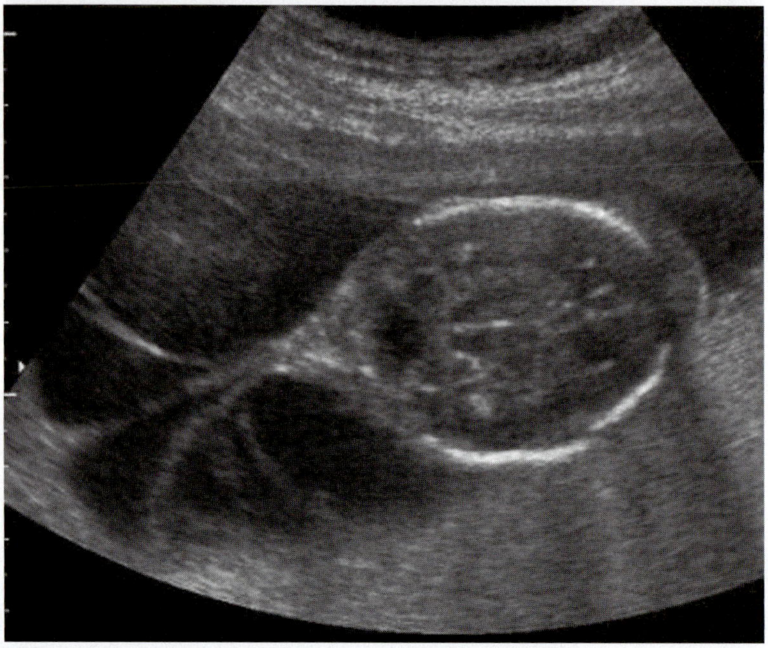

C

FIGURE 2-333, cont'd **(B)** Transverse view through the fetal abdomen shows severe thickening of the soft tissues around the abdomen as well as small cystic hygromas *(arrow)*. **(C)** Large septate cystic hygromas, typical of Turner syndrome.

affected fetuses die in utero; thus, third-trimester diagnosis of this abnormality is unusual.

HEREDITY

The pattern of inheritance for this syndrome usually is sporadic. This abnormality is *not* known to be associated with advanced maternal age.

NATURAL HISTORY AND OUTCOME

Most fetuses with the full XO syndrome are miscarried in the first trimester, prior to prenatal diagnosis, or have large cystic hygromata with severe lymphedema, leading to death later in gestation. Those who survive have regression of the cystic hygromata, resulting in webbing of the neck at that site. Associated coarctation of the aorta usually requires intervention.

Long-term survival is associated with ovarian dysgenesis and relatively short stature. Occasional abnormalities include hearing impairment and mental retardation.

Suggested Reading

Linden MG, Bender BG, Robinson A: Intrauterine diagnosis of sex chromosome aneuploidy. *Obstet Gynecol* 87:468–475, 1996.

Mostello DJ, Bofinger MK, Siddiqi TA: Spontaneous resolution of fetal cystic hygroma and hydrops in Turner syndrome. *Obstet Gynecol* 73:862–865, 1989.

Robinow M, Spisso K, Buschi AJ, Norman A, Brenbridge AG: Turner syndrome: sonography showing fetal hydrops simulating hydramnios. *AJR Am J Roentgenol* 135:846–848, 1980.

Saller DN, Canick JA, Schwartz S, Blitzer MG: Multiple-marker screening in pregnancies with hydropic and nonhydropic Turner syndrome. *Am J Obstet Gynecol* 167:1021–1024, 1992.

Wenstrom KD, Williamson RA, Grant SS: Detection of fetal Turner syndrome with multiple-marker screening. *Am J Obstet Gynecol* 170:570–573, 1994.

Tumors

CYSTIC HYGROMA/LYMPHANGIOMA

DESCRIPTION AND DEFINITION

Lymphangiomata and cystic hygromata are abnormalities of the lymphatic vessels, characterized by cysts within the soft tissues, usually in the nuchal region. When they occur in the lateral and posterior neck region, they often are associated with chromosomal abnormalities and hydrops. They can occur elsewhere—in the mediastinum, abdominal organs, or body surface—where they usually are isolated lesions, unrelated to chromosomal abnormalities.

ABNORMALITIES DETECTABLE BY ULTRASOUND

Nuchal translucency thickening is thought to represent small lymphatic anomalies occurring in the first trimester. These have a high association with chromosomal abnormalities. Nuchal translucency thickening and nuchal cystic hygromata are considered a spectrum of the same condition.

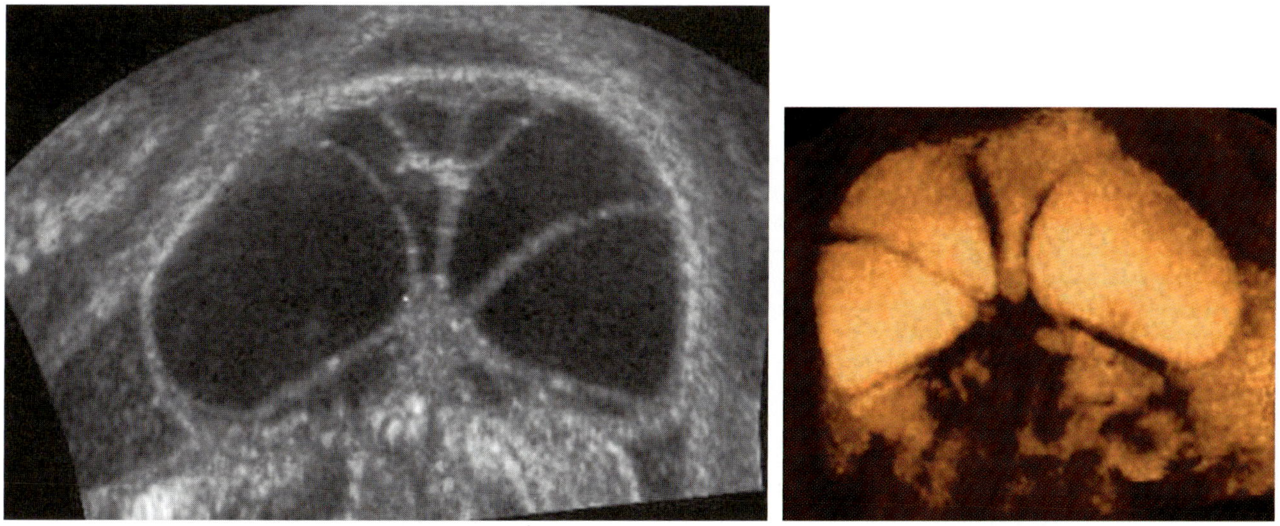

A B

FIGURE 2-334 (A) Three-dimensional reconstructed view of the entire septate hygroma. (B) Inverse mode shows the entire cystic hygroma as a cast.

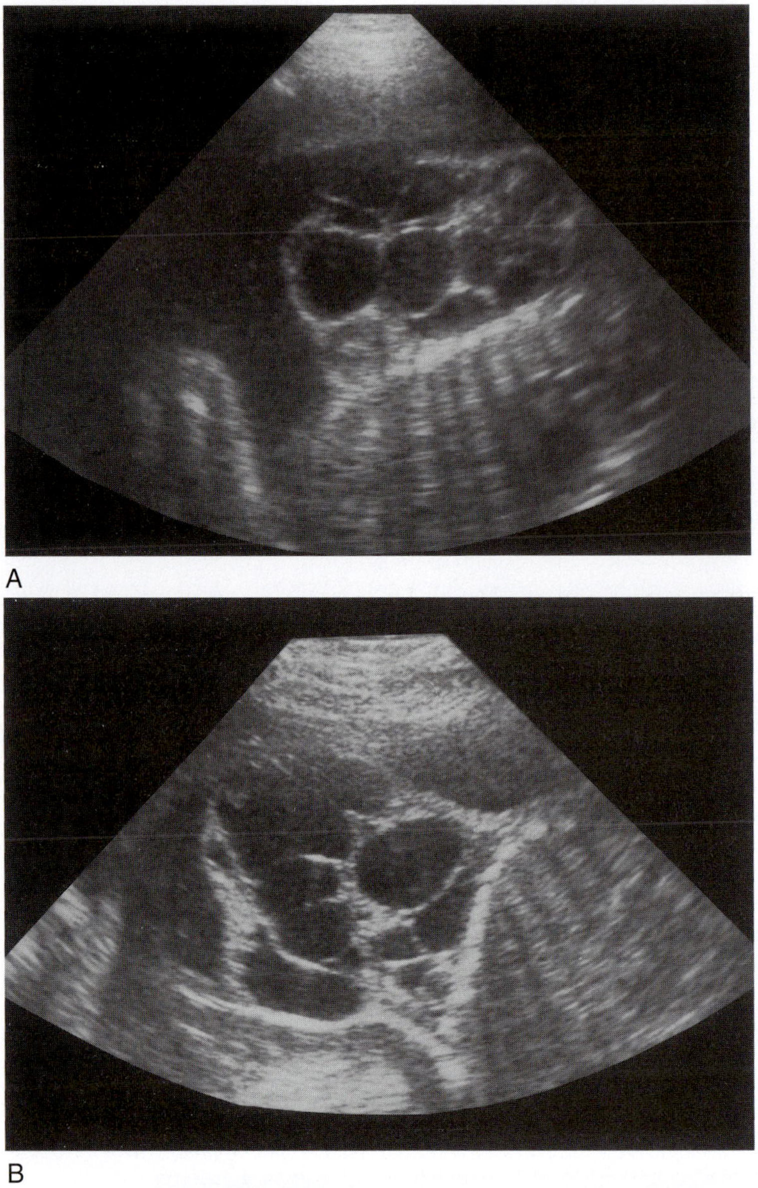

FIGURE 2-335 Longitudinal (A) and transverse (B) views through the fetal axilla show a large, multiseptate cystic mass, consistent with lymphangioma.

Nuchal cystic hygromata (second trimester) are fluid masses at the back of the fetal neck that vary in size, can be septate or simple, and often are parts of chromosomal syndromes.

Large, septate cystic hygromata are seen in second-trimester fetuses with Turner syndrome and can cause the following:

- Hydrops
- Severe skin edema, possibly the result of lymphangiectasia
- Pleural effusions
- Ascites

Isolated, nonnuchal cystic hygromata and lymphangiomata usually are cystic, with septa. They are not associated with other anomalies or chromosomal syndromes. They can occur anywhere on the fetal body, including the abdomen, chest, retroperitoneum, and limbs.

MAJOR DIFFERENTIAL DIAGNOSES

Nuchal cystic hygromata can be confused with other conditions, including the following:

- Amniotic band syndrome
- Encephalocele

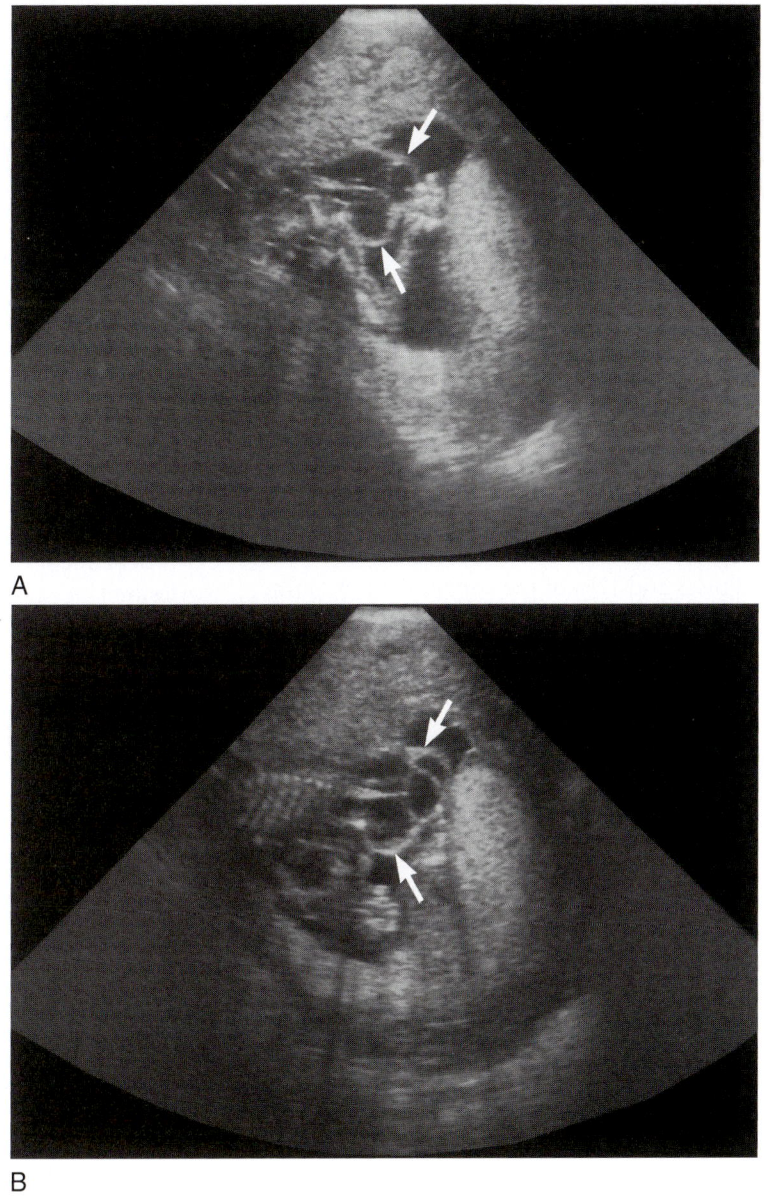

FIGURE 2-336 (A, B) Views of the fetal shoulder show a multiseptate cystic mass *(arrows)* located at the side of the neck, consistent with a lymphangioma.

Chromosomal syndromes associated with nuchal cystic hygromata include the following:

Down syndrome

Trisomy 18 (Edwards' syndrome)

XO syndrome (Turner syndrome)

Nuchal thickenings mimicking cystic hygromata are present among many nonkaryotypic abnormalities (see Chapter 1, p. 50, for differential diagnosis, nuchal thickening).

Differential diagnosis of nonnuchal cystic hygromata depends on the location of the tumor. When a lymphangioma occurs on the surface of the fetus, such as on the anterior abdominal wall, buttock, or scalp, the differential diagnosis includes the following:

Amniotic band syndrome

Encephalocele

Hemangioma

Omphalocele

Teratoma

Tumors of the extremities or skin can be associated with the following:

Klippel-Trenaunay-Weber syndrome

Proteus syndrome

Anterior neck lesions can be confused with the following:

- Branchial cleft cyst
- Goiter
- Thyroglossal duct cyst
- Teratoma

ULTRASOUND DIAGNOSIS

Nuchal cystic hygroma can be diagnosed in the first trimester. The incidence of chromosomal anomalies associated with the presence of first-trimester cystic hygromas is very high (≈50%). Regardless of karyotype, cystic hygromas can improve over time. In one study, cystic hygroma regressed in 10% of chromosomally abnormal fetuses and 17% of the euploid fetuses. Some nuchal translucency abnormalities may even disappear completely during gestation. The presence of septa or hydrops makes resolution or normal outcome unlikely. In the event of a normal karyotype and resolution of the nuchal mass, follow-up scans are recommended to identify anomalies not visible early in gestation, such as heart, CNS, and skeletal defects, as well as genetic syndromes.

Isolated cystic hygromata (with the exception of nuchal hygromata) typically have later onsets and are most often diagnosed in the third trimester, although occasionally they are detected in the second trimester. They can enlarge or shrink over the course of gestation. Follow-up scans are important to track the course of the hygromata and plan for postnatal resection.

HEREDITY

Nuchal cystic hygromata and nuchal lucencies may be part of a syndrome (as noted in Major Differential Diagnoses). In that case, the inheritance pattern would follow that of the syndrome.

Isolated cystic hygromata occur sporadically.

NATURAL HISTORY AND OUTCOME

The presence of a nuchal lucency anomaly may indicate an associated severe abnormality, such as a chromosomal defect. Among 134 cases of cystic hygromata (Malone et al.), 51% were chromosomally abnormal, and 34% had major anomalies, mostly cardiac and skeletal. Overall, survival with normal outcome occurred in 17% of cases.

In the Tanriverdi study, 53% of fetuses (mean gestational age 14.4 weeks) had other sonographically detected anomalies, most commonly hydrops, and 50% of those karyotyped were aneuploid. The overall fetal adverse outcome rate was 69%.

Although some fetuses with nuchal cystic hygromata that are nonseptate and associated with a normal karyotype do well, the fetus still can have one of many syndromes, such as Noonan syndrome, Pena Shokeir syndrome, multiple pterygium syndrome, cardiac defects, and many others. A normal outcome represents a minority of cases overall.

The outcome of fetuses with *isolated* cystic hygromata located in regions other than the neck is dependent on surgical removal of the local lesion.

Suggested Reading

Achiron R, Yagel S, Weissman A, et al: Fetal lateral neck cysts: early second-trimester transvaginal diagnosis, natural history and clinical significance. *Ultrasound Obstet Gynecol* 6:396–399, 1995.

Benacerraf BR, Frigoletto FD Jr: Prenatal sonographic diagnosis of isolated congenital cystic hygroma, unassociated with lymphedema or other morphologic abnormality. *J Ultrasound Med* 6:63–66, 1987.

Bernstein HS, Filly RA, Goldberg JD, Golbus MS: Prognosis of fetuses with a cystic hygroma. *Prenat Diagn* 11:349–355, 1991.

Bronshtein M, Bar-Hava I, Blumenfeld I, et al: The difference between septated and nonseptated nuchal cystic hygroma in the early second trimester. *Obstet Gynecol* 81:683–687, 1993.

Ganapathy R, Guven M, Sethna F, Vivekananda U, Thilaganathan B: Natural history and outcome of prenatally diagnosed cystic hygroma. *Prenat Diagn* 15;24:965–968, 2004.

Gandhi SV, Howarth ES, Krarup KC, Konje JC: Noonan syndrome presenting with transient cystic hygroma. *J Obstet Gynaecol* 24:183–184, 2004.

Giacalone PL, Boulot F, Deschamps F, et al: Prenatal diagnosis of a multifocal lymphangioma. *Prenat Diagn* 13:1133–1137, 1993.

Goldstein I, Jakobi P, Shoshany G, et al: Late-onset isolated cystic hygroma: the obstetrical significance, management, and outcome. *Prenat Diagn* 14:757–761, 1994.

Hoffman-Tretin J, Koenigsberg M, Ziprkowski M: Antenatal demonstration of axillary cystic hygroma. *J Ultrasound Med* 7:233–235, 1988.

Malnofski MJ, Poulton TB, Nazinitsky KJ, Hissong SL: Prenatal ultrasonographic diagnosis of retroperitoneal cystic lymphangioma. *J Ultrasound Med* 12:427–429, 1993.

Malone FD, Ball RH, Nyberg DA, et al., FASTER Trial Research Consortium: First-trimester septated cystic hygroma: prevalence, natural history, and pediatric outcome. *Obstet Gynecol* 106:288–294, 2005.

McCoy MC, Kuller JA, Chescheir NC, et al: Prenatal diagnosis and management of massive bilateral axillary cystic lymphangioma. *Obstet Gynecol* 85:853–856, 1995.

Pandya PP, Brizot ML, Kuhn P, Snijders RJM, Nicolaides KH: First-trimester fetal nuchal translucency thickness and risk for trisomies. *Obstet Gynecol* 84:420–423, 1994.

Pijpers L, Reuss A, Stewart PA, Wladimiroff JW, Sachs ES: Fetal cystic hygroma: prenatal diagnosis and management. *Obstet Gynecol* 72:223–224, 1988.

Podobnik M, Singer Z, Podobnik-Sarkanji S, Bulic M: First-trimester diagnosis of cystic hygromata by transvaginal sonography. *Ultrasound Obstet Gynecol* 2:124–125, 1992.

Rasidaki M, Sifakis S, Vardaki E, Koumantakis E: Prenatal diagnosis of a fetal chest wall cystic lymphangioma using ultrasonography and MRI: a case report with literature review. *Fetal Diagn Ther* 20:504–507, 2005.

Reichler A, Bronshtein M: Early prenatal diagnosis of axillary cystic hygroma. *J Ultrasound Med* 14:581–584, 1995.

Ruano R, Aubry JP, Simon I, et al: Prenatal diagnosis of a large axillary cystic lymphangioma by three-dimensional ultrasonography and magnetic resonance imaging. *J Ultrasound Med* 22:419–423, 2003.

Tanriverdi HA, Ertan AK, Hendrik HJ, Remberger K, Schmidt W: Outcome of cystic hygroma in fetuses with normal karyotypes depends on associated findings. *Eur J Obstet Gynecol Reprod Biol* 118:40–46, 2005.

Tanriverdi HA, Hendrik HJ, Ertan AK, Axt R, Schmidt W: Hygroma colli cysticum: prenatal diagnosis and prognosis. *Am J Perinatol* 18:415–420, 2001.

Thomas RL: Prenatal diagnosis of giant cystic hygroma: prognosis, counselling, and management. Case presentation and review of the recent literature. *Prenat Diagn* 12:919–923, 1992.

Trauffer PML, Anderson CE, Johnson A, et al: The natural history of euploid pregnancies with first-trimester cystic hygromas. *Am J Obstet Gynecol* 170:1279–1284, 1994.

Ville Y, Lalondrelle C, Doumerc S, et al: First-trimester diagnosis of nuchal anomalies: significance and fetal outcome. *Ultrasound Obstet Gynecol* 2:314–316, 1992.

Zalel Y, Shalev E, Ben-Ami M, Mogilner G, Weiner E: Ultrasonic diagnosis of mediastinal cystic hygroma. *Prenat Diagn* 12:541–544, 1992.

HEMANGIOMA

DESCRIPTION AND DEFINITION

Hemangioma is a common, benign, vascular tumor that can occur in visceral organs and on the skin, particularly in the head and neck region. These tumors are vascular hamartomata, some of which can have a lymphangiomatous component. Hemangiomata are some of the most common benign neoplasms in infancy and are readily detectable in utero, particularly the giant hemangiomata.

ABNORMALITIES DETECTABLE BY ULTRASOUND

Polyhydramnios

Hemangiomata seen sonographically usually are solid in appearance, although they can be complex. They are vascular lesions, with varying degrees of vascularity seen by Doppler (depending on flow rates).

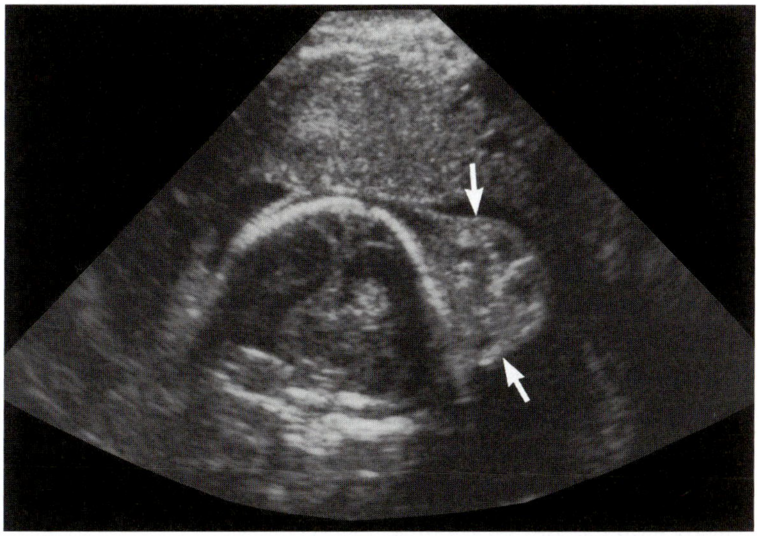

FIGURE 2-337 Coronal view of the fetal head shows a large echogenic mass emanating from the scalp *(arrows)*. This was found to be a hemangioma at birth.

MAJOR DIFFERENTIAL DIAGNOSES

Differential diagnosis depends on the location of the tumor.

When the tumor involves the neck area, the differential diagnosis includes the following:

- Branchial cleft cyst
- Cystic hygroma
- Encephalocele
- Goiter
- Teratoma
- Thyroglossal duct cyst

When a hemangioma occurs on the surface of the fetus, such as on the anterior abdominal wall, buttock, or scalp, the differential diagnosis includes the following:

- Amniotic band syndrome
- Encephalocele
- Lymphangioma
- Omphalocele
- Teratoma

Tumors of the extremities or skin can be associated with the following:

- Klippel-Trenaunay-Weber syndrome
- Proteus syndrome

Cord hemangiomata can be confused with the following:

- Allantoid cysts
- Hematomata of the cord
- Omphalomesenteric cysts
- Teratomata of the cord

Hemangiomata can occur in the viscera, such as the heart, in which cases the differential diagnosis includes the following:

- Rhabdomyoma
- Teratoma

ULTRASOUND DIAGNOSIS

Many cases of fetal hemangioma present for sonography as a result of polyhydramnios.

Widespread, cutaneous vascular hamartomatosis has been described at 24 weeks' gestation as a severely deforming abnormality involving much of the subcutaneous tissue of the fetus. Other reports of antenatally diagnosed hemangiomata cite involvement of the anterior abdominal wall at 38 weeks' gestation (in which case a previous 15-week scan had been normal), the fetal face at 32 weeks' gestation (in which case an 18-week scan had been normal), and the scalp at 30 weeks' gestation (in which case a 15-week scan had been normal). Several cases of facial, neck, and limb lesions have been reported, mostly in the third trimester. Intracardiac and hepatic lesions have been described.

Although many localized hemangiomata are discovered in the third trimester, a severe, diffuse hemangioma involving large portions of the fetal body or limb can be diagnosed earlier—in the mid-to-late second trimester. Hemangiomata also can be tumors involving the umbilical cord and placental surface. They are most often echogenic, with some incidence of cord edema. A hemangioma of the umbilical cord has been reported by our group as a complex mass seen at 33 weeks' gestational age. Chorioangiomata most often occur on the fetal surface of the placenta.

HEREDITY

Hemangiomata occur sporadically.

NATURAL HISTORY AND OUTCOME

The outcomes of pregnancies complicated by fetal hemangiomata are highly variable, depending on the size of the hemangioma and the degree of involvement of the fetus. Small hemangiomata are incidental findings and are easily managed after birth. Large hemangiomata, involving extensive parts of the fetal body, are life threatening and, in many cases, lethal.

Suggested Reading

Arienzo R, Ricco CS, Romeo F: A very rare fetal malformation: the cutaneous widespread vascular hamartomatosis. *Am J Obstet Gynecol* 157:1162–1163, 1987.

Boon LM, Enjoiras O, Mulliken JB: Congenital hemangioma: evidence of accelerated involution. *J Pediatr* 128:329–335, 1996.

Bulas DI, Johnson D, Allen JF, Kapur S: Fetal hemangioma: sonographic and color flow Doppler findings. *J Ultrasound Med* 11:499–501, 1992.

Gembruch U, Baschat AA, Gloeckner-Hoffmann K, Gortner L, Germer U: Prenatal diagnosis and management of fetuses with liver hemangiomata. *Ultrasound Obstet Gynecol* 19:454–460, 2002.

Grundy H, Glasmann A, Burlbaw J, et al: Hemangioma presenting as a cystic mass in the fetal neck. *J Ultrasound Med* 4:147–150, 1985.

Marler JJ, Fishman SJ, Upton J, et al: Prenatal diagnosis of vascular anomalies. *J Pediatr Surg* 37:318–326, 2002.

Maynor CH, Hertzberg BS, Kliewer MA, Heyneman LE, Carroll BA: Antenatal ultrasonographic diagnosis of abdominal wall hemangioma: potential to simulate ventral abdominal wall defects. *J Ultrasound Med* 14:317–319, 1995.

McGahan JP, Schneider JM: Fetal neck hemangioendothelioma with secondary hydrops fetalis: sonographic diagnosis. *J Clin Ultrasound* 14:384–388, 1986.

Meizner I, Bar-Ziv J, Holcberg G, Katz M: In utero prenatal diagnosis of fetal facial tumor—hemangioma. *J Clin Ultrasound* 13:435–437, 1985.

Pennell RG, Baltarowich OH: Prenatal sonographic diagnosis of a fetal facial hemangioma. *J Ultrasound Med* 5:525–528, 1986.

Platt LD, Geierman CA, Turkel SB, Young G, Keegan KA: Atrial hemangioma and hydrops fetalis. *Am J Obstet Gynecol* 141:107–109, 1981.

Pott Bartsch EM, Paek BW, Yoshizawa J, et al: Giant fetal hepatic hemangioma. Case report and literature review. *Fetal Diagn Ther* 18:59–64, 2003.

Shih JC, Ko TL, Lin MC, Shyu MK, Lee CN, Hsieh FJ: Quantitative three-dimensional power Doppler ultrasound predicts the outcome of placental chorioangioma. *Ultrasound Obstet Gynecol* 24:202–206, 2004.

Suma V, Marini A, Gamba PG, Luzzatto C: Giant hemangioma of the thigh: prenatal sonographic diagnosis. *J Clin Ultrasound* 18:421–424, 1990.

Yoshida S, Kikuchi A, Naito S, et al: Giant hemangioma of the fetal neck, mimicking a teratoma. *J Obstet Gynaecol Res* 32:47–54, 2006.

Zhou QC, Fan P, Peng QH, Zhang M, Fu Z, Wang CH: Prenatal echocardiographic differential diagnosis of fetal cardiac tumors. *Ultrasound Obstet Gynecol* 23:165–171, 2004.

NEUROBLASTOMA

DESCRIPTION AND DEFINITION

Neuroblastoma is considered one of the most common abdominal tumors among neonates. It most often occurs in the fetal adrenal gland or along the spine. If the tumor is identified early, it may be found as an isolated lesion. However, in many cases, it is found later in early childhood, after metastases have occurred. Prenatal diagnosis of a neuroblastoma is extremely important to achieve early treatment and prevent metastases.

ABNORMALITIES DETECTABLE BY ULTRASOUND

Fetal adrenal neuroblastoma is characterized by a cystic, solid, or complex mass in the region of the adrenal gland, directly above the level of the kidney and under the diaphragm. Fetal neuroblastoma has been identified along the spine.

MAJOR DIFFERENTIAL DIAGNOSES

The differential diagnosis of a fetal adrenal lesion includes the following:

Adrenal cyst

Adrenal hemorrhage

Extralobar subdiaphragmatic sequestration of the lung

Hydronephrotic upper pole of the duplex collecting system

Liver cyst

Liver mass, such as a hamartoma, on the undersurface or posterior aspect of the liver

Lymphangioma of the retroperitoneum

ULTRASOUND DIAGNOSIS

The earliest prenatal ultrasound diagnosis of neuroblastoma has been established in the third trimester. There have been reports of normal second-trimester scans in fetuses identified as having neuroblastoma in the third trimester.

HEREDITY

Although neuroblastomata most often occur sporadically, there is a familial tendency. Therefore, neuroblastoma is thought to have a hereditary form.

NATURAL HISTORY AND OUTCOME

When identified in utero, neuroblastomata are associated with an excellent outcome. Prenatal metastases are unusual.

When a neuroblastoma is discovered after birth in a symptomatic child, metastases have often occurred, and the outcome is uncertain.

We recently found an echogenic mass next to the fetal spine, between the fetal spine and the right kidney, in a 39-week fetus undergoing a biophysical profile. This mass elevated the lower

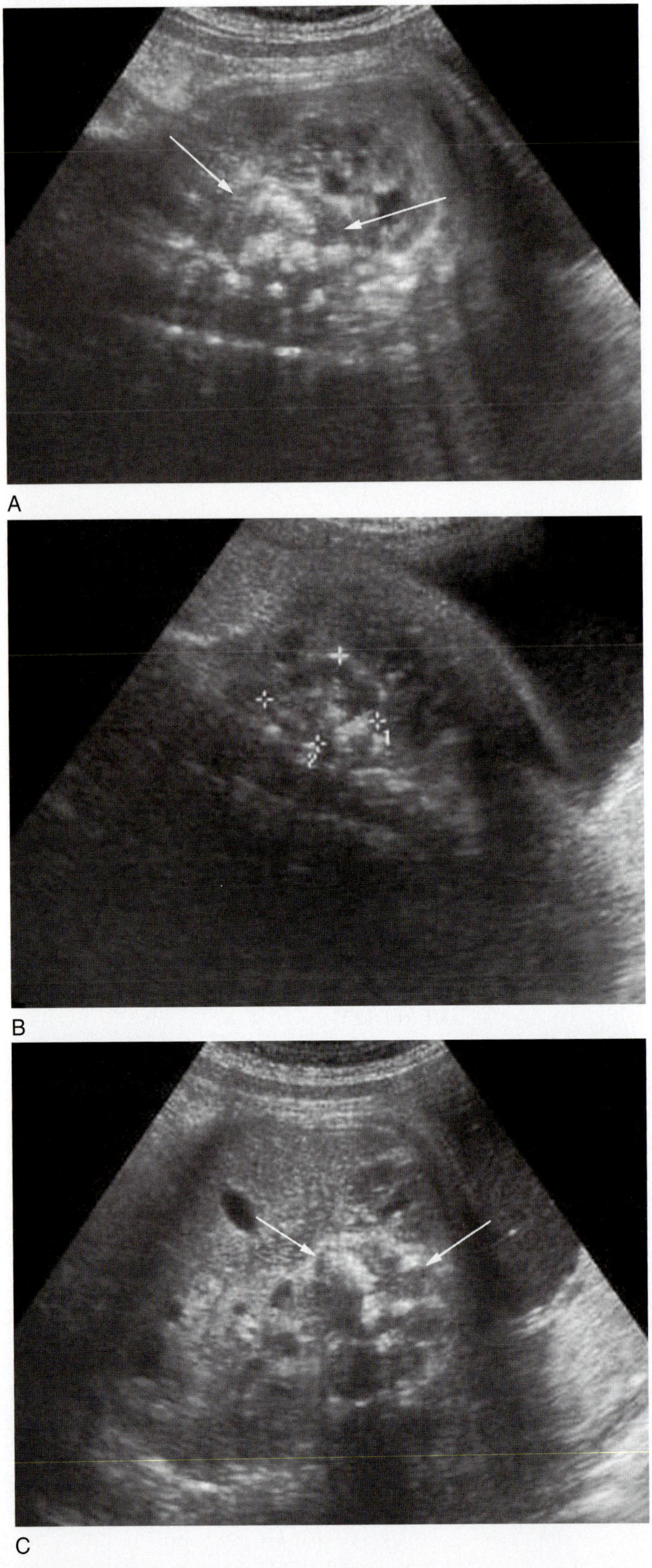

FIGURE 2-338 (A) Longitudinal view of the fetal kidney in a term fetus shows that the kidney is displaced away from the spine by a partly calcified mass *(arrows)*, subsequently proven to be a rapidly expanding neuroblastoma. (B) Mass indicated by the calipers. (C) Transverse view through the fetal abdomen shows the location of the mass *(arrows)* between the kidney and the spine.

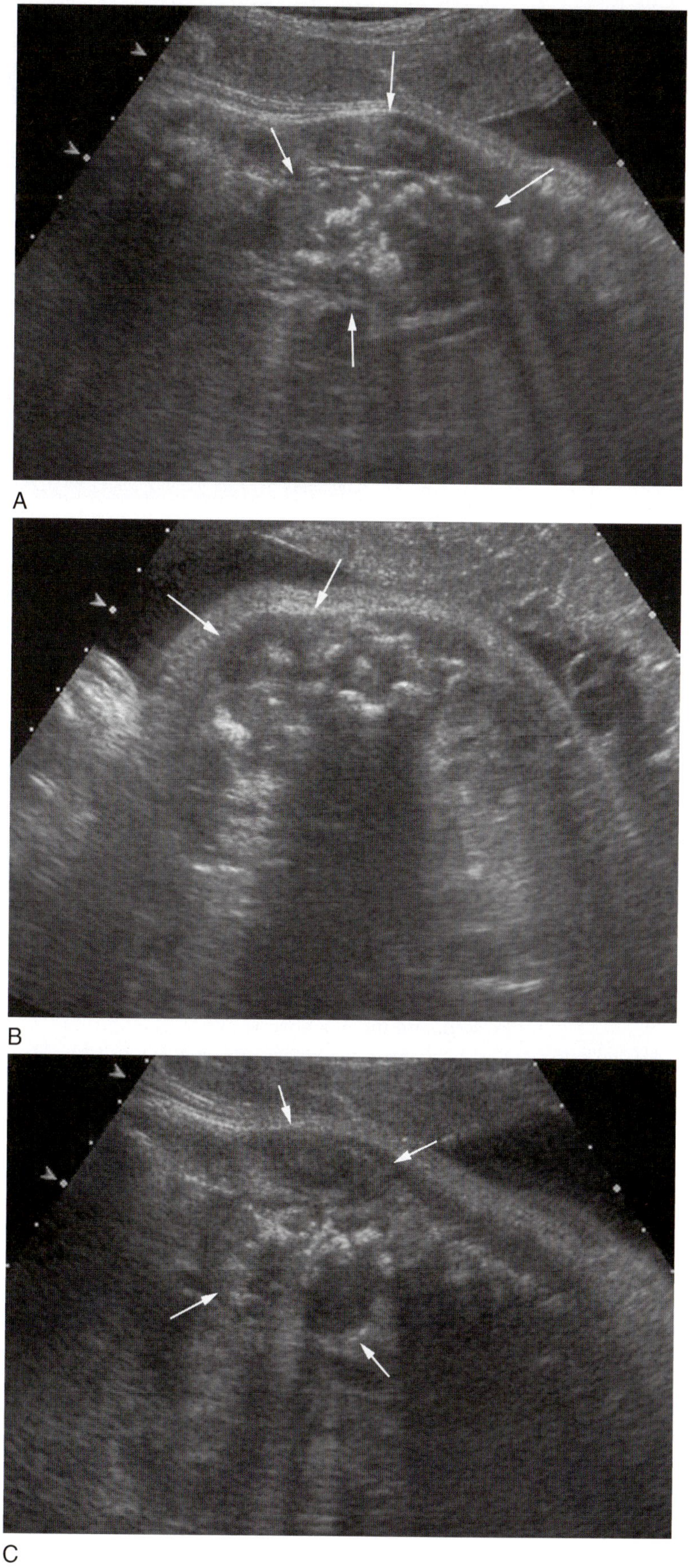

FIGURE 2-339 (A) One week later, the neuroblastoma has progressed significantly to involve the paraspinous muscles. Note that the tumor has expanded beyond the rib cage into the paraspinous muscles *(arrows)* on this longitudinal view through the flank. (B) Transverse view through the fetal back shows involvement of the paraspinous muscles *(arrows)* with the neuroblastoma. (C) Longitudinal view of the back of the fetus at the level of the tumor shows the bilobed nature of the tumor *(arrows)* both inside the rib cage and protruding out into the paraspinous muscles. *Continued*

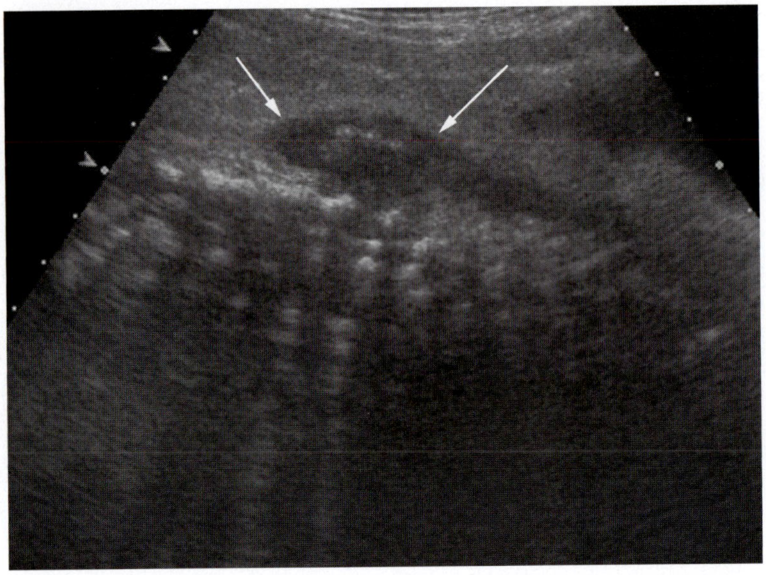

D

FIGURE 2-339, cont'd (D) Longitudinal view of part of the tumor *(arrows)* that is outside the thoracic spine. The fetus was delivered shortly after this image was taken and underwent immediate treatment of the tumor, with an excellent result.

pole of the kidney away from the spine. The mass was rapidly progressing; in the course of 10 days, it had traversed the ribcage at the level of the spine and posterior elements and involved the paraspinous muscles and the spinal canal. Progression of the mass prompted delivery, and the newborn had partial paralysis of the lower extremities at birth. With intensive chemotherapy, the tumor and paralysis regressed, and the newborn recovered.

Suggested Reading

Amundson GM, Trevenen CL, Mueller DL, Rubin SZ, Wesenberg RL: Neuroblastoma: a specific sonographic tissue pattern. *AJR Am J Roentgenol* 148:943–945, 1987.

Atkinson GO, Zaatari GS, Lorenzo RL, Gay BB, Garvin AJ: Cystic neuroblastoma in infants: radiographic and pathologic features. *AJR Am J Roentgenol* 146:113–117, 1986.

de Luca JL, Rousseau T, Durand C, Sagot P, Sapin E: Diagnostic and therapeutic dilemma with large prenatally detected cystic adrenal masses. *Fetal Diagn Ther* 17:11–16, 2002.

Ferraro EM, Fakhry J, Aruny FE, Bracero LA: Prenatal adrenal neuroblastoma: case report with review of the literature. *J Ultrasound Med* 7:275–278, 1988.

Fowlie F, Giacomantonio M, McKenzie E, Baird D, Covert A: Antenatal sonographic diagnosis of adrenal neuroblastoma. *J Can Assoc Radiol* 37:50–51, 1986.

Giulian BB, Chang CCN, Yoss BS: Prenatal ultrasonographic diagnosis of fetal adrenal neuroblastoma. *J Clin Ultrasound* 14:225–227, 1986.

Granata C, Fagnani AM, Gambini C, et al: Features and outcome of neuroblastoma detected before birth. *J Pediatr Surg* 35:88–91, 2000.

Grando A, Monteggia V, Gandara C, Ruano R, Bunduki V, Zugaib M: Prenatal sonographic diagnosis of adrenal neuroblastoma. *J Clin Ultrasound* 29:250–253, 2001.

Ho PTC, Estroff JA, Kazakewich H, et al: Prenatal detection of neuroblastoma: a ten-year experience from the Dana-Farber Cancer Institute and Children's Hospital. *Pediatrics* 92:358–364, 1993.

Houlihan C, Jampolsky M, Shilad A, Prinicipe D: Prenatal diagnosis of neuroblastoma with sonography and magnetic resonance imaging. *J Ultrasound Med* 23:547–550, 2004.

Nagasako H, Ijichi O, Shinkoda Y, et al: Fetal ultrasonography to prevent irreversible neurological sequelae of neonatal neuroblastoma. *Pediatr Hematol Oncol* 21:157–160, 2004.

Romero R: *Prenatal diagnosis of congenital anomalies.* East Norwalk, CT, 1988, Appleton & Lange.

Rubenstein SC, Benacerraf BR, Retik AB, Mandell J: Fetal suprarenal masses: sonographic appearance and differential diagnosis. *Ultrasound Obstet Gynecol* 5:164–167, 1995.

Suresh S, Indrani S, Vijayalakshmi S, Nirmala J, Meera G: Prenatal diagnosis of cerebral neuroblastoma by fetal brain biopsy. *J Ultrasound Med* 5:303–306, 1993.

Tanaka S, Tajiri T, Noguchi S, et al: Prenatally diagnosed cystic neuroblastoma: a report of two cases. *Asian J Surg* 26:225–227, 2003.

TERATOMA

DESCRIPTION AND DEFINITION

Teratomata are tumors that originate from any of the three germinal layers (ectodermal, mesodermal, and endodermal tissue). They can occur in the brain, oropharynx, sacral area, chest, abdomen, or gonads and commonly include adipose tissue, bone, nerve tissue, respiratory elements, and cartilage. Solid, cystic, or complex (combination of solid and cystic elements), these tumors have a disorganized appearance and can be quite vascular.

ABNORMALITIES DETECTABLE BY ULTRASOUND

Teratomata are associated with polyhydramnios.

1. If they occur in the brain, teratomata can expand the head dramatically, destroying much of the brain and replacing it with a rapidly growing complex mass.
2. If they arise from the palate and pharynx, teratomata "epignathus" tumors can extend through the oral and nasal cavities as a solid or complex mass, invading the base of the brain, oropharynx, mouth, and nose.
3. Teratomata arising from the presacral region can grow both intraabdominally and externally to large sizes. Sacrococcygeal teratomata can be cystic, solid, or both, and they may be quite vascular. They can cause hydrops from the extreme vascularity of the lesion.
4. Teratomata arising from the mediastinum or pericardium most often are solid and can cause hydrops from compression of the mediastinal structures.
5. Teratomata arising from the umbilical cord can grow to very large sizes, similar to sacrococcygeal teratoma. The appearance is that of a complex mass in the umbilical cord.
6. Teratomata may arise in the fetal pelvis from an ovary, giving the appearance of a solid pelvic mass.

Occasional Findings:

Hydrops (most common finding), secondary to presence of large vascular tumor

Cardiac abnormalities

Umbilical hernias

Facial clefts

MAJOR DIFFERENTIAL DIAGNOSES

Intracranial:

Aneurysm of the vein of Galen

Brain anomalies

Choroid plexus papilloma

Craniopharyngioma

Intracranial hemorrhage

Multiple porencephalic cysts

Neuroblastoma

Retinoblastoma

Schizencephaly

Tumors

Epignathus:

Conjoined twins

Encephalocele

Neck hemangioma

Sacrococcygeal:

Anterior or posterior meningoceles

Conjoined twins

Hemangioma

Lymphangioma

Neuroectodermal cyst

Mediastinal:

Bronchogenic cyst

Cardiac rhabdomyoma

Pulmonary cystic adenomatoid malformation

Pulmonary sequestration

Cord:

Allantoid cysts

Hemangioma of the cord

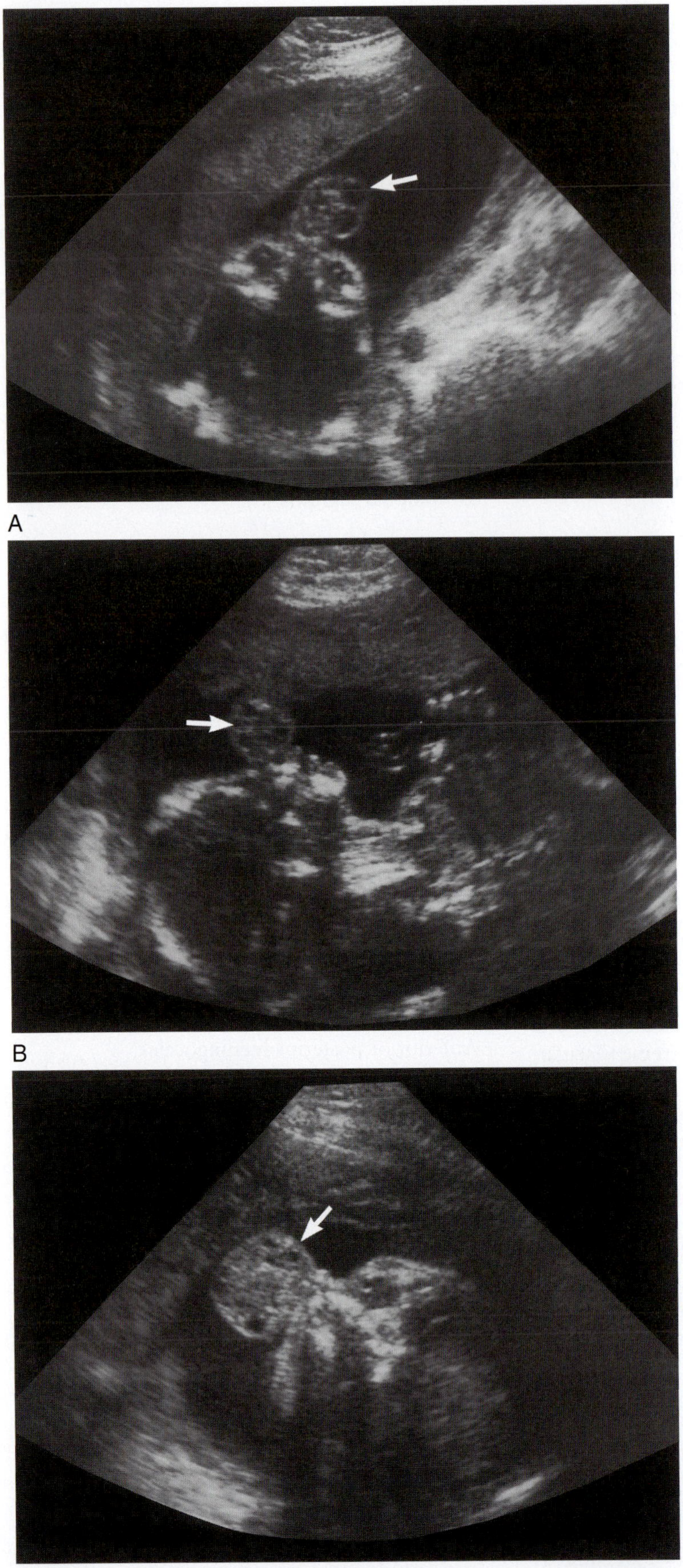

FIGURE 2-340 Transverse (A) and longitudinal (B) views through the level of the fetal nose reveal a nasal teratoma *(arrows)*, detected in the mid second trimester. (C) Follow-up scan, taken a few weeks later, shows growth of the teratoma *(arrow)*. This mass was successfully removed at birth.

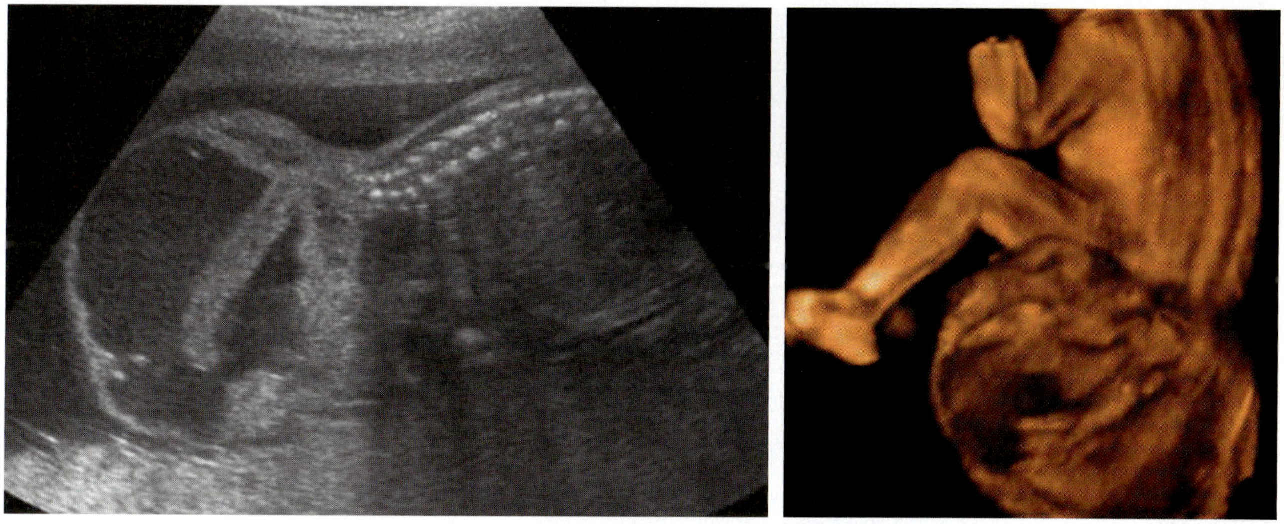

A B

FIGURE 2-341 **(A) View of the fetal buttock and lower spine shows a large cystic sacrococcygeal teratoma. (B) Three-dimensional surface rendering of the same fetus shows the fetus sitting on the large sacrococcygeal teratoma.**

Hematoma of the cord

Omphalomesenteric cysts

ULTRASOUND DIAGNOSIS

Ultrasound diagnosis of a teratoma usually occurs in the late second or third trimester because the tumor enlarges with gestational age. Many patients present because of size greater than dates, secondary to polyhydramnios associated with the tumor.

Intracranial: Diagnosis of intracranial teratomata has been established in the mid second trimester, based on detection of a large intracranial mass at 20 weeks' gestation.

Epignathus: Usually a late second-trimester or early-third trimester diagnosis, it often is prompted by polyhydramnios and a large mass emanating from the fetal mouth or face. A teratoma can occur in the cervical region or thyroid area, and it can present as a large facial or neck mass, similar to epignathus teratoma.

Sacrococcygeal: Prenatal diagnosis has been reported as early as the late first trimester/early second trimester. Follow-up ultrasound examination is required because these masses can grow rapidly and cause congestive heart failure from the vascularity and shunting within the tumor.

Mediastinal: Intrapericardial or mediastinal teratomata, which are uncommon, cause enlargement of the mediastinum by a cystic or solid mass. Usually, the mass eventually causes hydrops. Intrathoracic teratoma usually is a third-trimester diagnosis.

HEREDITY

These tumors occur sporadically.

NATURAL HISTORY AND OUTCOME

Teratomata involving the brain, face, oropharynx, or chest usually are fatal. Sacrococcygeal teratomata often have good outcomes, provided they can be removed successfully after birth.

Suggested Reading

Adzick NS, Crombleholme TM, Morgan MA, Quinn TM: A rapidly growing fetal teratoma. *Lancet* 349:538, 1997.

Alter DN, Reed KL, Marx GR, Anderson CF, Shenker L: Prenatal diagnosis of congestive heart failure in a fetus with a sacrococcygeal teratoma. *Obstet Gynecol* 71:978–981, 1988.

Bader R, Hornberger LK, Nijmeh LJ, et al: Fetal pericardial teratoma: presentation of two cases and review of literature. *Am J Perinatol* 23:53–58, 2006.

Bloechle M, Bollmann J, Wit J, et al: Neuroectodermal cyst may be a rare differential diagnosis of fetal sacrococcygeal teratoma: first case report of a prenatally observed neuroectodermal cyst. *Ultrasound Obstet Gynecol* 7:64–67, 1996.

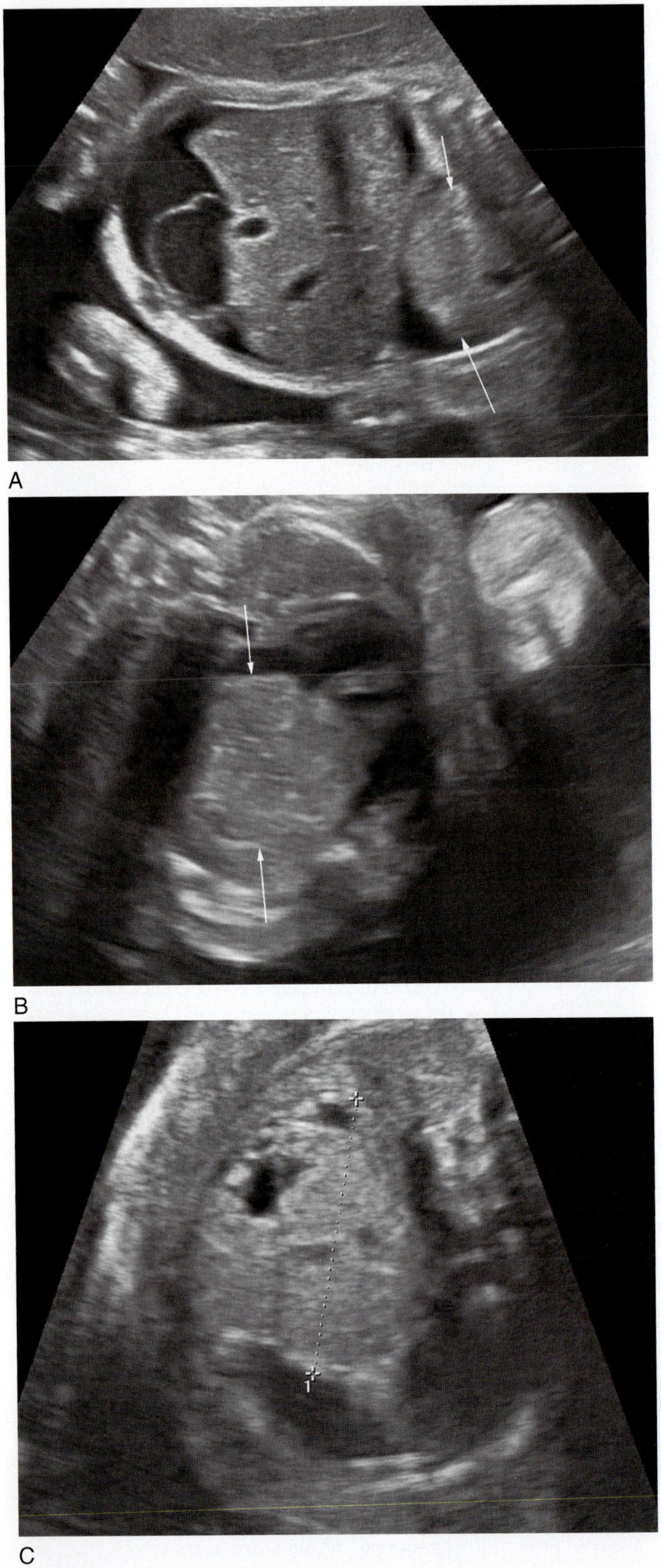

FIGURE 2-342 (A) View of the fetal chest and abdomen of a hydropic fetus shows ascites around the liver. Arrows indicate the pericardial teratoma responsible for the hydrops. (B, C) Transverse view through the fetal chest show the large teratoma *(arrows)* in the pericardium causing compression of the heart.

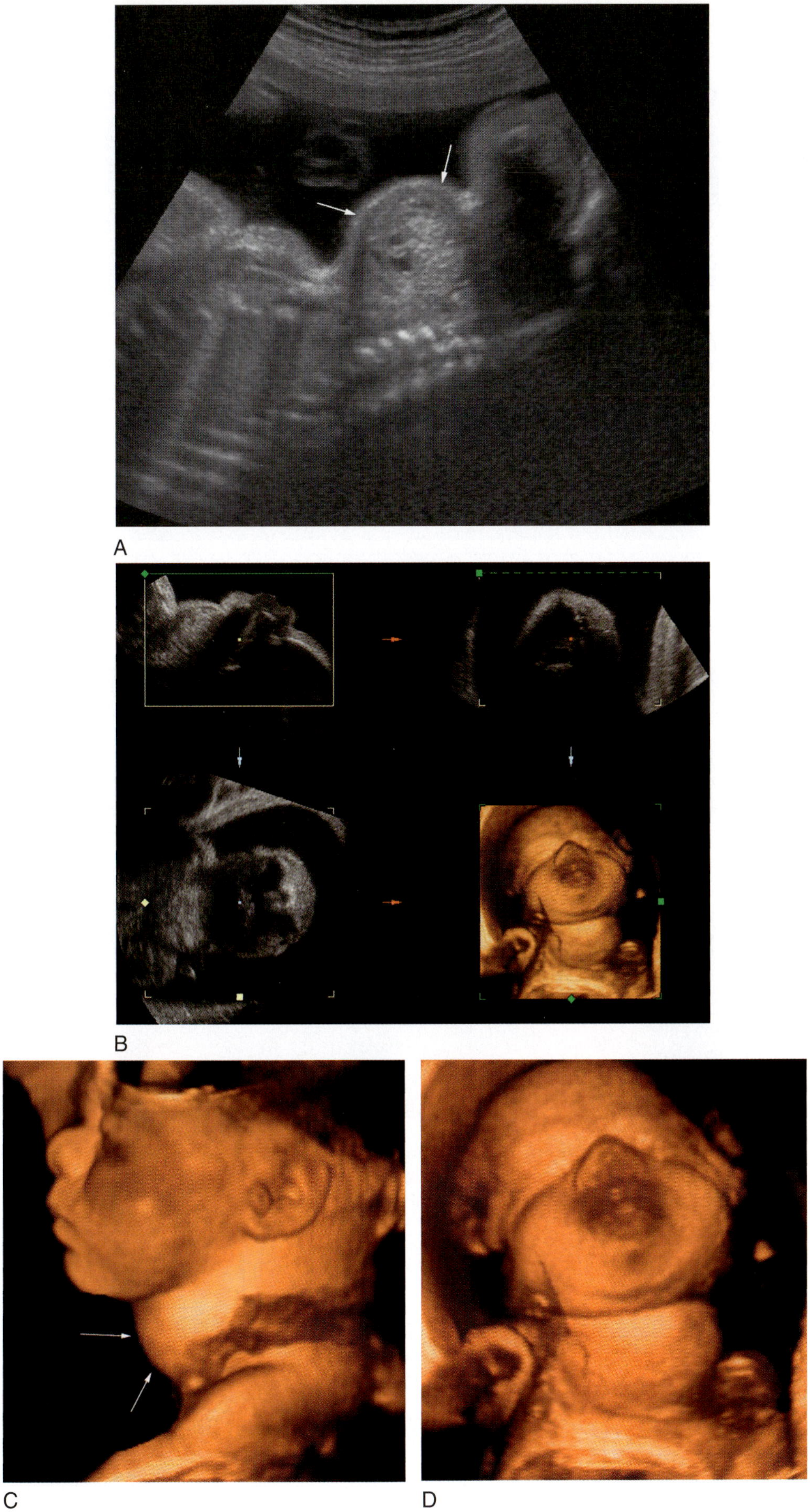

FIGURE 2-343 (A) Longitudinal view of a third-trimester fetus with a large neck mass *(arrows)* that proved to be a thyroid teratoma. (B) Three-dimensional multiplanar display of the enlarged fetal neck. (C, D) Three-dimensional volume displays of the surface of the fetal neck show the hyperextended neck resulting from the tumor *(arrows)*.

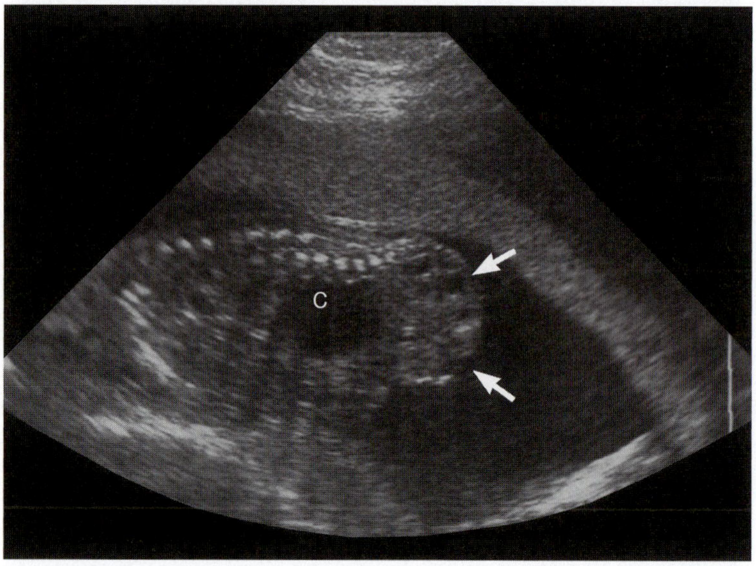

FIGURE 2-344 Longitudinal view of the fetal buttock and lower spine of a fetus with a sacrococcygeal teratoma *(arrows)*. A cystic component *(C)* is noted internally, above the solid component.

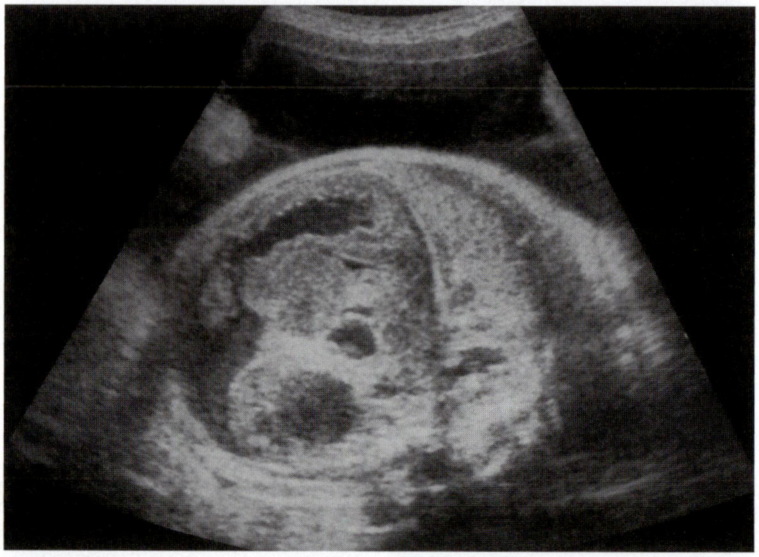

FIGURE 2-345 Transverse view through the abdomen of a third-trimester fetus shows a huge intraabdominal complex mass that was determined to be a sacrococcygeal teratoma. The teratoma is completely intra-abdominal, with very mature elements suggesting fetus in fetu.

Bonilia-Musoles F, Machado LE, Raga F, Osborne NG, Bonilla F Jr: Prenatal diagnosis of sacrococcygeal teratomas by two- and three-dimensional ultrasound. *Ultrasound Obstet Gynecol* 19:200–205, 2002.

Borges E, Lim-Dunham JE, Vade A: Fetus in fetu appearing as a prenatal neck mass. *J Ultrasound Med* 24:1313–1316, 2005.

Chen CP, Shih JC, Huang JK, Wang W, Tzen CY: Second-trimester evaluation of fetal sacrococcygeal teratoma using three-dimensional color Doppler ultrasound and magnetic resonance imaging. *Prenat Diagn* 23:602–603, 2003.

Chervenak FA, Isaacson G, Touloukian R, et al: Diagnosis and management of fetal teratomas. *Obstet Gynecol* 66:666–671, 1985.

Chervenak FA, Tortora M, Moya FR, Hobbins JC: Antenatal sonographic diagnosis of epignathus. *J Ultrasound Med* 3:235–237, 1984.

Clement K, Chamberlain P, Boyd P, Molyneux A: Prenatal diagnosis of an epignathus: a case report and review of the literature. *Ultrasound Obstet Gynecol* 18:178–181, 2001.

Dolkart LA, Balcom RJ, Eisinger G: Intracranial teratoma: prolonged neonatal survival after prenatal diagnosis. *Am J Obstet Gynecol* 162:768–769, 1990.

Fox DB, Bruner JP, Fleischer AC: Amplitude-based color Doppler sonography of fetus with sacrococcygeal teratoma. *J Ultrasound Med* 15:785–787, 1996.

Gross SJ, Benzie RJ, Sermer M, Skidmore MB, Wilson SR: Sacrococcygeal teratoma: prenatal diagnosis and management. *Am J Obstet Gynecol* 156:393–396, 1987.

Hogge WA, Thiagarajah S, Barber VG, Rodgers BM, Newman BM: Cystic sacrococcygeal teratoma: ultrasound diagnosis and perinatal management. *J Ultrasound Med* 6:707–710, 1987.

Langer JC, Harrison MR, Schmidt KG, et al: Fetal hydrops and death from sacrococcygeal teratoma: rationale for fetal surgery. *Am J Obstet Gynecol* 160:1145–1150, 1989.

Lees RF, Williamson BRJ, Brenbridge ANAG, Buschi AJ, Teja K: Sonography of benign sacral teratoma in utero. *Radiology* 134:717–718, 1980.

Lipman SP, Pretorius DH, Rumack CM, Manco-Johnson ML: Fetal intracranial teratoma: US diagnosis of three cases and a review of the literature. *Radiology* 157:491–494, 1985.

Merhi ZO, Haberman S, Roberts JL, Sobol-Benin G: Prenatal diagnosis of palatal teratoma by 3-dimensional sonography and color Doppler imaging. *J Ultrasound Med* 24:1317–1320, 2005.

Mintz MC, Mennuti M, Fishman M: Prenatal aspiration of sacrococcygeal teratoma. *AJR Am J Roentgenol* 141:367–368, 1983.

Montz FJ, Horenstein J, Platt LD, et al: The diagnosis of immature teratoma by maternal serum alpha-fetoprotein screening. *Obstet Gynecol* 73:522–525, 1989.

Ogamo M, Sugiyama T, Maeda Y, et al: The ex utero intrapartum treatment (EXIT) procedure in giant fetal neck masses. *Fetal Diagn Ther* 20:214–218, 2005.

Paes BA, DeSa DJ, Hunter DJS, Pirani M: Benign intracranial teratoma—prenatal diagnosis influencing early delivery. *Am J Obstet Gynecol* 143:600–601, 1982.

Palo P, Penttinen M, Kalimo H: Early ultrasound diagnosis of fetal intracranial tumors. *J Clin Ultrasound* 22:447–450, 1994.

Patel RB, Gibson JY, D'Cruz CA, Burkhalter JL: Sonographic diagnosis of cervical teratoma in utero. *AJR Am J Roentgenol* 139:1220–1222, 1982.

Perez-Aytes A, Sanchis N, Barbal A, et al: Nonimmunological hydrops fetalis and intrapericardial teratoma: case report and review. *Prenat Diagn* 15:859–863, 1995.

Richards SR: Ultrasonic diagnosis of intracranial teratoma in utero: a case report and literature review. *J Reprod Med* 32:73–75, 1987.

Roman AS, Monteagudo A, Timor-Tritsch I, Rebarber A: First-trimester diagnosis of sacrococcygeal teratoma: the role of three-dimensional ultrasound. *Ultrasound Obstet Gynecol* 23:612–614, 2004.

Romero R: *Prenatal diagnosis of congenital anomalies.* East Norwalk, CT, 1988, Appleton & Lange.

Seeds JW, Mittelstaedt CA, Cefalo RC, Parker TF Jr: Prenatal diagnosis of sacrococcygeal teratoma: an anechoic caudal mass. *J Clin Ultrasound* 10:193–195, 1982.

Sherer DM, Abramowicz JS, Eggers PC, et al: Prenatal ultrasonographic diagnosis of intracranial teratoma and massive craniomegaly with associated high-output cardiac failure. *Am J Obstet Gynecol* 168:97–99, 1993.

Sherer DM, Woods JR Jr, Abramowicz JS, et al: Prenatal sonographic assessment of early, rapidly growing fetal cervical teratoma. *Prenat Diagn* 13:1079–1084, 1993.

Sherowski RC, Williams CH, Nichols VB, Singh KB: Prenatal ultrasonographic diagnosis of a sacrococcygeal teratoma in twin pregnancy. *J Ultrasound Med* 4:159–161, 1985.

Sheth S, Nussbaum AR, Sanders RC, Hamper UM, Davidson AJ: Prenatal diagnosis of sacrococcygeal teratoma: sonographic-pathologic correlation. *Radiology* 169:131–136, 1988.

Shipp TD, Shamberger RC, Benacerraf BR: Prenatal diagnosis of a grade IV sacrococcygeal teratoma. *J Ultrasound Med* 15:175–177, 1996.

ten Broeke EDM, Verdonk GW, Roumen FJME: Prenatal ultrasound diagnosis of an intracranial teratoma influencing management: case report and review of the literature. *Eur J Obstet Gynecol Reprod Biol* 45:210–214, 1992.

Trecet JC, Claramunt V, Larraz J, et al: Prenatal ultrasound diagnosis of fetal teratoma of the neck. *J Clin Ultrasound* 12:509–511, 1984.

APPENDIX 2-1

Growth Restriction Syndromes

	Skull/Spine Abnormalities	Central Nervous System Abnormalities	Facial Abnormalities	Thickened Nuchal Lucency/Cystic Hygroma	Extremity Abnormalities
Cornelia de Lange syndrome	Brachycephaly	Microcephaly	Micrognathia	Nuchal thickening/ cystic hygroma	Micromelia (upper and lower extremities), ulna dysplasia, contractures of upper extremities
Noonan syndrome	Hemivertebrae		Hypertelorism, low-set ears	First-trimester lucency, second-trimester cystic hygromata, may lead to hydrops	
Russell-Silver syndrome			Prominent forehead, micrognathia		Limb asymmetry, short long-bones
Seckel syndrome		Microcephaly	Severe micrognathia, prominent nose		
Smith-Lemli-Opitz syndrome		Microcephaly, occasional cerebellar hypoplasia, occasional ventriculomegaly, occasional ACC, occasional holoprosencephaly	Occasional micrognathia, occasional cleft palate, occasional cataracts, occasional hypertelorism	Nuchal thickening	Clenched hands, valgus feet
Beckwith-Wiedemann syndrome			Macroglossia		
Maternal diabetes		Anencephaly, neural tube defects, caudal regression syndrome			
Perlman syndrome				First-trimester lucency/cystic hygroma	

ACC, Agenesis of the corpus callosum; *ASD,* atrial septal defect; *IUGR,* intrauterine growth restriction; *VSD,* ventricular septal defect.

Abnormal Digits	Cardiac Defects	Genitourinary or GI Abnormalities	Growth	Other
Syndactyly (upper and lower extremities), oligodactyly	Cardiac defects, VSD, ASD	Undescended testicles, hypospadias	IUGR (onset >20 wk)	
	Cardiac defects, VSD, ASD, pulmonic stenosis	Micropenis, cryptorchidism	Short stature (late or postnatal onset)	
Syndactyly (second and third toes), clinodactyly (fifth finger)			IUGR onset in second trimester	
Dislocated joints (esp. at radial heads), flexion deformities at hips and knees			Early-onset IUGR	
Syndactyly (second and third toes), postaxial polydactyly	Cardiac defects	Hydronephrosis, cystic kidneys, hypoplastic kidneys, micropenis, cryptorchidism, hypospadias, ambiguous genitalia	Late-onset IUGR	
	Occasional cardiomegaly	Enlarged kidneys, omphalocele, occasional enlarged pancreas, occasional hypospadias and cryptorchidism	Organ hypertrophy	Occasional placental molar appearance, polyhydramnios
	Cardiac defects	Renal anomalies		Polyhydramnios
	Cardiac defects	Enlarged kidneys, renal tumors, ascites, visceromegaly	Organ hypertrophy, macrosomia	Polyhydramnios

APPENDIX 2-2

Facial Anomalies

	Central Nervous System Abnormalities	Facial Abnormalities	Extremity Abnormalities
Branchio-oculo-facial syndrome	Occasional microcephaly	Microphthalmia, anophthalmia, pseudo-cleft lip, occasional orbital cyst, occasional cataract, occasional cleft palate, occasional ear abnormality	
Cerebrocosto-mandibular syndrome	Occasional microcephaly, occasional brain abnormality, occasional neural tube defect	Micrognathia, occasional choanal atresia	Occasional hypoplasia of the bones of upper extremities, occasional club feet
Fraser syndrome	Occasional microcephaly, occasional hydrocephalus and neural tube defect	Nose abnormalities, cryptophthalmos, ear abnormalities, occasional facial cleft and hypertelorism	
Goldenhar syndrome	Occasional ventriculomegaly	Mandible hypoplasia, asymmetry of jaw soft tissues, microphthalmia, ear abnormalities, occasional facial cleft	
Median cleft face	Occasional agenesis of corpus callosum, occasional lipoma of the corpus callosum, occasional frontal encephalocele	Malformed nose, hypertelorism, occasional microphthalmia	
Nager syndrome		Severe micrognathia, mandibular hypoplasia, cleft palate, occasional cleft lip, malformed low-set ears	Short radial ray, occasional limb reduction defects, occasional club feet
Oral-facial-digital syndrome 1 (OFD1)	Hydrocephalus, vermian hypoplasia, ACC, porencephaly	Median facial cleft, occasional facial asymmetry	
Oral-facial-digital syndrome II (Mohr)	Occasional ventriculomegaly, occasional porencephaly, occasional encephalocele, occasional lipoma, ACC, and other brain defects	Micrognathia, facial clefts, broad nasal bridge, bifid nasal tip, multiple tongue tumors	
Pierre Robin syndrome		Micrognathia, cleft palate	
Shprintzen syndrome	Microcephaly, occasional holoprosencephaly	Micrognathia, facial cleft, occasional Pierre Robin sequence (micrognathia and cleft palate)	Short long-bones
Stickler syndrome		Micrognathia, cleft palate, cataracts	Club feet
Treacher Collins syndrome		Micrognathia, abnormal orbits with ocular fissures slanted downward, hypoplastic zygomata, malformed ears with absent or low-set hypoplastic auricles and skin tags, choanal atresia, cleft palate	

ACC, Agenesis of the corpus callosum; *IUGR*, intrauterine growth restriction; *VSD*, ventricular septal defect.

Abnormal Digits	Spine Abnormalities	Cardiac Defects	Genitourinary or Gastrointestinal Abnormalities	Thoraco-abdominal Abnormalities	Other
Occasional polydactyly			Occasional renal agenesis		IUGR
	Hemivertebrae, occasional scoliosis	Occasional VSD	Occasional renal anomalies, occasional omphalocele	Narrow chest, decreased ossification of ribs, rib anomalies	Cystic hygroma/ nuchal thickening, polyhydramnios
Syndactyly			Genital abnormalities, urinary tract abnormalities, renal agenesis, occasional ascites	Laryngeal stenosis or atresia	
	Cervical/ thoracic hemivertebrae	Occasional cardiac defects	Occasional unilateral renal anomalies	Occasional unilateral lung anomalies	Polyhydramnios
		Occasional cardiac defects			
Thumb hypoplasia, digit abnormalities, occasional syndactyly, occasional clinodactyly					Polyhydramnios
Shortening of digits, clinodactyly, polydactyly, syndactyly			Adult-type polycystic kidney disease		
Polysyndactyly, bifid hallux, clinodactyly of fifth digit					
					Polyhydramnios
		Cardiac defects	Occasional cryptorchidism, occasional hypospadias	Occasional umbilical hernia	
					Polyhydramnios

APPENDIX 2-3

Brain Anomaly Syndromes

	Central Nervous System Abnormalities	Facial Abnormalities	Thickened Nuchal Lucency/Cystic Hygroma
Aicardi syndrome	Ventriculomegaly, ACC, interhemispheric cyst, occasional Dandy-Walker abnormality, occasional cortical heterotopia	Asymmetric orbits	
Gorlin syndrome	Macrocephaly, ventriculomegaly, calcification of the falx, occasional agenesis of the corpus callosum	Prognathism, cleft lip and palate, frontal bossing, occasional hypertelorism	
Hydrolethalus	Ventriculomegaly, neural tube defect	Micrognathia, cleft lip and palate, low-set ears, microphthalmia	Thickened nuchal translucency
Joubert	Dandy-Walker variant, occipital encephalocele, ventriculomegaly	Micrognathia	Thickened nuchal fold
Meckel-Gruber syndrome	Ventriculomegaly, microcephaly, posterior encephalocele, cerebellar hypoplasia, agenesis of the corpus callosum, Dandy-Walker abnormalities, Arnold-Ciari malformation	Micrognathia, cleft palate, microphthalmia	
Miller-Dieker syndrome (lissencephaly, type I)	Lack of normal gyri, mild ventriculomegaly, prominent sylvian fissure, underdeveloped corpus callosum, late-developing microcephaly		
Neu-Laxova syndrome	Microcephaly, lissencephaly, absent corpus callosum, hypoplastic cerebellum and cerebrum, occasional Dandy-Walker malformation, occasional ventriculomegaly, occasional hydranencephaly, occasional spina bifida	Micrognathia, hypertelorism with protruding eyes and absent lids, cataracts, microphthalmia, occasional facial clefting	
Septo-optic dysplasia	Absent cavum septi pellucidi, communication between frontal horns, ventriculomegaly, agenesis or thinned corpus callosum, occasional schizencephaly	Occasional craniofacial anomalies	
Walker-Warburg	Microcephaly, agyria, lissencephaly, ventriculomegaly, occipital encephalocele, Dandy-Walker, agenesis of the corpus callosum	Microphthalmia, cataracts, occasional cleft lip	
X-linked hydrocephalus	Ventriculomegaly of the lateral ventricles with a normal fourth ventricle		

ACC, Agenesis of the corpus callosum; *IUGR,* intrauterine growth restriction; *VSD,* ventricular septal defect.

Extremity Abnormalities	Abnormal Digits	Skeletal Abnormalities	Cardiac Defects	Miscellaneous Abnormalities	IUGR
		Occasional hemivertebrae			
	Short fourth metacarpal	Misshapen ribs, scoliosis, vertebral abnormalities			
Club feet	Postaxial polydactyly of the hands, hallux duplication		VSD, endocardial cushion defect	Hypospadias, polyhydramnios	
	Polydactyly			Multicystic kidneys	
	Polydactyly		Cardiac defects	Cystic dysplasia of the kidneys, cryptorchidism, oligohydramnios (due to renal dysplasia)	
			Cardiac defects	Renal dysplasia, duodenal atresia, cryptorchidism, polyhydramnios	IUGR
Short limbs, edema of hands and feet, flexion contractures	Syndactyly of fingers	Short neck	Occasional cardiac defects	Hypoplastic genitals, abnormal skin with swollen subcutaneous tissue and ichthyosis	Severe, early-onset IUGR
				Occasional genital abnormalities	
Adducted thumbs flexed over palms					

APPENDIX 2-4

Limb Abnormalities

	Central Nervous System Abnormalities	Facial Abnormalities	Thickened Nuchal Lucency/ Cystic Hygroma	Extremity Abnormalities
Adams-Oliver syndrome	Occasional encephalocele, occasional acrania, occasional microcephaly	Occasional facial cleft		Transverse limb defects, occasional club feet
Ectrodactyly–ectodermal dysplasia–clefting (EEC) syndrome	Occasional semilobar holoprosencephaly	Cleft lip with or without cleft palate, facial cleft, occasional choanal atresia, occasional micrognathia occasional malformed ears	Occasional cystic hygroma	
Fanconi anemia	Occasional ventriculomegaly, occasional absence of the corpus callosum, occasional microcephaly	Occasional microphthalmos	Thickened nuchal translucency	Short radial ray
Femoral hypoplasia–unusual facies syndrome		Micrognathia, cleft palate, low-set ears		Short, bowed femurs (bilateral or unilateral), variable hypoplasia of the humeri, club feet
Femur–fibula–ulna (FFU) syndrome				Hypoplasia or aplasia of the femur and fibula, absence of the arm, para-axial hemimelia of the ulna and fibula with lesser involvement of the humerus
Freeman-Sheldon syndrome (whistling face)	Microcephaly	Sloping forehead, small nose, deep-set eyes, long philtrum		Ulna deviation of the hands with flexion deformity of the fingers, contractures of hip and knee, club feet
Holt-Oram syndrome			Thickened nuchal translucency	Phocomelia, radius hypoplasia, ulna and humerus abnormalities, more severe on left side
Larsen syndrome		Depressed nasal bridge, cleft palate, hypertelorism, occasional cleft lip		Hyperextension at knees, dislocations at elbows, hips, and knees; club feet
Multiple pterygium syndrome (lethal type)	Occasional microcephaly, occasional ventriculomegaly	Micrognathia, cleft palate, hypertelorism	Neck edema, consistent with cystic hygroma	Flexion contractures of all joints of extremities

ASD, Atrial septal defect; *IUGR,* intrauterine growth restriction; *VSD,* ventricular septal defect.

Abnormal Digits	Other Skeletal Anomalies	Cardiac Defects	Genitourinary Abnormalities	Gastro-intestinal Abnormalities	Miscellaneous Anomalies	IUGR
Transverse limb (digital) defects of hands and feet, occasional syndactyly	Decreased ossification of areas of the skull	Occasional cardiac defects				
Syndactyly, ectrodactyly			Megaureter, ureterocele, hydronephrosis, renal aplasia, genital abnormalities			
Thumb and digit abnormalities		Occasional cardiac defects	Renal, ureter, and genital abnormalities	Occasional gastrointestinal obstruction		
	Vertebral abnormalities, sacral dysplasia		Urinary tract abnormalities			
Abnormal digits, absence of the fingers						
	Kyphoscoliosis		Incomplete descent of testes			IUGR
Absent thumbs, syndactyly	Clavicle abnormalities	Cardiac defects, ASD, VSD				
	Dysraphia, scoliosis, vertebral abnormalities	Occasional heart defects			Occasional tracheomalacia	
	Small chest, occasional vertebral body abnormalities	Occasional heart defects	Occasional hydronephrosis		Hydrops, pterygia involving cervical, chin area, axillary, antecubital popliteal, and ankle joints, polyhydramnios	

Continued

APPENDIX 2-4

Limb Abnormalities—cont'd

	Central Nervous System Abnormalities	Facial Abnormalities	Thickened Nuchal Lucency/ Cystic Hygroma	Extremity Abnormalities
Roberts syndrome	Microcephaly, occasional ventriculomegaly, occasional craniosynostosis, occasional encephalocele	Micrognathia, cleft lip and palate, hypertelorism, occasional microphthalmia, occasional cataracts	Occasional cystic hygromata	Severe hypomelia of limbs (more severe in upper limbs), short radial ray, absence or hypoplasia of humerus, femur, tibia, and fibula, flexion contractures of all joints of extremities
Thrombocytopenia–absent radius (TAR) syndrome	Occasional vermian hypoplasia	Occasional micrognathia, occasional cleft palate		Bilateral absence of radius with hypoplasia or absence of ulna, abnormal humerus, abnormal lower extremities, absence of fibulae, dislocations of lower extremities

ASD, Atrial septal defect; *IUGR,* intrauterine growth restriction; *VSD,* ventricular septal defect.

Abnormal Digits	Other Skeletal Anomalies	Cardiac Defects	Genitourinary Abnormalities	Gastro-intestinal Abnormalities	Miscellaneous Anomalies	IUGR
Oligodactyly, syndactyly		Occasional heart defect	Cryptorchidism, occasional renal abnormalities, occasional abnormal genitalia		Occasional polyhydramnios	IUGR
Thumbs are always present!		Occasional heart defects, including tetralogy of Fallot, ASD	Occasional renal anomalies			

APPENDIX 2-5

Skeletal Dysplasias

	Skull Abnormalities	Central Nervous System Abnormalities	Facial Abnormalities	Extremity Abnormalities
Achondrogenesis, types I and II (Parenti-Fraccaro and Langer-Saldino)	Large skull, poorly ossified skull (type I)		Micrognathia	Limb shortening (more severe in type I, more variable in type II)
Achondroplasia, heterozygous	Frontal bossing, increased BPD	Megalocephaly, occasional mild ventriculomegaly	Frontal bossing, depressed nasal bridge	Mild to moderately short femur and humerus, short trident hand
Atelosteogenesis, type I (lethal chondrodysplasia)			Depressed nasal bridge, micrognathia, hypertelorism	Gross shortening and deficient ossification of all limbs, markedly foreshortened humerus and femur, proximal flaring of humerus and femur, bowed radius, ulna, and tibia, absent fibula, club feet
Camptomelic dysplasia	Occasional large BPD	Ventriculomegaly	Cleft palate, micrognathia, hypertelorism, occasional depressed nasal bridge	Marked bowing of femur and tibia that may mimic a fracture, hypoplastic fibula, occasional club feet
Chondrodysplasia punctata, non-rhizomelic type (Conradi-Hunermann)			Depressed nasal bridge, occasional microphthalmia	Asymmetric shortening of extremities, abnormally early calcification of the proximal and distal epiphyses of the humerus and femur
Chondrodysplasia punctata, rhizomelic type	Brachycephaly	Ventriculomegaly, microcephaly	Hypertelorism, cataracts, depressed nasal bridge, occasional cleft palate	Symmetric, proximal shortening of humerus and femur
Cleidocranial dysostosis			Midface hypoplasia, hypertelorism, occasional cleft palate and nasal hypoplasia, occasional micrognathia	Normal long bones!
Diastrophic dysplasia			Micrognathia, cleft palate	Shortening of all long bones, with femurs measuring below 5th percentile, hitchhiker thumb, club feet
Ellis-van Creveld syndrome		Occasional Dandy-Walker malformation		Short long-bones, occasional club feet
Hypochondroplasia	Occasional mild frontal bossing	Macrocephaly	Occasional cataracts	Slightly short long-bones of all limbs (mainly in the third trimester)

ACC, Agenesis of the corpus callosum; *BPD,* biparietal diameter; *IUGR,* intrauterine growth restriction.

Abnormal Digits	Other Skeletal Anomalies	Narrow Chest	Cardiac Defects	Genitourinary Abnormalities	Miscellaneous
	Short, flared ribs, poorly ossified iliac bones, especially spine (and skull)	Narrow chest			Polyhydramnios, hydrops, thickened nuchal lucency
Trident hand with fingers of similar lengths	Accentuated lumbar lordosis				Occasional thickened nuchal translucency
	Abnormal vertebral bodies, thoracic platyspondyly with coronal clefts, narrow thoracic cage	Narrow chest			Polyhydramnios
	Bell-shaped, narrow chest, hypoplastic scapula	Narrow chest	Occasional cardiac defects	Ambiguous genitalia in males, occasional large kidneys, occasional hydronephrosis	Occasional nuchal translucency
	Spinal kyphoscoliosis, vertebral abnormalities		Occasional cardiac defects		
	Abnormal epiphyseal echogenicity			Occasional hypospadias and cryptorchidism	Occasional diaphragmatic hernia
	Shortening or absence of the clavicle, hypoplastic iliac bones with normal long bones, delayed mineralization of the pubic bone				
	Kyphoscoliosis		Cardiac defects		Polyhydramnios
Polydactyly of the hands, occasional polydactyly of the toes	Narrow thorax with short ribs, (short long-bones)	Narrow chest	Cardiac defects, including septal defects	Occasional cryptorchidism, occasional renal agenesis	Thickened nuchal translucency
Occasional postaxial polydactyly of the feet	Occasional narrowing of the spinal canal in the lumbar region				

Continued

APPENDIX 2-5

Skeletal Dysplasias—cont'd

	Skull Abnormalities	Central Nervous System Abnormalities	Facial Abnormalities	Extremity Abnormalities
Hypophosphatasia of the lethal type	Marked demineralization of the calvaria, soft-appearing skull with increased visualization of the brain			Short, bowed, demineralized bones with fractures
Jeune thoracic dystrophy (asphyxiating thoracic dysplasia)				Short long-bones (second or third trimester)
Kniest syndrome (metatropic dwarfism, type II)			Cleft palate, occasional cataracts	Short long-bones with bowing and irregular epiphyses (third trimester)
Majewski syndrome		Occasional small cerebellar vermis	Facial cleft	Short limbs, with shortening of all long bones
Metatropic dysplasia	Enlarged BPD	Occasional ventriculomegaly		Markedly shortened limbs with disproportionately long hands and feet, shortened femur, metaphyseal flaring
Osteopetrosis of the lethal type		Ventriculomegaly		Shortened long-bones
Short rib–polydactyly syndromes, types I and III				Severe micromelia with metaphyseal flaring
Spondyloepiphyseal dysplasia congenita			Flat facies	Slightly short long-bones, although limbs may not be short, lag in mineralization of epiphyses of long bones, flared epiphyses, club feet
Thanatophoric dysplasia, type I		Ventriculomegaly, occasional ACC	Small facies, depressed nasal bridge, full forehead	"Telephone receiver," very short long-bones (particularly the femur), fibulae shorter than tibiae
Thanatophoric dysplasia, type II	Cloverleaf-shaped skull	Occasional ACC		Curved, short long-bones (although femora are straighter than those found in type I)

Abnormal Digits	Other Skeletal Anomalies	Narrow Chest	Cardiac Defects	Genitourinary Abnormalities	Miscellaneous
	Marked demineralization of the calvaria, bowed tubular bones that are short and demineralized with multiple fractures				Thickened nuchal translucency
Occasional polydactyly	Short, horizontal ribs, narrow chest	Narrow chest			Occasional thickened nuchal translucency
	Lumbar kyphoscoliosis with platyspondyly				Inguinal hernia
Preaxial and postaxial polydactyly of the hands and feet	Narrow thorax with short ribs	Narrow chest		Occasional renal abnormalities	Polyhydramnios
	Long and narrow thorax, platyspondylia with progressive kyphoscoliosis	Narrow chest			
	Increased bone density, bone fractures				IUGR
Polydactyly	Extremely short ribs, underossified and distorted vertebral bodies	Narrow chest	Cardiac defects, including transposition of the great vessels, endocardial cushion defect, double-outlet right ventricle	Hypoplastic or polycystic kidneys, ambiguous genitalia	Imperforate anus, intestinal atresia
	Short neck and spine with platyspondylia and narrow intervertebral distances, kyphoscoliosis, lordosis, no ossification of the pubis, calcaneus, or talus				
	Narrow and short ribs with a small chest, platyspondyly	Narrow chest	Occasional cardiac defects	Occasional hydronephrosis	Polyhydramnios, occasional thickened nuchal translucency
	Mild platyspondyly	Narrow chest	Occasional cardiac defects	Occasional hydronephrosis	Occasional thickened nuchal translucency

APPENDIX 2-6
Craniosynostosis

	Skull Abnormalities	Central Nervous System Abnormalities	Facial Abnormalities	Extremity Abnormalities
Antley-Bixler syndrome	Craniosynostosis, abnormally shaped skull, frontal bossing	Occasional ventriculomegaly	Micrognathia, midface hypoplasia, choanal atresia	Radiohumeral synostosis, joint contractures, bowed bones (esp. femur), rockerbottom feet
Apert syndrome (acrocephalosyndactyly, type I)	Craniosynostosis, brachycephaly, acrocephaly, flat occiput	Agenesis of the corpus callosum, mild ventriculomegaly	High forehead, flat face, hypertelorism	Occasional upper extremity long-bone abnormalities
Carpenter syndrome (acrocephalosyndactyly, type II)	Craniosynostosis, brachycephaly, acrocephaly		Depressed nasal bridge, micrognathia, low-set ears	
Crouzon syndrome (craniofacial dysostosis type I)	Craniosynostosis, abnormally shaped skull, occasional cloverleaf skull	Occasional ventriculomegaly, occasional agenesis of the corpus callosum	Beaked nose, micrognathia, hypertelorism or hypotelorism, occasional cleft lip and palate	
Pfeiffer syndrome (acrofacial dysostosis)	Craniosynostosis, brachycephaly, acrocephaly, occasional cloverleaf skull	Occasional ventriculomegaly	Depressed nasal bridge, hypertelorism, occasional choanal atresia	
Saethre-Chotzen syndrome	Craniosynostosis (coronal suture)		Facial asymmetry caused by unilateral coronal synostosis	

ASD, Atrial septal defect; *VSD*, ventricular septal defect.

Abnormal Digits	Skeletal Anomalies	Cardiac Defects	Genitourinary Abnormalities	Miscellaneous Anomalies
		Occasional cardiac anomalies	Occasional renal anomalies, occasional ambiguous genitalia	Polyhydramnios, decreased fetal activity
Syndactyly (osseous and cutaneous); particularly of second, third, and fourth fingers; broad thumb and hallux	Fusion of cervical vertebrae at C5–C6	Occasional cardiac defects, such as tetralogy of Fallot	Occasional cystic kidneys, occasional hydronephrosis, occasional cryptorchidism	Abnormal nuchal lucency (first trimester), occasional diaphragmatic hernia
Clinodactyly, syndactyly, polydactyly, preaxial polydactyly of feet or wide hallux		Cardiac defects, such as ASD, VSD, tetralogy of Fallot, transposition of the great arteries	Hypogonadism, cryptorchidism	Omphalocele
Broad thumb and hallux, partial syndactyly	Occasional fused vertebrae	Occasional cardiac anomalies		Occasional tracheal abnormalities
Duplicated hallux, syndactyly hands and feet				

APPENDIX 2-7

Miscellaneous Syndromes

	Central Nervous System Abnormalities	Abnormal Facies	Thickened Nuchal Lucency/Cystic Hygroma	Abnormal Digits
Cystic fibrosis				
Fryns syndrome	Ventriculomegaly, Dandy-Walker malformation, agenesis of the corpus callosum	Micrognathia, cleft lip and palate, broad nasal bridge, abnormal ear shape, occasional microphthalmia	Cystic hygroma	Distal digital hypoplasia
Infantile polycystic kidney disease		Micrognathia		
Jarcho-Levin syndrome (spondylothoracic dysplasia)	Occasional neural tube defect	Occasional cleft palate	Thickened nuchal translucency	

VSD, Ventricular septal defect.

Skeletal Anomalies	Cardiac Defects	Thoracoabdominal/ Genitourinary Abnormalities	Miscellaneous
		Hyperechogenic bowel (second and third trimesters), dilated loops of bowel (second and third trimester), fixed and mildly dilated loops of small bowel without obstruction (second trimester), meconium peritonitis	Polyhydramnios
	Occasional cardiac defects, such as VSD	Diaphragmatic hernia, renal cysts, intestinal malrotation, uterine abnormalities, cryptorchidism, hypospadias	Occasional hydrops, polyhydramnios
	Congenital heart defects, such as VSD	Hepatic cysts (not usually seen on prenatal sonogram), enlarged, echogenic kidneys with lack of normal architecture	Severe oligohydramnios (variable onset)
Multiple abnormalities of vertebral bodies, particularly the thoracic spine, short spine, short neck, lordosis, kyphoscoliosis, crab-like flaring or absence of some of the ribs		Occasional cryptorchidism, occasional abnormal genitals, occasional hydronephrosis	Protuberant abdomen (because of short spine), occasional single umbilical artery

APPENDIX 2-8

Soft-Tissue Anomalies

	Fetal Surface Anomalies	Skull Abnormalities	Central Nervous System Abnormalities	Abnormal Facies	Extremity Abnormalities
Alpha-thalassemia					
Aplasia cutis congenita (ACC)	Skin irregularities, snowflake effect in amniotic fluid				
Harlequin syndrome	Thick anterior membrane, consistent with desquamated skin, "snowflake" effect in amniotic fluid			Large, wide-open, oval mouth, tiny nose, protuberant eyes	Swollen hands and legs, fixed flexion of extremities
Klippel-Trenaunay-Weber syndrome	Multiple cutaneous hemangiomata			Occasional asymmetric facial hypertrophy	Limb hypertrophy, long-bone asymmetry
Marfan syndrome				Occasional cataracts, occasional cleft palate	Tall stature (although the abnormal biometry is difficult to detect)
Osteogenesis imperfecta, type II	Thickened nuchal translucency, hydrops	Severe demineralization of the skull			Limb shortening and angulation, bone cortical surface wrinkling caused by severe fractures of all bones

IUGR, Intrauterine growth restriction.

Other Skeletal Anomalies	Cardiac Defects	Genitourinary Abnormalities	Gastrointestinal Abnormalities	Miscellaneous Anomalies	IUGR
	Cardiomegaly		Hyperechoic bowel	Severe hydrops, ascites, subcutaneous edema with cord edema, pericardial or pleural effusions, hepatosplenomegaly, oligohydramnios or polyhydramnios	
			Occasional pyloric atresia		
				Decreased fetal activity	IUGR
			Occasional gastrointestinal tract involvement with hemangiomata	Occasional retroperitoneum visceral involvement with hemangiomata, occasional lymphangiectasia	
Occasional scoliosis, occasional hemivertebrae	Cardiac abnormalities, focusing on the ascending aorta, aortic valves, and (less commonly) the pulmonary artery or descending aorta, occasional cardiac dysrhythmia		Occasional diaphragmatic hernia		
Bell-shaped or narrow chest caused by rib fractures				Decreased fetal movements	

Continued

APPENDIX 2-8

Soft-Tissue Anomalies—cont'd

	Fetal Surface Anomalies	Skull Abnormalities	Central Nervous System Abnormalities	Abnormal Facies	Extremity Abnormalities
Proteus syndrome	Large cystic spaces in the soft tissues of the limbs	Occasional craniosynostosis	Macrocephaly	Occasional ocular abnormalities	Limb enlargement, with large cystic spaces in the soft tissues, overgrowth (localized or overall), macrodactyly
Tuberous sclerosis	Fibroangiomatous skin lesions (probably not detectable on prenatal sonogram)		Brain lesions, particularly involving the basal ganglia and periventricular region		

IUGR, Intrauterine growth restriction.

Other Skeletal Anomalies	Cardiac Defects	Genitourinary Abnormalities	Gastrointestinal Abnormalities	Miscellaneous Anomalies	IUGR
		Occasional renal anomalies		Focal lymphangiomata or hemangiomata	
Cystic bone changes (probably not detectable on prenatal sonogram)	Cardiac rhabdomyomata	Renal angiomyolipomata (probably not detectable on prenatal sonogram)			

APPENDIX 2-9

Sequences and Associations

	Central Nervous System Abnormalities	Abnormal Facies	Extremity Abnormalities	Abnormal Digits	Other Skeletal Anomalies
Amniotic band sequence (location of abnormalities depends upon location of band)	Encephalocele, asymmetric anencephaly	Micrognathia, facial clefting	Asymmetric constriction or amputation of limbs (limb–body wall defects), club feet, asymmetric constriction of limbs	Asymmetric constriction or amputation of digits, clenched hands	
Arthrogryposis	Occasional ventriculomegaly, occasional lissencephaly, occasional agenesis of the corpus callosum, occasional vermian agenesis, occasional microcephaly	Occasional facial defects, occasional cataracts	Fixed extremities, arms most often flexed, hyperextended knees, club feet	Clenched hands with overlapping index fingers	Poor ossification of long bones suggesting osteoporosis
Cardiosplenic syndrome: asplenia (bilateral right sidedness)					
Cardiosplenic syndrome: polysplenia (bilateral left-sidedness)					
Caudal regression syndrome	Occasional NTD	Occasional facial cleft	Femoral hypoplasia, club feet, flexion contractures of the lower extremities		Agenesis or dysgenesis of the sacrum, abnormal lumbar vertebral bodies, pelvic deformities
Cerebro-oculo-facio-skeletal (COFS) syndrome	Microcephaly, ACC	Micrognathia, cataracts, microphthalmia	Contracture of all extremities, rockerbottom feet		
CHARGE association	Occasional mild ventriculomegaly, occasional Dandy-Walker variant	Hypoplastic nose, malformed ears, occasional micrognathia, occasional cleft lip and palate, occasional hypertelorism, occasional microphthalmia	Polyhydramnios	Occasional polydactyly or other hand anomalies	

ACC, Agenesis of the corpus callosum; *ASD*, atrial septal defect; *NTD*, neural tube defect; *TE*, tracheo-esophageal; *VSD*, ventricular septal defect.

Cardiac Defects	Thoracic Anomalies	Genitourinary Abnormalities	Gastrointestinal Abnormalities	Miscellaneous Anomalies
	Limb–body wall defects		Gastroschisis, omphalocele, limb–body wall defects	Extensive multisystem abnormalities
		Renal defects		Fetus often immobile, thickened nuchal translucency or cystic hygroma, polyhydramnios
Severe cardiac defects, right-sided cardiac apex, anomalous pulmonary venous return, bilateral superior vena cava, endocardial cushion defect, transposition of the great arteries, single ventricle, pulmonic stenosis	Bilateral, trilobed lungs	Renal anomalies	Right-sided stomach, midline liver	Thickened nuchal translucency
Complex cardiac defects, azygous continuation of the inferior vena cava, anomalous pulmonary venous return, dextrocardia, bilateral superior vena cava, endocardial cushion defect	Bilateral, bilobed lungs		Right-sided stomach, midline liver	Thickened nuchal translucency
Occasional cardiac defects	Occasional pulmonary hypoplasia	Occasional renal agenesis or anomaly	Occasional imperforate anus	Decreased movement of lower extremities, thickened nuchal translucency
Cardiac defects, including tetralogy of Fallot, double-outlet right ventricle, endocardial cushion defect, VSD, ASD	Occasional hemivertebrae	Micropenis and small scrotum, undescended testicles, occasional renal anomalies	Occasional anal atresia, occasional omphalocele, occasional TE fistula	Polyhydramnios, occasional cystic hygroma

Continued

APPENDIX 2-9

Sequences and Associations—cont'd

	Central Nervous System Abnormalities	Abnormal Facies	Extremity Abnormalities	Abnormal Digits	Other Skeletal Anomalies
Congenital adrenal hyperplasia					
Congenital high airway obstruction syndrome (CHAOS)					
Cloacal exstrophy sequence	NTD		Occasional lower limb abnormalities		Occasional widened synthesis pubis
Holoprosencephaly sequence (alobar)	Absent inner hemispheric fissure of third ventricle and olfactory bulb, single central ventricle, fused thalami, occasional microcephaly or macrocephaly, occasional dorsal cyst	Cyclopia, hypotelorism, cebocephaly, maxillary hypoplasia or absent premaxilla with hypotelorism, cleft lip and palate			
Idiopathic arterial calcification of infancy					
Klippel-Feil sequence		Low-set ears, facial asymmetry, occasional cleft palate			Cervical vertebral anomalies, short neck, occasional rib defect, occasional Sprengel abnormality, occasional scoliosis
Megacystis–microcolon–intestinal hypoperistalsis syndrome					

ACC, Agenesis of the corpus callosum; *ASD*, atrial septal defect; *NTD*, neural tube defect; *TE*, tracheo-esophageal; *VSD*, ventricular septal defect.

Cardiac Defects	Thoracic Anomalies	Genitourinary Abnormalities	Gastrointestinal Abnormalities	Miscellaneous Anomalies
		Ambiguous genitalia appearing as a phallus in a female fetus, occasional enlarged adrenals		Thickened nuchal translucency
	Enlarged echogenic lungs, inverted diaphragm, dilated tracheobronchial tree		Ascites	Hydrops, nuchal edema/thickening, oligohydramnios
		Cystic structures in fetal pelvis, absent bladder, genital abnormalities, occasional anomalous kidneys	Ventral wall defect, elephant trunk-like mass protruding from anterior abdominal wall, occasional ascites	Oligohydramnios, occasional single umbilical artery
				Thickened nuchal translucency
Pericardial effusion and calcification of the great vessels	Calcification of main arteries and hydrops in third trimester			Hydrops, polyhydramnios
Occasional cardiac defect		Occasional renal anomaly		
		Megacystis with keyhole appearance of posterior urethra, hydronephrosis	Enlarged stomach, occasional omphalocele	Oligohydramnios or polyhydramnios

Continued

APPENDIX 2-9

Sequences and Associations—cont'd

	Central Nervous System Abnormalities	Abnormal Facies	Extremity Abnormalities	Abnormal Digits	Other Skeletal Anomalies
MURCS association	Occasional cerebellar cysts	Occasional facial and external ear anomalies, occasional micrognathia, occasional cleft lip and palate	Occasional upper limb abnormalities		Vertebral abnormalities C5–T1, occasional rib deformities, occasional scapular abnormalities
Opitz syndrome	Occasional ACC, occasional ventriculomegaly, occasional vermian hypoplasia	Hypertelorism, cleft lip and palate, micrognathia			
Pena Shokeir syndrome		Micrognathia, depressed nasal bridge, hypertelorism, occasional cleft palate	Multiple contractures and ankylosis of limbs, ulna deviation of hands, club feet	Camptodactyly, clenched hands	
Pentalogy of Cantrell	Occasional NTD, occasional exencephaly	Occasional facial defects	Occasional club feet		
Prune-belly syndrome					
Renal agenesis (potter or oligohydramnios sequence)	Occasional ventriculomegaly, occasional NTD		Occasional sirenomelia, occasional absent radius		Narrow chest from compression, occasional vertebral defects
Scimitar syndrome					
Sirenomelia		Potter facies	Fusion and severe deformities of lower extremities		Multiple abnormalities of the lower spine
VATER association	Occasional spinal dysraphia		Radial ray abnormalities, short or absent radius, abnormal hands, occasional lower extremity anomalies	Occasional polydactyly, occasional syndactyly	Hemivertebrae, other vertebral abnormalities, scoliosis

ACC, Agenesis of the corpus callosum; *ASD,* atrial septal defect; *NTD,* neural tube defect; *TE,* tracheo-esophageal; *VSD,* ventricular septal defect.

Cardiac Defects	Thoracic Anomalies	Genitourinary Abnormalities	Gastrointestinal Abnormalities	Miscellaneous Anomalies
		Renal agenesis or ectopia, hypoplasia of the uterus and part of the vagina		
Occasional cardiac defects		Hypospadias, cryptorchidism, occasional renal anomalies		
Occasional cardiac anomalies	Hypoplastic lungs	Cryptorchidism		Polyhydramnios
Cardiac defects, including tetralogy of Fallot	Large abdominal wall defect, consisting of omphalocele and ectopia cordis		Large abdominal wall defect, consisting of omphalocele and ectopia cordis	Thickened nuchal translucency, occasional cystic hydroma
		Distended bladder and ureters, megalourethra, cryptorchidism		Oligohydramnios
Occasional complex cardiac defects		Absent kidneys	Narrow chest (from compression), occasional TE fistula, occasional imperforate anus, occasional duodenal atresia	Occasional single umbilical artery, oligohydramnios
Dextroposition of the heart, anomalous pulmonary vein draining into the inferior vena cava, occasional cardiac defects	Dextroposition of the heart, small right lung			
Cardiac defects	Abdominal wall defects, chest deformities, lung hypoplasia	Bilateral renal agenesis, absent genitals	Abdominal wall defects, imperforate anus	Single umbilical artery, oligohydramnios
Occasional cardiac defects	TE fistula	Hydronephrosis, cystic kidneys, occasional genital defects	Anal atresia	Occasional single umbilical artery

APPENDIX 2-10

Teratogens

	Skull and Central Nervous System Abnormalities	Abnormal Facies	Skeletal Anomalies
Acetazolamide			
Acetyl salicylic acid (aspirin) [anticoagulant]	Intracranial hemorrhage		
Alcohol	Microcephaly	Ear deformities, low forehead, depressed nasal bridge, micrognathia, cleft lip and palate, ophthalmic abnormalities	
Aminopterin (antifolate)	Incomplete skull ossification, ventriculomegaly, microcephaly, NTD, anencephaly	Micrognathia, low-set ears, facial cleft	Club feet, fibula hypoplasia
Amitriptyline [tranquilizer, antidepressant]		Micrognathia	Limb reduction, hand and foot abnormalities
Antithyroid agents			
Azathioprine [anticancer agent]			
Carbamazepine (Tegretol) [anticonvulsant]		Cleft lip	Club feet
Carbon monoxide	Cerebral atrophy, ventriculomegaly		
Chlordiazepoxide (Librium) [tranquilizer, antidepressant]	Microcephaly		
Chlorpheniramine	Ventriculomegaly		Hip dislocation
Chlorpropamide	Microcephaly	Ear abnormalities	Dysmorphic hands
Ciprofloxacin	Ventriculomegaly		
Clomiphene (Clomid) [hormone]	Microcephaly, meningomyelocele, anencephaly	Facial cleft	Club feet
Cocaine	Cranial defects		Limb reduction anomalies
Codeine	Ventriculomegaly	Facial cleft	Dislocated hip, musculoskeletal malformations
Cortisone [hormone]	Ventriculomegaly	Cleft lip and palate, cataract	Club feet
Cyclophosphamide [anticancer agent]		Depressed nasal bridge	
Cytarabine [anticancer agent]	Anencephaly		
Dextroamphetamine	Exencephaly		
Estrogen [hormone]		Eye and ear anomalies	Limb reductions
Ethosuximide [anticonvulsant]	Ventriculomegaly, meningomyelocele	Facial cleft, hypertelorism, nasal hypoplasia	Short neck, hip dislocation
Fluorouracil [anticancer agent]			Radial aplasia

ASD, Atrial septal defect; *NTD,* neural tube defect; *VSD,* ventricular septal defect.

Abnormal Digits	Cardiac Defects	Thoracic, Genitourinary, and Gastrointestinal Abnormalities	IUGR	Miscellaneous
			IUGR	Sacrococcygeal teratoma
			IUGR (occasional)	
	Cardiac and visceral malformations		IUGR	
Thumb hypoplasia, syndactyly			IUGR	
		Fetal goiter		
Polydactyly	Pulmonary valvar stenosis	Hypospadias	IUGR	
	ASD	Ambiguous genitalia		
				Stillbirth
	Cardiac defects	Duodenal atresia		
Polydactyly		Genital anomalies (females), gastrointestinal anomalies		
Syndactyly, polydactyly	Cardiac defects	Esophageal atresia, hypospadias		
	Cardiac disease	Renal abnormalities	IUGR	Placental abruption
	Cardiac defects	Respiratory malformations, pyloric stenosis		
	VSD, coarctation of the aorta		IUGR	
Ectrodactyly, syndactyly	Tetralogy of Fallot			
Lobster-claw deformities	Tetralogy of Fallot		IUGR	
	Cardiac defects			
	Cardiac disease			
	Cardiac defects			
		Esophageal and duodenal abnormalities		

Continued

APPENDIX 2-10

Teratogens—cont'd

	Skull and Central Nervous System Abnormalities	Abnormal Facies	Skeletal Anomalies
Fluoxetine (Prozac) [tranquilizer, antidepressant]			
Fluphenazine [tranquilizer, antidepressant]	Poor ossification of the frontal bone	Facial cleft	Poor ossification of frontal bone
Haloperidol [tranquilizer, antidepressant]			Limb deformities
Hydantoin [anticonvulsant]	Microcephaly (occasional) holoprosencephaly (occasional)	Hypertelorism, depressed nasal bridge, cleft lip and palate	Rib anomalies
Hyperthermia	Microcephaly, NTD	Facial defects	
Imipramine [tranquilizer, antidepressant]	Exencephaly	Cleft palate	Limb reduction abnormalities
Indomethacin			Phocomelia
Maternal phenylketonuria (PKU)	Microcephaly		
Meclizine [anticonvulsant]			
Meprobamate [tranquilizer, antidepressant]			Limb defects (bilateral)
Methotrexate [hormone]	Abnormal frontal bone, NTD, microcephaly	Low-set ears, mandibular hypoplasia	Abnormal frontal bone, club feet
Metronidazole (Flagyl) [antibiotic]	Possible increased risk of neuroblastoma	Midline facial defects	
Nortriptyline [tranquilizer, antidepressant]			Limb reduction
Oral contraceptives [hormone]			Vertebral anomalies (VATER), limb abnormalities (VATER)
Phenantoin [anticonvulsant]	Microcephaly	Broad nasal bridge, short nose, low-set ears, cleft lip and palate, hypertelorism	
Phenothiazine [tranquilizer, antidepressant]			Club feet
Phenylephrine		Ear abnormalities, eye abnormalities	Hip dislocation, club feet
Phenylpropanolamine			Hip dislocation
Procarbazine [anticancer agent]	Cerebral hemorrhage		
Progestin [hormone]	Ventriculomegaly, anencephaly, spina bifida	Cataract	Limb abnormalities
Propranolol			

ASD, Atrial septal defect; *NTD,* neural tube defect; *VSD,* ventricular septal defect.

Abnormal Digits	Cardiac Defects	Thoracic, Genitourinary, and Gastrointestinal Abnormalities	IUGR	Miscellaneous
				Occasional cluster of minor abnormalities, third-trimester exposure: preterm delivery, poor neonatal adaption, respiratory distress, jitteriness, low birth weight
Hypoplasia of the distal phalanges	Cardiac defects (occasional)	Genitourinary defects (occasional)	IUGR	
			IUGR	
		Diaphragmatic hernia, renal cystic disease		
	Closure of ductus arteriosus			Stillbirth, fetal hemorrhage
	Cardiac defects (tetralogy of Fallot)			
	Hypoplastic left heart			
	Cardiac defects	Respiratory defects		
Syndactyly	Dextrocardia		IUGR	
	Cardiac defects (VATER)	Tracheoesophageal fistula, esophageal atresia, anal atresia (VATER), genital anomalies		
Hypoplastic distal phalanges	Cardiac defects		IUGR	
Syndactyly				
Syndactyly		Umbilical hernia		
Polydactyly		Pectus excavatum		
Oligodactyly				
Thumb abnormalities	Tetralogy of Fallot, truncus arteriosis, VSD	Hypospadias		
	Bradycardia		IUGR	Small placenta

Continued

APPENDIX 2-10

Teratogens—cont'd

	Skull and Central Nervous System Abnormalities	Abnormal Facies	Skeletal Anomalies
Quinine [antibiotic]	Ventriculomegaly	Facial defects	Vertebral anomalies, dysmelia
Radiation (large dosage)	Microcephaly, spina bifida	Facial defects	
Smoking			
Tetracycline [antibiotic]			Impaired bone growth, enamel hypoplasia (teeth), limb hypoplasia
Thalidomide [hormone]		Microtia	Spinal malformations, limb reduction abnormalities
Thioguanine [anticancer agent]			
Trimethadione [anticonvulsant]	Microcephaly	Broad nasal bridge, low-set ears, cleft lip and palate	Hand and foot malformations
Valproic acid [anticonvulsant]	Microcephaly, meningomyelocele, septo-optic dysplasia	Low-set ears, facial cleft, depressed nasal bridge, micrognathia, cataracts	Absent radial ray
Warfarin (Coumadin) [anticoagulant]	Encephalocele, anencephaly, spina bifida	Choanal atresia, nasal hypoplasia, depressed nasal bridge, cataracts	Skeletal abnormalities, scoliosis, stippled epiphyses, rhizomelia

ASD, Atrial septal defect; *NTD,* neural tube defect; *VSD,* ventricular septal defect.

Abnormal Digits	Cardiac Defects	Thoracic, Genitourinary, and Gastrointestinal Abnormalities	IUGR	Miscellaneous
	Cardiac defects			
			IUGR	
	Cardiac defects		IUGR	Perinatal death, abruption, prematurity, low birth weight
		Hypospadias		
	Cardiac defects	Duodenal atresia		
Missing digits			IUGR	
	Cardiac defects, VSD, ASD	Esophageal atresia	IUGR	
	Tetralogy of Fallot	Urogenital defects	IUGR	
	Cardiac defects		IUGR	

APPENDIX 2-11

Chromosomal Anomalies

	Skull Abnormalities	Central Nervous System Abnormalities	Abnormal Facies	Nuchal Lucency/Cystic Hygroma	Abnormal Positions Of Limbs Or Extremities	Extremity Abnormalities
Cri du chat syndrome (distal 5p deletion)		Microcephaly, cerebellar anomalies, ventriculomegaly, encephalocele	Micrognathia, hypertelorism, nasal bone hypoplasia	Nuchal thickening, cystic hygroma		
Deletion 4p (Wolf-Hirschhorn syndrome)	Cranial asymmetry	Microcephaly, agenesis of the corpus callosum, occasional Dandy-Walker cyst and periventricular brain cystic areas	Micrognathia, hypertelorism, cleft lip and palate		Club feet	
Deletion 11q (Jacobsen syndrome)	Trigonocephaly	Microcephaly, occasional ventriculomegaly, occasional holoprosencephaly	Hypertelorism, depressed nasal bridge, micrognathia, ear malformations, occasional facial cleft	Occasional nuchal thickening	Joint contractures	
DiGeorge syndrome		Microcephaly, occasional brain anomalies	Micrognathia, facial cleft, occasional Pierre Robin syndrome	Nuchal thickening		Short long-bones
Tetrasomy 12p (Pallister-Killian syndrome)		Cerebellar hypoplasia, ventriculomegaly	Facial dysmorphism, hypertelorism, low-set ears	Nuchal thickening		Femoral and humeral shortening (micromelia)
Triploidy		Ventriculomegaly, agenesis of corpus callosum, Dandy-Walker malformation, holoprosencephaly, meningomyelocele	Hypertelorism, microphthalmia, micrognathia	Nuchal translucency thickening, cystic hygroma	Club feet	
Trisomy 9		Microcephaly, cerebellar anomalies, ventriculomegaly, NTD	Cleft lip and palate, micrognathia, microphthalmia	Nuchal thickening	Flexion deformities of the fingers, abnormal positioning of feet	

IUGR, Intrauterine growth restriction; *NTD,* neural tube defect; *VSD,* ventricular septal defect.

Abnormal Digits	Other Skeletal Anomalies	Cardiac Defects	Thoracic Anomalies	Genitourinary Abnormalities	Gastrointestinal Abnormalities	IUGR	Miscellaneous
		Cardiac defects, cardiomegaly				IUGR	Hydrops
Occasional polydactyly		Cardiac defects, including VSD		Hypospadias, cryptorchidism, occasional bladder exstrophy and renal anomalies	Diaphragmatic hernia	IUGR	
Occasional fifth finger clinodactyly		Cardiac defects		Hypospadias, cryptorchidism, occasional renal anomalies		IUGR	
		Cardiac defects		Occasional cryptorchidism, occasional hypospadias	Occasional umbilical hernia		
Clinodactyly of the fifth digit		Cardiac defects	Trunk edema, hydrops	Bilateral hydronephrosis	Diaphragmatic hernia, omphalocele		Polyhydramnios
Syndactyly of third and fourth fingers		Cardiac defects		Hydronephrosis, hypospadias	Omphalocele	Severe, early- onset IUGR affecting the skeleton more than the head	High-resistance umbilical artery Doppler waveform, enlarged placenta or small, prematurely calcified placenta
		Cardiac defects		Multicystic kidneys, hydronephrosis, hydroureter, cryptorchidism	Diaphragmatic hernia	IUGR	

Continued

APPENDIX 2-11

Chromosomal Anomalies—cont'd

	Skull Abnormalities	Central Nervous System Abnormalities	Abnormal Facies	Nuchal Lucency/Cystic Hygroma	Abnormal Positions Of Limbs Or Extremities	Extremity Abnormalities
Trisomy 10			Hypertelorism, cleft lip and palate, micrognathia	Nuchal thickening		Polydactyly (preaxial), syndactyly of toes, club feet
Trisomy 13 (Patau syndrome)		Holoprosencephaly, ventriculomegaly, enlarged cisterna magna, microcephaly, agenesis of the corpus callosum, NTD	Cleft lip and palate, midface hypoplasia, cyclopia, hypotelorism, microphthalmia	Nuchal thickening	Flexion deformity of fingers	Radial aplasia
Trisomy 18 (Edward syndrome)		Agenesis of corpus callosum, choroid plexus cysts, posterior fossa abnormalities, occasional meningomyelocele, occasional ventriculomegaly	Micrognathia, low-set ears, microphthalmia, hypertelorism, occasional cleft lip and palate	Nuchal thickening, cystic hygroma	Clenched hand with overlapping index finger, club feet, rockerbottom foot	Short radial ray
Trisomy 21 (Down syndrome)	Brachycephaly	Ventriculomegaly	Flat facies, small ears, nasal bone hypoplasia	Nuchal thickening		Short humerus and femur
Trisomy 22			Cleft lip and palate	Occasional neck webbing		
XO (Turner syndrome)				Large cystic hygroma		Short femur

Abnormal Digits	Other Skeletal Anomalies	Cardiac Defects	Thoracic Anomalies	Genitourinary Abnormalities	Gastrointestinal Abnormalities	IUGR	Miscellaneous
		Cardiac defect		Cryptorchidism		IUGR	
Polydactyly		Echogenic cordae tendineae, cardiac defects		Echogenic enlarged kidneys	Omphalocele, hyperechoic bowel		
		Cardiac defects		Hydronephrosis, cryptorchidism	Omphalocele, diaphragmatic hernia	IUGR	Polyhydramnios
Clinodactyly, hypoplasia of middle phalanx of fifth digit, sandal foot	Wide iliac angle	Cardiac defects, VSD, atrioventricular canal , tetralogy of Fallot, echogenic intracardiac focus		Pyelectasis	Hyperechogenic bowel, duodenal atresia		
Occasional hypoplastic digits		Cardiac defects		Renal anomalies	Gut abnormalities, imperforate anus		
		Cardiac defects, coarctation of the aorta	Hydrops, pleural effusion, ascites, severe lymphedema consistent with lymphangiectasia	Horseshoe kidneys			

3

Sonographic Fetal Findings with Borderline Significance:

The Grey Zone in Fetal Diagnosis

Bryann Bromley, MD, and Beryl R. Benacerraf, MD

Sonography has been instrumental in the prenatal diagnosis of fetal structural defects. Major structural anomalies are straightforward to identify and have a reasonably well-defined prognosis. With improvements in technology, however, we are faced with sonographic findings that are not anatomic defects but variations in anatomy that can have a normal or an abnormal outcome. These findings have a more subjective quality to their identification and can vary with fetal position and transducer settings, and they even may change over the course of gestation. In addition, many carry a wide variety of potential outcomes, ranging from children who are completely normal to those with karyotypic abnormalities and impaired mental function.

This "grey zone" in fetal diagnosis includes "minor markers" for aneuploidy. These markers are the result of variations in anatomy that, depending on ethnicity, carry a statistical association with an abnormal chromosome complement but otherwise are not generally associated with adverse perinatal outcome. Examples of these markers are the echogenic intracardiac focus and choroid plexus cysts. Other markers, such as hyperechoic bowel, may be the hallmark of a variety of underlying problems, such as cystic fibrosis (CF), congenital infection, and growth restriction, and yet the majority of fetuses with this finding are normal.

Whenever these findings are present on a prenatal sonogram, the sonologist must know the possible outcomes and must be able to explain the finding within the paradigm of "risk assessment" so that proper counseling can be provided. Pregnancy is a difficult time for many patients, and risk assessment is not an easily understood concept. The mention of anything other than "normal" will prompt concern in most patients, and it is our task to be able to counsel people in a rational and compassionate manner. Therefore knowledge of the sonographic findings and their clinical significance is crucial for the practicing fetal sonologist and sonographer.

Suggested Reading

Doubilet PM, Copel JA, Benson CB, Bahado-Singh RO, Platt LD: Choroid plexus cyst and echogenic intracardiac focus in women at low risk for chromosomal anomalies: the obligation to inform the mother. *J Ultrasound Med* 23:883–885, 2004.

Filly RA: Echogenic intracardiac foci and choroid plexus cysts. *J Ultrasound Med* 23:1135–1138, 2004.

Filly RA, Benacerraf BR, Nyberg DA, Hobbins JC: Choroid plexus cyst and echogenic intracardiac focus in women at low risk for chromosomal anomalies. *J Ultrasound Med* 23:447–449, 2004.

FETAL ECHOGENIC INTRACARDIAC FOCUS (EIF)

PREVALENCE

EIF is seen in 5% to 8% of euploid Caucasian fetuses. A similar prevalence is seen among African-American fetuses. The finding is more common in fetuses of Asian ancestry, in which 30% of euploid fetuses have an EIF. The EIF may resolve over the course of gestation.

ETIOLOGY

Sonographic findings are due to mineralization of the papillary muscle.

SONOGRAPHIC FINDINGS

The diagnosis of EIF is made when a discrete echogenic "dot" as bright as bone is seen within the cardiac ventricle. Most (88%) are located in the left ventricle. Technical factors, such as image settings, angle of insonation, and moderator band, can result in overdiagnosis or underdiagnosis. This finding usually is most visible if the four-chamber view of the heart is pointing directly toward or away from the ultrasound beam (parallel). In the fetus whose heart is oriented perpendicular to the beam, the EIF may be masked and not detectable.

OTHER CONSIDERATIONS

Aside from the relationship to aneuploidy, EIF is a benign finding and is not associated with an increased risk for structural heart defects. The added significance of multiple foci or foci in the right ventricle or both ventricles remains to be established.

DIFFERENTIAL DIAGNOSIS

Rhabdomyoma

Fetuses with rhabdomyomas usually have more extensive echogenic areas in the heart compared with fetuses with a discrete EIF. These tumors typically are located on the septum or in the atria.

ANEUPLOIDY

EIF has a statistical association with trisomies 21 and 13. Roberts et al. have reported the pathologic presence of an EIF in 16% of fetuses with trisomy 21 and 39% of fetuses with trisomy 13. As an *isolated* finding, the presence of an EIF carries a likelihood ratio between 1.4 and 2 for Down syndrome.

MANAGEMENT STRATEGIES

The finding of EIF should prompt a detailed structural survey, including a search for other makers of aneuploidy, such as the nuchal fold, nasal bone, hyperechoic bowel, pyelectasis, and long-bone length. As an *isolated* finding, the individual risk for Down syndrome can be calculated using the Bayes theorem. The revised risk

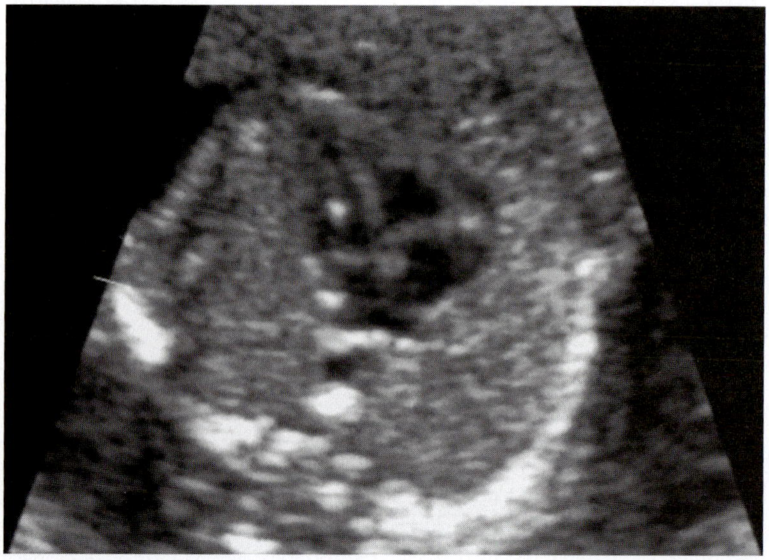

FIGURE 3-1 Four-chamber view of the heart of a second-trimester fetus shows an echogenic intracardiac focus within the left ventricle.

is obtained by multiplying the a priori risk by the likelihood ratio. In a patient at low a priori risk, the presence of this finding would not result in a revised risk that would warrant amniocentesis. These likelihood ratios are not applicable to the fetus of Asian ancestry and should not be used for risk modification in those patients. In the presence of other markers or structural defects, amniocentesis may be warranted.

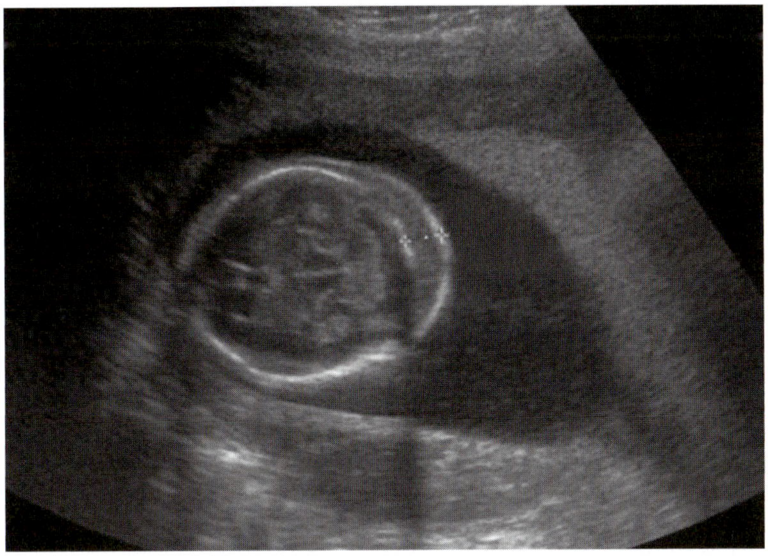

FIGURE 3-2 Transverse view of the fetal head of a second-trimester fetus with Down syndrome. Note the thickened nuchal fold *(calipers)* typical of this aneuploidy.

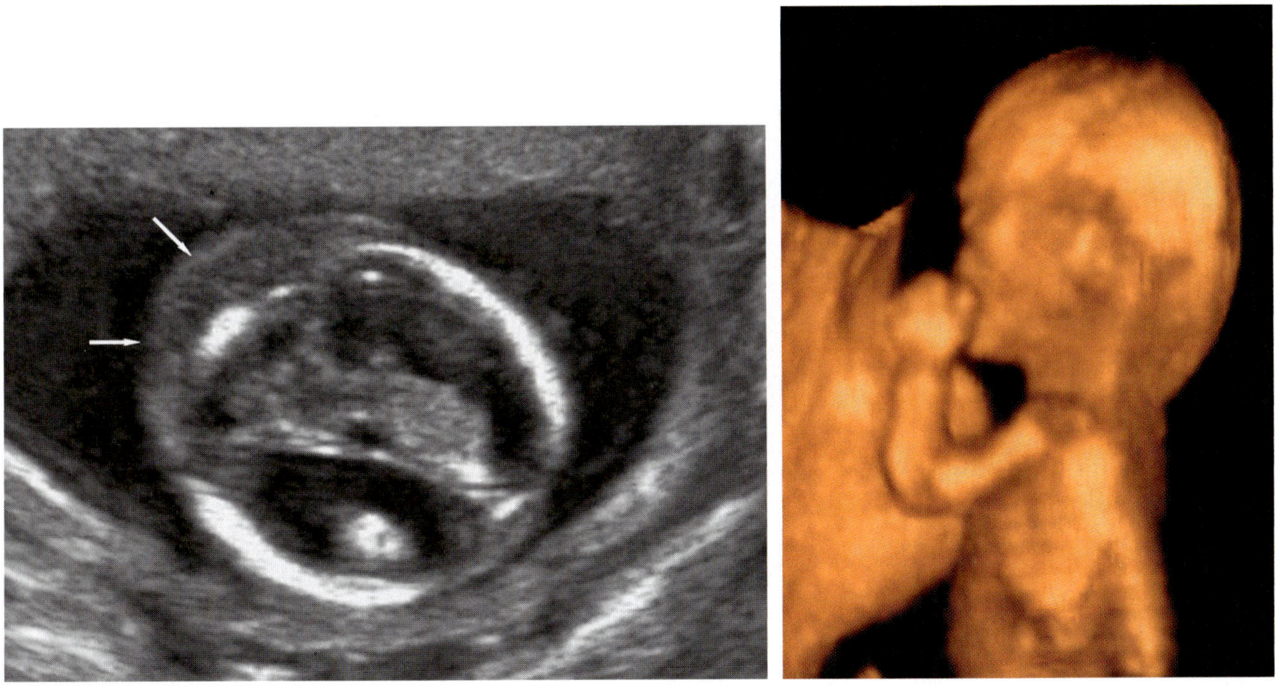

A B

FIGURE 3-3 (A) Oblique view of the fetal head of a 15-week fetus with Down syndrome shows mild ventriculomegaly and nuchal thickening *(arrows)*. (B) Three-dimensional surface rendering of the same 15-week fetus with Down syndrome shows nuchal thickening.

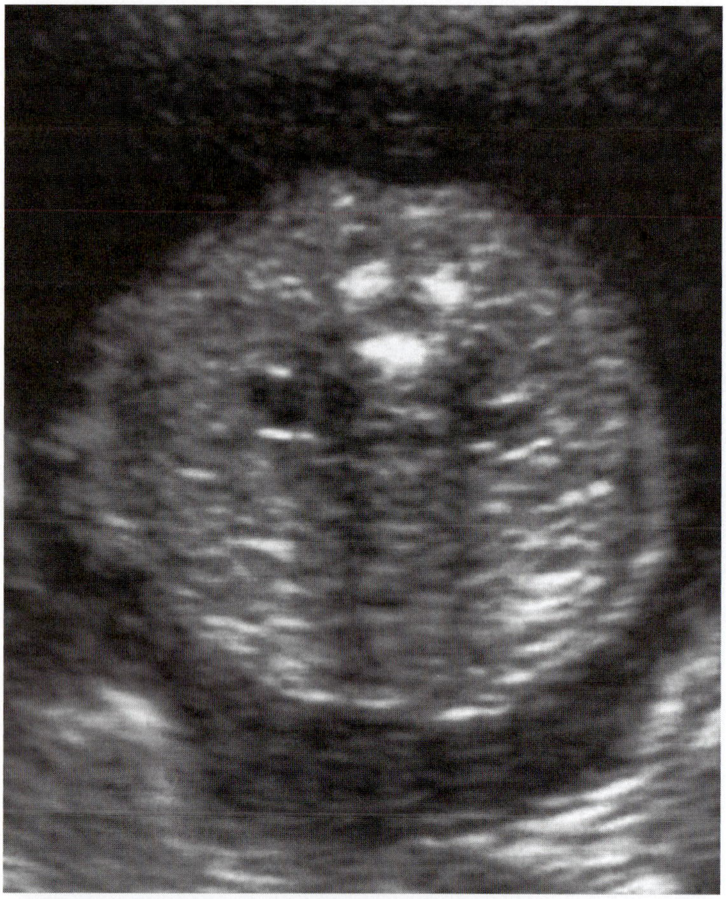

FIGURE 3-4 Transverse view of the fetal kidneys shows mild pyelectasis in a fetus with Down syndrome.

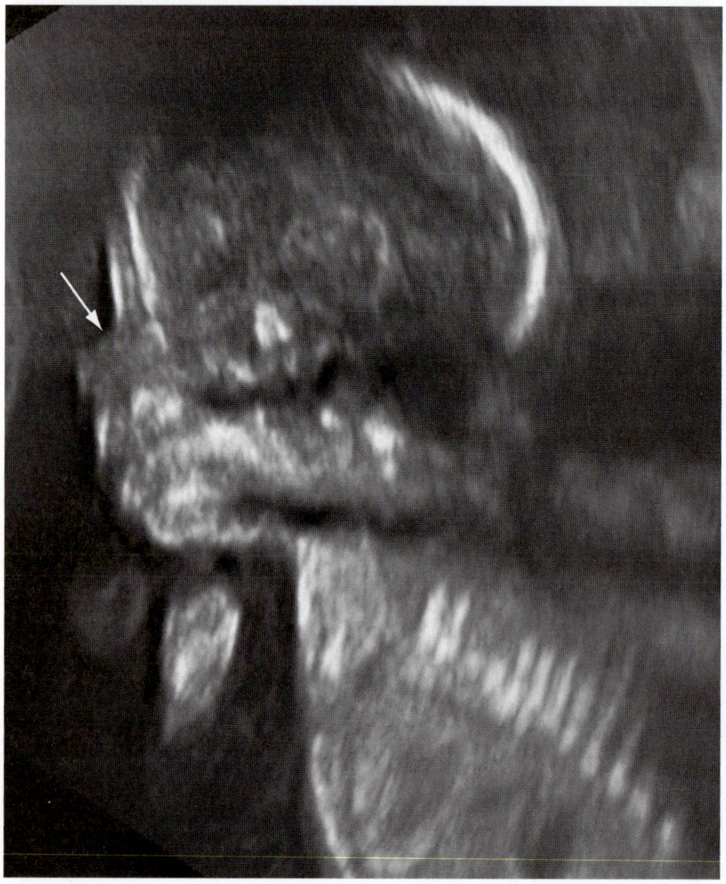

FIGURE 3-5 Profile view of an 18-week fetus with Down syndrome shows absent nasal bone ossification *(arrow)*.

Suggested Reading

Bromley B, Lieberman E, Laboda L, Benacerraf BR: Echogenic intracardiac focus, a sonographic sign for Down syndrome? *Obstet Gynecol* 86:998–1001, 1995.

Bromley B, Lieberman E, Shipp TD, Benacerraf BR: The genetic sonogram: a method of risk assessment for Down syndrome in the midtrimester. *J Ultrasound Med* 21:1087–1096, 2002.

Brown DL, Roberts DJ, Miller WA: Left ventricular echogenic focus in the fetal heart: pathologic correlation. *J Ultrasound Med* 13:613–616, 1994.

Lehman CD, Nyberg DA, Winter TC, Kapur RP, Resta RG, Luthy DA: Trisomy 13 syndrome: prenatal ultrasound findings in a review of 33 cases. *Radiology* 194:217–222, 1995.

Nyberg DA, Souter VL, El-Bastawissi A, Young S, Luthhardt F, Luthy DA: Isolated sonographic markers for detection of fetal Down syndrome in the second trimester of pregnancy. *J Ultrasound Med* 20:1053–1063, 2001.

Roberts DJ, Genest D: Cardiac histopathology characteristics of trisomies 13 and 21. *Hum Pathol* 23:1130–1140, 1992.

Shipp TD, Bromley B, Lieberman E, Benacerraf BR: The frequency of the detection of fetal echogenic intracardiac foci with respect to maternal race. *Ultrasound Obstet Gynecol* 15:460–462, 2000.

Wax JR, Donnelly J, Carpenter M, et al: Childhood cardiac function after prenatal diagnosis of intracardiac echogenic foci. *J Ultrasound Med* 22:783–787, 2003.

Wax JR, Mather J, Steinfeld J, Ingardia C: Fetal intracardiac echogenic foci: current understanding and clinical significance. *Obstet Gynecol Surv* 55:303–311, 2000.

Wax JR, Philput C: Fetal intracardiac echogenic foci: does it matter which ventricle? *J Ultrasound Med* 17:145–146, 1998.

Winn VD, Sonson J, Filly RA: Echogenic intracardiac focus: potential for misdiagnosis. *J Ultrasound Med* 22:1207–1214, 2003.

CHOROID PLEXUS CYST (CPC)

PREVALENCE

CPCs are found in 1% to 2% of euploid second-trimester fetuses and generally resolve by 28 weeks' gestation.

SONOGRAPHIC FINDINGS

A CPC is a discrete echolucency within the choroid plexus. CPCs tend to be <10 mm in diameter and may be unilateral or bilateral. "Spongy" or "heterogeneous" choroids are not considered CPCs, and care must be taken not to confuse the corpus striatum along the medial wall of the choroid with CPCs.

ANEUPLOIDY

CPCs are seen in 30% to 50% of fetuses with trisomy 18 (see Chapter 2, Trisomy 18, p. 490).

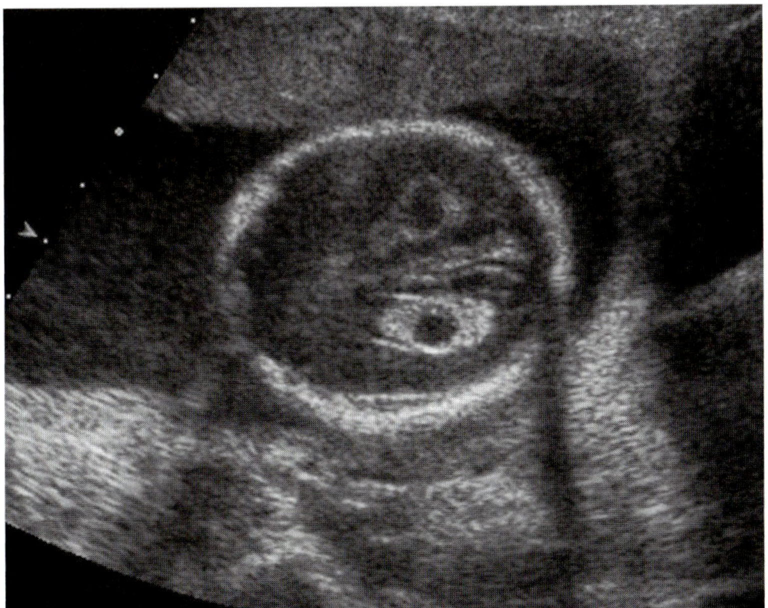

FIGURE 3-6 Transverse view through the fetal choroid plexus shows bilateral cysts in a euploid fetus.

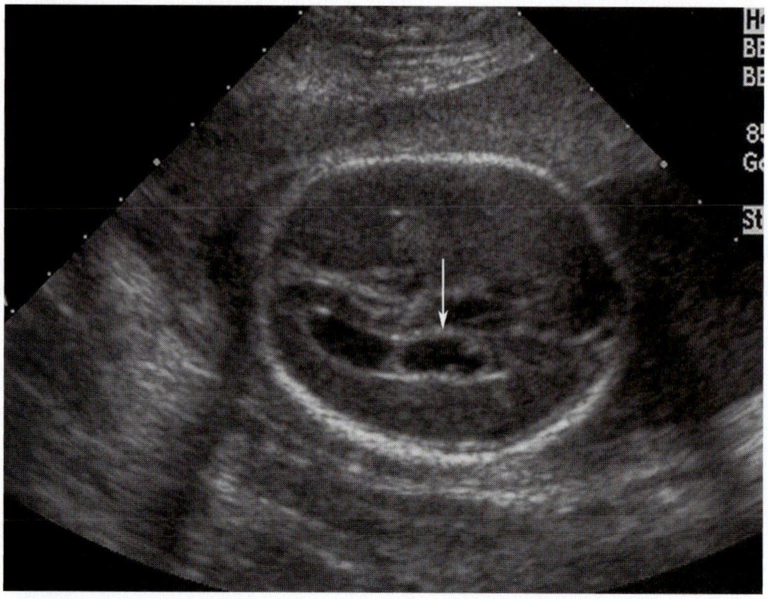

FIGURE 3-7 **Axial view of the fetal head at 24 weeks' gestation shows a choroid plexus cyst *(arrow)* in a fetus with trisomy 18.**

The overwhelming majority of fetuses with trisomy 18 have other sonographic markers suggesting aneuploidy. They include abnormalities of the posterior fossa, face, heart, neural tube, anterior abdominal wall, and extremities. The presence of CPC does not confer an increased risk for trisomy 21; the prevalence of CPC is the same in fetuses with and those without trisomy 21. Many investigators, including our group, have *not* found cyst size or laterality to be helpful in distinguishing affected from normal fetuses. Importantly, resolution of CPC does not necessarily reflect a normal karyotype.

MANAGEMENT STRATEGIES

The finding of a CPC should prompt a detailed structural survey that includes special attention to the cardiac anatomy and documentation of widely open hands (fetuses with trisomy 18 tend to have clenched fists). A search for all markers of aneuploidy is recommended. The survey must be performed ≥18 weeks' gestation because we have noted that lower sensitivity in detection of trisomy 18 is related to earlier gestational age. In the setting of an *isolated* CPC, correlation with a priori risk, preferably based on first-trimester screening or quadruple serum screen, is recommended. No other intervention or follow-up is necessary in most cases unless the patient is at increased risk for aneuploidy on the basis of other parameters.

Gross et al. performed a meta-analysis of publications on this issue and reported that the incidence of trisomy 18 was 0.27% (1/374) in fetuses with isolated CPCs. Isolated CPCs seen in the midtrimester have not been shown to be associated with any significant neurocognitive delays in early childhood.

Suggested Reading

Benacerraf BR, Harlow B, Frigoletto FD Jr: Are choroid plexus cysts an indication for second-trimester amniocentesis? *Am J Obstet Gynecol* 162:1001–1006, 1990.

Benacerraf BR, Miller WA, Frigoletto FD Jr: Sonographic detection of fetuses with trisomies 13 and 18: accuracy and limitations. *Am J Obstet Gynecol* 158:404–409, 1998.

Bernier FP, Crawford SG, Dewey D: Developmental outcome of children who had choroid plexus cysts detected prenatally. *Prenat Diagn* 25:322–326, 2005.

Bromley B, Lieberman E, Benacerraf BR: Choroid plexus cysts: not associated with Down syndrome. *Ultrasound Obstet Gynecol* 18:232–235, 1996.

Coco C, Jeanty P: Karyotyping of fetuses with isolated choroid plexus cysts is not justified in an unselected population. *J Ultrasound Med* 23:899–906, 2004.

Gross SJ, Shulman LP, Tolley EA, et al: Isolated fetal choroid plexus cysts and trisomy 18: a review and meta-analysis. *Am J Obstet Gynecol* 172:83–87, 1995.

Gupta, JK, Cave M, Lilford RF, et al: Clinical significance of fetal choroid plexus cysts. *Lancet* 346:724–729, 1995.

Nava S, Godmilow L, Reeser S, Ludomirsky A, Donnenfeld AE: Significance of sonographically detected second-trimester choroid plexus cysts: a series of 211 cases and a review of the literature. *Ultrasound Obstet Gynecol* 4:448–451, 1994.

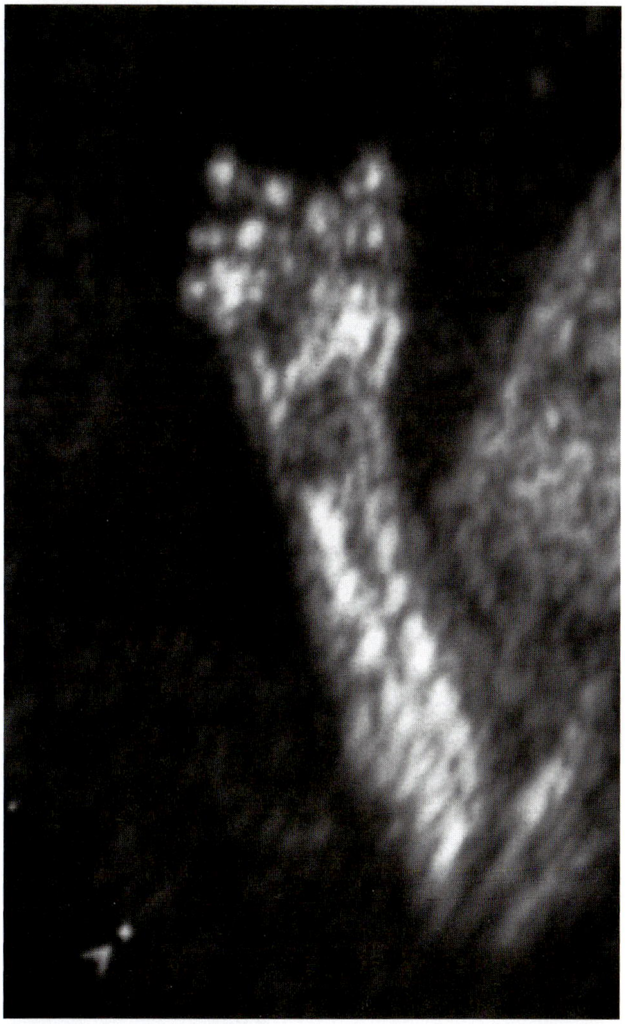

A

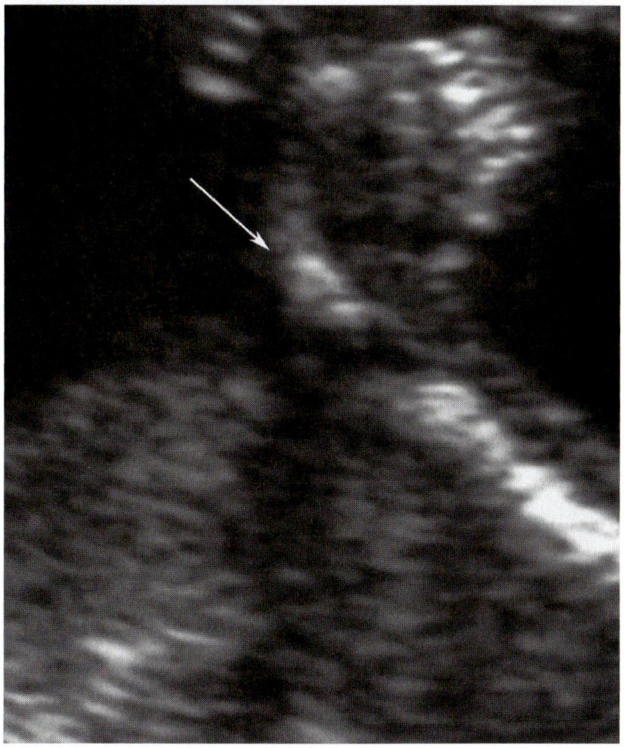

B

FIGURE 3-8 (A) View of the hand of a fetus with trisomy 18 shows the characteristic clenched fist and overlapping index finger. (B) Fetal arm of an early second-trimester fetus with trisomy 18. Note the abnormally short ulna *(arrow)* and absent radius with club hand. The hand is angled radially because of the forearm abnormality.

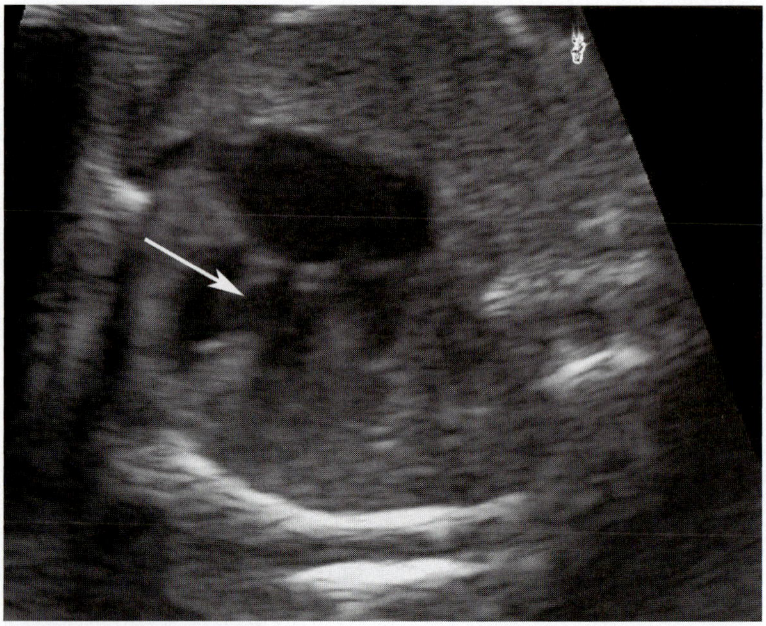

FIGURE 3-9 Four-chamber view of the heart of a 25-week fetus with trisomy 18 shows a large ventricular septal defect *(arrow)*.

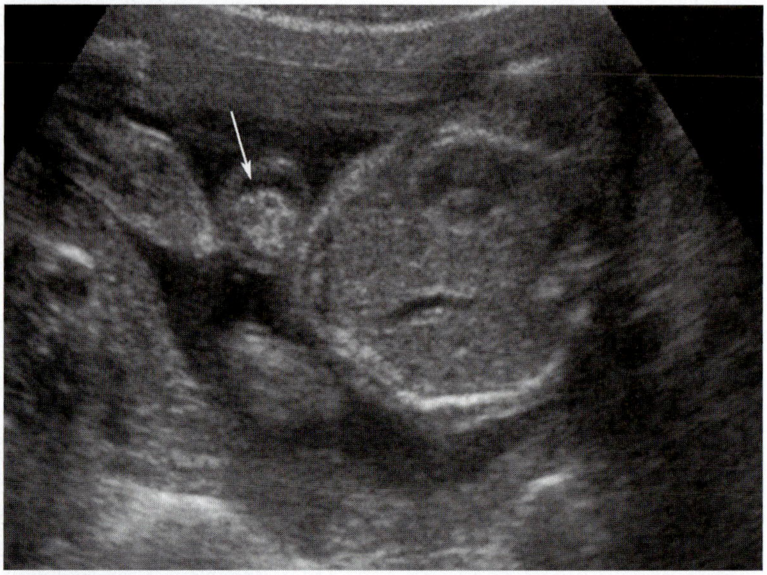

FIGURE 3-10 Transverse view of the fetal abdomen shows a small bowel containing omphalocele *(arrow)*, typically seen in trisomy 18.

HYPERECHOIC BOWEL (HB)

PREVALENCE

HB is seen in 0.2% to 0.6% of second-trimester fetuses.

SONOGRAPHIC FINDINGS

The fetal bowel is considered hyperechoic when the echogenicity is comparable to that of bone. The presence of this finding should not be entertained unless the clinician, using a transducer with a frequency of 3.5 to 5 MHz, finds that the bowel looks consistently echogenic. Higher-frequency transducers make normal bowel appear bright. Additionally, some postprocessing settings may display the bowel as echogenic and may need to be removed for accurate

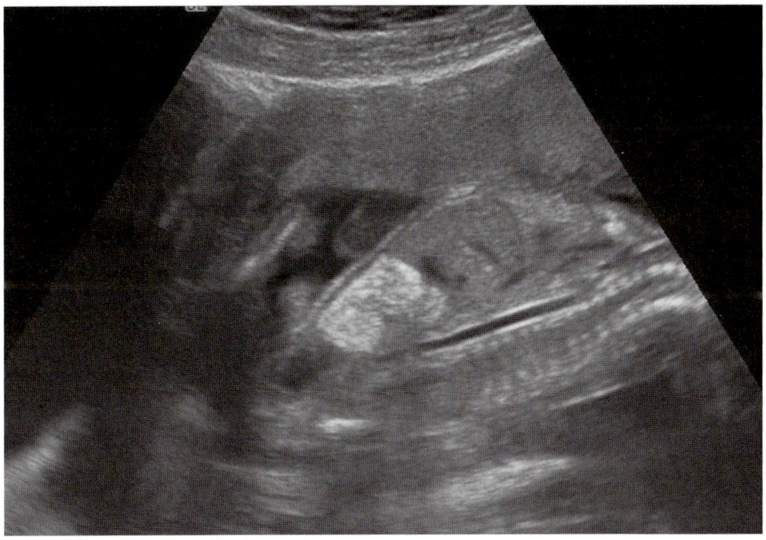

FIGURE 3-11 Longitudinal scan of a midtrimester fetal abdomen shows that the fetal bowel is as bright as the adjacent bone and therefore meets the criterion for hyperechoic bowel.

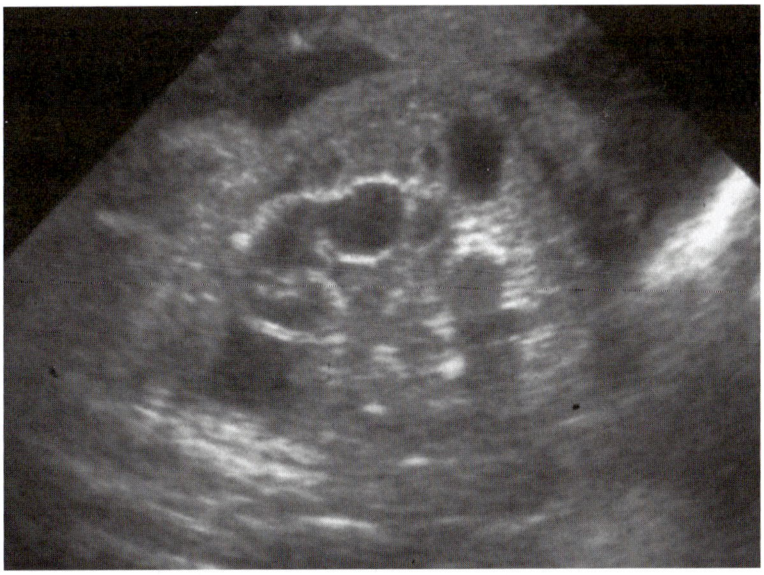

FIGURE 3-12 Late second-trimester fetus with cystic fibrosis. Note the dilated loop of bowel with a hyperechoic wall, characteristic of cystic fibrosis.

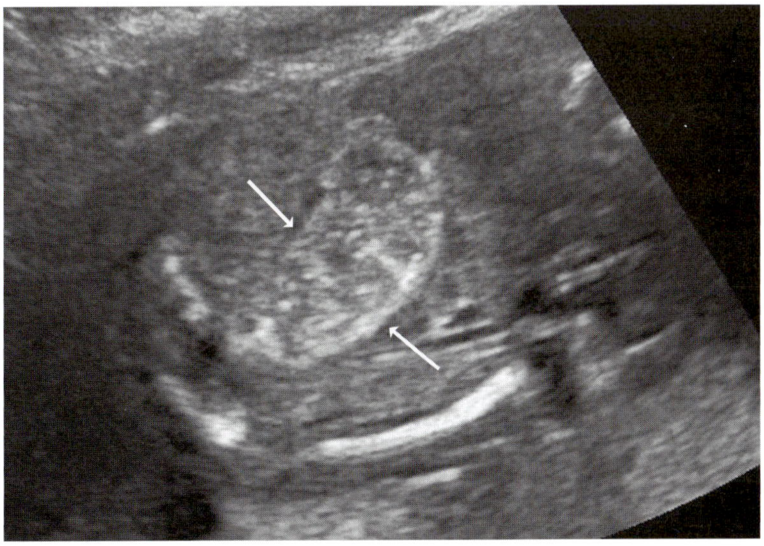

FIGURE 3-13 View of the lower abdomen of a 22-week fetus with a dilated loop of distal colon containing intraluminal calcifications. Note that the hyperechogenicity is confined to the lumen of a dilated loop of bowel *(arrows)*. This finding is characteristic of a vesicorectal fistula in a fetus with imperforate anus and should not be confused with hyperechoic bowel.

assessment of bowel echogenicity. Bowel hyperechogenicity may be transient, and reassessment of this finding at a later date can be falsely reassuring. It is important to evaluate the bowel loops to determine whether any bowel dilation is associated with hyperechogenicity, a finding that suggests CF.

ASSOCIATED ANOMALIES

HB has been associated with an increased risk for aneuploidy, most commonly Down syndrome, CF, congenital infection with cytomegalovirus (CMV) and toxoplasmosis, bowel abnormalities, early-onset growth restriction, and impending fetal death. There is also an association between intraamniotic bleeding and hyperechoic fetal bowel, most likely resulting from fetal swallowing of blood-tinged amniotic fluid. HB in the second trimester should not be confused with echogenic, colonic meconium in the third trimester, which is a normal sonographic finding not associated with any adverse outcome.

Down Syndrome

In a study of 94 fetuses with Down syndrome, Nyberg et al. noted that 7% had HB. This group also showed that as an *isolated* finding, HB carries a likelihood ratio of 6.7 for Down syndrome. A revised risk for aneuploidy can be calculated using the Bayes theorem.

Cystic Fibrosis (CF)

Approximately 5% to 10% of fetuses with HB have CF. Muller et al. studied 209 fetuses with HB. These investigators evaluated 8 mutations and found that 3.3 % of fetuses with HB had CF. This rate is 84 times higher than the background rate of CF in that population. In a study of 346,000 pregnancies evaluated over 10 years, Scotet et al. noted that 9.9% of fetuses with HB had CF. The calculation of risk for CF depends on the probability of this autosomal recessive disease, taking into account all relevant information, including genetic tests on both parents. This risk can be calculated using Bayesian methods; however, the calculations can be quite complex, and referral to a geneticist is recommended.

Growth Restriction

We have shown that approximately 16% of fetuses with HB have growth restriction. The majority of these have early growth restriction that is already evident on the midtrimester scan, and, in our experience, the combination of HB and growth restriction is associated with only a 25% survival. This is similar to the experience of Ghose et al., who reported a 10% incidence of growth restriction among fetuses with HB, only 34% whom survived.

Congenital Infection

McGregor et al. found a 4% prevalence of infection that included both CMV and toxoplasmosis.

Primary Bowel Abnormalities

HB has been associated with bowel abnormalities including obstruction and meconium cysts.

OUTCOME

Overall, 68–80% of fetuses with HB seen in the second trimester have normal outcome. Patel et al. followed up 103 fetuses with HB and no observable abnormalities on discharge from the hospital. There was no evidence of any serious long-term bowel pathology associated with isolated fetal echogenic bowel, once the above-mentioned abnormalities have been excluded.

MANAGEMENT STRATEGIES

If HB is suspected on a midtrimester scan it is important to verify transducer frequency and post processing settings so as not to 'overcall' its presence. A detailed structural survey is recommended, as well as a search for additional markers of aneuploidy. In cases of *isolated* HB, a revised risk of aneuploidy can be calculated using Bayes theorem with a likelihood ratio of 6.7. Meticulous attention must be paid to dating parameters to ensure appropriate growth. Additionally, a serum evaluation for congenital infection and CF is recommended. Risk calculations for CF depend on the population being studied and are quite complex, hence referral to a geneticist is advised.

A follow-up scan in the third trimester is recommended to assess growth and to watch for the development of potential bowel abnormalities.

Suggested Reading

Al-Kouatly HB, Chasen ST, Streltzoff J, Chervenak FA: The clinical significance of fetal echogenic bowel. *Am J Obstet Gynecol* 185:1035–1038, 2001.

Bromley B, Doubilet P, Frigoletto FD Jr, Krauss C, Estroff JA, Benacerraf BR: Is fetal hyperechoic bowel on second-trimester sonogram an indication for amniocentesis? *Obstet Gynecol* 83:647–651, 1994.

Corteville JE, Gray DL, Langer JC: Bowel abnormalities in the fetus—correlation of prenatal ultrasonographic findings with outcome. *Am J Obstet Gynecol* 175:724–729, 1996.

Font GE, Solari M: Prenatal diagnosis of bowel obstruction initially manifested as isolated hyperechoic bowel. *J Ultrasound Med* 17:721–723, 1998.

Ghose I, Mason GC, Martinez D, et al: Hyperechogenic fetal bowel: a prospective analysis of sixty consecutive cases. *BJOG* 107:426–429, 2000.

MacGregor SN, Tamura R, Sabbagha R, et al: Isolated hyperechoic fetal bowel: Significance and implications for management. *Am J Obstet Gynecol* 173:1254–1258, 1995.

Muller F, Dommergues M, Aubry MC, et al: Fetus-placenta-newborn. Hyperechogenic fetal bowel: an ultrasonographic marker for adverse fetal and neonatal outcome. *Am J Obstet Gynecol* 173:508–513, 1995.

Muller, F, Dommergues M, Simon-Bouy B, et al: Cystic fibrosis screening: a fetus with hyperechogenic bowel may be the index case. *J Med Genet* 35:657–660, 1998.

Nyberg DA, Resta RG, Luthy DA, Hickok DE, Mahony BS, Hirsch JH: Prenatal sonographic findings of Down syndrome: review of 94 cases. *Obstet Gynecol* 76:370–377, 1990.

Nyberg DA, Souter VL, El-Bastawissi A, Young S, Luthhardt F, Luthy DA: Isolated sonographic markers for detection of fetal Down syndrome in the second trimester of pregnancy. *J Ultrasound Med* 20:1053–1063, 2001.

Ogino S, Wilson RB, Grody WW: Bayesian risk assessment for autosomal recessive diseases: fetal echogenic bowel with one or no detectable CFTR mutation. *J Med Genet* 41:e70, 2005.

Patel Y, Boyd PA, Chamberlain P, Lakhoo K: Follow-up of children with isolated fetal echogenic bowel with particular reference to bowel-related symptoms. *Prenat Diagn* 24:35–37, 2004.

Paulson EK, Hertzberg BS: Hyperechoic meconium in the third trimester fetus: an uncommon normal variant. *J Ultrasound Med* 10:677–680, 1991.

Scotet V, De Braekeleer M, Audrezet MP, et al: Prenatal detection of cystic fibrosis by ultrasonography: a retrospective study of more than 346,000 pregnancies. *J Med Genet* 39:443–448, 2002.

Sepulveda W, Leung KY, Robertson ME, Kay E, Mayall ES, Fisk NM: Prevalence of cystic fibrosis mutations in pregnancies with fetal echogenic bowel. *Obstet Gynecol* 87:103–106, 1996.

Sepulveda W, Nicolaides P, Mai AM, Hassan J, Fisk NM: Is isolated second-trimester hyperechogenic bowel a predictor of suboptimal fetal growth? *Ultrasound Obstet Gynecol* 7:104–107, 1996.

Sepulveda W, Reid R, Nicolaidis P, Prendiville O, Chapman RS, Fisk NM: Second-trimester echogenic bowel and intraamniotic bleeding: association between fetal bowel echogenicity and amniotic fluid spectrophotometry at 410 nm. *Am J Obstet Gynecol* 174:839–842, 1996.

MECONIUM PERITONITIS (MP)

PREVALENCE

MP is rare in the fetus.

ETIOLOGY

Intraperitoneal calcifications are likely due to a sterile chemical reaction secondary to a bowel perforation in utero. A subsequent inflammatory response results in calcifications, ascites, and occasionally cyst formation. The underlying etiology for bowel perforation includes congenital anomalies such as atresias, volvulus, and intussusceptions. MP has been reported secondary to viral infections such as CMV, hepatitis, and parvovirus. Although MP often is associated with CF in the *neonate,* this is less often the case in prenatally diagnosed cases of MP. Casaccia et al. reported that approximately 7% of fetuses with MP had CF. Overall, these investigators found that 13% of neonates with a prenatal diagnosis of an intestinal anomaly had CF.

SONOGRAPHIC FINDINGS

MP is characterized by small, punctate, linear calcifications in the fetal abdomen. They often are seen on the surface of the liver or surrounding a pseudocyst. Transient ascites and polyhydramnios may be present.

OUTCOME

The outcome depends on the inciting etiology. Bowel perforation and ascites may resolve completely during the course of gestation. Our group has reported several cases of MP with no sequelae in the newborn, including no surgical intervention. In contrast, Eckoldt et al. reported a series of 11 fetuses with MP, 10 of whom required immediate surgical intervention after birth.

MANAGEMENT STRATEGIES

When a prenatal diagnosis of MP is suspected, parental carrier testing for CF is recommended. In addition, evaluation for infectious etiologies is warranted and should include hepatitis. Sonographic follow-up of the fetus is helpful to assess interval change.

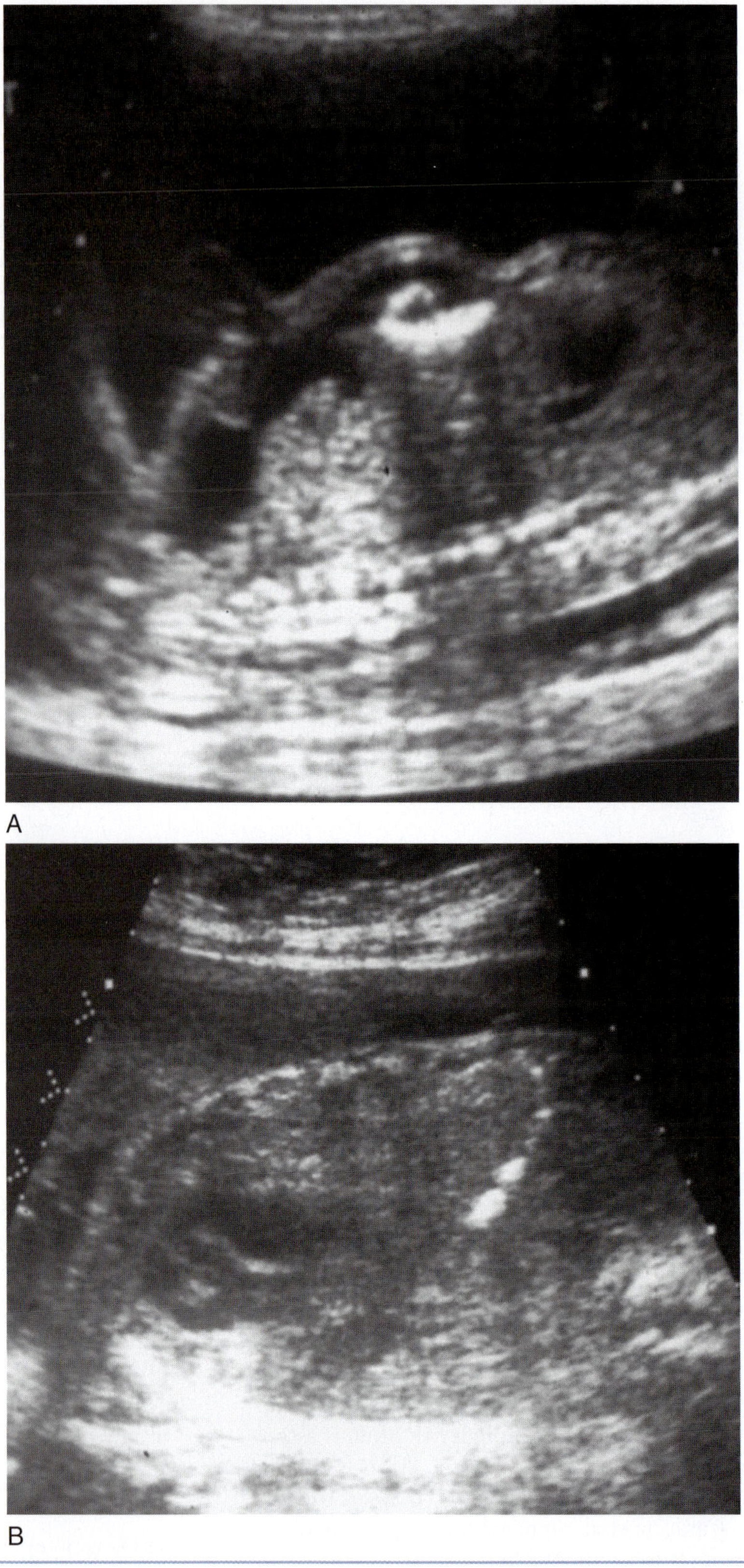

FIGURE 3-14 (**A**) Longitudinal view of the fetal abdomen of a second-trimester fetus with meconium peritonitis. Note the ascites and large clump of calcium located anterior to the fetal liver. The acoustic shadowing of the calcification should aid in distinguishing this entity from hyperechoic bowel. (**B**) View of the same fetal liver in the third trimester shows residual calcification on the surface of the tip of the liver, secondary to meconium peritonitis. The previously seen ascites has resolved. These calcifications are located on the surface of the liver, implicating meconium peritonitis as an etiology.

Suggested Reading

Casaccia G, Trucchi A, Nahom A, et al: The impact of cystic fibrosis on neonatal intestinal obstruction: the need for prenatal/neonatal screening. *Pediatr Surg Int* 19:75–78, 2003.

Eckoldt F, Heling KS, Woderich R, Kraft S, Bollmann R, Mau H: Meconium peritonitis and pseudo-cyst formation: prenatal diagnosis and post-natal course. *Prenat Diag* 23:904–908, 2003.

Estroff JA, Bromley B, Benacerraf BR: Fetal meconium peritonitis without sequelae. *Pediatr Radiol* 22:277–278, 1992.

Leikin E, Lysikiewicz A, Garry D, Tejani N: Intrauterine transmission of hepatitis A virus. *Obstet Gynecol* 88:690–691, 1996.

Pletcher BA, Williams MK, Mulivor RA, Barth D, Linder C, Rawlinson K: Intrauterine cytomegalovirus infection presenting as fetal meconium peritonitis. *Obstet Gynecol* 78:903–905, 1991.

Zerbini M, Gentilomi GA, Gallinella G, et al: Intrauterine parvovirus B19 infection and meconium peritonitis. *Prenat Diagn* 18:599–606, 1998.

FETAL LIVER CALCIFICATION (FLC)

PREVALENCE

FLCs are seen in 1:1000–1750 second-trimester fetal scans.

ETIOLOGY

Multiple etiologies include infectious (most commonly CMV), ischemic insults, and idiopathic causes.

SONOGRAPHIC FINDINGS

Hepatic calcifications appear as punctate echogenic foci in the liver parenchyma. They also may be perivascular or located on the peritoneal surface. Simchen et al. reported no correlation between the location or number of lesions with infection, aneuploidy, or additional anomalies.

DIFFERENTIAL DIAGNOSIS

The differential diagnosis of FLC includes MP and hepatic tumors. MP is associated with a peripheral pattern of calcifications lining the liver surface. A hemangioma usually is a mass lesion rather than an isolated calcification.

ASSOCIATED ANOMALIES

Simchen et al. described 61 fetuses with hepatic calcifications, of whom 40 (65%) had additional sonographic anomalies. The most frequent major anomalies reported were central nervous system anomalies, cardiac anomalies, cystic hygromas, skeletal abnormalities, and hydrops fetalis. Minor markers associated with liver calcifications included EIF and HB. Intrauterine growth restriction also was associated with FLC. This study was performed on a referral population, and therefore the rate of associated anomalies and aneuploidies may be higher than what would be expected in the general population.

Cystic Fibrosis

Surface calcifications (possibly resulting from meconium peritonitis) have been associated with CF.

Congenital Infection

A variety of different infectious etiologies have been associated with FLC. The most common is CMV. Other infectious etiologies, such as parvovirus, varicella, toxoplasmosis, and herpes, have been associated with FLC.

ANEUPLOIDY

In a study of 61 fetuses with FLC, Simchen et al. reported 11 cases (18%) of aneuploidy, most commonly trisomies 18, 13, and 21. Of the 11 fetuses with chromosomal anomalies, 10 had other sonographic features suggesting aneuploidy. The one aneuploid fetus with no associated findings had a single calcification, and trisomy 21 was diagnosed after birth.

OUTCOME

Isolated liver calcifications have a good prognosis once congenital infection and aneuploidy are deemed to be unlikely. Kyung-Eun et al. reported that these calcifications may resolve during the course of gestation.

MANAGEMENT STRATEGIES

The finding of a hepatic calcification should prompt a detailed structural survey, including cardiac evaluation and sonographic markers for aneuploidy. Specific attention to sonographic findings associated with congenital infection, such as intracranial calcifications, is warranted. Correlation with a priori risk based on quadruple serum screening or

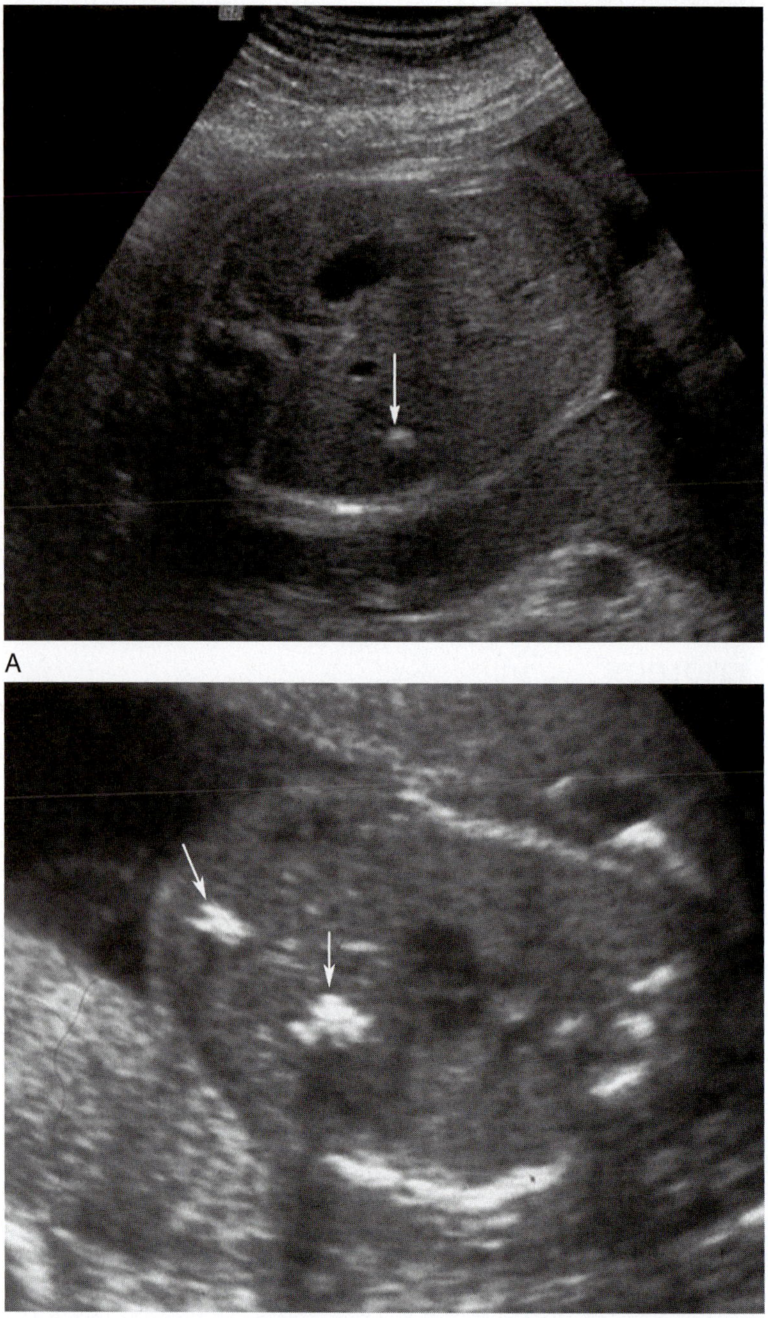

A

B

FIGURE 3-15 (A) Transverse scan through the fetal abdomen at the level of the stomach shows an isolated hepatic calcification *(arrow)* within the right lobe of the liver. (B) Transverse scan through the fetal abdomen of an early second-trimester fetus shows multiple liver calcifications *(arrows)* with associated acoustic shadowing. Both of these fetuses had a normal outcome.

first-trimester risk assessment is recommended, although no specific likelihood ratio has been established for FLC. Serum evaluation for congenital infection is recommended. Carroll and Maxwell suggest that in the setting of surface calcifications, CF carrier testing in the high-risk population should be considered.

In the case of isolated fetal intrahepatic calcification, the outcome usually is good. In our own study of 25 fetuses with isolated hepatic calcifications, one fetus who developed multiple hepatic calcifications and microcephaly in the third trimester died of CMV infection. The remaining 24 fetuses (96%) became normal children, without sequelae.

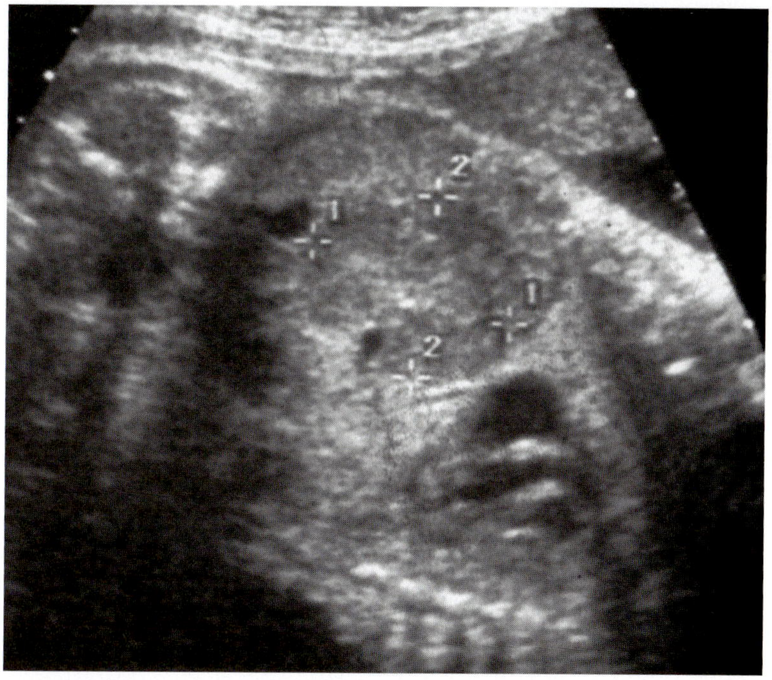

FIGURE 3-16 Longitudinal view of the fetal chest and abdomen shows a mass in the fetal liver (indicated by electronic calipers). There is some increased echogenicity in the center of the mass, but a mass such as this hemangioma should not be confused with simple fetal liver calcifications.

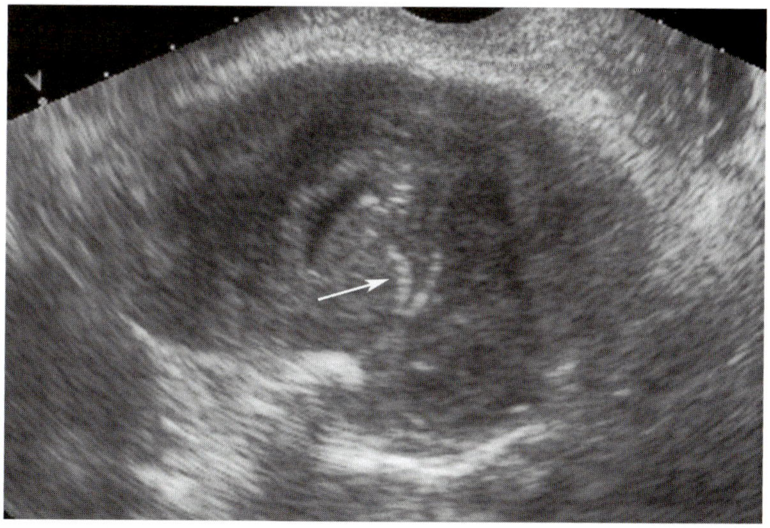

FIGURE 3-17 Oblique transvaginal view of the head of a third-trimester fetus with a congenital infection. Note the characteristic linear fan-like calcifications *(arrow)* in the basal ganglia often seen with cytomegalovirus infections. The finding of intrahepatic calcification should prompt a careful evaluation of the fetal brain for calcifications.

Suggested Reading

Achiron R, Seidman DS, Afek A, et al: Prenatal ultrasonographic diagnosis of fetal hepatic hyerechogenicities: clinical significance and implications for management. *Ultrasound Obstet Gynecol* 7:251–255, 1996.

Bronshtein M, Blaser S: Prenatal diagnosis of liver calcifications. *Obstet Gynecol* 86:739–743, 1995.

Carroll SG, Maxwell DJ: The significance of echogenic areas in the fetal abdomen. *Ultrasound Obstet Gynecol* 7:293–298, 1996.

Kyung-Eun J, Eun Kyung Lee, Kwon TH: Isolated echogenic foci in the left upper quadrant of the fetal abdomen. Are they significant? *J Ultrasound Med* 23:483–488, 2004.

Simchen MJ, Toi A, Bona M, Alkazaleh F, Ryan G, Chitayat D: Fetal hepatic calcifications: prenatal diagnosis and outcome. *Am J Obstet Gynecol* 187: 1617–1622, 2002.

Stein B, Bromley B, Michlewitz H, Miller W, Benacerraf B: Fetal liver calcifications: sonographic appearance and postnatal outcome. *Radiology* 197:489–492, 1995.

FETAL INTRAABDOMINAL UMBILICAL VEIN VARIX (FIUV)

PREVALENCE

Intraabdominal umbilical vein varix is an uncommon finding that typically is seen in the late second and early third trimesters of pregnancy.

ETIOLOGY

This finding is thought to be secondary to weakness of the umbilical vein wall and subsequent venous dilation resulting in a varix.

SONOGRAPHIC FINDINGS

FIUV is a vascular lesion generally seen as localized dilation of the intraabdominal portion of the umbilical vein. Although this is often a subjective finding, criteria that have been proposed to diagnose FIUV include focal dilation >9 mm, varix 50% greater than intrahepatic portion of umbilical vein, and varix >2 SD of mean for gestational age. Color Doppler is useful in distinguishing FIUV from other right-sided abdominal cysts.

DIFFERENTIAL DIAGNOSIS

The differential diagnosis of FIUV includes urachal cyst, choledochal cyst, and ovarian cyst. These are best distinguished from FIUV using Doppler studies.

ASSOCIATED ANOMALIES

Rahemtullah et al. reported additional sonographic findings, including multiple malformation syndromes, cardiac defects, and diaphragmatic hernia, in 35% of cases. Fetal hydrops and anemia have been reported in conjunction with FIUV.

ANEUPLOIDY

In a study by Fung et al., 9.9% of fetuses with FIUV had chromosomal anomalies; the most common were trisomies 21 and 18. The majority of those with chromosomal anomalies (89%) had associated sonographic findings in addition to FIUV.

OUTCOME

Outcomes are based on small case series and reviews of the available literature. In the series of Fung et al. that included 91 patients with FIUV, 54% of *all* the fetuses had a normal outcome. In the subgroup of 62 fetuses with apparently *isolated* FIUV, 74% had a normal outcome. Three cases of anomalies were identified after birth, including an abnormal ear, a branchial cleft cyst, and mild aortic stenosis. Five (8%) intrauterine fetal deaths occurred between 28 and 39 weeks' gestation. These authors speculate that the higher risk for adverse outcome is associated with an earlier diagnosis (<26 weeks' gestation).

MANAGEMENT STRATEGIES

Once FIUV is identified, a detailed anatomic survey that includes a meticulous cardiac examination is recommended. Karyotyping should be considered if other anomalies are present. The fetus should be evaluated sonographically in the third trimester to assess for possible thrombosis. The fetal course is unpredictable, and demise has occurred even with close monitoring.

Suggested Reading

Estroff JA, Benacerraf BR: Fetal umbilical vein varix: sonographic appearance and postnatal outcome. *J Ultrasound Med* 11:69–73, 1992.

Fung TY, Leung TN, Leung TY, Lau TK: Fetal intra-abdominal umbilical vein varix: what is the clinical significance? *Ultrasound Obstet Gynecol* 25:149–154, 2005.

Prefumo F, Thilaganathan B, Tekay A: Antenatal diagnosis of fetal intra-abdominal umbilical vein dilatation. *Ultrasound Obstet Gynecol* 17:82–85, 2001.

Rahemtullah A, Lieberman E, Benson C, Norton M: Outcome of pregnancy after prenatal diagnosis of umbilical vein varix. *J Ultrasound Med* 20:135–139, 2001.

Sepulveda W, Mackenna A, Sanchez J, Corral W, Carstens E: Fetal prognosis in varix of the intrafetal umbilical vein. *J Ultrasound Med* 17:171–175, 1998.

Valsky DV, Rosenak D, Hochner-Celnikier D, Porat S, Yagel S: Adverse outcome of isolated fetal intra-abdominal vein varix despite close monitoring. *Prenat Diag* 24:451–454, 2004.

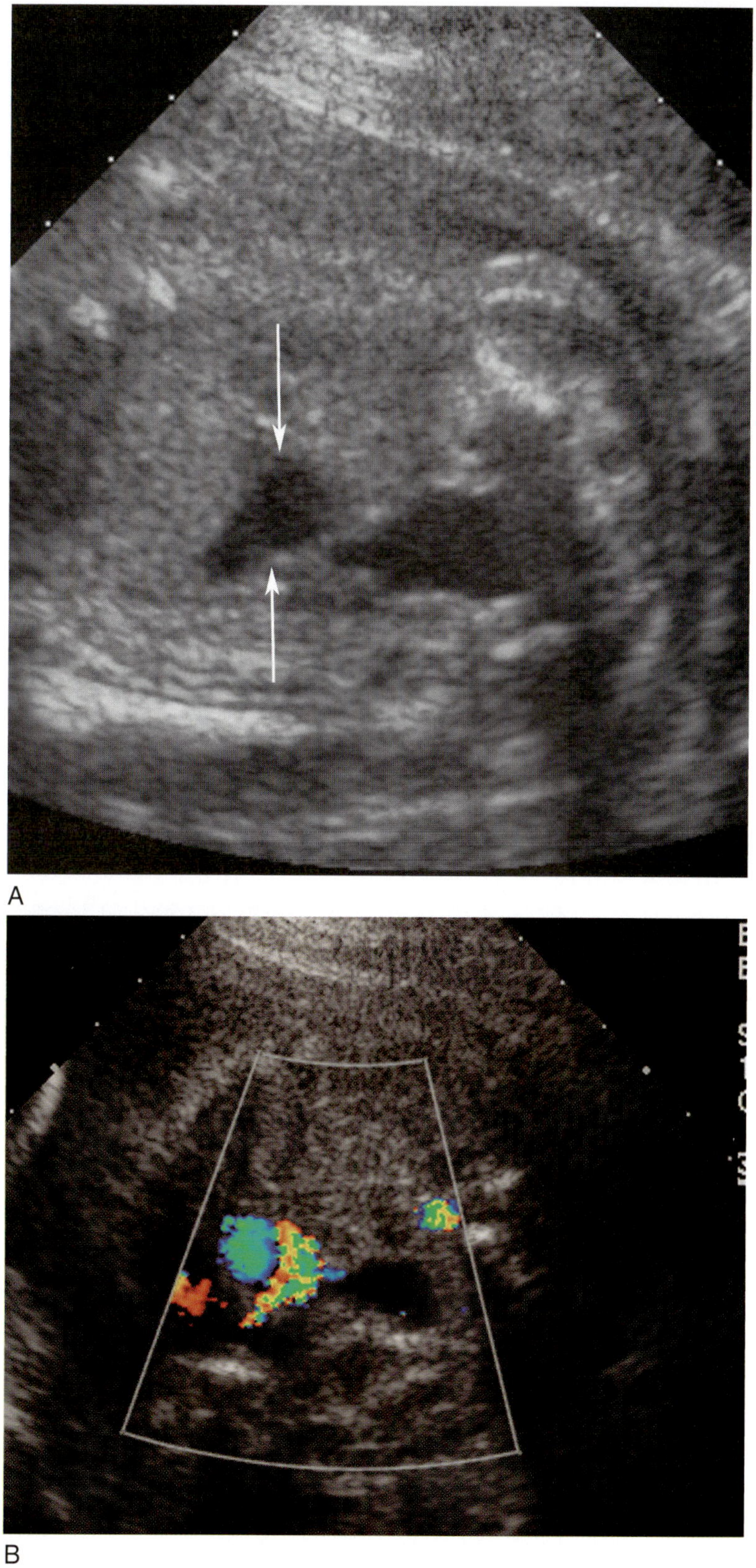

FIGURE 3-18 (A) Dilation of the umbilical vein *(arrows)* as it enters the fetal abdomen directly above the bladder. This is the characteristic appearance of an umbilical vein varix. (B) Adding color Doppler in this area shows the vascular nature of this finding.

PERSISTENT RIGHT UMBILICAL VEIN (PRUV)

PREVALENCE

PRUV occurs in 1:476 pregnancies and usually is noted in the second or third trimester.

ETIOLOGY

During early gestation, the right umbilical vein and portions of the left umbilical vein between the liver and sinus venosus regress. The remaining portion of the left umbilical vein, the left portal vein, and ductus venosus remain. Occasionally, however, the right umbilical vein fails to regress. When this occurs, the right umbilical vein may completely replace the left umbilical vein, or they may coexist.

SONOGRAPHIC FINDINGS

Findings are identified on axial scan through the fetal abdomen at the level of the stomach. The umbilical vein passes laterally and to the right side of the gallbladder so that the gallbladder is between the vein and the stomach. The umbilical vein connects to the right portal vein and curves toward the stomach.

ASSOCIATED ANOMALIES

Hill et al. observed PRUV in 33 of 15,237 consecutive obstetric ultrasounds. Six (18.2%) of these 33 fetuses with PRUV had additional congenital malformations, which included dysplastic kidneys, cardiac defects, hemivertebrae, caudal regression, club feet, cleft lip and palate, intrauterine growth retardation, anencephaly, and asplenia syndrome.

ANEUPLOIDY

As an isolated finding, this abnormality is not known to increase the risk of chromosomal abnormalities.

OUTCOME

As an *isolated* finding, PRUV likely is of little significance, and no follow-up is generally

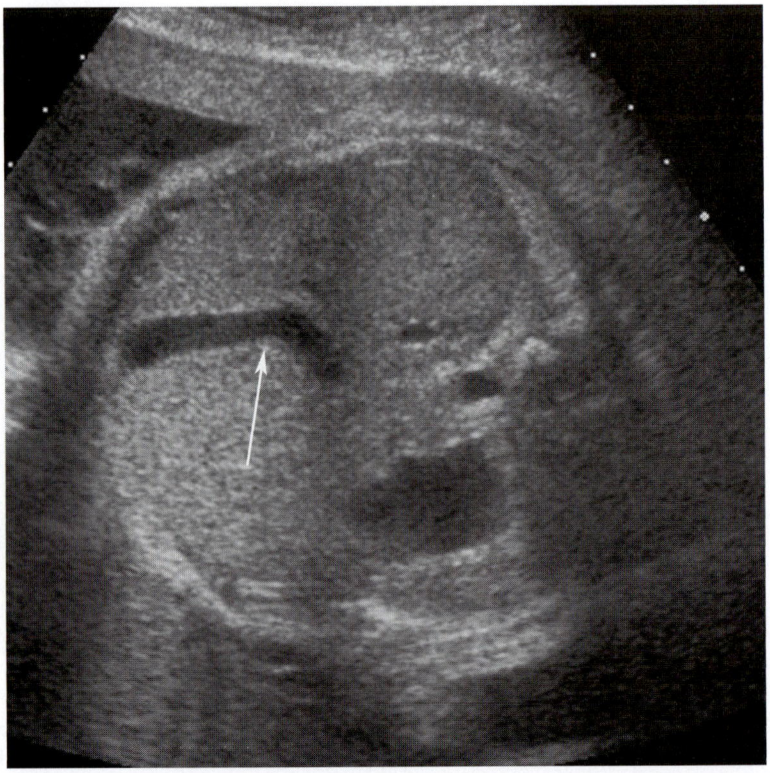

A

FIGURE 3-19 (A) Axial scan through the abdomen of a third-trimester fetus shows the persistent right umbilical vein *(arrow)* coursing toward the fetal stomach. *Continued*

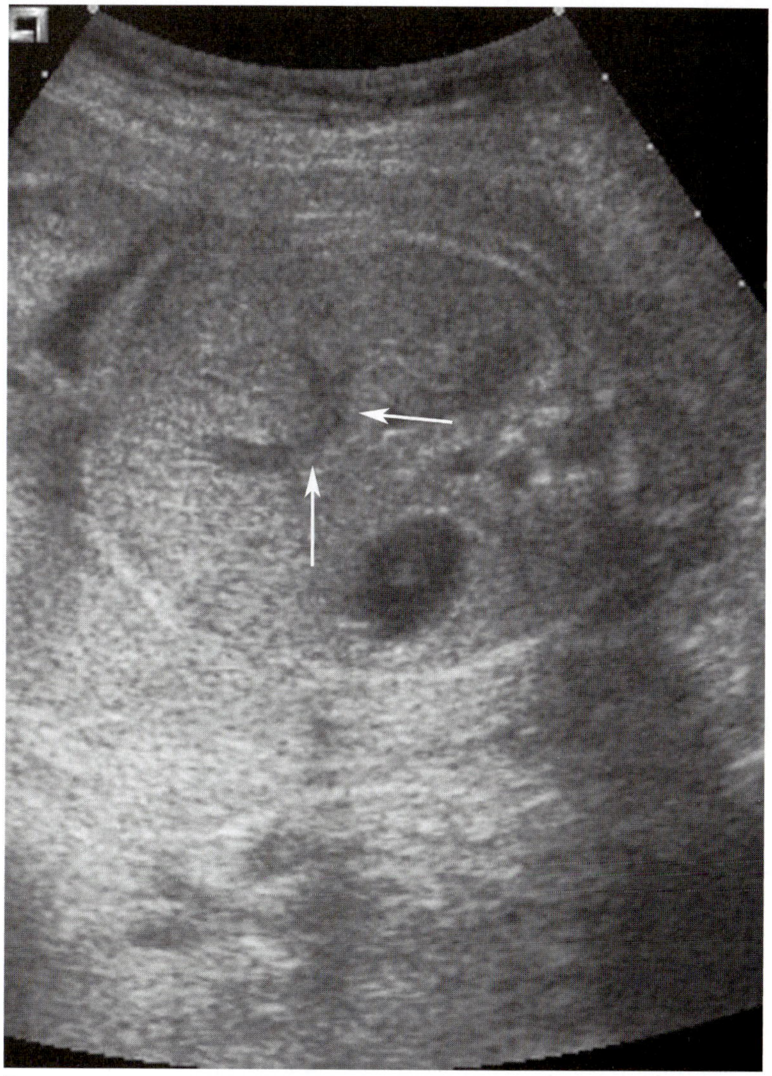

B

FIGURE 3-19, cont'd (**B**) Comparison view of the umbilical vein of a normal fetus. Note the orientation of the umbilical vein *(arrows)* as it courses away from the stomach bubble.

recommended. Kirsch et al. reported on nine cases of isolated intrahepatic PRUV in which no sequelae were identified after birth, except for one newborn who was noted to have hypospadias.

MANAGEMENT STRATEGIES

Fetuses with PRUV should undergo a detailed structural survey, including a detailed view of the fetal cardiac anatomy.

Suggested Reading

Hill LM, Mills A, Peterson C, Boyles D: Persistent right umbilical vein: sonographic detection and subsequent neonatal outcome. *Obstet Gynecol* 84:923–925, 1994.

Kirsch CFE, Feldstein VA, Goldstein RB, Filly RA: Persistent intrahepatic right umbilical vein: a prenatal sonographic series without significant anomalies. *J Ultrasound Med* 15:371–374, 1996.

Shen O, Tadmor OP, Yagel S: Prenatal diagnosis of persistent right umbilical vein. *Ultrasound Obstet Gynecol* 8:31–33, 1996.

Wolman I, Gull I, Fait G, et al: Persistent right umbilical vein: incidence and significance. *Ultrasound Obstet Gynecol* 19:562–564, 2002.

SINGLE UMBILICAL ARTERY (SUA)

PREVALENCE

SUA is seen in 1% of singleton pregnancies and 5% of twin gestations.

ETIOLOGY

The etiology is thought to be related to atrophy of a previously normal umbilical artery, most likely secondary to thrombosis.

SONOGRAPHIC FINDINGS

SUA usually is identified in the midtrimester as part of an anatomic survey. The number of vessels in the umbilical cord is most easily evaluated at the cord insertion site into the fetus, using color Doppler flow to demonstrate the vessels as they course around the bladder. Alternatively, a transverse section of a free loop of

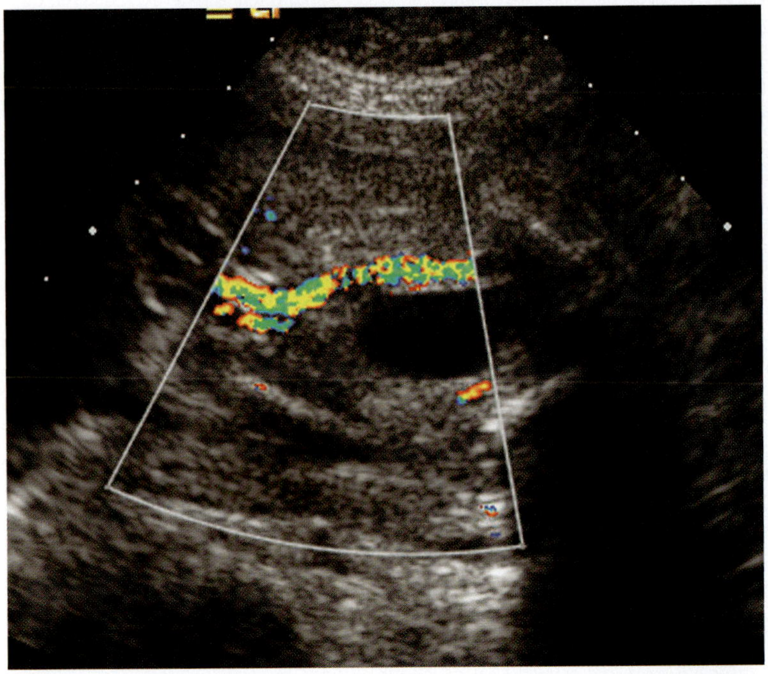

A

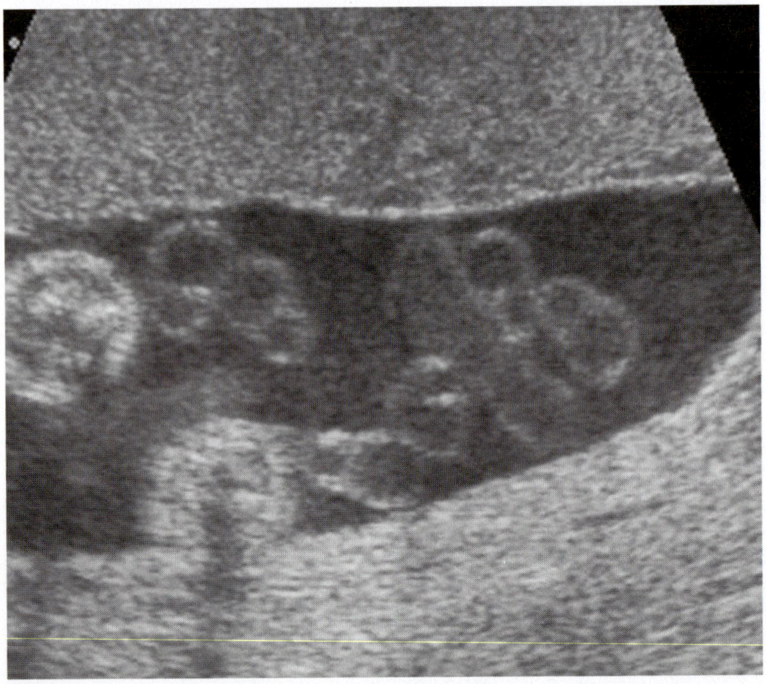

B

FIGURE 3-20 (A) Color Doppler shows single umbilical artery coursing around the fetal bladder in the midtrimester. (B) Cross-section of an umbilical cord shows the single umbilical artery in a midtrimester fetus.

cord can demonstrate the finding. The umbilical arteries may normally fuse toward the placenta, giving the appearance of a normal three-vessel cord at the fetal end but only two vessels at the placental insertion.

ASSOCIATED ANOMALIES

SUA is associated with other anomalies in 13% to 46% of fetuses. There is no specific pattern of malformation associated with SUA; however, cardiac and renal anomalies are most common. The side of the existing artery is equally distributed and is not associated with the risk of associated malformation.

ANEUPLOIDY

An *isolated* SUA does not appear to have an increased risk of aneuploidy. In fetuses with additional anomalies, the risk of aneuploidy, particularly trisomies 13 and 18, is high. The risk of trisomy 21 does not appear to be increased with SUA.

GROWTH

SUA has been linked to an increased risk of growth restriction, stillbirth, and preterm birth. This association has primarily been reported in fetuses with other congenital anomalies.

OUTCOME

The outcome of fetuses with an isolated SUA is good. Of note, however, Chow et al. reported that 7% of fetuses with an "isolated" single umbilical artery diagnosed prenatally have additional abnormalities identified after birth.

MANAGEMENT STRATEGIES

A detailed structural survey is indicated for fetuses with SUA. Special attention should be paid to the cardiac survey, kidneys, and hands because of the risk of trisomy 18. Markers for aneuploidy should be evaluated if the fetus is in the appropriate gestational age window. Correlation with maternal serum screening for aneuploidy is recommended, with special attention to the risk of trisomy 18. Amniocentesis should be considered if other risk factors or sonographic findings are present. Follow-up evaluation in the third trimester to assess interval growth is recommended.

Suggested Reading

Benirschke K, Kaufman P: *Pathology of the human placenta,* ed 2. New York, 1990, Springer-Verlag.

Blazer S, Sujov P, Escholi Z, Bar-Hava I, Bronshtein M: Single umbilical artery—right or left? Does it matter? *Prenat Diagn* 17:5–8, 1997.

Budorick NE, Kelly TF, Dunn JA, Scioscia AL: The single umbilical artery in a high-risk patient population. What should be offered? *J Ultrasound Med* 20:619–627, 2001.

Chow JS, Benson CB, Doubilet PM: Frequency and nature of structural anomalies in fetuses with single umbilical arteries. *J Ultrasound Med* 17:765–768, 1998.

Pierce BT, Dance VD, Wagner RK, Apodaca CC, Nielsen PE, Calhoun BC: Perinatal outcome following fetal single umbilical artery diagnosis. *J Matern Fetal Med* 10:59–63, 2001.

Thummala MR, Raju TN, Langenberg P: Isolated single umbilical artery anomaly and the risk for congenital malformations: a meta-analysis. *J Pediatr Surg* 33:580–585, 1998.

UMBILICAL CORD CYST IN THE FIRST TRIMESTER

PREVALENCE

Umbilical cord cyst is seen in 2% to 3% of first-trimester scans. Umbilical cord cysts seen in the first trimester tend to resolve by the second trimester.

ETIOLOGY

True umbilical cord cysts are remnants of either the allantois or the omphalomesenteric duct. Pseudocysts have no epithelial lining and are localized edema of Wharton jelly.

SONOGRAPHIC FINDINGS

The first-trimester umbilical cord cyst appears as a small echolucency without color flow along the umbilical cord. These cysts usually measure 3 to 6 mm and may be single or multiple. Sonographic differentiation of a true cyst from a pseudocyst is not possible.

ASSOCIATED ANOMALIES/ ANEUPLOIDY

Ross et al. reported on a series of 29 fetuses with umbilical cord cysts in the first trimester and noted that 26% had fetal anomalies, including

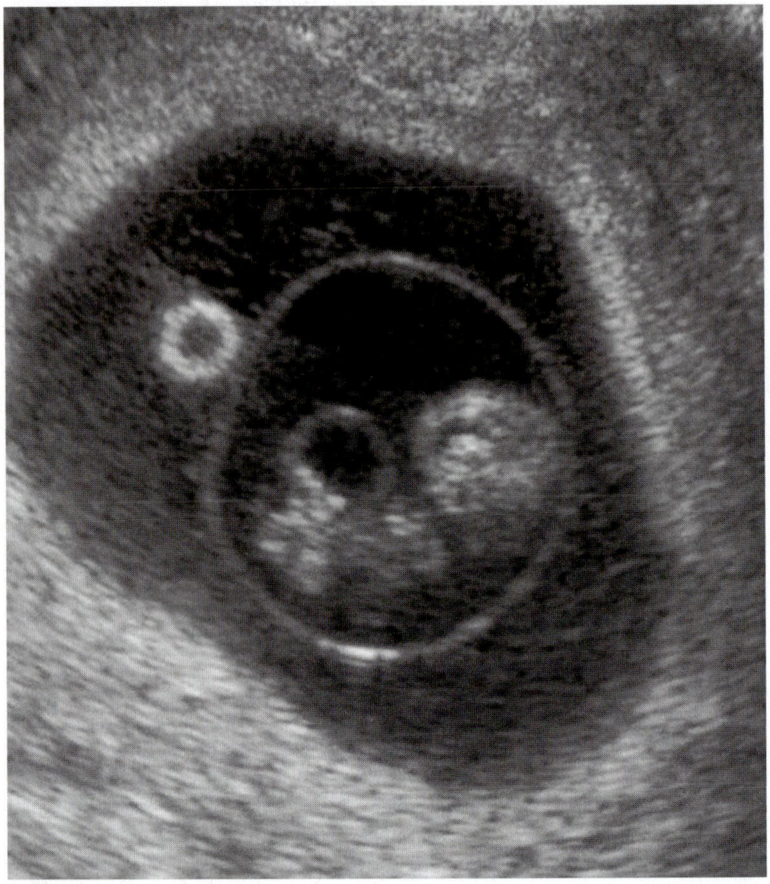

FIGURE 3-21 Umbilical cord cyst seen in the first trimester. Note that the yolk sac is separate from the intra-amniotic structures.

trisomy 18. The outcome may be worse if the cyst is located at either end of the cord (placental or fetal insertion), eccentrically with relation to the long axis of the cord, or if present beyond 12 weeks' gestation. Ghezzi et al. reported on 24 cases of umbilical cord cysts identified between 7 and 14 weeks' gestation. The cysts were single in 18 cases and multiple in six. All fetuses with a single umbilical cord cyst were born without structural anomalies and without features suggestive of chromosomal abnormalities. Of the fetuses with multiple cord cysts, four were spontaneously aborted (two of whom had trisomy 18), one had an obstructive uropathy, and one was a normal newborn.

OUTCOME

Ross et al. reported a normal outcome in 74% of fetuses noted to have a first-trimester umbilical cord cyst. Ghezzi et al. and Sepulveda et al. reported 100% normal outcome for single cysts. Multiple cysts were associated with a poorer outcome, with 83% of pregnancies ending in a spontaneous abortion or with aneuploidy.

MANAGEMENT STRATEGIES

Patients with a first-trimester umbilical cord cyst should undergo risk assessment for aneuploidy either in the first trimester or by serum screening. A detailed structural survey at 18 to 20 weeks, including a search for markers of aneuploidy, is recommended. Fetuses with a single umbilical cord cyst that resolves in the first trimester without additional risk factors and with a normal comprehensive structural survey do not require further evaluation.

Suggested Reading

Ghezzi F, Raio L, DiNaro E, Franchi M, Cromi A, Durig P: Single and multiple umbilical cord cysts in early gestation: two different entities. *Ultrasound Obstet Gynecol* 21:213–214, 2003.

Ross JA, Jurkovic D, Zosmer N, Jauniaux E, Hacket E, Nicolaides KH: Umbilical cord cysts early in pregnancy. *Obstet Gynecol* 89:442–445, 1997.

Sepulveda W, Leible S, Ulloa A, Ivankovic M, Schnapp C: Clinical significance of first trimester umbilical cord cysts. *J Ultrasound Med* 18:95–99, 1999.

INCOMPLETE FUSION OF THE CEREBELLAR VERMIS

PREVALENCE

Incomplete fusion of the cerebellar vermis varies with gestational age. In a study of 897 euploid fetuses between 14 and 18 weeks, our group reported that the fourth ventricle appeared to communicate with the cisterna magna in 56% of fetuses at 14 weeks, decreasing to 23% at 15 weeks and 6% at 17 weeks. By 18 weeks, this finding is considered abnormal.

ETIOLOGY

The cerebellar vermis is formed by fusion of the cerebellar hemisphere superiorly at approximately gestational week 9. This fusion continues inferiorly, with completion of development of the vermis at approximately week 15 or 16.

SONOGRAPHIC FINDINGS

Findings consist of a connection between the fourth ventricle and the cisterna magna attributable to a yet undeveloped inferior cerebellar vermis.

DIFFERENTIAL DIAGNOSIS

Dandy Walker Variant:

The diagnosis of a Dandy-Walker variant cannot be made reliably before 18 weeks' gestation because normal development of the vermis is not complete until this time. Incomplete development of the cerebellar vermis normally seen in the young fetus is indistinguishable from a true Dandy-Walker variant. Although reports of a first-trimester diagnosis are available, all suggest confirmatory follow-up later in gestation.

NATURAL HISTORY

Our group reported on a series of 897 euploid fetuses undergoing second-trimester amniocentesis who had a normal structural survey for stage and in whom the posterior fossa was seen sonographically. Of the 897 fetuses, 147 had a visible connection between the fourth ventricle and the cisterna magna. The younger the fetus, the more likely we were to see a connection between the fourth ventricle and the cisterna

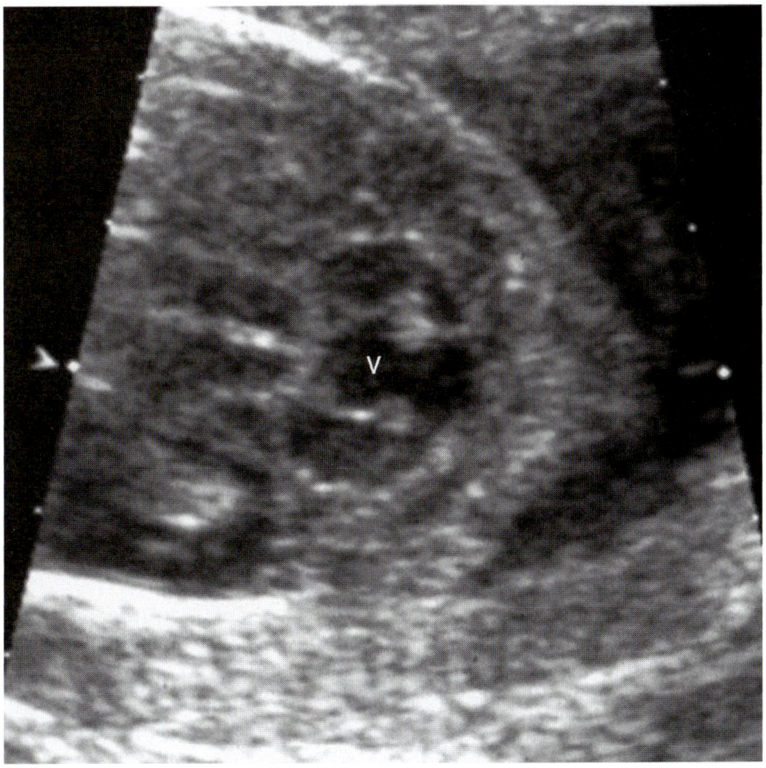

A

FIGURE 3-22 (A) Transverse view through the fetal posterior fossa in the early second trimester shows a communication between the fourth ventricle *(V)* and the cisterna magna, because the vermis is not completely formed.

Continued

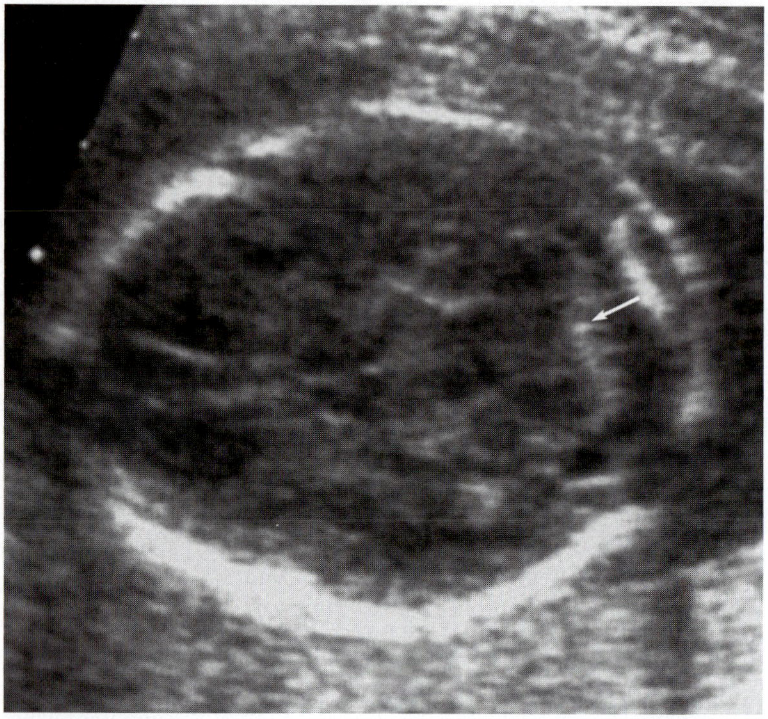
B

FIGURE 3-22, cont'd (B) Follow-up scan of the same fetus several weeks later shows that the posterior fossa now is normal, with complete development of the vermis *(arrow).*

magna (see Prevalence). Follow-up scans were performed at the discretion of the referring obstetrician and were available in 79% of fetuses. All but one had closure of the cerebellar vermis by 18 weeks' gestation. One fetus had a persistent communication diagnosed as a Dandy-Walker variant on follow-up prenatal scans as well as postnatal computed tomography.

MANAGEMENT STRATEGIES

A connection between the cisterna magna and the fourth ventricle in a fetus <18 weeks' gestation is likely a normal part of development. The finding should prompt a detailed evaluation after 18 weeks' gestation to identify a fetus with a true Dandy-Walker variant.

Suggested Reading

Bromley B, Nadel AS, Pauker S, Estroff JA, Benacerraf BR: Closure of he cerebellar vermis: evaluation with second trimester ultrasound. *Radiology* 193:761–763, 1994.

Lemire RJ, Loeser JD, Leech RW, Ellsworth A Jr: *Normal and abnormal development of the human nervous system.* Hagerstown, MD, 1975, Harper & Row.

Nizard J, Bernard JP, Ville Y: Fetal cystic malformations of the posterior fossa in the first trimester of pregnancy. *Fetal Diagn Ther* 20:146–151, 2005.

MILD PYELECTASIS

PREVALENCE

The prevalence of pyelectasis varies with criteria for positivity. Mandell et al. reported that 2.8% of euploid fetuses have a renal pelvis anteroposterior diameter (APD) 4 mm between 15 and 20 weeks. Pyelectasis is more common in male fetuses and more prevalent in third-trimester fetuses. Maternal oral hydration is not a major factor in fetal pyelectasis.

SONOGRAPHIC FINDINGS

Pyelectasis is identified by an echolucent fluid collection within the renal pelvis. Mild pyelectasis is considered present when the anterior posterior diameter (APD) of the renal pelvis measures at least 4 mm between 16 and 20 weeks' gestation, 5 mm between 20 and 30 weeks, and 7 mm between 30 and 40 weeks. In a meta-analysis, Lee et al. considered pyelectasis to be in the mild category if APD was ≤7 mm in the second trimester and ≤9 mm in the third trimester. In addition, for pyelectasis to be considered mild, no caliectasis and no change in echotexture or thinning of the renal parenchyma should be present. The bladder should appear normal. The presence of any of these additional features or greater degrees of dilation may reflect more significant renal pathology.

ANEUPLOIDY

Pyelectasis is seen in approximately 25% of fetuses with Down syndrome. As an *isolated* finding, mild pyelectasis carries a likelihood ratio of 1.5 for Down syndrome. A revised risk for aneuploidy is calculated using Bayes theorem, and amniocentesis is recommended only when the revised risk exceeds the commonly accepted threshold for offering karyotyping.

RENAL CONSIDERATIONS

Overall, children with mild pyelectasis are at greater risk for postnatal pathology compared with those without pyelectasis. In a meta-analysis by Lee et al., 11.9% of fetuses with mild pyelectasis had postnatal pathology. Postnatal outcomes include various obstructive processes and reflux.

Several different methods for determining thresholds of renal pelvis dimensions for use in evaluating the need for postnatal follow-up have been proposed.

In a study by Mandell et al. from our laboratory, we found that all fetuses requiring surgery had renal pelvis measurements ≥5 mm between 15 and 20 weeks, ≥8 mm between 20 and 30 weeks, and ≥10 mm between 30 and 40 weeks.

Adra et al. studied 68 cases of pyelectasis. Using a threshold of 8 mm for renal pelvis APD after 28 weeks, they reported sensitivity, specificity, and positive and negative predictive values for urinary tract abnormalities of 87%, 41%, 67%, and 70%, respectively. Although the sensitivity for detection of fetal renal abnormalities was high, the specificity in this study was rather low. The sensitivity and specificity obviously depend on the threshold used for renal pelvis APD.

Ouzounian et al. found that a threshold of 8 mm throughout gestation had 91% sensitivity and 72% specificity in predicting subsequent hydronephrosis. Use of a threshold of ≥5 mm yielded sensitivity of 100%, although specificity was only 24%. On this basis, they recommended that a threshold 5 mm at any gestational age warranted follow-up evaluation of fetal kidneys after birth.

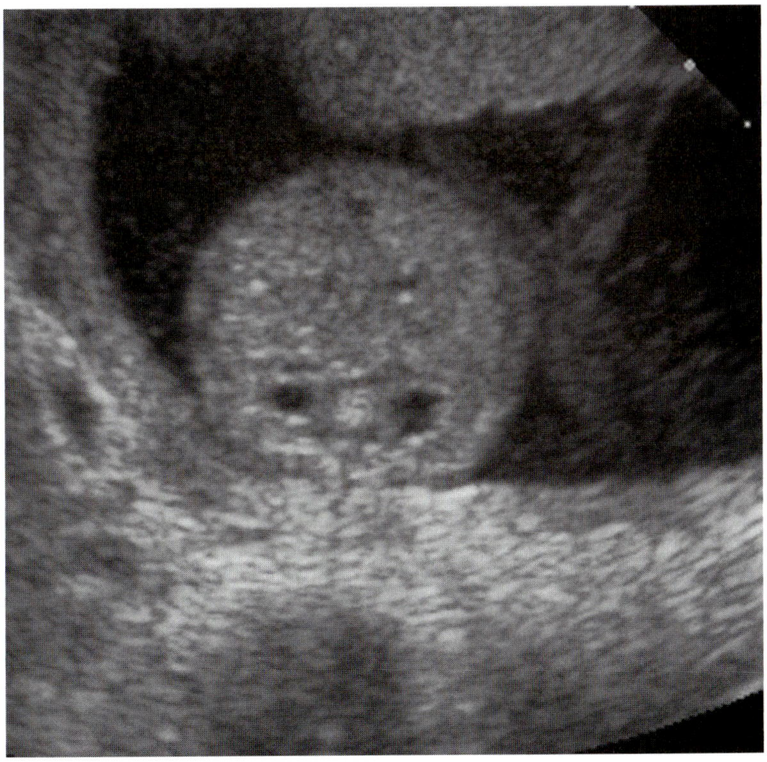

FIGURE 3-23 Transverse view of the fetal abdomen in the second trimester shows mild dilation of the fetal renal pelvis consistent with mild pyelectasis.

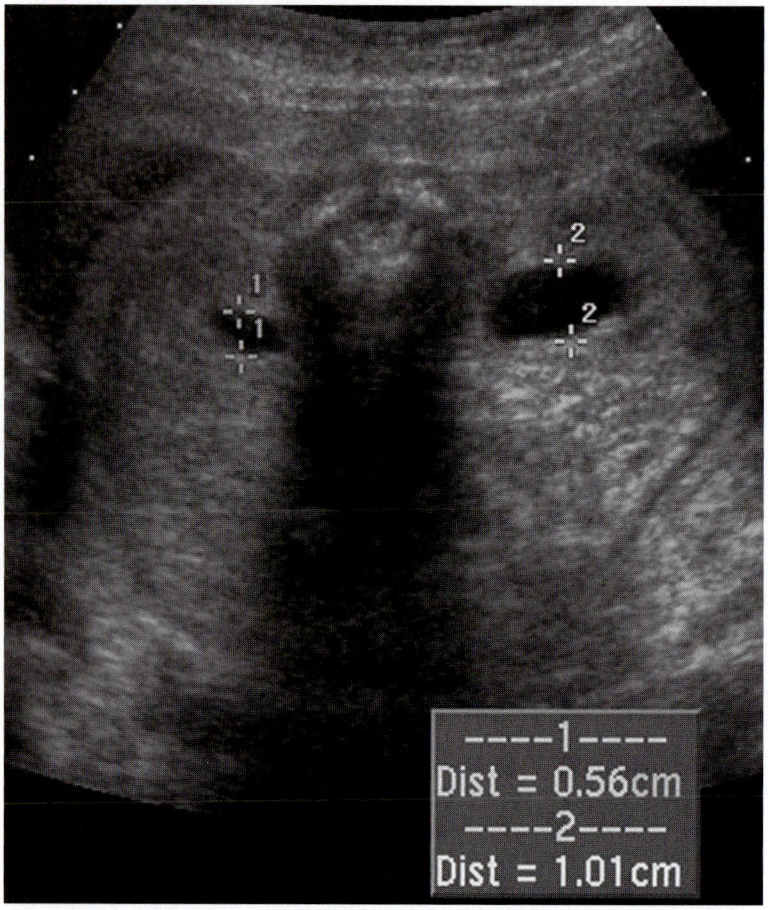

FIGURE 3-24 Prone transverse view of the fetal abdomen in the third trimester shows that one renal pelvis measures >10 mm, which is abnormal. The contralateral kidney has a anteroposterior diameter measurement of 5.6 mm and is considered normal for this late gestational age.

Prenatal ultrasound performed in the third trimester as opposed to earlier in pregnancy may be more predictive of postnatal outcome.

MANAGEMENT STRATEGIES

When mild pyelectasis is identified in the second trimester, a detailed structural survey is recommended, as is a search for additional markers of aneuploidy. In cases of isolated mild pyelectasis, using Bayes theorem with a likelihood ratio of 1.5 will provide a revised risk assessment for Down syndrome. In fetuses with isolated mild pyelectasis, karyotype is not indicated unless the revised risk estimate exceeds the commonly accepted threshold for offering amniocentesis. A follow-up scan in the third trimester is recommended to refine any recommendations for postnatal follow-up and management.

Suggested Reading

Adra AM, Mejides AA, Dennaoui MS, Beydoun SN: Fetal pyelectasis: is it always "physiologic"? *Am J Obstet Gynecol* 173:1263–1266, 1995.

Benacerraf BR, Mandell J, Estroff JA, Harlow BL, Frigoletto FD Jr: Fetal pyelectasis, a possible association with Down syndrome. *Obstet Gynecol* 76:58–60, 1990.

Bromley B, Lieberman E, Shipp TD, et al: The genetic sonogram: a method of risk assessment for Down syndrome in the midtrimester. *J Ultrasound Med* 21:1087–1096, 2002.

Lee RS, Cendron M, Kinnamon DD, Nguyen HT: Antenatal hydronephrosis as a predictor of postnatal outcome: a meta-analysis. *Pediatrics* 118:586–593, 2006.

Mandell J, Blyth BR, Peters CA, Retik AB, Estroff JA, Benacerraf BR: Structural genitourinary defects detected in utero. *Radiology* 178:193–196, 1991.

Nyberg DA, Souter VL, El-Bastawissi A, Young S, Luthhardt F, Luthy DA: Isolated sonographic markers for detection of fetal Down syndrome in the second trimester of pregnancy. *J Ultrasound Med* 20:1053–1063, 2001.

Ouzounian JG, Castro MA, Fresquez M, Al-Sulyman OM, Kovacs BW: Prognostic significance of antenatally detected fetal pyelectasis. *Ultrasound Obstet Gynecol* 7:424–428, 1996.

ECHOGENIC KIDNEYS WITH NORMAL AMNIOTIC FLUID VOLUME (AFV) AND NO ADDITIONAL ANOMALIES

PREVALENCE

Echogenic kidneys are rare in the fetus.

ETIOLOGY

The etiology depends on the final diagnosis. Increased echogenicity of the renal parenchyma can be the result of different types of cystic renal disease or dysplastic changes, or it can be a normal variant.

SONOGRAPHIC FINDINGS

The kidneys are considered echogenic when the echogenicity of the renal parenchyma is greater than that of the liver. In many cases, AFV and bladder are normal. This finding is generally observed in the second or third trimester.

DIFFERENTIAL DIAGNOSIS

This finding can be a normal variant, although a variety of cystic renal diseases have been implicated, including autosomal recessive polycystic kidney disease, autosomal dominant polycystic kidney disease, Finnish nephrosis, Meckel-Gruber syndrome, trisomy 13, Beckwith-Wiedemann syndrome, and other syndromes of fetal overgrowth.

OUTCOME

Perinatal outcome is primarily dependent on the associated AFV. In general, moderate-to-severe oligohydramnios is associated with poor fetal outcome. Normal, mildly decreased, or mildly increased AFV often is associated with survival and potentially normal renal function.

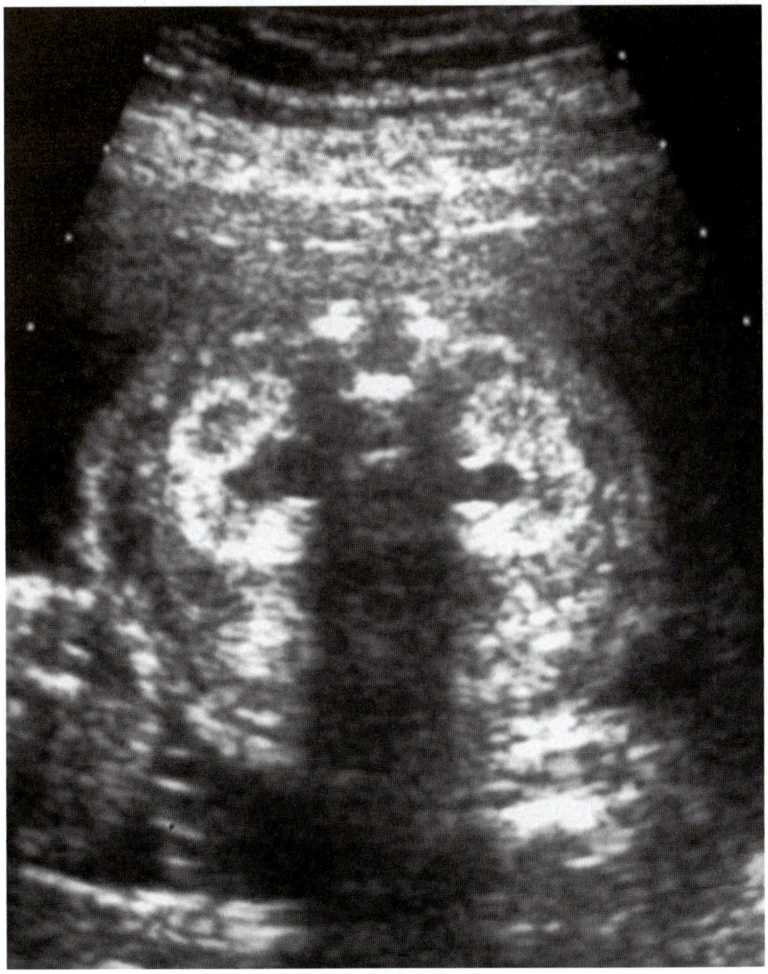

FIGURE 3-25 Transverse view through both kidneys of a fetus with increased renal echogenicity and a normal amniotic fluid volume.

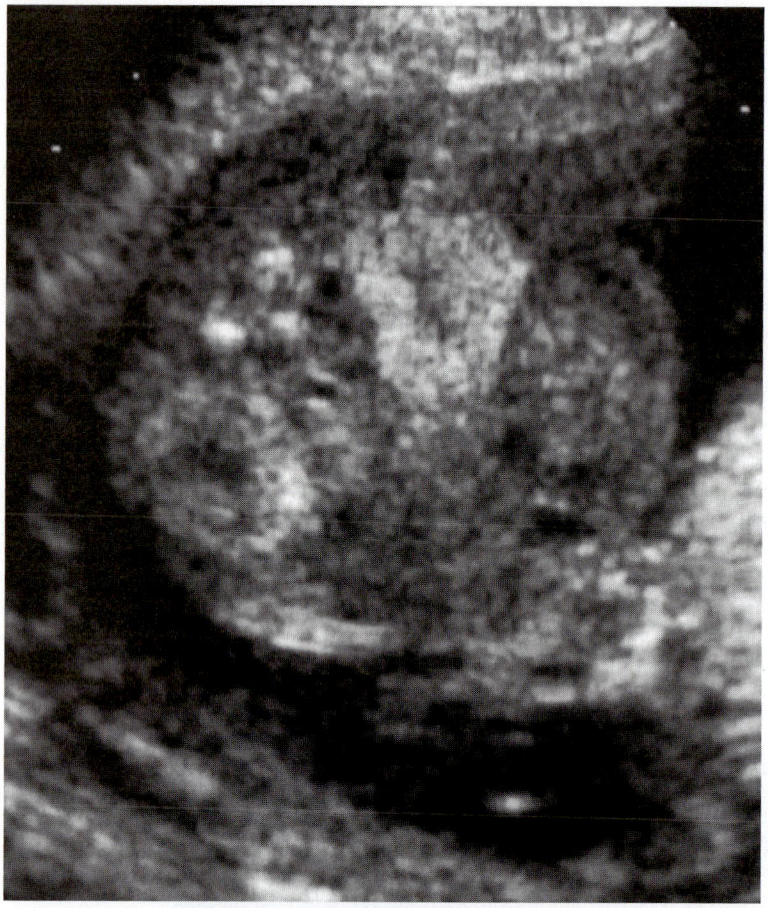

FIGURE 3-26 Transverse view of a second-trimester fetus with echogenic kidneys and a very high amniotic fluid alpha-fetoprotein, indicative of Finnish nephrosis.

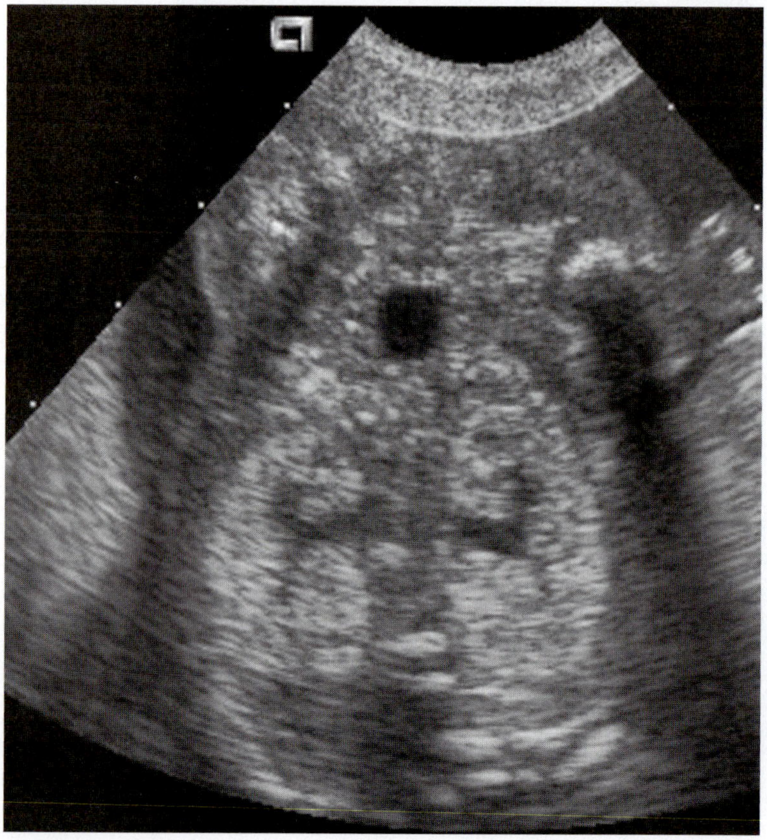

FIGURE 3-27 Coronal view of the fetal kidneys in an early second-trimester fetus with autosomal recessive polycystic kidney disease. There still is some amniotic fluid present and urine in the fetal bladder attributable to the early gestational age.

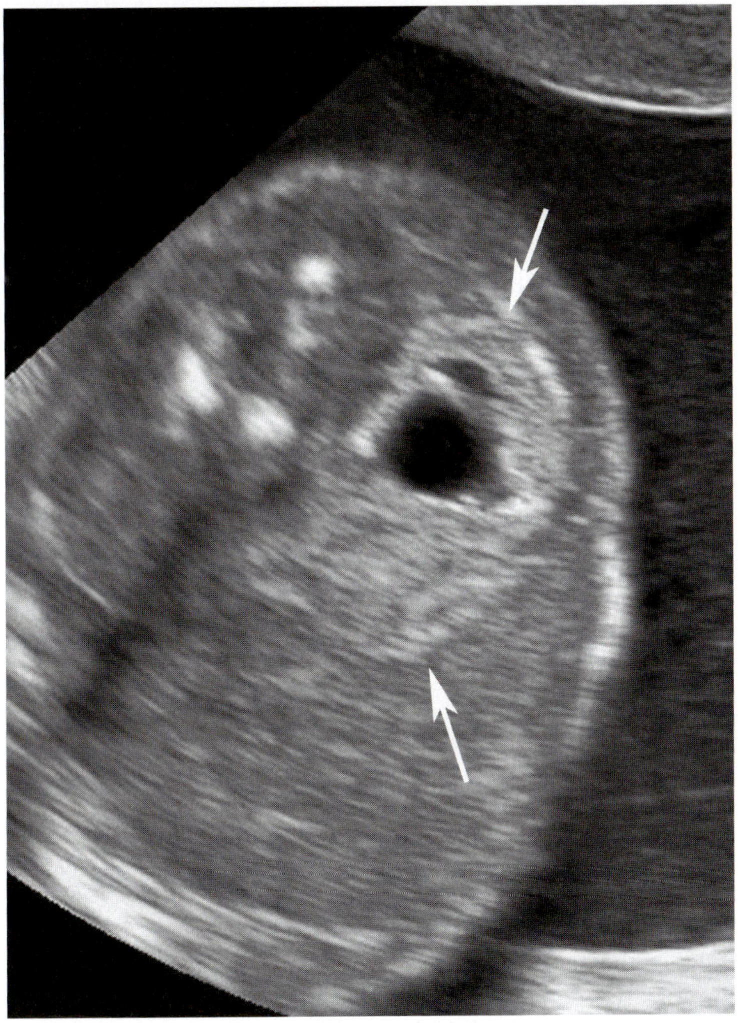

FIGURE 3-28 Oblique view of an echogenic kidney *(arrows)* with some cystic areas, suggesting dysplastic changes. This 18-week fetus had trisomy 13.

In a study of 19 fetuses with hyperechoic kidneys, our group found that 15 (79%) of 19 newborns had a functional or sonographic renal anomaly, and 74% of the fetuses survived. Fourteen of 19 had bilateral renal hyperechogenicity, and five had unilateral renal hyperechogenicity. Four (24%) of 19 were normal newborns with normal postnatal renal sonograms and renal function, indicating that this finding may be a normal variant. Five of the group died. Four of these five had autosomal recessive kidney disease, and one had bilateral multicystic dysplastic kidneys. Ten (53%) survived but had abnormalities on neonatal ultrasound. These included unilateral renal dysplasia (3), unilateral multicystic dysplastic kidney and contralateral hyperechoic kidney (2), hydronephrosis (2), and renal dysfunction of unknown type (3). Those that did not survive had associated oligohydramnios.

Carr et al. described the long-term outcome of a subset of fetuses with bilateral hyperechoic kidneys with preservation of the medullary pyramid architecture and normal amniotic fluid volume. Seven cases were available for follow-up over 3 years. Renal echogenicity resolved in four cases but persisted in the other three fetuses. Serum creatinine and electrolyte levels were normal in all cases. Mashiach et al. studied seven fetuses with hyperechoic kidneys and normal amniotic fluid volume. Three had autosomal dominant polycystic kidney disease, and one had autosomal recessive polycystic kidney disease. Two others had multifactorial renal dysplasia on autopsy, and one fetus had normal kidneys.

MANAGEMENT STRATEGIES

Increased renal echogenicity should prompt a detailed structural survey of the fetus, including markers for aneuploidy and continued prenatal sonographic monitoring for development of additional renal changes and amniotic fluid volume fluctuations. If the AFV remains normal and associated syndromes and aneuploidy are deemed unlikely, the newborn probably will survive, and the finding may either be clinically insignificant or represent nonlethal renal disease. If, on the other hand, oligohydramnios develops even late in the third trimester, the outcome is bleak. Autosomal recessive polycystic kidney disease may not result in decreased AFV until the third trimester.

Suggested Reading

Carr MC, Benacerraf BR, Estroff, JA, Mandell J: Prenatally diagnosed bilateral hyperechoic kidneys with normal amniotic fluid: postnatal outcome. *J Urol* 153:442–444, 1995.

Estroff JA, Mandell J, Benacerraf BR: Increased renal parenchymal echogenicity in the fetus: importance and clinical outcome. *Radiology* 181:135–139, 1991.

Mashiach R, Davidovits M, Eisenstein B, et al: Fetal hyperechogenic kidney with normal amniotic fluid volume: a diagnostic dilemma. *Prenat Diagn* 25:553–558, 2005.

EXTENSIVE AMNION–CHORION SEPARATION AFTER 17 WEEKS' GESTATION

PREVALENCE

Extensive amnion–chorion separation is rare after 17 weeks' gestation, although focal or limited separation of these membranes occurs more commonly.

ETIOLOGY

Extensive amnion–chorion separation generally occurs in patients who have undergone amniocentesis, although a minority of affected pregnancies have not undergone an invasive procedure. This finding has been reported in association with collagen abnormalities.

SONOGRAPHIC FINDINGS

Free-floating sheets of amnion are seen surrounding the fetus. Amnion–chorion separation is deemed to be extensive when free-floating membranes are visualized extending at least three fourths of the way around the gestational sac. Sometimes the fetus appears tightly enveloped by the loose and collapsed amnion. The fetus may be extruded from the amniotic cavity into the chorionic space, with amniotic membrane sheets floating at the base of the umbilical cord.

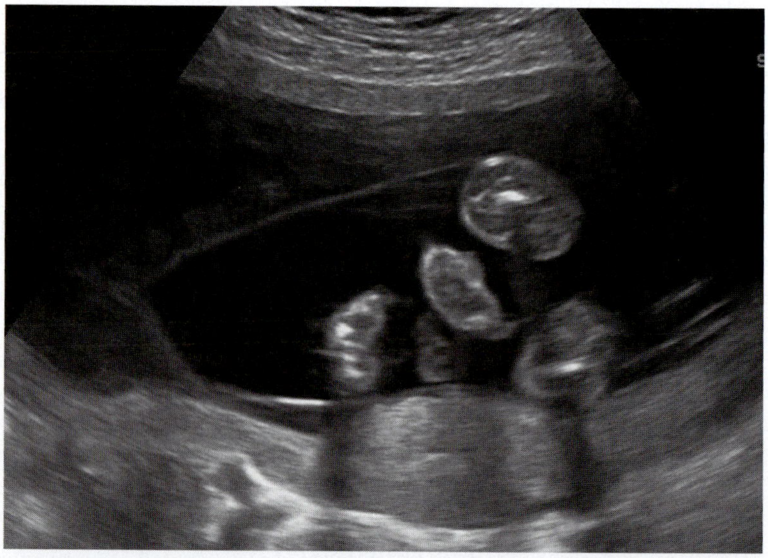

FIGURE 3-29 Complete separation of the amnion from the uterine side wall in a patient with extensive amnion–chorion separation. Note that the extremities are contained within the amniotic cavity, which is reduced in size because of separation of the amnion from the chorion.

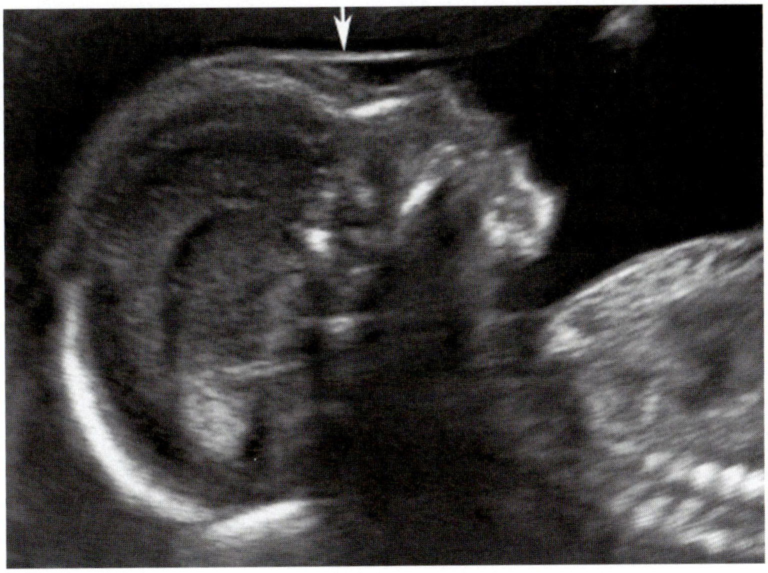

FIGURE 3-30 View of the fetal profile shows that the amnion *(arrow)* is in close proximity to the fetal nose. The fetus is enveloped by amniotic membrane, with collapse of the intraamniotic cavity.

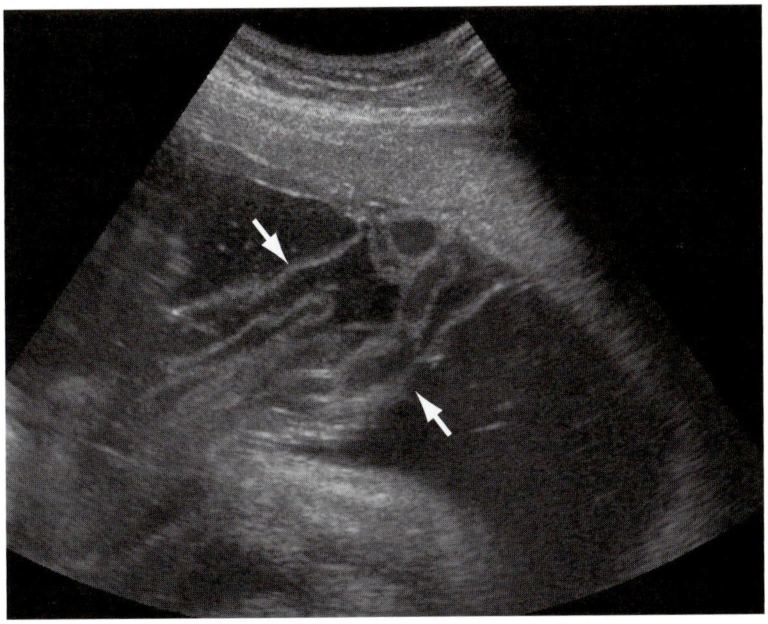

FIGURE 3-31 View of the fetal umbilical cord insertion site into the placenta of a third-trimester fetus with complete amnion–chorion separation. Note that the entire amniotic membrane *(arrows)* is collapsed around the cord insertion into the placenta, because the fetus is completely extruded into the chorionic space.

NATURAL HISTORY

Amnion–chorion separation is common prior to 14 weeks' gestation. As gestation progresses, the amnion fuses to the chorion. Fusion should be complete by 17 weeks' gestation. Complete amnion–chorion separation is considered abnormal beyond 17 weeks' gestation.

ASSOCIATED ANOMALIES

Potential defects associated with amnion–chorion separation are those caused by an amniotic band-type phenomenon, such as limb amputation defects and club feet. The loose amnion is thought to represent a spectrum of amniotic bands that developed later in gestation.

OUTCOME

In a study of 20 live fetuses with extensive amnion–chorion separation after 17 weeks' gestation, we noted that 13 (65%) fetuses had previously been subject to amniocentesis and 7 (35%) had not. Three fetuses had Down syndrome, two of whom had amnion–chorion separation prior to amniocentesis. All three of these fetuses had other markers suggesting aneuploidy; two of these pregnancies were electively terminated. Four fetuses died in utero between 24 and 25 weeks' gestation. It is hypothesized that membrane separation leads to amniotic band formation with subsequent compromise of the fetal umbilical cord.

In our population of 20 cases, 14 pregnancies resulted in live newborns, one with trisomy 21. Thirty-five percent of pregnancies delivered at term, and another 35% delivered prematurely because of a variety of perinatal complications, including growth restriction, oligohydramnios, and abruptio placentae.

MANAGEMENT STRATEGIES

If an extensive amnion–chorion separation is identified after 17 weeks' gestation, a detailed structural survey is recommended, including meticulous evaluation of the extremities. Because this finding is associated with an increased risk of trisomy 21, a search for markers and correlation with a priori risk assessment by serum screening or first-trimester risk analysis is recommended. Amniocentesis is technically more difficult to perform when the amnion is not fused to the chorion, but karyotypic analysis still may be indicated. Whether the risk of pregnancy loss is greater when amniocentesis is performed in the setting of extensive amnion–chorion separation has not been determined.

Suggested Reading

Abboud P, Mansour G, Zejli A, Gondry J: Chorioamniotic separation after 14 weeks' gestation associated with trisomy 21. *Ultrasound Obstet Gynecol* 22:94–95, 2003.

Benacerraf BR, Frigoletto FD Jr: Sonographic observation of amniotic rupture without amniotic band syndrome. *J Ultrasound Med* 11:109–111, 1992.

Bromley B, Shipp TD, Benacerraf BR: Amnion-chorion separation after 17 weeks gestation. *Obstet Gynecol* 94:1024–1026, 1999.

Stoler JM, Bromley B, Castro MA, Cole WG, Florer J, Wenstrup RJ: Separation of amniotic membranes after amniocentesis in an individual with the classical form of EDS and haploinsufficiency for COL5A1 expression. *Am J Med Genet* 101:174–177, 2001.

Ulm B, Ulm MR, Bernaschek G: Unfused amnion and chorion after 14 weeks gestation: associated fetal structural and chromosomal abnormalities. *Ultrasound Obstet Gynecol* 13:392–395, 1999.

4

Fetal Anomalies and Syndromes Associated with Monochorionic Twins

Thomas D. Shipp, MD, and Beryl R. Benacerraf, MD

Monozygotic twinning occurs in approximately 1 in 200 births, and this incidence remains relatively constant throughout the world. It is independent of race, maternal age, heredity, and fertility-enhancing treatments.[1–3] Because this type of twinning clearly is responsible for most of the morbidity and mortality of twin gestations, this chapter focuses on the malformations and syndromes associated with monozygotic twinning.

Although the incidence of monozygotic twinning at *birth* is 1 in 200, the incidence at *conception* is considerably higher. There is a threefold higher rate of monozygotic twins among spontaneous abortions compared with livebirth twins; the ratio of monozygotic to dizygotic twins is 17:1 in spontaneous abortions versus 0.8:1 in livebirths.[3] Most of these spontaneous abortions are attributable to early, lethal, structural defects that have a marked increased frequency among monozygotic twins. The excess of malformations among monozygotic twins most likely is related to the etiology that gives rise to monozygotic twinning, which is itself an aberration in development.

Although twins have a 14% incidence of perinatal mortality, monochorionic twins (the most common type of monozygotic twins) have a 25% incidence of perinatal mortality.[1] Hence, there is great interest in determining the zygosity and placentation of twins early in pregnancy so that pregnancies at increased risk for complications may undergo close monitoring, both for the presence of malformations and for the other complications of monozygotic twinning.

ZYGOSITY, CHORIONICITY, AND AMNIONICITY

All dizygotic twins are dichorionic and diamniotic, indicating separate placentae, chorions, and amnions. The presence of two separate placentae or of different fetal genders is a good indication that the twins are dichorionic–diamniotic. A difficulty arises, however, when there is one placental mass in twins of the same gender. Placentae can be located on opposite sides of the uterus, or they can be located side by side and thus appear fused. In most cases, however, they are separate and lack vascular connections.

Conversely, monozygotic twins may be associated with one of four different types of twinning, directly dependent on the time of splitting of the early zygote or embryo.[2,4]

1. If monozygotic twins split before the fifth day after conception, dichorionic–diamniotic twins will occur, and they will be indistinguishable sonographically from dizygotic twins. From 10% to 15% of dichorionic–diamniotic twins originate from a monozygotic twinning process in which division of the embryonic cells occurs during the first 4 days of gestation.[1]
2. Most monozygotic twins are monochorionic–diamniotic, representing 20% of spontaneous twins in the United States. This type of twinning involves a single placenta and two amnions and occurs when splitting of the early embryonic cells or embryo takes place between days 4 and 8 postconception.[1]
3. If the embryo divides early during the second week of gestation, monochorionic–monoamniotic placentation results. This occurs in 2% to 3% of monozygotic twins and is associated with a high mortality rate (50%).
4. Embryos dividing at the end of the second week of gestation will be conjoined.[2]

Several studies have demonstrated high accuracy in the sonographic differentiation between dichorionic–diamniotic twins and monochorionic–diamniotic twins, particularly in the first trimester. Before 12 weeks' gestation, it is easy to identify the thicker membrane separating dichorionic twins, because each has its own placenta with its chorionic sac and amnion. Later in gestation, the thickness and appearance of the membrane remain extremely helpful in distinguishing a dichorionic–diamniotic pregnancy (four layers of membrane) from a monochorionic–diamniotic pregnancy (two thin layers).[5] Several authors have introduced various signs, including the lambda or "twin peak" sign, as a prediction of chorionicity in twin pregnancies.[6–15] The determination of chorionicity in the first trimester is reported to be at least 95% and up to 99.3% sensitive; whereas in the second trimester, the accuracy may be reduced to 90%.[16–18] It is lower still in the third trimester because of the difficulty in determining membrane thickness and identifying the "twin peaks" as pregnancy progresses. Three-dimensional sonography may be helpful in determining chorionicity and amnionicity.[19]

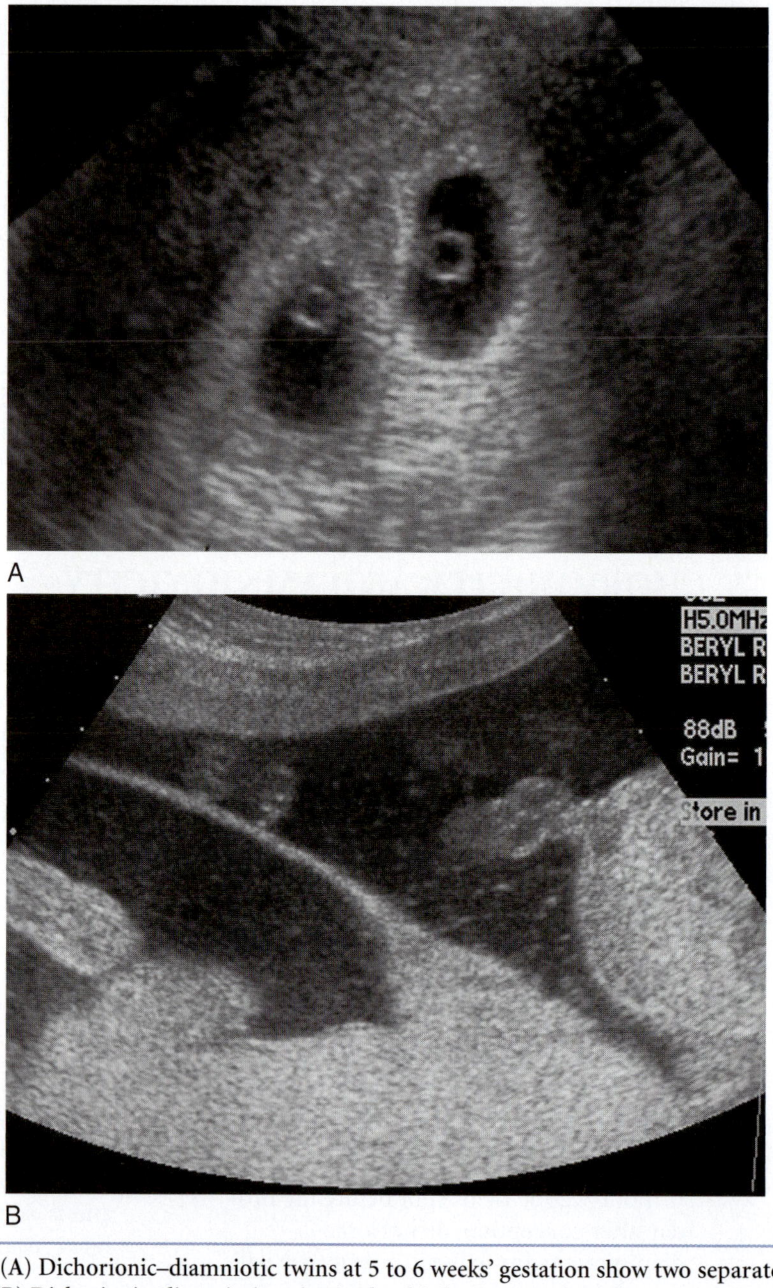

FIGURE 4-1 (**A**) Dichorionic–diamniotic twins at 5 to 6 weeks' gestation show two separate chorions and two yolk sacs. (**B**) Dichorionic–diamniotic twins in the third trimester show the twin peak sign at the base of the thick membrane, typically seen with this type of twinning.

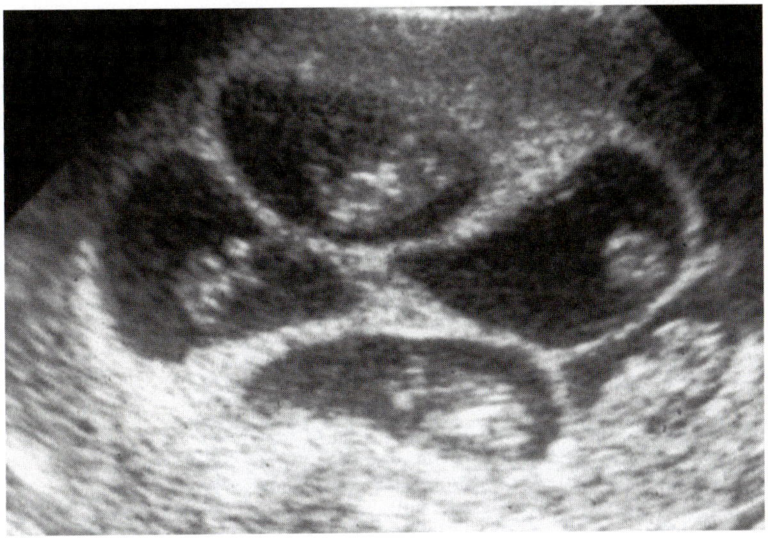

FIGURE 4-2 Quintuplet pregnancy at 8 weeks shows five chorions and five fetuses.

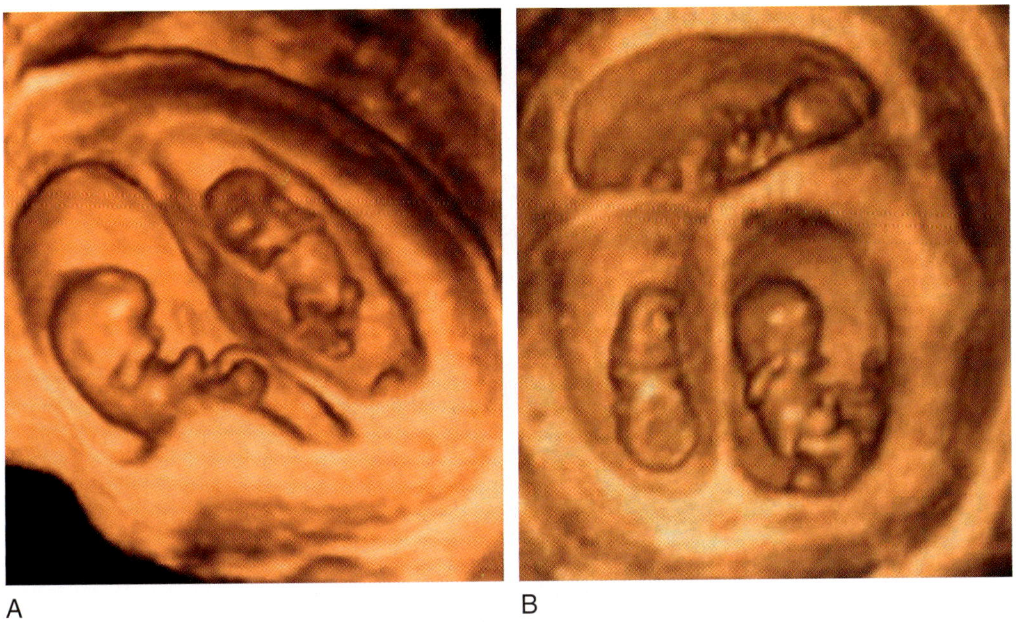

FIGURE 4-3 (A) Dichorionic–diamniotic twin pregnancy in the first trimester seen with three-dimensional surface reconstruction. Two separate chorions are well seen. (B) Three-dimensional surface reconstruction of trichorionic–triamniotic triplet pregnancy in the first trimester shows three different chorions.

The intertwin membrane for monochorionic–diamniotic twins is thin, made up of only two layers of amnion. Sometimes in the first trimester, it is difficult to identify the *amniotic* membrane dividing two amniotic sacs within a single chorion. In these cases, it is helpful to count the number of yolk sacs, which is equal to the number of amniotic sacs.[20,21] When a membrane is not visible sonographically, the notion of monoamniotic twins must be entertained. Nonvisualization of a separating membrane, however, cannot establish a definitive diagnosis of monoamniotic twins without further evaluation of the fetal environment. Serial scans can be integral to making the correct assessment. In many cases in which a separating membrane is not visualized, severe oligohydramnios is present in one amniotic sac and polyhydramnios is present in the other.[22] This is commonly seen in severe twin-to-twin transfusion syndrome, when the amniotic membrane cannot be visualized because it is fixed against one twin. Suspended within the oligohydramniotic sac, the twin with severe oligohydramnios appears to be stuck to the wall of the uterus.

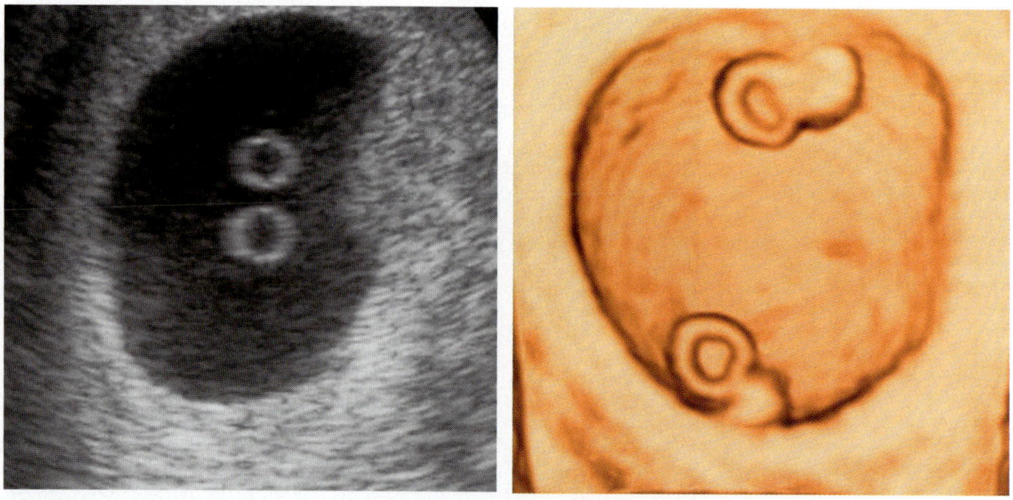

A B

FIGURE 4-4 (A) Monochorionic–diamniotic twin pregnancy shows a single chorion with two yolk sacs. The presence of two yolk sacs is highly suggestive that this pregnancy has two amnions. (B) Three-dimensional surface rendering of a 6-week monochorionic–diamniotic pregnancy shows two embryos adjacent to their own yolk sacs. Even though the amniotic membrane dividing them is not identified, it is presumed to exist because of the presence of two yolk sacs.

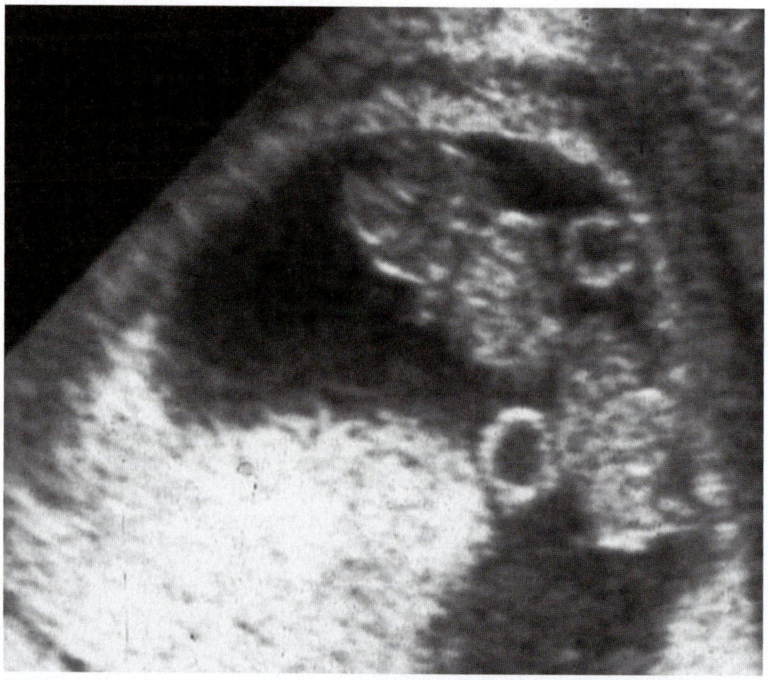

A

FIGURE 4-5 (A) Monochorionic–diamniotic twin pregnancy at 8 weeks shows two embryos and two yolk sacs. The thin amniotic membrane surrounding each embryo is not yet identified.

Continued

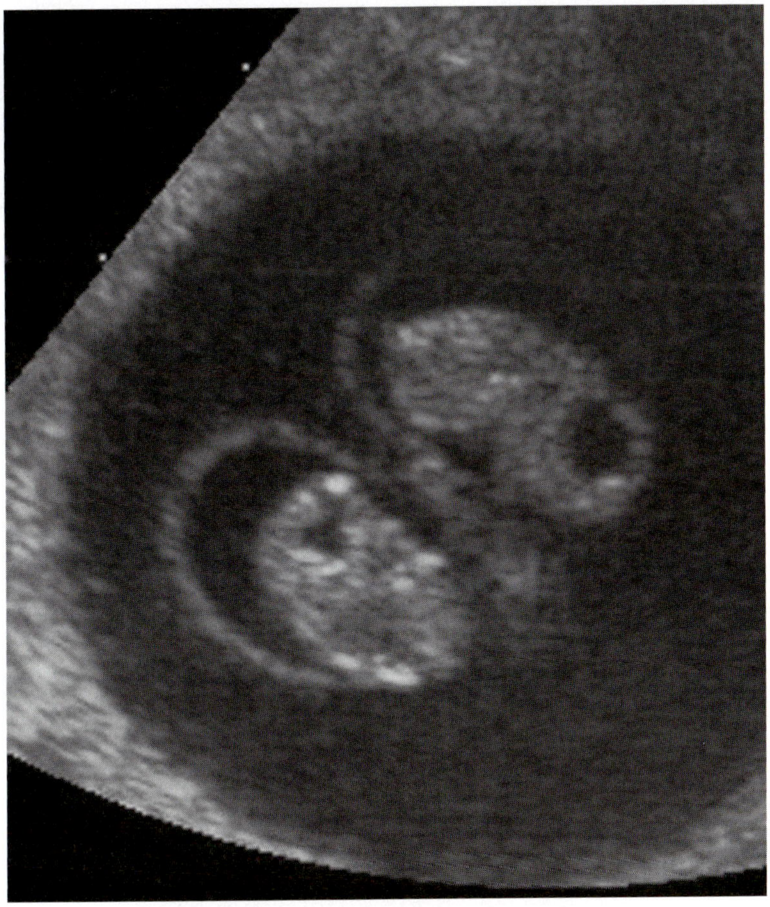

B

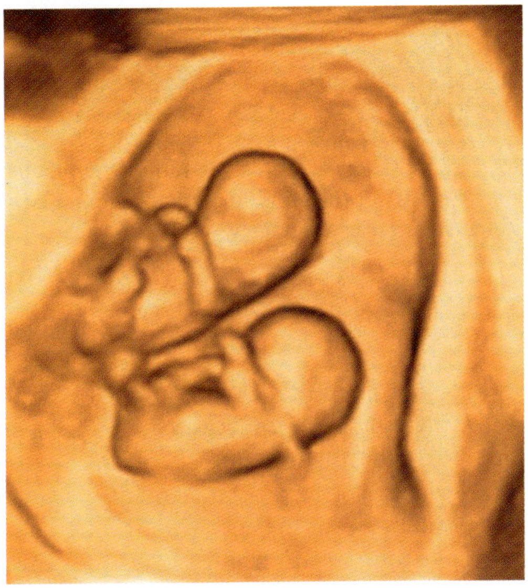

C

FIGURE 4-5, cont'd (B) Monochorionic–diamniotic twin pregnancy in the early first trimester, seen transvaginally at high frequency, shows the actual amniotic membrane surrounding each embryo. (C) Monochorionic–diamniotic twin pregnancy at 10 weeks shows two fetuses in the same chorion. The amniotic membranes are not well seen with three-dimensional surface reconstruction.

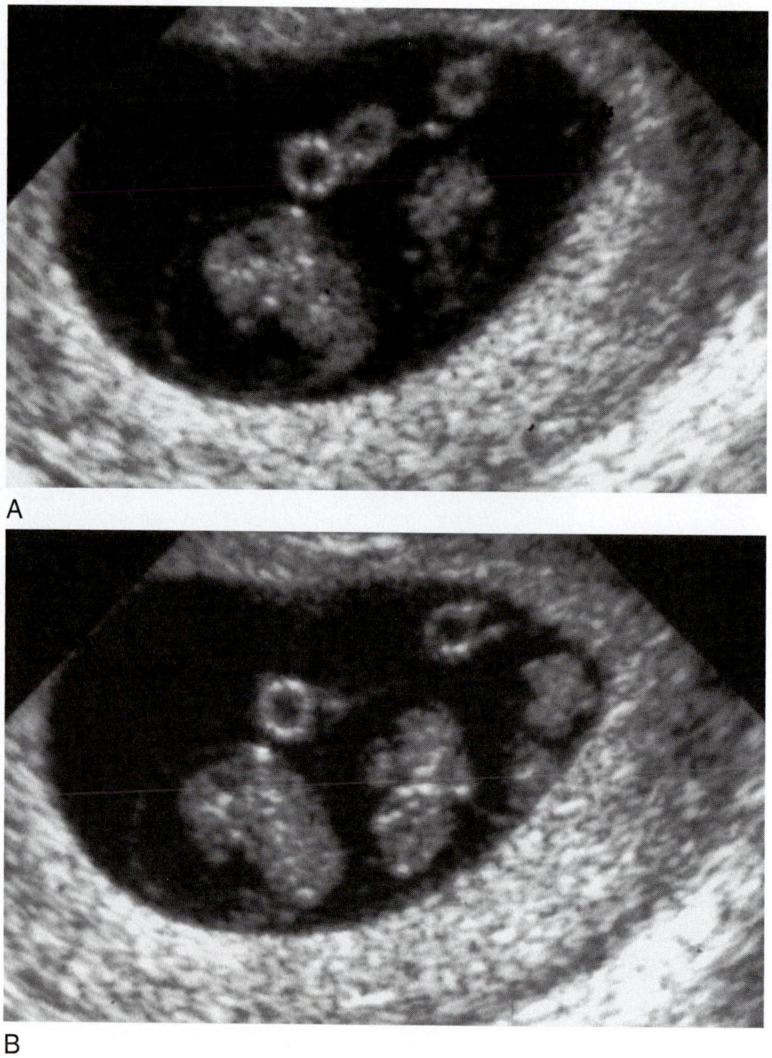

FIGURE 4-6 (A, B) Monochorionic–triamniotic triplet pregnancy shows three different embryos and three different yolk sacs. Part of the amniotic membrane can be seen occasionally. The presence of the three yolk sacs indicates a triamniotic pregnancy.

Monochorionic–monoamniotic twins are distinguished by the fact that both fetuses are free-floating.[23–26] In addition, if the pregnancy is monoamniotic, evidence of cord entanglement can be visualized sonographically and with Doppler instrumentation to confirm the diagnosis.[27] The diagnosis of monochorionic–monoamniotic twinning is imperative. The extremely high mortality rate (50%) and the 25% risk of neurologic injury to surviving fetuses after the death of a co-twin underscore the need for close monitoring and early delivery.[1,21,27] Multiple potential therapies have been attempted in monochorionic–monoamniotic twin pregnancies to improve the outcome. They have included medical amnioreduction, surgical amnioreduction, and fetal reduction, as with cord ligation. These therapies all have shown mixed success. The improved antenatal diagnosis, close surveillance, and early delivery all likely contribute to the reported improved survival rate noted over the past 75 years.[28]

Monoamniotic twinning also can occur if the dividing amniotic membrane of diamniotic twins is torn, possibly resulting in cord entanglement and amniotic band syndrome, with an overall perinatal mortality rate of 44%.[29,30] This situation can be caused iatrogenically during the performance of single-puncture amniocenteses in both amniotic sacs, in which case the membrane would be torn as the needle crosses it.

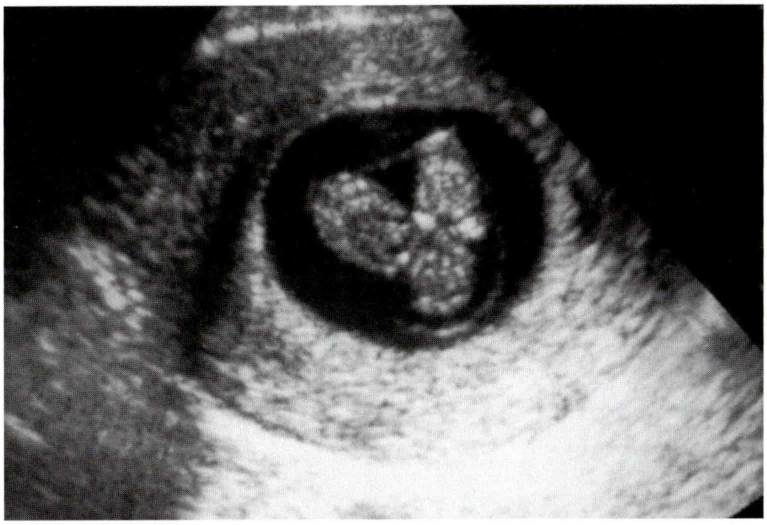

A

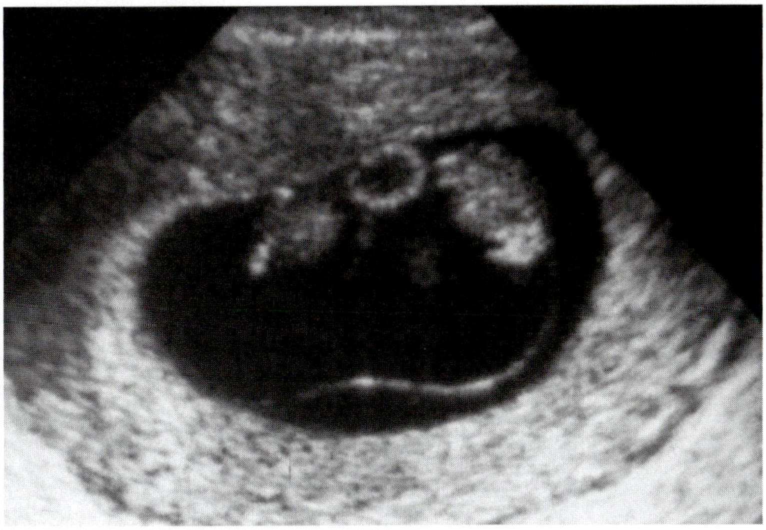

B

FIGURE 4-7 (A, B) Monochorionic–monoamniotic twin pregnancy in the first trimester shows two fetuses within one amnion. There is only one yolk sac, and the single amniotic membrane is seen surrounding the embryos (B).

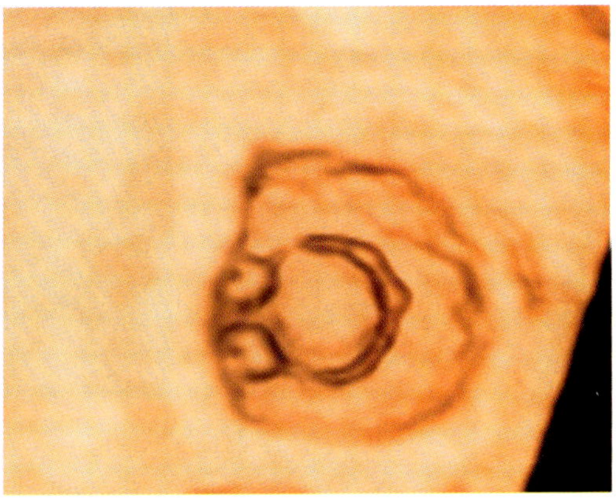

FIGURE 4-8 Monochorionic–monoamniotic twin pregnancy at 6 weeks seen with three-dimensional reconstruction. Note the two small embryos adjacent to a single, large yolk sac. Because of the large size of the yolk sac, this pregnancy had a poor prognosis and did not survive.

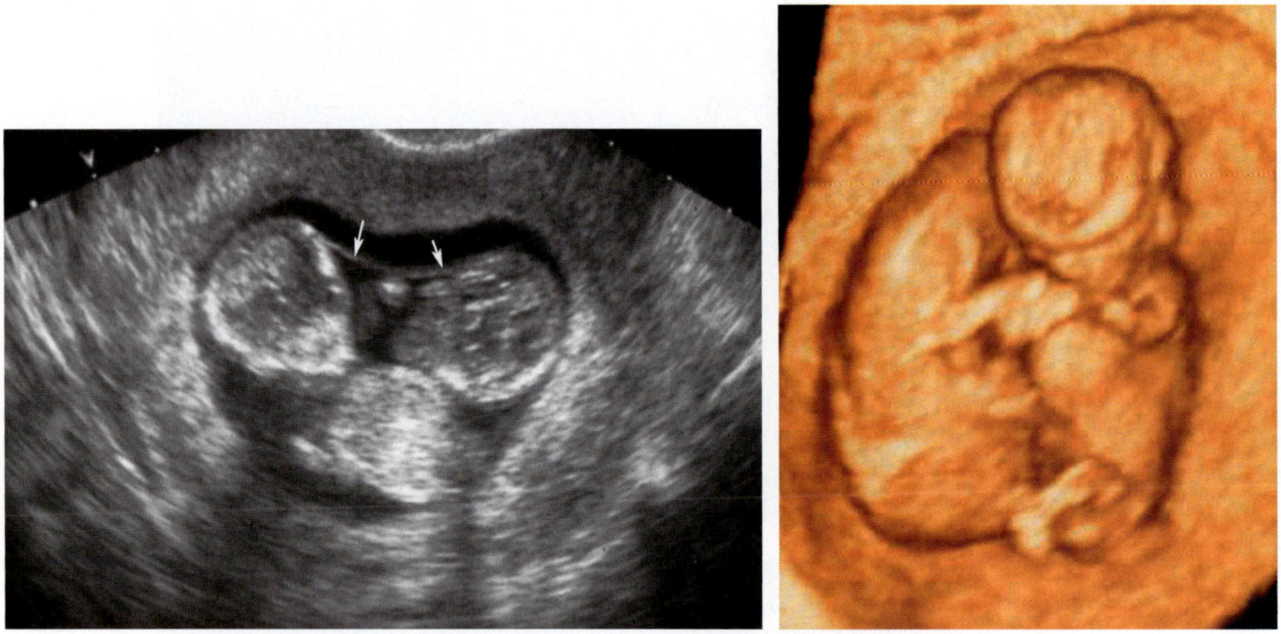

A B

FIGURE 4-9 (A) Later first-trimester monochorionic–monoamniotic pregnancy shows part of the two fetuses, including both heads, with the single amnion draped over the heads *(arrows)*. (B) Monochorionic–monoamniotic twin pregnancy in the later first trimester shows the two fetuses in close proximity to each other. The membranes are not visualized with three-dimensional surface reconstruction.

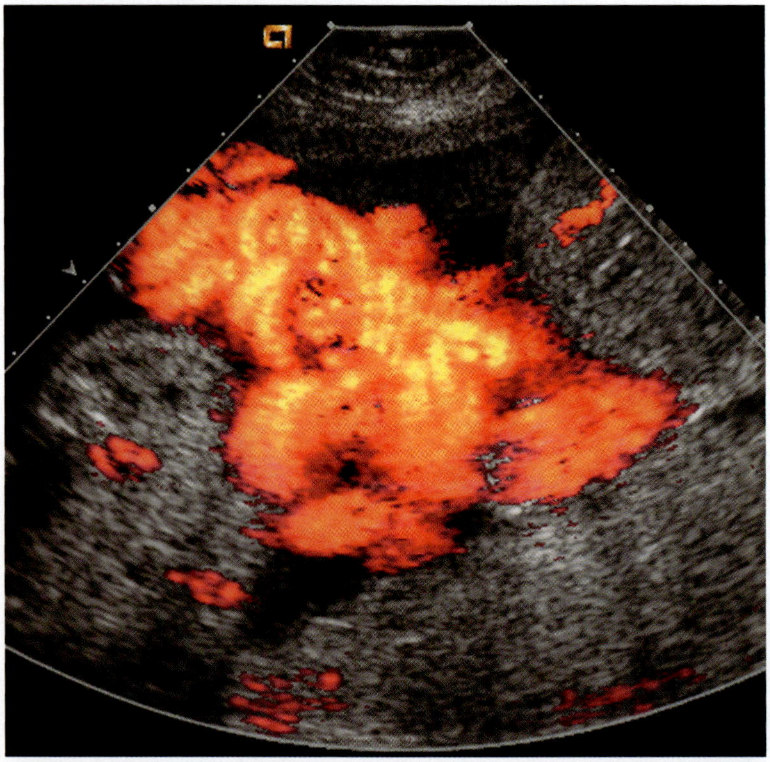

FIGURE 4-10 Third-trimester monochorionic–monoamniotic twin pregnancy, with entanglement of the two cords shown with power Doppler.

FETAL MALFORMATIONS IN MONOZYGOTIC TWINS

Monozygotic twins have an increased incidence of fetal malformations. These are thought to be related to the anomalous process of this type of twinning, which is considered an aberration in morphogenesis.[3] Incompletely separated or conjoined twins occur exclusively in monozygotic twinning and are discussed in the section on Conjoined Twins.

Several malformations appear to occur excessively in monozygotic twins compared with singletons or dizygotic twins. These anomalies include exstrophy of the cloaca, sirenomelia, VATER (**v**ertebral defects, **a**nal atresia, **t**racheoesophageal fistula, **e**sophageal atresia, and **r**adial and **r**enal dysplasias) association, anencephaly, situs defects, and holoprosencephaly.[3,31,32] Commonly, the concordance of malformations among monozygotic twins is only 10% to 20%, with most malformations being nonconcordant with the monozygotic co-twin. Reports of concordant abnormalities in twins include Prader-Willi syndrome, Goldenhar syndrome, multicystic dysplastic kidneys, gastroschisis, pentalogy of Cantrell, cystic fibrosis, cloacal exstrophy, and body stalk abnormalities (early embryo cleavage disorder).[33–37] Although having a pregnancy with a fetus that has a major anomaly is associated with an increased risk for preterm delivery, the neonatal outcome of the fetus without an anomaly does not seem to be affected by the presence of the anomalous twin.[38]

The more common, nonconcordant malformations include all types, such as neural tube defects, renal anomalies, limb defects, and others.[39–45] In particular, there can be rare occurrences when monozygotic twins appear to be of different sexes. One report describes gonadal dysgenesis in a monozygotic twin pair. In this case, the twins were discordant for phenotypic sex, and the "female" member showed gonadal dysgenesis and chromosomal mosaicism.[46] At least 25 cases of monozygous heterokaryotypic twins have been documented.[45,47] The most common heterokaryotype represents a postzygotic, nondisjunction event at the time of twinning. In this case, one karyotype is XY; in the second twin, the Y becomes lost, resulting in a Turner female (45XO). A similar case was reported in a triplet monozygotic pregnancy, in which one female presented with features of Turner syndrome and a 45XO chromosome constitution was detected in skin fibroblasts, although the lymphocytes of all three fetuses were 46XY. Again, this suggested a mitotic nondisjunction occurring in early embryonic development, leading to monosomy X in one cell line of the affected triplet.[48] A similar scenario was noted in a pair of monozygotic twins discordant for sex; the phenotypic female was a mosaic Turner, and her male twin had a normal karyotype.[49] Monozygotic twins discordant for partial trisomy 1 also have been described.[50] Among 22 cases of monozygotic twins with Down syndrome, there were four discordant pairs in which only one twin had Down syndrome.[45] Because of these occurrences, karyotyping of the fetuses in both amniotic sacs (even in a well-documented, monochorionic–diamniotic pregnancy) is recommended.

Selected feticide is a well-established management option for patients with dichorionic twin gestations, only one of which has a malformation. This procedure can be easily accomplished, with excellent outcome for the survivor. In dichorionic–diamniotic discordant twins, selective termination of one twin reportedly carried a pregnancy loss rate of 8.3% (13/156 patients) when the procedure was performed using potassium chloride.[51–53] When this procedure was attempted in monochorionic twins, however, there was a 100% loss rate, indicating that monochorionic placentation is a contraindication to selective reduction.[51] Determining chorionicity early in pregnancy, when this can be more confidently assessed, is crucial for the management of such fetal malformations that may be identified later in pregnancy.

DEATH OF ONE CO-TWIN

A complication especially important among monozygotic twins is the death of one of the fetuses. When this happens in dichorionic–diamniotic pregnancies, in most cases the co-twin continues to develop normally with minimal risk. When this process occurs in monochorionic–diamniotic twins, however, the surviving twin is at grave risk for fetal death. If it does not die, this twin is at a high risk for structural damage caused by passage of thromboplastic material from the circulation of the dead twin into the surviving co-twin. One theory is that this could result in disseminated intravascular coagulation, with severe damage to multiple organ systems.[54–58] Another possible etiology for this damage is emboli from the deceased co-twin's circulation gaining access to the survivor. A third hypothesis suggests that, secondary to complete circulatory collapse of the dead twin, a massive transfusion occurs from the live twin into the dead twin, leaving the live twin with severe and acute hypovolemia and its attendant sequelae.[59,60]

Any of these scenarios can lead to severe injury to the live twin, secondary to the death of its co-twin. These injuries include limb amputation, microcephaly, hydrocephalus, porencephalic cysts or hydranencephaly, hemifacial microsomia (Goldenhar syndrome) aplasia cutis, renal cortex necrosis, intestinal atresia, and anterior abdominal wall defects, such as gastroschisis. These abnormalities are caused by vascular disruptions, the most severe of which affect the brain and cause porencephaly and microcephaly.[54–58]

Whether even immediate delivery of the surviving twin would improve outcome for those monochorionic pregnancies experiencing death of one twin is unclear.[61] Karageyim Karsidag et al.[62] reported disseminated intravascular coagulation and multicystic encephalomalacia in the surviving neonate despite delivery within 30 minutes of the monochorionic co-twin demise.

When infarction of the organs of the live twin occurs after death of the co-twin, the resulting malformations can be accurately detected sonographically. Patten et al.[57] reported a series of six sonographically normal fetuses who, after the deaths of their monochorionic co-twins, developed ventriculomegaly, porencephaly, cerebral

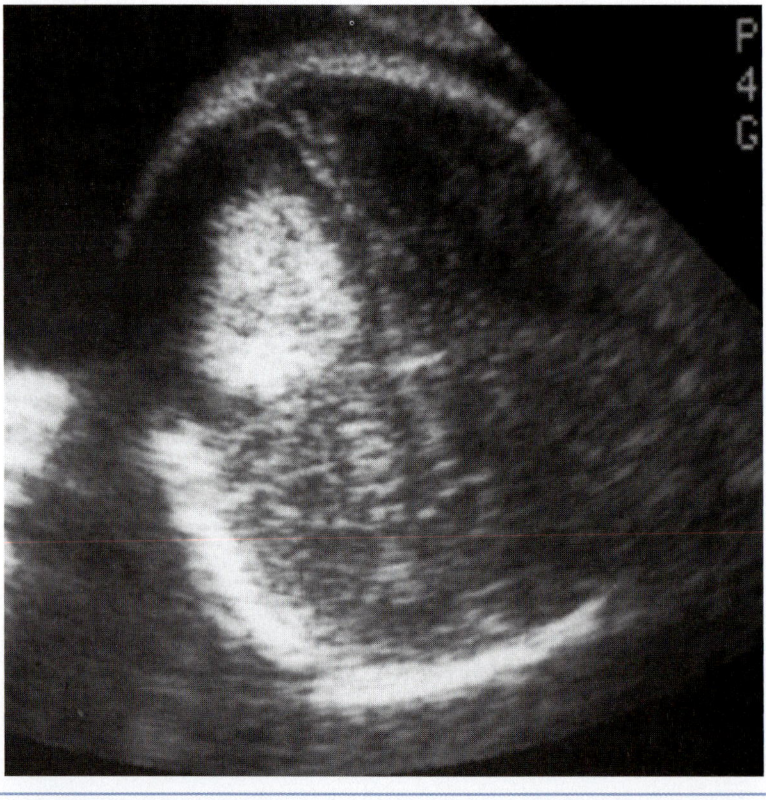

FIGURE 4-11 Coronal view of the fetal head of a monochorionic–diamniotic twin shows a large intracerebral hemorrhage in a pregnancy complicated by severe twin-to-twin transfusion syndrome.

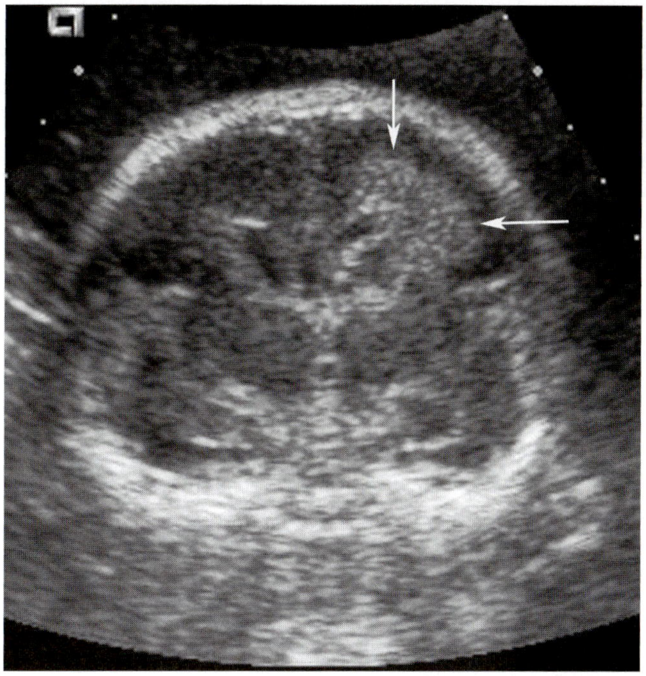

FIGURE 4-12 Coronal view of a second-trimester fetus with an intracranial bleed *(arrows),* unilaterally surrounding the frontal horn of the lateral ventricle. This type of lesion is common among fetuses with a demised monochorionic twin.

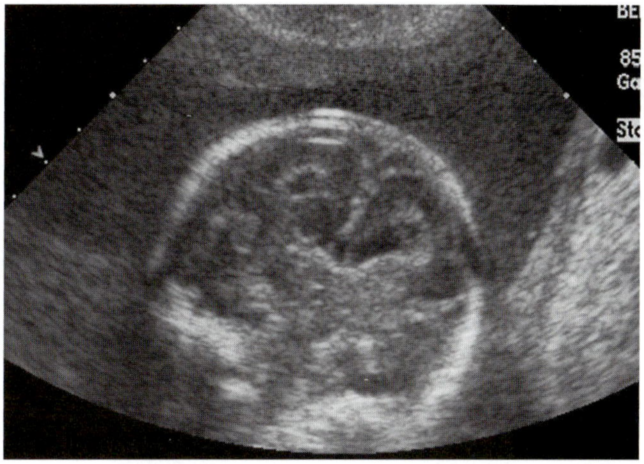

FIGURE 4-13 Monochorionic–diamniotic twin, after the co-twin succumbed to twin-to-twin transfusion syndrome. Note the periventricular leukomalacia, consistent with injury around the frontal horns.

atrophy, microcephaly, small bowel atresia, and renal cortical necrosis. Each surviving twin had neurodevelopmental delay at the time of follow-up studies. Progression of severe brain abnormalities could be visualized on serial ultrasound studies. Thus sonographic recognition of the infarction syndrome in a monochorionic twin pregnancy with the death of a co-twin carries a poor prognosis. Simonazzi et al.[63] demonstrated utility of fetal neurosonography among surviving fetuses after the demise of the monochorionic co-twin. The findings noted in the surviving fetuses were intracranial hemorrhage, brain atrophy, porencephaly, and periventricular echogenicities that evolved into polymicrogyria.

When pregnancy continues after the death of one twin, close monitoring of the surviving twin is necessary if extreme prematurity or immature lungs preclude immediate delivery. Disseminated intravascular coagulation can affect the mother carrying a dead fetus or twin. Therefore, when fetal death occurs later in pregnancy, maternal coagulation factors should be monitored for the duration of the pregnancy.

CONJOINED TWINS

The incidence of conjoined twins is approximately 1 in 50,000 pregnancies, with a 3:1 female preponderance. Although males are more common among monozygotic twins, 70% of conjoined twins are females.[45]

This condition represents an incomplete division of the embryonic disk that occurs at least 12 days after fertilization.[2] Eight main classifications of conjoined twins can be subdivided into those with ventral or dorsal unions. Among those with ventral unions, *thoracopagus twins* are joined at the thorax and share the chest and upper abdominal organs. This is the most common type of fusion, occurring in 70% of conjoined twins. *Omphalopagus twins* are joined at the abdomen, sharing the anterior abdominal wall and umbilicus, and often are associated with an omphalocele and a six-vessel cord. *Ischiopagus twins* are joined at the ischium, with union of the lower abdomen and genitourinary

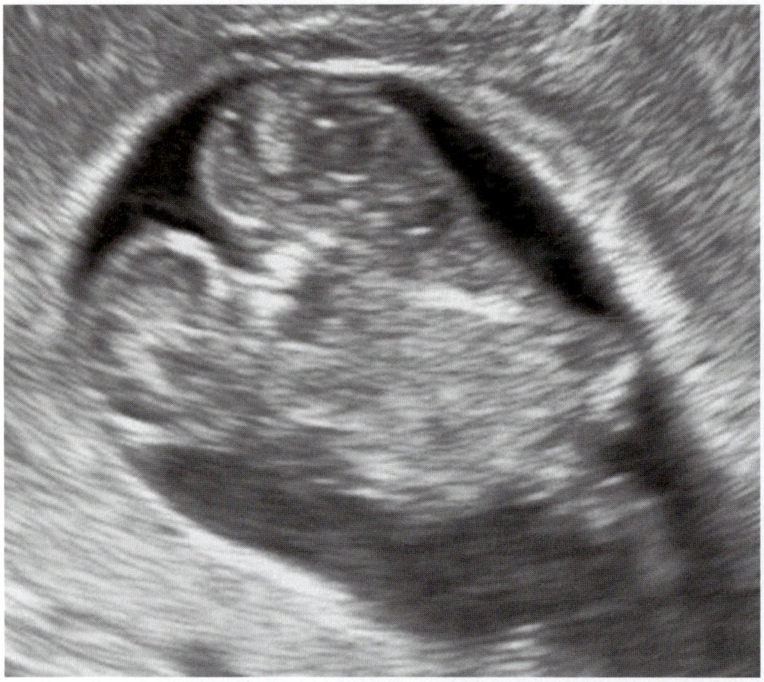

A

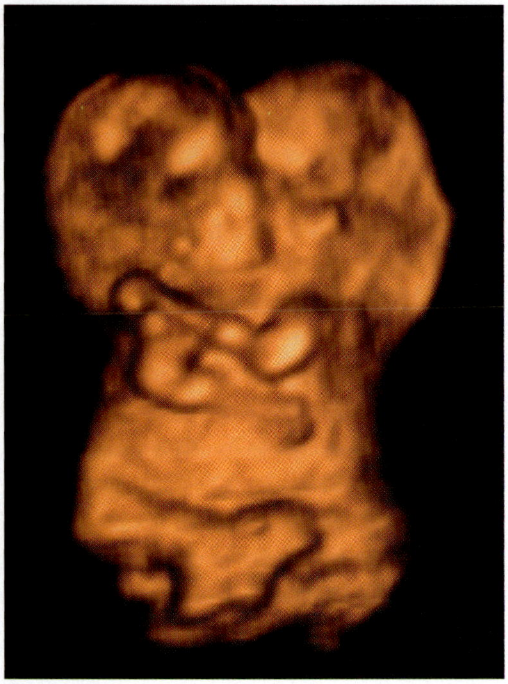

C

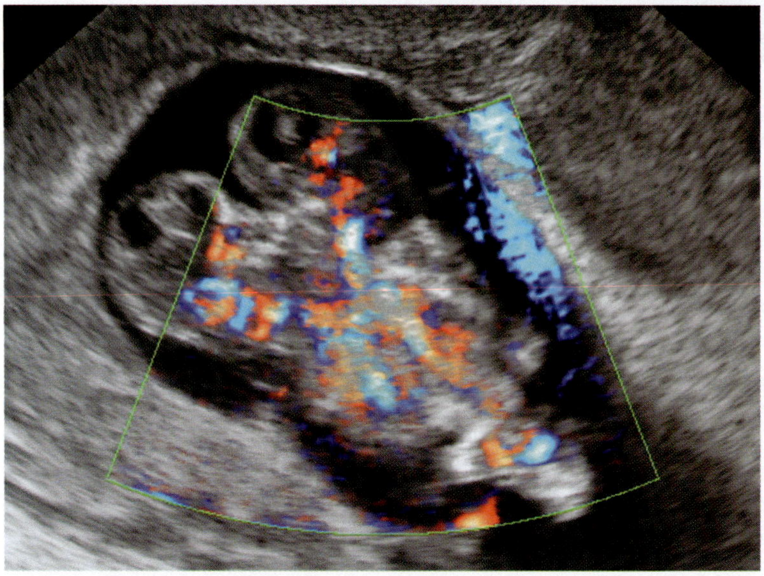

B

FIGURE 4-14 (A) A 10-week set of conjoined twins, joined throughout the entire thorax and abdomen. (B) Longitudinal view of the same 10-week twins, using color Doppler to display the vascular mapping in the areas of joining. (C) Three-dimensional surface rendering of the same 10-week twin set shows that the fetuses are extensively joined at the entire ventral aspect, including the chests and abdomens.

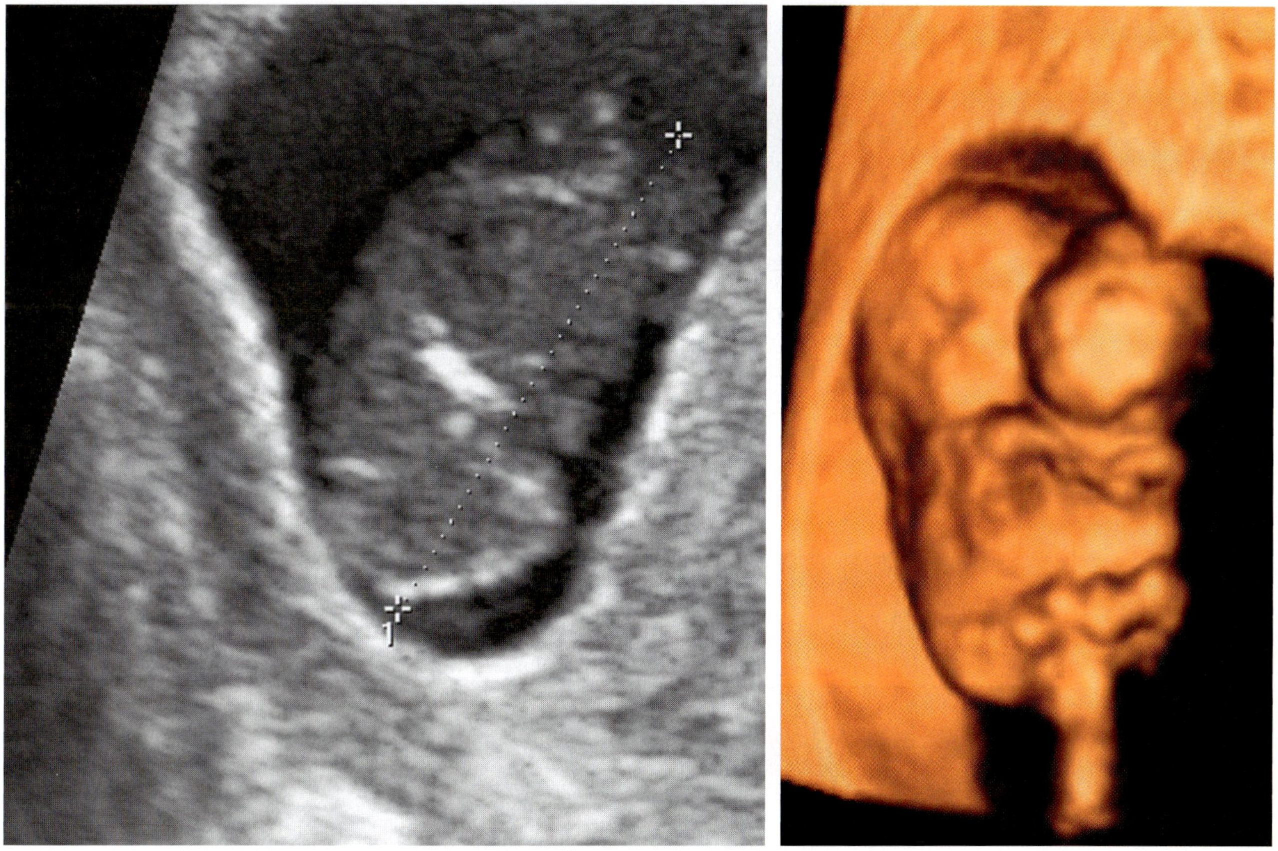

A B

FIGURE 4-15 (A) Nine-week failed pregnancy with a dead fetus (indicated by the calipers). The anatomy visualized in two dimensions did not permit accurate interpretation of abnormalities. (B) Surface rendering of the same failed pregnancy shows that the pregnancy actually represented a set of extensively conjoined twins. Note that they are joined along the entire ventral aspect, including both chests and abdomens. This detail was not well seen with standard two-dimensional imaging.

systems. *Cephalopagus twins* are joined from the top of the head to the umbilicus. Lateral unions, such as *parapagus twins,* involve union of the pelvis and variable degrees of the trunk. Dorsal unions, which include *pygopagus twins,* are joined at the sacrum and coccyx and share a common anus. *Craniopagus twins* are joined at the cranium, lying at right angles to each other. *Rachipagus twins* involve union of the vertebral column.[64]

Conjoined twins are easily detectable by sonographic studies.[65–73] Not only are they abnormal in their points of joining, but often they have associated congenital defects, such as cardiac malformations, gastrointestinal anomalies, and other anomalies. The point of joining and the associated malformations often are obvious anatomically. Also, conjoined twins tend to be in peculiar positions that often would be impossible if the twins were not fused, with hyperextended heads and intertwined limbs. Careful sonographic examination of each organ can establish the point of joining. Transvaginal and/or three-dimensional sonography may assist with the sonographic evaluation and diagnosis of conjoined twins, especially in the first trimester, when diagnosis is preferable.[74–76]

Although separation of conjoined twins can be accomplished, particularly when they are joined by a small and pliable area or through the liver or hip, such separation in twins who share a heart or who are extensively joined often is either impossible or associated with too poor a prognosis to attempt. Various severe forms of

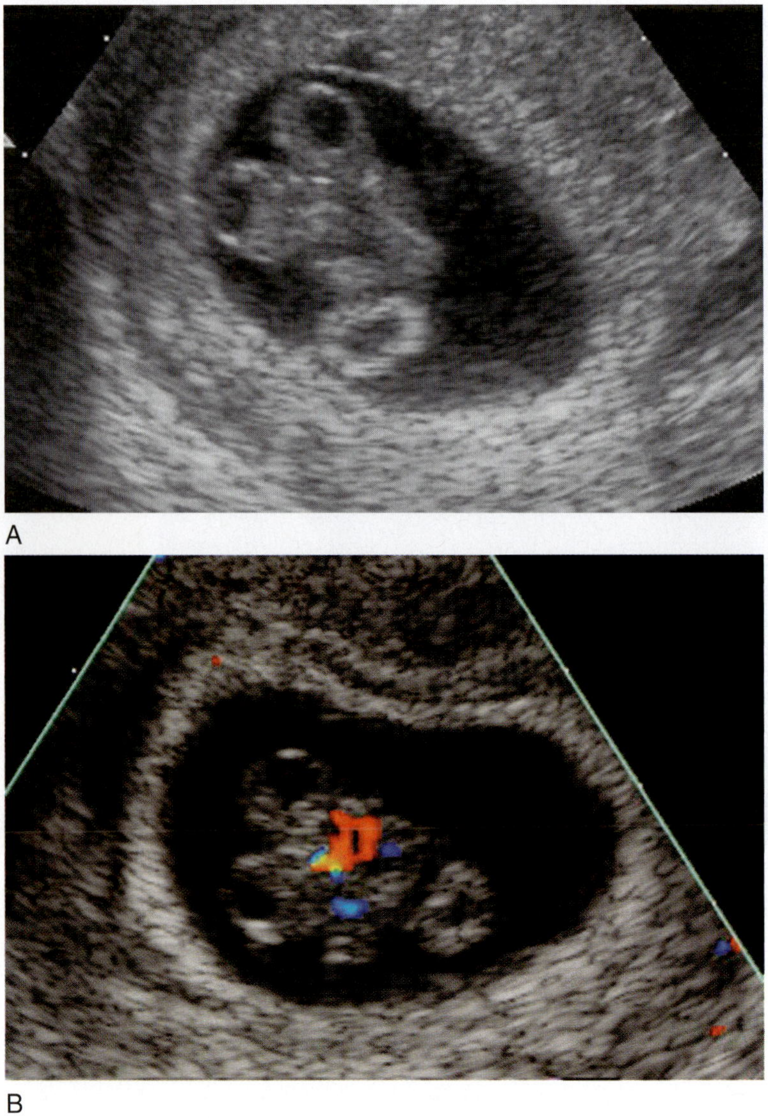

FIGURE 4-16 (**A**) Seven-week conjoined twins show a single yolk sac and two heads (indicated by the two cystic areas). (**B**) Color Doppler of the same conjoined twins shows the activity of the shared heart.

conjoined twins may be joined at more than one point in the classification scheme.[77–83] These include cephalothoracopagus janiceps, in which a single head and face is present, with two bodies and as many as eight extremities. Another scenario is two heads and a single body, as may be seen in dicephalus dipus dibrachius. A duplicate face can occur, with a partly duplicated head but a single body.

First-trimester diagnosis of conjoined twins has been reported in several studies.[73,82] Early diagnosis is most desirable, particularly considering the extremely poor prognosis associated with this type of twinning. Especially in cases involving a duplicated face, partly duplicated head, and single body, careful evaluation of the heart, brain, and face is necessary to make the correct diagnosis. Whenever the diagnosis of conjoined twins is made, a multidisciplinary approach is needed to determine the likelihood of postnatal viability. Consultations with pediatric and cardiac surgeons are indicated. Only then can realistic postnatal plans be made.

Text continued on p. 621

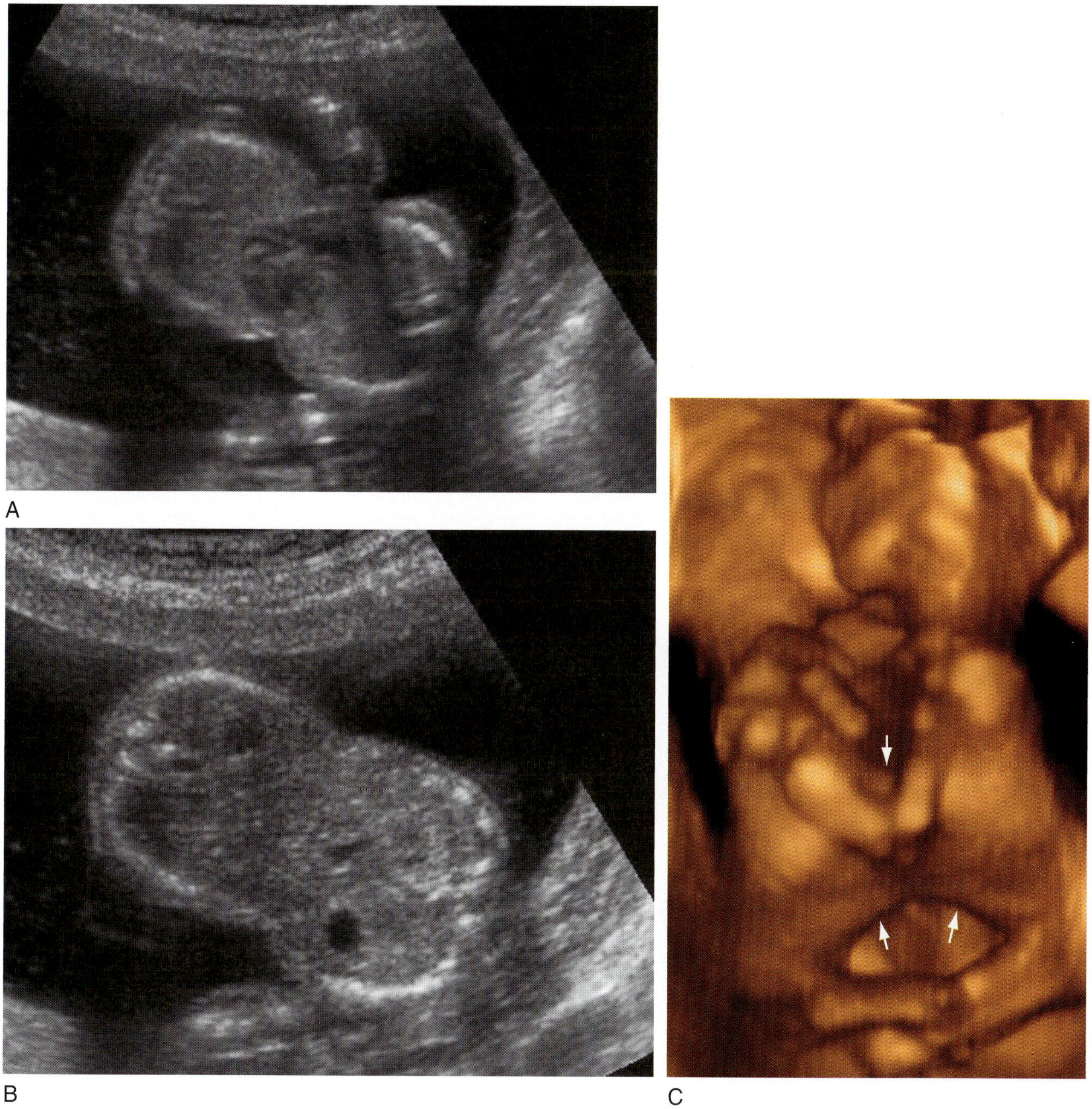

FIGURE 4-17 (A) Twenty-week set of conjoined twins, imaged transversely across the joined chests, shows the single, shared heart. The heart was extensively malformed, and safe separation of the twins was deemed not possible. (B) Transverse view through the joined abdomens of the same fetuses shows that the liver is shared, but the two stomach bubbles are separate. (C) Surface rendering of the same case shows that the fetuses are facing each other because of extensive sharing of the heart and liver. Arrows indicate the extent of the joining of these fetuses.

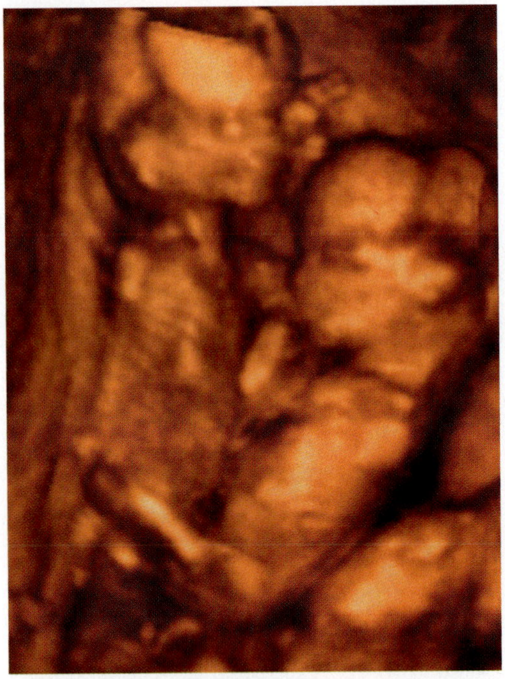

FIGURE 4-18 Eighteen-week conjoined twins sharing a liver and a portion of the pelvis.

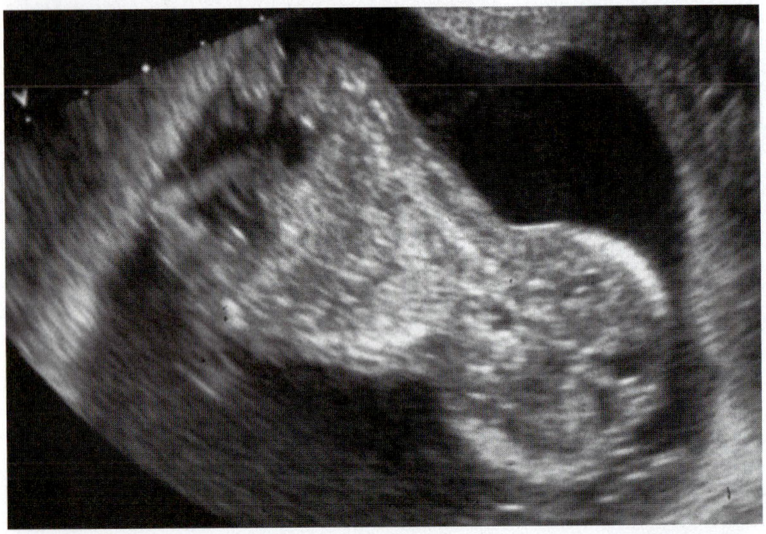

A

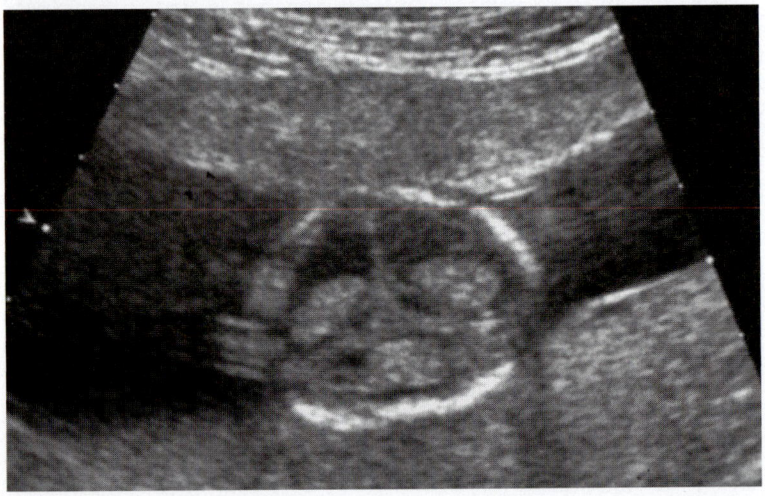

B

FIGURE 4-19 (A) Late first-trimester conjoined twins show a widened but single head, with duplication of the body. There are four lower extremities but only two upper extremities. (B) Transverse view of the fetal head of the same twin pair shows partial duplication of the brain and an unusual head shape.

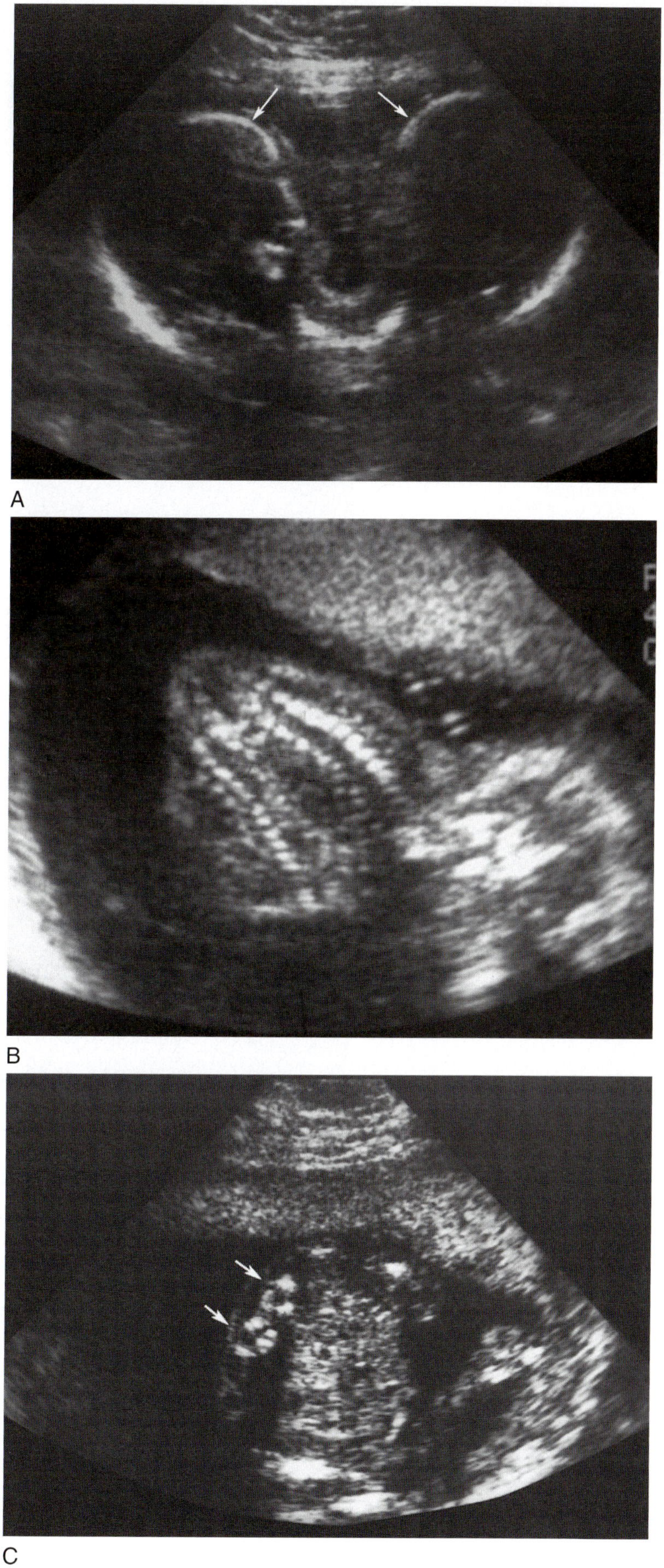

FIGURE 4-20 (A) View of a conjoined twin pair with two heads and only a partially duplicated body in dicephalus dipus dibrachius conjoined twins. Arrows indicate the two separate heads. (B, C) Coronal and transverse views through the duplicated spines *(arrows)* of the same twin pair show that the spines are side by side.

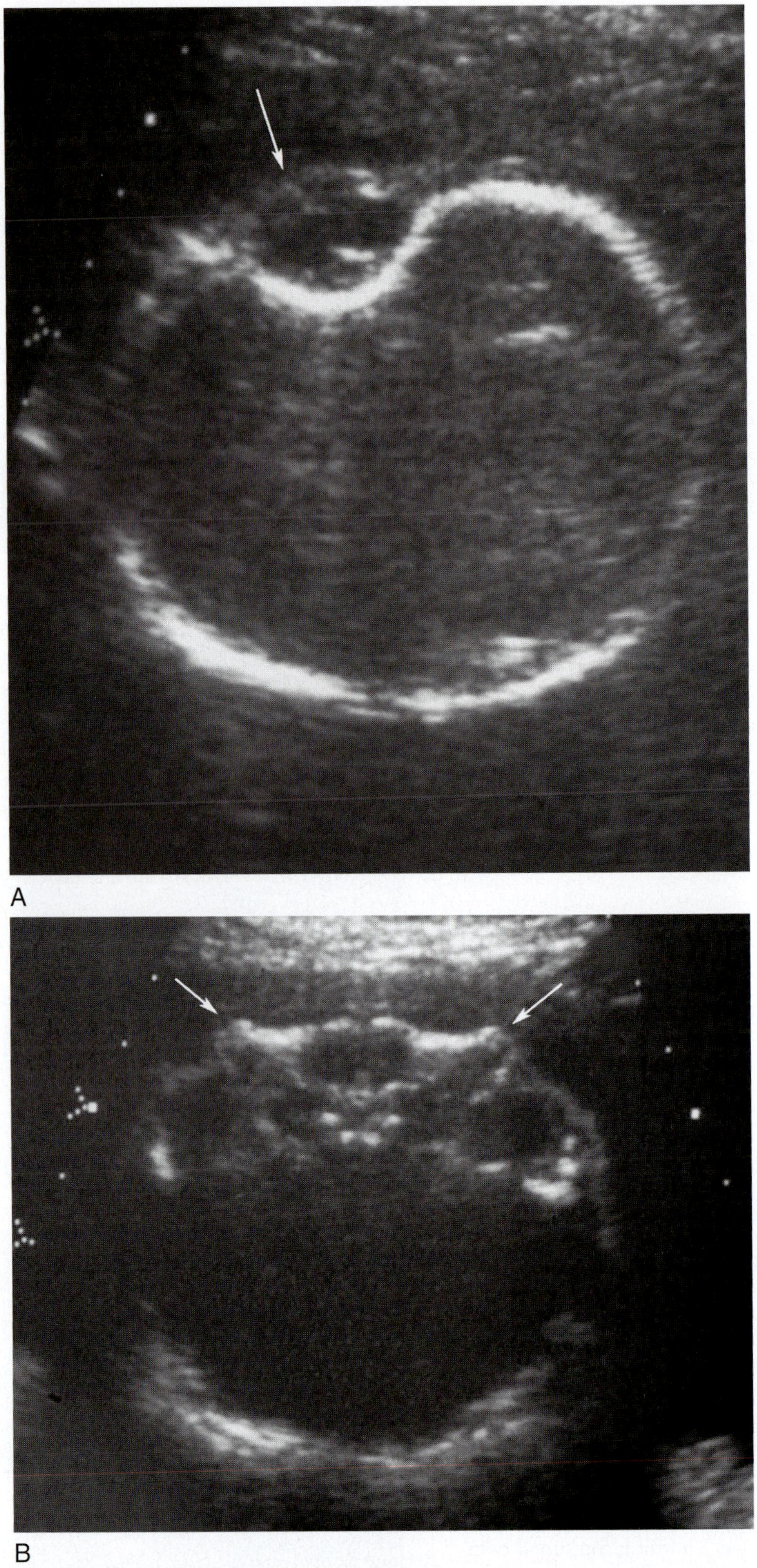

FIGURE 4-21 (A) Transverse view through the head of a fetus with a partially duplicated face. Note the double orbit in the center of the face *(arrow)*. (B) Transverse view through the fetal face, at a slightly different level, shows two noses *(arrows)* slightly below the central orbit. There also is an orbit on either outer side of these noses, consistent with a duplicated face.

ACARDIA

Acardia is a rare malformation of monozygotic twins that occurs in approximately 1 in 35,000 deliveries and 1 in 100 monozygotic twins.[1] Acardia results from an artery-to-artery placental shunt, whereby the arterial pressure of one twin overpowers that of the other twin early in gestation. The arterial blood flow of the second twin is reversed, such that the arterial blood from the first twin perfuses the second twin, whose blood then flows in reverse through the arterial system. Because of this flow reversal, most of the perfusion of the recipient twin involves the lower, rather than the upper, part of body, usually resulting in disruption and deterioration of the upper portion of that twin and the persistence of the lower part of the body. This alteration or reversal in the circulation of the recipient twin is responsible for the multiple anomalies that develop in that twin. In most cases, the head and upper body of the recipient twin do not develop, resulting in an isolated, malformed lower body with a huge amount of edema and no heart. This complication of monozygotic twins affects both monochorionic–monochorionic and monochorionic–diamniotic twins. A physiologic description—twin reversed arterial perfusion (TRAP) sequence—has been used for this scenario.[84]

Classification of the acardiac twin depends on the part of the body that develops.[85,86] *Acardius anceps* is the most highly developed form, consisting of some brain tissue and face, body, and extremities, but no heart. *Acardius acephalus* twins occur in 60% to 75% of cases and represent the most common single type; they are headless, exhibiting only the lower portions of the trunk and lower extremities. *Acardius acormus* is the rarest form, characterized by only a head and no body. *Acardius amorphus* is simply a mass of tissue that is unrecognizable, resembling a teratoma.

Prenatal diagnosis of acardiac twins is possible as early as 9 weeks' gestation and has been reported several times in the first trimester.[87–90] Because it is usually seen with a live, normal-appearing twin in the same pregnancy, care must be taken not to mistake an acardiac twin for a dead twin in the first trimester. The acardiac twin often looks like an amorphous lump of tissue that can be mistaken for a hydropic, dead fetus. Acardiac twins, however, tend to twitch and move, despite the absence of cardiac activity. They also have the characteristic appearance of a widened and edematous upper pole, without an identifiable head in most cases. The diagnosis can be confirmed by Doppler studies, which show reversal of flow through the umbilical artery of the acardiac twin, with arterial blood flowing toward this twin rather than away from it.[91–93]

Polyhydramnios often is a complication of acardiac twin pregnancies. The normal co-twin, who is perfusing the entire mass of tissue, may develop cardiomegaly, hydrops, high-output failure, or intrauterine growth restriction, all of which represent complications of being the

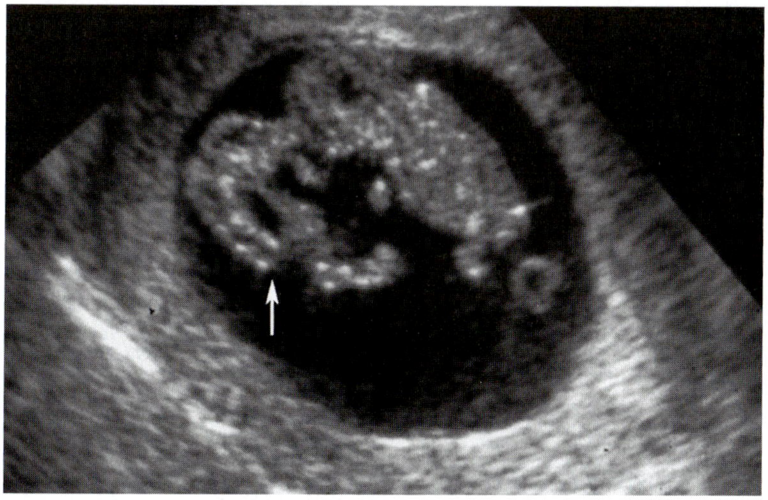

FIGURE 4-22 First-trimester monochorionic twin pair, one of whom is an acardiac twin *(arrow)*. Note the unusual outer contour of this abnormal twin compared with its normal counterpart.

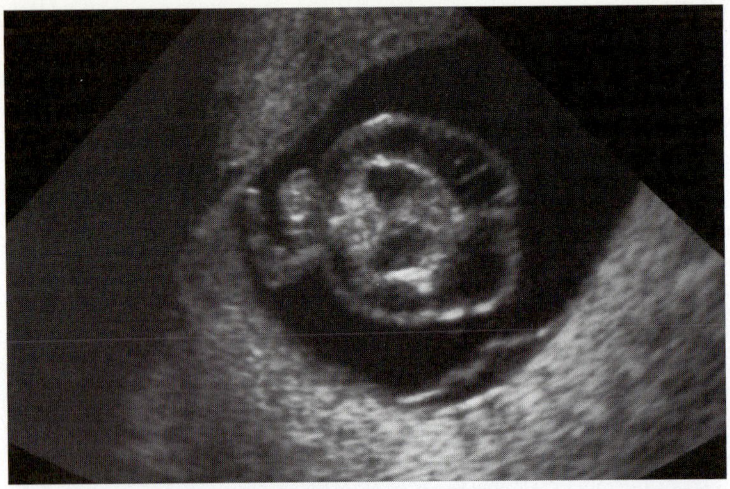

A

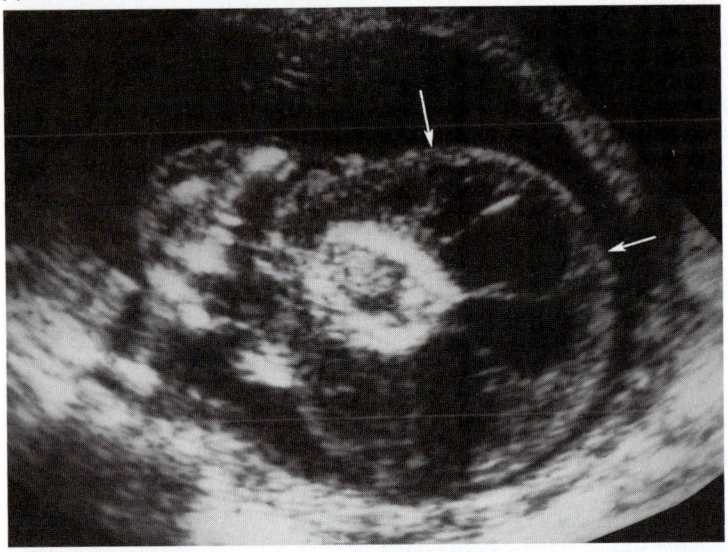

B

FIGURE 4-23 (A) First-trimester longitudinal view of a first-trimester acardiac fetus shows a severely edematous body with absent head and rudimentary lower extremities. (B) Second-trimester acardiac fetus shows the large upper pole of the fetus with an absent head and severe, septate cystic areas *(arrows)* involving the upper part of the body. This appearance is typical of an acardiac fetus. (C) Second-trimester acardiac fetus. There are large cystic areas throughout the soft tissues. A small amount of ascites is present within the body of the fetus, which has no head or chest. (D) Very large, late second-trimester acardiac fetus shows tremendous swelling of the soft tissues compared with the relatively small skeleton of the fetus. Note the ascites or pleural fluid present within the fetus. The co-twin of this very large acardiac fetus did not survive because of congestive heart failure.

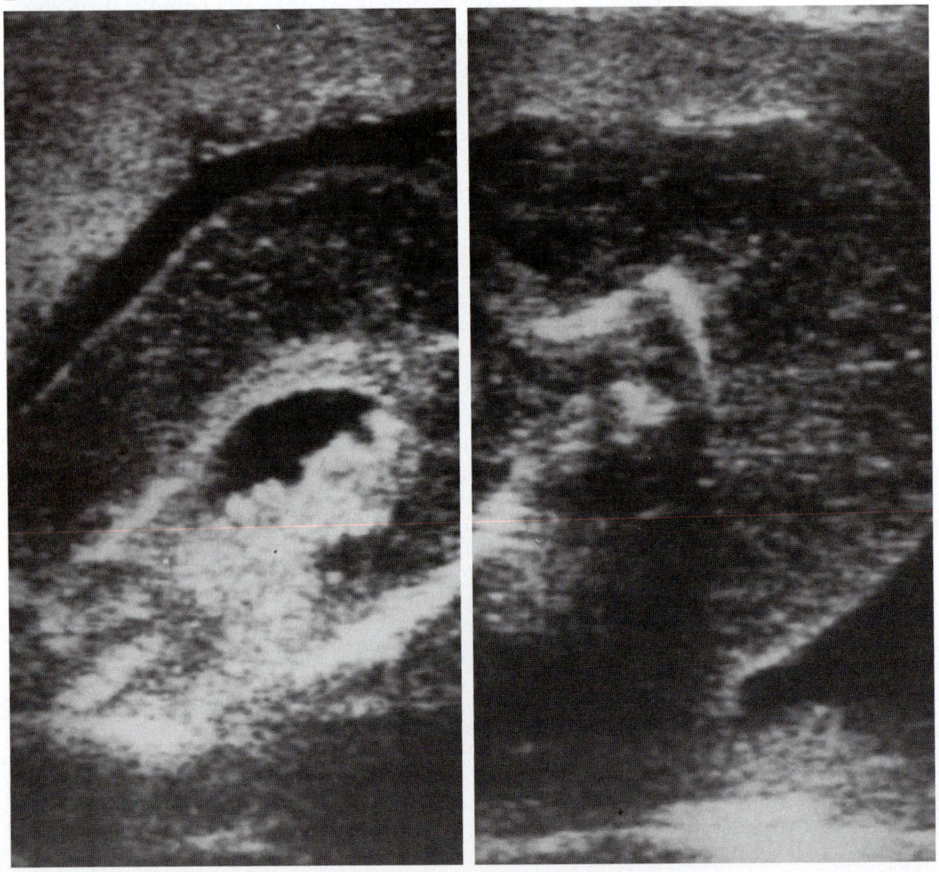

C D

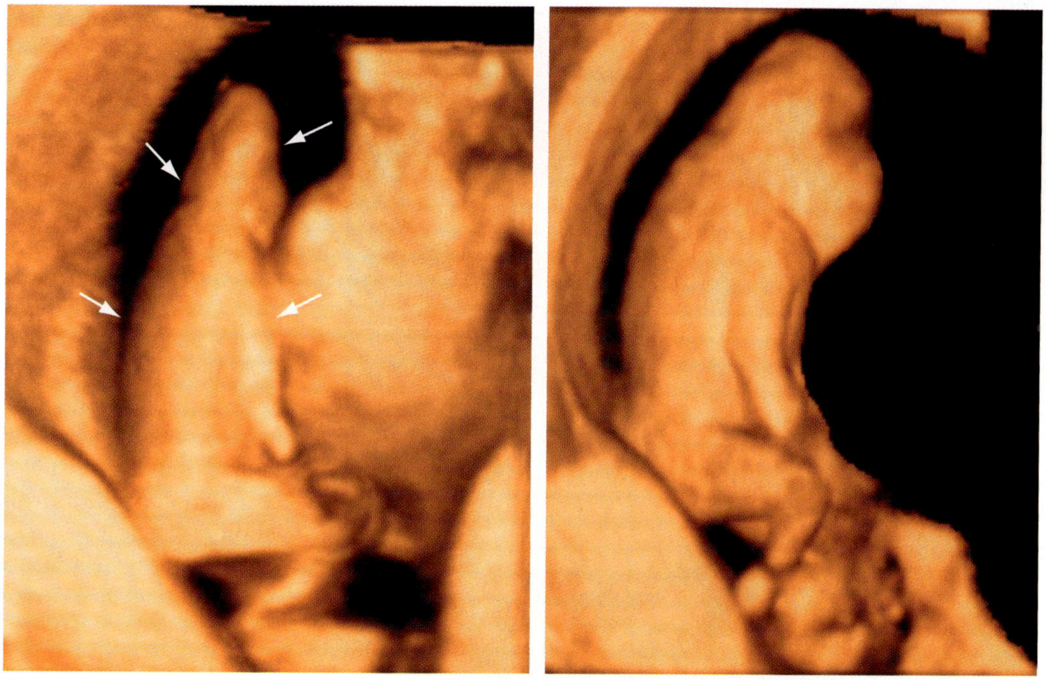

A B

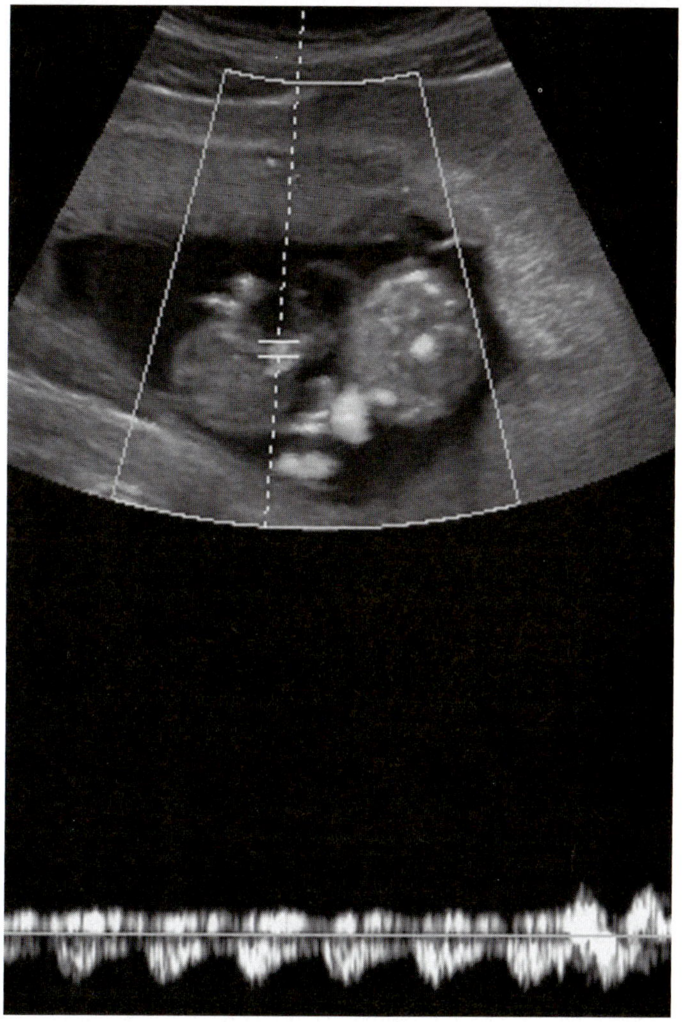

C

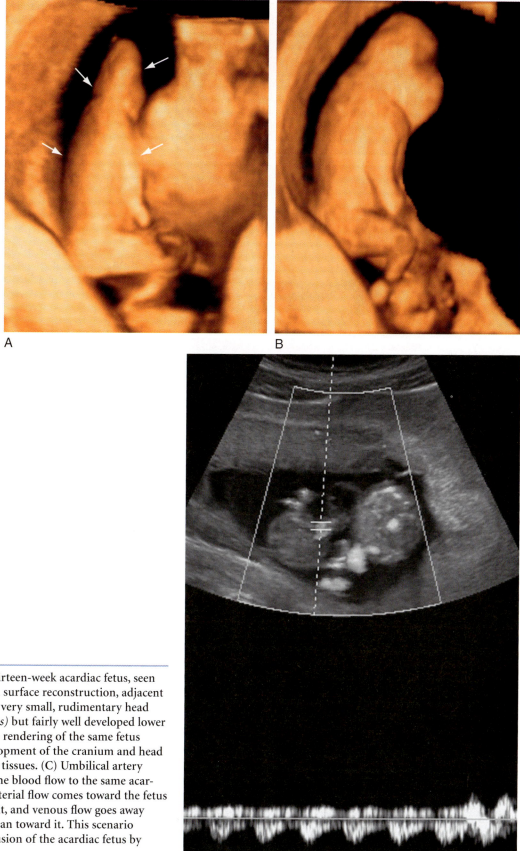

FIGURE 4-24 (A) Thirteen-week acardiac fetus, seen with three-dimensional surface reconstruction, adjacent to its co-twin. Note the very small, rudimentary head and upper body *(arrows)* but fairly well developed lower extremities. (B) Surface rendering of the same fetus shows the lack of development of the cranium and head and swelling of the soft tissues. (C) Umbilical artery Doppler waveform of the blood flow to the same acardiac twin shows that arterial flow comes toward the fetus rather than away from it, and venous flow goes away from the fetus rather than toward it. This scenario indicates reversed perfusion of the acardiac fetus by its co-twin.

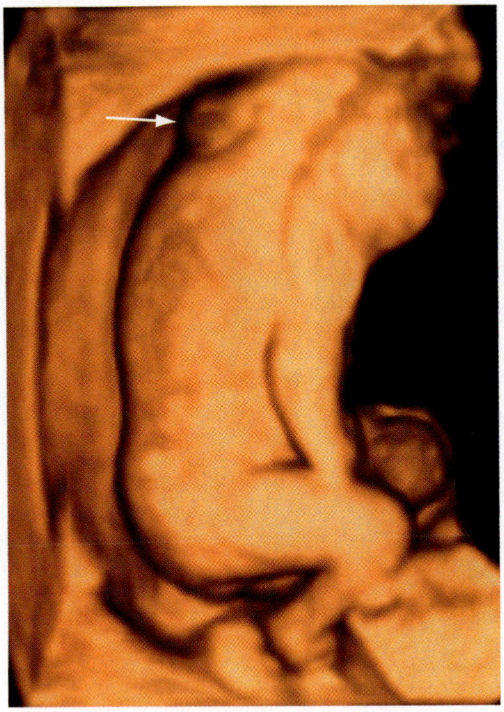

FIGURE 4-25 Second-trimester acardiac fetus shows severe deformities. Note the rudimentary head. Three-dimensional surface rendering shows fairly well developed lower extremities but a rudimentary head with a small encephalocele *(arrow)*.

pump twin for a large mass of tissue. Therefore the presence of an acardiac twin is associated with a high risk of morbidity and mortality for the pump twin. Factors associated with an increased risk for pregnancy loss include an acardiac twin–to–pump twin size ratio >50%, polyhydramnios, and preterm labor.[94,95]

The presence of an acardiac twin carries a nearly 50% risk of mortality for the normal twin.[95] Therefore, serial ultrasound studies are required to determine the optimal timing of delivery.[96,97] Occasionally, there will be spontaneous cessation of the umbilical blood flow in the acardiac twin, with an excellent outcome for the pump twin.[98] Many different techniques have been reported for treatment of TRAP sequence, including embolization of the acardiac twin, hysterotomy with delivery of the acardiac twin, hysterotomy with umbilical cord ligation, endoscopic umbilical cord ligation, endoscopic laser coagulation of the acardiac twin, thermocoagulation of the acardiac twin, and radiofrequency ablation of the acardiac twin.[91–106]

Quintero et al.[94] reviewed 74 patients with TRAP sequence and found that 65 of the 74 patients were candidates for surgical therapy for umbilical cord occlusion. There was no statistical significant difference in perinatal survival among those who underwent umbilical cord occlusion (65%) and those who did not undergo such treatment (43%). In subgroup analysis, perinatal outcome did appear improved if the dividing membrane was not disrupted during the surgical procedure. A unified treatment regimen has not been established. Additional data are required to determine which fetuses would benefit from therapy. Conservative management may be possible for those without the risk factors for loss.[94,95,107,108] In a literature review, Tan and Sepulveda[109] concluded that intrafetal ablation of the acardiac twin is superior to various umbilical cord ligation techniques.

TWIN-TO-TWIN TRANSFUSION SYNDROME

Vascular anastomoses are common among monochorionic placentae. Monochorionic–monoamniotic placentae have significantly more artery-to-artery anastomoses than monochorionic–diamniotic placentae. This may explain the much lower incidence of twin-to-twin transfusion syndrome among those with monochorionic–monoamniotic placentae.[110] Uncompensated artery-to-vein anastomoses within the placenta of monochorionic twins can lead to twin-to-twin transfusion syndrome or the oligohydramnios–polyhydramnios sequence.[1] Although most monochorionic placentae contain vascular anastomoses, only 15% actually result in twin-to-twin transfusion syndrome, which is typified by the small donor twin having oligohydramnios and the larger recipient twin having polyhydramnios. The donor twin can develop such severe oligohydramnios, or anhydramnios, that it becomes stuck, pinned to the side of the gestational sac by its membrane. The co-twin, with its increased perfusion, usually develops severe polyhydramnios and a large bladder secondary to the increased perfusion, and it is larger in comparison to the recipient twin's biometry. Twin-to-twin transfusion syndrome usually is a second-trimester diagnosis but has been detected in the first trimester.[111]

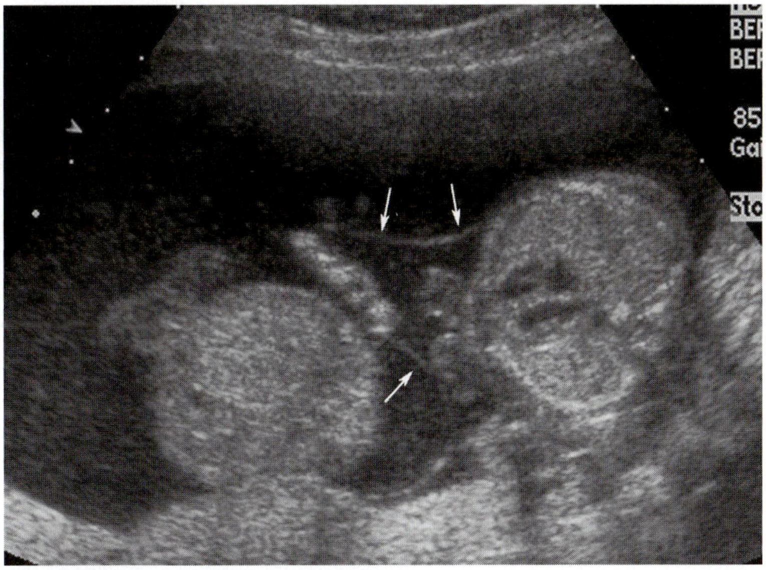

A

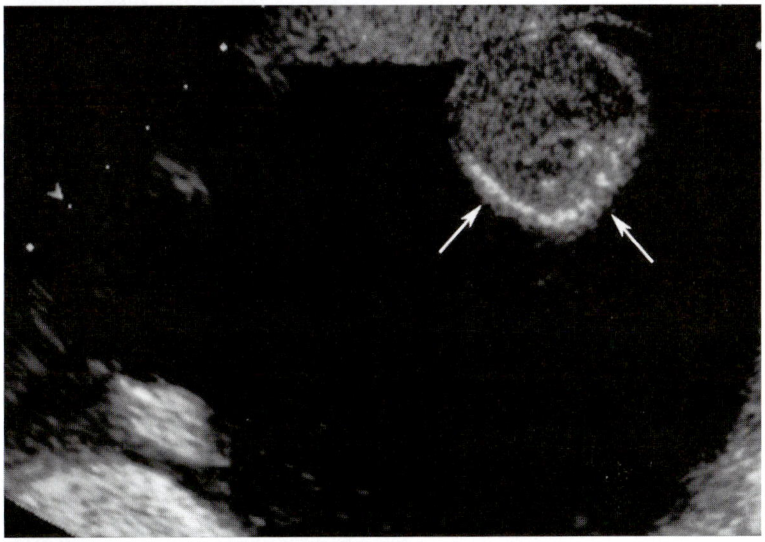

B

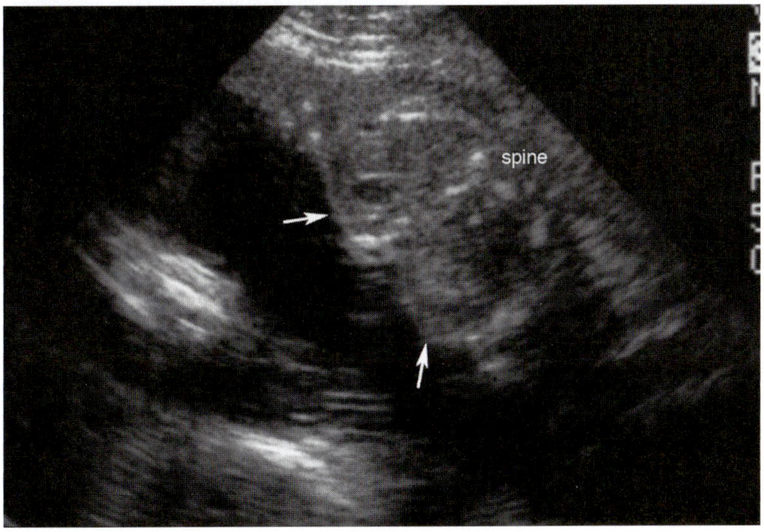

C

FIGURE 4-26 (A) Monochorionic–diamniotic twin pregnancy with moderate polyhydramnios and moderate oligohydramnios in this twin pair developing twin-to-twin transfusion syndrome. Arrows indicate the amniotic membrane draped over the small parts of the fetus in the oligohydramniotic sac. (B) Second-trimester monochorionic–diamniotic twin pair shows severe twin-to-twin transfusion syndrome. One of the fetuses is suspended from the anterior aspect of the uterus by its amniotic membrane (not visualized). This twin is "stuck" *(arrows)* and appears to defy gravity. (C) Late second-trimester twins with twin-to-twin transfusion syndrome seen in transverse view through the fetal abdomen of the stuck twin. The spine is labeled on the image, and the anterior abdominal wall of the fetus *(arrows)* is confined by the invisible, "stuck" amniotic membrane. This fetus appears to defy gravity, as it is imprisoned in its oligohydramniotic sac. *Continued*

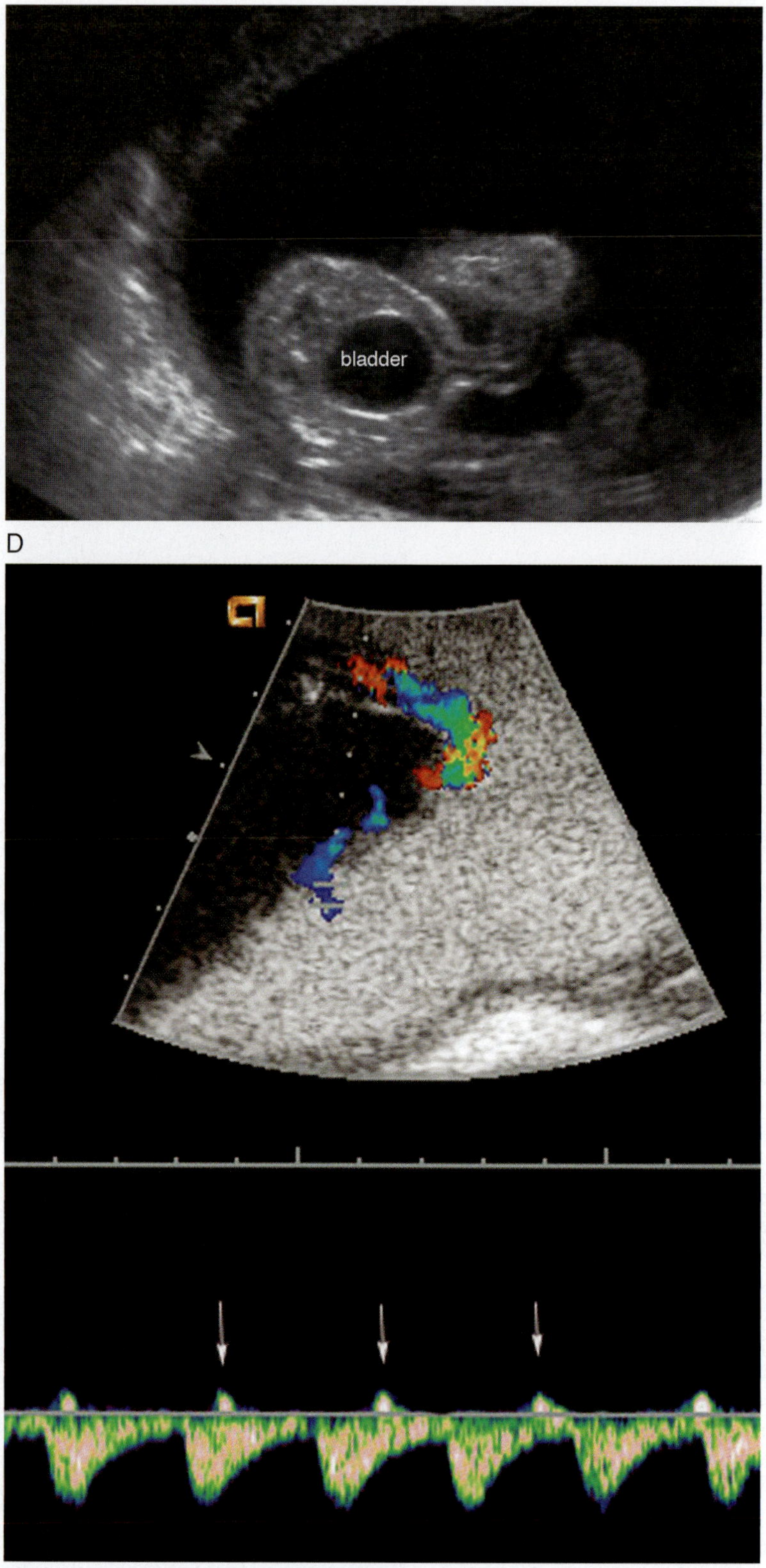

D

E

FIGURE 4-26, cont'd (D) Recipient twin in a monochorionic–diamniotic twin pregnancy with twin-to-twin transfusion syndrome. Note the distended bladder and large amount of amniotic fluid, typical of the recipient twin, as a result of fluid overload. (E) Typical artery-to-artery anastomoses in monochorionic twins, seen on the surface of the placenta. The Doppler window is located on the surface of the placenta and shows two sets of arterial pulses at different rates *(arrows)*.

The mortality rate of twin-to-twin transfusion is as high as 70% but varies by gestational age.[1] In twin-to-twin transfusion syndrome occurring before 20 weeks' gestation, the mortality rate is >90%. After 20 weeks, survival rates improve. The later the manifestation of this disorder, the better the prognosis.[112,113]

Although the vascular communications of the placenta cannot be seen sonographically in most cases, a number of sonographic findings are typical of twin-to-twin transfusion syndrome.[113–115] These sonographic findings include monochorionic placentation, with the membrane being particularly adherent to the fetus in the severely oligohydramniotic sac, thus obscuring the identification of this separating membrane. Most often, the oligohydramniotic twin is considerably smaller than its co-twin. A structural survey can be difficult to perform on the smaller twin because of its unusual distorted position in the uterus. Often, little fluid can be seen in the fetal bladder because of decreased perfusion of the kidneys and decreased urine production in the fetus. The co-twin usually is moving freely in a large, polyhydramniotic sac. Often, this co-twin's bladder is distended as a result of increased perfusion of the kidneys and polyuria, and the fetal heart may be slightly enlarged, indicating an increased risk for congestive heart failure. Recipient twins have been shown to develop decreased ventricular function and tricuspid regurgitation.[116] In severe cases, this fetus will develop nonimmune hydrops, which carries an extremely poor prognosis. Umbilical artery Doppler profiles usually are abnormal in both twins. However, Doppler studies were not able to differentiate between donor and recipient twins or to provide data prognostic of outcomes.[117] Identification of artery-to-artery anastomoses by color Doppler and pulse wave Doppler showing bidirectional flow has been associated with improved perinatal survival.[118]

Twin-to-twin transfusion syndrome is an extremely complex, dynamic, physiologic state. In our laboratory, several cases of severe twin-to-twin transfusion syndrome with a stuck twin developed at <20 weeks' gestation, and the process completely reversed later in gestation. The stuck twin became the polyhydramniotic twin, and the previous recipient twin became the donor. This reversal of the hemodynamic process of twin-to-twin transfusion syndrome carries an extremely poor prognosis. All the fetuses in our study died.[119] A poor prognosis in such cases now has been documented by others.[120]

Because of the dismal outcome in twin-to-twin transfusion syndrome, many attempts have been made to find treatments that would improve the prognosis. Most centers have treated twin-to-twin transfusion syndrome with multiple aggressive amniocenteses of the polyhydramniotic sac, with a resultant improvement in survival rates. Liters of fluid can be removed every few days in an attempt to normalize the amounts of amniotic fluid in both sacs.[121–125] Some studies have shown an improvement in outcome with this management technique, with an overall neonatal survival rate of 50%, including resolution of hydrops fetalis.[121,122] One study reported a 69% survival rate using serial amniocenteses in pregnancies complicated by twin-to-twin transfusion syndrome, compared with a rate of 16% among similar pregnancies managed only expectantly.[124] One study of fetuses with twin-to-twin transfusion syndrome conducted by Elliott et al.[125] revealed that 60% of hydropic fetuses who received serial amniocenteses had resolution of their hydrops. The perinatal survival rate was 79% in those cases. This contrasts dramatically with the nearly 100% mortality reported without therapy before 20 weeks' gestation.[125]

In the past 15 years or so, many investigators have evaluated various treatment options for twin-to-twin transfusion syndrome. Ville et al.[126] reported percutaneous endoscopic laser coagulation of the communicating placental vessels in 1995. Their preliminary report showed a 53% survival rate to delivery, and 71% of pregnancies had at least one survivor when treated with laser. Hecher et al.[127] compared endoscopic laser coagulation of communicating placental vessels with serial amniocenteses in severe twin-to-twin transfusion syndrome using data from centers where one or the other technique was used. They found a similar overall survival rate, 61% versus 51% for the laser and amniocentesis groups, respectively. However, the rate of abnormal neurosonographic findings was significantly higher (18%) among the amniocentesis group compared with 6% in the laser group.[127] Quintero et al.[128] have proposed a staging system of twin-to-twin transfusion based on sonographic and Doppler parameters. All stages have polyhydramnios and oligohydramnios, using criteria of ≥8 cm deepest vertical pocket for polyhydramnios and ≥2 cm vertical pocket for oligohydramnios. Stage I is diagnosed when bladder fluid is present in the donor's bladder. Stage II has absence of bladder fluid in the donor's bladder. Stage III adds an abnormal Doppler waveform with absent or reverse end-diastolic flow in the umbilical artery, absent or reverse flow in the ductus venosus, or pulsatile flow in the umbilical vein. Stage IV is associated with the presence of hydrops fetalis. Stage V is present when there is a demise of one or both twins.[128] This staging system has been validated by some, but not all, laboratories.[129,130] Quintero et al. used this staging system to determine when therapy would improve outcome. Overall, they identified at least one surviving infant in 67% of those treated by serial amniocentesis and 83% of those treated with selective laser photocoagulation of the communicating placental vessels. Intact neurologic survival was 51% in the serial amniocentesis group and 79% in the laser group. The authors, however, suggest that patients with stage I or II likely would have favorable outcomes with serial amniocentesis, especially if diagnosed at >22 weeks. Stage II at <22 weeks, stage III, and stage IV probably would benefit from selective laser photocoagulation of communicating placental vessels.[131] A randomized controlled trial comparing endoscopic laser surgery and serial amnioreduction was concluded early after interim analysis documented a statistically significant benefit for the laser group. The laser group had a 76% rate of survival of one twin up to 28 days of age versus 56% for the amnioreduction group. The authors concluded that, at <26 weeks, endoscopic laser coagulation is the most effective first-line treatment.[132] Two hundred consecutive pregnancies with severe twin-to-twin transfusion syndrome treated with laser at a median gestational age of 20.7 weeks were evaluated for survival on the basis of stage of disease. The survival of at least one twin was 93%, 83%, 83%, and 70% for stages I, II, III, and IV, respectively.[133] Fetal cardiac function also may be improved after selective laser ablation of placental communicating vessels; however, this has been shown not to be the case after amnioreduction.[134,135]

Other aggressive management schemes for these pregnancies have been proposed. Fetal umbilical cord ligation under ultrasound guidance has been attempted.[136,137] Although feasible, this remains a highly experimental procedure. In a study by Quintero et al.,[138] percutaneous umbilical cord ligation was accomplished in 11 of 13 cases, including cases of acardiac twins and of twin-to-twin transfusion syndrome. Seven of the 11 pregnancies resulted in living offspring. Other larger and more recent data have involved the evaluation of pregnancy and infant outcome with 80 consecutive cord coagulation in pregnancies with twin-to-twin transfusion syndrome, severe discordant growth, and TRAP sequence. Using laser or bipolar coagulation, the survival rate was 83%.[139] A randomized trial of amnioreduction versus septostomy has been reported as a treatment for those with twin-to-twin transfusion syndrome. The survival rates were similar for the two treatment groups, 78% versus 80% for amnioreduction and septostomy groups, respectively. Those undergoing septostomy were more likely to require a single procedure for treatment.[140]

The management of severe twin-to-twin transfusion syndrome with selective feticide is extremely dangerous because damage to the surviving twin is likely to occur. Although selective feticide has been performed successfully in twin-to-twin transfusion syndrome, there are several reports of umbilical artery steal syndrome resulting from the death of one twin.[59,141–144] Results have included one case of distal gangrene of the toes, with malformation of the foot, and one case of abrupt onset of microcephaly in twins surviving the spontaneous deaths of their donor twins.[141,142]

The incidence of velamentous cord insertions reportedly is increased in twin-to-twin transfusion syndrome, compared with other twinning situations.[145,146] In a study by Fries et al.,[146] 11 of 38 cases of monochorionic–diamniotic twins revealed evidence of twin-to-twin transfusion syndrome. The incidence of a velamentous cord insertion of one twin among these 11 was 63.6%, compared with 18% of those without twin-to-twin transfusion syndrome. Fries et al. suggested that a velamentous cord insertion may contribute to the development of the disparity in amniotic fluid volumes as a result of the easily compressed, membranously inserted cord.[126] In general, velamentous insertion is particularly common in single or fused twin placentae and may result from asymmetric expansion of the placenta. Large-volume amniocentesis has proved to be successful in these cases, possibly by reducing compression on the cord insertion. Monochorionic–diamniotic twin gestations that have velamentous cord insertions have a significantly increased risk for birth weight discordance, indicating an increased need for prenatal detection and monitoring of such pregnancies.[147]

CONCLUSION

The etiology of monozygotic twinning is unknown and probably represents a malformation in and of itself. It is associated with an increased incidence of major malformations, poor outcome, and placental vascular abnormalities leading to morbidity and mortality. Frequent ultrasonographic evaluation of monochorionic pregnancies is required to maximize survival, particularly in pregnancies demonstrating some of the complications. Occasionally, in cases of severe anomalies, intervention may be necessary to provide a chance for survival. In addition to the malformations and vascular anomalies described for monozygotic twins, an excess of perinatal mortality is caused by prematurity.

References

1. Benirschke K, Kim CK: Multiple pregnancy (first of two parts). *N Engl J Med* 288:1276–1284, 1973.
2. Blickstein I, Keith LG: *Multiple pregnancy: epidemiology, gestation, & perinatal outcome,* ed 2. New York, 2005, Taylor & Francis.
3. Jones KL: *Smith's recognizable patterns of human malformation,* ed 6. Philadelphia, 2006, Elsevier.
4. Benirschke K, Kaufmann P, Baergen R: *Pathology of the human placenta.* China, 2006, Springer.
5. Barss VA, Benacerraf BR, Frigoletto FD: Sonographic determination of chorion type in twin gestation. *Am J Obstet Gynecol* 179:779–783, 1985.
6. Sepulveda W, Sebire NJ, Hughes K, Kalogeropoulos A, Nicolaides KH: Evolution of the lambda or twin-chorionic peak sign in dichorionic twin pregnancies. *Obstet Gynecol* 89:439–441, 1997.
7. Sepulveda W, Sebire NJ, Hughes K, Odibo A, Nicolaides KH: The lambda sign at 10–14 weeks of gestation as a predictor of chorionicity in twin pregnancies. *Ultrasound Obstet Gynecol* 7:421–423, 1996.
8. Scardo JA, Ellings JM, Newman RB: Prospective determination of chorionicity, amnionicity, and zygosity in twin gestations. *Am J Obstet Gynecol* 173:1376–1380, 1995.
9. Hertzberg BS, Kurtz AB, Choi HY, et al: Significance of membrane thickness in the sonographic evaluation of twin gestations. *AJR Am J Roentgenol* 148:151–153, 1987.
10. Kurtz AB, Wapner RJ, Mata J, Johnson A, Morgan P: Twin pregnancies: accuracy of first-trimester abdominal US in predicting chorionicity and amnionicity. *Radiology* 185:759–762, 1992.
11. Mahony BS, Filly RA, Callen PW: Amnionicity and chorionicity in twin pregnancies: prediction using ultrasound. *Radiology* 155:205–209, 1985.
12. Monteagudo A, Timor-Tritsch IE, Sharma S: Early and simple determination of chorionic and amniotic type in multifetal gestations in the first fourteen weeks by high-frequency transvaginal ultrasonography. *Am J Obstet Gynecol* 170:824–829, 1994.
13. Finberg HJ: The "twin peak" sign: reliable evidence of dichorionic twinning. *J Ultrasound Med* 11:571–577, 1992.
14. Townsend RR, Simpson GF, Filly RA: Membrane thickness in ultrasound prediction of chorionicity of twin gestations. *J Ultrasound Med* 7:327–332, 1988.
15. D'Alton ME, Dudley DK: The ultrasonographic prediction of chorionicity in twin gestation. *Am J Obstet Gynecol* 160:557–561, 1989.
16. Lee YM, Cleary-Goldman J, Thaker HM, Simpson LL: Antenatal sonographic prediction of twin chorionicity. *Am J Obstet Gynecol* 195:863–867, 2006.
17. Stenhouse E, Hardwick C, Maharaj S, Webb J, Kelly T, Mackenzie FM: Chorionicity determination in twin pregnancies: how accurate are we? *Ultrasound Obstet Gynecol* 19:350–352, 2002.
18. Carroll SG, Soothill PW, Abdel-Fattah SA, Porter H, Montague I, Kyle PM: Prediction of chorionicity in twin pregnancies at 10-14 weeks of gestation. *BJOG* 109:182–186, 2002.
19. Kupesic S, Benoit B, Kurjak A, Bjelos D: Three-dimensional ultrasound in the imaging of multifetal pregnancy. *Ultrasound Rev Obstet Gynecol* 1:301–306, 2001.
20. Bromley BR, Benacerraf BR: Using the number of yolk sacs to determine amnionicity in early first trimester monochorionic twins. *J Ultrasound Med* 14:415–419, 1995.
21. Bilardo CM, Arabin B: Prenatal diagnosis of cord entanglement in monoamniotic multiple pregnancies. *Ultrasound Rev Obstet Gynecol* 1:365–371, 2001.
22. Filly RA, Goldstein RB, Callen PW: Monochorionic twinning: Sonographic assessment. *AJR Am J Roentgenol* 154:459–469, 1990.
23. Townsend RR, Filly RA: Sonography of nonconjoined monoamniotic twin pregnancies. *J Ultrasound Med* 7:665–670, 1988.
24. Nyberg DA, Filly RA, Golbus MS, Stephens JD: Entangled umbilical cords: a sign of monoamniotic twins. *J Ultrasound Med* 3:29–32, 1984.
25. Belfort MA, Moise KJ, Kirshon B, Saade G: The use of color flow Doppler ultrasonography to diagnose umbilical cord entanglement in monoamniotic twin gestations. *Am J Obstet Gynecol* 168:601–604, 1993.
26. Abuhamad AZ, Mari G, Copel JA, Cantwell CJ, Evans AT: Umbilical artery flow velocity waveforms in monoamniotic twins with cord entanglement. *Obstet Gynecol* 86:674–677, 1995.
27. Roqué H, Gillen-Goldstein J, Funai E, Young BK, Lockwood CJ: Perinatal outcomes in monoamniotic gestations. *J Matern Fetal Neonatal Med* 13:414–421, 2003.
28. Shveiky D, Ezra Y, Schenker JG, Rojansky N: Monoamniotic twins: an update on antenatal diagnosis and treatment. *J Matern Fetal Neonatal Med* 16:180–186, 2004.

29. Gilbert WM, Davis SE, Kaplan C, et al: Morbidity associated with prenatal disruption of the dividing membrane in twin gestations. *Obstet Gynecol* 78:623–630, 1991.
30. Megory E, Weiner E, Shalev E, Ohel G: Pseudo-monoamniotic twins with cord entanglement following genetic funipuncture. *Obstet Gynecol* 78:915–918, 1991.
31. Chitrit Y, Zorn B, Filidori M, Robert E, Chasseray JE: Cloacal exstrophy in monozygotic twins detected through antenatal ultrasound scanning. *J Clin Ultrasound* 21:339–342, 1993.
32. Lipitz S, Meizner I, Yagel S, et al: Expectant management of twin pregnancies discordant for anencephaly. *Obstet Gynecol* 86:969–972, 1995.
33. Filion R, Grignon A, Boisvert J: Antenatal diagnosis of ipsilateral multicystic kidney in identical twins. *J Ultrasound Med* 4:211–212, 1985.
34. Gorczyca DP, Lindfors KK, Giles KA, et al: Prenatally diagnosed gastroschisis in monozygotic twins. *J Clin Ultrasound* 17:216–218, 1989.
35. Baker ME, Rosenberg ER, Trofatter KF, Imber MJ, Bowie JD: The in utero findings in twin pentalogy of Cantrell. *J Ultrasound Med* 3:525–527, 1984.
36. Shih JC, Shyu MK, Hwa SL, et al: Concordant body stalk anomaly in monozygotic twinning—early embryo cleavage disorder. *Prenat Diagn* 16:467–470, 1996.
37. Schinzel AA, Smith DW, Miller JR: Monozygotic twinning and structural defects. *J Pediatr* 95:921–930, 1979.
38. Alexander JM, Ramus R, Cox SM, Gilstrap LC III: Outcome of twin gestations with a single anomalous fetus. *Am J Obstet Gynecol* 177:849–852, 1997.
39. Coleman BG, Grumbach K, Arger PH, et al: Twin gestations: monitoring of complications and anomalies with US. *Radiology* 165:449–453, 1987.
40. Hashimoto B, Callen PW, Filly RA, Laros RK: Ultrasound evaluation of polyhydramnios and twin pregnancy. *Am J Obstet Gynecol* 154:1069–1072, 1986.
41. Alien SR, Gray LJ, Frentzen BH, Cruz AC: Ultrasonographic diagnosis of congenital anomalies in twins. *Am J Obstet Gynecol* 165:1056–1060, 1991.
42. Edwards MS, Ellings JM, Newman RB, Menard MK: Predictive value of antepartum ultrasound examination for anomalies in twin gestations. *Ultrasound Obstet Gynecol* 6:43–49, 1995.
43. Kuller JA, Coulson CC, McCoy C, et al: Prenatal diagnosis of renal agenesis in a twin gestation. *Prenat Diagn* 14:1090–1092, 1994.
44. McNamara MF, McCurdy CM, Reed KL, Philipps AF, Seeds JW: The relation between pulmonary hypoplasia and amniotic fluid volume: lessons learned from discordant urinary tract anomalies in monoamniotic twins. *Obstet Gynecol* 85:867–869, 1995.
45. Benirschke K, Kim CK: Multiple pregnancy (second of two parts). *N Engl J Med* 288:1329–1335, 1973.
46. Karp L, Bryant JI, Tagatz G, Giblett E, Fialkow PJ: The occurrence of gonadal dysgenesis in association with monozygotic twinning. *J Med Genet* 12:70–78, 1975.
47. Nieuwint A, Van Zalen-Sprock R, Hummel P, et al: "Identical" twins with discordant karyotypes. *Prenat Diagn* 19:72–76, 1999.
48. Dallapiccola B, Stomeo C, Ferranti G, diLecce A, Purpura M: Discordant sex in one of three monozygotic triplets. *J Med Genet* 22:6–11, 1985.
49. Schmidt R, Sobel EH, Nitowsky HM, Dar H, Alien FH: Monozygotic twins discordant for sex. *J Med Genet* 13:64–79, 1976.
50. Watson WJ, Katz VL, Albright SG, Rao KW, Aylsworth AS: Monozygotic twins discordant for partial trisomy 1. *Obstet Gynecol* 76:949, 1990.
51. Evans MI, Goldberg JD, Dommergues M, et al: Efficacy of second-trimester selective termination for fetal abnormalities: international collaborative experience among the world's largest centers. *Am J Obstet Gynecol* 171:90–94, 1994.
52. Chitkara U, Berkowitz RL, Wilkins IA, et al: Selective second-trimester termination of the anomalous fetus in twin pregnancies. *Obstet Gynecol* 73:690–694, 1989.
53. Tabsh KMA: A report of 131 cases of multifetal pregnancy reduction. *Obstet Gynecol* 82:57–60, 1993.
54. Kilby MD, Govind A, O'Brien PMS: Outcome of twin pregnancies complicated by a single intrauterine death: a comparison with viable twin pregnancies. *Obstet Gynecol* 84:107–109, 1994.
55. Enbom JA: Twin pregnancy with intrauterine death of one twin. *Am J Obstet Gynecol* 152:242–249, 1985.
56. Weeks AD, Davies NP, Sprigg A, Fairlie FM: The sequential in utero death of heterokaryotic monozygotic twins. A case report and literature review. *Prenat Diagn* 16:657–663, 1996.
57. Patten RM, Mack LA, Nyberg DA, Filly RA: Twin embolization syndrome: prenatal sonographic detection and significance. *Radiology* 173:685–689, 1989.
58. Jung JH, Graham JM Jr, Schultz N, Smith DW: Congenital hydranencephaly/porencephaly due to vascular disruption in monozygotic twins. *Pediatrics* 73:467–469, 1984.
59. Jou HJ, Ng KY, Teng RJ, Hsieh FJ: Doppler sonographic detection of reverse twin-twin transfusion after intrauterine death of the donor. *J Ultrasound Med* 5:307–309, 1993.
60. Benirschke K: The contribution of placental anastomoses to prenatal twin damage. *Hum Pathol* 23:1319–1320, 1992 (editorial).
61. Nicolini U, Pisoni MP, Cela E, Roberts A: Fetal blood sampling immediately before and within 24 hours of death in monochorionic twin pregnancies complicated by single intrauterine death. *Am J Obstet Gynecol* 179:800–803, 1998.
62. Karageyim Karsidag AY, Kars B, Dansuk R, et al: Brain damage to the survivor within 30 min of co-twin demise in monochorionic twins. *Fetal Diagn Ther* 20:91–95, 2005.
63. Simonazzi G, Segata M, Ghi T, et al: Accurate neurosonographic prediction of brain injury in the surviving fetus after the death of a monochorionic cotwin. *Ultrasound Obstet Gynecol* 27:517–521, 2006.

64. Spitz L, Kiely EM: Conjoined twins. *JAMA* 289:1307–1310, 2003.
65. Sakala EP: Obstetric management of conjoined twins. *Obstet Gynecol* 67:21S–25S, 1986.
66. Apuzzio JJ, Ganesh V, Landau I, et al: Prenatal diagnosis of conjoined twins. *Am J Obstet Gynecol* 148:343–344, 1984.
67. Kalchbrenner M, Weiner S, Templeton J, Losure TA: Prenatal ultrasound diagnosis of thoracopagus conjoined twins. *J Clin Ultrasound* 15:59–63, 1987.
68. Sanders SP, Chin AJ, Parness LA, et al: Prenatal diagnosis of congenital heart defects in thoracoabdominally conjoined twins. *N Engl J Med* 313:370–374, 1985.
69. Wood MJ, Thompson HE, Roberson FM: Real-time ultrasound diagnosis of conjoined twins. *J Clin Ultrasound* 9:195–197, 1981.
70. Earth RA, Filly RA, Goldberg JD, Moore P, Silverman NH: Conjoined twins: prenatal diagnosis and assessment of associated malformations. *Radiology* 177:201–207, 1990.
71. Schmidt W, Heberling D, Kubli F: Antepartum ultrasonographic diagnosis of conjoined twins in early pregnancy. *Am J Obstet Gynecol* 139:961–963, 1981.
72. Hurren AJ, Sommerville AJ, Warren VF: Antenatal diagnosis of a set of conjoined twins presenting with unusual ultrasound findings. *J Clin Ultrasound* 16:672–674, 1988.
73. Skupski DW, Streltzoff J, Hutson JM, et al: Early diagnosis of conjoined twins in triplet pregnancy after in vitro fertilization and assisted hatching. *J Ultrasound Med* 14:611–615, 1995.
74. Bonilla-Musoles F, Machado LE, Osborne NG, et al: Two-dimensional and three-dimensional sonography of conjoined twins. *J Clin Ultrasound* 30:68–75, 2002.
75. Vural F, Vural B: First trimester diagnosis of dicephalic parapagus conjoined twins via transvaginal ultrasonography. *J Clin Ultrasound* 33:364–366, 2005.
76. Schmid O, Hagen A, Sarioglu N, et al: Early diagnosis of conjoined twins by real-time three-dimensional ultrasound—case report and review of the literature. *Ultraschall Med* 27:384–388, 2006.
77. Chen CP, Lee CC, Liu FF, et al: Prenatal diagnosis of cephalothoracopagus janiceps monosymmetros. *Prenat Diagn* 17:384–388, 1997.
78. Hartung RW, Yiu-Chiu V, Aschenbrener CA: Sonographic diagnosis of cephalothoracopagus in a triplet pregnancy. *J Ultrasound Med* 3:139–141, 1984.
79. Kokcu A, Ustun C, Alper T, Baris YS, Coksenim S: Case report: dicephalus dipus dibrachius conjoined twins diagnosed prenatally. *J Matern Fetal Med* 4:285–288, 1995.
80. Weingast GR, Johnson ML, Pretorius DH, et al: Difficulty in sonographic diagnosis of cephalothoracopagus. *J Ultrasound Med* 3:421–423, 1984.
81. Nolan R, Ling F, Langlotz H, Fletcher A: Cephalothoracopagus janiceps disymmetros twinning. *J Ultrasound Med* 9:593–598, 1990.
82. Fontanarosa M, Bagnoli G, Ciolini P, Spinelli G, Curiel P: First trimester sonographic diagnosis of diprosopus twins with craniorachischisis. *J Clin Ultrasound* 20:69–71, 1992.
83. Brenbridge AN, Kraft JL, Teja K: Sonographic findings in the prenatal diagnosis of cephalothoracopagus syncephalus: a case report. *J Reprod Med* 32:59–62, 1987.
84. Malhotra N, Sinha A, Deka D, Roy KK: Twin reversed arterial perfusion: report of four cases. *J Clin Ultrasound* 32:411–414, 2004.
85. Gibson JY, D'Cruz CA, Patel RB, et al: Acardiac anomaly: review of the subject with case report and emphasis on practical sonography. *J Clin Ultrasound* 14:541–545, 1986.
86. Napolitani FD, Schreiber I: The acardiac monster: a review of the world literature and presentation of 2 cases. *Am J Obstet Gynecol* 80:582–587, 1960.
87. Shalev E, Zalel Y, Ben-Ami M, Weiner E: First-trimester ultrasonic diagnosis of twin reversed arterial perfusion sequence. *Prenat Diagn* 12:219–222, 1992.
88. Zucchini S, Borghesani F, Soffriti G, et al: Transvaginal ultrasound diagnosis of twin reversed arterial perfusion syndrome at 9 weeks' gestation. *Ultrasound Obstet Gynecol* 3:209–211, 1993.
89. Stiller RJ, Romero R, Pace S, Hobbins JC: Prenatal identification of twin reversed arterial perfusion syndrome in the first trimester. *Am J Obstet Gynecol* 160:1194–1196, 1989.
90. Langlotz H, Sauerbrei E, Murray S: Transvaginal Doppler sonographic diagnosis of an acardiac twin at 12 weeks gestation. *J Ultrasound Med* 10:175–179, 1991.
91. Crade M, Nageotte MP, MacKenzie ML: The acardiac twin: a case report using color Doppler ultrasonography. *Ultrasound Obstet Gynecol* 2:364–365, 1992.
92. Benson CB, Bieber FR, Genest DR, Doubilet PM: Doppler demonstration of reversed umbilical blood flow in an acardiac twin. *J Clin Ultrasound* 17:291–295, 1989.
93. Al-Malt A, Ashmead G, Junge N, et al: Colorflow and Doppler velocimetry in prenatal diagnosis of acardiac triplet. *J Ultrasound Med* 10:341–345, 1991.
94. Quintero RA, Chmait RH, Murakoshi T, et al: Surgical management of twin reversed arterial perfusion sequence. *Am J Obstet Gynecol* 194:982–991, 2006.
95. Moore TR, Gale S, Benirschke K: Perinatal outcome of forty-nine pregnancies complicated by acardiac twinning. *Am J Obstet Gynecol* 163:907–912, 1990.
96. Fouron JC, Leduc L, Grigon A, et al: Importance of meticulous ultrasonographic investigation of the acardiac twin. *J Ultrasound Med* 13:1001–1004, 1994.
97. Mack LA, Gravett MG, Rumack CM, et al: Antenatal ultrasonic evaluation of acardiac monsters. *J Ultrasound Med* 1:13–18, 1982.
98. Cox M, Murphy K, Ryan G, et al: Spontaneous cessation of umbilical blood flow in the acardiac fetus of a twin pregnancy. *Prenat Diagn* 12:689–693, 1992.

99. McCurdy CM Jr, Childers JM, Seeds JW: Ligation of the umbilical cord of an acardiac acephalus twin with an endoscopic intrauterine technique. *Obstet Gynecol* 82:708–711, 1993.
100. Foley MR, Clewell WH, Finberg HJ, Mills MD: Use of the Foley Cordostat grasping device for selective ligation of the umbilical cord of an acardiac twin: a case report. *Am J Obstet Gynecol* 172:212–214, 1995.
101. Ginsberg NA, Applebaum M, Rabin SA, et al: Term birth after midtrimester hysterotomy and selective delivery of an acardiac twin. *Am J Obstet Gynecol* 167:33–37, 1992.
102. Fries MH, Goldberg JD, Golbus MS: Treatment of acardiac-acephalus twin gestations by hysterotomy and selective delivery. *Obstet Gynecol* 79:601–604, 1992.
103. Platt LD, DeVore GR, Bieniarz A, Benner P, Rao R: Antenatal diagnosis of acephalus acardia: a proposed management scheme. *Am J Obstet Gynecol* 146:857, 1983.
104. Arias F, Sunderji S, Gimpelson R, Colton E: Treatment of acardiac twinning. *Obstet Gynecol* 91:818–821, 1998.
105. Rodeck C, Deans A, Jauniaux E: Thermocoagulation for the early treatment of pregnancy with an acardiac twin. *N Engl J Med* 339:1293–1295, 1998.
106. Tsao KJ, Feldstein VA, Albanese CT, et al: Selective reduction of acardiac twin by radiofrequency ablation. *Am J Obstet Gynecol* 187:635–640, 2002.
107. Sullivan AE, Varner MW, Ball RH, Jackson M, Silver RM: The management of acardiac twins: a conservative approach. *Am J Obstet Gynecol* 189:1310–1313, 2003.
108. Weisz B, Peltz R, Chayen B, et al: Tailored management of twin reversed arterial perfusion (TRAP) sequence. *Ultrasound Obstet Gynecol* 23:451–455, 2004.
109. Tan TY, Sepulveda W: Acardiac twin: a systematic review of minimally invasive treatment modalities. *Ultrasound Obstet Gynecol* 22:409–419, 2003.
110. Umur A, van Gemert MJC, Nikkels PGJ: Monoamniotic- versus diamniotic-monochorionic twin placentas: anastomoses and twin-twin transfusion syndrome. *Am J Obstet Gynecol* 189:1325–1329, 2003.
111. Sharma S, Gray S, Guzman ER, Rosenberg JC, Shen-Schwarz S: Detection of twin-twin transfusion syndrome by first trimester ultrasonography. *J Ultrasound Med* 14:635–637, 1995.
112. Gonsoulin W, Moise KJ Jr, Kirshon B, et al: Outcome of twin-twin transfusion diagnosed before 28 weeks of gestation. *Obstet Gynecol* 75:214–216, 1990.
113. Bromley B, Frigoletto FD Jr, Estroff JA, Benacerraf BR: The natural history of oligohydramnios/polyhydramnios sequence in monochorionic diamniotic twins. *Ultrasound Obstet Gynecol* 2:317–320, 1992.
114. Brown DL, Benson CB, Driscoll SG, Doubilet PM: Twin-twin transfusion syndrome: sonographic findings. *Radiology* 170:61–63, 1989.
115. Danskin FH, Neilson JP: Twin-to-twin transfusion syndrome: what are appropriate diagnostic criteria? *Am J Obstet Gynecol* 161:365–369, 1989.
116. Simpson LL, Marx GR, Elkadry EA, D'Alton ME: Cardiac dysfunction in twin-twin transfusion syndrome: a prospective, longitudinal study. *Obstet Gynecol* 92:557–562, 1998.
117. Pretorius DH, Manchester D, Barkin S, Parker S, Nelson TR: Doppler ultrasound of twin transfusion syndrome. *J Ultrasound Med* 7:117–124, 1988.
118. Tan TYT, Taylor MJO, Wee LY, Vanderheyden T, Wimalasundera R, Fisk NM: Doppler for artery-artery anastomosis and stage-independent survival in twin-twin transfusion. *Obstet Gynecol* 103:1174–1180, 2004.
119. Bromley B, Benacerraf BR: Acute reversal of oligohydramnios-polyhydramnios sequence in monochorionic twins. *Int J Gynecol Obstet* 55:281–283, 1996.
120. Wee LY, Taylor MJO, Vanderheyden T, Wimalasundera R, Gardiner HM, Fisk NM: Reversal of twin-twin transfusion syndrome: frequency, vascular anatomy, associated anomalies and outcome. *Prenat Diagn* 24:104–110, 2004.
121. Wax JR, Callan NA, Perlman EJ, Feng TI, Blakemore KJ: The stuck twin phenomenon: experience with serial therapeutic amniocentesis. *J Matern Fetal Med* 1:239–244, 1992.
122. Urig MA, Clewell WH, Elliott JP: Twin-twin transfusion syndrome. *Am J Obstet Gynecol* 163:1522–1526, 1990.
123. Saunders NJ, Snijders RJM, Nicolaides KH: Therapeutic amniocentesis in twin-twin transfusion syndrome appearing in the second trimester of pregnancy. *Am J Obstet Gynecol* 166:820–824, 1992.
124. Mahony BS, Petty CN, Nyberg DA, et al: The "stuck twin" phenomenon: ultrasonographic findings, pregnancy outcome, and management with serial amniocentesis. *Am J Obstet Gynecol* 163:1513–1522, 1990.
125. Elliott JP, Urig MA, Clewell WH: Aggressive therapeutic amniocentesis for treatment of twin-twin transfusion syndrome. *Obstet Gynecol* 77:537–540, 1991.
126. Ville Y, Hyett J, Hecher K, Nicolaides K: Preliminary experience with endoscopic laser surgery for severe twin-twin transfusion syndrome. *N Engl J Med* 332:224–227, 1995.
127. Hecher K, Plath H, Bregenzer T, Hansmann M, Hackelöer BJ: Endoscopic laser surgery versus serial amniocenteses in the treatment of severe twin-twin transfusion syndrome. *Am J Obstet Gynecol* 180:717–724, 1999.
128. Quintero RA, Morales WJ, Allen MH, Bornick PW, Johnson PK, Kruger M: Staging of twin-twin transfusion syndrome. *J Perinatol* 19:550–555, 1999.
129. Taylor MJO, Govender L, Jolly M, Wee L, Fisk NM: Validation of the Quintero staging system for twin-twin transfusion syndrome. *Obstet Gynecol* 100:1257–1265, 2002.
130. Duncombe GJ, Dickinson JE, Evans SF: Perinatal characteristics and outcomes of pregnancies complicated by twin-twin transfusion syndrome. *Obstet Gynecol* 101:1190–1196, 2003.
131. Quintero RA, Dickinson JE, Morales WJ, et al: Stage-based treatment of twin-twin transfusion

syndrome. *Am J Obstet Gynecol* 188:1333–1340, 2003.

132. Senat M-V, Deprest J, Boulvain M, Paupe A, Winer N, Ville Y: Endoscopic laser surgery versus serial amnioreduction for severe twin-to-twin transfusion syndrome. *N Engl J Med* 351:136–144, 2004.
133. Huber A, Diehl W, Bregenzer T, Hackelöer B-J, Hecher K: Stage-related outcome in twin-twin transfusion syndrome treated by fetoscopic laser coagulation. *Obstet Gynecol* 108:333–337, 2006.
134. Barrea C, Alkazaleh F, Ryan G, et al: Prenatal cardiovascular manifestations in the twin-to-twin transfusion syndrome recipients and the impact of therapeutic amnioreduction. *Am J Obstet Gynecol* 192:892–902, 2005.
135. Barrea C, Hornberger LK, Alkazaleh F, et al: Impact of selective laser ablation of placental anastomoses on the cardiovascular pathology of the recipient twin in severe twin-twin transfusion syndrome. *Am J Obstet Gynecol* 195:1388–1395, 2006.
136. Lemery DJ, Vanlieferinghen P, Gasq M, et al: Fetal umbilical cord ligation under ultrasound guidance. *Ultrasound Obstet Gynecol* 4:399–401, 1994.
137. De Lia JE, Kuhlmann RS, Harstad TW, Cruikshank DP: Fetoscopic laser ablation of placental vessels in severe previable twin-twin transfusion syndrome. *Am J Obstet Gynecol* 172:1202–1211, 1995.
138. Quintero RA, Romero R, Reich H, et al: In utero percutaneous umbilical cord ligation in the management of complicated monochorionic multiple gestations. *Ultrasound Obstet Gynecol* 8:16–22, 1996.
139. Lewi L, Gratacos E, Ortibus E, et al: Pregnancy and infant outcome of 80 consecutive cord coagulations in complicated monochorionic multiple pregnancies. *Am J Obstet Gynecol* 194:782–789, 2006.
140. Moise Jr KJ, Dorman K, Lamvu G, et al; A randomized trial of amnioreduction versus septostomy in the treatment of twin-twin transfusion syndrome. *Am J Obstet Gynecol* 193:701–707, 2005.
141. Hecher K, Ville Y, Nicolaides KH: Fetal arterial Doppler studies in twin-twin transfusion syndrome. *J Ultrasound Med* 14:101–108, 1995.
142. Sherer DM, Abramowicz JS, Jaffe R, et al: Twin-twin transfusion with abrupt onset of microcephaly in the surviving recipient following spontaneous death of the donor twin. *Am J Obstet Gynecol* 169:85–88, 1993.
143. Mahone PR, Sherer DM, Abramowicz JS, Woods JR Jr: Twin-twin transfusion syndrome: rapid development of severe hydrops of the donor following selective feticide of the hydropic recipient. *Am J Obstet Gynecol* 169:166–168, 1993.
144. Wittman BK, Farquharson DF, Thomas WDS, Baldwin VJ, Wadsworth LD: The role of feticide in the management of severe twin transfusion syndrome. *Am J Obstet Gynecol* 155:1023–1026, 1986.
145. Reisner DP, Mahony BS, Petty CN, et al: Stuck twin syndrome: outcome in thirty-seven consecutive cases. *Am J Obstet Gynecol* 169:991–995, 1993.
146. Fries MH, Goldstein RB, Kilpatrick SJ, et al: The role of velamentous cord insertion in the etiology of twin-twin transfusion syndrome. *Obstet Gynecol* 81:569–574, 1993.
147. Hanley ML, Ananth CV, Shen-Schwarz S, Smulian JC, Lai YL, Vintzileos AM: Placental cord insertion and birth weight discordancy in twin gestations. *Obstet Gynecol* 99:477–482, 2002.

Index

Note: Italic numbers refer to figures.

A

B

I

J

K

Q

R

S

T